The Nature of Disease

PATHOLOGY FOR THE HEALTH PROFESSIONS

SECOND EDITION

The Nature of Disease

PATHOLOGY FOR THE HEALTH PROFESSIONS

SECOND EDITION

Thomas H. McConnell, MD, FCAP
Clinical Professor of Pathology
University of Texas Southwestern Medical Center
Dallas, Texas

Contributing Editors

Vera A. Paulson, MD, PhD
Pathology Resident
Brigham and Women's Hospital
Boston, Massachusetts

Mark A. Valasek, MD, PhD
Assistant Professor of Pathology
University of California San Diego
San Diego, California

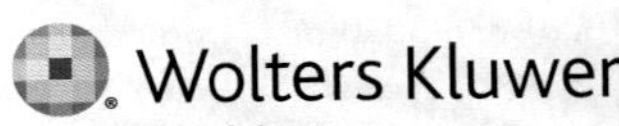
Wolters Kluwer Health | Lippincott Williams & Wilkins

Philadelphia • Baltimore • New York • London
Buenos Aires • Hong Kong • Sydney • Tokyo

Acquisitions Editor: David B. Troy
Development Editor: Laura Bonazolli
Marketing Manager: Leah Thomson
Product Development Editor: Eve Malakoff-Klein
Designer: Teresa Mallon
Art Direction: Jennifer Clements, LWW; Craig Durant, Dragonfly Media Group
Compositor: S4Carlisle Publishing Services

Second Edition

351 West Camden Street
Baltimore, MD 21201

2001 Market Street
Philadelphia, PA 19103

Printed in China

9 8 7 6 5 4 3 2

Library of Congress Cataloging-in Publication Data

McConnell, Thomas H., author.
The nature of disease : pathology for the health professions / Thomas H. McConnell ; contributing editors, Vera A. Paulson, Mark A. Valasek. — Second edition.
p. ; cm.
Includes bibliographical references and index.
ISBN 978-1-60913-369-6
I. Paulson, Vera A., editor. II. Valasek, Mark A., editor. III. Title.
[DNLM: 1. Pathology. QZ 4]
RB113
616.07—dc23

2013024270

THIS BOOK IS DEDICATED TO:

Marianne Harper McConnell
1939–2013

My wife of 50 years
She lighted no new lamp of learning, scaled no mighty peak, nor strove for achievement in any conventional way. Yet of those who are left only to memory, ask anyone who knew her: "Who do you remember with greatest admiration, respect and love?" and her name will surely be near the top.

Reviewers

We gratefully acknowledge the generous assistance of the reviewers whose names appear in the list that follows. These individuals were kind enough to provide input on different aspects of this text; their comments helped shape its final form.

Margy Blankenship
Chair, Health Division
Kentucky Community & Technical College System
Somerset, KY

Gerald Callahan
Associate Professor
Microbiology, Immunology, and Pathology
Colorado State University
Fort Collins, CO

David Derrico
Assistant Clinical Professor, Nursing
University of Florida
Gainesville, FL

Bertha C. Escobar-Poni
Associate Professor, Pathology and Human Anatomy
School of Medicine
Loma Linda University
Loma Linda, CA

Jacquelyn Harris
Medical Department Chair
Bryan College
Springfield, MO

Lisa Hight
Associate Profesor, Biology
Baptist College of Health Sciences
Memphis, TN

Jody LaCourt
Senior Teaching Specialist
University of Minnesota
Minneapolis, MN

Mark Lafferty
Science Department Chair
Delaware Technical and Community College
Wilmington, DE

Rene Lapierre
Coordinator, "Soins Paramédicaux"
Collège Boréal
Ontario, Quebec, Canada

Susan Leftwich Sale
Level Coordinator, Faculty
Riverside School of Professional Nursing, Riverside School of Health Careers
Newport News, VA

Steve Moon
Instructor, Allied Medicine
College of Medicine, The Ohio State University
Columbus, OH

John Olson
Lecturer
Arizona State University
Phoenix, AZ

Alisa Petree
Instructor/Clinical Coordinator
Medical Laboratory Technician
McLennan Community College
Waco, TX

Christine Recktenwald
Assistant Teaching Professor
College of Nursing at University of Missouri—St. Louis
St. Louis, MO

Vickie Roettger
Profesor
Missouri Southern State University
Joplin, MO

Sandra A. Sieck
Program Director
UW-L-Gunderson-Mayo PA Program
LaCrosse, WI

J. Steve Smith
Biology Department
Universityof West Florida
Pensacola, FL

Becky J. Socha,
Adjunct Faculty
Merrimack College
North Andover, MA

Gina Stephens
Program Chair, Medical Business Administrative Technologies
Georgia Northwester Technical Colleage
Rome, GA

Wanda Thuma-McDermond
Associate Professor of Nursing
Messiah College
Mechanicsburg, PA

Karen Tombs-Harling
Dean, Academic Affairs
Harrisburg Area Community College
Harrisburg, PA

Sheila Trahan
Academic Department Chair, Allied Health
Lamar Institute of Technology
Beaumont, TX

Preface

This Second Edition of ***The Nature of Disease*** *(TNOD)* is, like the first edition, written for a particular audience: students in the health professions.

In this edition, I combine three important features to bring students a unique learning experience.

- First, *my writing style is deliberately casual*. It is a narrative (storyteller) style, which is less formal than the stiff prose that populates similar textbooks. My experience shows that it makes reading and learning easier.
- Second, *each chapter opens with a review of normal anatomy and physiology*. Given that pathology and pathophysiology are nothing more than normal anatomy and physiology gone wrong, a brief review prepares the reader for the disease discussions that follow.
- Third, *each chapter focuses on one or more case studies*, which bind the material together and make it more memorable.

Classroom Vetted

TNOD literally grew out of a classroom. When I joined the academic community in 1997 after a career in the laboratory business, the classroom was an alien place to me. I puzzled over the fact that the students I taught, who were of the very highest quality, still had trouble grasping the material. I began to pay more attention to the textbooks available, and learned the student perspective of most pathology texts: they are difficult to read.

Much of the difficulty springs from the fact that most pathology books are compilations written by multiple authors, each with a certain writing style and with differing views about the relative importance of things. Their style is generally formal. The text doesn't flow, and reading is bare of enjoyment. I avoid these problems by bringing a single point of view and a natural writing style that is easy to read and remember.

Approach

Having spent much of my professional life communicating with busy physicians buried in a blizzard of paper, I know that brevity, manner, and style are the essence of written communication. *TNOD* adopts a deliberately casual narrative style, which served me well in medical practice. It makes reading easier, holds the reader's attention, and enhances understanding and recall of important points without sacrificing scientific relevance.

TNOD focuses on answering the most important questions that students have about every disease—definition of the condition, its cause, how the anatomy and physiology change and evolve, how it is diagnosed and treated, and the outlook. Along the way, the text uses a number of devices to deepen understanding, retain interest, and enhance recall:

- *Much of the molecular and microscopic detail typically found in similar textbooks has been eliminated.* Each chapter focuses on the essentials necessary to build a broad, fundamental understanding, with supporting detail where relevant.
- *New terms are boldfaced and defined at their first use in the narrative.* This practice alerts the reader to the importance of the new term, which is defined in the same sentence, or the one immediately following. Terms of secondary importance are italicized.
- *Selected important phrases are italicized for emphasis.* For example, in Chapter 7, Disorders of Blood Cells, the following italicized phrase emphasizes the threat of colon cancer: . . . *until proven otherwise, the cause of iron deficiency anemia in adult men or postmenopausal women is occult (undetected) bleeding from the gastrointestinal tract.*
- *The narrative is sprinkled with quotations—serious, whimsical, or humorous—to humanize the material and make the subject matter more memorable.* For example, Chapter 9, Disorders of the Heart, begins with a line from country and western singer Tim McGraw's tune, "Where the Green Grass Grows": ". . . *another supper from a sack, a ninety-nine cent heart attack*. . . ." This snippet of lyric speaks volumes about the American diet and heart disease, and students invariably enjoy and remember it.
- History of Medicine *boxes further humanize the narrative by presenting historical anecdotes that put in its historical perspective.* For example, in Chapter 23,

Disorders of Daily Life, the box titled *French Food, Fast Food, Fat Food* discusses the history of restaurants, the development of fast food in America, and the devastating rise of obesity in America since World War II. Study of the history of medicine makes the scienctific points memorable in a way not achievable otherwise.

Cases

Each chapter is built around one or more real-life cases. Learning about disease, its development, and its effects is an academic exercise, which requires orderly study using textbooks, lectures, seminars, journals, lab experiments, and so on.

Another important tool in understanding this subject is case studies. The case-study method for learning medicine is as old as medical science. A case study is the "story" of a particular patient and the course of their condition over a period of time. Cases humanize and particularize medicine in a way that no other method can. Diseases occur in people, and people vary greatly from one to another. Every disease occurs in someone of a certain age, sex, and ethnicity; someone who lives a certain lifestyle, and who, for good or ill, has found a certain niche in life. Every one of these characteristics relates in some way to the condition from which they are suffering when we meet them in the chapters.

Cases are chosen to illustrate a point, usually about disease behavior, diagnosis, or treatment. Typically they are written in the past tense, do not use the patient's real name, and follow a certain form, (discussed in detail below). Individualizing disease by presenting it in living, breathing, flesh-and-blood form enhances learning.

The idea is to make the story memorable, the better from which to learn, by telling the story as it actually happened and by including the unadorned facts, some of which may not be flattering to patients or caregivers. In this book, we have condensed cases to their essence, which means I have eliminated unimportant detail. And in some cases, I have added a bit of fiction to the illness to add teaching value. I am confident you will find these memorable, because all of them are real people in some disguise.

Many TNOD cases are supplemented by "What if . . .?" alternative scenarios that are posted online at thePoint.com. This feature is entitled *The Road Not Taken—An Alternative Scenario*. Because most of the cases are derived from autopsy material, I have added a twist to some of them, which imagines a better outcome for the patient had the case unfolded in a different way. For example, in *Chapter 8, Disorders of Blood Vessels*, the case is that of a man found dead in his office. He had a history of high blood pressure, obesity, lack of exercise and tended not to take his antihypertension prescription drugs. The alternative scenario imagines the patient behaving differently—losing weight, taking his blood pressure medicine regularly, exercising, and watching his diet—and living happily ever after.

Organization

Although this textbook is unique in many ways, it is organized in a familiar fashion: it presents general pathology and pathophysiology first and follows with discussions of disorders of organ systems.

Part 1, *Mechanisms of Health and Disease*, opens with a chapter titled *Health and Disease*, which discusses the nature of disease—that is, the intimate relationship between form and function in health and in illness. This chapter also emphasizes the difference between the disease itself and the signs and symptoms it produces. The failure of healthcare professionals and their patients to appreciate this distinction accounts for a great deal of medical misdirection and misunderstanding. The remaining chapters in Part 1 deal with pathologic forces that can affect any part of the body: the life and death of cells, inflammation and repair, immune disorders, infections, neoplasia, and aberrations of fluid balance and blood flow.

Part 2, *Disorders of Organ Systems,* expands on the understanding established in Part 1 by discussing conditions of the various organs and organ systems. Along the way, the narrative is stitched together with liberal use of cross-references to other material. In early chapters cross-references steer the reader to more detailed discussion in later chapters. In later chapters they recall earlier discussion of basic concepts. For example, in Chapter 17, Disorders of the Female Genital Tract and Breast, the discussion of dysplasia of the cervix calls on the reader to understand the concept of metaplasia, which was defined and discussed initially in Chapter 2.

Part 3, *Disorders of the Stages and States of Life,* fuses knowledge gained in Parts 1 and 2 into discussions of disorders associated with states of being. We suffer differently as we progress from fetus, to neonate, to child, to adult, and to old age. Foremost we are prisoners of our genes—some grant partial exemption from risk, others are the outright cause of disease. To a lesser extent we are prisoners of environment and habit.

We benefit from careful diet, exercise and helpful stress. Or we suffer from harmful stress malnutrition, obesity, indolence, tobacco use or illicit drug abuse. We are always at risk of trauma and the problem of pain is universal.

Art Program

No textbook of pathology can succeed without a first-rate art program. Line art simplifies the structures and concepts depicted by distilling them to their basic, most easily recognizable forms, while photographs show anatomic structures as they appear in real life. *The Nature of Disease* is richly illustrated with both.

Text discussions are augmented by more than 560 full-color figures. In keeping with the core notion that anatomic form and function go hand in hand, this textbook contains more gross clinical photographs of patients and pathologic photographs of organs, tissues and cells than comparable texts. Each photograph illustrates a critical point and is intended to speak for itself. The guiding principle in developing medical line art is that good art should be understandable at a glance, or with minimal study. Our line drawings have been designed to be esthetically pleasing and to guide the reader's thought without refering to the text or to read a lengthy legend.

A full description of each of the text's features as well as the online resources can be found in *Chapter Features: A Guided Tour*, which begins on the next page.

Instructor Resources

In addition to the student resources (see *Digital Connections* on page xiii) instructors also have access to the following teaching tools:

- PowerPoint slides with accompanying lecture notes
- Image bank of figures from the text
- Answers to Chapter Challenge review questions in the text
- Test generator with more than 2,000 questions

Summary

I trust you will learn by study of the material. But more than that, I hope you will enjoy reading it. I have spent a great deal of time and energy to make the science clear and the reading easy. This book is larded with humanity in order to make the science easy to grasp and retain. My hope is that this distinctive approach will entertain and will give disease a human face.

So, here it is; judge for yourself. And after you have judged, I want you to tell me what you think. This is no idle invitation—please send your comments, suggestions, praise, or criticism to me at thmiii@gmail.com

Thomas H. McConnell, MD, FCAP
Dallas, Texas

Chapter Features: A Guided Tour

Each chapter content begins with a discussion of *normal anatomy and physiology*, providing just the right amount of information to support the disease discussions that follow. The disease discussions are the core of each chapter and consist of a narrative examination of the many disorders that may arise.

The discussion of normal anatomy and physiology and of diseases and disorders is enhanced by the following features:

The *Contents* list outlines major headings and subheadings—providing an at-a-glance look at the material covered and its organization.

Contents

Case Study "I didn't give it a second thought." The case of Ling C.

THE NORMAL LIVER
The Liver Is a Ducted Gland Organized into Lobules
The Liver Has Diverse Functions

THE LIVER RESPONSE TO INJURY
Jaundice and Cholestasis Typically Occur Together
Cirrhosis Is Patterned Scarring of the Liver

METABOLIC LIVER DISEASE
Non-Alcoholic Fatty Liver Disease Is Very Common
Hemochromatosis Is Surprisingly Common
Wilson Disease Is a Disorder of Copper Metabolism
Hereditary Alpha-1 Antitrypsin Deficiency Causes Liver Disease and Emphysema

DISEASE OF INTRAHEPATIC BILE DUCTS
Prolonged Biliary Obstruction Causes Secondary Biliary Cirrhosis
mary Biliary Cirrhosis Is an Autoimmune Disease

Chapter Objectives

After studying this chapter, you should be able to complete the following tasks:

THE NORMAL LIVER
1. Explain the function and structure of the liver circulatory systems.

THE LIVER RESPONSE TO INJURY
2. Discuss the complications associated with liver injury.

VIRAL HEPATITIS
3. Compare and contrast the transmission route, incubation time, clinicopathologic syndromes associated with, and diagnostic findings of HAV, HBV, and HCV, and briefly comment on the clinical significance of infection with HDV and HEV.

NON-VIRAL INFLAMMATORY LIVER DISEASE
4. Name the nonviral causes of inflammatory liver disease.

Chapter Objectives follow the chapter outline and are sorted and displayed according to the headings under which they are discussed.

The *Case Study* that opens each chapter's content (some chapters contain more than one) is presented in the usual clinical fashion:

- *Chief Complaint*. The problem that stimulated the patient to seek care.
- *Clinical History*. The timeline of signs and symptoms relating to the current illness.
- *Physical Examination and Othe Data*. Physical, laboratory and imaging data.
- *Clinical Course*. The story of treatment, further diagnosis, and recovery or death.

Case Study

"My life is running out of my nose." The case of Elear

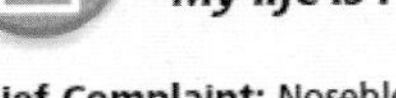

Chief Complaint: Nosebleed

Clinical History: Eleanor B., a 52-year-old professor of anthropology, presented to the emergency room of a large metropolitan hospital with a severe nosebleed. "I never have nosebleeds. This takes the cake; it just won't stop. My life is running out of my nose!"

Questioning revealed that she had been feeling unusually tired for much of the last year. "I seem to wear out at even the smallest tasks. Last week I stopped for a rest on a park bench on my way home. That's never been necessary before."

Physical Examination and Other Data: Eleanor was pale and her skin contained numerous pinpoint

Table 7.1

Value	Units
HGB	gm/d
HCT	%
RBC*	10^6 c
MCV	fL
MCHC	g/dL
MCH	pg

Two of every three deaths are premature; they are related to the loafer's heart, smoker's lung and drinker's liver.

DR. THOMAS J. BASSLER, PATHOLOGIST; QUOTED BY JAMES FIXX IN THE COMPLETE BOOK OF RUNNING (RANDOM HOUSE, 1977)

Brief *Quotations* help to illustrate the main idea of each chapter in an entertaining and informative way.

Case Study Revisited. The case and its outcome is reviewed discussed at the end of the chapter to reinforce the science discussed in the chapter.

Case Study Revisited

"My life is running out of my nose." The case of Elear

Eleanor died of bone marrow failure caused by one of the myeloproliferative syndromes: primary myelofibrosis. Malignant myeloid cells stimulated scar-like proliferation of fibrous tissue that replaced her bone marrow, forcing her spleen and liver to take over blood cell production (extramedullary hematopoiesis). This type of blood cell production, however, is not efficient. As a result, she was anemic and had a very low platelet count. On the initial visit, her WBC count was slightly elevated due to the presence of malignant cells. At the time of her death, however, each of her major cell lines was affected: platelet and leukocyte cell counts were very low, and she was severely anemic, even before her final, fatal hemorrhage. Let's discuss each of these elements.

findings were co
blood and lungs
esophagus.

- *Platelets:* Note tl
tion the platelet
a severe noseble
(*petechiae*, whic
induced bleedin
with platelets, w
her final admissi
the platelet cour
thrombocytopen
ulcer combined
esophageal hem
- *Erythrocytes:* Wh

Chapter Challenge

CHAPTER RECALL

1. A 67-year-old male is diagnosed with prostate cancer. In addition to surgery, he will receive antiandrogen (antitestosterone) therapy. What side effects (similar to those of aging) can be expected due to this therapy?
   A. Muscle wasting
   B. Decreased libido
   C. Abdominal adiposity
   D. All of the above
2. Aging is due in part to the accumulation of cellular damage. Which of the following is an important cause of cellular damage?
   A. Accelerated DNA repair
   B. Decreased telomerase activity
   C. Free ra
   D. All of t
3. An 88-yea
ences urin
cultures t
negative.
symptoms
   A. Increas
   B. Increas
   C. Increas
   D. Increas
4. Heritable
cause diff
position t

Chapter Challenge. Finally, each chapter ends with the *Chapter Challenge*, a comprehensive list of noncase questions and tasks that covers all of the chapter material. Answers are provided in the instructor's material.

Chapters are sprinkled with two types of questions, visual reminders of key points, and special boxed features.

Case notes. These are case-related questions that pertain to the relationship between the case and the topic at hand. For example, in *Chapter 9, Disorders of the Heart*, there is a discussion on the principle mechanisms of heart disease (e.g., pump failure, obstructed flow, etc.). The patient, Willard, suffered from stenosis of the aortic valve. Case Note 9.3 is "Which of the five principle mechanisms of heart disease did Willard have?" Answers are posted online.

Case Notes

12.3 One of Ling's symptoms from the episode of hepatitis 30 years earlier was yellow skin. 1) What is the name of that condition? 2) What is the name of the increased blood compound? 3) Where does it originate?

Pop Quiz. At the end of each major chapter heading is a list of questions related to the material covered under the heading. These are short, straightforward queries designed to solidify knowledge while it is fresh and readily available by quick restudy. Answers are posted online.

Pop Quiz

12.1 True or false? The liver produces all plasma proteins.
12.2 Name the two blood supplies of the liver.
12.3 What cells are responsible for portal blood filtration?

Remember This! **All refraction errors are caused by abnormal shape of the globe or cornea, or stiffness of the lens.**

Remember This. Within narrative sections,these highlighted statements emphasize the most important ideas, or suggest other ways to hep you remember key facts.

The Clinical Side presents supplemental information designed to highlight the patient side of a topic. For example, in *Chapter 9, Disorders of the Heart*, the box title is *Lifestyle and Coronary Artery Disease*. The box asks, *What Can the Average Joe or Jane Do to Prevent a Heart Attack?*, then briefly provides an answer, elements of which are sprinkled throughout the chapter narrative.

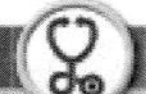

The Clinical Side

LIFESTYLE AND CORONARY ARTERY DISEASE

What can the average Joe or Jane do to pevent a heart attack?

- Giving up cigarettes is at the top of the list—nothing else comes close.
- Regular exercise, even a small amount, helps.
- Maintain a healthful weight.
- Reduce intake of foods high in saturated fat, such as burgers, full-fat cheeses, butter, and ice cream, as well as foods high in *trans* fats.

Evidence suggests that moderate consumption of alcohol can lessen the risk of cardiovascular disease.

Molecular Medicine presents additional insight into disease at the molecular level. Topics are simple molecular mechanisms that are easy to grasp and supplment understanding of chapter material. For example, in *Chapter 8, Disorders of Blood Vessels*, the box title is *A Tale of Two Sources of Cholesterol*. The box briefly discusses the sources of blood cholesterol and the molecular mechanisms of cholesterol-lowering drugs.

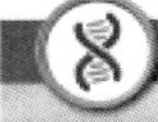

Molecular Medicine

A TALE OF TWO SOURCES OF CHOLESTEROL

Traditionally, the two major influences on the cholesterol in your body are said to be "food and family." It is true that genetics and the environment do determine your blood levels of cholesterol, but more accurately, your body acquires cholesterol either from the diet (by absorbing it from the intestine) or by synthesizing it (in the liver). These two sources of cholesterol require different drugs to treat high cholesterol. Statin drugs target liver synthesis of cholesterol by inhibiting an enzyme (HMG-CoA-reductase) in the cholesterol synthesis pathway. A newer drug, ezetimibe, blocks the molecular transporter in the small intestine that is responsible for absorbing dietary cholesterol.

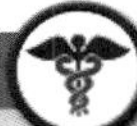

The History of Medicine

"...A DISORDER OF THE BREAST, MARKED WITH STRONG AND PECULIAR SYMPTOMS"

Coronary artery ischemia is the most common potentially fatal disease of people living in the United States and other developed Western nations. Whereas infectious diseases, diabetes, and many other illnesses were described in antiquity, CAD is a relatively recent discovery.

The typical chest pain of myocardial ischemia was first clearly described by English physician William Heberden (1710–1801). In 1768 he wrote: "There is a disorder of the breast, marked with strong and peculiar symptoms, considerable for the kind of danger belonging to it, and not extremely rare . . . [which causes a] sense of stran-

History of Medicine boxes present interesting stories about the development of medical science. For example, it is well-established today that coronary artery disease is common and fatal and is accompanied by clinical signs and symptoms known even to the average person on the street. It is easy to assume this has always been the case, but the History of Medicine box in *Chapter 9, Disorders of the Heart*, points out that chest pain and death were attributed to coronary artery disease only 100 years ago.

Digital Connections: Reinforcing and Enhancing Learning

Visit thePoint.lww.com thePoint and reinforce your learning with the following:

- Answers to Case Note questions
- Answers to Case Note and Pop Quiz questions
- Glossary of Key Terms

Animations, supplemental box content, supplemental case studies, and "The Road Not Taken" (an alternative ending for selected chapter case studies) enhance your learning and expand your understanding. In addition to the resources above, you can access the following on thePoint.com

Chapter 1:

- Animation: Acute Inflammation
- Animation: The Cell Cycle
- Animation: Wound Healing

Chapter 3:

- Animation: The Immune Response
- The Road Not Taken: Case Study Alternative Scenario
- Molecular Medicine: Detecting Autoimmune Antibodies
- The Clinical Side: Coombs Test

Chapter 4:

- Animation: The Chain of Infection
- The Road Not Taken: Case Study Alternative Scenario
- Supplemental Case Study: "A spider bit me." The case of D.W.
- History of Medicine: Who was Syphilus?
- History of Medicine: The Tuskegee Syphilis Experiment
- Lab Tools: How Do I Know If a Patient with a Genital Ulcer Has Syphilis?
- Lab Tools: Serologic Tests for Syphilis (STS)
- History of Medicine: The Discovery of Antibiotics
- History of Medicine: The History of Tuberculosis

Chapter 5:

- The Road Not Taken: Case Study Alternative Scenario
- Supplemental Case Study: "I have a chest cold that won't go away." The Case of Tina D.
- History of Medicine: Where There's Smoke, There's Cancer

Chapter 6:

- Animation: Hemostatis
- The Road Not Taken: Case Study Alternative Scenario

- Supplemental Case Study: "She's gone." The case of Rita B.
- Lab Tools: Mixing Blood and Water

Chapter 7:

- Animation: Oxygen Transport
- The Road Not Taken: Case Study Alternative Scenario
- Lab Tools: Measurement of Total Red Cell Mass
- History of Medicine: "The Royal Disease"

Chapter 8:

- Animation: Hypertension
- The Road Not Taken: Case Study Alternative Scenario

Chapter 9:

- Animation: The Cardia Cycle
- Animation: Congestive Heart Failure (CHF)

Chapter 10:

- Animation: Asthma, Gas Exchange
- The Road Not Taken: Case Study Alternative Scenario

Chapter 11:

- Animation: Digestion of CHO
- Animation: General Digestion

Chapter 12:

- Animation: Cirrhosis

Chapter 13:

- Animations: Diabetes, Hormone Control (Insulin and Glucose Metabolism)
- The Road Not Taken: Case Study Alternative Scenario
- Supplemental Case Study: "He drinks; I don't." The case of Charisa M.

Chapter 14:

- History of Medicine: President John F. Kennedy and Addison Disease

Chapter 15:

- Animation: Renal Function
- The Clinical Side: Measurement of Glomerular Filtration Rate

Chapter 17:

- The Road Not Taken: Case Study Alternative Scenario
- The Clinical Side: The Difference Between Absolute and Relative Risk
- The Clinical Side: Long-Term Estrogen Replacement Therapy

Chapter 19:

- Animation: Action Potential
- Animation: Nerve Synapse, Stroke
- History of Medicine: Strokes in United States Presidents

Chapter 20:

- History of Medicine: Braille
- The Clinical Side: Diagnosing Glaucoma

Chapter 21:

- Animation: The Immune Response
- The Road Not Taken: Case Study Alternative Scenario
- History of Medicine: John D. Rockefeller, Sr.'s Hair

Chapter 22:

- The Road Not Taken: Case Study Alternative Scenario
- History of Medicine: The History of DNA
- Lab Tools: Laboratory Diagnosis in Genetic Disease
- Molecular Medicine: Meiosis—From 46 Chromosomes to 23 and Back Again
- The Clinical Side: Diagnosis of Cytogenetic Defects

Chapter 23:

- The Road Not Taken: Case Study Alternative Scenario
- History of Medicine: Benjamin Franklin and Lead Toxicity
- The Clinical Side: Metabolic Rate and Aging

Chapter 24:

- The Clinical Side: Eat Less, Live Longer?

Acknowledgments

There was a time when I paid little attention to Acknowledgments pages in books. That was before I became an author and realized how critical are the contributions of people whose names are not on the cover.

The first edition of TNOD would not have occurred but for a chain of unlikely events that led me into academia after a career as a practicing pathologist. It began in June 1997 when I answered the phone to hear the voice of Lynn Little, a former employee I'd not heard from in years. He was calling in his capacity as Chairman of the Medical Laboratory Sciences department in the UT Southwestern Allied Health Sciences School (now the School of Health Professions). Lynn asked if I would be interested in teaching the required pathology course. Being somewhat at loose ends at the time, and having narrowly chosen private practice over academia 30 years earlier, I leapt at the chance.

Then came the task of assembling course materials from the archives in the pathology department of UT Southwestern Medical School. Beni Stewart, guru in the photography lab, and Beverly Shackelford, Supervisor of Education Programs, guided me through a huge collection of microscopic slides and photo images and helped me assemble the rudiments of a course.

Next I created an outline for students, which after a few years evolved into a ring-bound textbook. Soon word spread, other institutions began wanting to use my materials and before long I found myself in the publishing business. This was time-consuming, so I decided to mail copies to about two dozen publishers. One landed at Lippincott Williams and Wilkins. Several other publishers were interested, but it didn't take long for Lippincott to rise to the top of the heap by virtue of plainly evident professionalism.

Then came the formal editorial process, completely new to me, which proved to be one of the best educational experiences in a lifetime of learning. David Troy, executive acquisition editor, oversaw the first edition and continued his role with this second edition.

In publishing a medical textbook many people are working independently on pieces of the whole. There are the text documents (in successive versions), the art and photographs (in separate successive versions), the design team and its work products, the compositors who assembled all into the final layout you are now examing, and the printers. Eve Klein, Senior Product Development Editor, kept us and our work organized and on time. This was no mean feat.

I fancied myself good with words until I got into the hands of professional editors. To an extent that would surprise those not familiar with the editorial process, this second edition is the product of the superb editorial skills of Development Editor Laura Bonazzoli. Laura collected and codified critiques of the first edition and suggested structural reorganization of the content of this second edition. On a smaller scale she made chapter-by-chapter detailed recommendations about sequence, organization, and emphasis. Later, as draft chapters emerged, her medical knowledge added materially to chapter scientific accuracy and completeness, and her skill with words and grammar greatly improved text flow and comprehension.

Finally, a few words about Vera Paulson, MD, PhD, and Mark Valasek, MD, PhD, products of the MD/PhD program at UT Southwestern. Their work is embedded on every page. I wrote the first and final drafts of each chapter, but they independently combed the intermediate drafts for scientific completeness and accuracy. Each also has knack for organizing thoughts and a way with words that greatly improved the final product.

Thomas H. McConnell, MD, FCAP
Dallas, Texas

Contents

Expanded Contents

PART 1

Mechanisms of Health and Disease

These chapters discuss basic disease processes and pathophysiology that can affect any tissue, organ, or system of organs.

Chapter 1 Health and Disease
- Pathology, epidemiology, signs, symptoms, syndromes, and other concepts of disease
- The effects of genetics and environment
- The meaning of "normal" and "abnormal"; test sensitivity and specificity; false-positive and false-negative tests; the effect of prevalence on test interpretation

Chapter 2 Cellular Pathology: Injury, Inflammation, and Repair
- Labile, stable, and permanent tissues; the role of stem cells
- Necrosis, apoptosis, and other cell changes in health and diseaase
- Acute and chronic inflammation and the body's response to injury
- Regeneration, scarring, and repair in the recovery from injury

Chapter 3 Disorders of the Immune System
- Epithelial barriers and other nonimmune protection; alien antigens and the reactions of the immune system
- Cells and organs of the lymphoid and immune systems
- Anaphylaxis, delayed immunity, and other immune reactions
- Allergy and autoimmune disease
- AIDS and other immunodeficiencies; avian tuberculosis and other opportunistic infections

Chapter 4 Infectious Disease
- Prions, viruses, bacteria, worms, ticks, and other varieties of infectious agents
- Leukocytosis, fever, and other effects of infection
- Leukocytosis, lymphocytosis, eosinophilia, and other characteristics of infections by particular agents
- Gonorrhea, *Chlamydia*, syphilis, hepatitis, and other transmitted infections

Chapter 5 Neoplasia
- Definitions of adenoma, sarcoma, carcinoma, lymphoma, and other types of neoplasms
- DNA mutations, proto-oncogenes, tumor suppressor genes, the importance of apoptosis
- Premalignant states, malignant clones, growth fraction, degrees of differentiation, tumor blood supply, invasion and metastasis, immune surveillance
- The importance of clinical history; grading, staging, biopsy, cytology, cell markers, paraneoplastic syndromes, other aspects of clinical behavior and assessment
- Surgery, radiation, chemotherapy, vaccination, and other immune treatments

Chapter 6 Disorders of Fluid, Electrolyte and Acid–Base Balance, and Blood Flow
- Hydrodynamic pressure, osmotic pressure, and the movement of fluid and blood
- Intracellulular and extracellular fluid, plasma and blood volume, other body fluid compartments
- Edema, acidosis, dehydration, electrolyte imbalances
- Hemostasis, hemorrhage, congestion, thrombosis
- Thromboembolism and infarction
- Hypovolemic, cardiac, and septic shock; collapse of blood circulation

CHAPTER

1

Health and Disease

Contents

Chapter Objectives

After studying this chapter, you should be able to complete the following tasks:

WHAT IS DISEASE?

1. Define disease, and compare and contrast acute and chronic disease.
2. Describe the relationship between structure and function.
3. Discuss disease progression from latent period to complications/sequelae.

HOW DO SCIENTISTS STUDY DISEASE?

4. Compare and contrast the terms "etiology," "pathogenesis," and "pathophysiology." Also compare and contrast the terms "idiopathic," "iatrogenic," and "nosocomial."
5. Define "epidemiology," "incidence," and "prevalence."

WHAT CAUSES AND INFLUENCES DISEASE?

6. Discuss the roles of environmental factors, genetic factors, and determinants of health in the disease process.

HOW IS DISEASE EXPRESSED?

7. Compare and contrast symptoms and signs.
8. List the types of tests that are used to study disease (consider anatomical and clinical pathology).

HOW ARE MEDICAL TESTS INTERPRETED?

9. Explain the meaning of the terms "mean," "normal range," and "standard deviation" as they relate to medical tests and the concepts of normal and abnormal.
10. List the factors that influence the use of diagnostic tests. How does disease prevalence and incidence affect a diagnostic test? How should these tests be administered (e.g., why administer a sensitive test first)?

Case Study

"My daughter has a fever and an earache." The ca

Chief Complaint: Fever and earache

Clinical History: Anne M. was a 21-month-old girl sitting in her mother's lap. Her mother told the nurse practitioner that Anne had had a runny nose for several days but no fever. She became feverish, however, during the afternoon and had been crying and tugging at her left ear. This is when her mother brought her to the emergency room.

Physical Examination and Other Data: The nurse practitioner found that Anne had a temperature of 103°F and a perforated left eardrum with pus in the external auditory canal. Crusted mucus was present in and around the nostrils. The remainder of the exam was unremarkable—there was no skin rash, the chest was clear, the neck was flexible and moving the head produced no reaction from the child, and the anterior cranial fontanel was flat and soft. The practitioner made a diagnosis of acute rhinitis (a "cold") and acute otitis media (a middle ear infection), swabbed the pus for culture by the lab, and wrote a prescription for an antibiotic.

Clinical Course:
returned her to th
feverish but seem
at the same time.
pediatrician for cc
neck was now stif
moved. The anteri
bulging. The pedi
two lumbar vertebrae to collect a sample of spinal fluid (a spinal tap). The cerebrospinal fluid was milky. Lab microscopic examination revealed that it contained many white blood cells and a few rod-shaped bacteria. A call to the laboratory revealed that the ear culture obtained the day before was growing a pure growth of the bacterium *Haemophilus influenzae*. The diagnosis became acute bacterial meningitis. Anne was admitted to the hospital and placed on high doses of intravenous antibiotics. She made a prompt recovery.

After you have read this chapter, you should be able to discuss this case in proper scientific terms and explain why the physical examination did not detect meningitis on the first visit, and why diagnosis became certain the next day.

Be careful about reading health books. You may die of a misprint.

MARK TWAIN (SAMUEL LANGHORNE CLEMENS), 1835–1910, AMERICAN NOVELIST AND HUMORIST

In this chapter we are going to introduce you to disease, how it develops from beginning to end, and how it affects our anatomy and the functioning of our organs. But what exactly is disease? How does it differ from health? What's more, how can you know if someone is unhealthy, and if unhealthy, how can you discover the cause? Then, once you know the cause, what can you do to correct the situation safely; what can you say about the patient's future?

What Is Disease?

A young man visits his physician for a routine checkup. He feels fine and has a completely normal physical exam—despite the fact that an undetected malignant tumor is growing in his lungs. Although this young man and his physician perceive him as healthy, he is certainly sick. That's because the terms *sickness* and *health* refer to a state characterized, not according to how a person feels, but according to whether or not disease is actually present. So what, precisely, is disease?

Disease is really nothing more than healthy anatomy (**structure**) and physiology (**function**) gone wrong. Put another way, **disease** is a condition resulting from anatomical distortion or physiologic dysfunction. This definition holds whether or not the distortion or dysfunction is perceptible. Sometimes disease will cause no obvious dysfunction or "dis-ease," especially in the early stages, as we saw with the young man above. Moreover, some distortions occur at the molecular level and may not be detectable even under a microscope. Another example is high blood pressure, which is a famously silent killer.

Structure and function are inseparably locked together. For example, bacterial infection of the mitral heart valve may erode a hole (a structural abnormality) in the valve (Fig. 1.1). With each ventricular contraction, the hole allows backflow of blood (a dysfunction) into the left atrium. This inefficiency causes the heart to perform extra

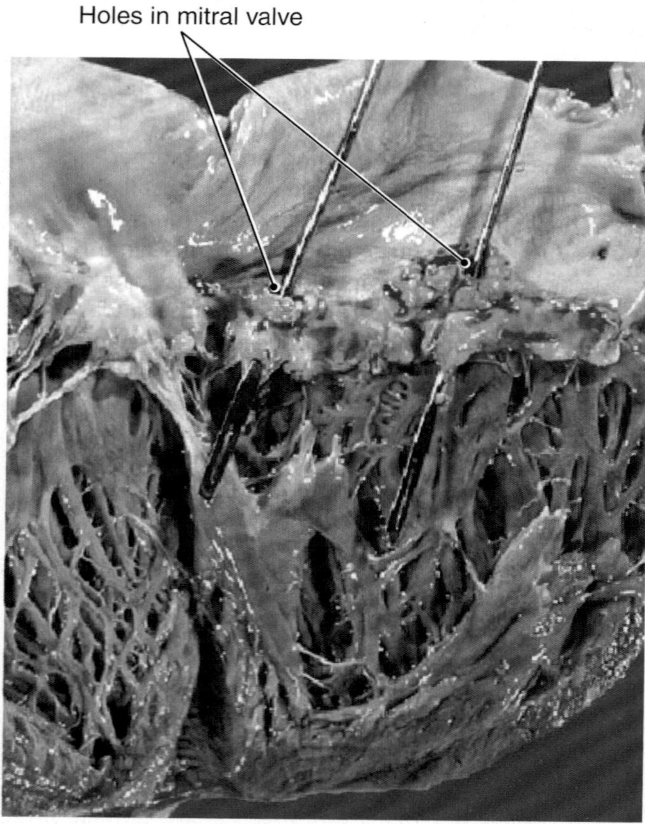

Figure 1.1 **Initial structural disorder.** Holes eaten into the mitral valve by bacteria are the initial structural defect. The result is regurgitation (backflow) of blood into the atrium—a functional disorder.

work to move the required amount of blood. This extra labor can lead to heart muscle exhaustion (heart failure), a functional disorder discussed in Chapter 9.

Likewise, a functional disorder may lead to structural change. For example, high blood pressure is a functional disorder that puts excessive strain on heart muscle as it struggles to eject blood against the elevated pressure in the arterial tree. This stress causes the left ventricular muscle to enlarge just like the skeletal muscles of a weightlifter doing gym exercises. The abnormally enlarged heart muscle is a structural disorder that has arisen from a functional disorder (Fig. 1.2).

Case Notes

1.1 Is the hole in Anne's eardrum a functional or a structural disorder?

Occasionally, medical science is unable to demonstrate a distortion or dysfunction responsible for a particular disease. When this occurs, it does not necessarily reflect the actual state of things in the body, but rather the limits of our technology. Patients with mental disorders, for

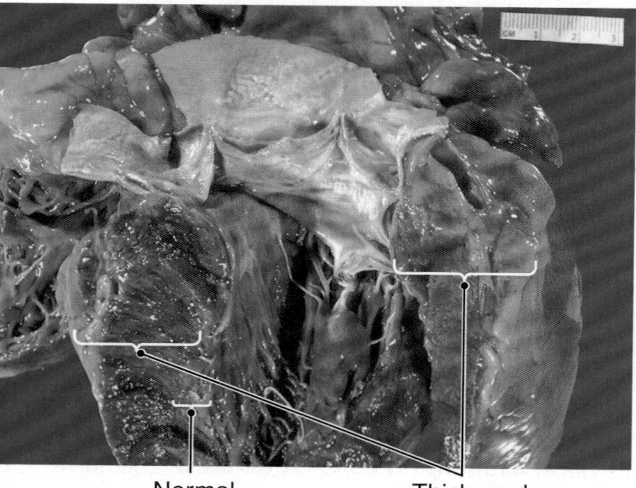

Figure 1.2 **Initial functional disorder.** High blood pressure is the initial functional disorder. Pumping against abnormally high pressure puts excess strain on the left ventricle. The result is thickening of heart muscle—a structural disorder.

example, have brain tissue that malfunctions in ways that are largely invisible to science. This is also true of certain other disorders. *Fibromyalgia*, for example, is a condition characterized by muscle and periarticular pain, tenderness, and stiffness that is not associated with any objective abnormality on medical imaging, blood analyses, or other investigations. *Irritable bowel syndrome* is another condition that illustrates the point. Patients suffer from diarrhea or constipation, abdominal pain, and bloating, but do not have any of the objective abnormalities associated with disease; labs, imaging studies, and physical findings are normal.

Apart from these exceptions, diseases present themselves by causing observable and measurable changes in the appearance (form) or performance (function) of cells, tissues, and organs. Alterations of form (such as a mass in the neck) and function (such as difficulty breathing) are assessed by collecting a medical history, performing a physical examination, and gathering objective data by laboratory tests, X-rays, and other means. We discuss this process later in this chapter, but you've already seen it reflected in the opening case study. Notice that the nurse practitioner first took a clinical history, and then performed a physical examination. She also sent a sample of tissue fluid to the laboratory for analysis.

All disease is either acute or chronic. **Acute** disease arises rapidly, is accompanied by distinctive clinical manifestations, and lasts a short time. For example, the bacterial infection in Anne's middle ear, acute otitis media, begins suddenly, is accompanied by characteristic ear pain and fever, and lasts a few days. **Chronic** disease usually begins slowly, with manifestations that are difficult to interpret. It persists for a long time, and generally cannot be prevented by vaccines or cured by medication. For example, the onset of wear and tear arthritis (called *osteoarthritis*) begins with vague stiffness or aches in certain joints, progresses slowly, cannot be cured (but can be treated), and lasts a lifetime.

The beginning of a disease is its **onset**, which may be facilitated by certain **predisposing factors**. These factors can be genetic or environmental. For example, heart disease may be promoted by certain genes inherited from an ancestor or by exposure to environmental toxins such as those in tobacco smoke. As discussed earlier, disease may be present but cause no apparent problems. This *subclinical* state may also be called the **latent period**. In infectious diseases, it is called the **incubation period** to reflect the fact that, although the person feels well, the infecting microorganism is rapidly reproducing within the body. Some disease, especially infectious disease, begins with a period of minor, nonspecific aches, dizziness, or other indications called the **prodromal period** that heralds the coming of more intense, specific indications of disease. For example, viral hepatitis often presents with loss of appetite, malaise, and mild fever that may persist for several days or longer before jaundice and other findings reveal the true nature of the problem.

After revealing itself, the condition may resolve with or without treatment. Alternatively, the condition may linger as chronic disease, which may wax and wane. When the disease is quiet, it is in **remission**; when it reappears, it is a **recurrence**. For example, after apparently successful treatment, breast cancer may disappear clinically only to reappear years, or decades, after initial treatment. A period of increased intensity of disease is an **exacerbation**. After the main illness has subsided, the patient enters a period of **recovery** during which health improves.

Sometimes a disease may quickly give rise to adverse consequences, which are called **complications**. For example, severe skin burns are often complicated by bacterial infections. In like manner, a disease may be associated with adverse outcomes at a later time, which are called **sequelae**. For example, repeated head trauma may lead to dementia later in life.

Case Notes

1.2 **Is Anne's meningitis an exacerbation or a complication of otitis media?**

Pop Quiz

1.1 True or false? A functional disorder can lead to a structural change.

1.2 True or false? Acute disease typically begins with manifestations that are difficult to interpret.

1.3 What is the scientific name for a period of vague, early manifestations that herald the coming of more pronounced disease?

1.4 What is the name for a short period of increased intensity of disease?

How Do Scientists Study Disease?

Two branches of medicine study disease as it occurs in individuals and in populations. Study of individuals elucidates functional and anatomic detail. Study of populations elucidates broad ethnic and geographic trends, modes of transmission, the influences of habits such as smoking, and the effects of age and sex, little of which can be gained by the study of individuals.

Pathology Is the Study of Disease in Individuals

Pathology is the scientific study of changes in bodily structure and function that occur as a result of disease. The term is derived from the Greek *pathos* meaning suffering, and *logos* indicating word or reason. The discipline of pathology has four main goals:

- To describe the **lesion** (the anatomic abnormality produced by the disease)
- To discover the **etiology** (cause) of the disease
- To understand the **pathogenesis** (natural history and development) of the disease process
- To explain the **pathophysiology** (the manner in which the incorrect function is expressed)

If the etiology is unknown, the disease is said to be **idiopathic** (from Greek *idio* meaning personal, thus of a personal, not commonly known, cause). For example, if a patient has a failing heart because of weak heart muscle and the cause of the weakness cannot be identified, the patient can be said to have idiopathic cardiomyopathy. In contrast, if the disease is a byproduct of medical diagnosis or treatment, it is said to be **iatrogenic** (from Greek *iatros* meaning physician). For example, if a patient develops a bladder infection after a catheter is inserted into the urinary bladder, the patient can be said to have iatrogenic cystitis. Finally, if a disease—especially an infection—originates while a patient is hospitalized, it is described as **nosocomial**, from Greek words meaning "to take care of disease." For example, a form of pneumonia caused by the *Staphylococcus* bacterium is commonly hospital acquired.

As an example of how these concepts fit together, consider an ordinary sunburn. The lesion is red, swollen, hot, painful skin. The etiology is excessive exposure to sunlight. The pathogenesis is absorption of high-energy ultraviolet (UV) rays, which injure skin. The pathophysiology is characterized by skin pain, swelling, redness, and warmth due to blood vessel dilation and increased blood flow, all of which are part of the reaction to the injury.

Case Notes

1.3 Is Anne's disease idiopathic?

Epidemiology Is the Study of Disease in Populations

Epidemiology is a discipline of medicine that studies the broad behavior of disease in large populations. One goal of epidemiology is to determine the **incidence** of a disease, which is the number of new cases of a particular disease that appear in a year, as well as the **prevalence**, which is the number of people with a certain disease at a given moment. For example, in 2009 the *incidence* of new prostate cancers in American men was approximately 192,000 cases. The *prevalence* of prostate cancer in American men was about 1.5%; that is, somewhat more than 1 in every 100 men had a history of prostate cancer. The **morbidity** rate is the number of people with an illness or complication of an illness and can be stated as either incidence or prevalence. The **mortality** rate is the number of people dying from a particular disease in a particular period of time.

Epidemiological methods are also used to identify factors that may increase an individual's likelihood of developing a specific disease. These factors are known as **risk factors**. For example, careful population studies have revealed that cigarette smoking is a risk factor for heart disease, and use of oral contraceptives is a risk factor for cervical cancer after five years of use. In contrast, protective factors are those that decrease risk. Engaging in regular physical activity is a protective factor in heart disease.

In addition, an epidemiologist may study a group of patients with a particular disease to determine what happens to them over time. This type of study helps epidemiologists establish a **prognosis**—the probability of recovery, death, or another outcome, for a disease. Probabilities are statistical likelihoods, and are often expressed as percentages. For example, the prognosis for many cancers is the percentage of patients expected to survive for a period of five, ten, or twenty years.

Pop Quiz

1.5 What is the scientific name for the cause of a disease?

1.6 What is the scientific name for a structural abnormality of disease?

1.7 True or false? The incidence of a disease is the number of new cases of a particular disease that appear in a year.

What Causes and Influences Disease?

When considering the origin of disease, it's important to distinguish between two types of factors: those that are capable of directly causing disease, and those that indirectly influence the initiation and progression of disease.

All Disease Is Due to Environmental Injuries and/or Genetic Defects

The causes of disease can be conceived of as a continuum. At one end of the continuum are diseases caused solely by environmental injury. At the opposite end are those caused solely by our genetic makeup. In the middle are the majority of diseases, those resulting from some combination of the two.

Environmental Injuries

The term *injuries* typically brings to mind physical trauma (burns, broken bones, etc.). But toxic molecules—from chemical poisonings to molecules released by infectious organisms—also commonly cause injuries. Cancer is also due to molecular injury: all cancers originate from damaged DNA. Such injurious forces are **environmental factors**; that is, they arise from the world in which we live. As we discuss below, our genetic makeup, age, gender, nutrition, and other factors can play a role in how we respond to injurious forces.

Genetic Defects

A genetic defect can be the sole cause of disease, such as cystic fibrosis, hemophilia, or sickle cell anemia. One of the most common genetic disorders is red–green colorblindness, which affects fully 7% of all males and is due to a defect in a clearly identified single gene. But most single gene (**monogenic**) diseases are rare. Diseases caused by the interaction of multiple genes (**polygenic**) are much more common, much less visible, and much more difficult to study. Not only certain diseases, but most human characteristics (traits) are polygenic. Hair and eye color, height, weight, intelligence, and facial features are examples. Important though they are, it is very difficult to identify the individual genes that make up the combination influencing, for example, intelligence. We don't know if it is closer to 100 or 1,000 genes, much less which genes are responsible and what role each plays. (See *The Clinical Side*, "The New Age of Personal Genomics.")

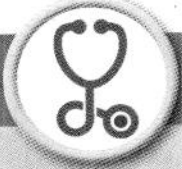

The Clinical Side

THE NEW AGE OF PERSONAL GENOMICS

In recent years, genetic technology companies have begun offering consumers an analysis of their personal genome that can identify genes that may predispose them to certain diseases. Even though anyone can purchase these genetic screenings, doing so may or may not be a good idea. In some ways it's like playing with dynamite. There is a lesson to be learned among families with Huntington chorea, an invariably fatal monogenic disease that begins to manifest in early to middle adulthood. Statistically speaking, the children of affected patients have a 50% chance of inheriting the disorder. Although these children could learn their fate from genetic analysis, many prefer not to know. For them there is wisdom in the saying, "Ignorance is bliss."

Consumers who do opt for genetic screening should have a thorough understanding of the benefits and drawbacks. It is advisable to speak with a doctor or genetic counselor before purchase of such tests and especially after results become available. Consumers should also have realistic expectations: studies show that most people who purchase personal gene tests do so with the expectation that they will change their evil ways if they are found to have a tendency to develop a certain disease. But the same studies show they don't change.

Multifactorial Diseases

Although genes are solely responsible for a few diseases and the environment accounts solely for many others, on the whole, both genetics and environment play a role in most. That is, *the majority of disease is multifactorial.* For example, some cancers develop because of inherited genetic mutations that predispose the patient to develop cancer, provided that environmental factors—like exposure to cigarette smoke—injure the patient's DNA. The fact that most disease is multifactorial means that most disease is not completely preventable in any individual. Again, cigarette smoking and lung cancer provide an excellent illustration of this tricky concept. Although 85% of all lung cancer deaths occur in smokers, 15% occur in lifelong nonsmokers, some of whom have had no significant exposure to secondhand smoke. So although eliminating all smoking would dramatically reduce lung cancer mortality within a population, avoiding smoking is not guaranteed to prevent lung cancer in any one individual.

Determinants of Health Can Indirectly Influence Disease

In addition to direct environmental and genetic causes, literally hundreds of factors in an individual's life can indirectly influence the initiation and progression of disease.

Recall Anne, from our case study, whose mother sought care for Anne's fever and ear pain. How do you think Anne's disease process might have been affected if her mother did not have access to the clinic—if, for example, she were a single mother working a minimum-wage job with no health insurance, and had waited a day or two to see if Anne's condition might resolve on its own, without the expense of medical care?

Access to quality healthcare is just one of many factors known to influence the development and progression of disease. Called *determinants of health*, these include personal, social, economic, and environmental factors that may not directly cause disease, but certainly play a role in its behavior. For instance, having social support—such as a loving family member who encourages you to see the doctor about that nagging cough—is a protective factor against disease, whereas living in a high-crime area—with limited options for safely engaging in walking, jogging, biking, and other types of outdoor physical activity—may promote obesity.

Pop Quiz

1.8 True or false? The majority of disease is monogenic.

1.9 True or false? A patient's ability to read and comprehend prescription-drug information is a determinant of health.

How Is Disease Expressed?

The nature of a disease is expressed by its symptoms, which are subjective and described by the patient during the medical history, and its signs, which are objective and are revealed during the physical, lab, X-ray, or other examination. The assembled facts then suggest the **diagnosis**, which is a name for the cause of the patient's problem. In considering the diagnostic process, it's important to keep in mind that although symptoms, signs, and test results may suggest a diagnosis, they may or may not suggest the *correct* diagnosis. It is helpful to think of such data as a roadmap, and the disease as the actual road. The roadmap may be incorrect, and the road may differ from what the map suggests.

Symptoms Are Subjective, and Signs Are Objective

Symptoms are complaints reported by the patient or by someone else on behalf of the patient. They therefore reflect a subjective experience of the disease. One of the most commonly reported symptoms is, of course, pain. Typically, the examiner asks the patient to describe the onset, duration, quality, and intensity of the pain, as well as what seems to exacerbate it and relieve it. Other common symptoms include fatigue, nausea, sensory impairment, and bowel dysfunction. All symptoms become part of the medical history.

Signs are objective data: observations by an examiner (e.g., registered nurse, nurse practitioner, physician assistant, or physician), lab data, imaging studies, electrocardiogram, and so on. For example, diarrhea reported by the patient is a symptom, but diarrhea observed by the examiner is a sign. Similarly, hearing loss reported by the patient is a symptom, but hearing loss demonstrated upon examination is a sign. Many signs can be detected only by the examiner. For instance, auscultation with a stethoscope may reveal heart, lung, or bowel sounds not detectible by the patient.

Notice that both symptoms and signs are *detectible* manifestations of disease. For example, a person may have a liver tumor that produces no symptoms and is too small to be palpated or seen. As noted earlier, in such cases the disease is said to be latent (or subclinical).

Case Notes

1.4 Name some symptoms and signs present on Anne's second visit.

Medical Tests Provide Data about Disease

Assessment of body tissues, fluids, and other components is a third way in which disease may make itself known. These studies are either anatomic or clinical.

Anatomic Pathology

Anatomic pathology is the study of structural changes caused by disease. Assessment of tissue specimens by the unaided eye is **gross examination**; assessment of magnified images of small structures is **microscopic examination**. The most basic and extensive gross examination is an **autopsy**, an after-death (postmortem) dissection of a body to determine the cause of death and other facts about the condition of the patient at the time of death. On a smaller scale, a **biopsy** is examination of living tissue, usually via microscope. For example, the study of tissues and cells in a breast biopsy or a Pap smear is an anatomic pathology procedure. Refer to *The Clinical Side*, "What Happens to a Biopsy Specimen," to see how tissue specimens are prepared for study.

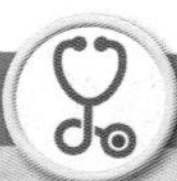

The Clinical Side

WHAT HAPPENS TO A BIOPSY SPECIMEN?

The word *biopsy* derives from Greek *bios* = life + *opsis* = sight. It is the obtaining of a piece of living tissue to discover the presence, cause, or extent of disease. The biopsy specimen is submitted to a pathologist or other medical professional for examination and diagnosis. Typically the specimen is placed in a fixative solution (usually formaldehyde) to prevent degeneration or bacterial growth and to ready the specimen for further study.

Examination occurs in two stages: gross and microscopic. The *gross examination* is study of the specimen with the unaided eye and includes the weight, size, shape, texture, color, and other features. The gross exam is followed by a microscopic study of all or carefully selected small pieces of the specimen.

In *microscopic study* of a biopsy, light shines upward from below the specimen and through it to the microscopist's eye. Microscopic study, therefore, requires slices of tissue thin enough to be transparent, usually less than one cell thick. But, just as a glass of water from the deep blue sea is almost colorless, in such thin slices there is not enough natural color present to make cells clearly visible. To solve this problem, dyes (stains) are added to color the cells. The finished result is somewhat like looking at a flag with the sun shining through from the backside.

Consider a specimen from a breast biopsy. The surgeon puts the raw lump of tissue in formaldehyde to preserve it and kill any bacteria that might cause decay during lab processing. A small sample is selected by the pathologist for further processing and is placed in a series of chemicals to soak out the fat and water, both of which render tissue fuzzy and blurry under the microscope. Next, the piece is immersed in hot paraffin wax, which soaks into the specimen to take the place of the missing fat and water. The paraffinized piece is chilled and becomes hard enough for very thin slicing by a highly precise instrument. A slice is laid flat on a slide and dipped in a series of chemicals to remove the paraffin, leaving behind on the slide surface an exceedingly thin layer of waterless, fat-free tissue; all that remains is protein, carbohydrate, and minerals. This is then dipped in a series of dyes that stain cell nuclei blue and cytoplasm red. Collagen, calcium, and other interstitial materials stain red or blue or a mixture of the two colors depending on individual characteristics. Places where fat and water used to be are empty and colorless.

Pathologists, or other specialists with microscopic expertise, study the tissue searching for patterns of disease—inflammation, degeneration, peculiar-looking cells, and so on.

In addition to ordinary microscopic study, special techniques can highlight certain cell characteristics and make them microscopically visible. An example is detection of estrogen-receptor molecules in breast cancer cells. The presence or absence of estrogen receptors is important in crafting the best therapy for breast cancer. The technique (called "immunohistochemistry") requires treating a thin slice of raw tumor tissue with antibodies and chemicals, the combination of which causes a colored precipitate to accumulate in breast cancer cells if estrogen receptors are present in them.

Clinical Pathology

Clinical pathology is the study of the functional aspects of disease by laboratory study of tissue, blood, urine, or other body fluids. Examples include blood glucose measurement to diagnose diabetes, or a culture of urine to detect bacterial infection. Clinical pathology extends from the lab to the bedside, too. A pathologist is practicing clinical pathology when he or she supervises the performance of a laboratory test, such as a blood aldosterone assay, and consults with another physician about the results.

A Syndrome Is a Collection of Symptoms, Signs, and Data

A distinctive collection of symptoms, signs, and data (anatomic or clinical) is a **syndrome**. For example, acquired immunodeficiency syndrome (AIDS) commonly includes profound fatigue (a symptom), and abnormally low counts of a particular type of T cell (a sign).

Sometimes, a particular syndrome may be caused by any of several different diseases. For example, *Cushing syndrome* (Chapter14) is a collection of symptoms, signs, and data attributable to chronic adrenocortical hormone (steroid hormone) excess. It is characterized by truncal obesity, a moon face, excess facial hair, easy bruising, skin striae (stretch marks), brittle bones, high blood glucose, and high blood cortisol, among many other features. Cushing syndrome is often due to medical treatment, but it can be due to adrenal, pituitary, or other disease.

Remember This! A syndrome is a distinctive collection of symptoms, signs, and test data.

Pop Quiz

1.10 Is an abnormality observed by a nurse a sign or a symptom?

1.11 True or false? A biopsy is an examination of a tissue specimen to determine the cause of death.

1.12 What is the name for a distinctive collection of symptoms, signs, and data?

How Are Medical Tests Interpreted?

We've said that one way disease expresses itself is by causing alterations in body tissues and chemicals that can be detected by medical tests. But when test results are in, how do clinicians interpret them in relation to disease? To answer that question, we first need to understand how to distinguish between normal and abnormal.

The Terms *Normal* and *Abnormal* Describe Observations and Measurements

In everyday conversation, we may refer to cancer or dementia as "abnormal," but clinicians do not use the terms *normal* and *abnormal* to describe health and disease. Rather, they use them to characterize observations and measurements. That's because medical test results vary greatly among healthy people, just as do height, weight, and other physical features. For example, a shoe size 15 EEE might be normal for a 6′10′, 350-lb man, but for a 5′2′, 105-lb woman it would be abnormal in the extreme. Neveretheless, even in a small woman, such a foot, though of a very abnormal size, would not necessarily indicate disease—it may function normally and be perfectly healthy. In the same way, healthy people may have unusually low, high, or otherwise abnormal test results even though they do not have a disease—the abnormal results merely reflect variation among individuals.

These variations of normal require that clinicians use an established definition of normal. For these purposes, **normal** means the usual result in healthy people. Likewise, **abnormal** means not the usual result in healthy people. It is true that most sick patients have abnormal test results, and most healthy patients have normal results. Nevertheless, sometimes sick patients have normal test results and sometimes healthy patients have abnormal test results; thus, applying the terms *normal* and *abnormal* only to observations and measurements is essential. Figure 1.3 depicts these concepts.

Qualitative versus Quantitative Tests

Qualitative tests are used to describe qualities, most commonly the presence, absence, or characteristics of a component, such as the shape of the heart as seen in a chest X-ray. For qualitative tests, the result is either normal (the expected result in healthy people) or abnormal (not the expected result in healthy people). For example, if a patient is suspected of having intestinal bleeding, stool can be tested for the presence or absence of blood. Either blood is present (abnormal) or it is not present (normal) and decisions can be made accordingly.

More commonly, a determination of normal or abnormal must be made for the results of *quantitative tests*, which measure quantities (amounts or numbers) of a component. For example, a quantitative test of kidney function might measure the amount of nitrogen in a patient's blood. This numerical data must then be compared to a standard. That is, for quantitative tests, a normal range must be established. Recall from above that normal is defined as the usual result in healthy people. But how do clinicians know what is usual?

Establishing Normal for Quantitative Tests

To establish normal for any particular quantity, epidemiologists perform statistical analysis of many results in a large number of presumably healthy people. These results

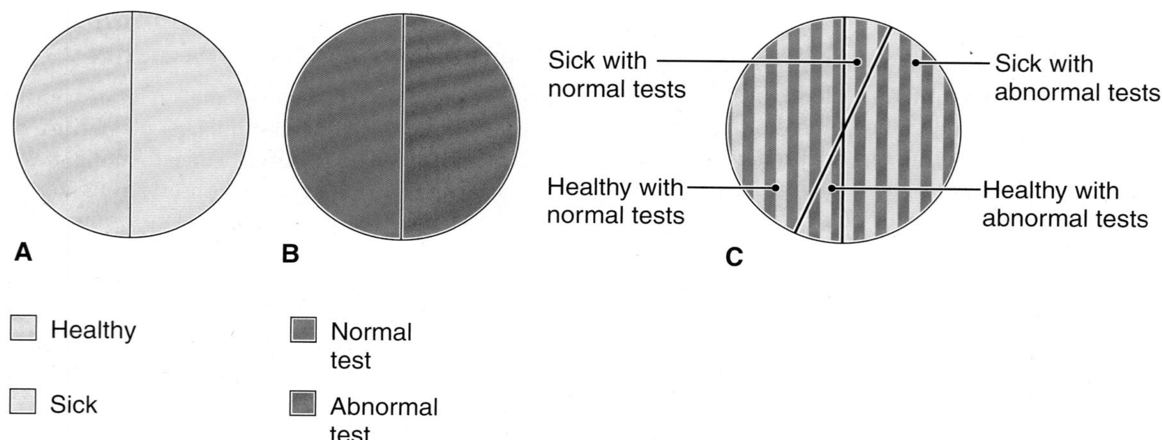

Figure 1.3 **Healthy or sick, normal or abnormal, and how they combine. A.** All patients are either healthy or sick. **B.** All measurements (tests) are either normal or abnormal. **C.** Some healthy patients have abnormal test results, and some sick patients have normal test results.

are averaged to determine the **mean** (average). Statistical formulas are also applied to the data to determine the **standard deviation**, a measure of the degree of natural variability of results; that is, the degree of variation from one normal person to another. When test results cluster tightly around the mean, the standard deviation is small. The test results for blood calcium levels, for example, have a small standard deviation because the body tightly controls blood calcium, and levels vary little from one person to another. On the other hand, when test results are widely scattered above and below the mean, as they are with blood glucose levels, the standard deviation is large.

To accommodate the natural variability of test results, epidemiologists use the mean and standard deviation to establish a normal *range*. By widespread agreement, the lower limit of the normal range is always set at two standard deviations below the mean, and the upper limit is set at two standard deviations above the mean. A graphic display of a hypothetical normal range study for blood glucose is shown in Figure 1.4. When normal is defined this way, the lowest 2.5% and highest 2.5% of results in presumably healthy persons are so far from the average that they are considered abnormal even though by definition the patient is healthy. Thus, by definition, 5% of presumably healthy people will have an abnormal test result.

Remember This! Healthy is not the same as normal; sick is not the same as abnormal.

As an example, let's presume we want to establish a normal range for blood glucose. We therefore ask 100 presumably healthy young adults to volunteer to have a blood glucose test. Those with signs or symptoms that suggest diabetes or those with a family history of diabetes are rejected. Those who are accepted are instructed not to eat or drink anything for four hours before the test. A blood glucose test is performed on each person, and the mean (average) and standard deviations are calculated for the group. If the average glucose in our group is 90 mg/dL, and one standard deviation (SD) is 10 mg/dL, then the normal range for fasting blood glucose levels would be from 90 minus 20 to 90 plus 20, or 70 to 110 mg/dL, as shown in Figure 1.4.

Positive versus Negative Results

When referring to tests for a particular disease, results are often referred to as *positive* if abnormal and *negative* if normal. The presumption is that positive suggests disease may be present, while negative suggests it is not. Presuming we know by other methods whether the patient is sick or well, test results for a particular disease are referred to as **true positive** if the test is positive and the patient actually has the disease. Conversely, the test is referred to as **false positive** if the test is positive but the patient does not have the disease. That is to say, a true positive test

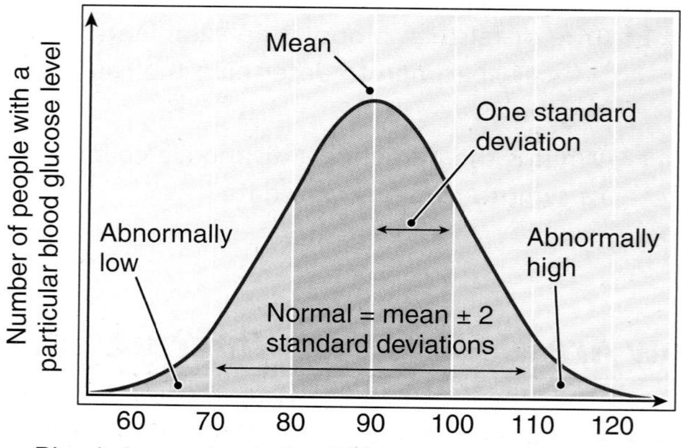

Figure 1.4 **The normal distribution curve.** Among healthy people who do not have diabetes, the greatest numbers of blood glucose levels are near the mean (90 mg/dL). A few people will have a blood glucose level below 70 mg/dL or greater than 110 mg/dL.

Table 1.1 Test Results: True and False Positive; True and False Negative

	Normal Test	Abnormal Test
HEALTHY	Healthy patient with normal test result: **True negative**	Healthy patient with abnormal test result: **False positive**
Example: People without diabetes	Normal fasting blood glucose level: *Diagnosis—no diabetes*	High fasting blood glucose level: *Perhaps patient not really fasting*
SICK	Sick patient with normal test result: **False negative**	Sick patient with abnormal test result: **True positive**
Example: People with untreated diabetes	Normal fasting blood glucose level: *Perhaps lab error*	High fasting blood glucose level: *Diagnosis—diabetes*

correctly indicates that disease is present, whereas a false positive test incorrectly suggests disease is present when, in fact, it is not. Likewise, negative results are referred to as **true negative** or **false negative**, depending on whether the test result correctly or incorrectly indicates that disease is absent. These combinations are depicted in grid form in Table 1.1.

Case Notes

1.5 Presuming that Anne's meningitis was present but not severe on the first visit, was Anne's soft, flat fontanel a true positive, false positive, true negative, or false negative test for meningitis?

The Extent of Abnormality

If a test is abnormal, the degree of abnormality is important—markedly abnormal results are more significant than are mildly abnormal ones. Disease is a continuum from mildly ailing to desperately ill, and test results vary accordingly. The greater the degree of abnormality, the more likely it is that the result means disease is present (the test is truly positive). For example, if the upper limit of normal blood glucose levels is 110 mg/dL, a patient with a fasting blood glucose level of 190 mg dL is much more likely to have diabetes than is a patient with a fasting blood glucose level of 120 mg/dL.

Test Sensitivity and Specificity Are Key Considerations

In addition to interpreting the values of test results as normal and abnormal, clinicians must be able to appreciate a test's sensitivity and specificity. The ability of a test to be positive in the presence of disease is test **sensitivity**. For example, a test is 99% sensitive if it is positive in 99 of 100 patients known to have the disease. Similarly, **specificity** is the ability of a test to be negative in the absence of the disease. A test is said to be 99% specific if it is negative in 99 of 100 persons known not to have the disease.

Case Notes

1.6 Presuming Anne had mild meningitis on the first visit, as a test for meningitis did the neck manipulation test lack sensitivity or specificity?

There is a trade-off between sensitivity and specificity. *Highly sensitive* tests are likely to be positive in patients with the condition or disease (truly positive), but they also have a tendency to be positive (falsely positive) in some healthy people, too. That is to say, if you screen for a certain condition using a highly sensitive test, the group with positive results will include most of the patients with the condition (you won't miss many), but mixed in will be a fairly large number of healthy patients who do not have the condition (their tests are falsely positive). Although this is less than ideal, the flip side is that you can be confident that those who had negative results are healthy (truly negative). That is to say, a negative result using a highly sensitive test is a very reliable indicator that the condition for which you are testing is *not* present. In the group with positive tests, you can sort out the false positives from the true positives by doing additional tests.

The opposite is true for *highly specific* tests—the test is likely to be negative in healthy patients who, of course, do not have the condition for which you are testing. The test may be negative, however, in some patients with the condition (their test is falsely negative). It follows that if you screen a group of patients using a highly specific test, you can be confident that those with positive tests have the condition (their test is likely to be a true positive, not a false positive). Nevertheless, the group with negative results will include some patients with disease, whom you can identify by further testing later.

Again, as a rule, highly sensitive tests are not very specific, and highly specific tests are not very sensitive. By way of example, consider home burglar alarms as a test for burglars. Alarms are very sensitive but not very specific—so although they do not miss many burglars, there are lots of false alarms. That is to say, burglar alarms have many false positives but few false negatives. By contrast, having a personal observer at home is much more specific but it is less sensitive. Rarely would an observer in the house falsely accuse someone of being a burglar unless they were unknown or unwelcome, but if the observer is out working in the back garden, then a burglar might not be detected.

Given that both sensitive and specific tests have drawbacks, which type of test does a clinician choose, and why? In the diagnostic process, the most effective strategy is this: first use a very sensitive test, and then follow up on patients who test positive by administering a very specific test. This is precisely the strategy used in many types of cancer screening. For example, sexually active women are routinely screened for cervical cancer using a Pap smear, which is a highly sensitive test; that is, it misses very few cases of cervical cancer (Fig. 1.5). A Pap smear is inexpensive, painless, and minimally invasive. The clinician collects a sample of cervical cells in a matter of seconds during a woman's routine pelvic exam. Nevertheless, because it is highly sensitive, Pap smear screening will result in false positives. So a diagnosis of—and treatment for—cervical cancer is not yet warranted for those women who test positive. Instead, these women undergo a second, highly specific test, a tissue biopsy. This second test is more invasive, more painful, more time consuming, and more expensive, so it is not practical as a screening test for presumably healthy women; it is, however, very useful to distinguish the true-positive smears (women with cancer) from the false-positive smears (women without cancer).

Remember This! Test first with highly sensitive tests; retest positives with highly specific tests.

Tests Vary in Their Predictive Value

The purpose of testing is to determine who has disease and who does not. The best test has high **predictive value**; that is, it accurately predicts who has and who does not have disease. Highly sensitive tests tend to have a lot of false positives, but very few false negatives. Therefore, *a negative result in a highly sensitive test has high predictive value.* Highly specific tests tend to have a lot of false negatives, but few false positives. Therefore, *a positive result in a highly specific test has high predictive value.* Another way to say this is that if a test has many true positives and few false positives, the predictive value of a positive test is high. Likewise, if a test has a great number of true negatives and few false negatives, the predictive value of a negative test is high.

For example, cardiac troponin I, a heart muscle protein that increases in blood as a result of a heart attack, normally circulates in blood in small amounts. Therefore, in a patient with chest pain and possible heart attack, increased cardiac troponin I is considered a positive test for cardiac

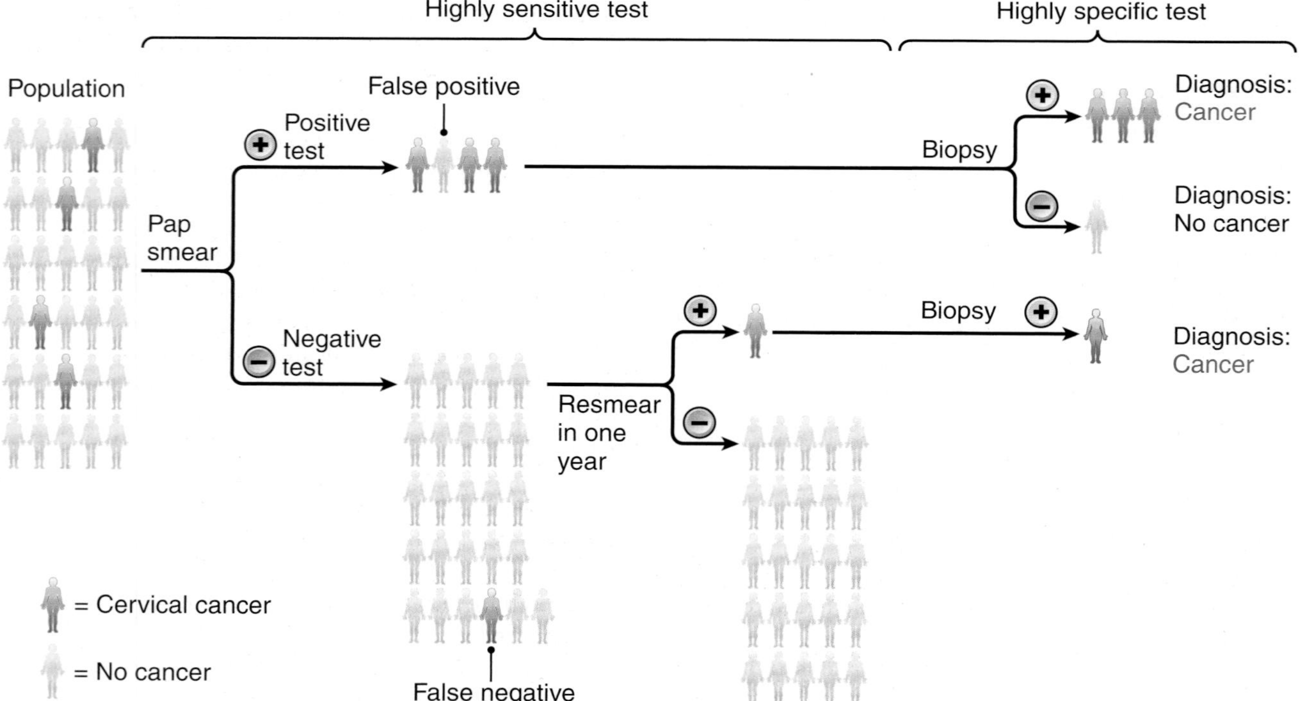

Figure 1.5 **Test sensitivity and specificity in the search for cancer of the cervix.** To detect cancer of the cervix, first use a highly sensitive test, the Pap smear, which is not likely to miss many cancers. Those who test positive by Pap smear are further investigated by cervical biopsy, a more specific test. Those who tested negative by Pap smear are retested by Pap smear the next year, which will likely identify false negatives missed on the first smear.

muscle damage and a reliable sign of a heart attack. Normal levels of cardiac troponin I suggest no cardiac muscle damage has occurred and the cause of the pain must be found elsewhere. Diagnostic use of cardiac troponin I as a tool to predict the presence or absence of heart muscle damage has shown that most patients with abnormally high cardiac troponin I have heart muscle damage. Conversely, the great majority of patients with normal cardiac troponin I do not have heart muscle damage. Thus, the predictive value of cardiac troponin I as an indicator of the presence or absence of heart muscle damage is high for both positive and negative tests, making cardiac troponin I a very widely used diagnostic test when heart muscle damage is suspected.

As discussed above, the degree of test abnormality is important—the greater the abnormality, the more likely is it that the result correctly suggests that disease is present. This means that a patient with very high cardiac troponin I is much more likely to have heart muscle damage (and more extensive damage) than is a patient with mildly elevated cardiac troponin I.

Disease Prevalence Influences a Test's Usefulness

How well a test performs (whether it has high or low predictive value) depends to a surprising degree on how many cases exist (the *prevalence*) in the group being tested. For example, consider the cardiac troponin I test just mentioned. The number of people having an acute heart attack is near zero among asymptomatic persons entering a shopping mall. Any positive test in such a group is very likely a false positive. On the other hand, the same test will be much more useful if performed in patients who present with chest pain to an emergency room because among such patients there are many having a heart attack. Therefore, in an emergency room population, a positive result is much more likely to be truly positive.

In medical diagnostic terms, a positive test is more likely to be truly positive (to have a high predictive value; to be a correct indication of disease) if there are a lot of people in the tested population who have the disease; that is, if the prevalence of disease is high in the tested population.

Case Notes

1.7 Is the prevalence of meningitis likely to be low or high in a group of infants with a tense, bulging fontanel?

Pop Quiz

1.13 True or false? All sick patients will have at least one abnormal test.

1.14 What percentage of the test results in healthy people fall within the mean plus and minus two standard deviations?

1.15 The ability of a test to be positive in the presence of disease is __________.

1.16 True or false? The best testing strategy is to start with highly sensitive tests and follow with highly specific ones.

Case Study Revisited

"My daughter has a fever and an earache." The case of Anne M.

Reviewing this case gives us an opportunity to review many of the terms and concepts covered in this chapter.

Anne's primary *symptom* on her first visit was pain, which she "reported" (through her mother) by crying and tugging on her ear. The nurse practitioner examined Anne and found the following *signs*, each of which can be thought of as a positive test: elevated temperature, runny nose and crusted nostrils, perforated left eardrum, and pus in the external auditory canal. Knowing that meningitis can be a *complication* of ear infection, the nurse also checked the flexibility of Anne's neck and the softness of her anterior fontanel. Both were normal; that is, they were negative tests. After examination the nurse practitioner concluded that the *diagnosis* was *acute* bacterial infection of the left middle ear (otitis media) with perforation of the tympanic membrane. The initial *etiology* was *acute* viral upper respiratory infection. The *pathogenesis* was swelling and mucus obstruction of the eustachian tube (abnormal *form*), which caused accumulation of fluid in the left middle

(continued)

"My daughter has a fever and an earache." The case of Anne M. (continued)

ear (abnormal *function*). This fluid became a culture medium for growth of resident bacteria from the throat and nose. As pus accumulated, pressure caused perforation of the eardrum. The hole became an obvious *lesion*.

When antibiotic treatment did not resolve the problem and Anne returned the next day, new symptoms and signs were present. New *symptoms* were sleepiness and jumpiness. New *signs* were positive tests for stiff neck and tense, bulging fontanel. Both were suggestively positive *screening* tests for meningitis. That is to say, their *predictive value* was not high enough to be reliable without further testing. Neither was *sensitive* enough to be positive the first day when, in retrospect, the meningitis was in an *incubation (latent) period*. This led to the decision to perform a spinal tap, a highly *sensitive* and *specific* test, which showed pus, a result with a high *predictive value*. The *etiology* of the otitis media and meningitis proved to be a bacterium, *Haemophilus influenzae*. The final *diagnosis* was *acute* bacterial meningitis.

The initial *prognosis* was guarded because bacterial meningitis is an extremely serious disease, sometimes fatal or the cause of permanent and serious *sequelae* such as deafness, mental retardation, or other problems. Nevertheless, with antibiotic therapy the disease was cured without *complications*, and the final *prognosis* was excellent.

Chapter Challenge

CHAPTER RECALL

1. A disease of unknown origin is more commonly referred to as
   A. iatrogenic.
   B. idiopathic.
   C. nosocomial.
   D. subclinical.

2. Which of the following is an example of anatomic pathology?
   A. Study of a breast biopsy specimen
   B. Study of a blood glucose level
   C. Study of the concentration of electrolytes (such as sodium) in urine
   D. Culture of phlegm (mucous) to detect microorganisms

3. A chronic disease differs from an acute disease because
   A. a chronic disease has distinct symptoms while an acute disease does not.
   B. a chronic disease (while it can be treated) will have long-term complications, while an acute disease has no long-term complications.
   C. a chronic disease has a slow onset with indistinct symptoms while an acute disease arises rapidly with distinctive symptoms.
   D. a chronic disease lasts a few days, while an acute disease lasts less than 24 hours.

4. A latent period
   A. occurs when a disease is present, but unaccompanied by signs and symptoms.
   B. is the onset/beginning of a disease.
   C. occurs when disease recurs.
   D. begins with nonspecific symptoms that herald the coming of more intense-specific symptoms.

5. True or false? A greater degree of abnormality does not increase the likelihood that disease is present.

6. Standard deviation is which of the following?
   A. A measure of the degree of natural variability of results
   B. Determined by measuring a value in the entire population (healthy and sick) to determine the normal range
   C. Always the same between different tests
   D. The averaged results

7. The natural history and development of the disease process is __________.
   A. Etiology
   B. Pathophysiology
   C. Pathogenesis
   D. Lesion

8. True or false? The cause of all disease is environmental injury or genetic defect.

9. The number of new cases per year is the ________________.
   A. Incidence
   B. Prevalence
   C. Occurrence
   D. Mortality rate

10. Heart disease is which of the following?
   A. Monogenic
   B. Polygenic
   C. Environmental
   D. Multifactorial

CONCEPTUAL UNDERSTANDING

11. Using examples from the text, describe the relationship between structure and function.

12. Compare and contrast signs and symptoms.

13. Sensitivity is to false positive as
   A. specificity is to false negative.
   B. specificity is to true positive.
   C. specificity is to true negative.
   D. predictive value is to false negative.

14. What roles do our environment and our genetics play in causing disease? Consider examples along the continuum.

15. Compare and contrast clinical and anatomic pathology.

APPLICATION

16. In screening a population for a lethal disease, what factors affect the type of test that you will choose? Consider sensitivity, specificity, prevalence, and predictive value.

17. Discuss health and sickness versus normal and abnormal in the context of true positive, false positive, true negative, and false negative.

CHAPTER

2

Cellular Pathology: Injury, Inflammation, and Repair

Contents

Chapter Objectives

After studying this chapter, you should be able to complete the following tasks:

CELL REPRODUCTION AND DIFFERENTIATION

1. Name and describe the various types of stem cells.
2. Explain the difference between labile, stable, and permanent cells.

CELL INJURY, DISEASE, AND DEATH

3. Discuss the various mechanisms of cell injury.
4. Compare and contrast the response to reversible injury (i.e., accumulations and adaptations) with the response to irreversible cell injury (i.e., apoptosis and necrosis).

THE INFLAMMATORY RESPONSE TO INJURY

5. Describe the cells and chemical mediators of the inflammatory process.
6. Compare and contrast acute and chronic inflammation.
7. Describe the systemic effects of inflammation.

REPAIR

8. Distinguish between parenchymal and fibrous repair.
9. Compare and contrast healing by first and second intention.
10. List factors that cause abnormal wound healing.

Case Study

"I cut my finger." The case of Marianne M.

Chief Complaint: Lacerated finger

Clinical History: Marianne M. was slicing an apple when she accidentally cut a finger. She applied pressure to stop the bleeding. A neighbor drove her to a physician's office immediately.

Physical Examination and Other Data: Marianne was an otherwise healthy-appearing middle-aged woman with a bloody towel wrapped around her left hand. Examination revealed a clean, 2 cm diagonal cut on the palmar surface of the left second finger at the proximal interphalangeal joint. The cut extended through the dermis and into subcutaneous fat but did not enter the joint. The wound was slowly oozing blo as it was at first,"

Clinical Course: washed with antib stitches. The finge splint applied to ir Marianne returnec removed. She was month. After the s that the scar was extend her finger. She was advised to do maximum stretch extension of the finger several times a day. One year after the accident, she was able to fully extend her finger in the course of normal activity.

To know truly is to know by causes.

FRANCIS BACON, 1561–1626, ENGLISH PHILOSOPHER AND SCIENTIST

Recall from Chapter 1 that most disease is due to cellular injury; that is, if we are sick, it is probably because our cells have been injured. **Inflammation** is the body's composite cellular reaction to injury. It limits the damage and initiates healing. **Repair** is the process of healing the injury by regenerating new cells to replace dead ones or by filling the void and closing the wound with scar tissue. Before exploring how cell injury, inflammation, and healing occur, let's review how cells reproduce.

Case Notes

2.1 **Will inflammation occur in Marianne's cut?**

Cell Reproduction and Differentiation

Maintenance of life requires replacement of injured or dead cells with new cells. But cells don't just spring into being. They have to start somewhere, and they start with self-reproduction: the division of one cell into two. Cell reproduction is necessary for growth from embryo to adult, but it is also important to maintain tissue health throughout life, because cells continually age and die and must be replaced.

Cell self-reproduction occurs in an orderly process known as the **cell cycle** (Fig. 2.1). The cycle starts with a single cell and proceeds through a series of steps known as **mitosis**, a process of organizing and dividing the nucleus into two daughter nuclei. Division of the cytoplasm is relatively simple: half the cytoplasm and organelles go to one new "daughter" cell and half to the other. But the nucleus is a special case: there is only one nucleus and its DNA must be organized into two *exactly* matching sets so that the DNA of each offspring cell will *perfectly* match the parent DNA. During mitosis the DNA in each chromosome duplicates itself, but the two identical sets remain attached in the center (Fig. 2.1, prophase). Then one set moves left, the other right, and the cytoplasm divides. Thus, one cell has become two. The DNA in each daughter cell is identical to the DNA of the parent cell, which ensures perpetuation of the original genetic code from one generation of cells to another. When mitosis ends there are two cells, each of which is back at the beginning point, ready for another ride on the cell cycle merry-go-round.

All Cells Arise from the Zygote

A **stem cell** is an unspecialized (undifferentiated) cell that in one mitotic cycle reproduces a copy of itself and creates a second, specialized (differentiated) cell (Fig. 2.2). The fertilized egg (zygote) is the granddaddy of all stem cells and of all other cells. It differentiates into three embryonic tissues: ectoderm, endoderm, and mesoderm.

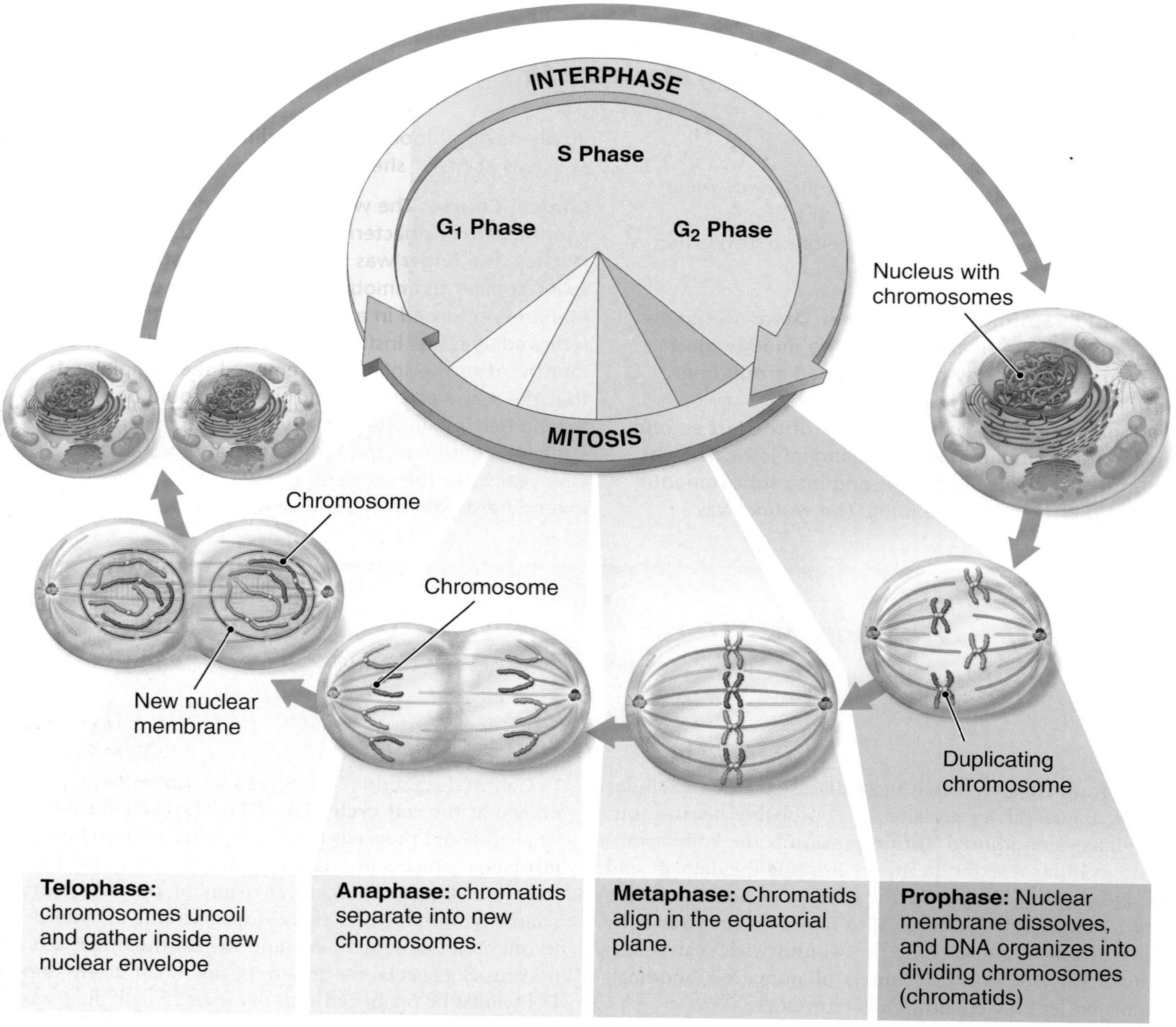

INTERPHASE
S Phase
G_1 Phase
G_2 Phase
MITOSIS
Nucleus with chromosomes
Chromosome
Chromosome
New nuclear membrane
Duplicating chromosome

Telophase: chromosomes uncoil and gather inside new nuclear envelope

Anaphase: chromatids separate into new chromosomes.

Metaphase: Chromatids align in the equatorial plane.

Prophase: Nuclear membrane dissolves, and DNA organizes into dividing chromosomes (chromatids)

Figure 2.1 **Mitosis.** Mitosis (division of the nucleus). After the nucleus divides the cytoplasm divides to complete the formation of two new cells. (Reprinted with permission from McConnell TH, Hull KL. *Human Form Human Function: Essentials of Anatomy & Physiology*. Baltimore, MD: Wolters Kluwer Health; 2011.)

From these three tissues, an entire organism evolves: trillions of cells differentiated into more than 200 specialized types. The three initial tissue types are the following:

- *Ectoderm*, which differentiates into hair, nails, and epidermis—the superficial layer of skin—and into brain and nerves
- *Endoderm*, which differentiates into the internal lining (mucosa) of the intestinal and respiratory tracts and into the liver and pancreas
- *Mesoderm*, which differentiates into the deep layer of skin (dermis), bone, skeletal muscle, blood vessels, smooth muscle (including the muscular wall of the gastrointestinal tract), pleura, peritoneum, pericardium, and the kidneys and gonads

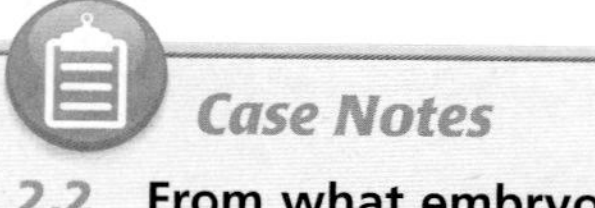

Case Notes

2.2 **From what embryologic tissue does Marianne's epidermis arise?**

Stem Cells Form Other Types of Cells

Stem cells are classified according to their power (potency) to develop into specialized cells. The most potent have the broadest powers: they can give rise to an entire organism or to any particular type of cell in the body. Such stem cells are *totipotent* stem cells (Latin *totus* = whole, and Latin *potens* = to be able). The zygote is such a cell.

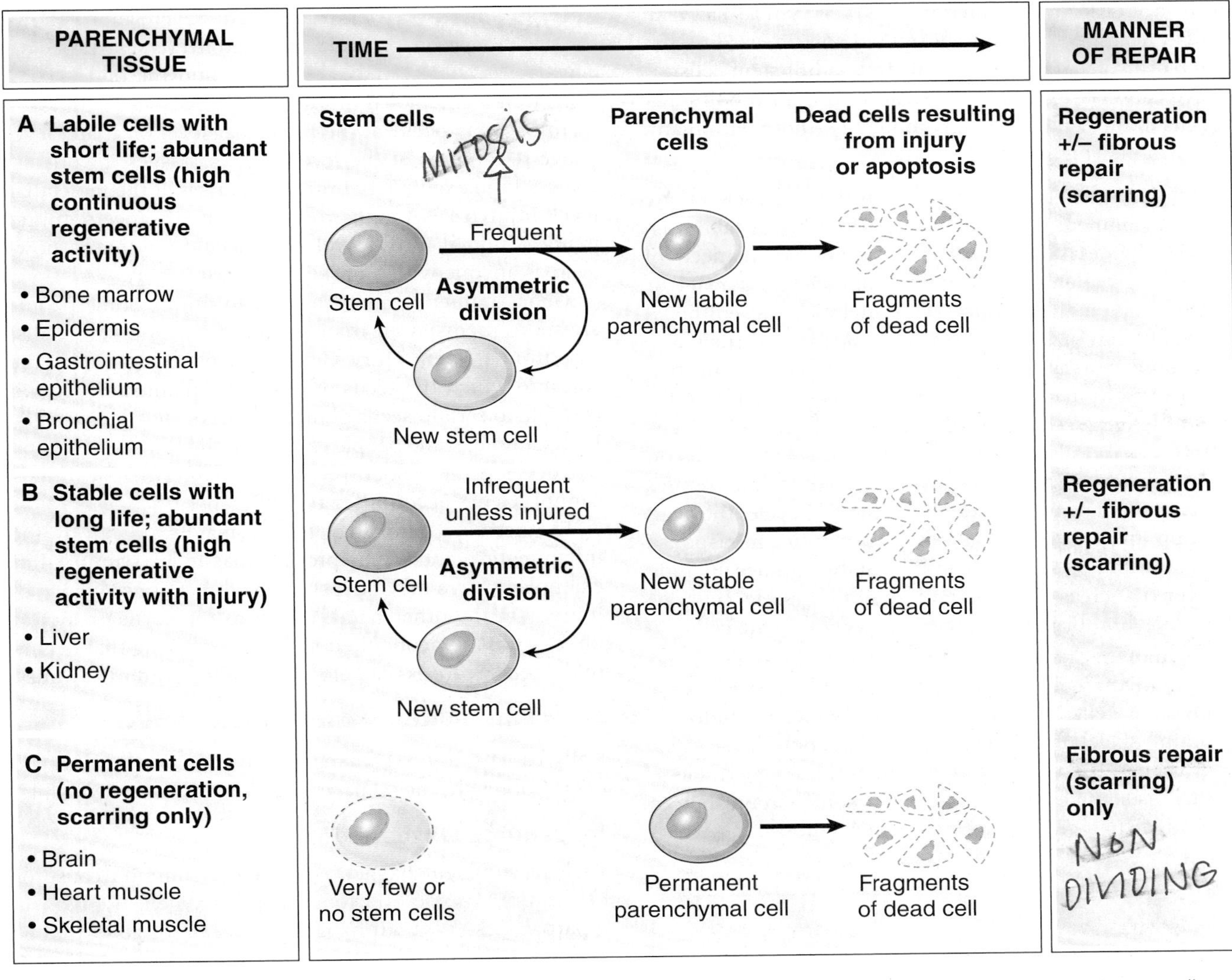

Figure 2.2 **Stem cells in the repair process. A.** Labile parenchymal tissues contain stem cells that continuously regenerate new stem cells and parenchymal cells to replace functional cells lost to injury (necrosis) or natural cell death (apoptosis). Labile tissues repair themselves by regeneration, or if the injury is great, by regeneration and scarring. **B.** Stable parenchymal tissues contain stem cells that reproduce rapidly only when stimulated by cell death resulting from injury. Stable tissues repair themselves by regeneration, or if the injury is great, by regeneration and scarring. **C.** Permanent tissues do not contain stem cells. They repair themselves by scarring only.

The first eight cells that arise from the zygote retain totipotency; that is, the capacity, if separated from the others, to reproduce an entire human being.

Subsequent stem cell generations beyond the initial eight cells become more specialized and less broadly potent. As the initial eight zygote cells divide, each differentiates into a more specialized version—the *pluripotent* stem cell (Latin *plur* = more, extra). Each pluripotent cell can produce any type of tissue—heart, brain, liver, skin, and so forth—but cannot form an entire new human being. These pluripotent stem cells are also called *embryonic stem cells*.

As division continues, pluripotent stem cells differentiate into less potent, more specialized *multipotent* stem cells. Each type of multipotent stem cell can produce a limited range of cell types. For example, *mesenchymal stem cells* can produce muscle, bone, ligament, or fat cells, while *hematopoietic stem cells* produce the many types of blood and bone marrow cells.

What sets stem cells apart from other types of cells is **asymmetric division** (Fig. 2.2). Contrary to nonstem cell division, a stem cell's two daughter cells are not alike. One daughter cell becomes a new stem cell to maintain the stem cell population; the other daughter cell becomes a more specialized cell.

Remember This! A stem cell divides asymmetrically into two different cells: one new stem cell and one new specialized cell.

Some Stem Cells Persist into Adulthood

Small numbers of multipotent stem cells, often referred to as *adult* stem cells, persist in adults to act as a ready reserve to replace dead or dysfunctional cells. A critical factor in human health is the ability of injured and diseased tissues to repair by generating new cells from adult stem cells.

We can classify body tissues according to the number of cells in the cell cycle at any moment—those with many, few, or none (Fig. 2.2):

- **Labile** tissues have many cells in the cell cycle at any given moment; in other words, the cells of labile tissues divide frequently. Labile tissues are in need of ongoing replenishment because of constant damage or environmental exposure. This includes the epithelial membranes of the skin, urinary tract, and GI tract, and all bone marrow cells. Replenishment comes from stem cells and from ordinary mitotic division of mature cells.
- **Stable** (*quiescent* or *quiet*) tissues have only a few cells in the cell cycle at any given moment. That is, cells do not divide very frequently. Although stable tissues generally have very few cells in the cell cycle, they can ramp up proliferation at a moment's notice in response to a stimulus, such as injury. Stable tissues include liver, pancreas, kidney, and smooth muscle cells, as well as fibroblasts and other connective tissue cells.
- **Permanent** (nondividing) tissues have very few or no cells in the cell cycle because they have very few or no stem cells. Permanent tissues—which include the brain, skeletal muscle, and cardiac muscle—cannot grow new tissue in response to injury. Nevertheless, there is some evidence that under some circumstances limited stem cell replacement can occur.

Case Notes

2.3 Is Marianne's epidermis a labile, stable, or permanent tissue?

Pop Quiz

2.1 True or false? Ectoderm is derived from the zygote and differentiates into hair, nails, and epidermis.

2.2 Asymmetric division is characteristic of what type of cell?

2.3 Distinguish between labile and permanent tissues.

Cell Injury, Disease, and Death

Mild injury or stress causes *reversible* adaptive cellular changes without cell death. These cellular adaptations constitute homeostasis in action, and return to normal once the injury or stress is relieved. Severe injury, however, causes pathologic cell death (an *irreversible* process). The process of cell injury or stress, and the body's reactions to it are depicted in Figure 2.3.

Injury may occur at the molecular level or at any level above it—that is, at the level of cells, tissues, or organs. Cancer is an example of injury that arises at the molecular level: injured DNA is the root cause of all cancers. Injury is not confined to the level of molecules and cells, however, as anyone with a broken bone can testify.

Genes influence how we react to injury. Some people are more predisposed than others to develop severe disease from a given injury. Genes may be thought of as the soil into which the seeds of injury are planted. Some soil is fertile to certain seeds of injury and less fertile to others. For example, some people can eat all the salt they like and not develop high blood pressure (Chapter 8), but others cannot. Genes account for the difference.

Furthermore, impaired health may result from the inflammation and repair process that follows injury. For example, an eye may be lost as the direct consequence of injury. On the other hand, injury to the cornea may not directly cost someone their sight, but scarring that occurs in the repair process can cloud vision long after the injury.

Cells Can Be Injured in Several Ways

Cells can be injured in many ways. Depending on the degree of insult, the damage may or may not be reversible.

Inadequate Oxygenation

Lack of sufficient oxygen is the most common cause of cell injury. **Anoxia** is a total lack of oxygen; **hypoxia** is a partial lack. Without oxygen, cells cannot generate energy, and without energy, cells die. Some tissues are more vulnerable to oxygen deprivation than others. Without oxygen, neurons in the brain and spinal cord begin to die after a few minutes, whereas muscle cells can survive for hours.

Inadequate blood flow is called **ischemia** (Greek, *iskhein* = keep back + *haima* = blood), and causes not only a lack of oxygen (hypoxia), but also decreased delivery of nutrients (e.g., glucose, amino acids) and accumulation of toxic waste products (e.g., CO_2, free radicals), which cannot be carried away.

Hypoxia or anoxia may occur in a number of clinical circumstances. The usual cause is ischemia caused by a *localized* block of tissue supplied by a single artery. *Generalized* hypoxia may be produced by lung disease, some kinds of poison, near drowning, suffocation, and other conditions. In generalized hypoxia, it is usually the brain that suffers first.

Short-term reversible cell damage due to hypoxia can be repaired by reoxygenation. For example, patients who have cardiac arrest suffer immediate brain hypoxia. If they are promptly resuscitated, however, they may avoid neurological damage.

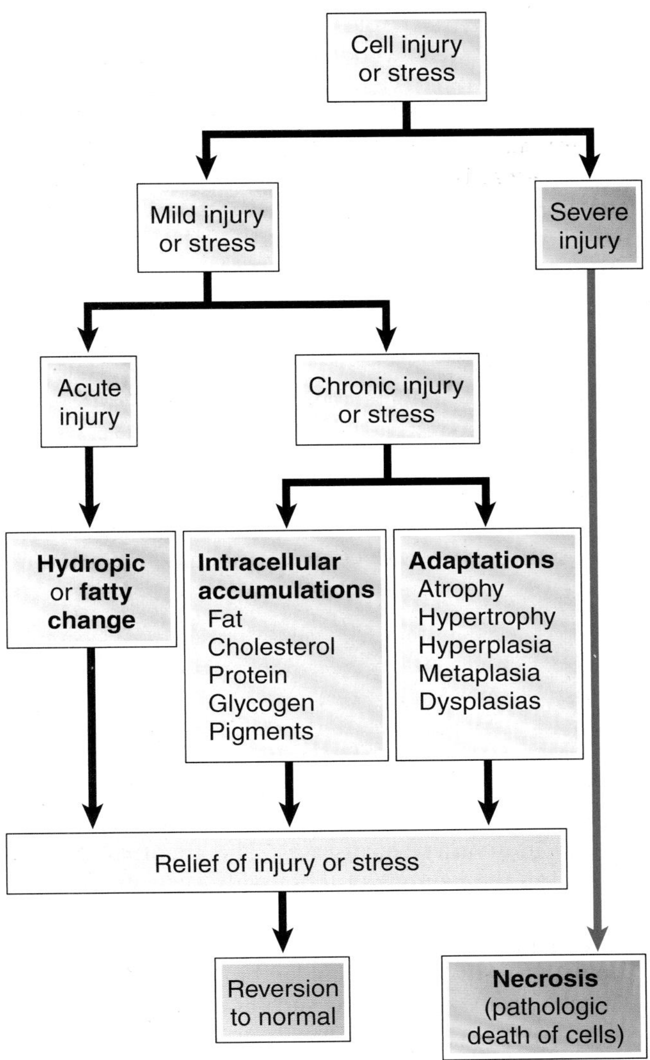

Figure 2.3 **Cell reactions to injury or stress.** Cells react in similar ways to mild chronic injury or unusual physiologic demand (stress). Severe injury leads to cell death.

Physical, Thermal, or Chemical Agents

Physical force or chemical agents can disrupt the structure of organs or tissues. Fatal hemorrhage and ischemia are the major consequences of physical force. Thermal injury can also occur; for instance, low temperatures may freeze the water in skin cells—a condition called **frostbite**. Cell death occurs when ice crystals rupture cell membranes. Low body temperature may also slow the heart's intrinsic pacemaker and cause cardiac arrest. Acids, alkalis, or heat may cause the death of skin, cornea, or mucosal surface cells.

Ionizing Radiation

Ionizing radiation is radiation strong enough to break (ionize) water (H_2O) into H^+ (hydrogen ion) and OH^- (hydroxyl ion). In *acute radiation injury*, the hydroxyl ion attaches to DNA and prevents cell reproduction. For cells that do not reproduce regularly—such as brain or liver cells—this is of little consequence. For cells that reproduce rapidly, however—such as blood cells in the bone marrow or gastrointestinal epithelial cells—it is a disaster. The white blood cell (WBC) count falls dramatically because WBCs live only a few days and must be replaced daily. Intestinal lining cells stop reproducing, and the lining sloughs away and is not replaced. Decreased WBC count and loss of intestinal epithelium leave the body vulnerable to infection.

Ionizing radiation is intentionally used to treat certain cancers; however, the amount (dosage) given to the patient is designed to avoid acute radiation injury. In rare instances, this treatment itself can cause another different type of cancer years later. The best example is breast angiosarcoma occurring after ionizing radiation therapy for breast carcinoma.

Chronic radiation injury causes DNA mutations that may result in neoplasia. An example is skin cancer, which can develop after years of exposure to excessive levels of ultraviolet (UV) radiation from the sun. Indeed, skin cancers due to UV exposure are so common as to not be included in most tabulations of cancer statistics.

Toxins

In a big enough dose, any natural or synthetic molecule, including water, can cause injury. Depending on the chemical, injury may occur in different organs and by different mechanisms. For example, heavy metals such as mercury and lead cause direct toxic injury to enzymes necessary for cell health. The effect of most toxic molecules is dose related. Fatal overdose of heroin is an example.

Microbes

Microbes can produce toxins that interfere with cell protein synthesis or cell oxygen utilization. For example, *Staphylococcus aureus* growing on unrefrigerated food produces a toxin that damages intestinal epithelial cells and causes food poisoning. The cell wall of some bacteria contains substances that are released into blood when the bacteria die. This can cause vascular collapse (shock) or widespread blood clotting inside of blood vessels (disseminated intravascular coagulation, Chapter 6). Viruses invade cells and kill from within by disrupting the cell or nuclear membrane or incite an immune system response that, while aimed at the virus, kills the cell.

Inflammation and Immune Reactions

Inflammation and immune reactions result from cell injury, but they may in turn cause injury themselves. Inflammatory cells release digestive enzymes designed to neutralize foreign agents, but they can also digest healthy tissue. Immune reactions injure cells directly by several mechanisms. For example, rheumatoid arthritis (RA) is an *autoimmune* disease in which the immune system is fooled into believing that the body's own cells (in the joint) are foreign and must be attacked.

Nutritional Imbalance

Nutritional imbalance can injure cells. Obesity, an epidemic in the developed world, is associated with cardiovascular disease, cancer, diabetes, and dozens of other ills. Conversely, cells may not receive enough calories, fluid, vitamins, or minerals to maintain good health.

Genetic and Metabolic Defects

Genetic diseases are discussed in detail in Chapter 22. Some genetic defects cause the accumulation of abnormal products, which can damage cells. For example, hemochromatosis is a genetic disease that causes a damaging accumulation of iron in cells.

Aging

Aging, discussed in detail in Chapter 24, causes progressive, mild injury that ultimately leads to cell death directly or renders cells less able to withstand other forms of injury.

Case Notes

2.4 Into which of the above categories does Marianne's injury fall?

Mild Injury or Stress Causes Reversible Cell Change

Whether or not cell injury is reversible depends on the duration and severity of injury or stress. Mild injury produces visible, reversible changes in cells, which revert to normal when the cause of injury disappears.

Acute Mild Injury or Stress

Acute mild injury causes brief, visible cell change. The most common cause is brief hypoxia or anoxia, though toxins may exert a similar effect.

The most common change is increased intracellular water, which is visible as **hydropic change** (*vacuolar degeneration*, Fig. 2.4A). This occurs because of a change in intracellular sodium concentration. Normally, extracellular sodium is higher than intracellular sodium. This concentration difference is maintained by the *sodium pump mechanism* of the cell membrane, which constantly pumps sodium out of the cell as fast as it seeps in. Lack of oxygen (hypoxia or anoxia) deprives the pump of its energy, damaging this mechanism and allowing sodium to seep across the membrane and into the cytoplasm. Because solutes attract water, a rise of intracellular solute (sodium) attracts water into the cytoplasm. Hydropic change is reversible if the injurious situation is corrected.

Mild acute injury also may cause an accumulation of fat, a condition called **steatosis** (Greek *steat* = fat, Fig. 2.4B). Steatosis is most common in liver cells because of the liver's premier role in fat metabolism. It is often observed in people who abuse alcohol. Unfortunately, steatosis (sometimes with inflammation) is now occurring commonly in young adults and even children as a result of obesity. Although reversible, longstanding steatosis of the liver can progress to cirrhosis and liver failure. Figure 2.5 compares a normal kidney and one with severe steatosis.

Chronic Mild Injury or Stress

Long-term mild injury or stress leads to changes that persist until the insult disappears. The two types of changes are: 1) intracellular accumulations, and 2) altered patterns of cell growth and differentiation.

Intracellular Accumulations

Water and fat may accumulate within reversibly injured cells as a result of mild, short-term injury. More prolonged injury is associated with other accumulations, including the following:

- *Cholesterol*: The most damaging intracellular accumulation is cholesterol in the cells of arteries in atherosclerosis (Chapter 8, Fig. 8.9).
- *Protein*: Normal body proteins are long molecules that must be folded into the appropriate shape for their function. Microscopically visible cytoplasmic accumulations of misfolded or otherwise abnormal proteins occur in a variety of diseases. The abnormal protein found in the neurons of those with Alzheimer disease (Chapter 19, Fig. 19.31) is an example.
- *Pigments*: The most widely occurring pigment accumulation is *lipofuscin*, a golden brown substance most notable in long-lived cells such as brain neurons, cardiac myocytes, and liver hepatocyte cells. Its presence indicates "wear-and-tear."
- *Environmental particles*: Inhaled particles from cigarette smoke or polluted air accumulate in respiratory cells and bronchial lymph nodes (Fig. 2.6) and contribute to a variety of respiratory diseases.

Altered Growth and Differentiation

Cells respond to chronic mild injury or stress, including the good stress of exercise, by making certain *adaptations*. When the source of the chronic injury or stress is removed, the cell, tissue, organ, or body part usually returns to normal.

Atrophy (Fig. 2.7) is decreased *size* and function of a cell, tissue, organ, or body part. In cells, it is an adaptive response to decreased demand or to increased stress as the cell shuts down its metabolic processes to conserve energy. *Physiologic atrophy* is a normal part of life. For example, the thymus gland atrophies almost totally by puberty, and muscles atrophy naturally with age. *Pathologic atrophy* typically is the result of disuse or lack of normal physiologic support. The bodies of underfed children are atrophic; organs deprived of blood and the nutrition it brings

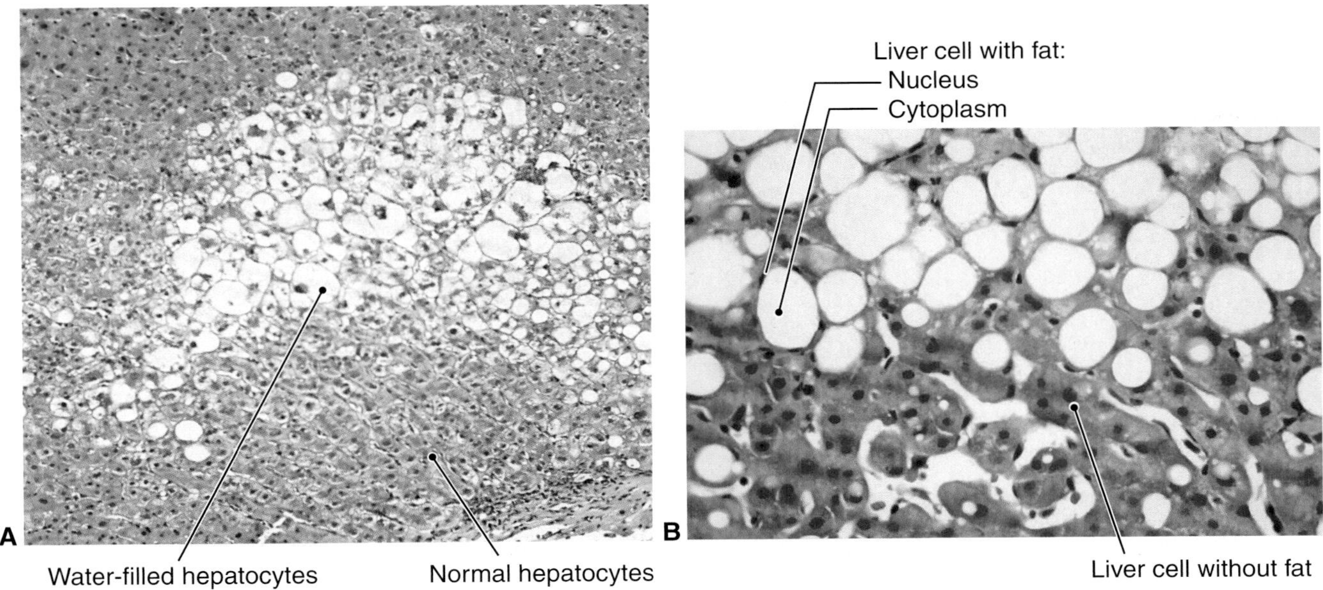

Figure 2.4 **Mild, reversible injury** (microscopic study). **A.** Liver with hydropic (vacuolar) change. **B.** Steatosis.

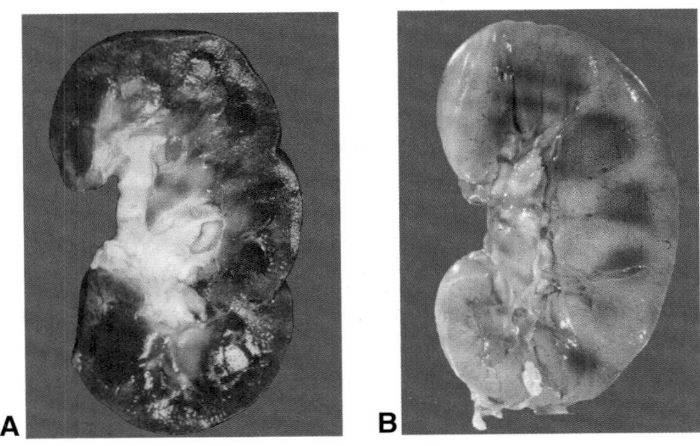

Figure 2.5 **Steatosis** (gross study). **A.** Normal kidney. **B.** Fatty change in a patient with toxic injury.

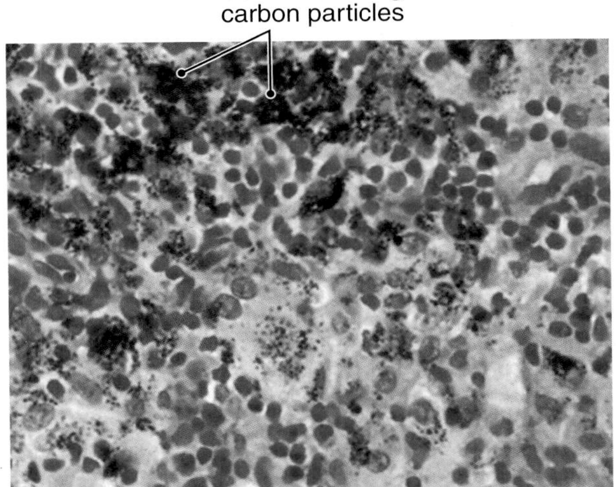

Figure 2.6 **Inhaled particles.** Bronchial lymph node filled with carbon particles. Biopsy from a chronic smoker at time of surgery for lung cancer.

will atrophy; paralyzed limbs atrophy from disuse; and the thyroid and the adrenals will atrophy if denied hormonal support from the pituitary.

The opposite of atrophy is **hypertrophy**: increased size and function owing to the increased *size* of individual cells. Hypertrophy is most often seen in muscle because muscle tissue has few stem cells, which means that muscle cannot meet increased demand by growing new cells; it must adapt by cell enlargement. Heart muscle hypertrophies in response to increased workload (Fig. 2.8).

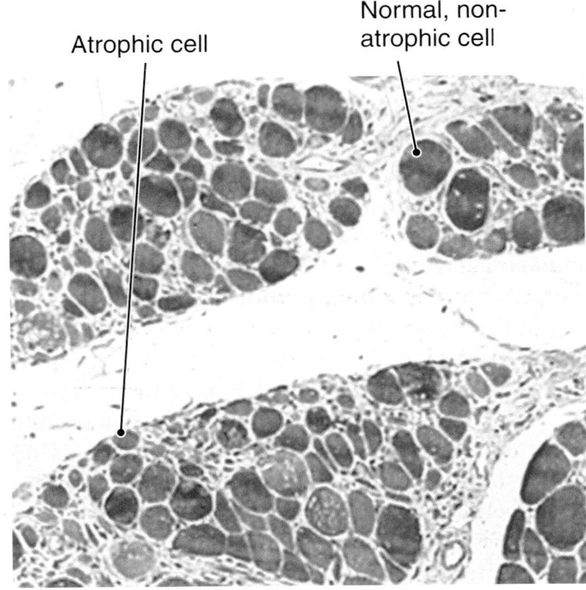

Figure 2.7 **Atrophy.** Muscle biopsy in a patient with chronic muscle inflammation. (Adapted with permission from Koopman WJ, Moreland LW. *Arthritis and Allied Conditions: A Textbook of Rheumatology. 15th ed.* Philadelphia, PA: Lippincott Williams & Wilkins; 2005.)

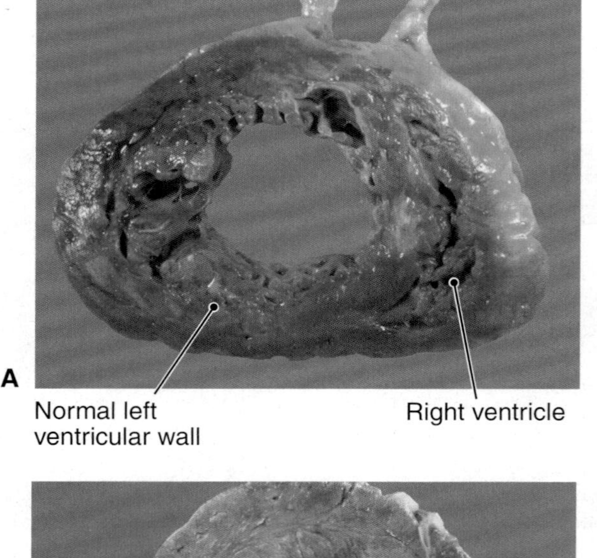

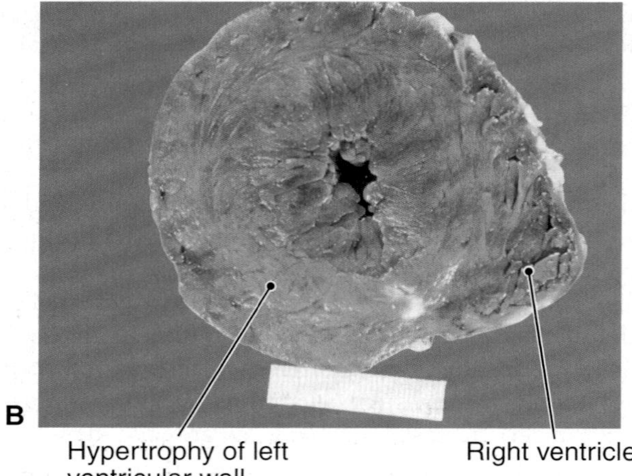

Figure 2.8 **Hypertrophy.** Cross sections of heart, viewed from above. **A.** Normal heart. Normal thickness of left ventricular wall. **B.** Hypertrophic left ventricle in a patient with severe, chronic hypertension. Ventricular wall is markedly thickened as a result of the increased size of individual muscle cells.

For example, ejecting blood from the left ventricle across a narrowed aortic valve has the same effect on left ventricular muscle cells as lifting weights has on the muscles of a weightlifter. Both are hard work.

Hyperplasia (Fig. 2.9) is the enlargement of a tissue or organ owing to an increase in the *number* of cells. Hyperplasia is sometimes due to hormonal stimulation. For example, overproduction of thyroid stimulating hormone by the pituitary will cause hyperplasia of the thyroid, and women's breast glands become hyperplastic with lactation. Chronic injury also can cause hyperplasia. The callused palms of someone doing hard work with their hands are nothing more than hyperplasia of the epidermis.

Sometimes, hypertrophy and hyperplasia occur together. Enlargement of the uterus in pregnancy is an example.

Metaplasia (Fig. 2.10) is a reversible change of one cell type into another caused by chronic injury. It is most common in epithelium, because epithelial cells are short-lived and are always being replenished from stem

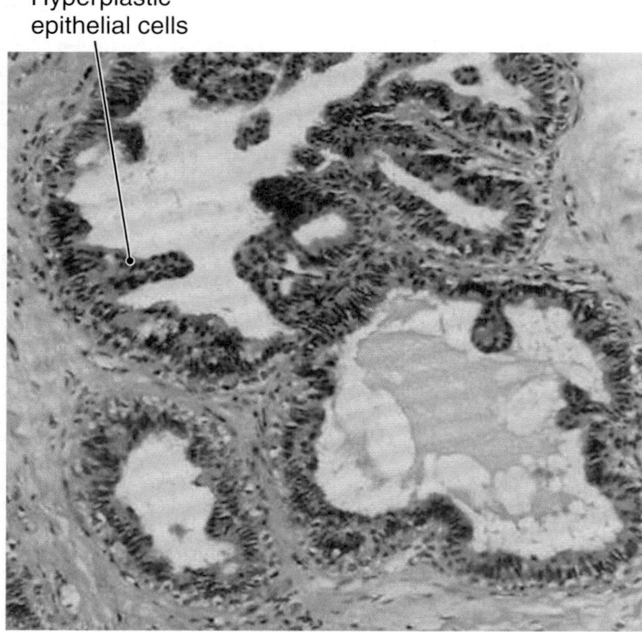

Figure 2.9 **Hyperplasia.** Breast biopsy with epithelial hyperplasia. Normally these ducts are lined by a single layer of cells.

cells (see the online case study for Chapter 2). Injured or stressed epithelial cells can mature into a different type of cell more suitable to existing conditions. For example, the respiratory epithelium in nonsmokers is tall columnar epithelium. In smokers, it changes into flat squamous epithelium, a simpler, more durable tissue better suited to defend against the noxious substances in smoke. Metaplastic epithelium reverts to normal when the injury stops.

Dysplasia literally means "disordered growth;" however, the term is also used to refer to a premalignant change of cells (Fig. 2.11). It usually occurs in epithelium, as the

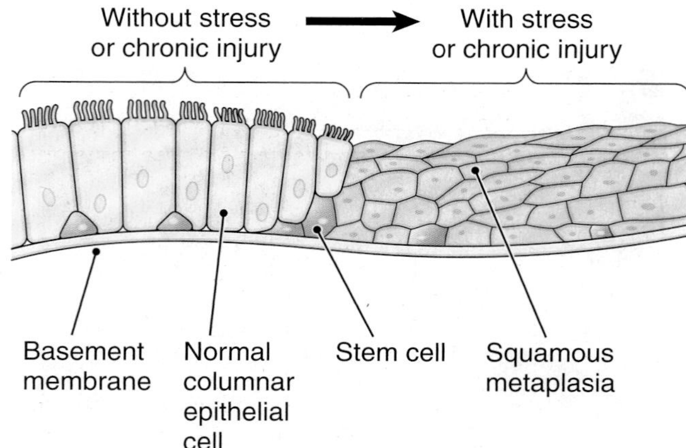

Figure 2.10 **Metaplasia.** Normal respiratory epithelium. Chronic injury such as smoking stimulates stem cells to produce squamous cells (right) instead of normal columnar epithelial cells (left). Normal columnar cells on the left have cilia and are not layered; squamous cells on the right have no cilia and are flat and layered.

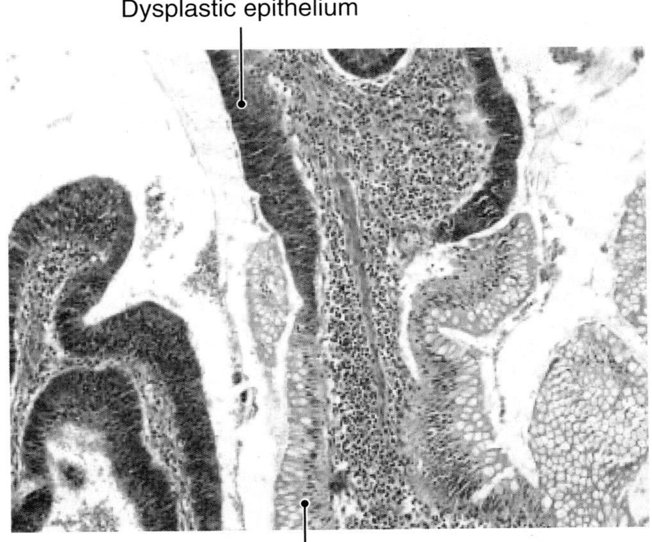

Figure 2.11 **Dysplasia.** Colonic epithelium. Above and left: Dysplastic epithelium. Below and right: Normal epithelium.

uniform appearance and orderly arrangement of cells is replaced by haphazardly arranged, enlarged, distorted cells with large, dark nuclei that reflect the chromosomal chaos within. Dysplasia is a milepost on the way to malignancy; however, it is not invasive and is usually reversible. Perhaps the best example is dysplastic cells detected by Pap smear performed at annual gynecologic exams.

Remember This! Dysplasia is a premalignant cell adaptation.

Severe Injury or Stress Causes Cell Death

Cells die because of injury or the passing of time. **Necrosis** (Greek *necros* = corpse) is the pathological death of cells due to injury (disease). Additionally, cells have a natural life span, and after living out their natural term of a few days, a few months, or a human lifetime, they die by "natural suicide" in a carefully regulated, orderly process called **apoptosis** (Greek *apo* = from, *ptosis* = falling; i.e., dropping out).

Necrosis

Necrosis is usually due to vascular ischemic hypoxia/anoxia in a contiguous block of cells, but in some circumstances it may occur in individual cells. There are four types of necrosis:

- **Coagulative necrosis** is characterized by a gel-like change in blocks of freshly dead cells. It is the most common type and occurs in **infarcts** (Fig. 2.12A), local blocks of necrotic tissue due to ischemia caused by impaired blood flow in the artery feeding the tissue. The name derives from the most common use of the word *coagulate*—to convert fluid into a solid mass, as when blood coagulates from fluid into a solid. Because cells die in place without anatomic disruption, gross and microscopic tissue architecture is preserved despite the fact that the tissue is dead. Microscopic study reveals a ghostly outline of cells and tissues (Fig. 2.12C). Solid organs like the liver, heart, and kidney are most often affected. For example, blockage of a coronary artery produces ischemia in downstream heart muscle cells, resulting in a myocardial infarct (commonly called a "heart attack").
- **Liquefactive necrosis** is cell death in which the dead tissue dissolves into fluid. Liquefaction occurs because dead cells are disrupted or dissolved. The most frequent type of liquefactive necrosis is produced by bacterial infection. Some bacteria incite severe cell damage and attract great numbers of WBCs that liberate digestive enzymes in an effort to kill the bacteria. In the process, dead cells are digested into the liquid commonly known as "pus" to form an **abscess**.
- **Caseous necrosis** is a variant form of coagulative necrosis with limited liquefaction and obliterated cellular detail. The most common cause is tuberculosis (TB) infection. *Caseous* means cheesy, and indeed the dead tissue is off-white, soft, pasty, and clumpy, like some varieties of cheese.
- **Fat necrosis** is a specialized form of liquefactive necrosis that occurs only in fat. It is especially common around the pancreas. Pancreatic disease (such as trauma or inflammation) liberates pancreatic digestive enzymes that convert pancreatic fat into glycerol and fatty acids. The fatty acids combine with calcium to form soap, which traps calcium as tiny deposits in the injured tissue where it is visible on X-rays. Fat necrosis can also occur in skin or any other fat, including the breast. This may pose a diagnostic challenge because breast cancers often contain calcium deposits.

Apoptosis

Apoptosis is the programmed, natural death of cells. The literal meaning in Greek is "falling away"; the term conjures up the imagery of leaves falling from a tree. It is something like cell suicide and is the product of a very specific, natural mechanism. Internal or external forces can activate the mechanism.

Apoptosis is important in embryological development. For example, the early embryonic hand has webbed fingers, but apoptosis of cells within the bands causes them to disappear.

Many pathologic processes also invoke apoptosis. An external, pathologic force that causes apoptosis is not the same as necrosis (even though cell death is the result), because necrosis does not invoke the apoptosis program. In such a circumstance, the external force activates "suicide" genes, inactivates other genes necessary to sustain cell life, and manufactures its own lethal cocktail of suicide substances that attack cell structures. Metabolism

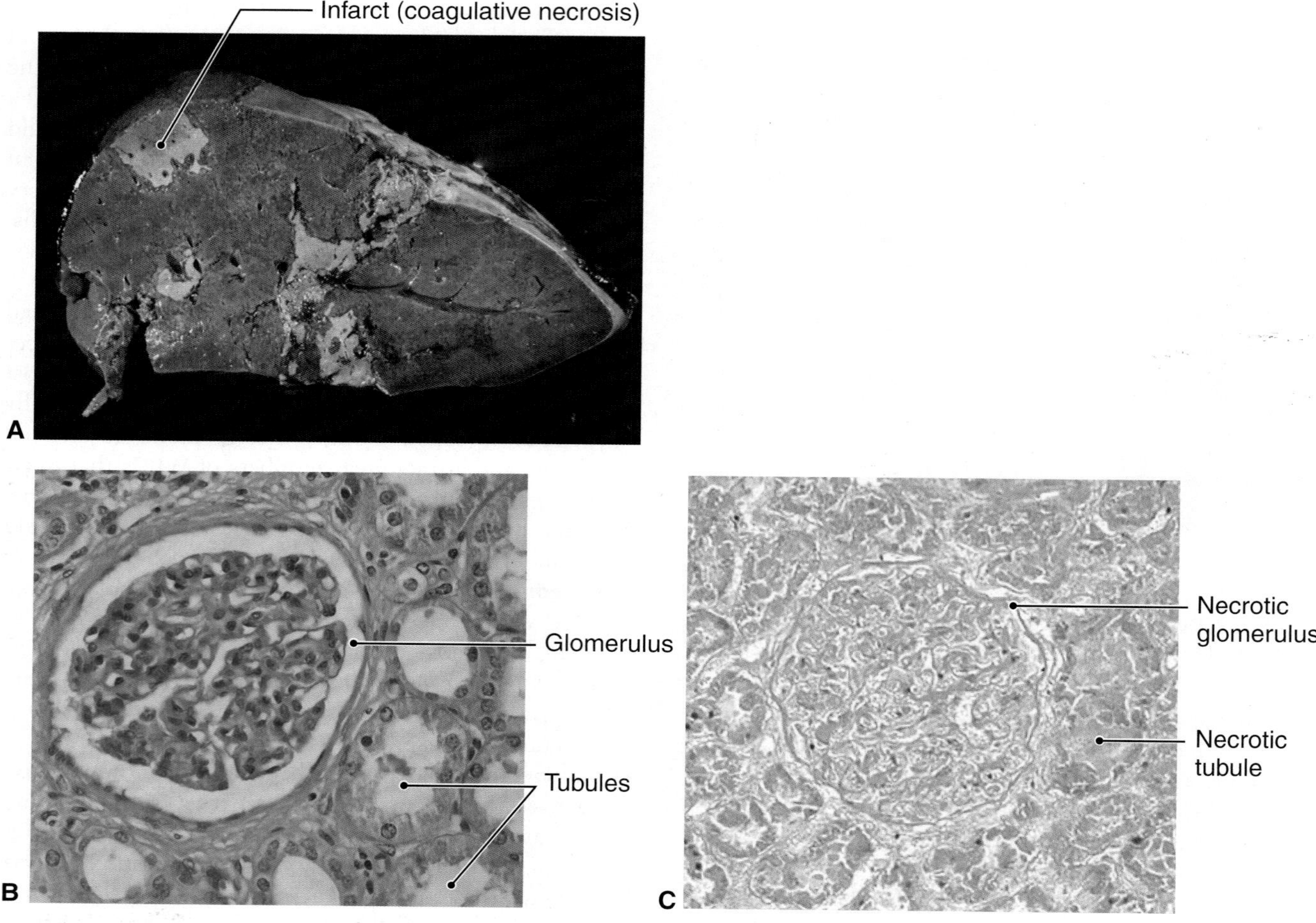

Figure 2.12 **Infarcts and coagulative necrosis. A.** Liver. Multiple infarcts. **B.** Kidney, normal glomerulus. **C.** Kidney, coagulative necrosis. Note that this freshly necrotic glomerulus retains a ghostly outline of normal tissue.

slows, and the cell shrivels and is ultimately ingested and digested by scavenger cells (macrophages). Some degenerative diseases, especially Alzheimer disease and other diseases of the nervous system, may be caused by pathologic apoptosis.

Remember This! Apoptosis is the programmed, natural death of single cells. Necrosis is pathological death, usually in blocks of cells.

Pop Quiz

2.4 True or false? The usual cause of hypoxia/anoxia is ischemia.

2.5 Name several causes of cell injury.

2.6 Name two indicators of reversible cell damage.

2.7 What type of accumulation occurs in the brain cells of patients with Alzheimer disease?

2.8 Distinguish between hyperplasia and hypertrophy.

2.9 Contrast metaplasia and dysplasia.

2.10 List the four types of necrosis.

2.11 Define infarct.

2.12 True or false? Necrosis and apoptosis usually involve blocks of contiguous cells.

The Inflammatory Response to Injury

Inflammation is the body's composite cellular and vascular reaction to injury (Fig. 2.13). **Acute inflammation** is the result of comparatively severe, short-term injury and

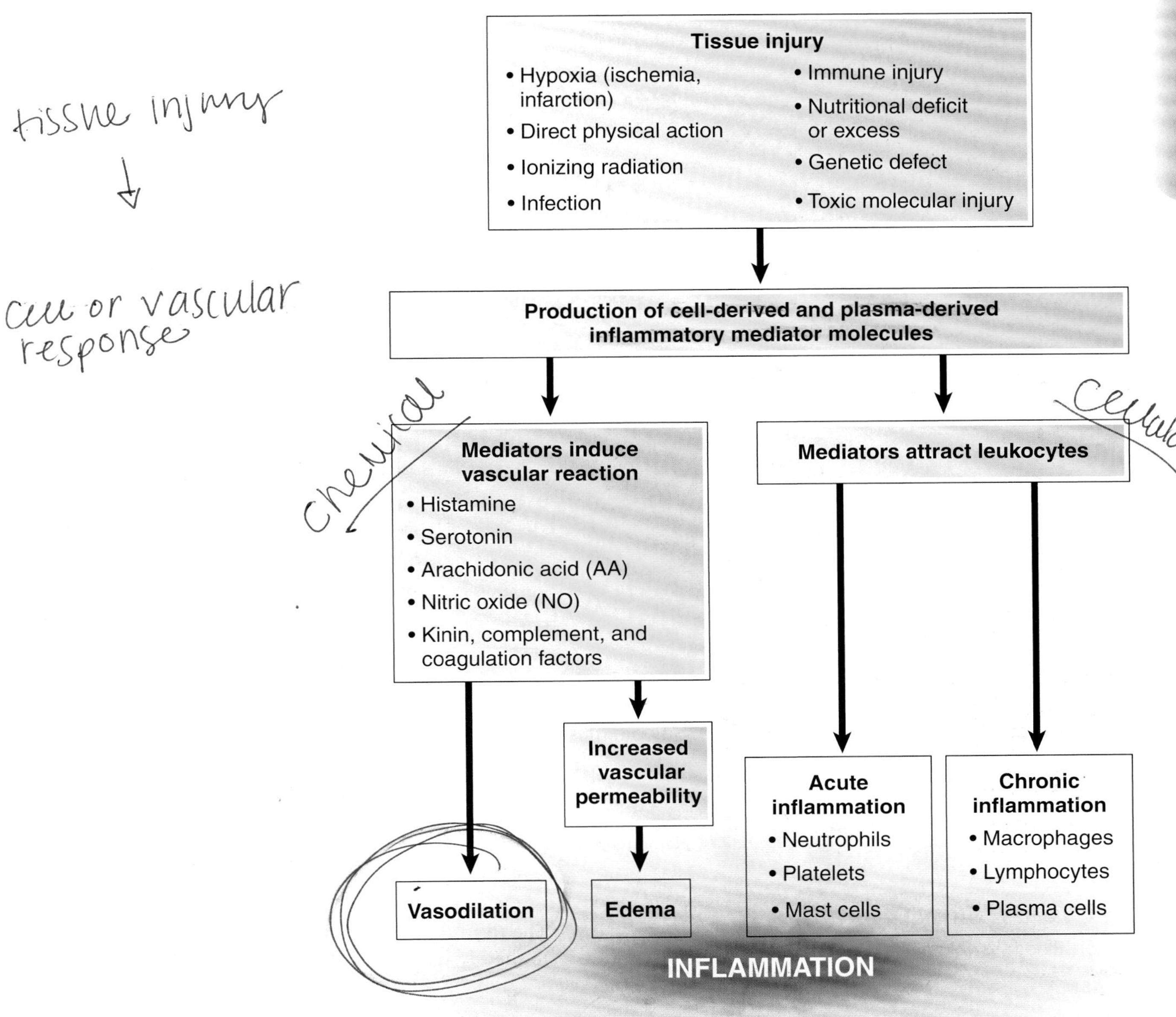

Figure 2.13 **The chain of events in inflammation.**

lasts a few hours or days. **Chronic inflammation** is the result of comparatively mild, longer-term injury and lasts weeks to years.

Inflammation is a protective response of local blood vessels, blood cells, plasma proteins, and cells in the tissue surrounding the injury. It occurs as a chain of events designed to limit the effect of injury, neutralize the offending force, and initiate the repair process. Though protective and essential to health, it can be deleterious. For example, fever is a beneficial aspect of inflammation, but it can rage out of control, with serious consequences that include death.

Leukocytes Are the Cells of Inflammation

As is illustrated in Figure 2.14 and detailed in Table 2.1, there are three types of **leukocytes** (*white blood cells, WBCs*): granulocytes, lymphocytes, and monocytes.

Granulocytes have a relatively small, multilobed nucleus and a large amount of cytoplasm, which contains large granules that are actually lysosomes filled with digestive enzymes. Granulocytes can crawl through tissues (*diapedesis*) and swallow microbes and other particulate matter (*phagocytosis*). They are the main cells in *acute* inflammation and acute *allergic* reactions.

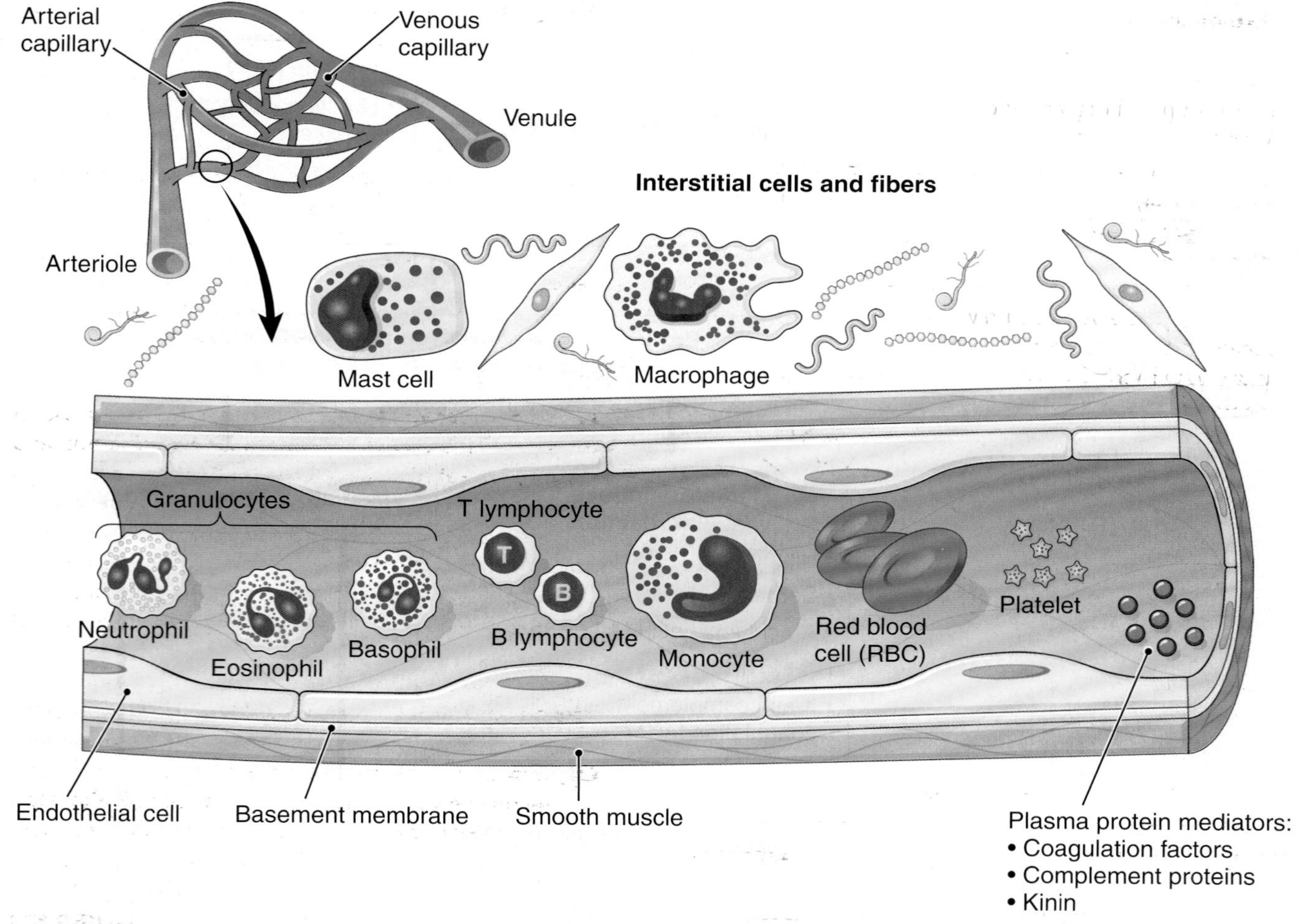

Figure 2.14 **Elements of the inflammatory response.**

Table 2.1	***Blood Components***
Whole Blood (% volume)	100%
PLASMA	**55%**
Water	90%
Protein	10%
FORMED ELEMENTS	**45%**
Red blood cells (RBCs)	99.9%
White blood cells (WBCs), platelets	0.1%
Formed Elements (count per mm³)	
RED BLOOD CELLS	**5,000,000**
PLATELETS	**250,000**
WHITE BLOOD CELLS	**7,500**
Granulocytes	70%
Neutrophils	67%
Eosinophils	<3%
Basophils	<1%
Lymphocytes	25%
Monocytes	5%

Granulocytes constitute about 70% of circulating WBC. The three types are named according to the color imparted to their lysosomes by a standard laboratory dye:

- **Neutrophils** have neutral (tan) granules and a segmented, multilobed nucleus. They are the main inflammatory cells in *acute* inflammation. Their main task is phagocytosis. Neutrophils also produce chemical messenger molecules that communicate to nearby cells or to distant organs.
- **Eosinophils** constitute less than 3% of circulating WBC. They have a bilobed nucleus and red cytoplasmic granules with anti-parasite properties. Eosinophils are the principal inflammatory cells in parasitic infections, such as intestinal worm infestation. They are also attracted to *allergic* reactions.
- **Basophils** are normally less than 1% of circulating WBCs. During *allergic* reactions, they attract other inflammatory cells, including large numbers of eosinophils. Their blue-purple granules contain histamine, which is responsible for the local signs of allergic reactions: swelling, itching, vascular congestion, and mucus production. A tissue cell with similar features is the **mast cell.**

Lymphocytes normally make up about 25% of circulating WBCs. They have a single large nucleus and scant cytoplasm with no granules. They are made in the bone marrow and migrate to lymphoid organs, where they mature. The two types of lymphocytes, **B cells** and **T cells**, are the main cells of the immune system and of *chronic* inflammation. B cells that are actively making antibodies have a distinctive appearance and are called **plasma cells**.

Monocytes normally account for about 5% of circulating WBCs. They are large cells with a large nucleus and a modest amount of cytoplasm with a few small granules. Monocytes are made in the bone marrow and, after migrating into tissue, mature into **macrophages**, which are voracious phagocytes.

Platelets are fragments of cytoplasm of a bone marrow cell, the *megakaryocyte*. Platelets are important in stopping hemorrhage, in blood clotting, and in inflammation.

Case Notes

2.5 Which type of leukocyte is most likely to migrate into Marianne's wound?

Chemical Signals Mediate the Inflammatory Process

Injured cells release chemical signals that work together to produce inflammation, reduce the consequences of the injury, and repair the damage. These chemical **mediators** are molecules that travel from one place to another to exert their effect. The three varieties are (Fig. 2.15) the following:

- **Autocrines** are signals that act back on the generating cell.
- **Paracrines** are molecules released by cells that act on *nearby* cells.
- **Hormones** (*endocrines*) are molecules released into the bloodstream to act on *distant* cells. Hormones released in inflamed tissue attract more inflammatory cells (leukocytes or WBCs) from nearby capillaries; circulate in blood to stimulate bone marrow to release additional leukocytes; and act on the brain to increase body temperature (fever).

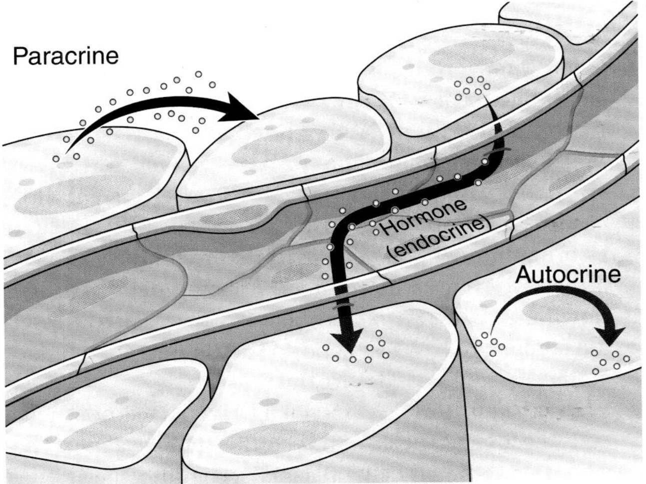

Figure 2.15 **Mediators of the inflammatory response.** Some mediators (autocrines) act back upon the cell that generates them; others act on nearby cells (paracrines), or enter the blood stream to act on the cells of distant organs (endocrines, or hormones).

Mediators may be derived from plasma, leukocytes, endothelial cells, or injured cells. Some are small molecules like histamine, whereas others are large proteins.

Cell-Derived Mediators

Histamine and *serotonin* are vasoactive amines stored in *basophils* and *mast cells*, which cause vasodilation and increased permeability of capillary walls.

Arachidonic acid (AA) and its derivatives are a family of compounds derived from components of damaged cell membrane. *Prostaglandins* are an important example. Compounds in the AA family cause vasodilation and increased capillary permeability, and mediate pain and fever. Some anti-inflammatory drugs exert their effect by blocking AA activity.

Nitric oxide (NO) is a gas released by endothelial cells. It causes vasodilation and also has bactericidal properties.

Cytokines are protein molecules secreted by cells that act to enhance immune reactions by attracting leukocytes, stimulating phagocytosis, and causing vasodilation. Some cytokines promote increased "stickiness" of vascular endothelial cells, which enables blood cells to attach to endothelial cells in order to escape from capillaries and migrate into tissues. Some molecules (**chemokines**) act as chemical attractants to lure WBCs toward the damage, a process known as **chemotaxis**.

Plasma-Derived Mediators

The **complement system** is a set of about two dozen proteins that react with one another in a chain reaction initiated by the immune system or by the presence of products derived from microbes. The products of complement interactions cause vasodilation, attract WBCs, and directly attack and destroy microbes.

The **kinin system** is closely related to the clotting system and consists of more than a dozen blood proteins that interact to generate molecules that cause vasodilation and increased endothelial cell permeability. *Bradykinin* (Greek *bradus* = slow + *kinesis* = movement) is activated by the coagulation system. It acts to strengthen and prolong the effect of other mediators, and enhances pain.

The **clotting system** is a set of about a dozen proteins that interact with one another in a complex cascade to cause blood to clot, a necessity in control of hemorrhage associated with injury. Activation of the clotting system also stimulates the kinin system and complement systems, enhancing their activity.

The Initial Inflammatory Response Is Vascular

Endothelial cells line all blood vessels and the heart chambers. By becoming more or less permeable, they act as gatekeepers in the flow of hormones, proteins, nutrients, and other essentials into and out of the bloodstream and tissues. Capillaries are formed of endothelial cells only. The walls of arterioles and arteries are formed of lining endothelial cells and smooth muscle, which can contract and relax to regulate blood flow.

Blood vessel dynamics are controlled by hormones and other chemical mediators, and by the autonomic nervous system. After injury, these mechanisms cause immediate, temporary *contraction* of local arterioles for a few seconds. This is followed by *dilation* of arterioles, which floods local capillaries with blood. The tissue becomes red and warm, a condition called **hyperemia** (Greek *hyper* = above + *haimia* = blood). The influx of blood dilates capillaries and stretches the endothelial cells, opening spaces in the seams between cells. Plasma leaks from blood into tissue, which swells as fluid accumulates, a condition called **edema**. An example is the quick redness and swelling from a slap in the face.

The physics of fluid flow becomes important as vasodilation occurs. Blood flows fastest in the center of a vessel because peripheral flow is slowed by wall friction. Larger, heavier cells (leukocytes) tend to travel in the slow-moving fluid along the wall. Furthermore, because dilated capillaries are much larger, increased *volume* of blood flows but the *speed* of flow is reduced. Slow-moving leukocytes along the capillary wall begin to stick to the lining endothelial cells, a process mediated by chemical mediators released from damaged cells near the capillary.

Remember This! Vascular reaction and inflammation occur in every injury.

Cellular Reaction Follows Vascular Reaction

As just noted, inflammatory mediators act on the endothelium and leukocytes to make them sticky. Platelets also adhere and release their own mediators to increase stickiness and to initiate the coagulation process, which generates strands of fibrin to bind leukocytes to the capillary wall. Via *diapedesis*, neutrophils wedge themselves between the stretched seams joining endothelial cells and crawl into the damaged area. They migrate into the heart of the damaged tissue by *chemotaxis*, like a bloodhound following an ever-stronger scent.

Complement, immune and other proteins released at the time of injury attach to injured cell or bacterial membrane and become identifier molecules that attract neutrophils. The neutrophil begins the process of phagocytosis by binding itself to the target and wrapping it in folds of cell membrane. The trapped target is then invaginated into the neutrophil to create a *phagocytic vacuole*, a bubble of neutrophil cell membrane that contains the target. The vacuole is then merged with a neutrophilic granule (lysosome). The result is destruction and dissolution of the target into harmless molecules.

Neutrophils and a few basophils and eosinophils accumulate rapidly in the first few hours. They are part of the acute inflammatory response and do their job and die within a few hours of leaving the blood. The tide of inflammatory mediators fades quickly if the injury was brief, and after about 48 hours neutrophils, basophils, and eosinophils begin to fade away and are replaced by lymphocytes and macrophages.

Case Notes

2.6 What is the name of the process by which leukocytes find their way into Marianne's injured tissue?

2.7 Other than bleeding, will a vascular reaction occur in Marianne's wound?

Acute Inflammation Follows Brief Injury

Acute inflammation follows *brief* injury and lasts a few hours or days. It usually results from microbial infection (especially bacterial infection), physical or chemical injury, or some immune reactions, such as the skin rash of poison ivy. It is characterized by vascular dilation, accumulation of edema, and infiltration of neutrophils, and usually resolves without scarring.

Phases of Acute Inflammation

Figure 2.16 presents a detailed look at the steps in the inflammatory sequence:

- *Before injury* (Fig. 2.16A): Blood flows rapidly and smoothly; most WBCs flow in the center of the stream. Endothelial cells are snugly fitted together.
- *Injury occurs; immediate vasoconstriction is followed shortly by vasodilation* (Fig. 2.16B): After instant, brief vasoconstriction (not illustrated), blood vessels dilate to bring more blood *volume* to the injured tissue. Nevertheless, even as more blood is being delivered, it is flowing at a slower *speed* because the dilated vessels are so enlarged. WBCs tend to "settle out" or "sludge" along the edges of the stream.
- *The vascular wall changes* (Fig. 2.16C): Endothelial cells become "sticky" and "leaky." Gaps appear between endothelial cells, plasma seeps into the injured site, and neutrophils adhere to "sticky" capillary walls.
- *Neutrophils migrate* (Fig. 2.16D): They crawl into the injured site through gaps between endothelial cells and accumulate at the injured site.

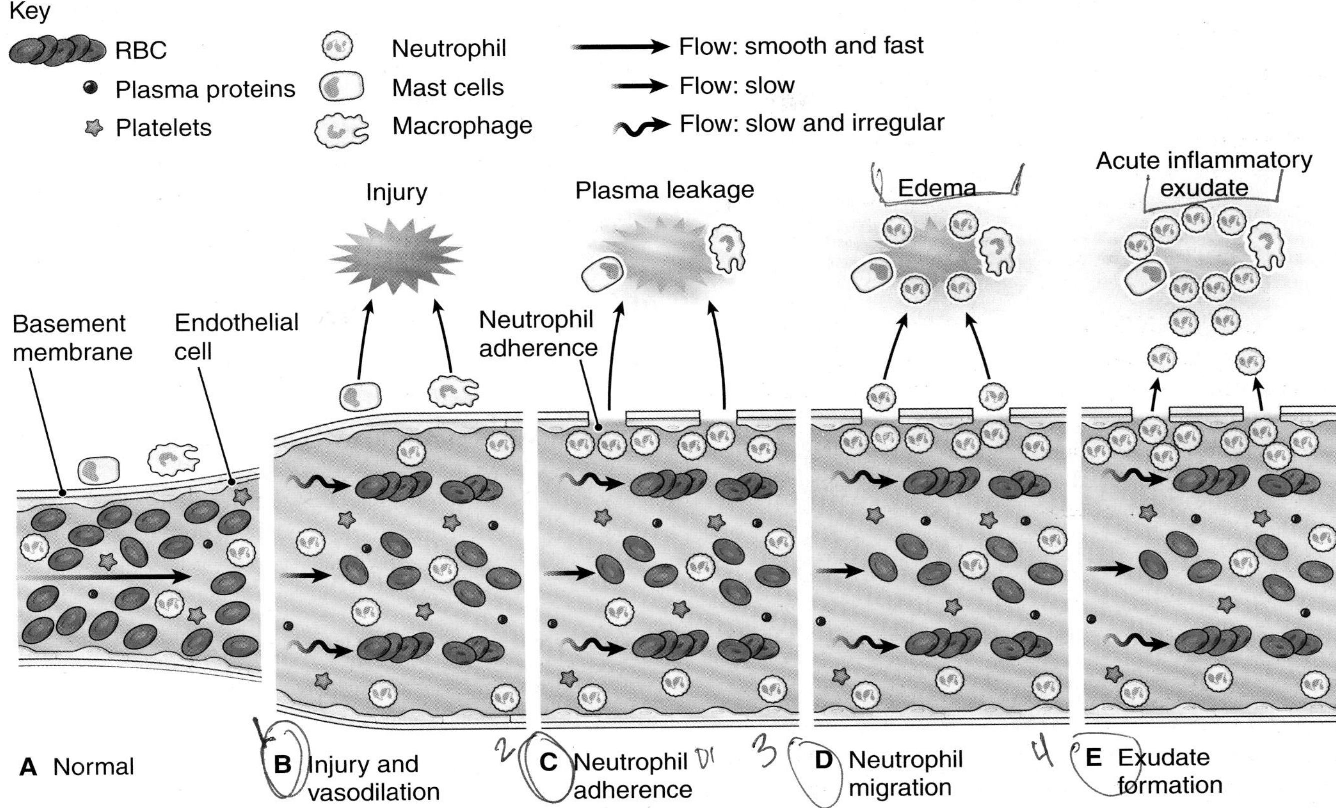

Figure 2.16 **The sequence of events in acute inflammation. A.** Normal capillary, blood cells, and cells in adjacent tissue. **B.** After injury, capillaries dilate and the *volume* of blood flow increases. Nevertheless, *speed* of flow is slow at the edges of the stream. Tissue macrophages and mast cell migrate toward the injury. **C.** Openings appear in the seams between injured endothelial cells, and plasma leaks into the injury site. Injured endothelial cells become "sticky" and neutrophils and platelets adhere to them. **D.** Plasma accumulates as edema fluid and the site swells. **E.** Accumulated edema and inflammatory cells combine to form an acute inflammatory exudate.

- *Exudate accumulates* (Fig. 2.16E): At the same time, inflammatory fluid (*exudate*) accumulates as plasma leaks through the vessel wall. Neutrophils continue to migrate into injured tissue, swimming upstream against the increasing gradient of *chemokines* and other molecules that spread outward from the injured site.

In the meantime, plasma in the edema fluid begins to clot, initiating the kinin and complement system reactions that combine to sustain the response.

Figure 2.17 shows the timing of these acute inflammatory events.

Characteristics of Acute Inflammation

Acute inflammation has four *clinical* characteristics, shown in Figure 2.18, which were first described by the Roman Celsus about 2,000 years ago:

- *Tumor*: swelling
- *Rubor*: redness
- *Calor*: heat
- *Dolor*: pain

Microscopically, acute inflammation (Fig. 2.19) is characterized by

- *injured cells* in various stages of reaction to injury—hydropic degeneration, necrosis, or other changes;
- *dilated capillaries* gorged with blood and neutrophils;
- an *accumulation of neutrophils*, which may be either sparse or dense according to the severity of injury. An exception is acute allergic reactions, which are characterized by dense accumulations of eosinophils.

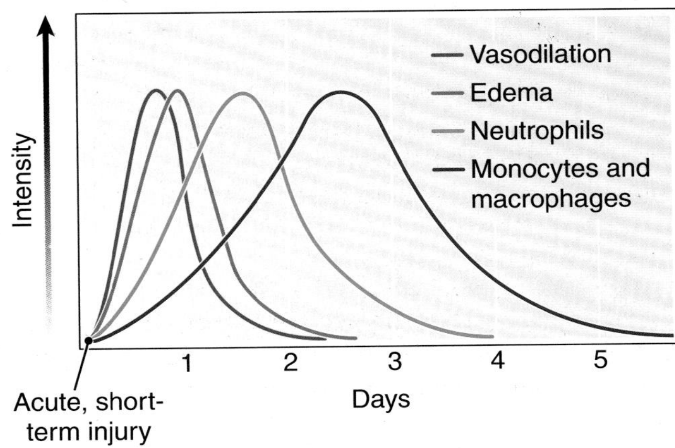

Figure 2.17 **The timing of acute inflammatory events.**

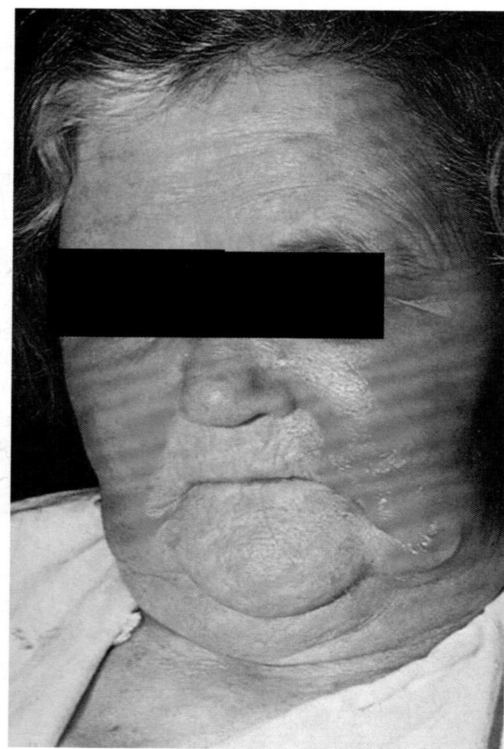

Figure 2.18 **The clinical picture of acute inflammation.** This patient has erysipelas (an acute bacterial skin infection). Intense inflammation (*rubor*) and moderate edema (*tumor*) are visible. Her unhappy expression makes it easy to imagine the heat (*calor*) and pain (*dolor*).

The accumulation of fluid and WBCs at the injured site is the **acute inflammatory exudate**, which may accumulate in several *anatomic patterns* in grossly visible inflammation:

- **Serous inflammation** is a pattern seen in mild, short-term inflammation. It is characterized by copious amounts of watery fluid that is low in protein compared to other inflammatory exudates and contains relatively few inflammatory cells. An example is the oozing fluid from a superficial skin burn.
- **Fibrinous inflammation** follows a somewhat more severe injury and is characterized by a thicker, wetter exudate that contains more neutrophils. The exudate contains coagulation factors that interact to form a stringy web of fibrin, which gives the process its name. Examples include the crust (scab) of a superficial skin injury and inflammation of mesothelial surfaces such as the lining of the pleura or pericardium (Fig. 2.20).
- **Suppurative (purulent, pyogenic) inflammation** occurs with severe acute injury and is associated with *liquefactive necrosis*. It is characterized by creamy fluid (**pus**) composed of necrotic debris, and overwhelming numbers of neutrophils. Certain bacteria, such as *Staphylococcus aureus*, are especially prone to cause purulent inflammation.

Resolution of Acute Inflammation

Most acute inflammation resolves (heals) quickly. It may linger, however, as an abscess or evolve into chronic inflammation if the offending cause persists. Scarring (discussed shortly) may occur in more severe cases.

Complete resolution is the usual outcome because most acute inflammation is associated with limited, short-term injury—sunburn, for example. Mildly injured tissue regenerates, molecular mediators are washed away, necrotic debris from severely injured cells are digested or phagocytized, blood vessels contract, and fluid is absorbed.

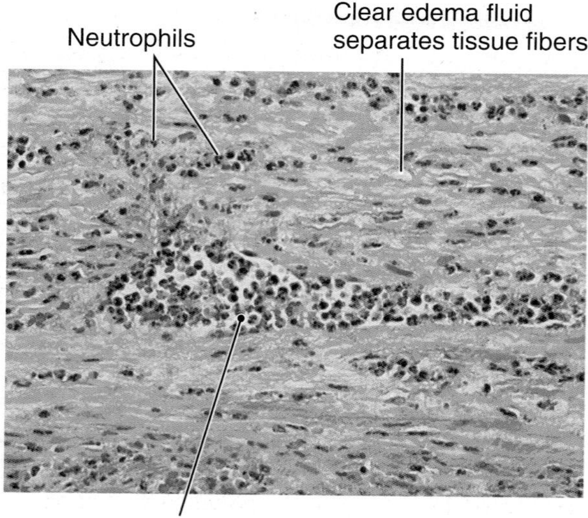

Figure 2.19 **Acute inflammatory exudate.** Microscopic study of the wall of an inflamed appendix. The capillary in the center is very dilated and packed with neutrophils. Neutrophils and edema fluid combine to form the inflammatory exudate.

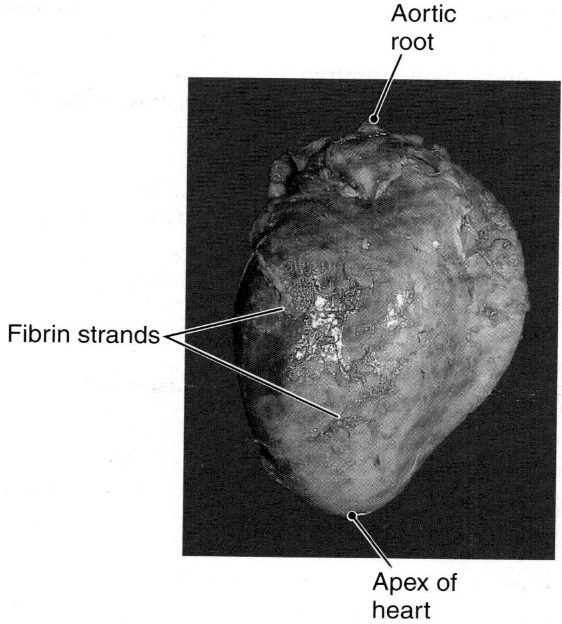

Figure 2.20 **Acute fibrinous inflammatory exudate.** Heart within the pericardial sac. Acute fibrinous pericarditis. The pericardium is covered by an acute inflammatory exudate containing stringy strands of fibrin.

Scarring may occur with severe or repeated acute inflammatory episodes if substantial tissue destruction occurs beyond the capacity of tissue to regenerate. A full thickness burn is an example.

Chronic inflammation may develop if the cause of the inflammation persists.

Chronic Inflammation Occurs with Persistent Injury

Chronic inflammation occurs when cell injury is persistent and moderate, usually not severe enough to cause necrosis.

Causes of Chronic Inflammation

Chronic inflammation is usually caused by one of the following:

- *Persistent infection.* Most infections are potent enough to incite the vigorous response of acute inflammation. Some microorganisms, however, are less immediately toxic and invoke a less intense, longer lasting, immune response. This includes the agent of TB, *Mycobacterium tuberculosis*; the agent of syphilis, *Treponema pallidum*; most parasites and fungi; and some viruses.
- *Autoimmune disease.* Autoimmune diseases are those in which the immune system mistakenly attacks the body's own tissues instead of some invading agent. All autoimmune disease is chronic and causes chronic inflammation. An example is rheumatoid arthritis.
- *Persistent exposure to injurious agents.* For example, chronic inflammation occurs in response to daily cigarette smoking.

Again, persistence of injury is the hallmark of chronic inflammation. An initial injury may evoke short-term acute inflammation, but if the injury persists, chronic inflammation will evolve. For example, a wood splinter beneath skin produces immediate, mild, acute inflammation. If it is contaminated with bacteria and is not removed, an abscess likely will occur. If the splinter remains longer than a week, the abscess will resolve by antibiotic therapy, rupture, or natural defenses. If it is not removed, chronic inflammation will develop; that is, the initial infiltrate of neutrophils will be replaced by an accumulation of lymphocytes, macrophages, new blood vessels, and scar tissue.

Characteristics of Chronic Inflammation

Chronic inflammation is less intense than acute, and therefore is usually not as hot, swollen, red, or tender. Moreover, some chronically inflamed tissue may be shrunken by scar, atrophy, or necrosis. For example, chronically inflamed muscle often becomes atrophic (Fig. 2.7).

Persistent injury invokes an immune response, which dispatches macrophages and lymphocytes to the site to bolster defense. Macrophages are phagocytic of bacteria and other foreign agents and cellular debris, and secrete cytokines that facilitate the overall inflammatory response. Lymphocytes have particular anti-microbial qualities, which are discussed in more detail in Chapter 3.

In **granulomatous inflammation**, a special type of chronic inflammation, sheets of macrophages aggregate around a central group of necrotic cells or an infectious microorganism to form tiny inflammatory nodules called **granulomas**. Adjacent macrophages aggregate to form huge cells with abundant cytoplasm that contains dozens of macrophage nuclei—**multinucleated giant cells** (Fig. 2.21). It is a feature of TB and a few other conditions.

Because the injury persists, the healing process also persists. Healing involves regeneration of injured or dead cells when possible, scarring if regeneration is incomplete or impossible, and ingrowth of new blood vessels (*angiogenesis*) to support the process. This process is discussed in detail shortly.

In summary, chronic inflammation features an abundance of lymphocytes and macrophages, few or no neutrophils, attempted regeneration of destroyed cells, scarring, and a rich supply of blood vessels.

Remember This! Chronic inflammation is a mixture of ongoing inflammation and healing.

Inflammation Has Effects beyond the Site of Injury

Inflammation, whether acute or chronic, has effects beyond the site of injury. The regional lymphatic system can

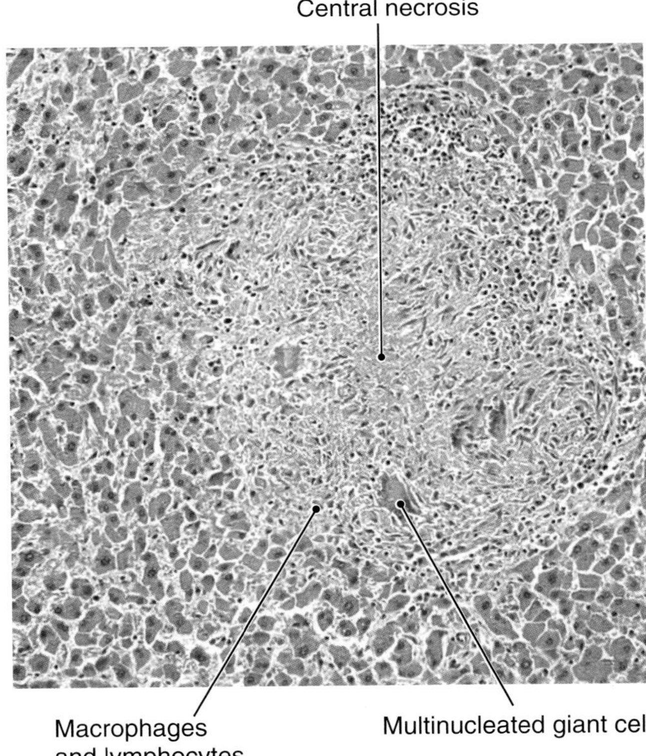

Figure 2.21 **Granulomatous inflammation.** Tuberculosis of the liver. Normal liver cells surround the granuloma, which is composed of a central core of necrotic tissue and a halo of lymphocytes and macrophages containing multinucleated giant cells.

become involved and inflammatory mediators seep into blood to produce general effects on the body.

Effect on the Lymphatic System

Tissue fluid from all of the body except the brain is drained by the lymphatic system. **Lymphangitis** is inflammation, usually bacterial infection, of lymph vessels. It is characterized by red streaks of tender, inflamed lymphatic vessels extending centrally from the infected site. In **lymphadenitis**, lymph nodes filtering fluid from an injured or infected site may themselves become infected. Often, an enlarged lymph node is not infected; rather, it is reacting to inflammatory products draining away from the infection or injury, a condition known as **reactive hyperplasia**. *Clinically*, the term **lymphadenopathy** is applied to enlarged or tender lymph nodes irrespective of suspected diagnosis.

Systemic Effects

Inflammatory mediators find their way into the bloodstream. From there, they influence the brain to produce fever, malaise, drowsiness, and poor appetite. They can also cause blood pressure to fall, suppress liver production of albumin, and cause the liver to produce **reactant proteins**. Reactant proteins can be assayed by simple laboratory tests, and are a useful diagnostic tool.

Among the more important acute reactant proteins is **C-reactive protein (CRP)**, made by the liver. Increased blood CRP is a reliable marker for inflammation, and increases with even minor degrees of inflammation. Low-grade inflammation caused by chronic injury is associated with atherosclerosis, cancer, obesity, Alzheimer disease, and other conditions. For example, an elevated level of CRP in an otherwise apparently healthy, nonobese patient has a strong association with atherosclerosis.

Inflammatory mediators also stimulate the liver to manufacture other proteins, notably **fibrinogen**, the coagulation protein that polymerizes into the meshwork of fibrin in a blood clot. A peculiar but useful effect of increased fibrinogen is that it causes red blood cells (RBCs) to settle rapidly in their own plasma, an effect measured by the **erythrocyte sedimentation rate (ESR)**. ESR and CRP are useful laboratory tools, as discussed in *The Clinical Side*, "Laboratory Indicators of Inflammation."

The Clinical Side

LABORATORY INDICATORS OF INFLAMMATION

Increased ESR and/or CRP indicates that inflammation is present somewhere in the body. Occasionally they may be the only indicators of inflammation.

ESR is a time-honored test widely used in office practice or in locations where easy access to laboratory services is not available. This old, simple, sensitive, cheap, and reliable test is performed by collecting whole blood in an anticoagulant, putting it into an upright standardized narrow tube and measuring how fast the RBCs settle to the bottom. Persons with an increased ESR have inflammation of some kind somewhere, the extent roughly proportional to the degree of ESR increase. ESR may be increased, however, by a very long list of noninflammatory conditions including pregnancy, anemia, and malignancy. Furthermore, although the test is easy to perform, it's also easy to make a mistake. For example, even the slightest vibration or tilting of the tube will produce falsely high results. Use of ESR has declined in recent years as improved CRP testing has become available, although ESR remains a useful diagnostic tool.

CRP rises and falls more quickly than ESR after an acute inflammatory event. CRP is, therefore, a better indicator of current inflammation. Additionally, it is a much more sensitive test, detecting inflammation that ESR may miss. For example, low-grade inflammation occurs in the fatty deposits in patients who are obese, and is reflected by increased CRP in obesity. Inflammation also plays an important role in the pathogenesis of atherosclerosis, and CRP is elevated in patients with atherosclerosis. What's more, CRP tends to rise in advance of the development of Type II diabetes mellitus. CRP detects this inflammatory reaction and therefore correlates with risks for obesity, atherosclerosis, and the development of Type II diabetes. As a result, elevated CRP levels parallel an increasing risk of heart attack, stroke, peripheral vascular disease, and diabetes. CRP may also be increased by high blood pressure, recent exercise, alcohol consumption, smoking, coffee consumption, pregnancy, oral contraceptives, and other factors.

Case Notes

2.8 Will Marianne's injury show typical signs of acute inflammation, and, if so, what are they?

Effects of Inflammation Due to Infection

Bacterial infection, as in a staphylococcal abscess, usually produces acute, pyogenic (suppurative, purulent) inflammation and increased numbers of neutrophils in blood (*neutrophilia*). Other types of bacteria may produce other reactions. For example, *syphilis* and *Lyme disease* are chronic infections caused by slender, corkscrew-shaped bacteria (spirochetes) that evoke a chronic inflammatory reaction.

Parasites such as intestinal roundworms invade tissue and stimulate an outpouring of eosinophils from the bone marrow into blood (*eosinophilia*). Protozoan parasites, by contrast, usually do not invade tissue and instead cause acute, superficial mucosal inflammation with little systemic effect. *Trichomonas vaginalis* infection of the vagina is an example.

Most *viral* infections, such as influenza, evoke a lymphocytic inflammation and increased lymphocytes in blood (*lymphocytosis*).

Pop Quiz

2.13 True or false? Acute inflammation is usually the result of a comparatively mild injury.

2.14 Neutrophils are the principal cell of which kind of inflammation?

2.15 Name the two sources of inflammatory mediators.

2.16 After injury, which comes first: cellular or vascular reaction?

2.17 Place the following in proper order: sticky endothelium, neutrophils leave blood, vasodilation, vasoconstriction.

2.18 Name the four clinical signs of acute inflammation.

2.19 Name some causes of chronic inflammation.

2.20 True or false? Lymphocytes are the main cells of acute inflammation.

2.21 Which is the most important cell in chronic inflammation?

2.22 Define lymphadenopathy.

2.23 True or false? CRP does not rise except in severe, long-term inflammation.

2.24 True or false? Most bacterial infections evoke a lymphocytic reaction.

Repair

Can honour set to a leg? No. Or an arm? No. Or take away the grief of a wound? No.

WILLIAM SHAKESPEARE (1564–1616), ENGLISH PLAYWRIGHT, HENRY IV, PART 1 (V.I)

Repair (Fig. 2.22) is the body's collective attempt to restore normal structure and function to the injured site, the wound. A **wound** is an injury resulting from short-term injury at a discrete site; for example, a surgical skin incision. Most wounds are minor—a skin scratch or a bruise, for example—and heal without treatment. Nevertheless, some wounds require medical management.

Repair consists of two processes:

- **Regeneration** is the complete, or nearly complete, restoration of normal anatomy and function by the regrowth of *normal functional cells* (**parenchyma**) and supporting tissue (**stroma**). Regeneration usually follows relatively mild injury and results in little or no scarring.
- **Healing** is a mix of regeneration and scarring, or scarring alone if regeneration is not possible. Tissue that cannot be replaced "good as new" by regeneration must be mended by **fibrous repair** (*scar formation*). Scarring occurs: 1) if the damage to tissue is so extensive that the supporting framework is destroyed (e.g., severe thermal burn of skin); or 2) if the injured tissue is composed of permanent cells, such as myocardium, skeletal muscle, or brain.

Many Cell Types Are Involved in Repair

Recall from our earlier discussion that the three types of tissue—*labile*, *stable*, and *permanent* (Fig. 2.2)—are identified according to their ability to regenerate new cells after injury. Stem cells regenerate parenchymal cells, but if the damage is too severe for repair by parenchymal cell regeneration alone, cells of the fibrous repair process complete the job. First, inflammatory cells secrete mediators that regulate other cells in the repair process. Macrophages are especially important. They linger longest at the site and act to stimulate growth of connective tissue cells.

The role of connective tissue cells in repair cannot be overstated. These cells hold the wound together and provide the framework (*stroma*) upon which parenchyma is rebuilt. The two elements of the stromal framework are the *basement membrane* and the *extracellular matrix*. Without stromal support, tissues cannot return to their normal configuration, and scarring occurs. The more severe the injury, the more likely it is that the stromal framework will be too damaged for regeneration of normal anatomy.

Remember This! Repair is either by regeneration of damaged parenchymal cells or by fibrous repair, or a mixture of both.

Fibrous Repair Generates Scar Tissue

Fibrous repair occurs in the following sequence (Fig. 2.23):

- *Cell migration and proliferation*—to provide raw material for repair
- *Angiogenesis*—the growth of new blood vessels to nourish the process
- *Scar development*—synthesis of collagen fibers to knit together disrupted tissue

Cell Migration and Proliferation

The healing process begins within hours of injury as leukocytes migrate into the wound to limit the damage

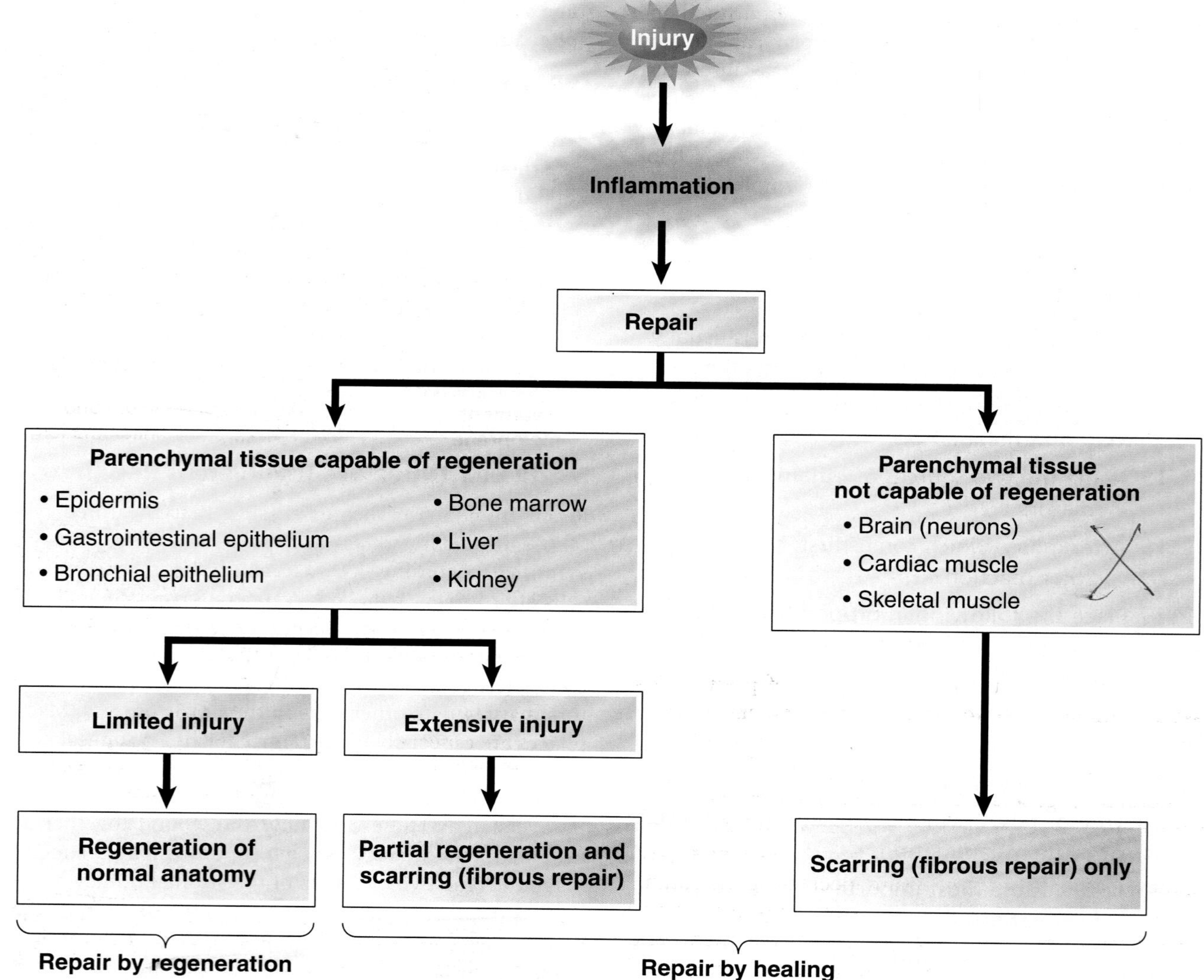

Figure 2.22 **The repair process.** In parenchymal tissues capable of regeneration (labile and stable tissues, those with stem cells), mild injury is repaired solely by regeneration. More severe injury is repaired by regeneration and scarring. In parenchymal tissues not capable of regeneration (permanent tissues, those with few or no stem cells), repair is by scarring only.

and begin clearing the site of debris and foreign material. Leukocytes attracted to the site produce cytokines that stimulate migration and proliferation of myofibroblasts into the injury site. At the same time, endothelial cells from nearby blood vessels begin to sprout angioblasts, which form into new capillaries. Myofibroblasts proliferate to fill space not occupied by regenerating parenchymal cells, synthesize collagen fibers to knit back together the disrupted tissue, and provide the permanent structure to support additional cell growth.

Growth of New Blood Vessels

Angiogenesis is the growth of new blood vessels into the wound. Vascular endothelial growth factor and other factors stimulate new vessels to sprout from existing vessels. Angiogenesis occurs in several smooth, interrelated steps, as is depicted in Figure 2.24.

- *Dissolution of the basement membrane* of the parent vessel(s) in the injured site by proteolytic enzymes released by inflammatory cells
- *Migration and proliferation of endothelial cells* through the defect and up the gradient of cytokines released by inflammatory cells and injured cells
- *Organization of a new capillary branch* as the tube of endothelial cells generates a basement membrane. Later in the healing process the new blood vessels enlarge to convey nutrients, cytokines, and hormones to the site.

Scar Development

Scar development occurs in several related and overlapping steps that deposit a network of collagen and other fibers to bind together the edges of the wound.

The initial phase in scar development is migration and proliferation of fibroblasts and new blood vessels into the

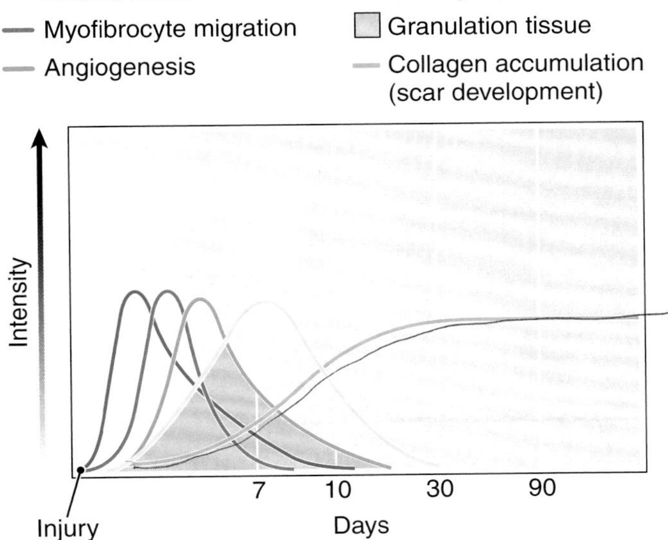

Figure 2.23 **The sequence of fibrous repair (scarring).** Even as the inflammatory process unfolds, fibrous repair begins. Myofibrocytes migrate into the wound and new blood vessels sprout to form granulation tissue, which fades as collagen is deposited and accumulates as a scar.

injured site. The result is development of **granulation tissue**, a fragile, easy-to-bleed, highly vascular mixture of capillaries, fibroblasts, residual edema, and small numbers of leukocytes (Fig. 2.25A). As the process unfolds, myofibroblasts generate a matrix of collagen and other fibers to bind together the edges of the wound and give it strength. The myofibroblasts then begin to contract, pulling the edges of the wound inward, decreasing the volume to be healed. If an epithelium is nearby, it regenerates and grows inward across the surface (Fig. 2.26). As the wound edges are pulled inward, fibroblasts produce collagen and other extracellular components to bind the wound firmly and give it strength. Fluid is gradually resorbed, inflammatory cells disappear, and the site becomes occupied by less cellular, more collagenous tissue. Blood vessels shrink or disappear as workload decreases. The result is a dense, relatively bloodless scar (Fig. 2.25B). Finally, the scar is reshaped (**remodeled**) as mechanical forces pull it into a configuration that eases stress on the wound. A fresh scar is tense and produces a noticeable sensation of tightness or deformity. After complete remodeling, however, a scar fits comfortably in the site, molded in conformity to surrounding tissue.

Wound Healing

Clinically, the repair process is called "wound healing." A **wound** is a visible injury, usually one due to trauma. Most wounds are minor—a skin scratch or bruise, for example—and heal without treatment. Nevertheless, some wounds require medical management. For more about management of wounds and scars, see *Molecular Medicine*, "Molecular Treatment and Prevention of Skin Scars."

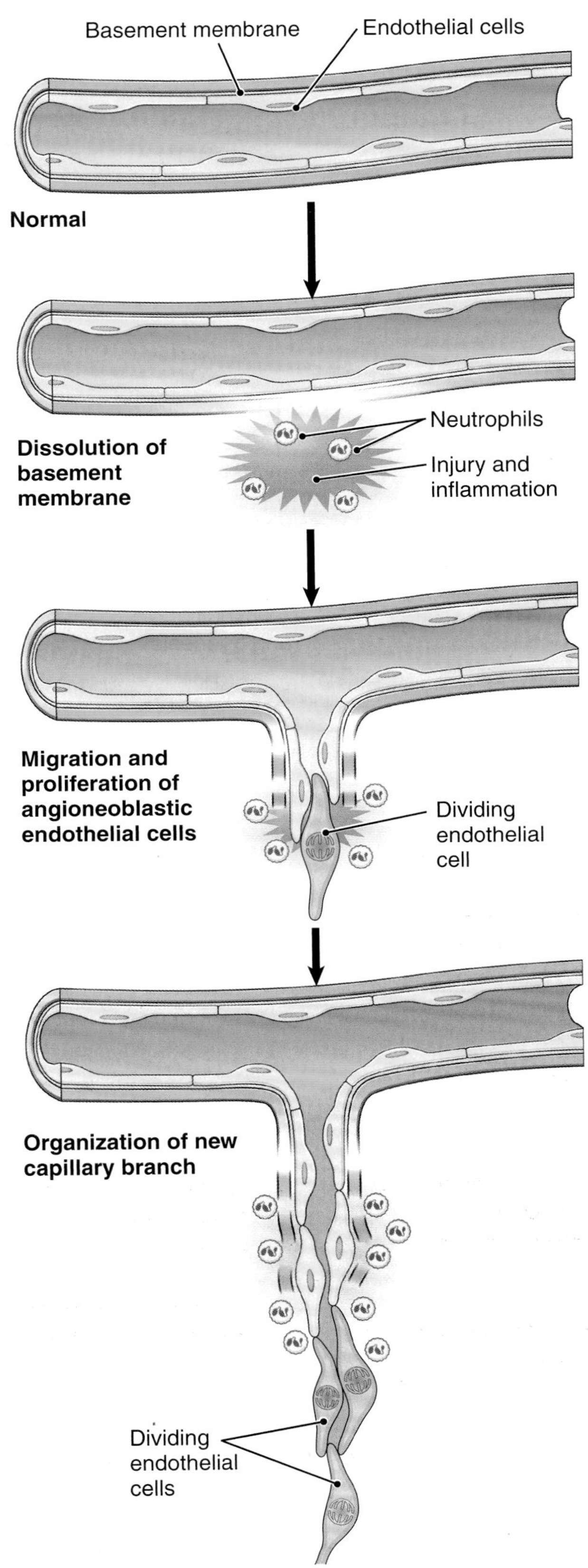

Figure 2.24 **Angiogenesis.** The basement membrane of injured capillaries dissolves, and endothelial cells migrate through the defect and into the injury, where they proliferate to form a new capillary.

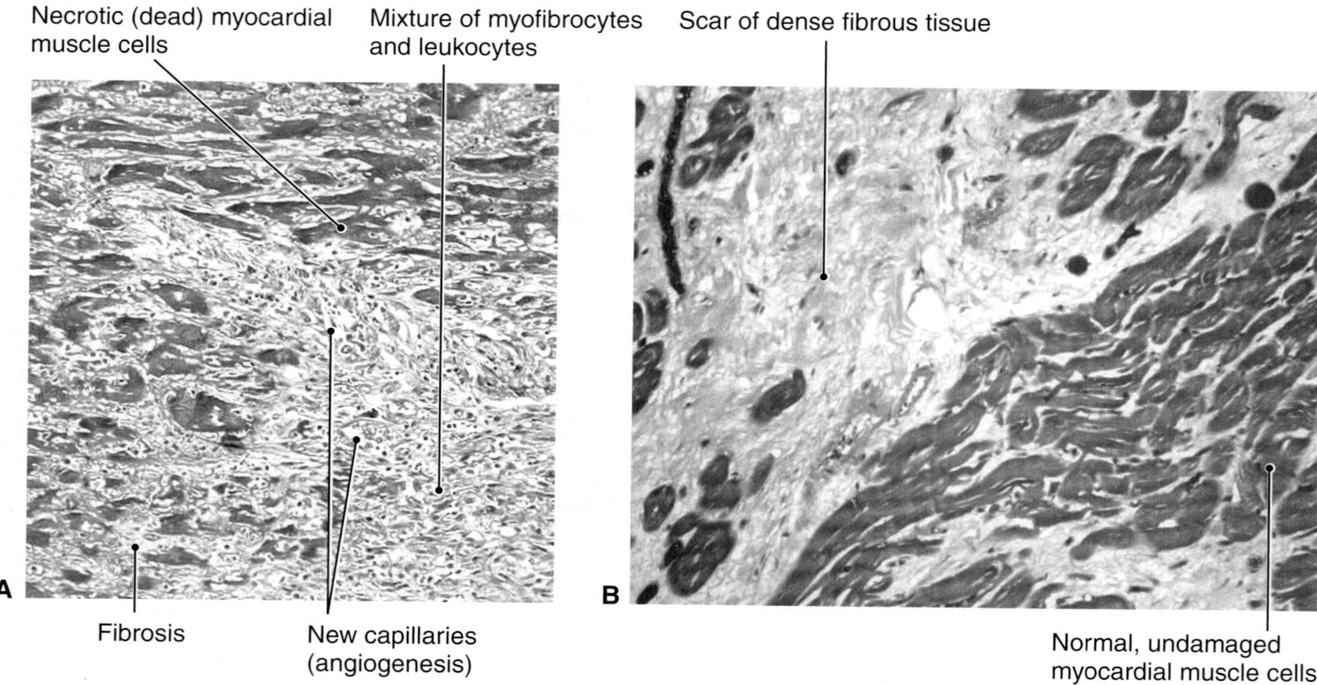

Figure 2.25 **Granulation tissue and scarring. A.** Granulation tissue in healing myocardial infarct. **B.** Scar tissue in healed myocardial infarct.

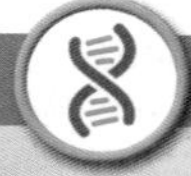

Molecular Medicine

MOLECULAR TREATMENT AND PREVENTION OF SKIN SCARS

Many methods are available to treat hypertrophic scars or keloid scars of skin (see Fig. 2.27), including compression therapy, occlusive dressings, radiation, and surgery. Recently, drug therapies have been added to the list. But what about everyday scars? Some of the biological processes at work in hypertrophic or keloid scars are present in everyday scars, most importantly increased (and altered) collagen production. Since collagen is produced by fibroblasts, therapeutic drugs can be used to decrease the number of fibroblasts or the amount of collagen produced by each fibroblast. For example, a traditional drug therapy is highly potent glucocorticoids (e.g., triamcinolone), which can be applied topically or injected into the site. A newer and promising approach relates to **transforming growth factor beta (TGFbeta)**, which is secreted by several types of cells in the repair process. TGFbeta promotes scar formation by stimulating production of collagen and proliferation of fibroblasts. Anti-TGFbeta therapy has minimized scars formation and has proven helpful in minimizing postburn scar formation. It may also be helpful in existing scars and chronic inflammatory conditions where fibrosis is a clinical problem.

The fundamentals of healing are the same in every wound. Nevertheless, it is instructive to compare differences between the healing of narrow and broad wounds (Fig. 2.26). Narrow wounds with closely approximated edges heal by what is called **first intention**; a surgical incision is an example. A freshly sutured wound has about 70% of normal tensile strength. After suture removal at one week, tensile strength is about 10%. Strength improves to about 75% at three months and after a year has returned to near normal.

Broad wounds with widely separated margins heal by **second intention**; deep skin burns or large intestinal ulcers are examples of this type of wound. Healing by second intention is much the same as healing by first intention. The volume of dead tissue to be removed is greater, and regeneration of the surface epithelium is slower because the wound is wider. The final volume of the scar may be as little as 10% of the original defect. In tissue covered by epithelium, new epithelial cells advance inward from the edges, first forming a thin membrane of immature cells that rest on underlying granulation tissue. They then differentiate into mature epithelium as the wound below matures into a scar.

Case Notes

2.9 Which, if any, parenchymal cells were damaged in Marianne's cut?

2.10 Will fibrous repair be necessary in the healing of Marianne's wound?

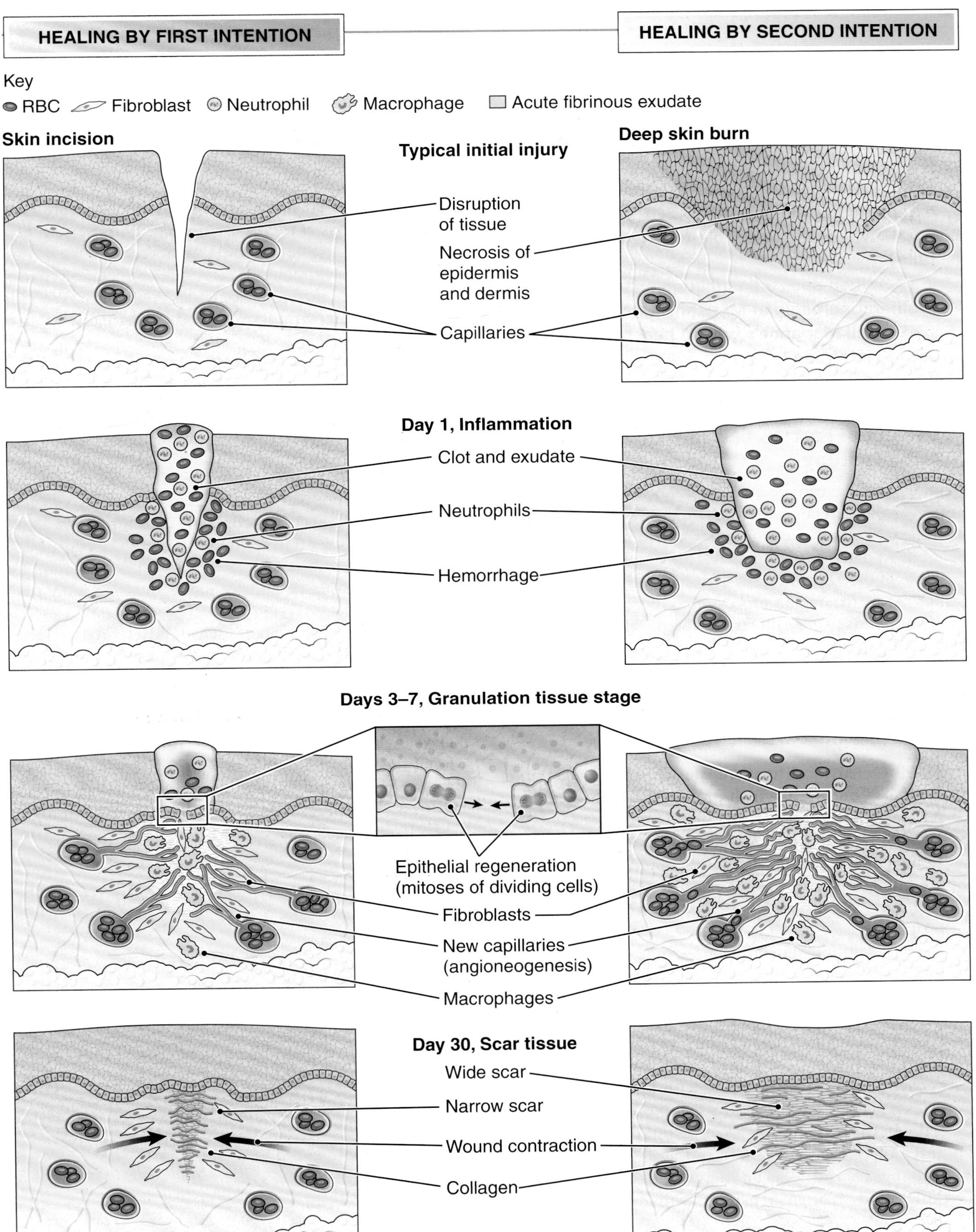

Figure 2.26 **Healing by first and second intention.** Left: Narrow wounds heal by first intention, usually in less than a week, and leave a small scar. Right: Wide wounds heal by second intention, have more inflammatory tissue, take several weeks to heal, and leave a larger scar.

Case Notes

2.11 Will granulation tissue appear in Marianne's wound?

2.12 Why does Marianne have trouble extending her finger?

2.13 Why is she later able to extend her finger fully?

2.14 When does inflammation and stem cell proliferation begin in Marianne's wound?

2.15 Will Marianne's wound heal by first or second intention?

A Variety of Factors Can Impair Wound Healing

Wound healing can be impaired. Local factors include infections and retained foreign bodies; systemic factors include vascular disease and poor nutrition. For example, wounds in patients with diabetes are notably slow to heal because of the vascular disease from which most diabetics suffer. Also, the repair process may become pathologic. The online case study illustrates the problem of impaired wound repair.

Host Factors

Local and general host factors may prevent a wound from healing normally.

- *Infection:* The most frequent cause of abnormal wound healing is infection, which prolongs the injury and interferes with healing at the same time.
- *Poor nutrition:* Deficiency of vitamin C or protein inhibits collagen synthesis. For example, elderly people are often poorly nourished because they may be poor, forgetful, or otherwise unable to feed themselves properly.
- *Steroids:* Anti-inflammatory glucocorticoids, widely used in therapy of autoimmune disease and other conditions, slow the growth of myofibroblasts and production of collagen, which binds wound edges together.
- *Poor blood supply:* Blood brings nutrition to the site and poor blood flow impairs healing. For example, as mentioned earlier, patients with long-standing diabetes usually have diseased small blood vessels, especially in the feet and legs. As a result, diabetic wounds heal slowly, especially those in the feet. Something as seemingly harmless as an ingrown toenail can be very difficult to treat in a patient with diabetic vascular disease.
- *Foreign bodies:* Pieces of metal, wood, glass, or bone may obstruct the tight closure of a wound and produce continued irritation and inflammation that may also encourage infection.
- *Mechanical factors:* Increased pressure or torsion may stress the wound so that a tight closure does not occur.

Wounds that do not heal properly may rupture (**dehiscence**) or may ulcerate. Dehiscence is most common when high tension is placed on an abdominal wound by sitting up in bed, coughing, vomiting, or sneezing. Smoking and diabetes increase the risk of dehiscence. Wounds may ulcerate if repair does not proceed normally.

Pathologic Wound Healing

Wound repair may create a problem rather than solving one. There are two main types of pathologic repair. Each is nonneoplastic, exuberant overgrowth of otherwise normal tissue.

A **keloid** (Fig. 2.27) is a hyperplastic scar that is prominent, raised, or nodular, and that contains excess collagen. Some patients, especially people of African heritage, have a genetic predisposition to keloid formation. Despite the fact that keloids may appear quickly and grow rapidly, they are not neoplastic and are rarely anything more than a cosmetic problem.

The second type of aberrant wound repair is a localized, highly vascular collection of persistent granulation tissue called **pyogenic granuloma**. Often these nodules of vascular tissue have lost their inflammatory infiltrate and edema fluid, giving them an exceptional vascularity that makes them look like a vascular tumor (*hemangioma*). One of the most noticeable sites for pyogenic granuloma is in the healing umbilicus of newborns, where it appears as a fleshy bleeding nodule that can appear alarming to the child's parents.

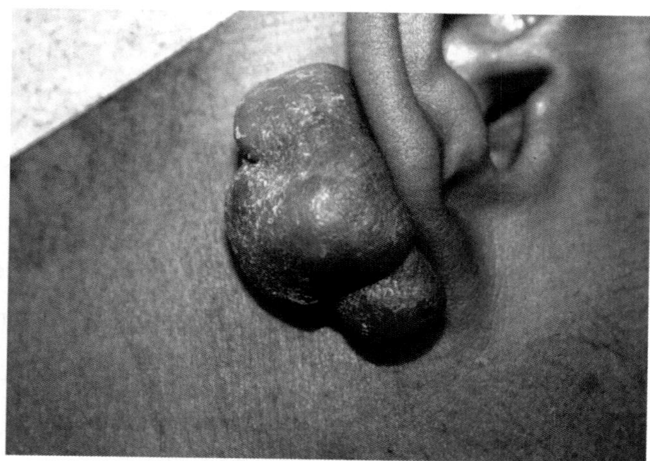

Figure 2.27 **Keloid of the ear lobe.** A keloid is hyperplastic scar. This one was successfully removed with good cosmetic effect and did not recur.

Pop Quiz

2.25 After inflammation, what is the first step in fibrous repair?

2.26 From where do new blood vessels originate in angiogenesis?

2.27 What is remodeling?

2.28 Fill in the blank. __________ cells are the main functional cells of an organ or tissue.

2.29 True or false? All repair requires some degree of regeneration.

2.30 True or false? Stable cells are not capable of regeneration.

2.31 What is the most abundant cell in fibrous repair?

2.32 What is the traditional name for the method of healing of broad wounds?

2.33 When is a healing wound most vascular?

2.34 In what disease state do diabetic wounds sometimes heal slowly?

Case Study Revisited

"I cut my finger." The case of Marianne M.

Revisiting this case gives us an opportunity to review many of the terms and concepts covered in this chapter.

It may seem odd to think of Marianne's cut as a disease or illness, but the sequence from injury to inflammation to repair occurs in her case exactly as heart muscle does after a heart attack.

The cut extended through epidermis, a labile tissue rich with stem cells; through the dermis, a supporting connective tissue without stem cells; and into fat, also a connective tissue without stem cells.

Cells at every level died of necrosis, which immediately liberated a flood of inflammatory mediators. Blood vessels in the dermis instantly contracted for a few seconds and then relaxed. The process of *hemostasis,* designed to stop bleeding, kicked in. Marianne applied pressure to assist hemostasis and sought medical help.

The wound was closed with stitches so that it could heal by first intention. Had no medical help been available and the wound left open, it would have healed by second intention, but it would have taken much longer and left a bigger scar.

Within the first hour, nearby blood vessels were dilated, the endothelial cells were sticky, and leukocytes were crawling through the seams between cells. Edema fluid was leaking through these same stretched seams and bringing plasma-derived mediators to the scene. Soon the process of angiogenesis began and new blood vessels budded from nearby existing ones.

At the same time, myofibroblasts and fibroblasts began to proliferate. By the second or third day, macrophages had largely replaced neutrophils. By the fourth or fifth day, the wound was filled with granulation tissue: richly vascular, warm, swollen with edema fluid and blood, and quite tender. In classic terms: *rubor, tumor, calor, dolor*.

All the while epidermal stem cells have been repaving the skin surface with new epidermis by asymmetrically dividing, creating one new epidermal cell and one new replacement stem cell.

By the end of the first week, fibroblasts are weaving a progressively thicker, stronger bond of collagen fibers to replace the weak hold of myofibroblast contraction. By the end of the second week, many of the blood vessels have disappeared and collagenous scar tissue continues to accumulate. At the end of the first month, the scar is pink and tight as fibroblast collagen production continues. At this point Marianne worried that she would never be able to fully straighten her finger, but diligent extension exercises stress the scar continually until, by the end of the year, the scar has remodeled to fit comfortably over the joint and full functionality has returned.

Chapter Challenge

CHAPTER RECALL

1. True or false? A multipotent stem cell has the ability to produce any kind of tissue.
2. Which of the following tissues is made of labile cells?
   A. Heart
   B. Bone marrow
   C. Liver
   D. Skeletal muscle
3. In what ways can cells be injured?
4. Which of the following is derived from the endoderm?
   A. Skin
   B. Kidney
   C. Pancreas
   D. Bone
5. Fill in the blank. __________ necrosis is characterized by the ghostly outline of cells that have died in place, their architecture preserved.
   A. Coagulative
   B. Liquefactive
   C. Caseous
   D. Fat
6. True or false? Lipofuscin is the "wear and tear" pigment.
7. Which of the following cells is the principal inflammatory cell in a parasitic infection?
   A. Lymphocyte
   B. Eosinophil
   C. Basophil
   D. Monocyte
8. True or false? Hormones are endocrines released into the bloodstream to act on nearby cells.
9. Which of the following characterize chronic inflammation?
   A. An abundance of lymphocytes and macrophages, few or no neutrophils, attempted regeneration of destroyed cells, scarring, and a rich supply of blood vessels.
   B. It is caused by a brief injury and lasts a few hours or days.
   C. It is characterized by vascular dilation, accumulation of edema, damaged cells, and infiltration of neutrophils.
   D. It is characterized by the clinical manifestations of tumor, rubor, calor, and dolor, and heals without scarring.
10. Copious amounts of water fluid, low in protein, are seen in ______________.
    A. Chronic inflammation
    B. Serous inflammation
    C. Fibrinous inflammation
    D. Suppurative inflammation
11. True or false? Multinucleated giant cells are found in TB.
12. True or false? Regeneration is the complete, or nearly complete, restoration of normal anatomy and function by the regrowth of normal functional cells.
13. A surgical incision heals by which of the following:
    A. First intention
    B. Second intention
    C. Regeneration
    D. Fibrous repair

CONCEPTUAL UNDERSTANDING

14. Using examples from the text, discuss the relationship between chronic injury/stress and the resulting adaptations.
15. Compare and contrast apoptosis and necrosis.
16. Explain how the physics of fluid flow in blood vessels influences the migration of leukocytes in the setting of inflammation.
17. Describe the timeline of angiogenesis.

APPLICATION

18. Jane, a 25-year-old female, was recently in a motor vehicle collision. Luckily she was wearing her seatbelt. Several months later, Jane had an X-ray that showed small calcifications in her breast. Explain what has occurred (rest assured Jane does not have breast cancer).
19. Sam, a 5-year-old male, was badly burned when he pulled a pot of boiling water off of the stove. What determines how well his injuries will heal?

Disorders of the Immune System

Contents

Chapter Objectives

After studying this chapter, you should be able to complete the following tasks:

NON-IMMUNE DEFENSE MECHANISMS

1. Name the two principal nonimmune defense systems.

LYMPHOID ORGANS AND THE LYMPHATIC SYSTEM

2. Describe the components of the lymphatic system and their function.

INNATE AND ADAPTIVE IMMUNITY

3. Compare and contrast innate and adaptive immunity.

CELLS OF THE IMMUNE SYSTEM

4. List the cells of the immune system and describe their role in immunity.

B LYMPHOCYTE (ANTIBODY)-MEDIATED IMMUNITY

5. Name the five types of antibodies and discuss the context in which they function.

T LYMPHOCYTE (DELAYED)-MEDIATED IMMUNITY

6. Explain the difference between MHC Type I and Type II display.

HYPERSENSITIVITY REACTIONS

7. Discuss the pathogenesis of the four types of hypersensitivity and give examples of each type.

ALLERGIC DISORDERS AND ATOPY

8. Using examples from the text, explain the pathogenesis of allergic and atopic reactions.

AUTOIMMUNE DISORDERS

9. Briefly discuss the immune mechanisms and clinical findings in rheumatoid arthritis, Sjögren disease, systemic sclerosis, inflammatory myopathy, and systemic lupus erythematosus.

AMYLOIDOSIS

10. Compare and contrast primary and secondary amyloidosis, and list the systemic effects of amyloidosis.

IMMUNITY IN TISSUE TRANSPLANTATION AND BLOOD TRANSFUSION

11. Explain the factors taken into consideration with regards to tissue transplantation and blood transfusion and the consequences of a mismatch.

IMMUNODEFICIENCY DISORDERS

12. Describe the deficiency of each of the following, and give examples of the organisms they are predisposed to: X-linked agammaglobulinemia, isolated immunoglobulin A (IgA) deficiency, thymic hypoplasia, and severe combined immunodeficiency.
13. Briefly discuss the phases of HIV/AIDS, and explain the role of infections, AIDS-defining neoplasms, and laboratory data in making the diagnosis.

Case Study

"She is still using." The case of Miriam K.

Chief Complaint: Fever and swollen glands

Clinical History: Miriam K., a 28-year-old single woman with no children, immigrated to the United States from Botswana three years before she was brought to the emergency room by a friend. Her primary complaints were fever and "swollen glands." Questioning revealed that over the last six months she had lost 25 lb and had a poor appetite, recurrent night sweats, and intermittent fever. She reported that she was well before leaving Botswana—an African nation in which in 2010 about 25% of adults were infected with HIV. She admitted having sex for money and said she used intravenous drugs but quit six months ago. Her friend said privately, however, "She is still using."

Physical Examination and Other Data: Physical exam revealed a lethargic, thin woman complaining of thirst and abdominal cramps. Enlarged lymph nodes were present in the cervical, axillary, and inguinal regions. Marks on her forearms suggested the possibility of self-injection. Lab studies in the emergency room showed her to be severely anemic (low red cell count), and to have low blood platelet and lymphocyte counts.

Clinical Course: Miriam was admitted to the hospital for evaluation. Further tests revealed that she had HIV proteins and anti-HIV antibodies in her blood. Blood platelet count was 90,000/mm^3 (normal: 150,000–450,000). Further study revealed antiplatelet antibodies covered her platelets. Her CD4+ lymphocyte (helper T cell) count was 295 cells/mm^3 (normal: >500). Small doses of steroids improved her low platelet count. She was transfused with two units of packed red blood cells, which corrected her anemia. She was discharged with diagnoses of "HIV infection; not yet AIDS" and "autoimmune thrombocytopenia." She was provided a starter pack of anti-HIV drugs, a prescription for more, and an appointment at a public-health clinic. She failed to fill the prescription or keep the clinic appointment.

Fourteen months later, Miriam appeared in the emergency room again complaining of shortness of breath. Chest X-rays showed bilateral pulmonary shadows suggestive of pneumonia. Her helper T cell count was 186/mm^3. She was given antibiotics and restarted on anti-HIV therapy. She was provided a clinic appointment but again failed to appear for follow-up care.

Her final appearance in the emergency room occurred 10 months later when she was brought in by staff from a homeless shelter. She was semicomatose. Caregivers reported that she suffered from severe memory problems, was unable to walk or feed herself, and had persistent coughing, diarrhea, painful urination, and weight loss. Clinical investigation revealed extensive bilateral pneumonia and severe urinary tract infection, but she died before a full workup was completed.

An autopsy was performed. The body was very thin. The lungs were severely congested and nearly airless. Microscopic study revealed that the air sacs were filled with *Pneumocystis jirovecii* a type of fungus. Given the degree of infection, there was relatively little inflammatory reaction against it. Abdominal lymph nodes were enlarged. The spleen was also enlarged and congested. Both kidneys were riddled with small abscesses. Urinary cultures reported postmortem showed overwhelming numbers of streptococci bacteria. The mucosa of the small and large intestine was extensively ulcerated. Microscopic study revealed evidence of cytomegalovirus infection in the intestinal epithelial cells. In the left frontal lobe of the brain was a 4-cm tumor, shown by subsequent study to be composed of B cells. Her cerebral cortex was mildly atrophied, and microscopic study revealed white matter lesions consistent with early multifocal leukoencephalopathy.

"She is still using." The case of Miriam K. (continued)

The final autopsy diagnoses were the following:

- AIDS with opportunistic pneumonia (*Pneumocystis jirovecii*)
- Multifocal leukoencephalopathy
- Mild cerebrocortical atrophy
- B cell lymphoma of the brain
- Streptococcal pyelonephritis
- Opportunistic infection of the small and large intestines (cytomegalovirus)

Immune: Having the capacity to withstand, impervious, resistant, unsusceptible.

ROGET'S II: THE NEW THESAURUS, THIRD EDITION, 1995

To be immune is to be protected. The word *immune* is derived from Latin *im* (without) + *munus* (duty) and is generally used to indicate exempt status. It was not a medical term until the 1880s, however, when it began to be used to describe becoming exempt from (immune to) contagious disease.

As understanding improved, it became clear that immunity applies to a much broader concept: molecular-level protection against anything alien or foreign to the interior of the body. In a phrase: *It's us against them.* "Us" is defined by each person's normal DNA and the proteins made in accordance with DNA instructions, which we refer to as **self**. With the exception of identical twins, every person on the planet is a singular package of proteins unlike any other. "Them" is the proteins of other living things—cat dander, bacteria, viruses, organs of other people, and so on—each of which is a product of *their* DNA and are **nonself** to other humans (Fig. 3.1). Although the proteins we consume as food are also nonself, the process of digestion breaks them down into their component amino acid molecules, which are too small to be recognized as nonself. Tumor cells are a special case: our very own DNA has become corrupted into nonself. Thus, every tumor, benign or malignant, produces alien proteins that are recognized by the immune system as nonself and are therefore subject to immune attack, an antineoplastic immune function referred to as *immune surveillance* (Chapter 5). **Immunity**, therefore, is a cellular and molecular mechanism to defend the body against nonself threats. See *The History of Medicine*, "Edward Jenner's Joy," which offers insight into the development of vaccination as a method of harnessing the immune system to prevent infection.

Defense against nonself threats requires the action of three major body systems:

- *Physical and chemical barriers* such as skin, mucus membranes, and gastric acid, which provide non-immune protection
- The *lymphatic system*, a branching network of lymphoid vessels and lymphoid organs, which houses immune cells
- The *immune system*, a cellular/molecular defense system. The key players are white blood cells (WBCs).

Case Notes

3.1 Are Miriam's cells self or nonself to another person?

3.2 Miriam is infected by HIV. Are HIV proteins self or nonself to Miriam's immune system?

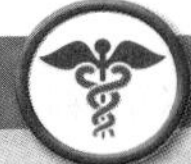

The History of Medicine

EDWARD JENNER'S JOY

The joy I felt at the prospect before me of being the instrument destined to take away from the world one of its greatest calamities (smallpox) was so excessive that I found myself in a kind of reverie.

EDWARD JENNER (1749–1823), ENGLISH SURGEON, UPON REALIZING THAT COWPOX VACCINATION COULD PREVENT SMALLPOX

The tale of Edward Jenner's discovery is well known, but in fact he was a latecomer to vaccination practice.

Smallpox is an infectious viral disease known since antiquity—the mummified remains of Egyptian pharaoh Ramses IV (d. 1156 BCE) bears evidence of it. As recently as 1967, smallpox caused epidemics resulting in two million deaths. A massive vaccination effort by the World Health Organization (WHO) led to eventual elimination of the disease: the last recorded case was in Somalia in 1977. The only remaining smallpox viruses are believed to be in two tightly guarded laboratories, one in Russia and the other in the United States.

Some evidence indicates that smallpox vaccination was practiced in India as early as 1500 BCE, and the Chinese may have engaged in similar practices in the 10th century. In 1716, Lady Mary Wortley Montagu, the wife of the British ambassador to the Ottoman Empire, witnessed physicians in Istanbul practicing smallpox vaccination by collecting pus from the sores of victims with mild cases of smallpox for inoculation into the skin of healthy people. A mild illness followed. Practitioners claimed permanent protection against smallpox. She brought the idea back to England and successfully inoculated her five-year-old son in 1721. The key to success, we now know, was that there are two varieties of the smallpox virus, *variola minor* and *variola major*. *Variola minor* infection caused a much less serious disease than *variola major*, which was often fatal or at least very debilitating. Physicians collected pus from *minor* victims and rubbed it into a scratch created on skin. The resulting illness conferred lifelong immunity and was usually mild because the virus was *minor* and the route of inoculation was skin rather than inhalation of droplets spewed by coughs of the severely ill. The practice spread widely. During the American Revolution, General George Washington regarded smallpox as a threat nearly equal to the English army and wisely demanded that his troops be inoculated.

Jenner's insight was an improvement in vaccination practice. It had long been observed that cowpox and smallpox were similar: both caused acute illnesses characterized by skin and mucus membrane eruptions, both were highly contagious, and both could be spread by skin-to-skin contact. What's more, it was known that dairymaids who had had cowpox did not catch smallpox. In May 1796 Jenner found a young dairymaid, Sarah Nelmes, with fresh cowpox sores. He collected some of the fluid from her lesions and on May 14, inoculated James Phipps, an eight-year-old boy. The youngster became mildly ill for a few days but quickly recovered. On July 1, Jenner inoculated the boy with smallpox. Today we shudder at the danger to which the boy was exposed, but medical ethics were different in the 18th century, and Jenner's daring move may well have saved the boy's life. No disease developed. Over the next two years, Jenner repeated his experiment on more patients and was always successful. He published his results in 1798, the practice of cowpox inoculation spread around the world, and smallpox infections and deaths plunged.

Non-Immune Defense Mechanisms

To cause harm, all nonself threats must first penetrate the *physical and chemical barriers* of the **nonimmune defense mechanisms** (Fig. 3.2):

- *Skin*: The surface layer of skin, the epidermis, is formed of layers of flat cells that shed daily, carrying microbes with them. Epidermal cells discourage microbial growth; they are dry and composed of dense, indigestible protein, and their pH is acidic. Disruption of the skin's

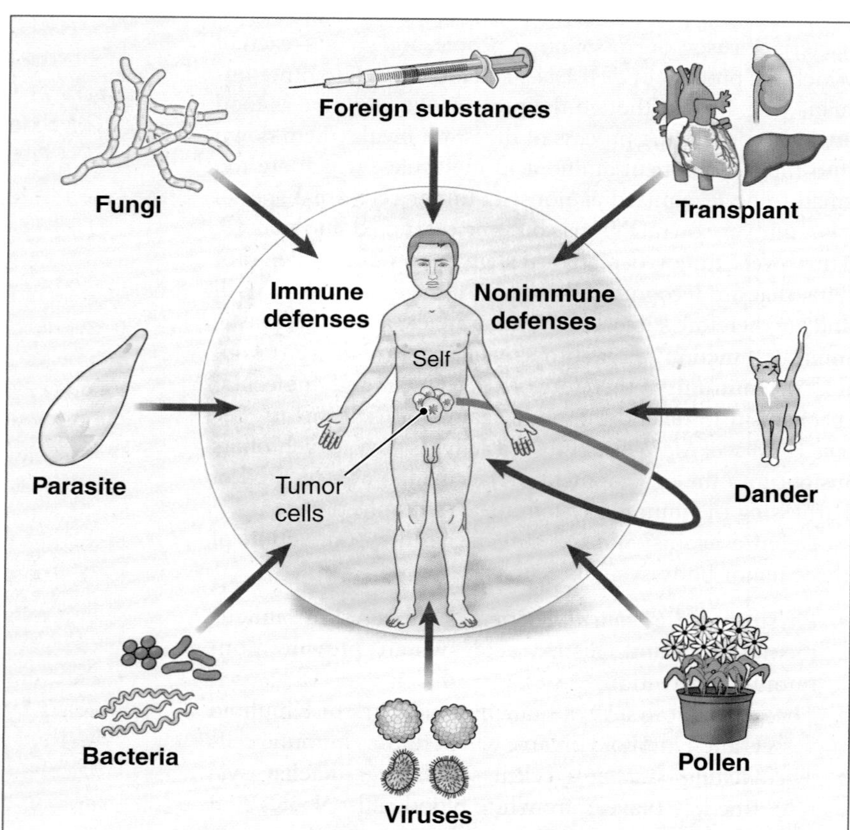

Figure 3.1 **Self and nonself.** Immune and nonimmune defenses protect self from external, alien, nonself substances. Neoplasms are nonself tissue that arise internally.

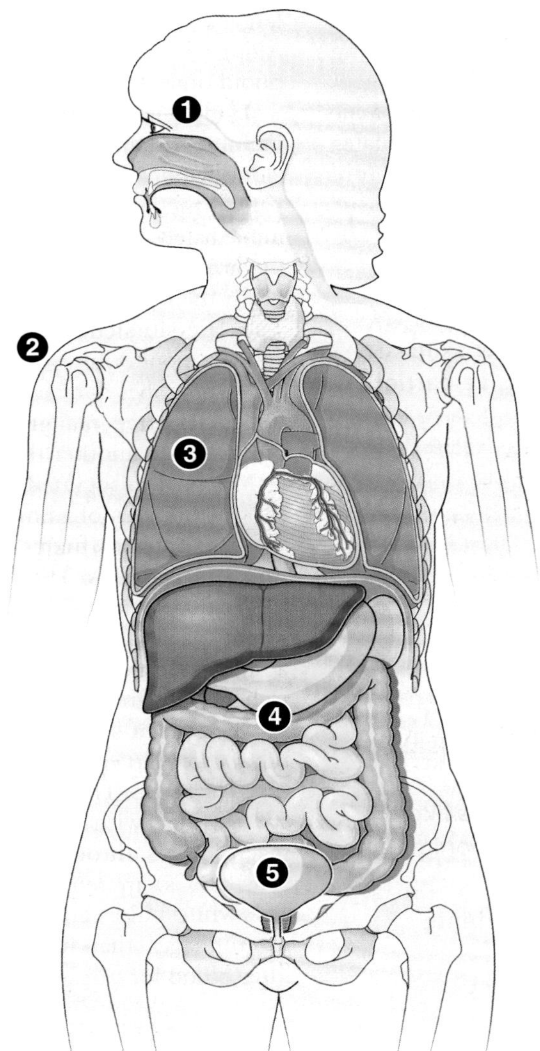

Figure 3.2 **Nonimmune defense mechanisms.**

physical integrity, however (e.g., by needle stick, burn, insect bite), may allow microorganisms to penetrate, and moist skin is more susceptible to invasion than dry.

- *Sclera*: The white of the eye is washed by tears, which have an antibiotic quality owing to lysozyme, an antibacterial enzyme, and is wiped clean every few seconds by blinks.
- *Body membranes:*
  - *Respiratory tract*: The respiratory tract is lined by a shoulder-to-shoulder army of tall, ciliated cells that shed regularly. Interspersed are mucin-secreting cells that provide a mucin film. With each breath, we inhale at least a few microorganisms, most of which are trapped by nasal and bronchial mucus. Those that reach the bronchi are swept upward to the throat by the bronchial cilia and are coughed out or swallowed. Anything that interferes with these mechanisms promotes respiratory infection. For example, alcohol impairs the sweeping motion of the bronchial cilia so that chronic alcoholics are prone to bacterial pneumonia; cigarette smoke has much the same effect.
  - *Gastrointestinal tract*: Like skin, the oral cavity, pharynx, and esophagus are lined by layers of flat cells that shed daily and resist bacterial penetration. The stomach and small and large bowel are lined by tall columnar cells that shed regularly. The intestinal tract is defended by multiple mechanisms, including a protective layer of mucus, gastric acid, pancreatic enzymes, and detergent bile salts. Gastrointestinal epithelial cells shed daily, making it difficult for organisms or particles to gain a strong grip.
  - *Genitourinary tract*: Also like skin, the vagina is lined by layers of flat cells that shed daily and resist bacterial penetration. Urine is normally sterile because it is acidic; it is also flushed constantly by a system designed to avoid retrograde flow.

In addition to these physical barriers, blood and tissue fluids are sifted continuously through various filtering apparatuses, each of which can capture and dispose of microbes. Blood passes through the spleen and bone marrow thousands of times a day, while tissue fluid percolates through lymph nodes (described below), which capture and destroy nonself material.

Case Notes

3.3 **Miriam stuck needles through her skin. Would this be a violation of a defensive barrier?**

Pop Quiz

3.1 True or false? Alcohol impairs the motion of cilia, predisposing alcoholics to respiratory infections.

3.2 True or false? Immune defense mechanisms are the first line of defense against microorganisms.

3.3 True or false? Filtering mechanisms like the spleen and the lymph nodes are nonimmune defense mechanisms.

3.4 Name a principal nonimmune defense system.

Lymphoid Organs and the Lymphatic System

Because of their role in preparing lymphocytes for their several roles in immunity (discussed below), *bone marrow* and the *thymus* are the **primary lymphoid organs**. The **lymphatic system** (Fig. 3.3) is a network of small **lymph vessels** and **secondary lymphoid organs**—tonsils, lymph nodes, and specialized nodules of lymphoid tissue in the respiratory and intestinal tracts. The *lymphatic system* has three functions:

- To house and support immune cells
- To filter tissue fluid for nonself content
- In the intestines only, to absorb dietary fat and deliver it into the blood (Chapter 11)

Lymphatic vessels originate in tissues as minute lymphatic capillaries, which absorb fluid from the intercellular space. This newly formed **lymph fluid** is identical to interstitial fluid, and contains water, electrolytes, and a little protein. It flows toward the chest through progressively larger vessels, which empty into large veins near the heart. Along the way it percolates through multiple small lymphoid organs called *lymph nodes*.

Lymph nodes are small lymphoid organs composed of immune system cells. About 500 lymph nodes are scattered along lymph channels in fat and other soft tissue in every part of the body. Prominent groups of lymph nodes occur immediately beneath the skin in the groin (*inguinal* nodes), the armpit (*axillary* nodes), and along the lateral neck beneath the ear and jaw (*cervical* and *submandibular* nodes). They are situated as the "sentry posts" of the lymphatic system, monitoring lymph fluid for microbes and trapping those microbes for destruction by immune cells. Lymph nodes also trap malignant tumor cells that spread from one tissue to another through lymphatic vessels.

Mucosal-associated lymphoid tissue (MALT) consists of nodules of immune system cells situated at sites where pathogens frequently enter the body—the respiratory and GI tracts. The **tonsils** are large masses of MALT tissue that form a ring around the opening of the throat at the back of the mouth. Nodules of MALT are also abundant in the bronchial tree, and in the small intestine (where they are called Peyer patches).

The **spleen** serves also as a secondary immune organ, but is not part of the lymphatic system. It has two main types of tissue. The *red pulp* is composed of broad venous spaces filled with slow-moving blood, lymphocytes, and macrophages, through which blood filters as old red blood cells (RBCs) are removed and nonself content is detected. The white pulp consists of nodules of lymphocytes and macrophages that function much like lymph nodes to filter blood for nonself-content.

Pop Quiz

3.5 True or false? The white pulp of the spleen is made of venous sinuses, while the red pulp is composed of lymphocytes.

3.6 MALT is lymphoid tissue present in the upper respiratory tract and ______________.

3.7 Lymph nodes serve as sentry posts monitoring the body for ______________ and ______________.

Innate and Adaptive Immunity

The immune system has two main divisions *innate* and *adaptive*.

Innate immunity (*natural* or *native* immunity) is present from birth and consists of cellular and molecular defense capabilities that have an evolved ability to attack *any* nonself substance. Innate immunity does not require prior exposure to nonself material for training or programming.

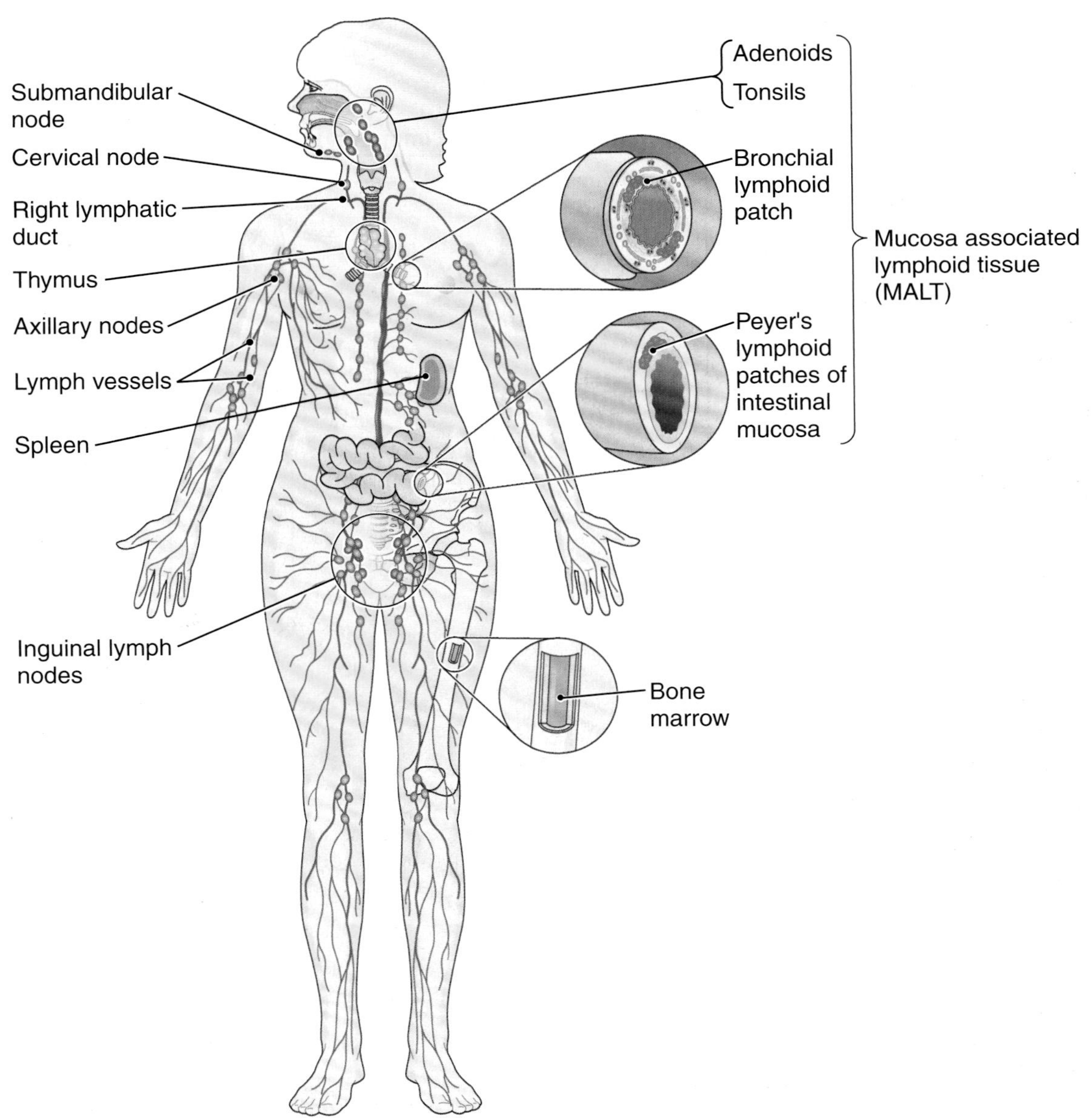

Figure 3.3 **Lymphoid organs and the lymphatic system.**

Response begins within minutes and is fast and broad, like a quick shotgun blast targeted at *any* invader. The inflammatory response (Chapter 2) is an important part of innate immunity. Recall that inflammation is the response to injury. It has many aspects, among them phagocytosis of invading microbes, cleaning up cellular debris, and initiation of the healing process. Nevertheless, *to the extent that inflammatory cells attack and destroy invading bacteria and other nonself agents, inflammation is an aspect of innate immunity.*

Adaptive immunity (*acquired* or *specific* immunity) is a somewhat slower, *programmable* system that interacts with invading nonself material, learns its characteristics, and manufactures a targeted, highly specific response designed to fight that *specific* invader. The response is then memorized for use again in the future. By convention, the phrase *"immune response"* refers solely to responses of the *adaptive* immune system. The varieties of adaptive immune responses are detailed in Figure 3.4.

An **antigen** is any substance capable of inciting an *adaptive* immune response. Almost all antigens are *nonself proteins*, though a few other large nonself molecules are capable of stimulating an adaptive immune response. In addition, some small, nonprotein molecules can stimulate an immune reaction by combining with a normal self-protein in such a way that the combination becomes nonself. Molecules that behave in this way are called **haptens**. For example, the skin rash of poison ivy is an immune reaction caused by a hapten, which combines with normal skin protein to turn the combination into a nonself antigen.

The initial reaction to antigen exposure—the **primary immune response**—takes about a week because the immune system has not previously encountered the antigen in question.

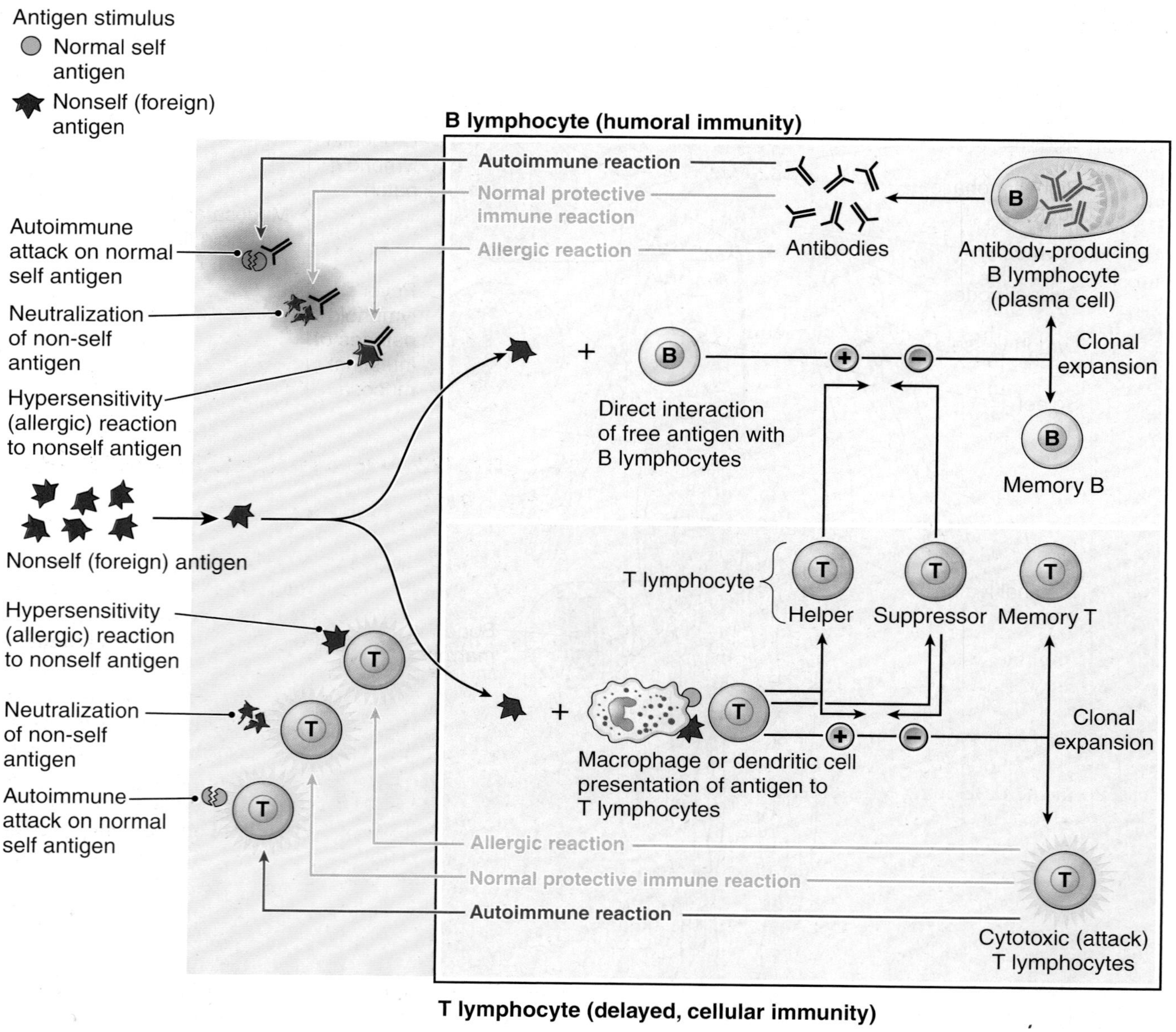

Antigen stimulus
Normal self antigen
Nonself (foreign) antigen

B lymphocyte (humoral immunity)

Autoimmune reaction
Normal protective immune reaction
Allergic reaction
Antibodies
Antibody-producing B lymphocyte (plasma cell)
Autoimmune attack on normal self antigen
Neutralization of non-self antigen
Hypersensitivity (allergic) reaction to nonself antigen
Direct interaction of free antigen with B lymphocytes
Clonal expansion
Memory B
Nonself (foreign) antigen
T lymphocyte
Helper
Suppressor
Memory T
Hypersensitivity (allergic) reaction to nonself antigen
Neutralization of non-self antigen
Autoimmune attack on normal self antigen
Macrophage or dendritic cell presentation of antigen to T lymphocytes
Clonal expansion
Allergic reaction
Normal protective immune reaction
Autoimmune reaction
Cytotoxic (attack) T lymphocytes

T lymphocyte (delayed, cellular immunity)

Figure 3.4 **The types and sequences of immune reactions.** Nonself antigen may react with B or T cells. In a **normal reaction (green)** B cells respond by producing memory cells and plasma cells, which secrete antibodies to attack and neutralize the nonself antigen. T cells respond normally by producing memory cells and cytotoxic cells that attack and neutralize the nonself antigen. T cells also produce helper and suppressor cells that modulate both B and T cell reactions. In an **autoimmune reaction (red)** the attacking antibodies or cytotoxic T cells mistakenly attack normal self tissue, causing tissue damage and inflammation. In an **allergic reaction (yellow)** the attacking antibodies properly attack the nonself antigen, but in an exaggerated manner that causes congestion and inflammation.

All *subsequent* exposures are **secondary immune responses**, which are much quicker because the immune system has memorized the first encounter and is able to spring into action instantly. This memory aspect of immunity is the scientific foundation for vaccinations against infection.

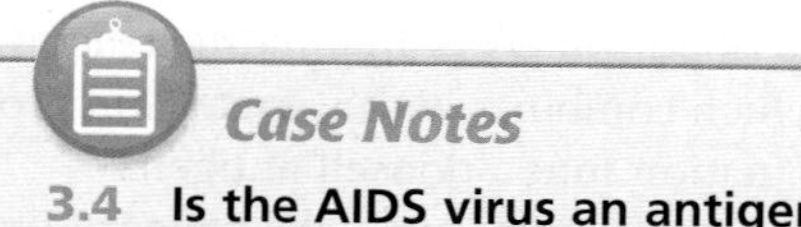

Case Notes

3.4 Is the AIDS virus an antigen or an antibody?

3.5 Are Miriam's antibodies self or nonself?

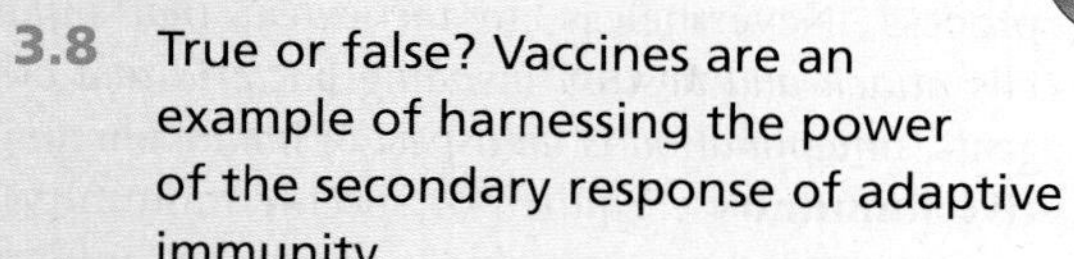

Pop Quiz

3.8 True or false? Vaccines are an example of harnessing the power of the secondary response of adaptive immunity.

3.9 True or false? Innate immunity requires programming.

3.10 Define antigen and antibody.

Cells of the Immune System

Because the inflammatory response is one aspect of innate immunity, every white blood cell (WBC) is in some sense an immune cell. *Macrophages, dendritic cells,* and *lymphocytes,* however, are the specialized (WBCs) of the immune system. They reside mainly in lymphoid organs.

Macrophages are large tissue phagocytic cells derived from blood monocytes, a type of WBC. Like all WBCs, monocytes circulate freely in blood and migrate into all tissues, where they roam widely and acquire a colossal appetite for ingesting and destroying microbes and other nonself antigens. In some organs they have acquired special names: *microglia* in the brain and *Kupffer cells* in the liver, for example. **Dendritic cells** are a second variety of tissue macrophage, which can evolve from monocytes or from lymphocytes (discussed next). Unlike macrophages, they remain fixed in place. They are concentrated in lymphoid organs and in tissues exposed to the environment: skin, the lining of the respiratory tract, and the lining of the GI tract. Dendritic cells and macrophages are also called **antigen presenting cells** because they capture antigens and prepare them for presentation to T lymphocytes, which mobilize the T cell immune system to identify and attack the antigen.

Lymphocytes are small WBCs that are the effector cells of the immune system. Lymphocytes circulating in blood comprise about 5% of all lymphocytes; the other 95% reside in lymphoid organs and other tissues. Primitive lymphocytes in the developing fetus differentiate into several populations. One line of fetal lymphocytes migrates to the thymus, where they mature into *T lymphocytes* or *T cells*. Another fetal lymphocyte line remains in the bone marrow where it matures into *B lymphocytes* or *B cells*. From the thymus and bone marrow, lymphocytes enter the blood stream and spread throughout the body, but especially to lymph nodes and other lymphoid organs. **T lymphocytes** comprise about two-thirds of blood lymphocytes and are the agents of *cellular* (delayed) *adaptive* immune response. **B lymphocytes** comprise about one-fourth of blood lymphocytes and are the agents of the *humoral* (antibody) *adaptive* immune response.

The third population of lymphocytes is **natural killer (NK) cells** (the only type of lymphocyte without the word *lymphocyte* in its name); these are effector cells of the *innate* immune system. They comprise about 10% of blood lymphocytes, but what they lack in numbers they make up for in speed and aggression. They do not require education and have an innate capacity to instantly recognize, attack, and kill virus-infected cells and tumor cells.

All lymphocytes look the same but they and other types of cells can be identified by distinctive clusters of proteins on their cell membranes called **cluster differentiation (CD) proteins** (they are commonly called CD *antigens* because, being proteins, they are capable of inciting an immune reaction in another person, to whom they are nonself). Laboratory identification of the CD type of immune cells is very helpful in the study of immune disease. For example, a cell with type 4 CD antigen is designated CD4+—the malignant T cells in a majority of T cell leukemias are CD4+ cells.

Pop Quiz

3.11 True or false? NK cells require immune programming to be effective.

3.12 What two immune cell types are able to migrate freely among blood and lymphoid organs?

B Lymphocyte (Antibody)-Mediated Immunity

B cells have their effect on nonself antigens by secretion of **antibodies** (Fig. 3.4), antiantigen proteins that circulate freely in blood and other body fluids. Because of its secretory nature, the B cell system is also termed **humoral immunity** after the ancient term for mythical substances, *humors*, thought to be circulating in the blood as the cause of all disease. Antibodies are produced only in response to *freely circulating* antigen from *extra*cellular threats such as bacteria, fungi, parasites, pollen, and injected foreign material. Upon antigen contact, B cells activate and are transformed into **plasma cells**, antibody-secreting B cells that reproduce a clone of identical cells (**clonal expansion**) to amplify their antibody producing power. Not all B cells secrete antibodies—some serve as **memory B cells**, which linger in the body, preprogrammed and ready to quickly multiply and release a flood of antibodies the next time the antigen appears. Antibody production is critically dependent on *helper T cells* (discussed below).

Antibodies are a type of protein known as **immunoglobulin** (or *gamma globulin*), which constitutes about 20% of plasma protein. Immunoglobulins are large proteins with a complex structure. The backbone of each is composed of two long molecules, the *heavy (H) chains*, and two shorter molecules, the *light (L) chains*.

The five classes (types) of immunoglobulin are G, A, M, D, and E (abbreviated IgG, IgA, etc.), each of which is defined by its heavy chain. IgG has a heavy chain type called *gamma;* IgA has an *alpha* heavy chain, and so on. Each immunoglobulin has two distinct regions: an unchanging backbone (the *constant fragment*, or F_C) and a fragment that varies according to the antigen to be attacked (the *variable* or *antibody fragment*, F_{AB}).

Each class of antibody has a unique molecular structure and serves a particular immune function:

- **IgG** is the smallest and most abundant immunoglobulin in blood. Its main duty is to neutralize microorganisms.

In response to antigen challenge, it is produced rather slowly and persists a very long time. It confers permanent immunity against reinfection (Fig. 3.5).

- **IgA** is most abundant in mucosal secretions where MALT tissue is abundant, especially the GI tract and respiratory membranes, which are open to the environment and exposed to many microorganisms. It is also present in high concentration in tears and in the milk of nursing mothers, from which it temporarily transfers mother's immunity.
- **IgM** is the largest immunoglobulin; hence its alternative name, *macroglobulin*. It attacks microorganisms and is produced rapidly, providing initial protection while IgG production is getting underway, after which levels fall markedly (Fig. 3.5).
- **IgD** does not appear in blood. It is bound exclusively to the cell membrane of B cells and participates in the process of activating B cells to recognize antigen and undergo clonal expansion.
- **IgE** appears in blood only in trace amounts. The bulk of it attaches to *mast cells*, the tissue version of blood basophils (a variety of WBC). It is important in allergic reactions such as hay fever or skin allergies (see *Type I hypersensitivity reactions*, below).

Antibodies are effective by: 1) neutralizing the function of the antigen; 2) causing cell death by rupturing the cell membrane (usually of a microbe) of which the antigen is a part; 3) inciting an inflammatory reaction to neutralize or digest the microbe; or 4) making the microbe more susceptible to phagocytosis by inflammatory cells.

Antibodies achieve their effect by attaching to the target antigen. The combination of antigen and antibody is called an **immune complex**. By further antigen-antibody agglomeration, immune complexes may become quite large and lodge in any tissue, where they incite acute inflammation (see *Type III hypersensitivity reaction*, below).

Most B cell immunity arises from endogenous (internal) production of antibodies by the person's own immune system (**active immunity**). Nevertheless, antibodies can be transferred passively (**passive immunity**) to confer temporary immunity, as in the case of antibody injections (gamma globulin injections) to prevent infection. Fetuses and newborn infants gain temporary immunity by passive transfer of antibody from mother to infant across the placenta and in breast milk.

Case Notes

3.6 Miriam had a lung fungus infection. Her B cell system, though weakened, presumably produced antifungal antibodies. To which immunoglobulin class did the *initial* antibody response belong?

3.7 Which element of the immune system produced her antiplatelet antibodies?

3.8 What type of cell produced the anti-HIV antibodies in Miriam's blood?

Pop Quiz

3.13 True or false? B cells do not require that an antigen presenting cell present antigen to them.

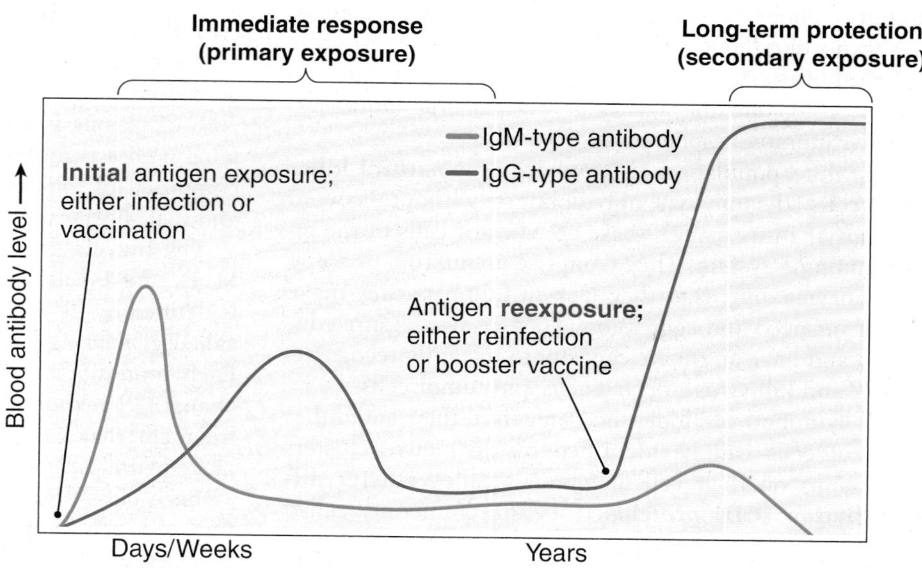

Figure 3.5 **Antibody response to antigen exposure.** On initial antigen exposure IgM-type antibody is produced first, providing quick protection but no permanent immunity. IgG-type antibody levels soon rise and provide additional immune defense and permanent immunity. On re-exposure IgG antibody rises quickly to prevent infection.

3.14 True or false? B cells react only with antigen attached to the surface of a cell.

3.15 True or false? B cells must have T cell support to function normally.

3.16 Which antibody does not circulate in blood?

Case Notes

3.9 Miriam's CD4+ blood lymphocyte count was low. What type of lymphocytes are they?

3.10 In which organ were Miriam's T cells educated?

3.11 Which variety of T cells attacked Miriam's HIV-infected cells?

3.12 Does the AIDS virus live inside or outside of Miriam's cells?

T Lymphocyte (Delayed)-Mediated Immunity

In contrast to B cells, which are activated only by freely circulating antigen, T cells are stimulated only by contact with antigen bound to a cell membrane—an *antigen presenting cell* (a macrophage or dendritic cell) must first react with the antigen (Fig. 3.4), bind it to its cell membrane, and then present it to the T cell for action. T cells then must migrate to the site of the offending antigen and attack it. This requires time, usually a few days—much longer than the minutes or hours for B cell response. Because the reaction is not immediate and because cells, not antibodies, effect the reaction, T cell immunity is also called **delayed immunity** or **cellular immunity**.

T cell subtypes (Fig. 3.4) differ according to function:

- **Cytotoxic T cells** are the effector cells of cellular adaptive immunity. They target and destroy cells that the immune system has identified as containing alien antigen, either a cancer cell or a cell infected by a virus. They are also active in the defense against some bacterial, fungal, and other infections. They also act to suppress unnecessary antibody production to prevent runaway reactions and autoimmune disease. Their CD antigen type is usually CD8+. These interact with Type I MHC display (discussed below).
- **Helper T cells** facilitate the immune activities of B cells and other T cells. Their CD antigen type is usually CD4+. These cells interact with Type II MHC display (discussed below).
- **Regulatory** or **suppressor T cells** modulate the immune response to shut down the immune response after successful defense to maintain immune homeostasis and prevent development of autoimmune disease (discussed below).
- **Memory T cells** enable the cellular immune system to mount a rapid secondary immune response.

Because viruses do their damage from within cells, antiviral defense is usually a job for T cells. To get into cells, however, viruses must travel freely through blood and extracellular fluids; therefore, viruses can stimulate antiviral antibody production by B cells. T cells are also stimulated by cells within which corrupted DNA is present, destroying them before they can become malignant. T cells also mediate immune rejection of tissue transplants.

An important part of immunity is the mechanism by which antigens are displayed to immune cells. This mechanism functions as a billboard that immune cells read in order to know what to do. This apparatus, the **major histocompatibility complex (MHC)**, is a glycoprotein complex on the surface of *all* cells except RBCs that allows immune cells to recognize the cell as self or nonself. MHC proteins were first discovered on leukocytes (WBCs) and are commonly known as **human leukocyte antigens (HLA)**. Every person, with the exception of identical twins, has a unique set of MHC antigens. See *Molecular Medicine*, "HLA Antigens," which explains their clinical importance.

Remember This! There are two major divisions of the adaptive immune system: The B cell system, which secretes antibodies to attack nonself antigen, and the T cell system, in which the T cells themselves attack.

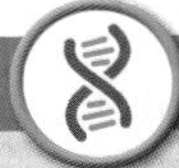

Molecular Medicine

HLA ANTIGENS

HLA antigens (also known as MHC antigens) are present on the surface of every cell except RBCs. Apart from their role in adaptive immunity, they have two other critical roles in medicine.

First, HLA antigens are the prime reason tissue transplants are rejected. As antigens, they are capable of inciting an immune reaction in *another* person if they are transplanted. For example, the HLA antigens in a transplanted heart are nonself to the recipient and incite the recipient's immune system to attack.

Second, HLA antigens tend to be associated with certain diseases. Each human has a different set, but they share common features that allow them to be sorted into subtypes. Certain HLA subtypes are associated with certain diseases, especially autoimmune genetic diseases. For example, people with HLA-B27 subtype have a much higher prevalence of rheumatic diseases. As a result, HLA typing can be used as a diagnostic tool in the investigation of some diseases.

There are two types of MHC—*class I* and *class II*. Class I MHCs are present on the surface of *every* body cell except RBCs. Class II MHCs occur only on macrophages and dendritic cells.

MHC I glycoproteins display antigens *synthesized inside* a virus-infected or cancerous cell. In healthy cells, MHC I glycoproteins display *normal* self-antigens, in effect displaying the message: "*This cell and all other cells like me are self; leave us alone.*" In contrast, cancerous or virus-infected cells synthesize *alien*, nonself proteins. In these unhealthy cells, MHC I glycoproteins display these nonself (but internally produced) antigens. The message is different: "*Alien antigen present inside; kill me.*"

The process works much the same for **MHC II** complexes, which are present on the surface of macrophages and dendritic cells, whose job is to capture and display *external* nonself antigen. The macrophage or dendritic cell grabs the antigen, from, say, an invading bacterium. It then displays the antigen using its MHC II glycoprotein. This display serves a function similar to a picture of the criminal on a Criminal Wanted poster with the message: "*Dangerous invader looks like this. Go find it and kill it.*"

The critical distinction between MHC I and II is this: the immune system attacks the cell with the MHC I display, but just reads the MHC II display and goes looking for something else to attack.

Because they play such an important role in presenting *nonself* antigens to the immune system, it is easy to forget that MHC glycoproteins *are antigens themselves* to the immune systems of *other* people. Indeed, they derive their name from their discovery as important antigens in transplant medicine. As such, they can be powerful adversaries in organ or tissue transplantation.

Remember This! An antigen is any substance capable of inciting an adaptive immune response. Almost all antigens are proteins. The term *antigen* is usually used instead of *protein* when discussing immunity.

Case Notes

3.13 Would Miriam's T cells attack free HIV in the extracellular space?

3.14 Would Miriam's innate or adaptive immune system or both react to the HIV virus?

3.15 Which type of MHC would have displayed antigens from the cytomegalovirus that infected cells in Miriam's intestine?

Pop Quiz

3.17 True or false? Class I MHC display occurs on the surface of *every* cell in the body except RBCs.

3.18 True or false? T cell activation is more complex and takes longer than B cell activation, and is therefore sometimes called "delayed immunity."

3.19 Name the four types of T cells.

Hypersensitivity Reactions

Hypersensitivity reactions are the result of an abnormally active immune system and are the cause of allergy and autoimmune disease.

The four mechanisms of hypersensitivity are:

- B cell mediated
  1. *Immediate* (Type I)
  2. *Cytotoxic* (Type II)
  3. *Immune complex* (Type III)
- T cell mediated
  4. *Cellular (delayed)* (Type IV)

Two features of hypersensitivity disease are especially important:

1. Antigens from the environment or from within the body may initiate the reaction.
2. Hypersensitivity disease is associated with certain HLA genotypes.

Type I Immune Reaction: Immediate Hypersensitivity

Immediate hypersensitivity (Fig. 3.6) is a reaction that occurs within a few minutes after an antigen combines with preformed antibody created by B cells from an earlier exposure. The earlier episode is the initial or *sensitizing exposure*, during which IgE antibodies are secreted by B cells and attach to mast cells (tissue basophils). The initial, sensitizing exposure produces no symptoms, but it sets the stage for a rapid reaction on subsequent exposure. On subsequent exposure, the antigen combines with IgE antibody already present on the surface of mast cells and triggers mast cell release of preformed vasoactive substances (e.g., histamine) and inflammatory mediators. The result is vascular dilation, congestion, mucus secretion, and inflammation.

Type I hypersensitivity reactions underlie most allergic disorders. Systemic reactions can include shock, suffocation, or death. Local reactions depend on site of entry and may take the form of a skin rash or swelling (urticaria, hives), nasal and conjunctival discharge (allergic rhinitis and conjunctivitis), or bronchial asthma (Chapter 10).

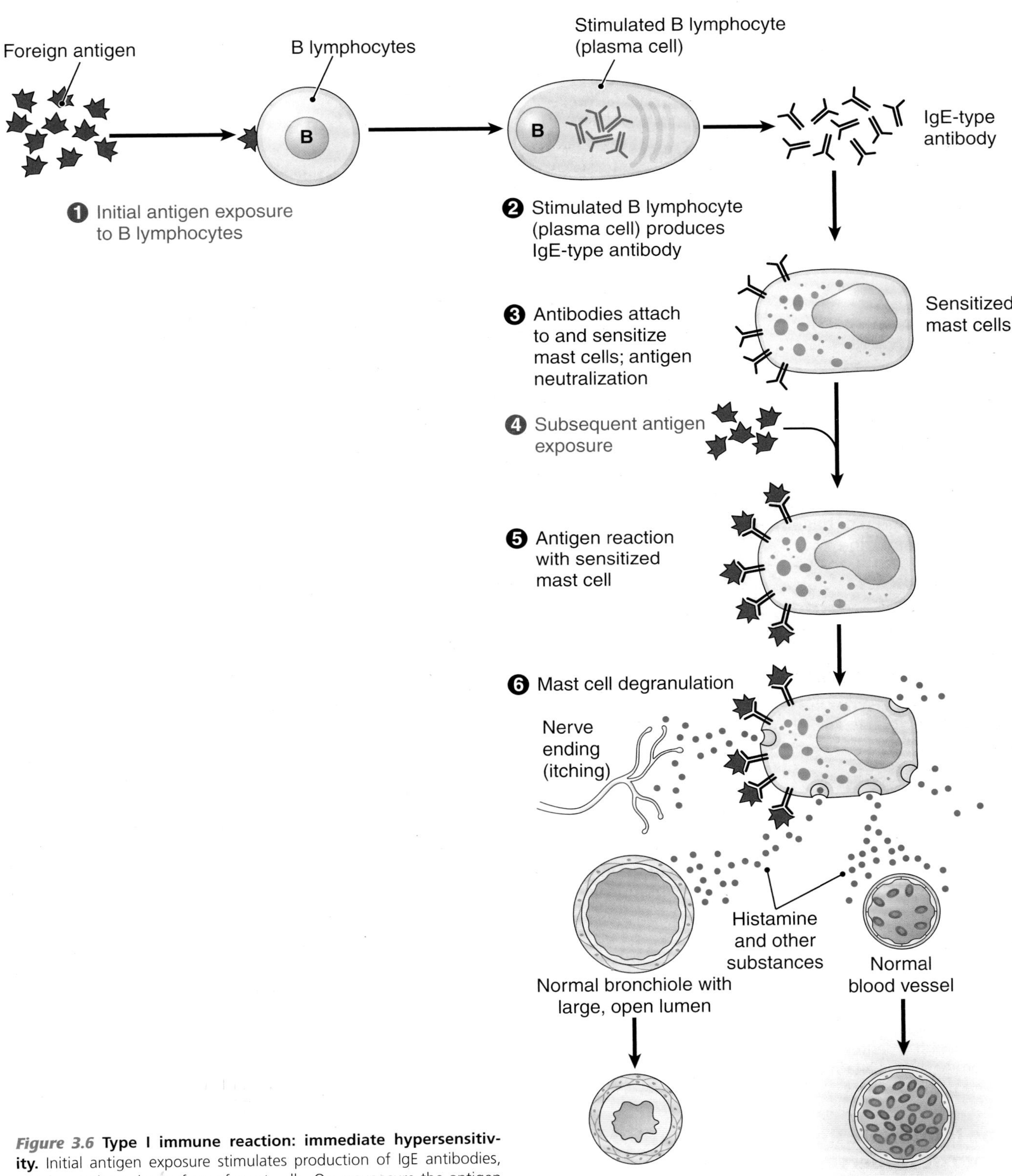

Figure 3.6 **Type I immune reaction: immediate hypersensitivity.** Initial antigen exposure stimulates production of IgE antibodies, which attach to the surface of mast cells. On reexposure the antigen combines with antibody on the mast cell surface to stimulate immediate release of histamine from mast cell cytoplasmic granules, which causes itching; bronchospasm, wheezing, and shortness of breath; and vasodilation and edema formation with low blood pressure, weakness, and tissue swelling.

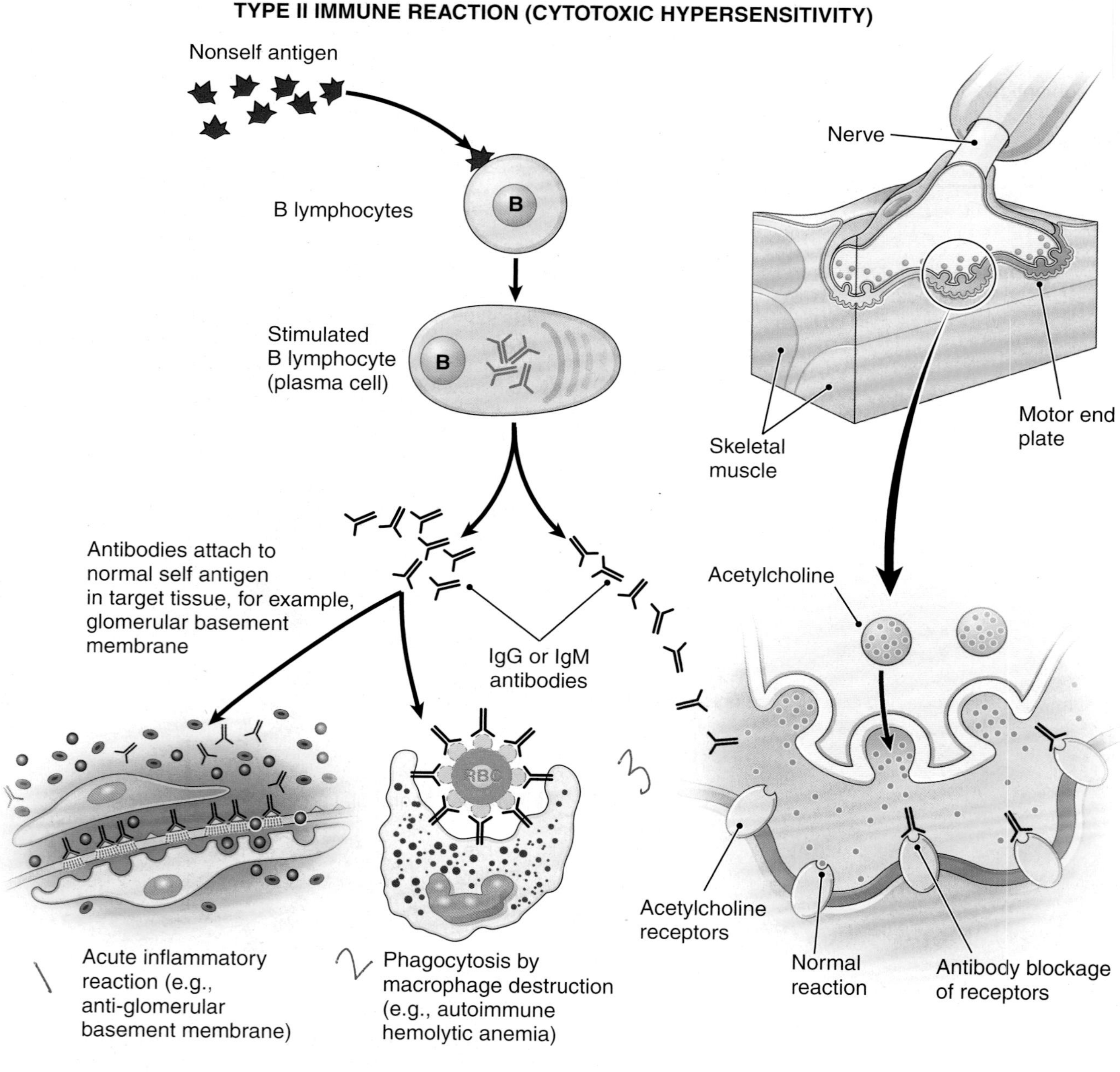

Figure 3.7 **Type II immune reaction: cytotoxic hypersensitivity. A.** Target tissue inflammation or cell death. Antibodies attach to target antigen, which is destroyed by inflammation (e.g., glomerular basement membrane) or phagocytosis (e.g., RBC). **B**. Interference with target cell function. Antibodies attach to target-cell receptors and interfere with function (e.g., blockage of signal transmission from nerve to muscle in myasthenia gravis).

Type II Immune Reaction: Cytotoxic Hypersensitivity

Cytotoxic hypersensitivity (Fig. 3.7) is caused by B cell production of antibodies that react with antigens on the surface membrane of cells, or with extracellular tissue components. For reasons usually unknown, normal self-antigens become seen as nonself by the immune system and become targets for immune attack. The antigen may be native to the cell or tissue component or may have become attached to it. Some reactions are initiated by molecules that act as *haptens* (discussed above), which convert self-protein into a nonself combination.

Cytotoxic reactions are mediated by IgG and IgM antibodies that form antigen-antibody complexes on the cell surface. These complexes may alter the cell's function or be enough to kill the cell by complement activation or by attracting NK cells or macrophages. Cell death is illustrated in Figure 3.7A. In this instance, RBCs are coated by antibody attached to a target antigen in the cell membrane. Red cell destruction (hemolysis) is the result (see the discussion of immune hemolytic anemia in Chapter 7). Altered cell function is illustrated in Figure 3.7B. In this instance antibodies bind to target-cell membrane receptors and block receptor function. For example, in myasthenia gravis (Chapter 18), an antibody attaches to acetylcholine receptors on the muscle side of the neuromuscular junction, preventing transmission of the nerve signal to muscle.

Type III Immune Reaction: Immune-Complex Hypersensitivity

Immune complex hypersensitivity is an immune reaction of B cells in which free/soluble antigen and antibody combine to form an immune complex that deposits in tissue, damaging it and inciting an inflammatory reaction (Fig. 3.8).

Systemic hypersensitivity occurs when the complex forms in blood and is deposited in tissue (Fig. 3.8A). The prototype is *serum sickness*, a reaction once common following the outdated practice of injecting humans with horse serum containing horse antitetanus antibody to obtain passive immunization against tetanus. Exposure to horse antigen triggers antibody production, which forms immune complexes with remaining injected horse antigen. The closest thing to it is *poststreptococcal glomerulonephritis* (Chapter 15), in which streptococcal antigens form immune complexes with naturally produced antistreptococcal antibodies and the complexes deposit in glomeruli. Several other autoimmune diseases are caused by systemic Type III reaction.

Local hypersensitivity reactions (Fig. 3.7B) are those in which the immune complexes form and remain at the site of antigen introduction. Most cases of autoimmune pneumonitis (*farmer's lung*) are local Type III reactions. Farmer's lung is caused by chronic inhalation of organic material such as hay mold (a fungus), which lodges in the lung and stimulates production of antifungus antibody that combines locally with the inhaled antigen to cause autoimmune pneumonia.

Type IV Immune Reaction: Cellular Hypersensitivity

Cellular (delayed) hypersensitivity reaction is different from the three other types because it is a T cell reaction. No antibodies are produced and the clinical reaction is delayed a few days after antigen contact.

As is illustrated in Figure 3.9, antigen is captured by antigen-presenting cells for presentation to T cells. T cells react to produce clone *cytotoxic T cells* to attack the invader, but which attack normal self-antigen instead. Clones of *suppressor T cells*, *helper T cells*, and *memory T cells* are also produced.

Certain infections, including infection by *Mycobacterium tuberculosis* (the bacillus that causes *tuberculosis*), incite a Type IV hypersensitivity reaction. In tuberculosis it is not the TB bacillus itself that causes the most tissue damage; it is the Type IV hypersensitivity reaction the bacillus initiates.

Contact dermatitis is the most common form of Type IV hypersensitivity disease. Common agents are poison ivy, latex gloves, and metallic jewelry. The skin reaction to these substances does not appear clinically for two to three days after exposure. Other diseases caused by Type IV hypersensitivity are *Type I diabetes mellitus*, *rheumatoid arthritis* (RA), *multiple sclerosis* (Chapter 19), and *Crohn disease* (Chapter 11). *Transplant rejection* is often a Type IV hypersensitivity reaction based on recipient intolerance of donor antigens in the MHC.

Case Notes

3.16 Miriam's low platelet count was due to antibodies attached to platelet surface membrane. Which variety of hypersensitivity does this represent: I, II, III, IV?

Pop Quiz

3.20 True or false? Type IV reactions account for allergies.

3.21 What is the name of an antigen bound to its antibody and circulating in blood?

3.22 What is the name of the hypersensitivity reaction in which an antibody attaches to a cell and injures it?

Allergic Disorders and Atopy

Allergy is any exaggerated but otherwise normal immune response to a foreign antigen regardless of the type of hypersensitivity reaction. An **allergen** is any substance (antigen) that induces an allergic reaction.

Atopy is allergy due to Type I hypersensitivity. The great majority of allergies are atopic, but some are mediated by other mechanisms. That is to say, all atopy is allergic, but not all allergy is atopic. For example, hypersensitivity pneumonitis (Chapter 10) is an allergic reaction that owes to Type III hypersensitivity, and poison ivy dermatitis (Chapter 21) is a Type IV delayed hypersensitivity reaction. Atopic disorders are very common and usually affect the nose (seasonal allergic rhinitis), skin (atopic dermatitis, Chapter 21), and airway (atopic asthma, Chapter 10).

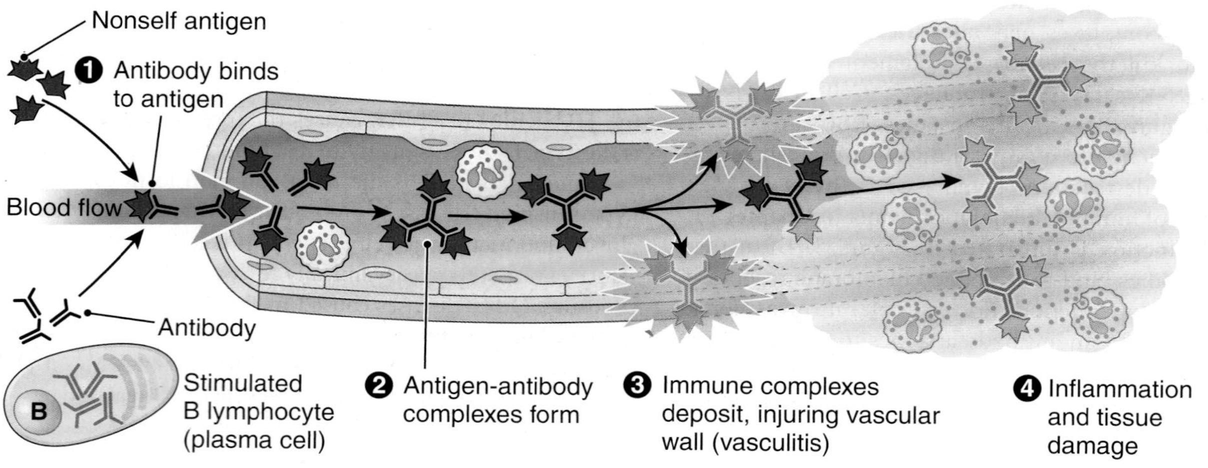

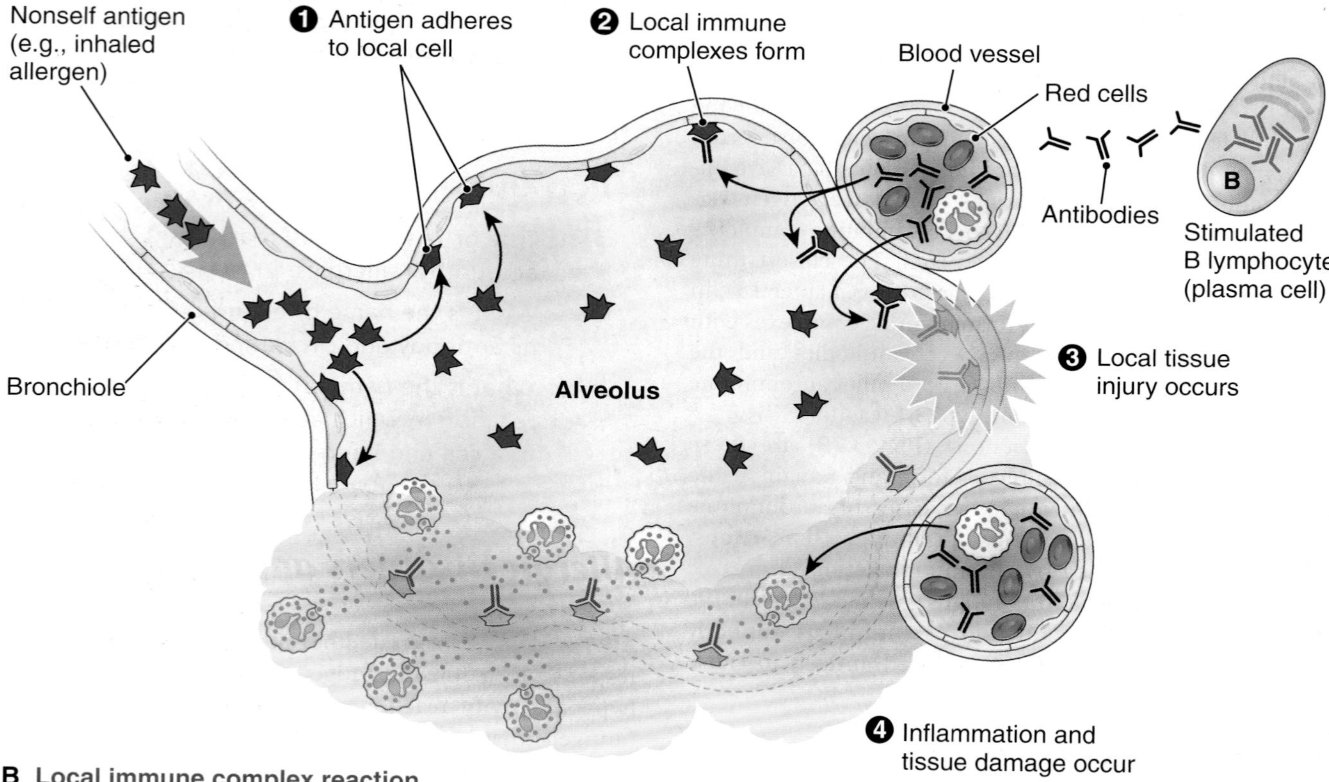

Figure 3.8 **Type III immune reaction: immune-complex hypersensitivity.** Antigen and antibody bind together to create an immune complex. **A**. Systemic immune complex reaction. In systemic autoimmune reactions, immune complexes cause vasculitis and widespread tissue damage. **B**. Local immune complex reaction. In local autoimmune reactions, immune complexes form and remain locally to cause damage (e.g., allergic pneumonia caused by inhaled antigens).

The etiology and pathogenesis of atopy is complex. Most of the data is epidemiologic and difficult to apply to an individual case. There is also a strong familial (genetic) tendency. The most common allergens are house dust, animal dander, fungus mold, and pollen from trees, grasses, and weeds. The skin of patients with atopic dermatitis is usually colonized by *Staphylococcus aureus* and improves with its elimination, but the pathologic mechanisms are not clear.

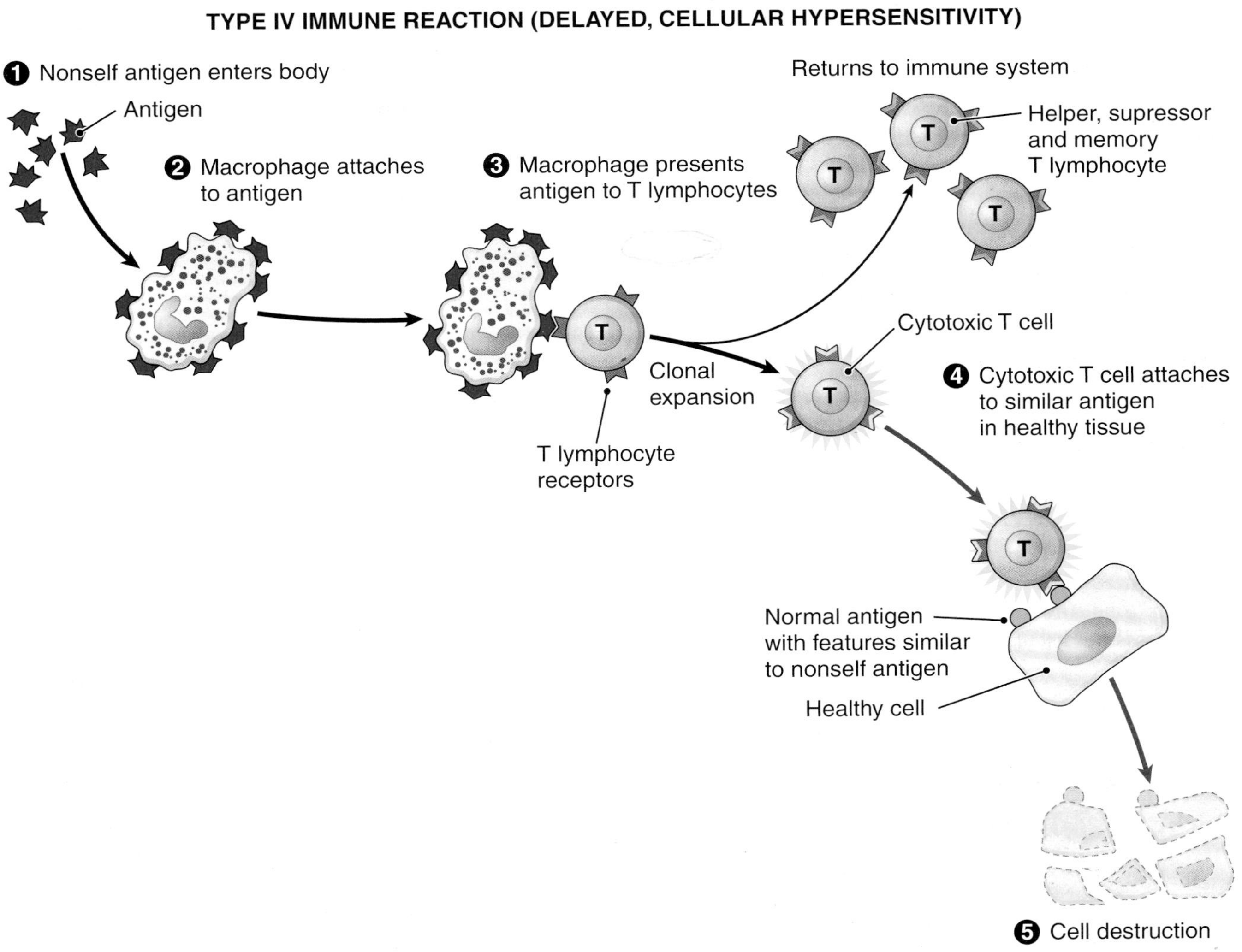

Figure 3.9 **Type IV immune reaction: cellular hypersensitivity.** Macrophages capture antigen and present it to T lymphocytes, thus programming (sensitizing) them. Some lymphocytes become cytotoxic T cells that attack the antigen wherever it is found; others become helper, suppressor and memory T cells.

The pathophysiology is explained above in Figure 3.6. Histamine released from Ig E-sensitized mast cells in skin, lungs, and GI mucosa causes the following:

- Local vasodilation (vascular congestion, erythema)
- Increased capillary permeability and edema
- Stimulation of nearby nerve endings (itching)
- Smooth muscle spasm in airways (wheezing) and GI tract (increased motility, urgency)
- Increases in salivary gland and bronchial gland secretion

Many atopic patients develop the *atopic triad*: rhinitis, dermatitis, and asthma. Symptoms tend to be seasonal and include rhinorrhea, sneezing, and nasal congestion; itchy, watery eyes; acute or chronic, itchy skin lesions; wheezing and shortness of breath. Asthma appearing before age 30 is likely atopic; after 30, other factors such as smoking are more important.

History is the most reliable guide to diagnosis. Blood eosinophil count is usually high. Skin testing with a panel of allergens may be valuable in some cases.

Treatment should begin by avoiding the allergen or removing it from the environment. Treatment of rhinitis is with a combination of antihistamines, decongestants, and nasal corticosteroids. Patients with atopic dermatitis may improve with dilute bleach baths to eliminate skin staphylococci. Treatment of atopic asthma relies on oral antihistamines, inhaled steroids, and other modalities discussed in Chapter 10. Some patients with severe atopy may require desensitization: graduated injections to build up tolerance.

Food allergy is an atopic, exaggerated immune response to dietary proteins. It is rare: less than 3% of suspected cases are genuine. The remaining 97%+ are nonimmune reactions to food (e.g., lactose intolerance, irritable bowel syndrome, infectious gastroenteritis), reactions to food additives or food contaminants, or other food intolerance. Almost any food or food additive can cause an allergic reaction, but the most common triggers in infants include milk, soy, eggs, peanuts, and wheat.

In older children and adults, nuts and seafood are the most common culprits.

Systemic effects of the histamine released by atopic reactions include vasodilation, which may cause a headache or a precipitous drop in blood pressure manifested as fainting or shock. Sudden vascular collapse may be fatal after antigen exposure (e.g., bee sting) in a previously sensitized patient. This type of severe, generalized atopic reaction is called **anaphylaxis**. It is an acute, life-threatening, IgE-mediated allergic reaction that occurs in previously sensitized people when they are reexposed to the sensitizing antigen. Severe vascular dilation causes the vascular space to become relatively underfilled and blood pressure falls, which may cause dizziness or fainting (*syncope*). Symptoms include difficult inspiration due to throat or laryngeal edema (*stridor*), dyspnea, wheezing, and hypotension. Diagnosis is clinical. Bronchospasm and upper airway edema are treated with inhaled or injected epinephrine (adrenalin) or related drugs. Airway maintenance may require emergency intubation. Hypotension requires IV fluids to expand vascular volume and vasopressors to reestablish vascular tone and increase vascular resistance (see the blood pressure discussion in Chapter 9).

Pop Quiz

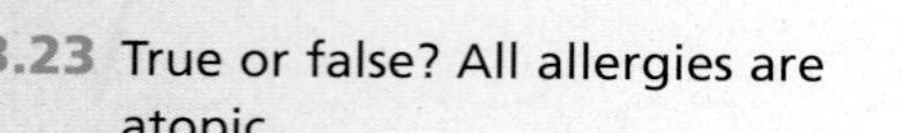

3.23 True or false? All allergies are atopic.

3.24 What preformed antibody mediates anaphylaxis?

Autoimmune Disorders

In **autoimmunity**, our own tissues—our very own self-antigens—become targets of the immune system. We become, in a sense, our own worst enemy. Historically, autoimmune diseases have been called *collagen-vascular diseases* or *connective tissue diseases* because blood vessels and connective tissues are often the target.

Autoimmune disease is common and affects about 2% of the U.S. population. Autoimmune antibodies are also commonly present in the blood of apparently healthy people, especially in older age groups. Clinical manifestations are extremely varied. Some diseases are confined to a single organ. Type I diabetes is an example: cytotoxic T cells attack the insulin-secreting beta cells of pancreatic islands of Langerhans. On the other hand, SLE is an example of multisystem autoimmune disease: B cell antibodies attack DNA and other cell elements, insuring that virtually any tissue can be affected. Table 3.1 lists selected systemic and organ specific autoimmune diseases.

What is it that goes so terribly wrong with our own tissues that self becomes alien and is attacked by the very immune system that is designed to protect us? In most instances, it is not self that changes, but the immune system.

- *Imperfect fetal B and T cell programming*. The whole of normal immune function hinges on self-tolerance; that is, the ability of the immune system to recognize self and not attack it. Loss of self-tolerance leads to autoimmune disease. Recall that T cells learn how to recognize self in the fetal thymus, and B cells learn in the bone marrow. But the process is not perfect, and *a few nontolerant T and B cells survive*. These potentially troublesome "time bomb" cells are held in check by suppressor T cells and other mechanisms. Autoimmune disease can occur if these nontolerant cells escape suppression. Alternatively, helper T cells can give them an exceptional, abnormal boost.
- *Inaccessible self-antigens*. Antigen that has been hidden from contact with immune cells since conception may become unmasked and attacked because hidden antigens were never initially designated as self in the embryo. *Sympathetic ophthalmitis* is an example. During normal embryogenesis, some ocular antigens are never processed by the immune system to be recognized as self. Ocular trauma or disease may expose these antigens to the immune

Table 3.1 Selected Autoimmune Diseases

Disease	B or T cell mediator	Hypersensitivity Type (I, II, III, IV)
SYSTEMIC DISEASES		
Systemic lupus erythematosus (SLE)	B	Immune complex (III)
Rheumatoid arthritis (RA)	T	Cellular
Immune thrombocytopenia	B	Cytotoxic (II)
ORGAN SPECIFIC DISEASES		
Type I Diabetes mellitus	T	Cellular (IV)
Poststreptococcal glomerulonephritis	B	Immune complex (III)
Farmer's lung	B	Immune Complex (III)

system, thereby stimulating production of antibodies that attack antigen in *both* eyes. It is the threat of autoimmune ophthalmitis in the *other* eye that prompts removal of sightless eyes that are severely diseased or traumatized.

- *Molecular mimicry*. The antigens in some infectious agent or other foreign protein may share antigenic molecular features that mimic certain self-antigens. Immune response directed at the foreign antigen also attacks the self-antigen like it (Fig. 3.10). Poststreptococcal rheumatic carditis (Chapter 9) is an example. Some streptococci have antigens similar to those found in the heart, and strep infection produces antistreptococcal antibodies that react with cardiac antigens. Other microbes are theorized to be the initiating agent for other autoimmune diseases.
- *Infection and inflammation*. Apart from molecular mimicry it appears that the tissue injury and inflammation that accompany infection may alter self-antigens in a way that makes them appear to be nonself. Inflammation is so much a part of autoimmune disease that it is a chicken versus egg question. Which came first, the autoimmune disease or the inflammation associated with some microbe?

No matter the mechanism, some patients are genetically more susceptible than others to autoimmune disease and can be identified by MHC/HLA genotyping. For example, the presence of HLA-B27 antigen is closely linked to certain rheumatoid diseases (Chapter 18).

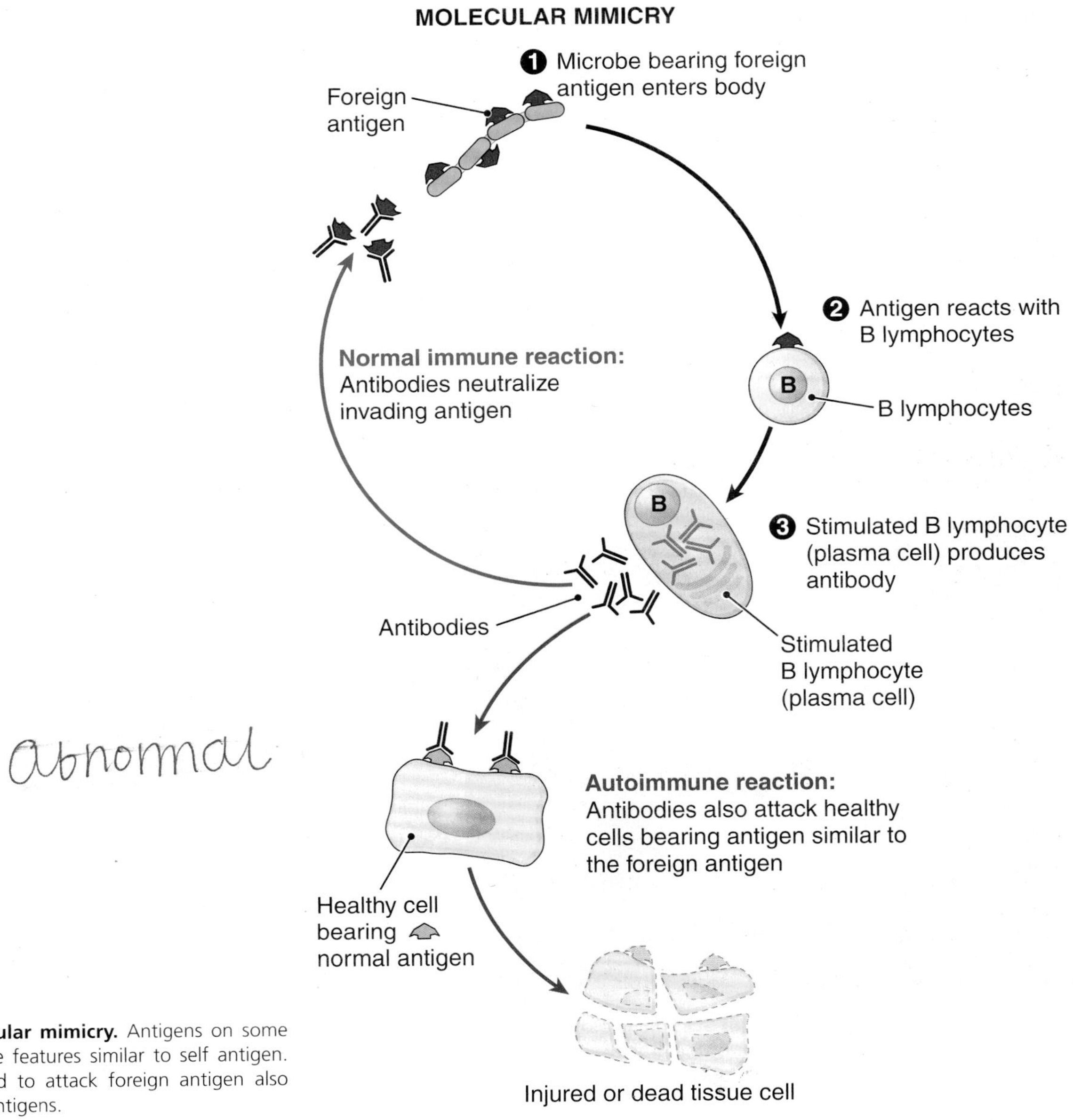

Figure 3.10 Molecular mimicry. Antigens on some microbes have some features similar to self antigen. Antibodies produced to attack foreign antigen also attack normal self antigens.

In the following discussion we will focus on a few autoimmune diseases, leaving the remainder to our discussion of autoimmune disease in various organ systems.

Remember This! Inflammation is the main consequence of an autoimmune reaction.

Case Notes

3.17 Does Miriam have an autoimmune disease, and if so, what is it?

Systemic Lupus Erythematosus

Systemic lupus erythematosus (SLE), (or *lupus*) is a multisystem autoimmune disease caused by immune complex (Type III) hypersensitivity. The name derives from its systemic nature and the characteristic red (erythematous) rash on the cheeks, which resembles the facial markings of a wolf (*Canis lupus*). The facial rash is commonly called a *malar* (cheek) or *butterfly rash* in medical texts because it spreads across the bridge of the nose from one cheek to the other like the wings of a butterfly (Fig. 3.11).

SLE has strikingly diverse manifestations that may affect any organ or tissue, especially the skin, serosal membranes, kidney, joints, and even the brain. It is unpredictable by nature, waxing and waning in intensity and manifestation. SLE is characterized by a multitude of antibodies to various organs and tissue components, but it is associated in particular with the presence of **antinuclear antibodies (ANA)** in blood or tissue, which may target DNA or RNA. The disease is fairly common, affecting about 1 in 2,500 people; 90% of patients are female, most of them 15 to 30 years old at time of diagnosis.

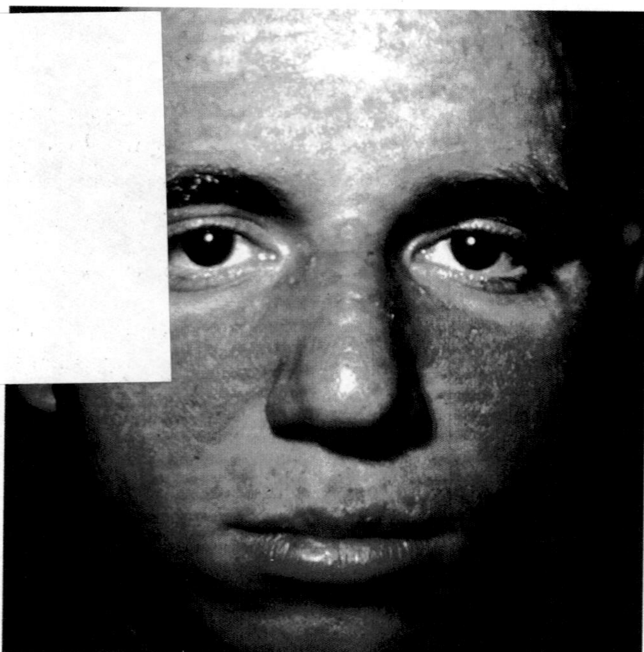

Figure 3.11 **Malar "butterfly" rash of SLE.** The photosensitive butterfly rash is a common manifestation of SLE. It may also occur as a skin disease (*discoid lupus erythematosus*) in patients who do not have systemic lupus.

If the only clinical feature present is the butterfly rash, the disease is referred to as **chronic discoid lupus erythematosus**, though ANAs may be present in blood.

Etiology and Pathogenesis

There is clear evidence of genetic influence—there is a very high chance that if one identical twin has SLE, the other will also; and a few genes have been identified that occur with increased prevalence in SLE. Sex hormones are also important: nine of ten cases occur in women. Chronic administration of certain drugs induces SLE in 15% to 20% of patients taking them. The most notable of these drugs are procainamide (a cardiac antiarrhythmic drug) and hydralazine (an antihypertensive drug). Remission occurs with drug withdrawal. Ultraviolet (UV) light may play a role: the malar butterfly rash is accentuated by sunlight and SLE patients tend to have other light-sensitive skin reactions.

In SLE, loss of self-tolerance is probably due to overactive helper T cells that stimulate B cell production of antiself antibodies. ANAs are the laboratory hallmark of SLE. The detection of ANA in a patient's blood is a very *sensitive* test for the presence of an autoimmune disease, but it is not highly *specific*. That is to say, almost every SLE patient has a positive ANA, but positive ANA may be seen in other autoimmune disease.

SLE is characterized by a variety of circulating autoantibodies against RBCs, platelets, lymphocytes, and other cells and against RNA, DNA, and other cell elements. These antibodies and their target antigens form circulating immune complexes that deposit in various tissues, especially arteries. The result is vasculitis with inflammation and necrosis, which can occur in any location and accounts for the great variability of clinical signs and symptoms in SLE. Antibodies may also form against certain substances used in some blood tests for syphilis, hence *false-positive test results for syphilis* (Chapter 4) *are regularly found in SLE*. About 10% of SLE patients develop *lupus anticoagulant*, an antibody that interferes with laboratory test of coagulation, which falsely suggests patients have a deficiency in coagulation. Actually, the contrary is true: patients with lupus anticoagulant are hypercoagulable and can be plagued with venous and arterial thromboses, thrombocytopenia, and spontaneous abortions.

Clinical and Pathologic Features

Figure 3.12 depicts the clinical findings in patients with SLE, which can affect virtually any tissue or organ. Anatomic lesions appear in the usual sites affected by immune complex hypersensitivity (see above). The following anatomic lesions are most common:

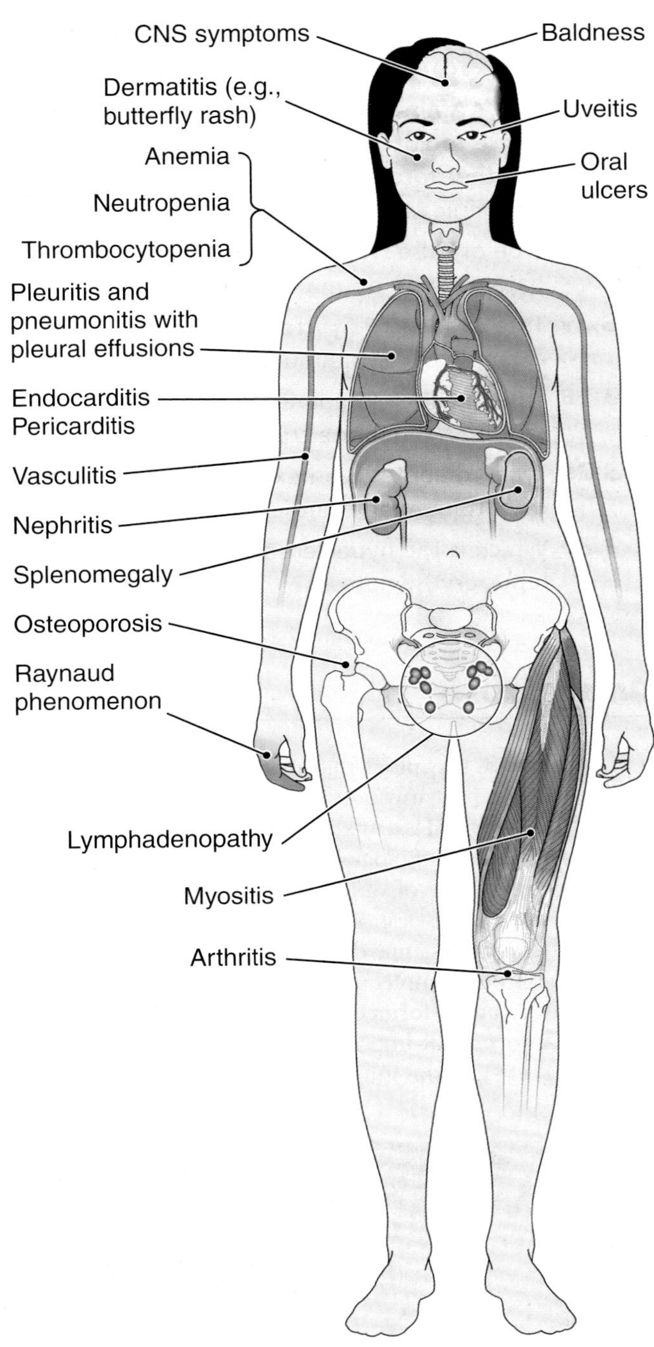

Figure 3.12 **Clinical findings in systemic lupus erythematosus (SLE).**

- *Cytopenia.* Red and white blood cells count and platelet count are usually low.
- *Acute necrotizing vasculitis* in any organ. Blood vessels in any organ may be involved, explaining the remarkable variety of signs and symptoms of SLE.
- *Skin lesions,* which may be exacerbated by exposure to sunlight (photosensitivity). Particularly characteristic is the butterfly-shaped rash mentioned earlier (Fig. 3.11).
- *Serous effusions and fibrinous exudates* of the pericardium and pleurae.
- *Myocarditis and cardiac valvular vegetations.*
- *Glomerulonephritis,* which is common and often severe.
- *Arthritis,* which may be clinically striking, though deforming lesions are rare.
- *Uveitis,* inflammation of the anterior chamber of the eye.
- *Brain involvement,* which is common and includes microinfarcts and organic psychosis or dementia.

Diagnosis and Treatment

Diagnosis is clinical and supported by laboratory presence of low RBC, WBC and platelet count, low blood complement levels, and the presence of ANA. The erythrocyte sedimentation rate (ESR) is high and blood C-reactive protein (CRP) is increased, each providing concrete evidence of underlying inflammation. Presentation can be subtle: fever of unknown origin, a small amount of protein in the urine, or psychosis. SLE is a notorious masquerader. Female sex raises the index of suspicion.

The clinical course of SLE is variable and unpredictable. Some patients have minimal problems, but others are seriously affected. Thirty percent die in the first 10 years after diagnosis. Sooner or later renal disease becomes a problem in most patients. Death often results from renal failure, infections, or diffuse central nervous system involvement.

Treatment of mild cases may require nonsteroidal anti-inflammatory drugs (NSAIDS) and little more. Antimalarial drugs may be added for moderate disease (they have an anti-inflammatory effect, although the mechanism is not clear). Severe disease requires steroids and antineoplastic drugs to suppress immune activity.

Other Autoimmune Diseases

Rheumatoid arthritis (RA) is an autoimmune disease affecting the lining membrane (synovium) of joints. RA also may affect extra-articular tissue such as heart, lungs, skin, and blood vessels. Most patients have a characteristic immune complex, *rheumatoid factor,* in their blood. We will defer discussion of RA and related disease to our discussion of bone and joint disease in Chapter 18.

Sjögren syndrome is a chronic autoimmune inflammatory disease of the lacrimal and salivary glands, which features dry eyes (*keratoconjunctivitis sicca*) and dry mouth (*xerostomia*). It mainly affects women over 40. Though usually localized, it can occur in association with other autoimmune disorders such as SLE or RA. Most Sjögren patients will have rheumatoid factor and other autoantibodies in their blood but will not have RA or other autoimmune disease. About one-third of patients will have extra-glandular involvement: pulmonary fibrosis, arthritis, or peripheral neuropathy. Diagnosis requires lip biopsy to document inflammation of small accessory salivary glands. Treatment is symptomatic. Cyclosporine (an immunosuppressant) eye drops are effective in increasing tear production.

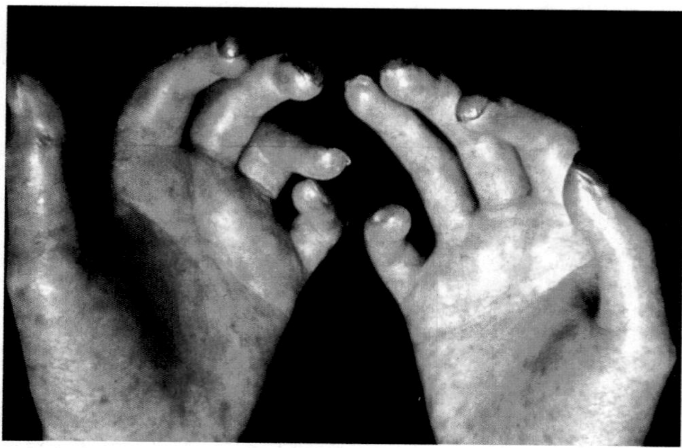

Figure 3.13 **Systemic sclerosis (scleroderma).** This crippling deformity of the hands results from severe skin sclerosis.

Systemic sclerosis (Fig. 3.13), historically called *scleroderma*, is a sometimes cripplingly severe disease featuring microvascular damage and inflammation and fibrosis of the supporting fibrous intercellular tissue (interstitium) of many organs, especially the dermis. Fibrosis, the hallmark of systemic sclerosis, may affect the GI tract, lungs, kidney, heart, skeletal muscle, and small blood vessels. The immune mechanism is not clear, but both T and B cell function appear to be abnormal. Mainly a disease of young women, it may prove devastatingly disfiguring, disabling, or fatal. Although it may manifest many of the features of SLE or RA, it is distinctive because of the striking skin disease and the near uniform presence of *Raynaud phenomenon* (Chapter 8), a condition resulting from spasm of small blood vessels that causes coldness, blanching, numbness, and pain in the fingers and toes. Patients with systemic sclerosis may have trouble swallowing (dysphagia) from esophageal involvement. In severe chronic disease, pulmonary fibrosis may prove fatal. Treatment is directed at complications as there is no effective treatment of the underlying disease.

Polyarteritis nodosa and other vasculitides are autoimmune diseases dominated by generalized blood vessel inflammation. We will defer our discussion to Chapter 8 and disorders of blood vessels.

The *inflammatory myopathies* are a varied group of disorders characterized by autoimmune skeletal muscle injury that occur alone or in conjunction with other autoimmune disease such as SLE or RA. Each disease differs from the others in detail, but all feature widespread muscle weakness, soreness, fatigue, lymphocytic inflammatory cell infiltrates in affected muscle groups, and laboratory evidence of autoimmune disease. We will defer our discussion to Chapter 18 and disorders of skeletal muscle.

Mixed connective tissue disease is a name sometimes applied to widespread autoimmune disease with a mix of features from SLE, RA, and inflammatory myopathy.

Pop Quiz

3.25 True or false? Molecular mimicry is due to antigens on microbes or other foreign proteins sharing common antigenic features with self-antigen.

3.26 True or false? ANAs are found only in patients who do not have SLE.

3.27 True or false? Polyarteritis nodosa is an example of autoimmune vasculitis.

3.28 True or false? Rheumatoid factor is a circulating immune complex.

3.29 Type I diabetes is an example of which type of autoimmune disease reaction?

3.30 Which is the hypersensitivity mechanism in lupus erythematosus?

Amyloidosis

Immune proteins may play a role in other diseases, though the diseases are not primarily autoimmune. One such disease is amyloidosis. **Amyloid** is a mixture of insoluble proteins, some of which may be immunoglobulin fragments. It deposits in the intercellular space of various organs, usually in conjunction with another disease. **Amyloidosis** is any dysfunction resulting from the systemic deposition of amyloid protein.

Normal protein molecules are folded in a particular manner. Amyloid is formed if misfolded protein becomes arranged into crystal-like molecules. Deposited between cells (Fig. 3.14) in the interstitial space, amyloid appears

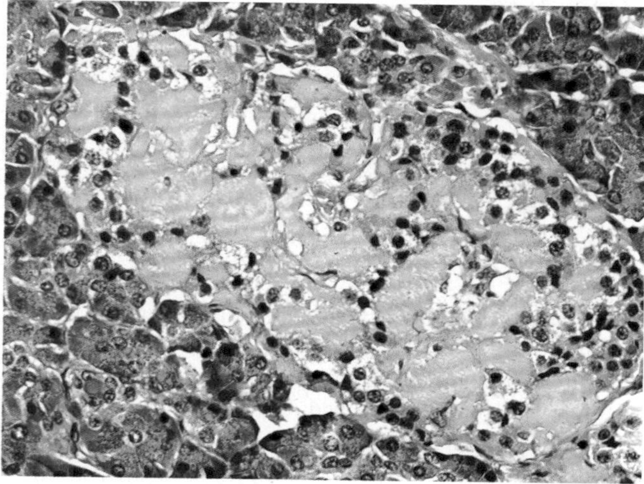

Figure 3.14 **Amyloidosis.** An islet of Langerhans in the pancreas of a patient with Type II diabetes mellitus. (Reprinted with permission from Mills SE. *Histology for Pathologists.* 3rd ed. Philadelphia, PA: Lippincott Williams & Wilkins; 2007.)

microscopically as a translucent, smooth, glassy material. Diagnosis of amyloidosis requires biopsy and microscopic diagnosis.

There are two categories of amyloid protein: 1) misfolded *mutant* proteins; and 2) misfolded *normal* proteins. Misfolded mutant proteins are the cause of primary (genetic, inheritable) amyloidosis. Misfolded normal proteins are the cause of amyloidosis secondary to some other disease. Normally, when proteins misfold, cell quality control mechanisms degrade them into waste products. If this mechanism is overwhelmed or does not function properly, amyloid accumulates.

The most common type of amyloidosis is light chain amyloidosis, a secondary amyloidosis associated with B cell malignancies such as multiple myeloma (Chapter 7). The lymphocytes in these malignancies secrete a great excess of abnormal immunoglobulin, which is degraded into its heavy and light chain components. The light chains deposit as amyloid in some patients. Other patients with light chain amyloidosis do not have B cell malignancy, but have excess abnormal immunoglobulin in their blood.

Reactive systemic amyloidosis occurs in conjunction with chronic inflammatory disease, such as RA. The amyloid protein is not an immunoglobulin but appears to be related to proteins produced during the inflammatory response.

Hereditary (primary) amyloidosis is rare and caused by one of several gene defects, the most common of which is **hereditary Mediterranean fever**. It occurs most often in people of Middle Eastern heritage and features increased production of inflammatory cytokines associated with fever and synovial, pleural, and peritoneal inflammation.

Amyloidosis of aging occurs in patients in their 70s and 80s. The heart is most often involved.

Local amyloid deposits occur locally in the islets of Langerhans in some patients with Type II diabetes, in some endocrine tumors, and in the brains of patients with Alzheimer disease.

Some amyloid deposits do little or no harm. Others may prove fatal. Symptoms are location dependent. Renal deposits may cause proteinuria or renal failure, while cardiac deposits may cause congestive heart failure. Diagnosis requires biopsy proof. Amyloidosis cannot be treated effectively; average survival is a few years.

Pop Quiz

3.31 Name the two general categories of amyloidosis.

3.32 Malignancy of what cell is responsible for the most common form of amyloidosis?

Immunity in Tissue Transplantation and Blood Transfusion

Successful transplantation usually requires that donor and recipient be as much alike antigenically as possible to avoid immune rejection of the donated organ. The closest donor matches of antigens have the fewest rejections and are most likely to be found in close relatives of the recipient. Excepting identical siblings, every transplant causes some degree of immune rejection, which can be diminished by careful matching of major histocompatibility complex (MHC/HLA) antigens and major (ABO) blood group types and carefully administered immunosuppressive therapy. MHC/HLA matching is more important for some transplants than others. The reasons are unclear. For example, kidney and bone marrow transplants require a very close match, whereas requirements for heart and liver transplants are less strict.

There are several varieties of transplantation. If the patient is both the donor and recipient (e.g., skin grafts, hair transplants) the graft is an **autograft**. A transplant between individuals is a **homograft** or **allograft** (e.g., heart, kidney, liver). Transplantation across species is a **xenograft**. Xenografting is poorly tolerated (e.g., monkey livers transplanted into humans), but some avascular tissue xenografts work well. For example, many heart valve replacements in humans are from swine (valves contain no blood vessels).

Despite the ever-present threat of rejection, transplants are widely successful. Kidney transplants have been successfully employed for 50 years. Liver, heart, lung, and pancreas transplants are increasingly successful. Bone marrow transplants are effective for bone marrow failure and some leukemias. Skin and limb transplants are also proving successful.

Transplant Rejection Is an Immune Phenomenon

All homografts cause some immune reaction. Both T and B cells play a role. The main threat is chronic T cell activity. Acute antibody-mediated B cell rejection is less common but more urgent.

Hyperacute rejection is a reaction that occurs within minutes or hours when *preformed* antibodies in the recipient's blood react immediately with graft vasculature. Immediate removal of the donated organ is necessary to avoid more widespread immune reaction.

Acute rejection usually occurs within a few weeks, owing to an immune vasculitis; however, it can occur later if immunosuppressive therapy fails. Both B and T cells are involved. Rejection may be avoided by prompt and aggressive administration of immunosuppressive drugs.

Chronic transplant rejection develops over a period of months to years and is mainly the result of prolonged T cell assault on donor cells. Chronic vasculitis, which deprives the organ of blood flow, is an important factor.

Graft versus host disease (GVHD) is an especially severe complication of bone marrow transplantation. Successful marrow transplantation requires pretransplant chemotherapy or radiation to suppress the *recipient's* immune system and the original bone marrow. With the recipient immune system suppressed, *donor* lymphocytes replace the immune system of the recipient. The result is a patient whose immune system belongs to the donor and sees every patient cell as alien and attempts to reject recipient (host) tissues, especially skin, GI epithelium, and liver. Acute GVHD features dermatitis, diarrhea, and jaundice. Chronic GVHD is characterized by dermal sclerosis, Sjögren syndrome, and immunodeficiency. Death from infection is a common result. There is no good treatment beyond steroids and symptomatic relief.

The best way to prevent rejection is careful antigen matching between donor and recipient. Because ideal matches are uncommon, pretransplant immunosuppression is helpful. Cyclosporine and related drugs are commonly employed. Administration of therapeutic anti-T cell antigens also can reduce the number of T cells available to attack the donated organ. But immunosuppression leaves the patient at risk for infection.

Blood Transfusion Is Temporary Liquid Tissue Transplantation

Blood is liquid tissue, so transfusion is tissue transplantation, though it is temporary because most transfused white cells die within a few days and red cells in a few months. Because RBCs are 1,000 times more common than WBCs and 100 times more common than platelets, successful blood transfusion depends primarily on RBC antigen compatibility between donor and recipient.

Every RBC carries antigens on its surface, which can be divided into three groups: major blood group antigens, minor blood group antigens, and Rh antigens.

ABO Blood Groups

Major blood group antigens are coded by autosomal dominant genes, one from each parent. Genes may be A or B or neither (O). Six genetic combinations (*genotypes*) are possible. *AA, AB, AO, BO, BB,* and *OO*. Because A and B are dominant over O, four blood groups (*phenotypes*) occur: A (*AA, AO*), B (*BB, BO*), AB (*AB*), and O (*OO*). Group prevalence in the United States is O: 45%; A: 41%; B: 10%; and AB: 4%. But percentages vary by ethnicity.

Every person has in their blood IgM-type **antibodies** to the major blood group antigens *not* on their RBCs (Fig. 3.15). Newborns do not have these antibodies. The antibodies develop owing to immune reaction to the presence of A and B antigens in food and bacteria. Plasma from blood group A develops anti-B antibody; group B has anti-A, group O has anti-A and anti-B; and group AB has neither anti-A nor anti-B.

The presence of these natural antibodies dictates which blood can be transfused into a patient. If group A red cells are mixed with plasma containing anti-A antibody (groups B and O), an antigen-antibody reaction will link (agglutinate) the RBCs into an unwieldy chain that assures RBC destruction if it occurs in the body. The same is true for B cells mixed into plasma containing with anti-B (groups A and O). Since blood group O contains no major blood group antigens, it can be transfused into patients of any type. Group O is, therefore, the *universal donor*. In contrast, because patients with group AB have no anti-A or anti-B in their plasma, they can receive blood of any of the four types: AB, A, B, or O. Group AB is, therefore, the *universal recipient*.

Case Notes

3.18 **We learn later that Miriam's blood was O positive. Could she have safely been transfused by type A or type B blood?**

The Rh Blood Group

The **Rh blood group system** is a second red cell antigen system. There are several Rh antigens, but only the d/D (recessive/dominant) antigen is clinically significant. Patients who have the dominant D allele (D/D or d/D) are Rh positive (Rh+). Patients who are d/d are Rh negative (Rh-). The environment contains no Rh antigen, so natural antibodies do not develop. About 85% of Americans are Rh positive. Percentages vary by ethnic group.

Anti-Rh antibodies develop only in Rh– patients exposed to Rh+ cells by transfusion or in the circumstance of an Rh– mother carrying an Rh+ fetus. In transfusion practice, donor and recipient blood are carefully tested for Rh characteristics (see crossmatch discussion below) to ensure that Rh characteristics are compatible. Patients who are Rh+ can receive Rh-positive or negative RBC by transfusion. Rh-negative patients, however, should not be given Rh+ blood because they will become sensitized and cannot receive a second Rh+ transfusion, and because testing might have missed anti-Rh antibodies, the presence of which could cause a severe hemolytic transfusion reaction.

Rh-related hemolytic reactions occur only if prior sensitization of an Rh-negative recipient has occurred. Strict blood bank practice has virtually eliminated Rh-related transfusion reactions. Nevertheless, Rh sensitization can occur in an Rh-negative woman carrying an Rh-positive child. The fetus's RBC leak into the maternal circulation at delivery and can stimulate the production of maternal anti-Rh antibodies. These antibodies are IgG-type, small enough to cross the placenta to attack the Rh+ fetal red

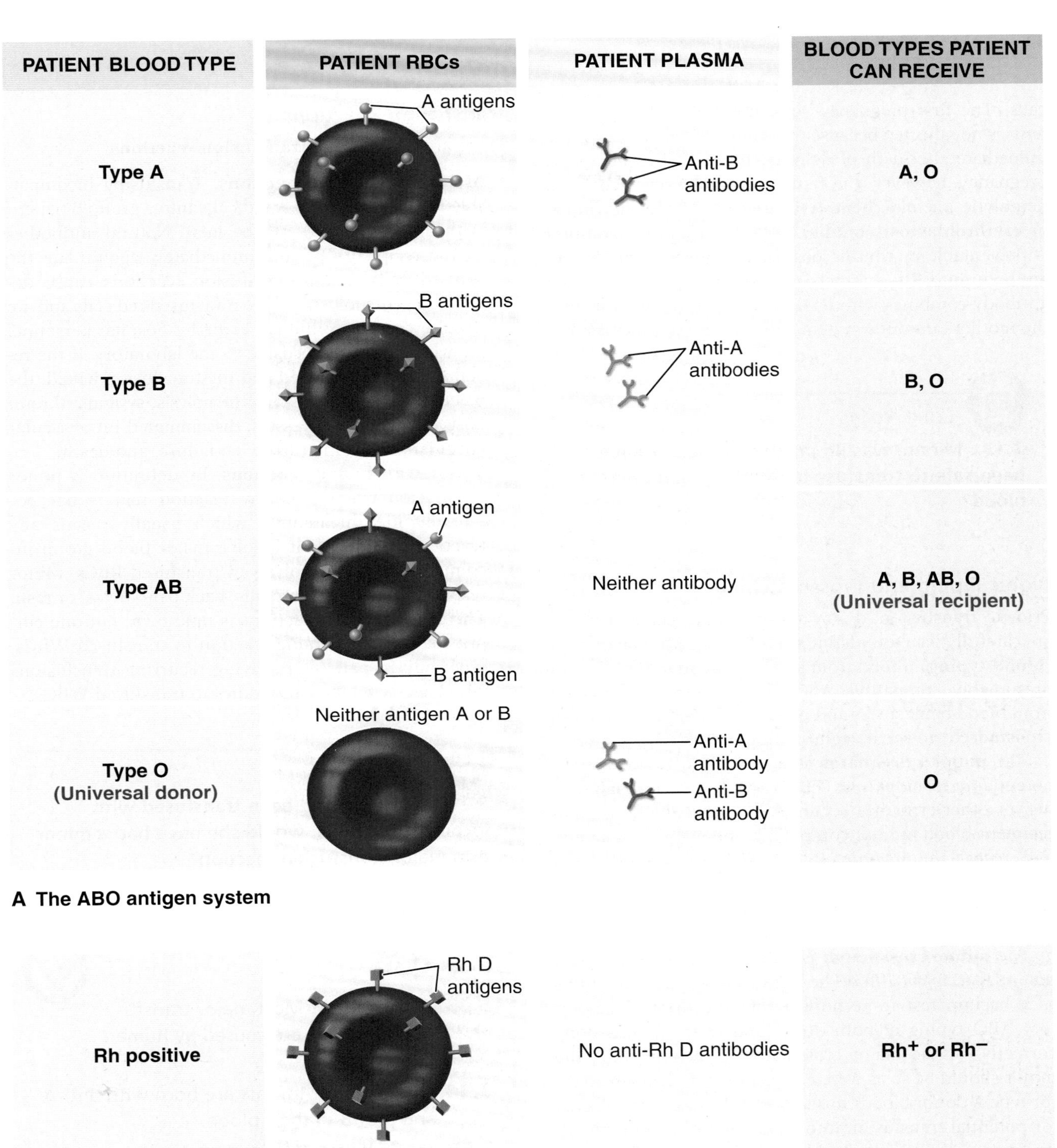

Figure 3.15 **Common blood groups. A.** ABO blood groups. An individual's plasma contains antibodies against A or B antigens not present on his or her erythrocytes. **B.** Rh blood groups. Antibodies against antigen Rh D are present only in Rh-negative people who have been exposed to Rh-positive blood from a transfusion or from an Rh-negative mother delivering an Rh-positive infant. (Reprinted with permission from McConnell TH, Hull KL. *Human Form Human Function: Essentials of Anatomy & Physiology*. Baltimore, MD: Wolters Kluwer Health; 2011.)

cells. The first pregnancy sensitizes the mother but the fetus is not affected because the "transfusion" occurs in the immediate aftermath of delivery. In any subsequent Rh+ pregnancy, however, the fetus may suffer severe or fatal hemolytic anemia (**hemolytic disease of the newborn**, or **erythroblastosis fetalis**). Nevertheless, the condition is preventable by routine postpartum injection of anti-Rh antibody into Rh– mothers delivering an Rh+ fetus. The antibody combines with fetal Rh antigen, masking it from the mother's immune system and preventing sensitization.

Case Notes

3.19 Miriam was Rh positive. Would it have been safe to transfuse her with Rh negative blood?

Blood Typing and Crossmatching

Prior to transfusion, donor and potential recipient blood are carefully tested to define the ABO and Rh type of each (**blood typing**). Blood from several potential donors with presumably compatible ABO and Rh types is selected from blood bank stores and mixed with recipient blood (a **crossmatch**) to see if agglutination occurs.

The **major crossmatch** is a mix of *donor RBCs* with potential *recipient plasma* (Fig. 3.16). If a clerical, lab testing, or other error has occurred such that the donor and recipient blood are not compatible, the major crossmatch will reveal the incompatibility. The major crossmatch is the key factor in determining compatibility because transfusing incompatible RBCs can be fatal (see discussion below).

The **minor crossmatch** is a mix of *donor plasma* with potential *recipient RBC*. The minor crossmatch functions as a backup test to reconfirm that the original laboratory ABO typing of both donor and recipient was done correctly—if the major crossmatch is incompatible, the minor should be so as well. For example, if through an error type A donor blood (mislabeled as B) has been selected for potential transfusion into a patient with type B blood, the major crossmatch would catch the error—the recipient, who is actually A but mislabelled B, will have anti-B antibodies that would agglutinate the proposed donor B cells. The minor crossmatch would also catch the error—the recipient's actual A cells would be agglutinated by the anti-A in the plasma of the proposed B donor. Transfusing blood incompatible by minor crossmatch is acceptable. There is little danger in transfusing incompatible *plasma* (e.g., type O blood containing anti-A and anti-B into a patient with type B blood) because the antibody is greatly diluted by the recipient's plasma. This is allowable practice in urgent situations when precisely matched blood is not readily available.

Transfusion Reactions

There are two types of **transfusion reactions**:

- **Major transfusion reactions**. Transfusing incompatible RBCs (e.g., group A red cells into a group B patient with anti-A plasma) can be fatal. Natural antibodies in the recipient's plasma immediately agglutinate the infused cells. Major transfusion reactions cause destruction (hemolysis) of the transfused red cells and are usually caused by human error by hospital personnel anywhere from the bedside to the laboratory. If the reaction is not recognized and the transfusion halted, the reaction may lead to severe hemolysis, systemic thrombosis of small blood vessels, disseminated intravascular coagulation (Chapter 6), renal failure, and death.
- **Minor transfusion reactions**. By definition, a minor transfusion reaction is any reaction that is not potentially life threatening, which usually means any reaction that does not involve major blood group incompatibility or hemolysis of transfused RBCs. Minor reactions include fever, chills, back pain, hives, or rash. The cause of most reactions is unknown, but one culprit may be an immune reaction to transfused WBCs, especially in patients receiving recurring transfusions who have developed antibodies to transfused WBCs.

Case Notes

3.20 If Miriam had been transfused with incompatible RBCs, would she have had a minor or a major transfusion reaction?

Pop Quiz

3.33 True or false? Most major transfusion reactions are caused by human error.

3.34 True or false? Infants are born with anti-A and anti-B in their blood.

3.35 True or false? An Rh positive mother can form antibodies against her Rh negative fetus?

3.36 True or false? Acute tissue transplant rejection is the result of both B and T cells.

3.37 Are B cells or T cells the main threat in tissue transplantation?

3.38 What mediates hyperacute rejection?

3.39 Which blood type is the universal donor?

3.40 The major crossmatch mixes recipient ________ with donor ________.

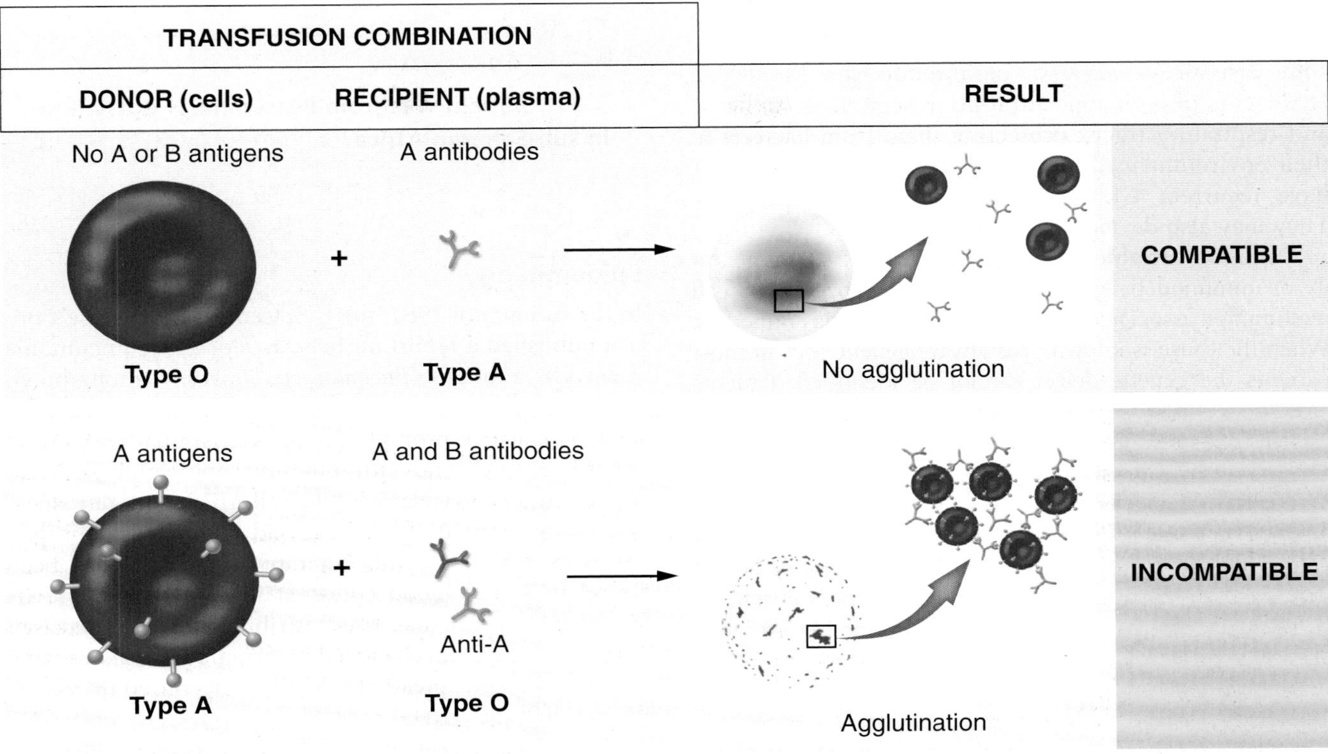

Figure 3.16 **The major crossmatch.** Donor blood cells are mixed with the recipient's plasma to check for compatibility (see text for *minor* crossmatch). A compatible transfusion combination will not result in an agglutination reaction. In this example, someone with type A blood can receive a transfusion with type O blood, but not vice versa. (Adapted with permission from McConnell TH, Hull KL. *Human Form Human Function: Essentials of Anatomy & Physiology*. Baltimore, MD: Wolters Kluwer Health; 2011.)

Immunodeficiency Disorders

Immunodeficiency diseases may be primary or acquired. Primary immunodeficiencies are caused by inherited genetic defects. Acquired deficiencies occur secondary to another disease (e.g., leukemia), and are much more common. AIDS (acquired immunodeficiency syndrome) is the most common of all immunodeficiency diseases.

In immunodeficiency, the entire immune system may be affected, or only subsets of T or B cells may be involved. In either situation, disease usually becomes apparent because of unusual or persistent infection. Organisms that ordinarily do not cause infection in people with healthy immune systems are the cause of many infections in immunodeficient patients. Such infections are called **opportunistic infections**. Figure 4.6 in Chapter 4 offers a summary of opportunistic pathogens and the sites they most often infect. Patients with deficiency in B cell function do not produce effective antibody response and usually suffer from infections from pyogenic bacteria, such as staphylococcus or streptococcus. Patients with defective T cell function are more prone to virus and fungus infections and are also vulnerable to the development of neoplasms as a result of failed immune surveillance.

Remember This! Immunodeficiency disease leads to infection and malignancy.

Inherited Immunodeficiency Disorders

Primary immunodeficiencies are a varied group of diseases that affect the development of mature B or T cells. Although many types have been identified, only a few are discussed here.

X-linked agammaglobulinemia (*Bruton Disease*) is an X-linked recessive defect of B cell development that is inherited according to Mendelian principles. Patients lack the ability to produce normal immunoglobulin. T cells are unaffected. It first comes to attention at about age six months, after the infant loses the benefit of passive maternal antibodies. Patients present with a history of recurrent infections: bronchitis, pneumonia, sinusitis, pharyngitis, and ear and GI infections. Infective bacteria are usually staphylococcus, streptococcus, or *Haemophilus*. Patients also tend to have intestinal parasites and certain viral infections. Some patients develop autoimmune disease, especially arthritis similar to RA. Treatment is monthly intravenous immunoglobulin injections.

Other than AIDS, the most common immunodeficiency is **isolated immunoglobulin A (IgA) deficiency**. It is caused by an autosomal recessive defect that occurs in about 1 in 700 persons of European descent but is rare in people of African or Asian heritage. Nevertheless, some cases occur as a result of viral infection. Recall that IgA occurs in high concentration in secretions of the GI and respiratory tracts, protecting them from bacteria in their environment. Deprived of this protection, patients have recurrent GI, sinus, and pulmonary infections. They may also develop lupus or rheumatoid arthritis.

Common variable immunodeficiency (CVID) is a family of immunodeficiency disorders characterized by B cell malfunction associated with low levels of plasma antibodies. When the cause is known, it is always genetic, but in most patients the genetic defect cannot be identified. Patients have common symptoms, including recurrent infections. Autoimmune disorders commonly occur.

Thymic hypoplasia (*DiGeorge syndrome*) is the embryonic failure of the thymus to develop. T cell function is deficient; B cell immunity is unaffected. Because development of the fetal thymus is closely related to nearby anatomic structures, these patients may also lack parathyroid glands and suffer from hypoparathyroidism (Chapter 14), and may have anomalies of the neck, face, ears, heart, and aorta. They suffer from viral, fungal, and protozoan infections. Thymus transplant is effective in some patients.

Severe combined immunodeficiency (SCID) is a group of inherited disorders affecting both B and T cell function. Many different gene defects have been identified as causative, and all are inherited in Mendelian fashion. Some are X linked and affect males only. Lymphoid tissues and the thymus are underdeveloped. Infections usually appear before six months of age. Patients suffer a wide range of infections, many of them caused by *Pneumocystis*, *Candida*, and other opportunistic microbes. Patients must be kept in strict isolation until bone marrow or stem cell transplantation.

Acquired Immunodeficiency Syndrome (AIDS)

AIDS is a grave immunodeficiency caused by infection with the human immunodeficiency virus (HIV), which infects T cells and related macrophages. Patients are prone to severe infection, secondary neoplasms, and nervous system symptoms. Keep in mind that there are acquired immunodeficiencies other than AIDS. For example, chemotherapy or radiation can devastate the immune system and cause immunodeficiency similar in some ways to the effect of HIV infection. Nevertheless, AIDS is by far the most common.

It is difficult to overstate the effect of the AIDS pandemic. As of 2013, 70 million people have been infected, causing 35 million deaths. Prevalence in sub-Saharan Africa is stunning. Over two-thirds of all persons living with AIDS are in sub-Saharan Africa, where in some nations in excess of 25% of the population is infected. Nevertheless, improved therapy and public health measures are having their effect. The trend of new infections and deaths is downward, but even so in 2010 there were 2.7 million new infections and 1.8 million deaths.

Case Notes

3.21 Miriam was from Botswana. Is Botswana in sub-Saharan Africa?

Epidemiology

In the summer of 1981, the U.S. Centers for Disease Control published a report on five cases of a rare pneumonia caused by a fungus (*Pneumocystis jirovecii*) among previously healthy young homosexual men in the Los Angeles area. The article prompted reports of similar cases from other U.S. cities, and within months, epidemiologists had identified the "new" disease we call AIDS. Still, retrospective study suggests the disease had originated more than 20 years earlier, in sub-Saharan Africa: HIV has been found in stored blood collected in Congo in 1959. Its worldwide spread has been attributed to the increased frequency of air travel and a concurrent increase in sexual promiscuity and spread of sexually transmitted infections (which includes AIDS).

Among *adolescents and adults*, five distinct groups are at risk for HIV infection. The relative prevalence of these groups varies substantially by nation and by socioeconomic factors. The groups are the following:

- Homosexual or bisexual men
- Intravenous drug abusers
- Patients with hemophilia (almost all of whom are men)
- Recipients of transfusions of human blood or blood components
- Heterosexual intimate contacts of intravenous drug users and others above

Of HIV-infected patients under age 13, the majority have been infected by transmission of virus from mother to infant.

The predominant mode of sexual spread varies geographically according to economic conditions. Homosexual spread is the prevalent mode in developed nations. In underdeveloped nations, heterosexual contact is the predominant mode of sexual spread because poor public health education and resources lead to higher rates of syphilis, gonorrhea, and other sexually transmitted diseases. HIV is carried in semen and enters mucosal barriers through genital abrasions, sores, or inflamed mucosa. Because of these factors, HIV passes more easily from men to women than the reverse.

Today, transmission by blood or blood products or by medical procedures is rare, although many hemophiliacs and some other transfusion recipients were infected before screening tests for HIV were devised in the early 1980s. The risk to healthcare workers is real but very small—about 0.3% of workers become infected when accidentally stuck by a needle used in an HIV-infected patient. Transmission in utero to the fetus occurs in about 25% of untreated mothers.

Case Notes

3.22 Into which of the risk groups above did Miriam fall?

Etiology and Pathogenesis

HIV is transmitted by close human contact that transfers body fluid, mainly semen and blood or blood products. Sexual transmission by males is via semen, females via vaginal secretions. Nonsexual transmission is usually via shared needles among intravenous drug abusers. Casual or indirect contact—toilet seats, dinnerware, handshakes, a kiss on the cheek, insect bites, and so on—does not transmit HIV.

The HIV virus infects only human cells; there is no animal reservoir. Like all viruses, HIV can reproduce only inside of cells by parasitizing intracellular mechanisms. HIV invades cells by attaching to the MHC complex and preferentially infects T cells and related macrophages with the CD4 type of MHC antigen (mainly *helper T cells*). Ordinarily DNA synthesizes RNA, but once inside CD4+ cells, in the reverse of normal, HIV RNA synthesizes abnormal DNA that merges with normal DNA to become part of a new, corrupted T cell DNA (Fig. 3.17). Later, the process is reversed and corrupted DNA produces new HIV RNA, which becomes the core of a new virus particle. New HIV viruses exit the dying cell to infect and kill other CD4+ cells, and the cycle continues until T cell function is devastated and the patient dies from AIDS-related opportunistic infection or malignancy.

Some infected CD4+ cells do not die but linger as a population of infected but inactive (*latent*) cells that can be stimulated to become active again and resume the cycle of T cell destruction. Latent cell replication is rekindled by the non-HIV infections that are common in HIV-infected patients. The new infection stimulates latent cells and renewed internal HIV replication.

B cell immunity is adversely affected because normal B cell function requires helper T cell support and helper T cells are the prime target of HIV. B cells are stimulated by HIV antigens and the antigens of the *cytomegalovirus (CMV), Epstein-Barr virus (EBV)*, and other infections that occur in AIDS. The stimulated B cells produce large amounts of ineffective antibody. The net result is that both T cell and B cell function is defective.

Despite the fact that neurons are not infected, *the nervous system is a major target of HIV infection. Microglia*, nervous system macrophages (Chapter 19) are infected, as are macrophages everywhere, but the mechanism by which nervous system damage occurs is unknown.

Case Notes

3.23 Which cell marker on which of Miriam's cells was targeted by HIV?

3.24 Could Miriam have gotten HIV from a mosquito bite?

3.25 Can we say with certainty that Miriam got AIDS from another infected person?

The Diagnosis of HIV and AIDS

AIDS and HIV infection are not the same. AIDS is a state of immune deficiency caused by HIV infection, but many with HIV infection are not affected severely enough to warrant a diagnosis of AIDS. HIV infection can be detected by laboratory tests that detect the presence of HIV viral antigens in blood or saliva or anti-HIV antibodies in blood.

Laboratory data *alone* can prove HIV infection only, but it cannot *prove* AIDS. AIDS is a *clinical* diagnosis proved by the presence of certain AIDS-related diseases with or without supporting lab data. This is a good time to recall that AIDS is a *syndrome* (Chapter 1): a constellation of *clinical* signs and symptoms.

AIDS is defined by the presence of certain clinical illnesses, some of which are listed below for illustrative purposes:

1. *Definitive, without* confirming laboratory data
   a) *Lymphoma of the brain* in a patient <60 years of age
   b) *Kaposi sarcoma* in a patient <60 years of age
   c) *Pneumocystis jirovecii* pneumonia
   d) *Cryptococcosis* (a fungus infection) in any organ other than the lung
   e) *Mycobacterium avium* (bird tuberculosis) infection in any organ other than lungs, skin, or lymph nodes
   f) *Progressive multifocal leukoencephalopathy* (a degenerative brain disease caused by the JC virus)
2. *Definitive, with* confirming laboratory data (HIV antigens or antibodies in blood, CD4+ lymphocyte [helper T cell] count <200 cells/microliter or <14% of peripheral blood lymphocytes)
   a) *Kaposi sarcoma* at any age
   b) *Lymphoma of the brain* at any age
   c) *Pulmonary tuberculosis*
   d) *Disseminated coccidioidomycosis* (a fungus infection)
3. *Presumptive, with* confirming laboratory data (as above)
   a) *CMV infection of the retina*
   b) *Pneumonia*, especially recurrent pneumonia
   c) *Toxoplasmosis* (a protozoan infection) *of the brain*

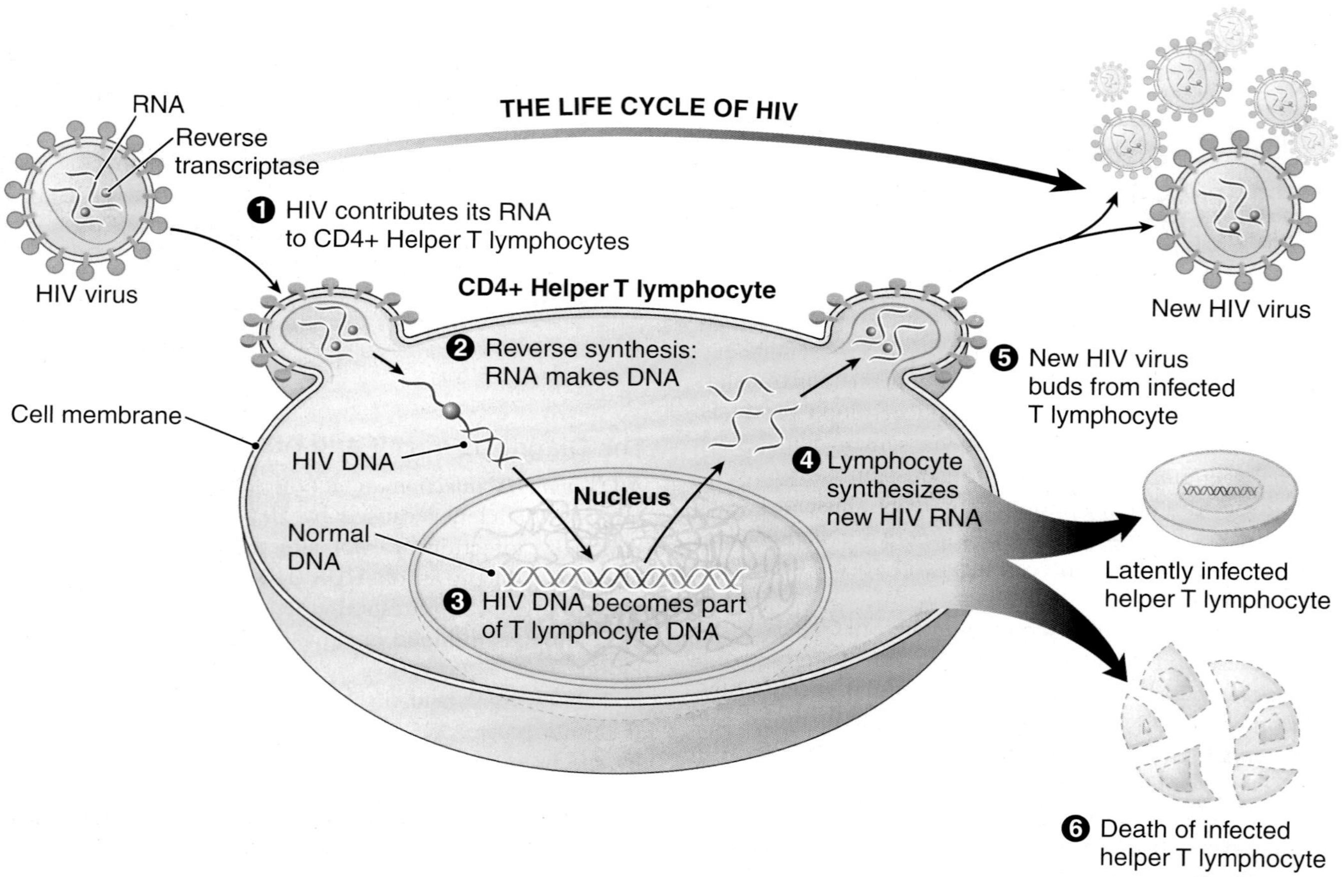

THE LIFE CYCLE OF HIV

RNA
Reverse transcriptase
HIV virus
1 HIV contributes its RNA to CD4+ Helper T lymphocytes
CD4+ Helper T lymphocyte
2 Reverse synthesis: RNA makes DNA
Cell membrane
HIV DNA
Nucleus
Normal DNA
3 HIV DNA becomes part of T lymphocyte DNA
4 Lymphocyte synthesizes new HIV RNA
5 New HIV virus buds from infected T lymphocyte
New HIV virus
Latently infected helper T lymphocyte
6 Death of infected helper T lymphocyte

Figure 3.17 **HIV infection of a T lymphocyte.** In the life cycle of HIV the virus merges with the T lymphocyte's cell membrane and injects its RNA into the cytoplasm, where, in a reverse of the usual process, new DNA is synthesized from RNA. This new HIV DNA is incorporated into the DNA of the T lymphocyte nucleus. The infected T lymphocyte then synthesizes new HIV RNA, which buds from the cell membrane as a new HIV virus, after which the infected T lymphocyte dies.

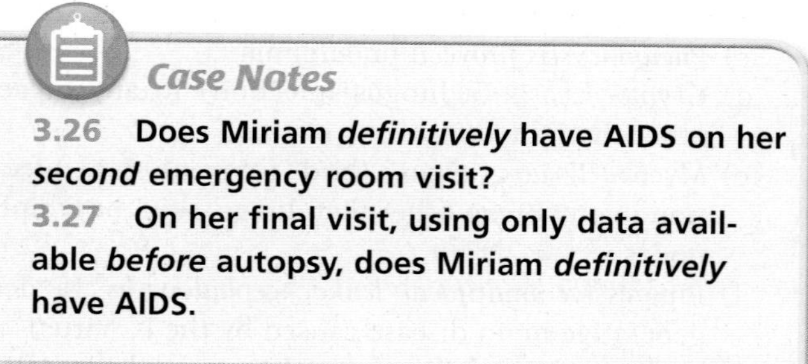

Case Notes

3.26 **Does Miriam *definitively* have AIDS on her *second* emergency room visit?**

3.27 **On her final visit, using only data available *before* autopsy, does Miriam *definitively* have AIDS.**

The Natural Progression of HIV Infection

HIV infection develops in three phases: 1) an acute viral syndrome; 2) a chronic (latent) infection in which most patients are asymptomatic; and 3) progression to clinical AIDS. Peripheral blood CD4+ helper T cell counts are a reliable guide to the progress of the disease—lower counts are usually associated with more advanced disease and a grimmer prognosis.

Immediately after HIV infection, patients are asymptomatic. Nevertheless, as is illustrated in Figure 3.18, after a few weeks most patients develop an acute "flu syndrome," with sore throat, muscle soreness (myalgia), fever, and rash, which resolves in a few weeks. In this phase HIV is present in blood in high concentration and CD4+ (helper T cell) cell counts may fall markedly. Nevertheless, CD4+ T cells soon replenish, the number of virus particles in blood falls to low levels, and anti-HIV antibodies appear in blood as the HIV infection enters a latent phase, during which the virus continues to reproduce. Latency usually lasts from 7 to 10 years with few symptoms. In some patients, latency lasts only two to three years. In rare patients, latency appears to last indefinitely and AIDS does not develop. During latency, CD4+ T cell counts in blood remain normal as dying CD4+ T cells are replenished by immune system reserves, and few clinical symptoms are present. Late in the latent period some patients may develop generalized enlargement of lymph nodes (*lymphadenopathy*). Absent treatment, a crisis phase appears as CD4+ T cell counts fall dramatically and HIV infection evolves into full-blown AIDS. At this time, AIDS-related opportunistic infections or malignancy appear and the diagnosis changes from HIV infection to AIDS (see discussion below). This predeath period

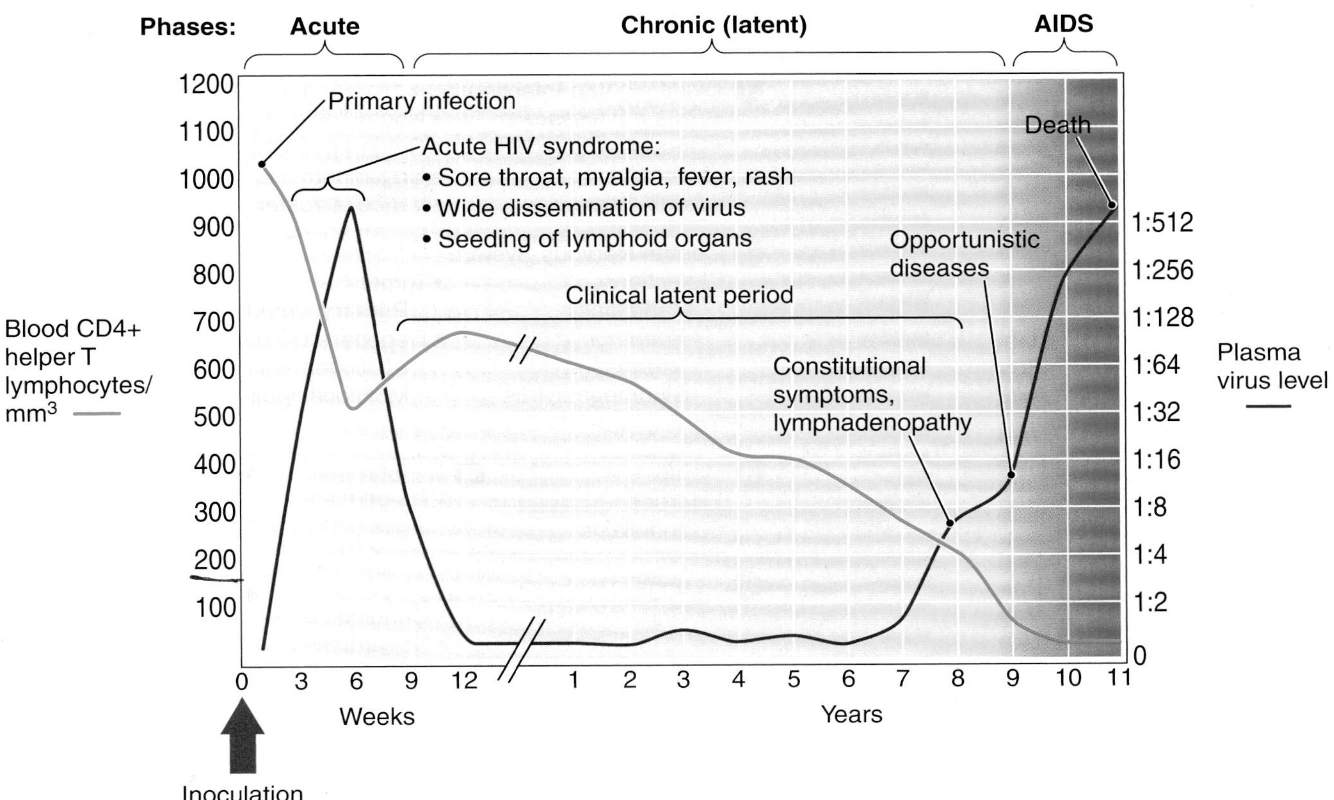

Figure 3.18 **Phases of HIV infection and AIDS.** Shortly after infection with HIV, a flu-like acute HIV syndrome occurs. Blood virus level is high, helper T cell (CD4+ lymphocytes) count falls, and the virus spreads widely. In the *latent period*, which may last for years, helper T cell levels are moderately depressed, and virus levels in blood are low. In the final *crisis phase* the CD4+ T cell count falls markedly. Opportunistic infections appear that are usually the cause of death.

is characterized by a near-complete breakdown of the immune system as opportunistic infections occur, especially in the lungs and GI tract; neurologic symptoms and dementia appear; and secondary neoplasms may develop.

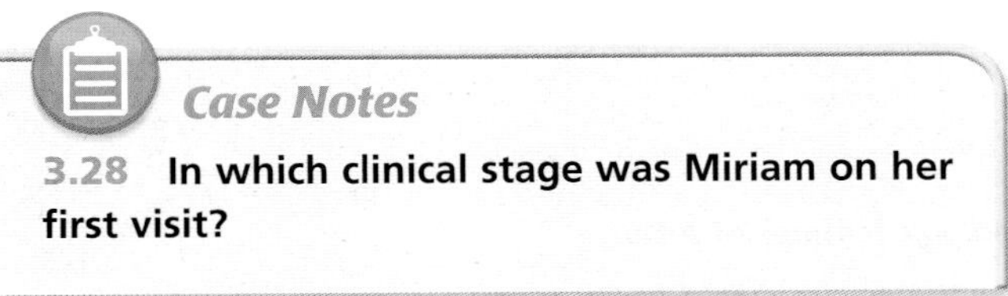

Case Notes

3.28 In which clinical stage was Miriam on her first visit?

Clinical Features

The clinical manifestations of HIV infection are minimal: the brief "flu syndrome" of acute infection and the lymphadenopathy of some patients in late latency. The following discussion outlines the clinical features of AIDS as seen in the United States (Fig. 3.19). Opportunistic infections and other features differ in other geographies according to local infectious patterns.

The typical U.S. patient is a young adult from one of the risk groups discussed earlier, who presents with fever, weight loss, diarrhea, palpable lymph nodes, infection, neurologic symptoms (including psychosis or dementia), and, perhaps, an AIDS-related secondary neoplasm. Two types of AIDS infections occur: those caused by pathogens that also affect patients with healthy immune systems, and those caused by opportunistic pathogens.

***Pneumocystis jirovecii* pneumonia** (Fig. 3.20) is a presenting opportunistic infection in many patients; others present with mucosal candidiasis, ulcerating oral herpes, disseminated CMV infection (especially retinitis or gastroenteritis), or disseminated tuberculosis. Early in the disease, ordinary *Mycobacterium tuberculosis* infections occur, but later the avian (bird) strain, *Mycobacterium avium*, predominates as opportunistic infections become more common. Brain and meningeal infections are common. Diarrhea is a constant problem and may result from a variety of organisms rarely seen in non-AIDS patients.

Because of failed immune surveillance, AIDS patients also have a high incidence of certain tumors, especially Kaposi sarcoma, B-cell lymphoma (Chapter 7), and cervical carcinoma. **Kaposi sarcoma** is a sluggish vascular tumor caused by a herpesvirus. Skin is most often affected. Another virus, the Epstein-Barr virus (EBV), may underlie the aggressive B-cell lymphomas that occur in some AIDS patients.

Nervous system involvement is demonstrable at autopsy in the majority of patients. About half have neurologic symptoms, including mental aberrations that may progress to a severe AIDS-related dementia, or *progressive*

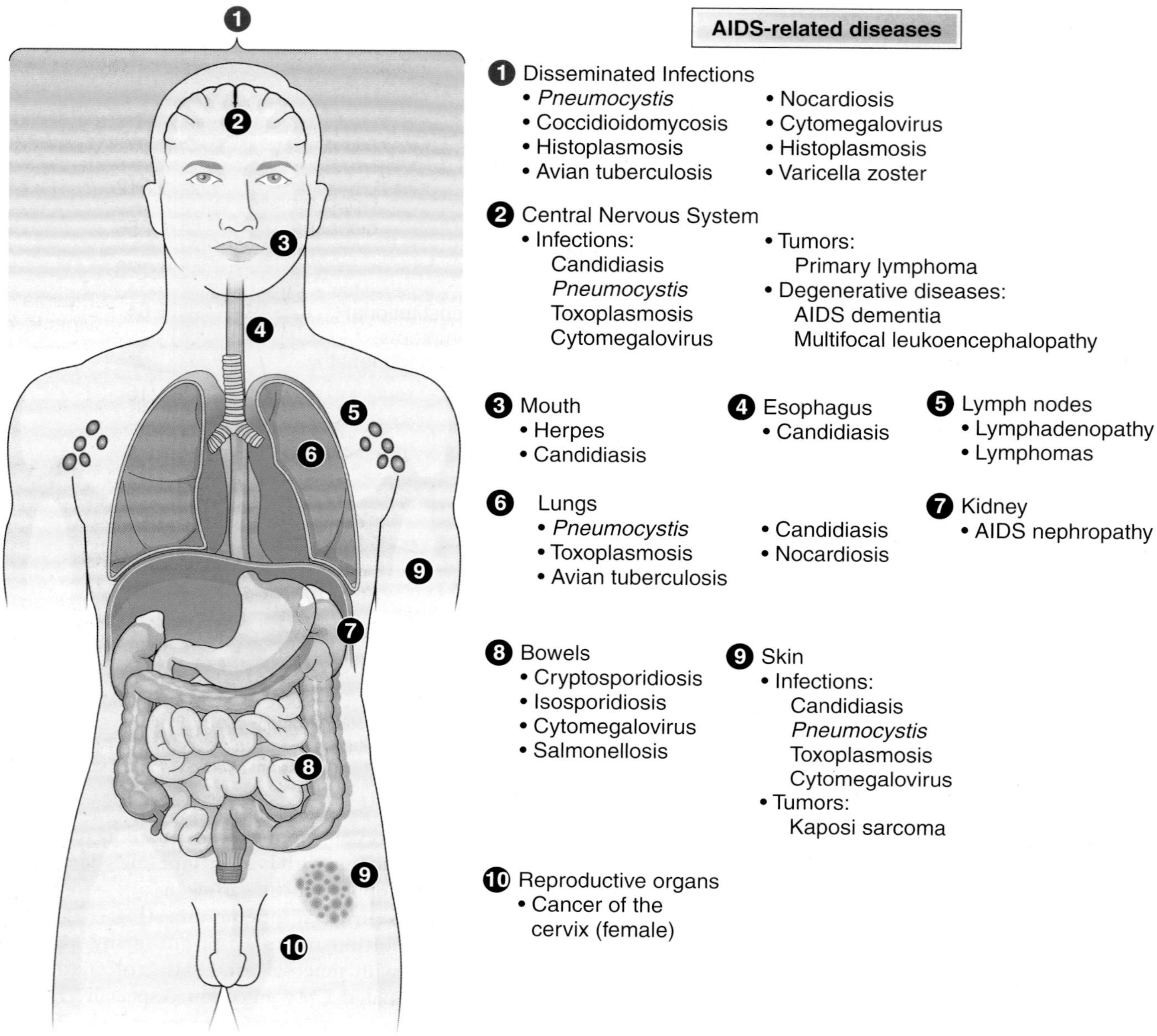

AIDS-related diseases

1. Disseminated Infections
   - *Pneumocystis*
   - Coccidioidomycosis
   - Histoplasmosis
   - Avian tuberculosis
   - Nocardiosis
   - Cytomegalovirus
   - Histoplasmosis
   - Varicella zoster
2. Central Nervous System
   - Infections:
     Candidiasis
     Pneumocystis
     Toxoplasmosis
     Cytomegalovirus
   - Tumors:
     Primary lymphoma
   - Degenerative diseases:
     AIDS dementia
     Multifocal leukoencephalopathy
3. Mouth
   - Herpes
   - Candidiasis
4. Esophagus
   - Candidiasis
5. Lymph nodes
   - Lymphadenopathy
   - Lymphomas
6. Lungs
   - *Pneumocystis*
   - Toxoplasmosis
   - Avian tuberculosis
   - Candidiasis
   - Nocardiosis
7. Kidney
   - AIDS nephropathy
8. Bowels
   - Cryptosporidiosis
   - Isosporidiosis
   - Cytomegalovirus
   - Salmonellosis
9. Skin
   - Infections:
     Candidiasis
     Pneumocystis
     Toxoplasmosis
     Cytomegalovirus
   - Tumors:
     Kaposi sarcoma
10. Reproductive organs
    - Cancer of the cervix (female)

Figure 3.19 **Clinical and pathologic features of AIDS.**

multifocal leukoencephalopathy (Chapter 19), a degenerative disease of white matter.

The gross and microscopic changes of HIV infection are neither specific nor diagnostic; rather, the findings are related to the secondary infections, neoplasms, and other consequences of HIV infection.

Case Notes

3.29 Which of the final autopsy diagnoses in Miriam is the only one not appearing on the list of AIDS-related infections?

Treatment

Treatment of HIV infection and AIDS is a complex matter with two main goals: to control the HIV virus and to control other infections. Once a patient is infected with HIV, the virus cannot be eliminated, though this remains a goal of research. Nevertheless, the virus can be controlled successfully by a combination of antivirus drugs given in high concentrations, a technique known as **highly active antiretroviral therapy (HAART)**. HAART limits virus proliferation, decreases the number and seriousness of opportunistic infections and other complications, and prolongs life. The control of opportunistic infections requires combinations of antibiotics and antiviral drugs.

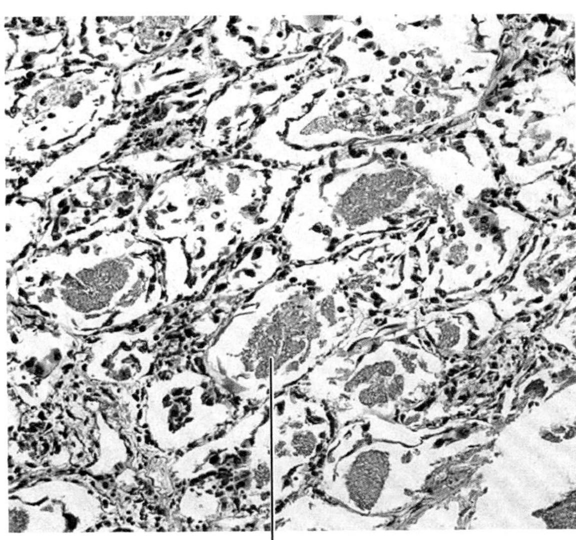

Figure 3.20 ***Pneumocystis jirovecii*** **pneumonia.** In this microscopic study of lung tissue, clouds of organisms fill the alveoli.

These drugs may have numerous and serious side effects and require continual monitoring.

With HAART anti-HIV therapy, the latency period can be extended almost indefinitely and the life expectancy for HIV patients approaches that of noninfected people.

Pop Quiz

3.41 True or false? Most immune deficiencies are acquired.

3.42 True or false? The HIV virus attacks both B and T cells directly.

3.43 True or false? HIV is spread mainly by semen and blood.

3.44 True or false? The diagnosis of AIDS depends primarily on finding AIDS-related disease.

3.45 Name in order the three phases of HIV infection.

3.46 What is the most common immunodeficiency other than AIDS?

3.47 Among adolescents and adults in developed countries, which is the most common risk group for HIV/AIDS?

3.48 What is the therapy that prolongs life in HIV infected individuals?

3.49 Why are AIDS patients at high risk for malignancy?

Case Study Revisited

"She is still using." The case of Miriam K.

Miriam engaged in prostitution and intravenous drug use, two AIDS-risky behaviors that frequently coincide. We will never know if she was infected by using a contaminated dirty needle or by semen. Nor do we know when she was infected. Given that she had been in the United States only three years, that the HIV latent period is 7–10 years, and that HIV prevalence in Botswana is high, it seems likely she was infected there.

Her first appearance in the emergency room was prompted by fever and lymphadenopathy ("swollen glands"). The staff correctly suspected HIV infection based on her history. Lab tests verified HIV infection, but no definitive AIDS-defining illness was detected. Being HIV positive with general lymphadenopathy put her late in the latent, pre-AIDS stage of infection. HIV can stimulate hypersensitivity reaction, which explained her autoimmune thrombocytopenia (low platelet count). The record does not reveal whether or not she was tested for drugs, but in view of her failure to take medication or keep appointments it seems very likely that she was "still using" as her friend said.

The disease took its usual course in untreated HIV infection, and she progressed to AIDS. As some AIDS patients do, she developed an autoimmune disorder: thrombocytopenia caused by antiplatelet antibodies. Her helper T cell population was devastated. Profound immunodeficiency developed, and multiple infections supervened, any one of which can be fatal. She died of overwhelming infection. We do not have predeath B and T cell counts, but her bacterial urinary tract infection indicates B cell failure, and

(continued)

"She is still using." The case of Miriam K. (continued)

the fungal pneumonia and viral intestinal infection indicate T cell failure, both of which are in keeping with AIDS pathophysiology. T cell failure also explains the development of a brain neoplasm—without T cell immunosurveillance, mutant DNA evolved into malignancy. That the brain is a prime HIV target is also proven by the presence of multifocal leukoencephalopathy, a degenerative disease of white matter. Atrophy of the cerebral cortex accounts for her memory problems.

Chapter Challenge

CHAPTER RECALL

1. A 42-year-old African American male presents to his doctor complaining of fatigue. He reports that he feels refreshed when he awakens in the morning, but becomes progressively more tired as the day continues. He denies shortness of breath, pallor, and recent weight loss. Tests reveal the he has myasthenia gravis caused by antibodies that bind to acetylcholine receptors of the neuromuscular junction, an example of what type of hypersensitivity?
   A. Immediate hypersensitivity (Type I)
   B. Cytotoxic hypersensitivity (Type II)
   C. Immune complex hypersensitivity (Type III)
   D. Cellular (delayed) hypersensitivity (Type IV)

2. Which of the following is an example of innate immunity?
   A. Secretion of mucus and detergent bile salts by the GI epithelia
   B. Filtering mechanisms like the spleen
   C. Attack of virus-infected cells by NK cells
   D. Production of antibodies by B lymphocytes

3. Which of the following statements about blood groups/transfusions is true?
   A. A major crossmatch is a mixture of donor RBCs with potential recipient plasma.
   B. Blood group genotypes are A, B, AB, and O.
   C. The agglutination of type-A RBCs transfused into a patient with type-B blood is an example of a minor transfusion reaction.
   D. Blood group AB is the universal donor.

4. A worried mother brings her daughter to the free clinic. She recently noticed a rash on her 10-year-old daughter's neck/chest. On closer exam, you observe the "rash" is raised, red, and in the shape of a heart, similar to the nickel heart on the little girl's necklace. What type of hypersensitivity reaction has occurred?
   A. Immediate hypersensitivity (Type I)
   B. Cytotoxic hypersensitivity (Type II)
   C. Immune complex hypersensitivity (Type III)
   D. Cellular (delayed) hypersensitivity (Type IV)

5. Which of the following is an antigen presenting cell localized to the skin, or other epithelial linings, and fixed in place?
   A. Kupffer cells
   B. Dendritic cells
   C. Plasma cells
   D. T lymphocytes

6. A 17-year-old Hispanic male presents to the ER in critical condition. He was playing baseball with his friends, when he complained of being stung by a bee. His teammates report that shortly after being stung, he began wheezing and complaining of difficulty breathing. He then abruptly collapsed on the field, and medics raced to his aid. What is the underlying etiology of his symptoms?
   A. Ig-E antibodies
   B. Immune complexes
   C. Activated T cells
   D. Cytotoxic antibodies

7. A 45-year-old African American female is observed to have a rash that extends from one cheek across the bridge of her nose and onto the other cheek. Her routine blood work reveals anemia and thrombocytopenia, and her urinalysis is positive for protein and blood (indicative of glomerulonephritis). Which of the following is true regarding her disease?
   A. Brain involvement is uncommon in her disease.
   B. The presence of ANA is highly specific and diagnostic of her disease.

C. Her disease may be due to starting hydralazine for elevated blood pressure.
D. Her disease is a vasculitis caused by Type II hypersensitivity.

8. A 40-year-old Caucasian male presents to the clinic with relapsing and remitting fever, chills, nonproductive cough, dyspnea, headache, and malaise. He has noticed that the symptoms always occur within one to two hours of working in his barn, and typically resolve one to two days later. You diagnose the patient with farmer's lung. What type of hypersensitivity does he suffer from?
A. Immediate hypersensitivity (Type I)
B. Cytotoxic hypersensitivity (Type II)
C. Immune complex hypersensitivity (Type III)
D. Cellular (Delayed) hypersensitivity (Type IV)

9. A 74-year-old Caucasian woman presents for a routine physical and is found to be anemic. Her colonoscopy a year ago was normal, and additional laboratory tests confirm that she is not iron deficient. Serum protein electrophoresis demonstrates a protein spike, and her kidney biopsy microscopically demonstrates a translucent, smooth, glassy material. Multiple myeloma is diagnosed. What is the etiology of her amyloidosis?
A. Hereditary amyloidosis
B. Misfolded mutant proteins
C. Reactive systemic amyloidosis
D. Light chain amyloidosis

10. A 33-year-old African American female presents to the clinic with fever, weight loss, diarrhea, and palpable lymph nodes. A full skin exam reveals several violaceous plaques that are determined to be Kaposi sarcoma. What stage of HIV/AIDS has she presented in?
A. Acute HIV infection
B. Definitive, without confirming laboratory data
C. Definitive, with confirming laboratory data
D. Presumptive, with confirming laboratory data

11. True or false? Scleroderma is characterized by the fibrosis of organ interstitium, and is commonly characterized by Raynaud phenomenon.

12. True or false? Homosexual spread of AIDS is the most common cause of infection in underdeveloped nations.

13. True or false? The immune system attacks the cell with MHC I display, but reads the cell with MHC II display to identify nonself antigens present in the body.

14. True or false? The skin rash of poison ivy is an immune reaction caused by a hapten.

15. True or false? Fetuses and infants gain temporary active immunity across the placenta and in breast milk.

16. True or false? The red pulp, which contains lymphocytes and macrophages, filters blood to remove old RBCs and detect nonself content while the white pulp filters blood for nonself content.

17. Match the following antibodies to their description and function:
i. IgA
ii. IgD
iii. IgE
iv. IgG
v. IgM
A. The smallest, most abundant immunoglobulin in blood; it confers permanent immunity against reinfection.
B. Antibody abundant in mucosal secretions where MALT tissue, tears, and in the milk of nursing mothers.
C. Largest immunoglobulin, providing initial antibody protection after infection.
D. Antibody bound exclusively to the cell membrane of B cells; activates B cells to recognize antigen and undergo clonal expansion.
E. The antibody important in allergic reactions (including Type I hypersensitivity).

18. Match the following cells to their function:
i. Memory T cells
ii. Cytotoxic T cells
iii. Suppressor T cells
iv. Helper T cells
A. The effector cells of cellular adaptive immunity; they carry the CD8 antigen and target cells with nonself molecules displayed on Type I MHC.
B. T cells facilitate the immune activities of B cells and other T cells; they carry a CD4 antigen, and interact with cells with Type II MHC display.
C. T cells that maintain immune homeostasis and prevent development of autoimmune disease.
D. T cells that enable the cellular immune system to mount a rapid secondary immune response.

19. Match the following immunodeficiencies with their clinical manifestations:
i. SCID
ii. Bruton Disease
iii. DiGeorge Syndrome
iv. CVID
v. Isolated IgA deficiency
A. X-linked recessive defect that prevents B cells from producing normal immunoglobulin. Beginning at six months of age, patients present with a history of recurrent infections: bronchitis, pneumonia, sinusitis, pharyngitis, and ear and

GI infections, by organisms including staphylococcus, streptococcus, *Haemophilus*, parasites, and viruses.

B. Autosomal recessive defect that causes recurrent GI, sinus, and pulmonary infections in patients. Labs show low IgA.

C. Predominately unknown cause in which there are low levels or plasma antibodies.

D. Failure of embryonic thymus to form that causes T cell deficiency, while B cell immunity is unaffected. Patients suffer from viral, fungal, and protozoan infections, and may have abnormalities of the neck, face, ears, and heart.

E. Several inheritance patterns. Patients have dysfunction of both B and T cells. Patients must remain in isolation as they suffer from a wide range of infections, including *Pneumocystis*, *Candida*, and other opportunistic microbes.

CONCEPTUAL UNDERSTANDING

20. What are the three functions of the lymphatic system?

21. How does a primary immune response differ from a secondary immune response?

22. List the four ways antibodies are effective against neutralizing an infectious agent.

23. What is the mechanism of hyperacute, acute, and chronic transplant rejection?

APPLICATION

24. A 42-year-old African American woman with a history of lupus calls the clinic to discuss her recent test for sexually transmitted infections. She is very upset as she has tested positive for syphilis, and asks you how this is possible as she has been in a monogamous relationship for the last 20 years. What advice do you have to offer her?

25. A 12-year-old child is undergoing a bone marrow transplant in two weeks. What treatment side-effects are to be expected?

26. Why do most infections occur most often in the epithelia, and what anti-infection mechanisms do epithelia employ?

27. A 25-year-old Hispanic male suffers trauma to his right eye. Surgeons are unable to salvage his eye, and it is removed. What immune mechanism dictates that the diseased eye be removed? What are other causes of autoimmune disease?

28. What special consideration should be made for a woman who is Rh negative when a blood transfusion is necessary?

CHAPTER

4

Infectious Disease

Contents

Chapter Objectives

After studying this chapter, you should be able to complete the following tasks:

THE BIOLOGY OF INFECTIOUS DISEASE

1. List the most common worldwide causes of death resulting from infection.
2. Briefly describe how organisms spread in tissue.
3. Name the three mechanisms that are responsible for causing damage to tissue.
4. Describe the cellular inflammatory reaction to bacteria, viruses, mycobacteria, fungi, parasitic worms, and protozoa.
5. List the clinical phases of infection that occur after an organism invades the body.

VIRUS INFECTIONS

6. Discuss the signs, symptoms, and pathogenesis of the following virus infections: rhinovirus;

adenovirus; respiratory syncytial virus, influenza; rotavirus; Norwalk virus; Coxsackie virus; measles; rubella; mumps; poliomyelitis; herpes simplex virus; herpes zoster virus; cytomegalovirus; human papillomavirus.

BACTERIAL INFECTIONS

7. Categorize the following bacteria according to shape, oxygen requirements, and staining characteristics, and describe the accompanying symptoms: staphylococcus; streptococcus; diphtheria; listeria, *Clostridium*; *Neisseria*; *Rickettsia*; *Bordetella pertussis*, *Pseudomonas*; campylobacter; Borrelia burgdorferi; mixed anaerobic infection; and tuberculosis.

FUNGAL INFECTIONS

8. Discuss how patient immune system functionality alters the types of fungal infections that patients acquire.

PARASITE INFECTIONS

9. Discuss the manifestations of the most common parasitic infections, including: protozoa (malaria, amebiasis, giardiasis), helminthes (intestinal nematodes, filariasis, schistosomiasis, tapeworms), and ectoparasites (lice, scabies).

SEXUALLY TRANSMITTED INFECTIONS

10. Using clinical presentations and pathological findings, distinguish amongst the most common sexually transmitted diseases.

LABORATORY TOOLS

11. Know the "gold standard," as well as the newer diagnostic tests available, when it comes to identifying infectious organisms.

Case Study

"I knew she was sick when she didn't want a cigarette." The case of Ruth R.

Chief Complaint: Cough and fever

Clinical History: Ruth R. was a 63-year-old retired bookkeeper. After attending a football game, she was brought to an urgent care clinic by her husband. He said, "I knew she was sick when she didn't want a cigarette in the car after the game." She complained of cough, scratchy throat, and fever, which had been gradually building for a day or two. She had been feeling "bum," and had spent most of the previous day in bed.

Past medical history was remarkable for mild, nondeforming chronic rheumatoid arthritis that was well controlled. She had smoked a pack of cigarettes a day for more than 40 years. She said she "doesn't believe in vaccinations" and had not had a flu shot.

Physical Examination and Other Data: The patient was a small, thin woman in moderate distress. Vital signs were: temperature 100.8°F (normal: 98.6°), heart rate 82 (normal: 72), respiratory rate 20 (normal: 14), and blood pressure 142/88 (normal: 120/80). Physical exam was remarkable only for distant breath sounds, mild barrel-chest deformity, and a few wheezes. Lab studies were unremarkable except for mild lymphocytosis in the peripheral blood. Chest radiograph revealed signs of moderate emphysema. No infiltrates were present.

Clinical Course: The nurse practitioner made a diagnosis of viral upper respiratory infection and, after conferring with a physician, resisted the patient's demand for a shot of penicillin. Aspirin, aerosol inhalations, and supportive care were prescribed.

She returned two days later, so weak she had to be rolled in a wheelchair. She complained of severe aching with high fever and chills. Temperature was 101.2°F; respirations 24; heart rate 112. She was flushed, her eyes were red and watery, and her breath sounds were wet and full of crackling rales. Chest radiograph revealed patchy infiltrates throughout both lungs. Laboratory studies were unremarkable except for a white blood count of 17,200/mm^3, mostly neutrophils.

A pulmonary consultant agreed that she had chronic obstructive pulmonary disease and influenza, likely complicated by bacterial pneumonia. She was hospitalized for ventilatory assistance, intravenous rehydration, and antibiotic therapy. Sputum culture grew a Gram-negative bacillus, which on further testing proved to be the bacterium *Haemophilus influenza*.

The hospital course was rocky. Her pneumonia worsened initially despite intense pulmonary therapy and intravenous antibiotics. She became hypoxic, obtunded, and disoriented. On the fourth hospital day she began to improve and was discharged to home on the tenth hospital day with advice to stop smoking and have an annual influenza vaccination.

For each illness that doctors cure with medicine, they provoke ten in healthy people by inoculating them with the virus that is a thousand times more powerful than any microbe: the idea that one is ill.

MARCEL PROUST (1871–1922), FRENCH NOVELIST

One of Charles Darwin's greatest insights was that life is a battle for survival. For most of human history, our fight has been a battle against infectious disease, and in many ways it still is. An **infectious disease** is one in which a transmissible (infectious) agent invades through physical barriers (such as skin or gastrointestinal [GI] mucosa) and overcomes innate and adaptive immune defenses to cause injury and disease.

Case Notes

4.1 **Name Ruth's infectious diseases.**

Infections are among the oldest and most common afflictions of humankind, as is illustrated in *The History of Medicine*, "Milestones in the Fight against Infectious Disease"; they remain a very serious problem today. The normal or expected rate of infection in a population or geographic area is the **endemic** rate. When cases occur at above normal rates, the infection is termed **epidemic**. Most governments require that healthcare providers report certain infections, including, but not limited to, hepatitis, HIV, measles, *sexually transmitted infection* tuberculosis (TB), and diarrhea caused by *E. coli*. Assembling reliable data, however, about the worldwide burden of infectious disease is difficult because so many infections go unreported. The U.S. Centers for Disease Control and Prevention (CDC) and the World Health Organization (WHO) offer the following overview (2011). Approximately 2 billion (~30% of world population) people are infected with the hepatitis B virus, making it (probably) the most *prevalent* of all infectious diseases. By contrast, in 2010 about 34 million were living with HIV/AIDS. The CDC and WHO offer no estimate of the number of people living with malaria, but they estimate 500 million new malaria infections (*incidence*) occur each year. Deaths from infectious disease are more reliably reported. Table 4.1 lists the most common causes of fatal infection worldwide, ranking them with other leading causes of death.

Only in the last few decades have chronic diseases such as cancer and heart disease surpassed infections as the first and second most common causes of death worldwide. Nevertheless, despite scientific and public health advances, taken as a whole, *infectious disease remains the number one cause of death worldwide*. Those who stand the least chance of surviving tend to be underprivileged, very young or very old, debilitated, or to have AIDS.

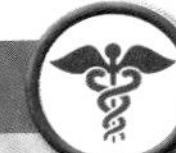

The History of Medicine

MILESTONES IN THE FIGHT AGAINST INFECTIOUS DISEASE

Microbiologic life existed on earth long before humans; we are interlopers in a microbial world, not the other way around. The staying power of microbes is proven; ours is not. That some illnesses are contagious (transferable from one person to another) is among the oldest facts of history, but it took centuries of painstaking experimentation to prove microbes cause infectious disease.

The Greeks did not know of microbes and believed that maggots on decaying animals sprang from spontaneous generation, a theory not disproved until the middle of the 17th century when Francisco Redi, an Italian physician, showed that maggots would not appear if a jar of meat was covered by cloth. About this time Anton von Leeuwenhoek, a Dutch textile merchant, using a combination of lenses designed for inspecting fabric, assembled a powerful microscope that he used to identify the first microscopic living things, which he called "animalcules," and we know as "protozoa."

The 19th-century French scientist Louis Pasteur, as an outgrowth of his studies on yeast and the fermentation of wine and beer, proved in 1865 that microbes could cause disease in humans and began to advocate cleanliness and sterilization as protective measures. Pasteur's cause was taken up by Joseph Lister, an English surgeon after whom Listerine mouthwash was named. Lister's advocacy of antiseptic surgery achieved dramatic results: the death rate for limb amputation, the most serious surgery of the time, fell from 40% to 3%.

In the latter part of the 19th century, Robert Koch, a German microbiologist, proved that specific microbes were associated with specific diseases. In 1897, Ronald Ross showed that mosquitoes carry malaria; in 1911, Peyton Rous proved that viruses can cause cancer; and in 1928, Alexander Fleming discovered the antibiotic qualities of penicillin.

Although we have known about infectious diseases, such as leprosy, since biblical times, new infections are discovered regularly—AIDS, hepatitis C, and Lyme disease were discovered in the 1980s and 1990s. In 2003, severe acute respiratory syndrome (SARS) was found to be caused by a virus previously known only in animals.

Table 4.1 Top Ten Causes of Death, All Ages, Worldwide, 2008, World Health Organization

Rank	Condition	Deaths
1	Ischemic heart disease	7,300,000
2	Cerebrovascular disease	6,200,000
3	Pneumonia	3,500,000
4	Chronic obstructive pulmonary disease	3,300,000
5	Diarrheal disease*	2,500,000
6	HIV/AIDS	1,800,000
7	Lung cancer	1,400,000
8	Tuberculosis	1,300,000
9	Diabetes	1,300,000
10	Traffic accidents	1,200,000
	All infections above	9,100,000

*Presumed infectious

Case Notes

4.2 Had Ruth died of pneumonia, would her cause of death rank high or low on the top ten list of worldwide causes of death?

The Biology of Infectious Disease

Our mouths, throats, lungs, intestines, skin, and other epithelial surfaces normally swarm with a mixture of organisms including potentially infectious agents. Not all such agents are capable of causing disease. Most exist in a quiet, **commensal** relationship with us; that is, they benefit but we are not harmed. Those that *can* cause disease are called **pathogens**. They infect us to ensure the survival of *their* species by gaining access to the shelter and nutrition *our* innards offer, usually at a high cost (sickness and death) to us. The infected person, plant, or animal is the **host**. Infectious agents are essentially **parasites**—organisms that live off of the host, the infected living thing. We rid our bodies of them using our immune systems, sometimes with the help of an armamentarium of antibiotics, and they in turn evolve into "superbugs" in accord with Darwinian survival of the fittest. It is a battle that never ends.

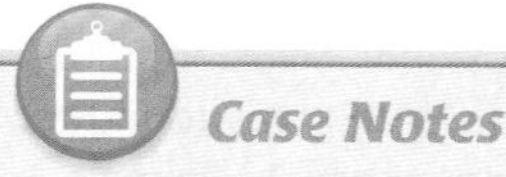

4.3 Name Ruth's pathogens.

The Characteristics of Infectious Agents Vary Greatly

Infectious agents are usually microscopic and are typically called **microbes** (Fig. 4.1). The smallest are protein molecules, so small they cannot be seen with an ordinary microscope. In contrast, the largest are intestinal worms, which may be an inch wide and several feet long. Many agents are not living things—a living thing is something that has its own metabolism and reproduces. Bacteria are living things. Viruses are not—they can reproduce but have no metabolism of their own; they obtain energy from the host, but produce no energy of their own.

Prions

Prions are mere molecules, a corrupted form of normal brain protein (*prion protein, PrP*), the function of which is still uncertain. They have no DNA or metabolism. They "reproduce" only by producing more corrupted PrP, much as a snowflake grows larger by adding more crystallized water. Prions cause chronic degenerative brain disease in humans (e.g., *Creutzfeldt-Jakob disease*) and animals (e.g., *mad cow disease*). Infection occurs by ingestion of contaminated tissue; from contaminated blood products/transplants (such as corneas); from hormones purified from infected people; and from contaminated surgical instruments. Some cases are caused by acquired gene mutations that create corrupted PrP without prior infection.

Viruses

Next up the scale of size and complexity are **viruses**, which are packets of nucleic acid encased in a protein coat (capsid). Viruses have no cell wall or nucleus and have no metabolism (they cannot capture, store, and burn energy). Therefore, they are obligate intracellular parasites that must invade the interior of a cell and hijack the cell's metabolism and reproductive machinery to produce their RNA or DNA. Outside of a cell, they can only exist but cannot multiply. Against viruses, conventional antibiotics (e.g., penicillin) are not effective because their effect relies on disrupting bacterial cell membrane or metabolism, neither of which viruses possess.

The *Baltimore system*, developed by Nobel Prize–winning biologist David Baltimore, classifies viruses according to whether their nucleic acid is DNA or RNA, whether it is single or double-stranded, and other details that are beyond the scope of this textbook.

Viruses are too small to be seen by conventional light microscopy and were therefore only theorized to exist until the development of electron microscopes in the 1930s. In some infected cells, however, they aggregate into clumps (*inclusion bodies*) large enough to be seen with normal light microscopy.

Virus infections are common and usually mild and transient, such as the common cold. Some, however, may persist for years or a lifetime as silent or smoldering

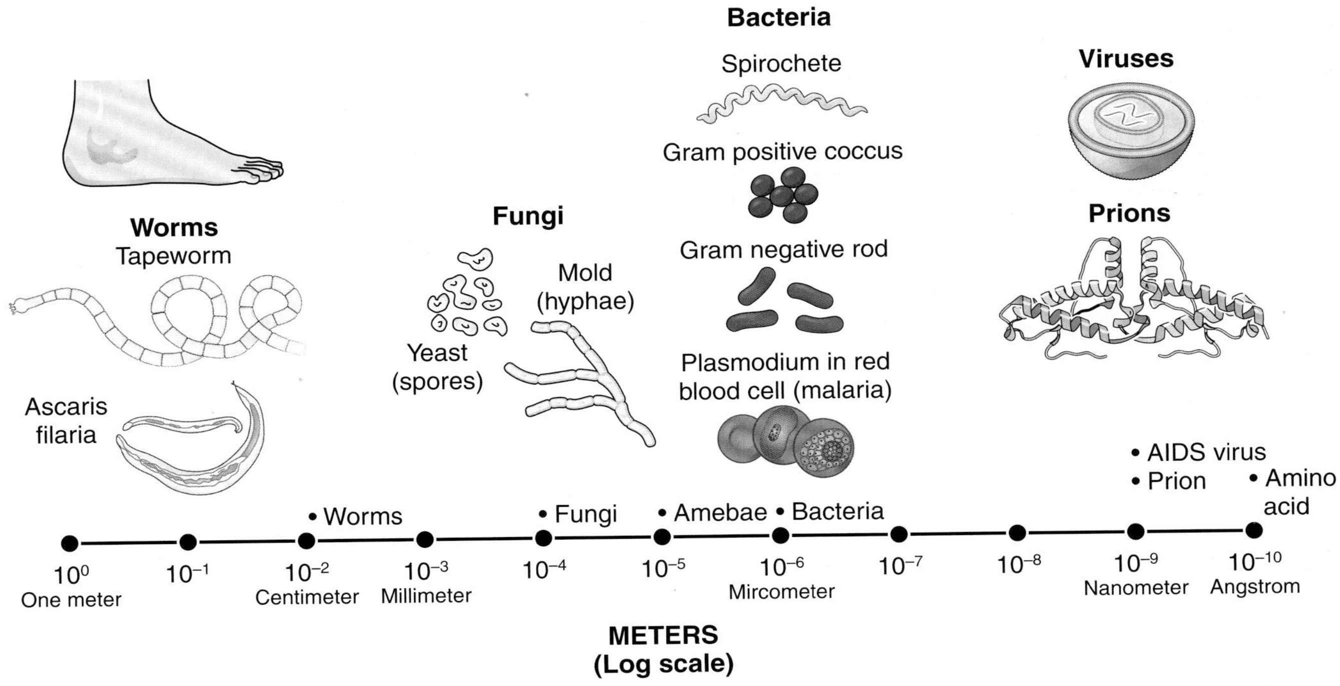

Figure 4.1 **Agents of infectious disease.** Arranged left to right in descending order of size (logarithmic scale).

infections (e.g., hepatitis B virus, human immunodeficiency virus [HIV]). Others are capable of transforming infected cells into tumor cells (e.g., the human papilloma virus causes cancer of the cervix).

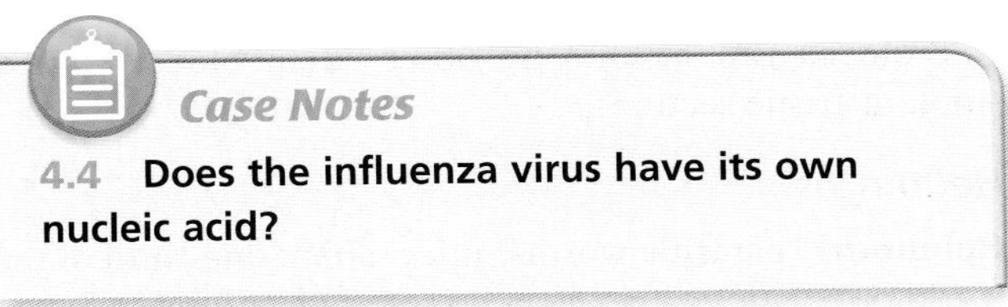
Case Notes

4.4 **Does the influenza virus have its own nucleic acid?**

Bacteria

Billions to trillions of bacteria populate the mouth, intestinal tract, and every square millimeter of skin surface. The intestine alone contains about 400 species of bacteria, most of which are *anaerobic* (they can live without oxygen). They live in symbiosis with us: we provide them a home and they produce vital substances we cannot live without (e.g., the majority of vitamin K is produced by intestinal bacteria, though leafy green vegetables provide a modest supplement).

Bacteria are much larger than viruses and can be seen by conventional light microscopy. They can live and reproduce outside of cells in body fluid or in any other environment that contains nutrients to support them (e.g., soil, water). They have a DNA, but no nucleus. They have a cell membrane and require energy to live, which makes them susceptible to antibiotics, many of which exert their effect by dissolving the cell wall or interfering with bacterial metabolism. A few bacteria are exceptions to these rules, most notably *Chlamydia*, an obligate intracellular parasite that lives in epithelial cells. *Chlamydia* is one of the most common *reportable* (to public health authorities) infectious agents, and will be discussed below in detail.

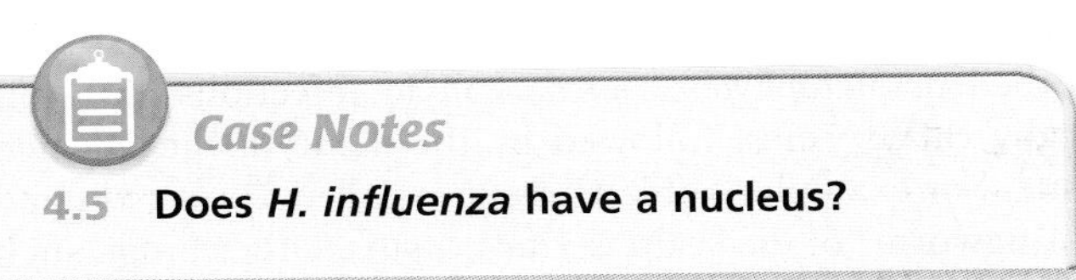
Case Notes

4.5 **Does *H. influenza* have a nucleus?**

Bacteria are classified according to shape, need for oxygen, and color after a standard stain. The **Gram stain** is the universal standard stain. Crystal-violet, a deep purple dye, is applied to a smear of sputum, urine, pus, urethral exudate, spinal fluid, or other substance thought to contain bacteria. Next a decolorizer is applied. Some bacteria retain the crystal-violet; others decolorize. Finally, a red counterstain is added to restain those bacteria that lost their crystal-violet stain to the decolorizer. Bacteria that retained their deep purple coloring are **Gram-positive**; those that lost it and restained red are **Gram-negative** (Fig. 4.2). Spherical forms are **cocci**, elongated forms are **bacilli**, and bacteria that are a combination of the two are referred to as **coccobacilli**. **Spirochetes** have a corkscrew shape. Bacteria that require oxygen are **aerobic**; those that do not are **anaerobic**.

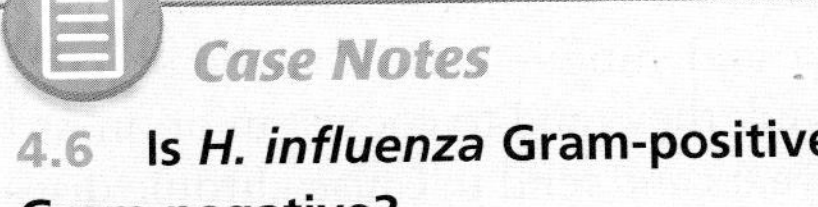
Case Notes

4.6 **Is *H. influenza* Gram-positive or Gram-negative?**

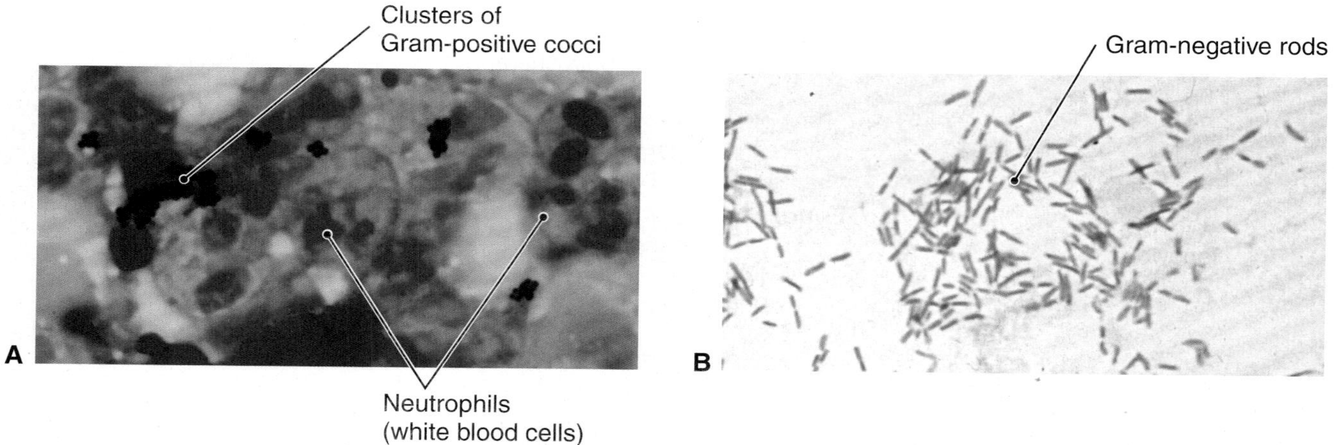

Figure 4.2 **Gram stain. A.** Gram-positive cocci (*Staphylococcus aureus*) in pus swabbed from an abscess (large, dark-red globules are white cell nuclei). **B**. Gram-negative bacilli (rods) (*Escherichia coli*) from a culture plate.

Fungi

Next up the scale of size and complexity are **fungi**. They have two distinctive forms: those that grow as long, branching, multicellular filaments (*hyphae*), which are known as **molds**, or those that grow as multicellular clusters of budding round forms (*spores*) called **yeast**. For some important fungal pathogens, the form of growth is temperature dependent. In cool temperature (e.g., on skin), they tend to grow as hyphae, but at body temperature deep infections occur in yeast form.

Infections of skin, hair, and nails are caused by species called *dermatophytes*. Dermatophyte infections are typically called *Tinea*, followed by the name of the infected site. For example, "athlete's foot" is called *Tinea pedis* and "ringworm" of the scalp is *Tinea capitis*. Other fungi, such as *Histoplasma capsulatum*, are associated with deep infections in the lungs or other viscera. Still other fungi are normal residents of skin and intestines (*Candida, Aspergillus*) but may cause disease in immunodeficient patients. *Pneumocystis jirovecii* is a very small fungus that causes serious pneumonia in persons with AIDS.

Fungi can often be seen on routine microscopic examination of tissue, scrapings, or fluid; however, special stains are sometimes necessary. Laboratory tests are available to test for the presence of antifungal antibodies in blood.

Parasites

Recall from above that we said that all infectious organisms are, in a certain sense, parasitic: they live in or on us at our expense. Here, however, we turn our attention to organisms that differ in two important ways from those discussed above. First, they are multicellular and usually larger than bacteria and fungi—many can be seen with the naked eye. Second, they tend to coexist in or on us for weeks, months, or years and tend to cause chronic disease rather than episodes of acute infection.

Protozoa

Protozoa are motile, single-cell, nucleated organisms that are capable of reproducing within cells (e.g., malarial protozoa in red blood cells) or extracellularly (e.g., intestinal amebae). They are responsible for much illness and death in developing countries. In industrialized nations, protozoa cause common, less serious disease such as vaginitis (*Trichomonas vaginalis*) and diarrhea (*Giardia lamblia*). Insects spread some protozoa, such as malaria; others, such as amebic dysentery, are spread by ingestion of fecally contaminated food.

Protozoa can be directly observed in blood smears, stool, or tissue sections.

Helminths

Helminths (parasitic worms) infect about one-third of the world population. They may be several feet long and may have very complex reproductive life cycles involving more than one host. For example, in *schistosomiasis*, the most serious of all helminth diseases, the schistosome worm passes through snails before infecting humans. A few intestinal helminths are of little consequence, but hundreds may consume enough blood to produce anemia. Most helminths infect the GI tract or liver; some infect blood or muscle.

Ectoparasites

Ectoparasites are small insect-like creatures that attach to or live in the skin (e.g., fleas, ticks, bedbugs, lice). They may cause local skin irritation from bites, but they also may transmit pathogens—ticks transmit the spirochete *Borrelia burgdorferi*, which causes *Lyme disease* (discussed below).

Infection Causes Injury

After infection, organisms cause damage by three mechanisms:

- *Direct cell contact or invasion*
- *Release of toxins* that circulate to cause cell death or damage at a distance, or release of enzymes that cause local damage
- *Provocation of an immune response* that, though directed at the pathogen, causes additional tissue damage

Virulence is the degree of harmfulness of a microbe. Viral virulence is an index of the damage viruses are capable of inflicting by entering cells and multiplying. They may kill the cell directly, incite an immune reaction that kills the cell or damages adjacent tissue, or transform the cell into a cancerous one. Most microbes, viruses included, exhibit a preference for a particular type of cell (**tropism**). For example, *rhinoviruses* (one cause of the common cold) proliferate best in cool tissue and infect the nasal mucosa because it is cooled by inhaled air. In addition, most viruses have surface protein receptors that attach to specific host cell surface proteins to gain entry into cells. For example, HIV has a specific protein that attaches to the CD4 protein receptor on the surface of helper T cells, enabling the virus to invade the cell. Some viruses kill cells; HIV is an example.

Bacterial virulence depends on the ability of the organism to attach to or invade the host cell or secrete a toxin. Some bacteria secrete glue-like *adhesins* that bind them to cells or fibers, whereas others have hair-like protein projections (pili) that latch onto tissue proteins. A bacterial **toxin** is any bacterial substance that contributes to illness. It can be a component of the cell membrane released as the organism dies (**endotoxin**), or it can be a product synthesized and excreted by the bacterium (**exotoxin**). Most endotoxins come from Gram-negative bacteria and can cause a form of vascular collapse called *endotoxic shock*. In contrast, bacterial exotoxins are secreted by living bacteria into the medium in which they grow. Often the medium is outside the patient (e.g., food) and the toxin is ingested, producing an immediate effect. For example, a common type of food poisoning features nausea, vomiting, and diarrhea caused by an exotoxin produced by staphylococci growing on unrefrigerated food. *Clostridium botulinum*, a Gram-positive, anaerobic bacillus, grows in contaminated canned or sealed food and synthesizes a neurotoxin that causes muscle paralysis (*botulism*).

Frequently, **host immunity** is the cause of tissue damage. For example, recall from Chapter 3 in our discussion of molecular mimicry that certain streptococcal antigens are so similar to human heart antigens that the immune response to strep throat is sometimes the cause of heart muscle autoimmune attack (e.g., rheumatic fever).

Inflammation Is the Usual Response to Infection

Viruses generally incite **chronic inflammation**, which is characterized by accumulation of lymphocytes and macrophages. Some viruses (e.g., *herpes*), however, cause cell death (**cytopathic reaction**) and others (e.g., *human papillomavirus*) cause abnormal cell growth (**cytoproliferative reaction**).

Bacteria usually incite suppurative (purulent) inflammation, usually called "acute inflammation," which is characterized by neutrophil infiltration, edema at the site, and an increased number of neutrophils in blood (neutrophilia). Masses of neutrophils and liquefactive necrosis combine to form pus. This type of pus-forming (pyogenic) reaction is usually produced by Gram-positive cocci such as *staphylococcus* or *streptococcus* or Gram-negative bacilli such as *E. coli* or *H. influenza*.

There are several noteworthy exceptions to the general rule that bacteria incite acute inflammation. The bacteria of two sexually transmitted infections (STI), *Chlamydia trachomatis*, the most common STI, and *Treponema pallidum*, the agent of *syphilis*, incite lymphocytic (or plasmacytic) inflammation. *Mycobacterium tuberculosis*, the agent of *TB*, and some fungus infections incite granulomatous inflammation, a special variety of chronic inflammation in which macrophages and lymphocytes predominate and aggregate into microscopic nodules (called *granulomas*).

Parasitic worm infections incite eosinophilic inflammation characterized by dense accumulations of eosinophils.

Notwithstanding all of the above, if infection persists, chronic inflammation and scarring will occur.

Case Notes

4.7 **What type of inflammatory reaction was incited by the influenza virus? By the *H. influenza* bacterium?**

Infectious Agents Spread in Certain Ways

Infections spread from point to point in a predictable manner, the various participants joined like links in a chain (Fig. 4.3). Infections are transmissible directly or indirectly from one living thing to another, from bird to bird, or bird to human, for example. Nonliving things do not become infected (although they can transmit infection [e.g., doorknob]). A bacterium may live and reproduce in soil, water, or potato salad, for example. The potato salad is *contaminated*, not infected.

Contagion is the spread of infection from one person (host) to another. Contagion can occur in almost any setting: at home or work or even in a hospital. Infection acquired outside of a hospital is a **community-acquired** infection. If acquired in a hospital, it is a **nosocomial** infection. For every pathogen there is a **reservoir**, a place where the pathogen exists and from which it spreads to

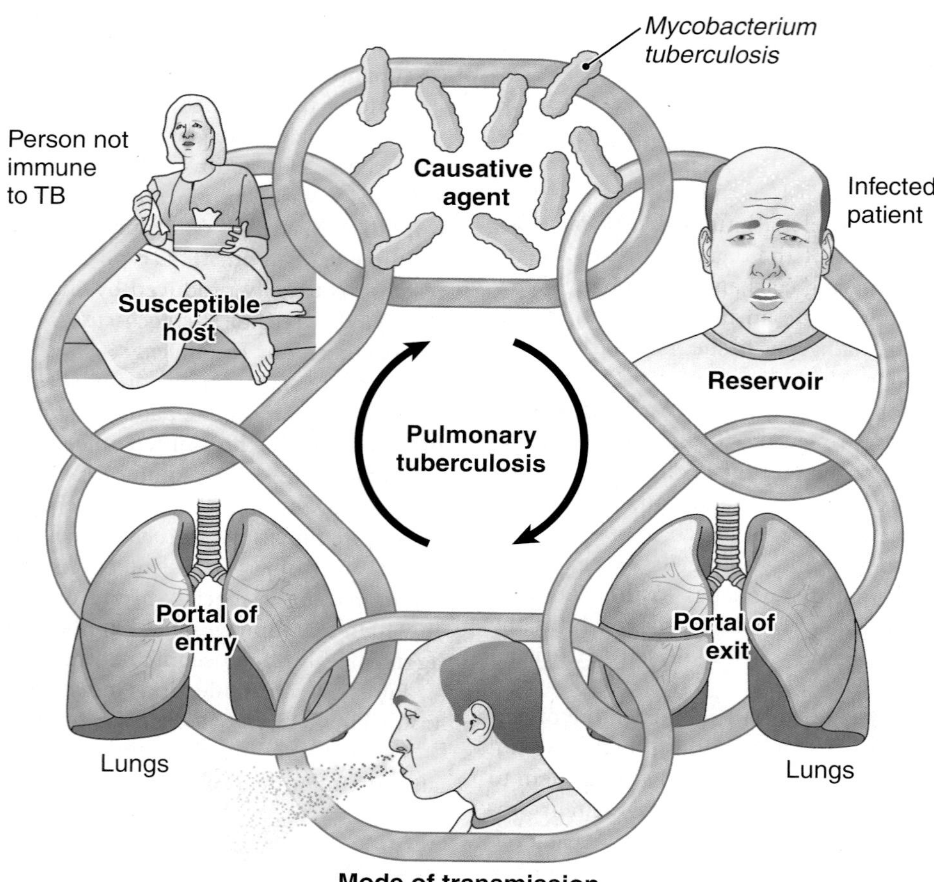

Figure 4.3 **Contagion.** The spread of infectious agents from one point to another.

new hosts. The reservoir may be food, water, soil, equipment, animals or animal products, or humans. The reservoir may be an obviously infected person, or it may be an asymptomatic **carrier**—a person or animal harboring the pathogen but suffering no obvious disease. Many people are asymptomatic carriers of hepatitis viruses.

The mode of transmission from reservoir to new host may be by the following:

- *Direct contact.* Sexual intercourse, for example, transmits certain diseases such as syphilis (a bacterial disease) or herpes (a viral disease). Most organisms penetrate through breaks in skin or sexual mucosa. Because few organisms are necessary to establish infection, skin needle sticks are a special hazard for people who use or abuse injected drugs and for healthcare workers.
- *Ingestion.* Ingestion of contaminated food is sometimes responsible, as in hepatitis A infection. The number of organisms is important. A larger dose is more likely to establish a new infection, and some organisms are more resistant to gastric acid than others.
- *Indirect contact.* Sometimes **fomites**—inanimate materials such as doorknobs, gloves, bed sheets, or handkerchiefs—carry the pathogen. In each instance, the host contaminates the fomite with feces, nasal secretions, cells, or other material.
- *Droplets.* Respiratory droplets from coughing or sneezing are the mode of transmission for most upper respiratory infections ("colds"), influenza, pneumonia, and mumps.
- *Vectors.* Insect vectors, intermediate carriers such as mosquitoes, often transmit malaria and other parasitic diseases.

Case Notes

4.8 What is the likely mode of contagion for Ruth's influenza and bacterial pneumonia?

Regardless of the mode of transmission, hands often play a role because they are in regular contact with the nose, mouth, genitalia, and other body parts. Frequent hand washing is effective in controlling the spread of infectious disease. This is especially true in restaurants and hospitals.

Not all people and pathogens are equal—some people are more susceptible to infection than others, and some pathogens are more contagious and more virulent than others. Immunodeficiency or impaired nonimmune defense mechanisms are common causes of infection. For example, severely burned patients lack intact skin to protect them and may subsequently acquire skin infections that invade the rest of the body, and AIDS patients have defective immunity that renders them especially susceptible to infection. Some people are genetically more susceptible or resistant to infection. For example, people of African heritage are resistant to one type of malaria because they lack the Duffy red blood cell antigen to which the malaria parasite must attach to enter the red cell.

Some organisms cause infection at the site of entry, whereas others enter lymph vessels and spread to lymph nodes; still others invade blood and spread widely to settle in a particular tissue (Fig. 4.4). For example, *Staphylococcus* from a skin infection might invade the lymphatic system to produce *lymphangitis* and then spread into the blood, which might carry organisms to the brain, causing a brain abscess. When blood is the main infected tissue, the condition is called **septicemia** or **sepsis**.

In tissues, microorganisms spread along planes of least resistance. For example, bacteria from a ruptured appendix can spread along the smooth surfaces of the peritoneum to cause an infection around the liver. In other infections, spread of organisms is confined to superficial epithelial surfaces. Bacterial throat infection (*pharyngitis*), caused by *Streptococcus* ("strep throat"), is an example.

The influenza virus exhibits tropism for the lungs. An agent may settle in tissue, however, at a point distant from

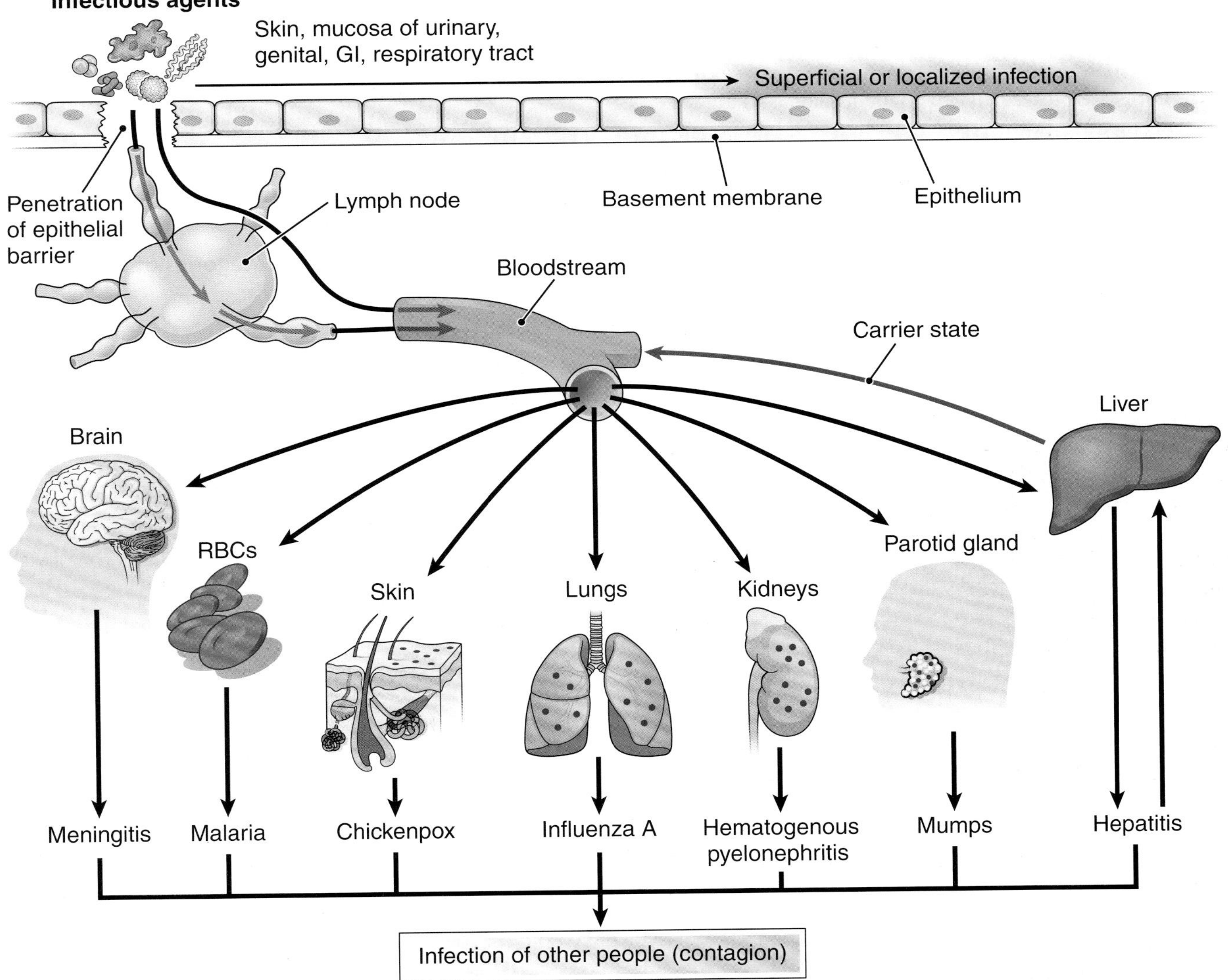

Figure 4.4 **Invasion and spread of infectious agents.** To infect and spread, agents (pathogens) must invade the body, usually by penetrating an epithelial barrier. After invading, most pathogens spread first through the lymphatic system before entering the blood and disseminating to distant organs.

the point of entry. For example, *Neisseria meningitidis* is a bacterium that usually lodges silently in the throat initially, but when it invades it has tropism for the meninges and causes bacterial meningitis.

Infection Runs a Natural Course

The natural course of infection is depicted in Figure 4.5. The initial event in every infection is the invasion of the organism into the body. The time between invasion and appearance of signs or symptoms is the **incubation period**, during which the organism attempts to proliferate. If the body's defenses are effective, no illness occurs. Otherwise, the organism multiplies to the point that it produces damage sufficient to cause signs and symptoms. After the incubation period, a **prodromal period** may occur in which the patient suffers from mild, nonspecific symptoms. Headache, loss of appetite, and fatigue are common prodromal symptoms. The prodrome is followed by the **acute phase** of the illness, a time of maximum acute, typical clinical signs and symptoms. Then follows a period of **convalescence**, during which symptoms fade. Finally, in the **recovery period**, no symptoms are present, but the patient may feel fatigued.

The picture, however, is not always so simple. If the patient's defenses are inadequate, the organism may continue to proliferate and invade the bloodstream, colonizing various organs. For example, if the brain coverings (meninges) are colonized, meningitis may occur and septicemia can cause shock, intravascular coagulation, or other calamity.

Although most infections are cleared completely by body defenses or medical therapy, some patients may regain good health but still harbor the organism. They are carriers, a potential source of infection for others.

Case Notes

4.9 What phase of illness was Ruth in when she felt "bum" before becoming acutely ill?

4.10 In what phase was Ruth upon discharge from the hospital?

Pop Quiz

4.1 True or false? Gram-positive organisms are purple while Gram-negative organisms are red-pink.

4.2 True or false? Virulence is the ability to cause disease.

4.3 True or false? Host immunity always decreases virulence.

4.4 True or false? Incubation time varies between diseases.

4.5 What are the major categories of infectious agents?

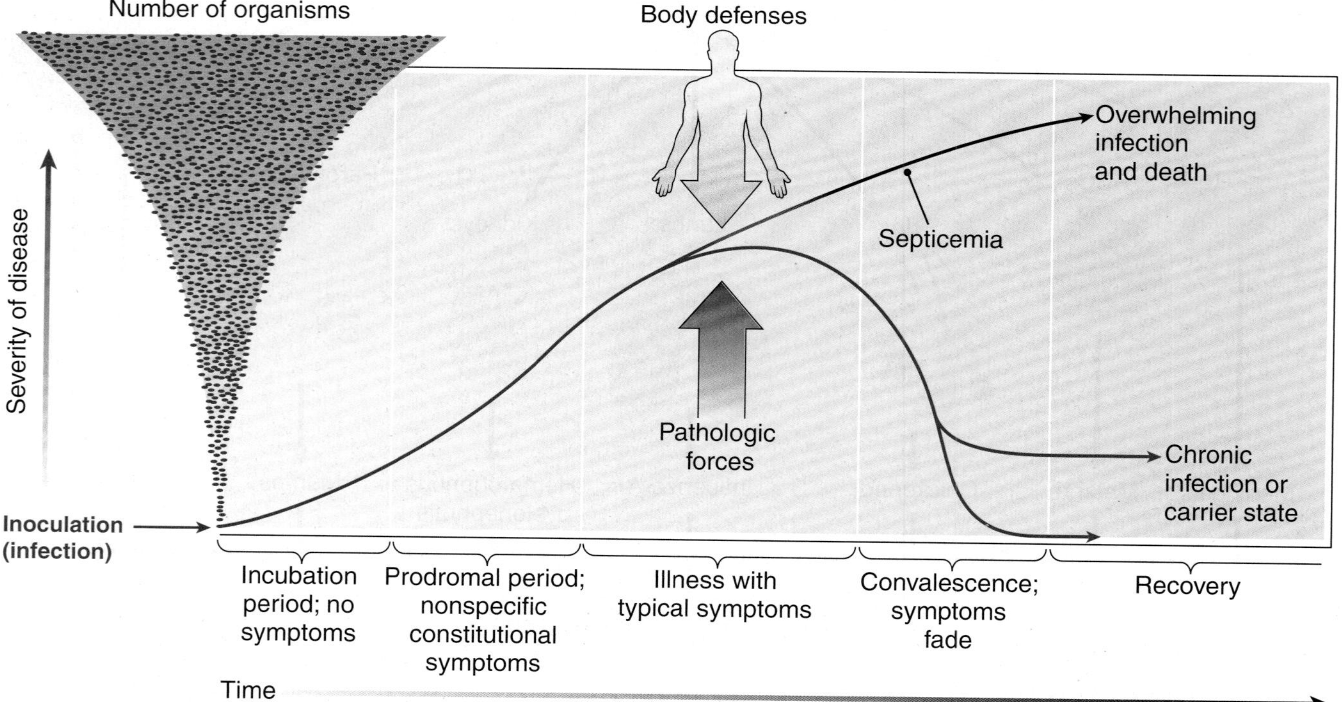

Figure 4.5 **The natural course of infection.**

4.6 Name the crucial differences between viruses and bacteria.
4.7 How does temperature affect the form of fungus?
4.8 What are ectoparasites?
4.9 How do infectious agents spread?
4.10 Define tropism.
4.11 An organism called *Bacillus cereus* grows in reheated rice and can cause food poisoning very quickly within four hours. Is it more likely that endotoxin or exotoxin causes this disease?
4.12 Eosinophilic inflammation is most likely caused by what type of infection?
4.13 Granulomas, or granulomatous inflammation, are most likely caused by what two types of organisms?
4.14 During which period of the natural course of an infection do the symptoms fade?

Virus Infections

Virus infections may be acute or chronic. In acute infection the virus is quickly neutralized and eliminated. In chronic infection the virus is not eliminated and is capable of producing sustained effects.

Acute Virus Infections Are Transient

Acute, transient virus infection is caused by dozens of viruses and hundreds of subtypes, too many to mention here. The usual result is an effective host immune response that eliminates the virus. Permanent immunity may or may not result. Permanent immunity occurs if there is one unchanging version of the virus; *mumps* is an example. If the virus mutates regularly into a new strain, however, such as occurs with influenza, last year's immune response is not effective in preventing this year's infection. Briefly discussed below are some of the more important acute virus infections, with references to discussion in other chapters.

Viruses Mainly Tropic for the Respiratory Tract

Rhinoviruses are a family of over 100 varieties that are the cause of about half of all cases of the **common cold**. The remainder of common colds owes to about a half-dozen other viruses, each with many varieties. Typical symptoms include sore throat, rhinorrhea, nasal congestion, sneezing, and cough. Primary transmission is person-to-person contact. Respiratory droplet transmission is possible, but less important. No vaccine is available. Treatment is supportive.

Adenovirus usually infects the upper respiratory tract, causing tonsillitis (similar to strep throat, discussed below), and often presents in combination with conjunctivitis. Adenovirus may also cause severe respiratory infections including croup, *bronchiolitis* (inflammation of small airways of the lung, Chapter 22) and pneumonia, ear infections, or gastroenteritis (the stomach flu). Treatment is largely directed at symptom management; no antiviral drugs are available.

Respiratory syncytial virus (RSV) is a major cause of lower respiratory tract infections during infancy and childhood. The most common cause of bronchiolitis and pneumonia in children under one year of age, it generally produces mild respiratory symptoms, though it can lead to severe respiratory illness requiring hospitalization. Treatment is supportive care.

The term "flu" is widely used to refer to a variety of mild respiratory illnesses, but **influenza** properly refers to an illness caused by *influenza viruses*. It is spread primarily by respiratory droplets, and, less often, by direct contact. Influenza causes widespread sporadic illness yearly during fall and winter in temperate climates. Epidemics in the United States occur about every two to three years. Worldwide pandemics of severe disease occur regularly but less often.

There are two clinically important types of influenza: A and B. Type B is less common and causes mild disease. Typical influenza A disease is a severe respiratory infection quite apart from the usual "cold." Symptoms include fever, chills, nasal congestion, cough, headache, myalgia, and malaise. Even healthy adults can be rendered bedfast for a week, and it can be fatal in elderly or debilitated patients or those in late pregnancy. Diagnosis is usually clinical and depends on local epidemiologic patterns. High-risk patients, their caregivers and household contacts, healthcare practitioners, all people over 50 years of age, and all children ages 6 months to 18 years should receive annual influenza vaccination. Annual vaccination is necessary because of constant mutations of the virus (*antigenic drift*). Antiviral treatment reduces the duration of illness by a day or so and should be given to high-risk patients.

Case Notes

4.11 **Was Ruth's infection more likely type A or type B influenza?**

Viruses Mainly Tropic for the Gastrointestinal Tract

Rotavirus is the most common cause of severe diarrhea among infants and young children. Transmission is by the fecal-oral route. It typically presents with vomiting, followed by four to eight days of watery diarrhea, accompanied by a low-grade fever. Dehydration is a common and severe side effect. Diagnosis is made by detection of virus in the stool. Treatment is supportive. Vaccination is effective.

The **norovirus** (Norwalk virus) causes about 90% of nonbacterial outbreaks of epidemic gastroenteritis around the world. Older children and adults are most often affected. It is transmitted by fecally contaminated food or water, by person-to-person contact, and by aerosolization. Outbreaks of norovirus are especially common on cruise ships, and in long-term care facilities, overnight camps, hospitals, prisons, and dormitories. It typically presents as 24 to 48 hours of nausea, abdominal pain, vomiting, and watery diarrhea. Lethargy, weakness, muscle cramps, headaches, and low-grade fever may also accompany the illness. The virus is usually self-limiting, and treatment is supportive. No vaccine is available.

Other Transient Virus Infections

Measles (*rubeola*) is a very highly contagious infection by the *measles virus*. It is spread through nasal and oral secretions. Measles is the most common cause of vaccine-preventable illness worldwide, in 2011 infecting about 20 million people and causing 160,000 deaths, mostly in children in developing nations. It is characterized by fever, cough, nasal congestion, conjunctivitis, a maculopapular rash, and rash-like (Koplik) spots on the buccal mucosa. Diagnosis is usually clinical. Treatment is supportive. Vaccination is effective.

Mumps is an acute, contagious infection caused by the *mumps virus*. It is characterized by painful swelling of the salivary glands, usually the parotids. It is less contagious than measles. The virus probably enters through the mouth or nose. Systemic spread may involve the gonads, brain or meninges, or the pancreas. Diagnosis is usually clinical. Treatment is supportive. Vaccination is effective.

Rubella (*German measles*) is a contagious virus infection by the *rubella virus* that may be asymptomatic or may cause a brief, mild febrile illness featuring adenopathy, rash, and constitutional symptoms. Less contagious than measles, it is spread by respiratory droplets. Infection early in the first trimester of pregnancy can cause spontaneous abortion or congenital defects. Diagnosis is clinical. Treatment is usually unnecessary. Vaccination is effective.

Poliomyelitis is an acute, contagious infection caused by the *poliovirus*. It is spread by oral-fecal contamination. Most infections cause no symptoms, but in about 1% the virus invades motor neurons in the brain or spinal cord, causing paralysis. Diagnosis is clinical, although laboratory detection is possible. Treatment is supportive. Vaccination is effective.

Hepatitis A virus is the cause of acute viral hepatitis (Chapter 12), an epidemic form of hepatitis transmitted by oral-fecal contamination.

Coxsackie viruses are classed into two subtypes, A and B. *Type A* infection is tropic for oral mucosa and skin. Children are most often affected. Infection causes painful blisters of the oral cavity (*herpangina*) and rash on the palms and soles, a syndrome called *hand-foot-and-mouth disease*. *Type B* infection is tropic for heart, lungs, pancreas, and nervous system and causes inflammation of those organs. Symptoms are usually mild. Treatment is supportive. No vaccine is available.

Some Viruses Cause Persistent Infection

Persistent virus infections are those in which the immune system does not eliminate the virus. The result can be recurrent flare-ups (*latent infection*), chronic tissue injury and inflammation (*productive infection*), or the transformation of normal tissue into a neoplasm (*transformative infection*). Some viruses ordinarily causing acute infection may cause persistent infection, and some persistent infections may have both productive and transformative effects.

Latent Virus Infections

Latent virus infections are those in which the virus persists in noninfectious form, but can periodically reactivate to cause recurrent disease and new infections. Members of the herpesvirus family cause almost all latent virus infections. Infection causes large clusters of virus particles to appear as nuclear inclusions, a diagnostic clue that can be seen in cells from infected tissue.

Herpes simplex virus (HSV) has two subtypes, *type 1* and *type 2*. Type 1 is usually associated with oral **cold sores**, and type 2 with **genital herpes**, although each type regularly infects either site. The diseases are the same, only the location is different. Both cause crops of small, painful blisters in skin or mucosa, which fade in a week or so without treatment. The virus invades the tips of sensory axons and travels up the axon to become latent in neuron nuclei in the spinal cord or brain. The virus has mechanisms to avoid immune recognition and can reactivate spontaneously, multiplying and traveling back out the axon to reinfect skin or mucosa again. Sometimes HSV can infect the cornea and inflict damage that results in blindness. Rarely, HSV will cause fatal encephalitis. No effective vaccine is available. Topical and oral antiviral compounds (e.g., acyclovir) may quicken resolution and lessen symptoms.

The **herpes zoster virus** or **varicella-zoster virus (VZV)** is closely related to HSV. The acute infection is **chickenpox**, an acute, systemic infection, usually affecting children. It typically begins with mild constitutional symptoms followed by clusters of weeping, crusted small skin blisters. Lesions may also appear in the mouth, eyes, and upper respiratory tract. In uneventful cases, the lesions disappear in two to three weeks. Adult infection or infection of immunocompromised hosts may be severe or fatal due to pneumonia or nervous system involvement. Diagnosis is clinical. Those at risk of severe complications may be treated with immune globulin or antiviral compounds.

After infection, VZV invades neurons and persists in the neuron nucleus and reactivates in the same way, causing local outcroppings of painful, small blisters (**shingles**) in the distribution of the infected nerve (the *dermatome*). In immunocompetent hosts, VZV recurs as shingles only once, but in immunocompromised hosts, it may recur in the same location many times. Vaccination is effective.

Cytomegalovirus (CMV) is a variety of herpesvirus that infects blood monocytes and related cells and causes a wide array of illnesses depending on host age and immune status. Route of transmission depends on age. It can cross the placenta to infect the fetus with devastating effect, or it can pass to the newborn through vaginal secretions or breast milk. In childcare settings it passes via saliva from child to child or to adults, and in adults it can be sexually transmitted. Acute infection can produce marked but short-lived T cell immunosuppression. Congenital infection may cause birth defects, hepatitis, or encephalitis. Newborn infection may cause severe hepatitis or pneumonia. In healthy children and adults infection is usually asymptomatic. When symptoms occur, the presentation mimics that of *infectious mononucleosis* (Chapter 22) and is called *CMV mononucleosis*. It is characterized by fever, atypical lymphocytosis, lymphadenopathy, and lab evidence of mild hepatitis. CMV infection in immunocompromised hosts is often severe and may occur as primary or latent infection. It is the most common *opportunistic infection* in AIDS patients, where its most frequent manifestations are pneumonia, retinitis, and colitis. Antiviral compounds may be effective. There is no effective vaccine.

Human immunodeficiency virus (HIV), the agent of AIDS, is discussed in detail in Chapter 3. HIV infects the nucleus of T cells and uses its RNA to make DNA, which it splices into host cell DNA and thereby takes over host cell metabolism. HIV/AIDS patients are especially vulnerable to **opportunistic infections**, infections by organisms that do not cause disease in people with healthy immune systems. Figure 4.6 depicts the various organisms that cause opportunistic infections and the sites most likely to be infected.

Productive Virus Infections

Productive infections are those in which the virus persists in infectious form, and continues to replicate and cause chronic injury. The most common types of chronic productive virus infection are caused by the **hepatitis B virus** and **hepatitis C virus**, the agents of distinctive types of chronic viral hepatitis, which are discussed in detail in Chapter 12. Each is associated with chronic, productive scarring of the liver (cirrhosis). Other viruses can cause chronic infection. For example, mutant, immune-resistant measles virus is the cause of *subacute sclerosing panencephalitis*, a severely debilitating brain infection.

Transformative Virus Infections

Transformative infections are those in which the virus persists in infectious form, and can stimulate the transformation of normal tissue into a neoplasm.

The **Epstein-Barr virus (EBV)** is the agent of *infectious mononucleosis* (IM), a short-term febrile illness of young adults that is discussed in Chapter 22. EBV is endemic in many populations and can produce chronic infection that has been linked to the development of some *non-Hodgkin lymphomas* (Chapter 7) and *nasopharyngeal carcinoma*, a tumor rare in the West, but more common in Asia and Africa. No vaccine is available.

There are over 100 types of **human papilloma virus (HPV)**, which preferentially infects skin and squamous mucosa. Most infections are asymptomatic and of no lasting consequence. Some types, however, cause skin warts (Chapter 21), others anogenital warts, and others dysplasia and cancer of the cervix (Chapters 5 and 17). Vaccines are available to prevent the HPV types that cause most cervical cancer.

Kaposi sarcoma associated herpesvirus (KSHV) is the agent of *Kaposi sarcoma*, a sluggishly malignant skin tumor that is endemic in the Mediterranean basin and Africa. An epidemic variety, however, is associated with HIV/AIDS and other immunosuppressed conditions (Chapter 3). This variety is the most common AIDS-defining neoplasm, and is more aggressive than the endemic variety.

Chronic *hepatitis B virus* infection is associated with an increased risk for development of hepatocellular carcinoma (Chapter 12).

Case Notes

4.12 Without an influenza vaccination, will Ruth's immune system protect her against another influenza infection next flu season? Why?

Pop Quiz

4.15 True or false? Vaccination against viruses has decreased the incidence of many virus diseases.

4.16 True or false? Vaccination against viruses increases cancer risk.

4.17 What virus is responsible for cold sores? Shingles? Infectious mononucleosis?

4.18 What virus is most likely to cause gastroenteritis on a cruise ship? The common cold during the school year? Involve the parotids and gonads?

4.19 Why are influenza vaccines recommended annually?

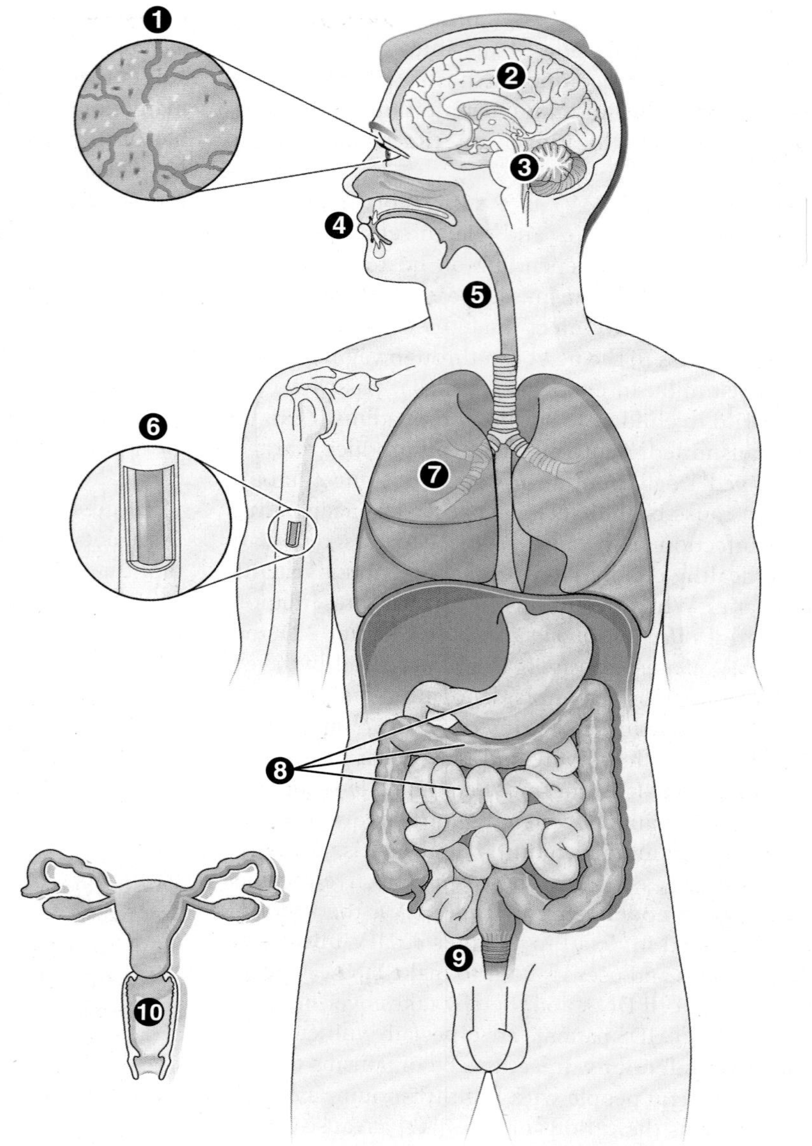

1. Chorioretinitis
   - Cytomegalovirus
2. Encephalitis
   - Cytomegalovirus
   - *Toxoplasma*
3. Meningitis
   - *Cryptococcus*
4. Stomatitis
   - *Candida*
5. Esophagitis
   - *Candida*
   - Cytomegalovirus
6. Bone marrow infections
   - *Mycobacterium avium*
7. Pneumonia
   - *Pneumocystis jirovecii*
   - *Mycobacterium avium*
8. Gastritis, enteritis, colitis
   - *Candida*
   - Cytomegalovirus
   - *Mycobacterium avium*
9. Proctitis
   - *Candida*
10. Vaginitis
   - *Candida*

Figure 4.6 **Opportunistic and AIDS-related infections.**

Bacterial Infections

Bacterial infections may be acute or chronic. In acute infection the bacterium is quickly neutralized and eliminated. In chronic infection the bacterium is not eliminated and is capable of producing sustained effects. Relatively few bacterial infections are chronic.

Staphylococci and Streptococci Are Gram-Positive

Gram-positive cocci are very common aerobic pathogens that cause acute, intense, pyogenic (pus-forming) infection.

Staphylococci

Staphylococci are Gram-positive cocci that cause acute, pyogenic infections. Staph grows in tight clusters and has characteristics that tend to cause localized, intense inflammation. *Staphylococcus aureus* is the most common pathogenic species and is distinguished from other, less virulent varieties by the presence in *S. aureus* of an enzyme called *coagulase*.

S. aureus causes skin abscesses and other infections, pharyngitis, bone infection, pneumonia, and heart valve infections, and is the major cause of infection in skin burns. Some varieties secrete exotoxins. One variety of *food poisoning* is caused by ingestion of unrefrigerated food contaminated with staph that produces an intestinal exotoxin. In menstruating women, staph can multiply in vaginal tampons and produce a systemic exotoxin that causes *toxic shock syndrome*, which features fever, aching, and diarrhea, followed in a few days by a sunburn-like rash. It can progress to sepsis.

S. aureus is spread by direct contact with skin or clothing. Many people harbor *S. aureus* in their nostrils. Diagnosis is by culture and Gram stain. Antibiotic treatment varies according to outcomes of laboratory tests to determine which antibiotics are likely to be most effective (*antibiotic sensitivity testing*, discussed below). Antibiotic-resistant strains have evolved, and some are now known to be resistant even to treatment with late-generation antibiotics such as methicillin. These varieties of *S. aureus* are referred to as *methicillin-resistant staphylococcus aureus (MRSA)* and are a growing threat to hospitalized patients.

Coagulase negative staph (e.g., *S. epidermidis*) is a normal resident of skin and an opportunistic pathogen that infects vascular and urinary catheters, artificial heart valves, and other medical device. Along with *S. aureus*, it is a common cause of endocarditis in intravenous drug users.

Streptococci

Streptococci also cause a wide variety of pyogenic infections of skin, pharynx, lungs, and heart valves (Fig. 4.7A). They tend to grow in twisted chains (Greek *streptos* = easily twisted) and to spread along surfaces and tissue planes. According to their metabolic, mitotic, and reproductive characteristics they are classified into genus and species, such as *S. pneumoniae* and *S. pyogenes*. For clinical purposes, however, they are more easily identified according to their antigenic properties (**groups A, B, D**, etc.) and according to the character of the hemolysis they cause (**alpha hemolytic** and **beta hemolytic**) when cultured on blood agar plates:

- **Alpha hemolytic**
  - *S. pneumoniae* (sometimes called the *pneumococcus*) is the cause of lobar pneumonia (Chapter 10). Vaccination is recommended for the infirm and elderly.
  - *Streptococcus mutans* is an anaerobic species that is a major cause of dental caries.
- **Beta hemolytic**
  - **Group A** streptococci typically cause infection of superficial surfaces such as pharynx or skin.
    - *Acute streptococcal pharyngitis* is a painful, superficial throat infection commonly called "strep throat."
    - Two types of group A skin infection occur. *Cellulitis* is a painful, superficial, edematous, erythematous infection of skin, subcutaneous tissue, and lymphatics. *Impetigo* is a superficial skin infection of young children (also caused by staph) that appears first as transient, small blisters, which break to form patches of red, "honey-crusted" lesions covered with dried exudate.
- **Group B** streptococci are a major cause of neonatal pneumonia, meningitis, and sepsis, and in adults are frequent culprits in urinary tract infections.
- **Group D** streptococci (also called **enterococci**) are anaerobic (the others are aerobic) *Enterococcus faecalis* and *Enterococcus faecium* are common commensal organisms in the human intestines. Under certain circumstances, however, they are capable of causing endocarditis, urinary tract infections, diverticulitis, and meningitis. A concerning feature of these enterococci is that some strains are resistant to vancomycin, the antibiotic of last resort if other treatment fails.

Streptococci can invade the bloodstream and spread widely to cause serious secondary infections (Fig. 4.7B), blood infections (*septicemia*), infection of the meninges (*meningitis*), or heart valves (bacterial *endocarditis*). Unlike staph, strep can stimulate autoimmune reactions in the kidney (glomerulonephritis, Chapter 15) or the heart (myocarditis and valvulitis in *rheumatic fever* [Chapter 9]).

Streptococci are also associated with noninfectious consequences (Fig. 4.7C). *Scarlet fever* (*scarlatina*), an intensely red skin reaction caused by an exotoxin, is an added feature in some infections. Streptococci can also stimulate the autoimmune reactions that are the cause of *rheumatic fever* (Chapter 9) and *glomerulonephritis* (Chapter 15).

Strep is spread by direct contact. Diagnosis is by Gram stain and culture characteristics. Antibiotic therapy is effective treatment.

Gram-Positive Bacilli Cause Diverse Infections

Staphylococci and streptococci cause a variety of infectious syndromes. In sharp contrast, Gram-positive bacilli cause illnesses closely identified with each species.

Corynebacterium Diphtheriae

Diphtheria is an acute pharyngeal or skin infection caused by *Corynebacterium diphtheriae*, an anaerobic, Gram-positive bacillus passed through respiratory droplets or skin contact. Some varieties produce an exotoxin. Skin infection produces no signature signs; however, skin ulcers may occur if exotoxin is produced. *C. diphtheria* is most widely known for the distinctive throat and upper respiratory syndrome (*diphtheria*) toxigenic strains cause in infected children. The classic illness begins with mild sore throat, difficulty swallowing, low-grade fever, and rapid heart rate and evolves into nausea, vomiting, chills, headache, and the development of a characteristic yellow, then gray inflammatory membrane in the tonsillar area. The membrane may extend into the airway and partially obstruct it or suddenly detach, causing complete and fatal obstruction. Local edema of throat structures may cause a swollen neck (bull neck), hoarseness, inspiratory high-pitched wheeze (stridor), and shortness of breath (dyspnea). Myocardial and neural tissue damage may occur secondary to exotoxin effect. Diagnosis is clinical and confirmed by culture. Treatment is with antitoxin and antibiotics. Vaccination is effective for prevention.

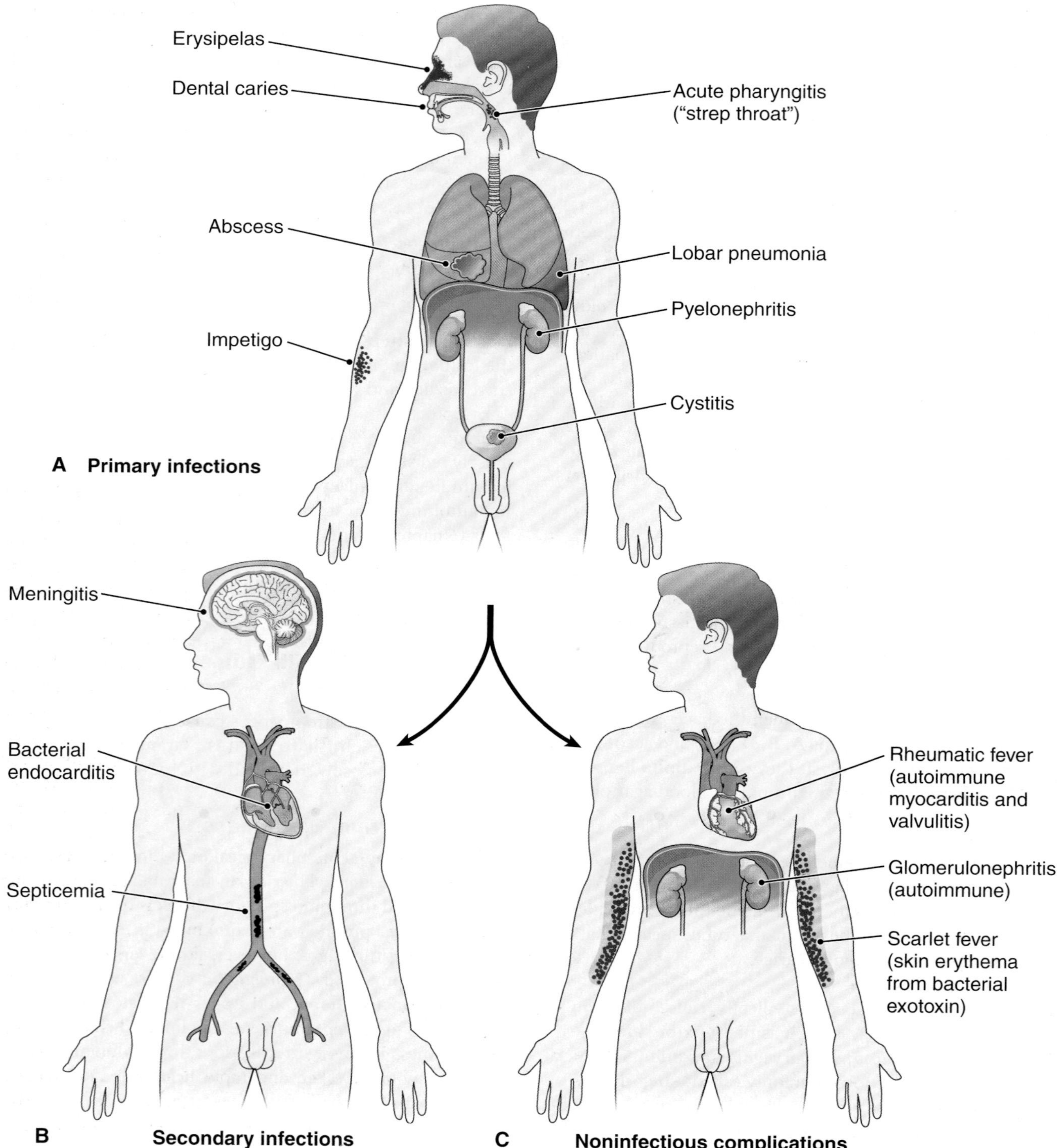

Figure 4.7 **Streptococcal diseases.**

Listeria Monocytogenes

Listeria monocytogenes is a Gram-positive bacillus that is ubiquitous in the environment, grows at refrigerator temperature, and causes food-borne infections through contaminated dairy products, raw vegetables, and raw chicken and other meats. **Listeriosis** features bacteremia, meningitis, encephalitis, and dermatitis. Pregnant women, the elderly, and the immunodeficient are especially vulnerable. Infected pregnant women are at risk for spontaneous abortion; their newborns are at risk for neonatal sepsis. Diagnosis is by laboratory culture. Antibiotic treatment is effective.

Bacillus Anthracis

Bacillus anthracis, the agent of **anthrax**, is a large, toxin-producing, encapsulated, aerobic or anaerobic Gram-positive bacillus that produces *spores* capable of lying dormant in soil for decades or longer. Spores can be made into a very fine powder that is easily disbursed and inhaled, making it an ideal bioterrorist weapon. Anthrax is a common and often fatal pathogen in cattle and farm animals, which acquire infection through inhalation of dust or by direct contact. It is transmitted to humans by contact with infected animals or their products. In humans, infection typically occurs through skin and causes itchy sores, often with black eschars (scabs). Inhalation infection is less common but far more dangerous: anthrax pneumonia is often fatal. It is sensitive to antibiotics. A vaccine is available.

Nocardia

Nocardia species are a family of Gram-positive, bacillus-like aerobes that grow in distinctive branched chains similar to fungal hyphae and are widely found in soil. **Nocardiosis** is an acute or chronic, typically disseminated infection caused by various species of *Nocardia*. Most infections occur in immunodeficient patients. Pneumonia is typical, but skin and nervous system infections are common. Diagnosis is by culture and special stains. Antibiotic treatment is usually effective.

Clostridia

Clostridium species are Gram-positive anaerobic bacilli that grow in animal feces and soil. Four *Clostridium* species cause significant human disease:

- *C. difficile* is a commensal anaerobe that normally lives in low numbers in the colon. Under some circumstances, often when oral antibiotics kill off the competition, it overgrows, releases toxins, and causes **pseudomembranous colitis**, a severe inflammatory disease of the colon (Chapter 11).
- *C. perfringens* is the agent of **gas gangrene**. It and related species cause diffuse infection and necrosis of soft tissues (*cellulitis*) and muscle (*myonecrosis*). Infection usually occurs when trauma implants the organism, which then thrives in necrotic tissue. It also occurs as a uterine infection associated with unsanitary induced abortion. Treatment is surgical drainage, debridement, and antibiotics.
- *C. tetani* is the agent of **tetanus**, an acute poisoning from a neurotoxin. It infects deep puncture wounds and releases a neurotoxin that causes severe muscle spasms and convulsions. It grows in puncture wounds and in the umbilical stump of newborns. Spasm of jaw muscles accounts for its common name *lockjaw*. Diagnosis is clinical. Treatment is with antitoxin. Childhood DPT vaccination (diphtheria, pertussis, and tetanus) provides protection against the toxin, but not against infection.
- *C. botulinum* is the agent of **botulism**, a paralytic poisoning. It grows in inadequately sterilized canned foods and releases a potent neurotoxin that blocks release of acetylcholine at the neuromuscular junction. Symptoms are symmetric cranial nerve paralysis and progressive descending paralysis of spinal nerves. Sensory nerves are not affected. Most cases are due to ingestion of the toxin in contaminated food. Some cases of infant botulism can be traced to honey—infants under age 12 months should not be fed honey. Wound botulism is uncommon but is a hazard of dirty needle use among intravenous drug abusers. Diagnosis is clinical and by laboratory identification of toxin. Treatment is supportive care supplemented by antitoxin. Under the trade name Botox®, the toxin is widely used cosmetically to temporarily remove skin wrinkles by paralyzing facial muscles.

Neisseria Are the Only Important Gram-Negative Cocci

N. meningitidis (**meningococcus**) is an important cause of meningitis (Chapter 19), especially in young children. It is typically carried in the throat of about 10% of the population and is spread by respiratory droplets. About a dozen subtypes exist. Immune response eliminates the subtype but provides no immunity to other subtypes. **Meningococcal meningitis** often occurs when people encounter new subtypes to which they are not immune, which typically occurs among children in daycare or school or in young adults living in college dormitories or military barracks. *N. meningitidis* occurs sporadically in the United States, but epidemics occur periodically in underdeveloped nations. Meningococcal meningitis and septicemia typically occur together. Symptoms are severe and include headache, nausea, vomiting, malaise, rash, multiple organ failure, shock, and disseminated intravascular coagulation. *Meningococcal meningitis is a life-threatening emergency.* Therefore, the diagnosis is presumptive and antibiotic treatment must begin instantly after obtaining spinal fluid for diagnostic examination and culture. Diagnosis is clinical with signs and symptoms of meningitis and is confirmed by spinal fluid and blood culture.

Early diagnosis and antibiotic therapy is critical. Although antibiotic treatment has greatly reduced mortality, the death rate is still about 10%. Vaccination is effective and recommended for those entering college or military service.

N. gonorrhoeae (*gonococcus*) is the cause of *gonorrhea*, a sexually transmitted infection discussed below.

Most Gram-Negative Bacilli Cause Intestinal and Respiratory Infections

There are a large number of Gram-negative bacillus species. *Helicobacter pylori, E. coli, Salmonella, Shigella,* and *Vibrio cholera* mainly cause gastrointestinal infections (Chapter 11), whereas *H. influenza* and *Legionella pneumophila* usually cause respiratory infections (Chapter 10). These are discussed in their respective chapters. *Haemophilus ducreyi* and *Chlamydiae* are Gram-negative bacilli that cause *sexually transmitted infections*, which are discussed as a separate topic at the end of this chapter. A few other gram negative species are discussed immediately below.

Bordetella Pertussis

Bordetella pertussis is a Gram-negative, short, thick bacillus that is the agent of **pertussis** or **whooping cough**, a highly communicable disease of children featuring paroxysms of severe coughing accompanied by a final inspiratory whistle—the "whoop." Illness, which typically begins as an ordinary upper respiratory infection in a child under five years of age, becomes progressively worse until severe coughing and inspiratory stridor occur. Asphyxia and death may follow, especially in infants. Diagnosis is by nasal or throat culture and quick lab tests to detect the organism. Antibiotic treatment is effective. Vaccination is preventive.

Pseudomonas Aeruginosa

Pseudomonas aeruginosa is an opportunistic pathogen that frequently causes hospital-acquired infections, particularly among burn victims, patients on ventilators, or any patient with a chronic, debilitating condition. *Pseudomonas* is very widely distributed and favors moist environments such as sinks, solutions, and toilets. Transmission to patients by healthcare workers is a special hazard in burn units and neonatal intensive care units. Many sites can be infected and infection is usually severe. *Pseudomonas* is also a common infection in the lungs of patients with cystic fibrosis (Chapter 22), and in immuno-compromised patients. Diagnosis is by culture. Antibiotic therapy requires careful selection because resistance is common.

Rickettsiae Are Transmitted by Insect Bites

The *Rickettsiae*, a group of obligate intracellular bacteria, are transmitted to humans by insect bites. Rickettsial diseases are caused by a family of Gram-negative, obligate intracellular coccobacilli. Most have an arthropod vector. Symptoms usually include sudden fever with severe headache, malaise, exhaustion, and a characteristic rash. Diagnosis is clinical and confirmed by specialized laboratory tests. Antibiotic therapy is effective.

R. rickettsii is one of a group of rickettsiae that are agents of **spotted fevers**, the most common of which is *Rocky Mountain spotted fever*. Named for the location of its initial discovery, it occurs mainly in the southeast United States and the Americas. Wood ticks and dog ticks are the natural reservoir and transmit disease by skin bite. Symptoms are high fever, headaches, and skin rash.

R. prowazeki is the agent of **epidemic typhus**. It is transmitted by body lice living on people who are in close quarters and do not change clothing regularly. It features prolonged high fever, severe headaches, and a skin rash.

R. tsutsugamushi is the agent of **scrub typhus**. The natural reservoir is rural rodents such as field mice. It is transmitted to humans by the bite of a type of mite commonly known as a *chigger*, or from person to person by body lice. Symptoms are fever, a primary bite lesion, a skin rash, and lymphadenopathy.

Spirochetes Are Corkscrew-Shaped

Spirochetes are flagellated, motile, very thin, corkscrew-shaped Gram-negative bacteria that are too thin to be seen by conventional light microscopy. Visualization requires special light microscopy technique.

Campylobacter Jejuni

Campylobacter jejuni is a common cause of enteritis. Infection typically is associated with consumption of undercooked poultry. Patients present with symptoms including abdominal pain, diarrhea (ranging from loose to bloody), fever, and malaise, all of which last from 24 hours up to a week or more. It responds to antibiotics, but is usually self-limiting. It can be associated with the development of transient paralysis (Guillain-Barré Syndrome, Chapter 19) approximately two to three weeks after infection.

Borrelia Burgdorferi

Lyme disease, named after the Connecticut town where it was first discovered in the 1970s, is caused by the spirochete *Borrelia burgdorferi*. It is transmitted from rodents to humans by the bite of a deer tick. About 20,000 cases are reported annually in the United States, most of them along the northeastern seacoast and around the Great Lakes.

Disease develops in three stages. Stage 1 begins with the tick bite. A red skin lesion with a pale center (*erythema migrans*) appears and spreads slowly, disappearing in four to eight weeks. Mild fever and lymphadenopathy may occur. Stage 2 infection features lymphadenopathy, recurrent fever, skin rash, joint and muscle pains, cardiac arrhythmias, and meningitis. Stage 3 is chronic disease, two to three years after the bite. It features arthritis, peripheral neuropathy, and meningitis. Symptoms may be mild or incapacitating. Early treatment with antibiotics is curative; however, later treatment is less successful.

Some Infections Are Caused by a Mixture of Organisms

Anaerobic infections are often caused by a mix of organisms, usually commensal bacteria resident at the site. For example, a mixture of oral anaerobes usually causes human bite infections. Anaerobic bacteria often live in abundance and in tissues where oxygen levels are low, mainly in the recesses of skin pores, gums, the crypts of tonsils, the vagina, and throughout the GI tract. These bacteria usually do not produce toxins. Nevertheless, infection may occur if equilibrium is upset by surgery, antibiotic use, poor blood supply, or tissue necrosis. Anaerobes also live in soil and other environmental sites and can cause disease by wound or food contamination.

Anaerobic infection often occurs as an abscess, which may seed other sites with infection by spread through the blood stream. For example, anaerobic bacteremia is the cause of some brain abscesses. Some cases of chronic sinusitis and otitis media are due to anaerobic infection. Dental and peritonsillar abscesses are also usually caused by oral anaerobes, and most tooth loss owes to chronic periodontitis caused by anaerobes living along the gumline. Aspiration of mouth or gastric contents into the lungs may cause anaerobic pneumonia or lung abscess, while bowel wall disruption may liberate intestinal anaerobes to cause liver or intraperitoneal abscesses.

Mycobacteria Cause Chronic Infection

Mycobacteria are a family of comma-shaped aerobic bacilli that cause chronic infection, TB foremost. Although they do not stain well by Gram stain, they stain easily with carbolfuchsin, a red dye (*Ziehl-Neelsen stain*), and hold fast to it so tightly that the dye cannot be washed away by strong acid (Fig. 4.8). Thus, they are referred to as **acid-fast**, a term widely used to denote all mycobacteria. *Mycobacterium tuberculosis* is the agent of human *TB* and *Mycobacterium leprae* is the agent of human *leprosy*. There are dozens of other varieties, but few are clinically important, with the exception of *Mycobacterium avium*, which infects birds, and *Mycobacterium bovinum*, which infects cattle. Both can infect humans. *Mycobacterium avium* is a frequent opportunistic pathogen in AIDS.

Mycobacterium Tuberculosis

Tuberculosis (TB) is a major chronic, progressive communicable disease caused by *Mycobacterium tuberculosis*.

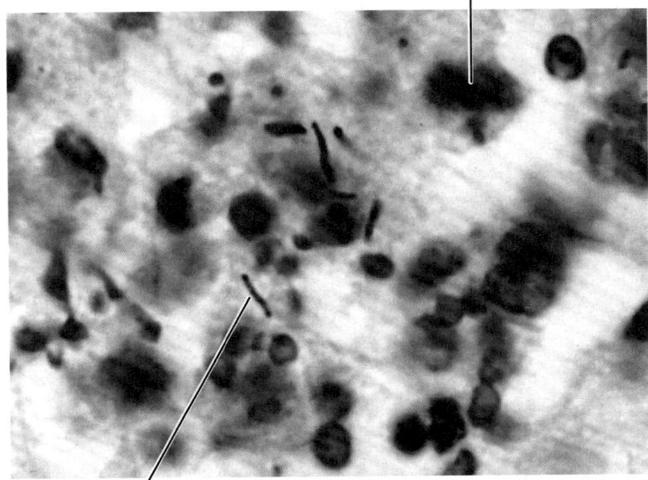

Figure 4.8 **Mycobacterium tuberculosis.** High-power microscopic study of acid-fast stain of sputum. Cells in the background are from the bronchi and mouth.

It occurs most commonly in the lungs and usually features a period of latency, sometimes for many years, following initial infection. Extrapulmonary sites (e.g., vertebrae, meninges) may also be infected. TB incites distinctive chronic granulomatous inflammation, which features a central area of semi-solid crumbly, necrotic tissue called **caseous necrosis** (Latin *caseus* = cheesy).

Epidemiology

Tuberculosis was known in ancient Egypt, and it continues to reside quietly in a latent state in nearly 2 billion people worldwide. The WHO reports that in 2011 there were about 8.7 million new TB cases (1 million of them in people with AIDS) and 1.4 million deaths. In the United States, TB infections rose in parallel with the AIDS epidemic. Since the mid-1990s, however, the incidence has declined to about 11,000 per annum in 2011.

Most new cases occur in immigrants. TB thrives amid poverty, crowding, and chronic debilitating illness. In the United States, TB is mainly a disease of the elderly, urban poor, and people with AIDS. Some ethnic groups have much higher susceptibility to infection—African Americans, Alaskan Inuit, Native Americans, Hispanics, and Southeast Asians. Also at increased risk are those with diabetes mellitus, lymphoma, chronic lung disease, malnutrition, alcoholism, and immunodeficiency. See *The History of Medicine*, "The History of Tuberculosis," available online at thePoint.com, which provides additional historical context.

Case Notes

4.13 Is Ruth more or less susceptible to TB than the average person?

Pathogenesis

Four points are central to understanding the pathogenesis of TB:

- Many are *infected*, but few are *diseased*. About 95% of infections are arrested in the lungs or bronchial lymph nodes by the immune system and become dormant without symptoms of disease. This initial infection is known as **primary TB**.
- In about 5% of initial infections, the immune system cannot control spread and infection immediately progresses to active disease, which is known as **primary progressive TB**.
- Almost 95% of clinical TB is **reactivation TB** (*secondary TB*), which arises from dormant *primary TB* because the patient has developed a chronic, debilitating disease such as diabetes, chronic lung disease, or malignancy.

- When reactivation TB occurs, by definition it is arising in someone who has been infected and *sensitized* by the original Type IV (T cell) hypersensitivity reaction (Chapter 3), which arrested the original infection. Later, when organisms reactivate, the sensitized immune system mounts an immediate Type IV immune reaction. The lesions of secondary TB are characterized by *granulomatous inflammation* (Chapter 2).

Figure 4.9 depicts the relationships among the different pathogenic pathways for development of TB. *Infection* occurs as organisms are seeded by airborne droplets from a diseased person into the lungs of a person not previously infected. The initial infection causes limited, asymptomatic damage before being stopped by cellular (Type IV) immunity. In many patients, however, the organisms are not killed but remain inactive, and may persist for many years until patient immunity declines and they reactivate as reactivation TB (secondary TB).

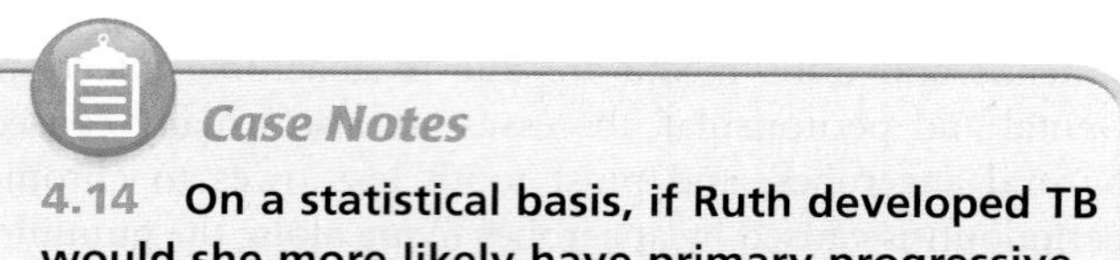

Case Notes

4.14 On a statistical basis, if Ruth developed TB would she more likely have primary progressive TB or reactivation TB?

Pathology

The initial pulmonary lesion of *primary TB* is usually a small focus of granulomatous inflammation with central caseous necrosis and multinucleated giant cells.

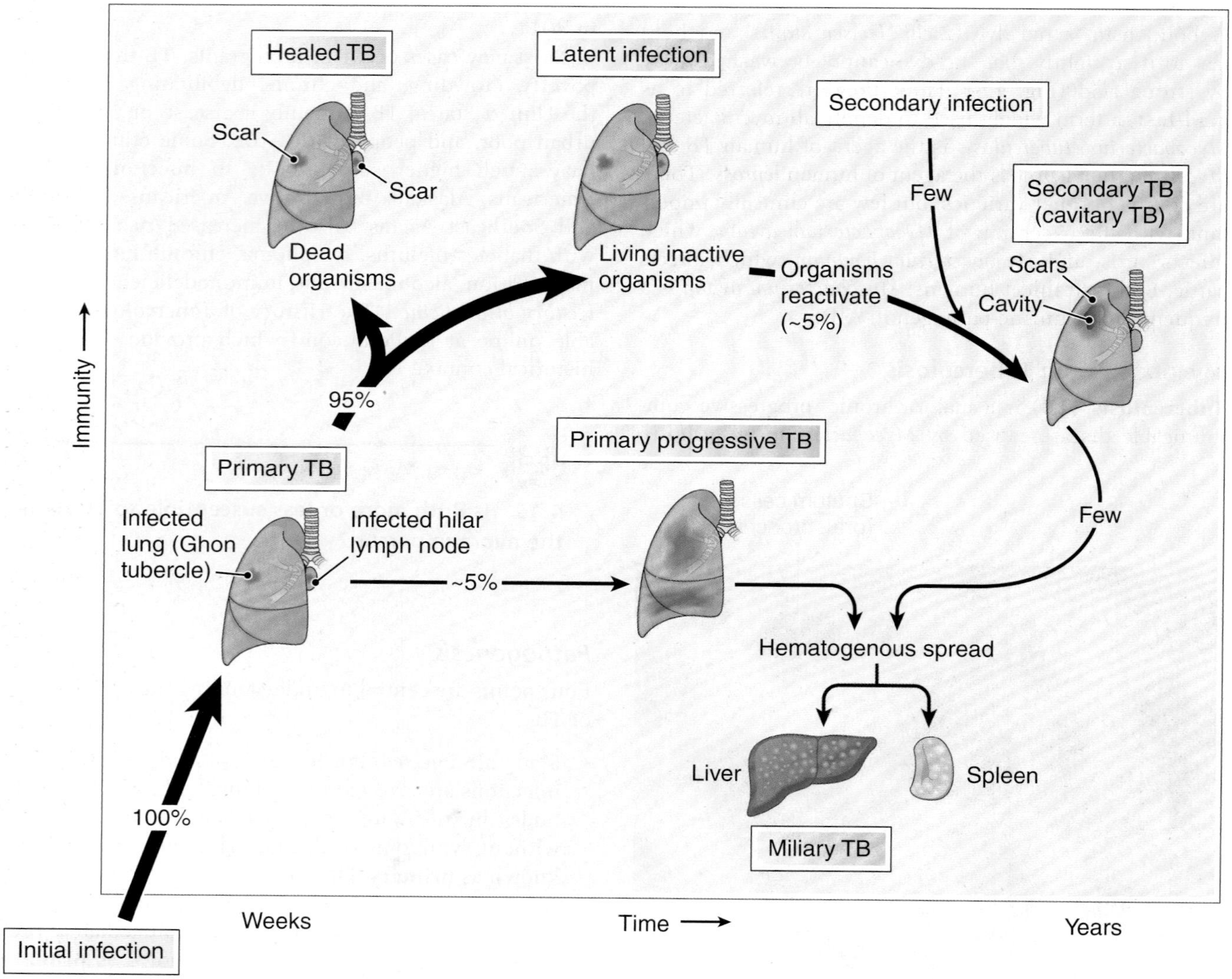

Figure 4.9 **The natural history of tuberculosis (TB).** Initial (primary) infection rarely progresses to disease because an effective immune response arrests the infection before it spreads beyond the initial site (Ghon tubercle), or beyond the lung and a few mediastinal (hilar) lymph nodes. Some initial infections (~5%) spread quickly and widely as *primary progressive TB*. Primary progressive TB produces many small lesions and is called *miliary* (seed-like) TB. Most clinical TB is *secondary TB* stemming from reactivation of dormant, old infections as microbes escape from their long containment by the immune system. A few cases of secondary TB arise from a second (new) infection.

Because 95% of such lesions are arrested by the immune system, with time the lesions scar and calcify to produce the typical lesions seen incidentally in patients dying of other disease or in chest X-rays. The initial lung lesion, called the **Ghon tubercle**, may be associated with similar lesions in infected mediastinal (hilar) lymph nodes—a combination known as the **Ghon complex** (Fig. 4.10).

Primary progressive TB usually occurs in children, in the immunodeficient, and in elderly or debilitated patients. Typically it occurs as extensive pulmonary TB, which sometimes is associated with widespread blood-borne spread to other organs, a pathological appearance known as **miliary TB** because various organs contain hundreds or thousands of tiny whitish lesions that look like millet seeds. Patients with primary progressive TB do not develop caseating granulomas like patients with reactivation TB, because in primary progressive TB the immune system has not been previously sensitized by infection.

Secondary TB (*reactivation TB*) accounts for about 95% of clinical TB. It is the pattern of disease that arises in previously infected and sensitized persons in whom the initial infection was contained by the immune system. This prior immune sensitization results in accumulation of macrophages and lymphocytes around foci of tubercle bacilli and necrotic tissue, which forms the **caseating granulomas** that are characteristic of reactivation TB.

Disease may develop within a few months of infection, but it more commonly occurs many years later, when patient resistance is weakened by some other condition and the original organisms reactivate, or (uncommonly) the patient is infected a second time. Secondary TB is almost always manifest by lesions in the apex of the lung (Fig. 4.11). The sensitized immune system of patients with reactivation TB causes the development of less numerous, larger lesions with central cores of caseous necrosis. Neglected cases may cavitate into airways, seeding bronchial tubes with millions of organisms, which spread more widely in the lungs and are coughed out as a cloud of infective organisms. Systemic spread to other organs may occur.

Diagnosis and Treatment

By its nature, primary infection is asymptomatic except in the 5% of patients in whom the initial infection overwhelms defenses (e.g., in those with AIDS) and becomes widespread as primary progressive TB.

The usual clinical onset of secondary TB is subtle. Low-grade fever, night sweats, mild malaise, weight loss, and poor appetite are hallmarks. In neglected cases, the patient gradually wastes away, accounting for the old name—*consumption*. As pulmonary disease progresses, patients begin to cough and produce sputum, which may be bloody.

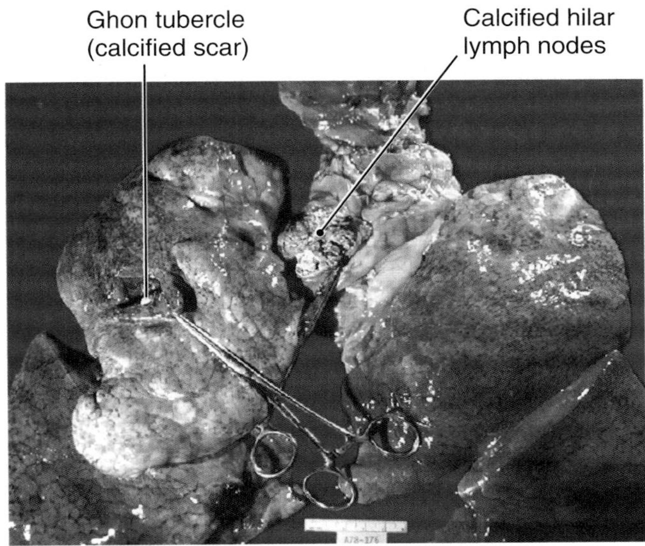

Figure 4.10 **Primary (healed) tuberculosis.** Forceps point to the Ghon tubercle. This infection was arrested after spreading to nearby hilar lymph nodes. Together these two lesions are known as the Ghon complex.

Clinical and chest X-ray findings may add up to a very high index of suspicion, but positive diagnosis rests on detection of acid-fast organisms in sputum cultures or smears or by other direct laboratory detection.

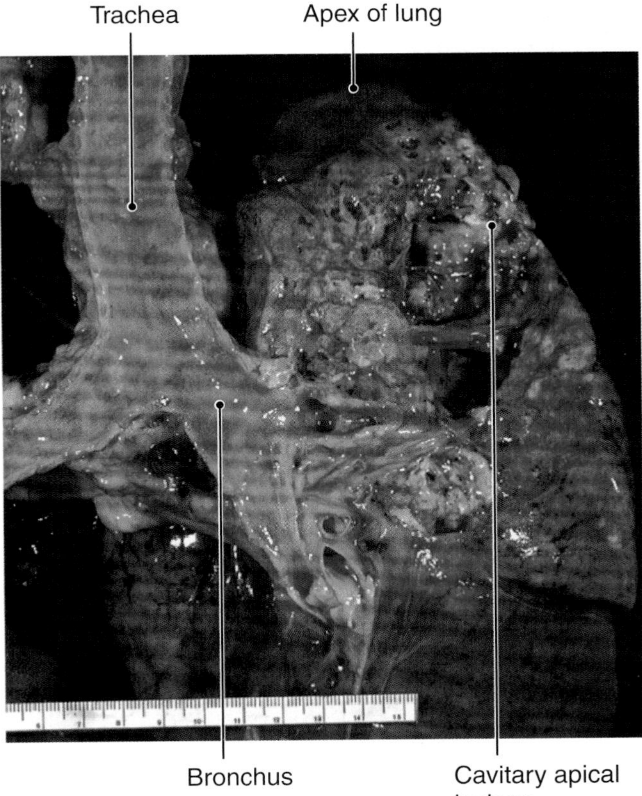

Figure 4.11 **Secondary pulmonary tuberculosis.** Most secondary pulmonary tuberculosis lesions occur in the lung apices.

The *purified protein derivative (PPD) test* (also known as the **Mantoux test**) is a skin test for *infection*. As it is positive in both latent and active cases, it is not diagnostic of active disease. The test is performed by injecting treated TB protein (tuberculin) into the patient's skin (see *The Clinical Side*, "The Mantoux Skin Test"). Previously infected patients have a positive test. Almost all patients with negative test results are not infected. A positive reaction means only that the patient has been infected, either a few weeks earlier or many years ago. The size of the reaction allows patients to be separated into groups based on their risk for developing active TB—smaller reactions indicate a greater risk for active disease. In a person with no risk factors, the injection site needs to swell to greater than 15 mm to count as a positive test.

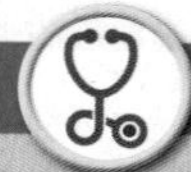

The Clinical Side

THE MANTOUX SKIN TEST (TUBERCULIN SKIN TEST, PPD TEST)

The Mantoux test is a skin test for prior infection and sensitization to the organism *Mycobacterium tuberculosis*. The test does not distinguish, however, between active and inactive infection. It is used to evaluate people with symptoms of TB or asymptomatic people who may have been exposed to TB. Some healthcare workers are screened at the beginning of their careers and regularly thereafter, to see if they convert from negative to positive, an occurrence that can indicate recent infection. Routine testing of persons at low risk is not recommended.

About two weeks after infection, the patient's immune system becomes sensitized enough to produce a positive skin test. A positive reaction is indicated by induration (firmness); erythema (redness) does not count. False-negative reactions may occur, for example, in AIDS or other immunodeficiencies, in sarcoidosis, in Hodgkin disease, and in overwhelming TB infection.

The test is performed by injecting a small amount of mycobacterium protein (PPD) into the skin of the volar surface of the forearm and observing the reaction between 48 and 72 hours later.

Results are interpreted according to the following table:

Interpretation of the Mantoux Test

Induration	Interpretation	Analysis
None	Negative	Not infected
5–10 mm	Positive	Infected; considered positive in patients at high risk for development of active TB. This group includes: • patients with AIDS, or on immunosuppression or steroid therapy; • persons with findings suggesting prior active pulmonary TB; and • people recently in contact with a patient with active TB.
10–15 mm	Positive	Infected; considered positive in patients at increased risk for developing active TB. This is a large and varied group, with preexisting risk factors for TB: • Recent immigrants • IV drug abusers • TB lab personnel • Residents of institutions such as prisons and nursing homes • Patients with chronic lung disease • Persons with malignancy or other debilitating disease
>15 mm	Positive	Infected; considered positive in healthy people with no known TB risk factors. Unlikely to develop active TB

The Mantoux skin test is mainly an epidemiological tool. In individual cases, it adds little value, for two reasons: 1) it is usually positive in diseased patients, but it is also positive in a large number of healthy people who have healed primary lesions only; and 2) false-negative tests are rather common: a test could be negative even in infected patients because immunity is compromised. It is generally used to identify exposures and therefore identify patients who may need to be followed with annual chest X-rays. In addition, a positive test may be helpful to exclude deep pulmonary fungus infections (Chapter 10), which can mimic pulmonary TB clinically.

Most TB occurs in poor, malnourished, immunodeficient or otherwise debilitated people, so the death rate is significant—about 10% among those with active disease and about 25% for those with disseminated disease. Because it is such a serious and widespread disease, public health considerations are paramount. Most patients can be treated at home provided they cover their mouth with each cough and restrict visitors. As many patients fail to follow treatment guidelines, public health personnel may monitor patients by personally delivering TB drugs and directly observing ingestion.

Case Notes

4.15 After recovery, Ruth was given a Mantoux test and reacted positive with induration of 13 mm. Does this mean she has active TB?

Mycobacterium Leprae

Leprosy is a chronic infection caused by *Mycobacterium leprae*, which has tropism for the low temperature found in peripheral nerves, skin, and the oral-respiratory mucous membranes. Before the development of effective treatment, people with leprosy became disfigured and disabled, and were shunned. It is now understood, however, that leprosy is poorly contagious, rarely causes death, and can be effectively treated.

Humans are the main natural reservoir for *M. leprae*. Armadillos are the only other confirmed reservoir. Infection is thought to be passed from person to person through nasal droplets and secretions. Casual contact does not seem to spread the disease. About half of people with leprosy appear to have contracted it through close, long-term contact with an infected person. Even after contact with the bacteria, most people do not become infected; healthcare providers often work for many years with people who have leprosy without contracting the disease. Most immunocompetent people who are infected with *M. leprae* do not develop leprosy because of effective immune response.

Annually about 250,000 new cases are reported worldwide, most from Africa, Southeast Asia, and South America. In the United States, about 150 new cases are reported each year. About 95% of people are naturally immune. For those who are not, how leprosy spreads is unclear. Spread in the United States may come from armadillos—20% of the wild population is infected. Contrary to prior notions, recent evidence suggests that new U.S. cases were not contracted while traveling abroad.

Leprosy affects mainly the skin and peripheral nerves. Nerve involvement causes numbness and weakness in areas controlled by the affected nerves. Recognizing skin lesions usually requires special expertise. Diagnosis is clinical and confirmed by biopsy. Treatment is with antimycobacterial drugs.

Pop Quiz

4.20 True or false? Anaerobic bacteria are present in the mouth and are responsible for aspiration pneumonia.

4.21 True or false? Staphylococcus and streptococcus are Gram-positive bacteria that can infect a number of different organs.

4.22 True or false? In testing for TB, a PPD test of less than 15 mm is always considered negative.

4.23 True or false? *Mycobacterium leprae* is the most virulent mycobacterium.

4.24 True or false? TB has no predilection for ethnic groups.

4.25 Are most cases of TB primary or secondary TB?

4.26 Gas gangrene is caused by which Clostridial species?

4.27 A new teenage mother refuses antibiotic treatment for her newborn. What is the newborn at risk for?

Fungus Infections

Fungi are nucleated cells with a cell wall. They grow in two forms: as multicellular filaments (*hyphae*) called **molds** or as single cells called **yeast**. Many pathogenic fungi are *dimorphic*—they are yeast at human body temperature and mold at room temperature.

A fungus is a **mycosis**. The four main clinical forms of fungal infection are the following:

1. *Superficial mycoses* are common and confined to skin, hair, and nails.
2. *Subcutaneous mycoses* involve the skin, subcutaneous tissues, and lymphatics and rarely spread further.
3. *Endemic mycoses* are caused by dimorphic fungi and produce serious systemic disease in otherwise healthy people.
4. *Opportunistic mycoses* can cause fatal systemic disease in the immunosuppressed, or less commonly in patients with implanted catheters or other medical hardware.

Candida Infections Are Usually Superficial and Minor

Candida are a group of fungi that usually live as commensals on skin and in the mouth, GI tract, and vagina. *C. albicans* is the most common of human fungal infections (**candidiasis**, or **moniliasis**). Most infections originate when normal flora breach the skin or mucosal barriers. Infection is usually confined to skin or mucosa, but may spread systemically as a much more serious illness, particularly in patients who have a low blood neutrophil count (neutropenia) due to leukemia, chemotherapy, bone marrow transplantation, or immunosuppression. The most common *C. albicans* infections are diaper rash and vaginitis. Skin infections tend to occur in skin folds and are red, weepy, and itchy. Vaginal candidiasis occurs most often when vaginal floral equilibrium is upset by hormone changes, such as in pregnancy, or as a result of antibiotic therapy for a nonvaginal infection. Symptoms are itching and white vaginal discharge. Diabetics and burn patients are particularly susceptible to superficial candidiasis. Bloodstream infection may occur with indwelling intravenous catheters. Diagnosis is by microscopic study of vaginal exudate or skin scrapings, or by culture. Papanicolaou (PAP) smears can sometimes identify yeast from cervical swabs during annual gynecologic exams. Antifungal drugs are effective.

Deep Mycoses Are More Serious

Blastomycosis (*Blastomyces dermatitidis*), **coccidioidomycosis** (*Coccidioides immitis*), **cryptococcosis** (*Cryptococcus neoformans*), and **histoplasmosis** are somewhat similar endemic diseases. Collectively they are referred to as the **deep mycoses**. The organisms are widespread in soil and dust or in areas with heavy bird droppings. Infection is acquired by inhalation; therefore, the lungs are the primary site of infection. As in TB, the initial lung infection may be arrested by the immune system and reignite later if the patient becomes debilitated or immunodeficient, or disseminated disease may occur with initial exposure. Immunosuppressed patients and patients with defective white cell function (e.g., leukemia) are most at risk. Diagnosis relies on chest X-ray suspicion, culture of sputum or other fluid, or direct detection by lab techniques. Antifungal drug therapy is effective in immunocompetent patients.

Patients who are immunosuppressed, on steroid therapy, or who have severe burns, diabetes, autoimmune disease, or impaired white cell function are also at risk for disseminated infection by *Aspergillus* (**aspergillosis**) and *Zygomycetes* (*Mucor* or *Rhizopus*), fungi that are widespread in nature. Depending on the clinical situation, antifungals may not be effective and surgical evacuation and debridement of the diseased tissue and its accompanying infectious organisms is sometimes required to remove the infection (e.g., mucormycosis of the nasopharynx and sinuses).

Pop Quiz

4.28 Name the endemic mycoses.

4.29 Mucor infection in the nasal passages of a diabetic patient is a surgical emergency. What is the main host factor that predisposes to many fungal infections including *Mucor*?

Parasite Infections

Recall that a parasite is an organism that lives in or on another organism and benefits by deriving nutrients for itself at the expense of the host. The worldwide burden of parasitic disease is enormous. Most cases occur in developing nations with limited healthcare resources, and the majority of cases probably go unreported. Estimates of the number of malaria cases range from 300 million to 2 billion. Table 4.2 presents broad-brush estimates of the prevalence and mortality of parasitic disease. Such statistics can vary, however, sometimes greatly, from one expert analysis to another.

Humans are parasitized by three varieties of parasites: *protozoa*, *worms*, and *ectoparasites*.

Protozoa Are Unicellular Motile Pathogens

Protozoa are unicellular, motile, microscopic pathogens with a nucleus. They are larger and more complex than are bacteria and fungi.

Malaria is caused by one of four species of tiny *Plasmodium* amoebae (Fig. 4.12), dozens of which can fit within a red blood cell (RBC). Transmission is from infected to noninfected persons by the bite of an infected mosquito. No immunity develops and reinfection may occur. At a minimum, hundreds of millions of people are infected annually, mostly in tropical climates, and about a million people die annually of it.

Malaria parasites invade RBCs and destroy them in hemolytic cycles as immature new organisms burst from infected red cells, causing episodes of hemolysis, fever, and

Table 4.2 Worldwide Human Parasitic Infections

Disease Category	People Infected (approx.)	Deaths per Year (approx.)
PROTOZOA	**2 BILLION**	**1 MILLION**
Leishmaniasis (WHO 2013)	12 million	Few thousands
Malaria (WHO 2009)	225 million	780,000
Amebiasis	50 million	40,000
Giardiasis	1 billion	Few thousands
HELMINTHS (WORMS)	**4 BILLION**	**1 MILLION**
Intestinal nematodes (WHO 2005)	2 billion	Few thousands
Filariasis (WHO 2013)	120 million	Few thousands
Schistosomiasis (WHO 2011)	240 million	250,000
Tapeworms	20 million	Few thousands

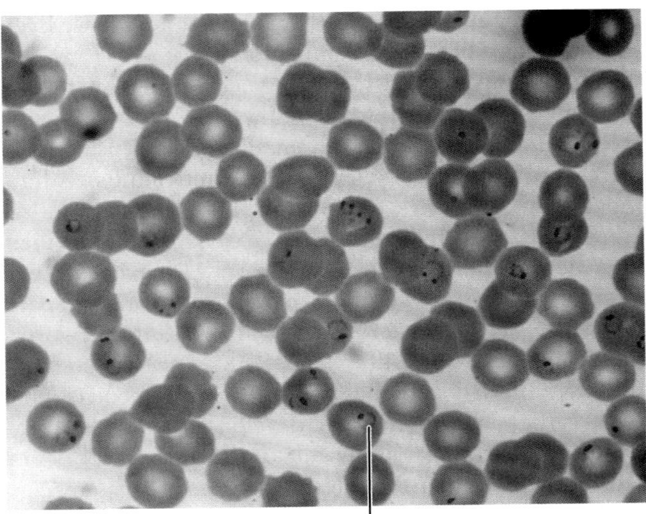

Figure 4.12 **The blood in malaria.** Red cells contain *Plasmodium* organisms.

jaundice every 48 to 72 hours as new generations of parasite reproduce. Splenomegaly is common. Ninety percent of fatal cases occur in sub-Saharan Africa. Children are especially vulnerable. Diagnosis is by seeing *Plasmodium* in peripheral RBCs. Treatment and drug prophylaxis are effective and vary, depending on the species and drug sensitivity. Antimalarial drug prophylaxis is effective for all types, but some drug-resistant strains now exist.

Amebiasis is infection by *Entamoeba histolytica*, a protozoan that infects hundreds of millions of persons annually on the Indian subcontinent, Mexico, and South America. Most cases (90%) are asymptomatic but symptomatic infection can be fatal. Infection is acquired through consumption of food contaminated by human feces that contains amebic cysts, which are capsules of amebae designed to survive in the environment. After ingestion, the amebae break out of the cyst in the intestine; some invade the colon mucosa and others form new cysts that are passed in feces. Invasion of bowel mucosa produces abdominal pain and diarrhea. Invasion into the portal blood often produces amebic liver abscesses, but brain, lung, and other organs may be involved.

Leishmaniasis is a chronic inflammatory disease of skin, mucous membranes, and viscera caused by species of *Leishmania*, a microscopic, intracellular protozoan that infects white blood cells (WBCs). It is transmitted from infected animals by sandflies and is most common in underdeveloped nations. Diagnosis is by visualization of the parasite in blood cells aspirated from the spleen, bone marrow, liver, or lymph node. Drug therapy is effective.

Trypanosomiasis is a disease caused by several varieties of *Trypanosoma*, microscopic protozoa that infect blood and are transmitted from human to human by insects. One variety, African trypanosomiasis, or sleeping sickness, is transmitted by the tsetse fly and causes intermittent fevers, enlarged lymph nodes and spleen, and progressive brain dysfunction. **Chagas disease** is a variety of trypanosomiasis occurring mainly in South America. It features periorbital edema, fever, hepatosplenomegaly and, later, myocardial infection. Cats are a natural reservoir. Transmission is by nocturnal bite of the "kissing bug"—quarter-inch brown insects with a long proboscis that nest near vertebrates and suck blood at night. Diagnosis and drug therapy for trypanosomal disease is similar to that for leishmaniasis.

The protozoan *Giardia* causes **giardiasis**. Annual incidence in the United States is about 2.5 million cases. Perhaps one billion people are infected worldwide. It is acquired by ingesting fecally contaminated water or unwashed vegetables or fruits. Most infections are asymptomatic, but some cause acute or chronic diarrhea. *G. lamblia* is not killed by water chlorination; it must be filtered out. Giardiasis is a common infection in campers who drink stream water, especially near cattle or human habitation. Diagnosis is by microscopic detection in feces or duodenal aspirate. Drug therapy is effective.

Cryptosporidiosis and **microsporidiosis** are infections caused by small protozoa, which may cause diarrhea in otherwise healthy people but are most notable as opportunistic intestinal pathogens in AIDS and other immunodeficiency states. Diagnosis is by microscopic detection in feces. Drug therapy is effective.

Trichomoniasis is a STI of the vagina or male genital tract with *Trichomonas vaginalis*, which is discussed below.

Helminths Are Worms

Worm (**helminth**) infections deserve special attention because they infect about 2.5 *billion* people. Prevention is the key to reducing helminth infections.

Most helminth infections are little more than a nuisance, but many patients are severely affected. Worms vary in length from a few millimeters to over a meter, and most migrate from the point of entry through various organs as they grow and mature. Many have complex life cycles that require passage through other hosts before reinfecting humans. *Peripheral blood eosinophilia is a hallmark of helminth infections.* Diagnosis is by detection of the worm or eggs by biopsy or stool examination. Treatment with specialized antihelminthic drugs is effective for all of the types discussed here.

Roundworm Infections

Roundworms (*nematodes*) infect either the intestines or subcutaneous tissues. The clinical presentation of roundworm infections varies greatly; however, most are accompanied by increased numbers of blood eosinophils (*eosinophilia*).

Filariasis (Latin *filum* = thread) is an infection by small (1–3 cm) roundworms transmitted by mosquitoes and found most commonly in Asia and Africa. The most common variety infests lymphatics and subcutaneous tissue and can cause massive lymphedema of the scrotum and legs (elephantiasis).

Intestinal roundworms are common in tropical climates but rarely cause serious problems. They live in the intestine and spread by oral-fecal contamination. **Ascariasis** is caused by intestinal infestation with the *Ascaris* species of large roundworms. It affects over one billion people worldwide. Transmission is by oral-fecal contamination. The life cycle is complex—ingested eggs hatch and larvae invade the intestinal mucosa to enter the blood, where they migrate to the lungs, crawl up the trachea, and are coughed out or swallowed. They reenter the intestine, where they attach to the mucosa and suck blood for nourishment. Most infections are asymptomatic but can be suspected by blood eosinophilia. Severe infections may cause intestinal bleeding, anemia, or intestinal obstruction.

Hookworms are intestinal roundworms that infect over one billion persons, mostly in tropical climates. Their life cycle is similar to that of *Ascaris* but they initially enter through skin and then infect the blood. Most infections are asymptomatic, but severe infestation may cause intestinal bleeding and anemia.

Pinworm infection, caused by *Enterobius vermicularis,* a small (1 cm) roundworm, is a very common pediatric infection in the United States. Transmitted by the oral-fecal route, pinworms live in the intestine and usually cause no symptoms; however, in some patients the worms crawl onto perianal skin and cause intense itching. Diagnosis can be made by pressing clear acetate tape to the perianal region and examining it microscopically for worms or eggs.

Trichinosis is infection by the *Trichina* roundworm, and is transmitted by eating inadequately cooked infected pork in which worm larvae are encysted. The ingested larvae mature in the intestine, invade blood, and spread to muscle, where they remain and cause muscle pain, fever, and periorbital edema.

Flatworm Infections

Flatworms (*flukes*) are *trematodes* that infect blood vessels, GI tract, lungs, or liver. They are categorized by the organs they infect—blood vessels, GI tract, liver, lungs, or brain.

Schistosomiasis *is by far the most important of all worm infections.* It is caused by one of several flukes from the *Schistosoma* family, which mainly infects the vasculature of the GI and genitourinary tract. Schistosomiasis affects about 4% of the world population, and is second only to malaria in terms of death and disability. It is most common in central Africa and other tropical climates. Eggs are passed in urine and stool into water, from whence larvae infect snails and mature before reentering water to invade the skin of humans and disseminate widely via blood. Severe infections are characterized by intense liver, intestinal, and bladder inflammation.

Tapeworms (*cestodes*) are segmented, ribbon-shaped worms that infect about 50 million people worldwide, most commonly in developing nations. Tapeworms cycle through three stages—eggs, larvae, and adults. Adults inhabit the intestines of the final host, humans. Adult tapeworms that infect humans are named after their intermediate host: the fish tapeworm (*Diphyllobothrium latum*), the beef tapeworm (*Taenia saginata*), and the pork tapeworm (*Taenia solium*). Eggs laid by adult tapeworms living in human intestines are excreted with feces into the environment and ingested by an intermediate host (e.g., cattle), in which larvae develop, enter the circulation, and encyst in the musculature (e.g., beef, pork) or other organs. When the intermediate host is eaten (e.g., undercooked steak), cysts are liberated by the digestive process and develop into adult tapeworms in the human intestines, and the cycle begins again. Though infection is common, infected people are often not ill, although they may suffer weight loss and minor abdominal discomfort and may become alarmed upon finding pieces of worm in their stool.

The *pork* tapeworm can cause severe illness if *eggs* (as opposed to larvae in muscle) are ingested from fecally contaminated food or drink. The eggs release a form of the worm that invades blood vessels and disseminates to deposit widely in many tissues as small (1 cm) cysts, *cysticerci* (**cysticercosis**). Cysticerci do not cause inflammation, but remain alive and create problems by mass effect. Severe infestation of the brain can cause seizures or death. Surgical removal may be necessary.

Echinococcosis (*hydatid disease*) is a tapeworm infection caused by larvae of several varieties of tapeworm passed back and forth between dogs and cows: cattle eat grass contaminated by dog feces; dogs eat cow flesh. Human infection occurs by ingestion of food contaminated by infected dog feces. Larvae invade blood vessels and lodge in deep organs, especially liver and lungs, where they may mature into large cysts (*hydatids*) several centimeters in diameter. Most infections are acquired in childhood but do not become symptomatic for many years. Symptoms relate to size of the cysts. Drug treatment is effective but surgical excision of some hydatids may be necessary.

Ectoparasites Live on Skin or Hair

An **ectoparasite** lives on the surface of the host.

Lice (*pediculosis*) are wingless, blood-sucking insects that infest the hair of the head, body, or pubis. They are discussed more fully in Chapter 21 (Fig. 21.19). *Head lice* live in scalp hair and are transmitted by close contact. In the United States, they occur predominantly in the hair of young schoolchildren, mainly girls. They do not transmit disease. *Body lice* live in clothing or furniture but feed on human blood. They are vectors for scrub typhus (discussed above). Pubic lice live in coarse genital hair, or sometimes beard or eyelashes. They do not transmit disease.

Scabies is an infestation of the skin mite *Sarcoptes scabiei*. It lives only in the skin of humans and is passed by direct contact. It causes intensely itchy (pruritic) red papules (small bumps) around the wrists, waistline, genitals, and the webs of the fingers. Diagnosis is clinical and by demonstration of the insect in skin scrapings. Treatment is with topical drugs.

Pop Quiz

4.30 True or false? Cooking pork prevents trichinosis.

4.31 True or false? Echinococcus infects the liver and is acquired by ingesting contaminated food.

4.32 What is the most common protozoal infection in the world? In the United States?

4.33 Schistosomes can infect which organs?

4.34 What skin surfaces are infected by scabies?

Sexually Transmitted Infections

The sexual revolution is over and the microbes won.

P. J. O'ROURKE (B. 1947), AMERICAN HUMORIST AND POLITICAL COMMENTATOR, IN "GIVE WAR A CHANCE"

Sexually transmitted infection (STI) is infection communicated by sexual contact. HIV/AIDS is an STI discussed in Chapter 3 because it primarily attacks the immune system.

Virtually any variety of organism can cause STI:

- *Viral STIs* include genital and anorectal warts caused by HPV, genital herpes, and HIV/AIDS.
- *Bacterial STIs* include syphilis, gonorrhea, and *Chlamydia* and *Mycoplasma* infections.
- *Parasitic STIs* include trichomoniasis, scabies (skin mites), and pediculosis (lice).

Other infections, not considered primary STIs, can be transmitted sexually, most notably viral hepatitis (Chapter 12). Gastrointestinal infections such as salmonellosis and shigellosis (Chapter 11) can be transmitted by oral or anal sex. A further point is that spread of some STIs creates open sores and mucosal lesions that facilitate the spread of other STIs. For example, heterosexually transmitted HIV/AIDS is more common in sub-Saharan Africa and Southeast Asia than in developed nations because of the higher prevalence of non-HIV STIs.

STI statistics usually underestimate the number of cases because many cases are asymptomatic and unknown to the patient; others are symptomatic but remain untreated because of ignorance, poverty, or shame, and still others are treated but unreported to health authorities. The most reliable data come from nations with a legal requirement that certain STIs must be reported to health authorities. For nonreportable diseases, data are based on expert estimates and some voluntary data from physician offices.

STIs stand apart from many other infections because of the following:

- Immunity against reinfection is often not achieved, making reinfection possible.
- Diagnostic testing is often not readily available or is expensive and slow.
- Many cases are treated syndromically; that is, treatment is directed at the organism most likely to produce the clinical findings at hand, and a definitive diagnosis is never established.
- Infection is often asymptomatic, especially in women, which increases the likelihood of transmission, including maternal-fetal transmission.
- More than one STI may be present at the same time.
- Patient follow-up and contagion tracing is often absent or uncertain.
- No cure is available for viral STIs such as HPV, genital herpes, or HIV/AIDS.

Important aspects of some sexually transmitted diseases are summarized in Table 4.3.

Diagnosis Is Often Difficult or Incomplete

Diagnosis of STIs depends upon the type of organism suspected. Bacteria such as *N. gonorrhoeae* (Fig. 4.13) can be easily detected in a smear of urethral fluid in a male or cervical swab in a female. On the other hand, demonstration of spirochetes in fluid expressed from a syphilitic chancre requires darkfield microscopy, which is usually available only in large STI clinics or public health laboratories.

Culture is not often helpful. Most STI organisms are difficult to culture in clinical settings because the organisms are fastidious and require exceptionally careful handling or elaborate laboratory technique.

Chlamydia and related organisms can be identified by DNA profile, which is usually slower and more expensive than circumstances usually allow.

Blood testing for antibodies is not useful except in syphilis. Antisyphilis antibodies remain present for a lifetime, so tests are useful only as an epidemiologic tool to prove the presence of current *or past* infection.

Table 4.3 Selected Sexually Infections (United States)

Condition	New Cases per Year, 2010	Agent	Lesions	Associated Conditions and Complications	Therapy
*Trichomoniasis***	~ 7,000,000 new infections, but only ~ 150,000 sought care	*Trichomonas vaginalis*	Males: urethritis, balanitis Females: vaginitis	None	Special antimicrobials
Human papilloma virus infection**	~ 6,000,000 new infections, but only ~ 375,000 sought care	*Human papillomavirus*	Either sex: condyloma acuminatum	Males: none Females: dysplasia or cancer of the vulva, vagina, cervix	Excision or destruction
Genital herpes **	~ 2,000,000 new cases, but only ~ 230,000 sought care	*Herpesvirus*	Genital and oral vesicles, ulcers	Adults: Recurrent eruptions. Neonates: fatal infection from mother	Antiviral drugs reduce frequency and duration of eruptions
Chlamydia infection	~ 1,200,000 new infections	*Chlamydia trachomatis*	Either sex: lymphogranuloma venereum Males: proctitis, urethritis, prostatitis, epididymitis Females: cervicitis, salpingitis	Males: urethral stricture Females: tubal obstruction, ectopic pregnancy, infertility Neonates: conjunctivitis, pneumonia	Antibiotics
Gonorrhea	~ 340,000 new infections	*Neisseria gonorrhoeae*	Either sex: urethritis, proctitis, pharyngitis Neonates: conjunctivitis Males: prostatitis, epididymitis Females: vulvovaginitis, cervicitis, salpingitis	Either sex: disseminated infection Males: urethral stricture Females: ectopic pregnancy, infertility.	Antibiotics
Syphilis	~ 46,000 new cases reported in various stages	*Treponema pallidum*	Either sex: *Primary*: chancre *Secondary:* skin disease, condyloma lata, lymphadenopathy	Either sex: *Tertiary*: dementia, aortic disease	Penicillin
HIV infection	~ 43,000 new cases	Human immunodeficiency virus	Either sex: Initial skin rash	Either sex: opportunistic infections, neoplasms	Anti-HIV drugs suppress but do not cure disease
Chancroid	Rare in the U.S., very common in Africa and SE Asia	*Haemophilus ducreyi*	Either sex: painful genital ulcers	Important cofactor in spread of AIDs in Africa and SE Asia	Antibiotics
Molluscum contagiosum infection	Very common, exact incidence unknown	*Molluscum contagiosum* virus	Either sex: small white papules on genitalia (or other sites, not always due to sexual contact)	None	None

*New case data for 2010, U.S. Centers for Disease Control and Prevention and other sources.

**Mandatory reporting is not required for these STI infections. The figures reported are best source estimates, some of which vary widely.

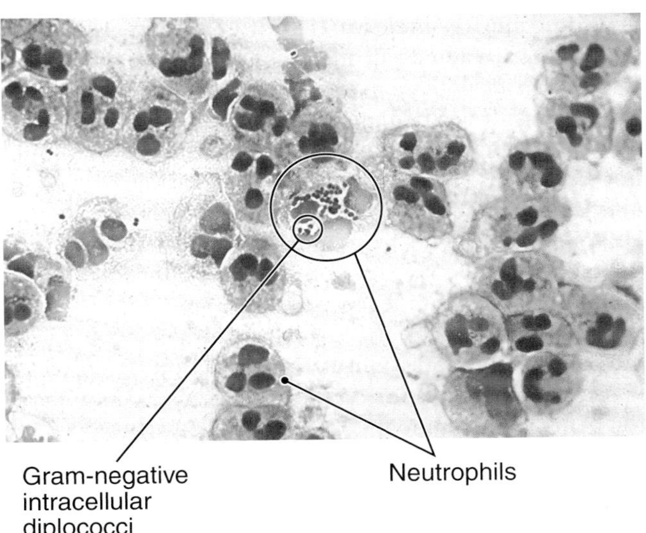

Figure 4.13 **Gram stain of urethral exudate in a case of gonorrhea.** Note numerous neutrophils and *intracellular* (phagocytized) Gram-negative (red) diplococci in the cytoplasm of a neutrophil.

Prevention of STI Requires Safe Sex Practices

Major developments in STI prevention are a multivalent vaccine for human papilloma virus (HPV), which is available for young women and men and a vaccine for hepatitis B.

The only certain way to prevent STI is by not having sex, a decidedly unpopular option. For those having sex, the best way to prevent STIs is to use a condom and have sex with only one person who is not having sex with others—limiting the number of sex partners is very important in the control of STI. These alternatives are not popular and widely ignored. For example, patients treated in STI clinics report an average of three partners in the prior three months and dozens of partners over their lifetime. Reinfection is common because of failure to follow safe sex practices.

Male and female condoms are effective at preventing transmission of most STIs, including HIV/AIDS, but many couples resist using them. Condoms, however, cannot prevent genital herpesvirus and human papillomavirus infection, or parasite infestation, which can be spread by pubic, groin, or other anatomic contact. Other protective devices (e.g., dental dams and female condoms, for oral sex) can also be used. After sexual contact, urination and thorough genital washing with soap and water also decrease the risk.

Reinfection Often Occurs

The usual treatment for bacterial STIs is antibiotics, which is usually successful. Antiviral drugs are effective in modifying the course of herpes and HIV/AIDS, but do not eliminate the infection. Highly active antiretroviral therapy (HAART) for the treatment of HIV infection has markedly improved the longevity of patients with HIV/AIDS. Currently, patients no longer commonly die of the infection itself. Instead, other concurrent diseases, such as hepatitis C-related liver disease (which causes cirrhosis), metabolic disease, cardiac disease, and others are increasingly becoming the predominant causes of morbidity and mortality in this patient population. Following STI treatment, reinfection is very common because of failure to use condoms or other devices and the practice of having sex with multiple partners, most of whom also have multiple partners. Antiparasitic drugs are usually effective in parasitic STIs.

Remember This! STIs are difficult to prevent only because of failure to follow safe sex practices.

Gonorrhea Is a Bacterial STI

Gonorrhea is an STI caused by the Gram-negative coccus *Neisseria gonorrhoeae* (Fig. 4.13). It infects about 340,000 people each year in the United States. It is second only to *Chlamydia* (discussed below) as a cause of STIs.

Infection in men usually causes acute urethritis, but the prostate and epididymis can also be involved (Chapter 16). Urethral strictures may develop. Infection in women is less symptomatic but may have consequences that are far more serious (Chapter 17). Acute infection may involve the vagina, cervix, or fallopian tubes and when symptomatic is characterized by vaginal discharge (*leukorrhea*), lower pelvic pain, and dysuria. About 1 in every 200 college-aged and young adult women is infected, and most are asymptomatic. Repeated infection is a consequence of unsafe sexual practices. Repeated infection, even if asymptomatic, can lead to chronic inflammation and scarring (*pelvic inflammatory disease*) that may cause infertility or ectopic pregnancy. Infected mothers can infect the fetus with gonorrhea as it passes through the vaginal canal.

Infection may also occur in the throat or anus (proctitis). Septicemia and disseminated infection may occur in immunodeficient patients. Neonatal infection can occur in the eyes of an infant passing through an infected birth canal. In developed nations, routine instillation of antibiotics in the eyes of newborns prevents disease, but gonococcal blindness continues to occur in some developing nations. Infection is diagnosed by Gram stain of exudate, culture, and other laboratory methods. Antibiotic treatment is effective. Treatment of sexual partners is necessary to prevent spread.

Trichomoniasis Is an Amebic STI

Trichomoniasis is a STI of the vagina or male genital tract with *Trichomonas vaginalis*, an ameba-like organism present normally in the vagina of about 10% of otherwise healthy women. New infections in either sex are often asymptomatic. Women are most often symptomatic and have a mild vaginitis featuring leukorrhea and burning that is often precipitated by a change in the vaginal environment that causes the organism to flourish. Risk factors include pregnancy and the loss of normal vaginal bacterial flora (which inhibit *T. vaginalis* growth) following antibiotic therapy for an unrelated condition. Infection also may cause urethritis, vaginitis, or occasionally cystitis, epididymitis, or prostatitis. Diagnosis is by microscopic examination of vaginal or urethral smears. Treatment with special antimicrobials is effective.

Chlamydia Infection Is the Most Common Sexually Transmitted Infection Worldwide

Chlamydiae are a group of Gram-negative obligate intracellular bacteria. The most important by far is *C. trachomatis*, which causes a sexually transmitted genitourinary infection. *C. trachomatis is the most common sexually transmitted disease (STI) in the world.* In 2008, over 1.2 million cases of chlamydial STI were reported in the United States, more than three times the number of gonorrhea cases. In the developing world, *C. trachomatis* is also the agent of *trachoma*, a common cause of blindness (Chapter 20).

Remember This! ***Chlamydia and gonorrhea are the most common causes of STI-related infertility.***

Genital infection by the L subtype of *C. trachomatis* causes **lymphogranuloma venereum**, a chronic, ulcerative venereal disease that is endemic in Asia, Africa, the Caribbean, and South America. The infection initially appears as a small lesion on genital mucosa or skin. Two to six weeks later, inguinal, pelvic, or perirectal lymph nodes enlarge and may rupture, creating chronic draining sinus tracts with scarring and strictures of the urethra, vagina, or rectum. Diagnosis is clinical. Antibiotics are effective treatment.

In women as in men, *Chlamydia* behaves much the same as gonorrhea. About 5% of college-age and young adult women are infected. Clinical diagnosis is challenging because many patients, men and women, are asymptomatic carriers. Although early detection is desirable because a single dose of antibiotic is curative, *Chlamydia* infection is difficult to prove. Most patients are treated based on clinical evidence, not laboratory proof.

Human Papillomavirus Is an STI That Causes Dysplasia and Cancer

Human papillomavirus (HPV) is a family of over 100 viruses that cause a variety of skin and genital lesions. Apart from largely innocuous *Trichomonas vaginalis* infections (discussed below), HPV is far and away the most common *serious* STI in the United States. Some types of HPV cause common skin warts, especially in children, and are passed by casual skin-to-skin contact. Other types are passed mainly by sexual contact and cause both benign and malignant genital neoplasms. HPV genital infection is common; perhaps 6 million new HPV infections are reported in men and women in the United States each year, but infection is probably much more widespread, with some authorities estimating that perhaps 5–10% of the U.S. adult population is infected at any given time. Rates are highest in young adults and decline rapidly in older adults, as the number of sexual partners declines. Recently developed vaccines promise to decrease infection rates.

Sexually transmitted HPV produces two different but related lesions in women (Chapter 17): **condyloma acuminatum** (*genital wart*) and *squamous carcinoma* of the vulva, vagina, or, most commonly, of the cervix. *Condyloma acuminatum* is the more common of these two lesions. It is a benign, cauliflower-like growth of the cervical, vaginal, or vulvar squamous mucosa. It should not be confused with the similar-appearing *condyloma lata* of secondary syphilis (discussed below). Genital HPV may be passed to infants at vaginal delivery, and infected infants may develop multiple, life-threatening papillomas of the upper respiratory tract.

In men (Chapter 16) *condyloma acuminatum* is the most common expression of HPV infection. Dysplasia is less common and occurs on the glans penis. Carcinoma of the penis is uncommon.

Condyloma and dysplasia may be removed by surgery, cryotherapy, electrocautery, or laser, or they may be treated topically by certain antimitotic chemotherapy drugs used in cancer treatments. Invasive carcinoma requires surgery

HPV vaccination is effective for prevention.

Syphilis Is a Chronic STI Caused by Treponema pallidum

Syphilis is a chronic sexually transmitted disease caused by the spirochete *Treponema pallidum*. It is communicated across minute breaks in skin or mucosa by sexual activity or, in the case of congenital syphilis, across the placenta from an infected mother.

Confirmed cases of syphilis must be reported to public health authorities. In 2011 about 46,000 new US cases were reported. This figure includes new cases diagnosed at each of the four stages of syphilis, not just fresh primary infections. Though the least common of sexually transmitted diseases, it is one of the most serious because untreated infection can cause dementia, severe disability, or death.

Clinical Features

Untreated syphilis develops through four stages: *primary, secondary, latent,* and *tertiary*. The hallmark lesion of **primary syphilis** is the **chancre**, a hard, moist, painless ulcer, illustrated in Figure 4.14, which appears at the site of implantation about two to four weeks after infection. The lesion, which teems with spirochetes, is usually on the penis; or sometimes on the scrotum, groin, anus, or mouth. With or without treatment, the chancre disappears in three to six weeks. Syphilis induces the immune system to produce antispirochete antibodies, which are useful in diagnosis, but *do not confer immunity against reinfection in the future, nor do they eliminate the current infection.*

In untreated syphilis, the *chancre* resolves spontaneously and is followed in most untreated patients by **secondary syphilis**, a combination of lymphadenopathy and skin lesions on the palms of the hands and the soles of the feet. These lesions also teem with infectious spirochetes. In moist areas of the body, such as the axillae, groin, inner thigh, and anogenital region, broad-based, cauliflower-like epidermal growths known as **condyloma lata** may develop.

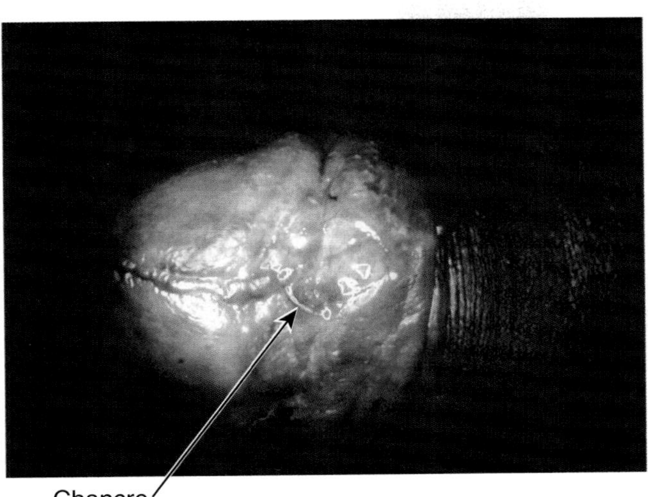

Figure 4.14 **Primary chancre of the penis.** Examination of fluid expressed from the lesion showed numerous spirochetes.

Latent syphilis is subclinical. In about one-third of untreated patients, the disease reemerges from latency 5 to 20 years later as **tertiary syphilis**. Most tertiary syphilis affects the cardiovascular system and usually presents as *syphilitic aortitis*. Inflammation of the aortic wall results in aneurysmal dilation of the proximal aorta. Dilation can stretch the aortic valve such that valve leaflets cannot close, and valvular insufficiency (regurgitation) occurs (Chapter 9).

The nervous system is infected (**neurosyphilis**) in all patients with tertiary syphilis, but only in about 10% does it become the main problem. In some patients the posterior (dorsal) nerve roots of the spinal cord are affected, which causes a sensory defect and abnormal gait, a syndrome known as **tabes dorsalis**. Finally, chronic infection of the brain may cause atrophy of the cerebral cortex, which produces a dementia known as **general paresis**.

T. pallidum can cross the placenta to cause **congenital syphilis**. Because signs of maternal syphilis may be difficult to detect, and because fetal effects may be devastating or fatal, serologic testing for syphilis is mandatory during pregnancy. Nearly half of all pregnancies in women with untreated syphilis end in spontaneous abortion.

Diagnosis and Treatment

Fluid expressed from the chancre of primary syphilis or the skin lesions of secondary syphilis contains spirochetes that can be demonstrated by a special microscopic technique.

Laboratory tests for antibodies are the mainstay of diagnosis. *T. pallidum* infection causes production of two types of antibodies in blood—those directed specifically against *T. pallidum* (*antitreponemal antibodies*) and other antibodies (*reagins*) that react with *cardiolipin*, a phospholipid present in human tissue and in *T. pallidum*.

Tests for **reagin antibodies** are widely used as initial screening tests because they are cheap, quick, and reliable. The most commonly used are the Venereal Disease Research Laboratory (VDRL) and rapid plasma reagin (RPR) tests. They usually become positive within six weeks of infection, remain positive in secondary syphilis, and disappear with successful treatment. They are usually not positive, however, in tertiary syphilis. False positive tests are fairly common, especially in the presence of systemic lupus erythematosus (SLE), rheumatoid arthritis (RA) or other autoimmune disease, pregnancy, and intravenous drug abuse.

Tests for **antitreponemal antibodies** are used as a follow-up to verify positive reagin tests. The test most often employed is the fluorescent treponema antibody (absorbed) test, the FTA-ABS. They, too, become positive within six weeks of infection, but they remain positive for life. Detection of *antitreponemal antibody* is a very reliable indication that the patient has syphilis or has had syphilis (treated or untreated) at some time. Although false-positive and false-negative test results occur in antitreponemal antibody tests, they are uncommon.

Neither antibody produces immunity nor fights the infection; they are merely used as passive markers of the disease.

Intramuscular injection of long-acting penicillin is curative.

Chancroid Is an STI Caused by Haemophilus ducreyi

Chancroid is infection of the genital skin or mucous membranes caused by *Haemophilus ducreyi*. It is characterized by painful papules, ulcers, and marked inguinal lymphadenopathy, which may progress to nodal abscess. It is rare in the United States. It occurs most frequently in Africa and Southeast Asia as genital ulcers among men who frequent prostitutes. The open sores are an important cofactor in the spread of heterosexual AIDS. Diagnosis is usually clinical because the organism is difficult to confirm by laboratory methods. Antibiotic treatment is effective.

Molluscum contagiosum Is an Innocuous, Self-Healing STI

Molluscum contagiosum is an innocuous, self-healing viral disease that causes eruptions of small (a few mm) white papules on the skin of the genitals or on the thighs or buttocks. Nonsexual transmission may occur. The eruptions look like small, white abscesses but without the redness and tenderness of an abscess, and they contain a pearly, cheesy material instead of pus. Lesions disappear spontaneously in a week or so. Treatment is not necessary.

Case Notes

4.16 **During Ruth's hospitalization, a routine RPR blood test for syphilis was positive. Does this mean Ruth has syphilis?**

Pop Quiz

4.35 What are the first and second most common sexually transmitted diseases in the United States?

4.36 What mode of transmission is responsible for the infections of Lyme disease?

4.37 How does each stage of syphilis manifest?

4.38 True or false? Chlamydia can be cured with a single dose of antibiotics.

4.39 True or false? Condyloma lata is a benign, cauliflower-like growth of the cervical, vaginal, or vulvar squamous mucosa caused by HPV.

4.40 True or false? Antisyphilis antibodies remain present for a lifetime.

4.41 True or false? Immunity against reinfection with STIs prevents patients from acquiring the same STI a second time.

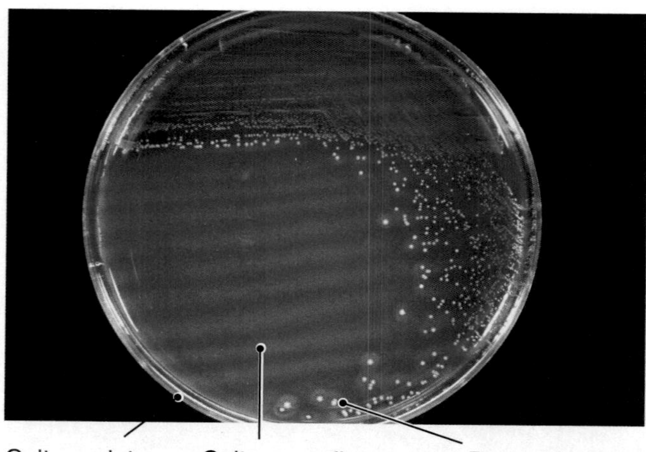

Figure 4.15 **Bacterial culture.** In this plate of culture material consisting of blood and agar, each colony consists of growth from a single bacterium. All of the colonies on this plate are similar and probably composed of the same organism. Individual colonies can be sampled for further identification and antimicrobial sensitivity testing.

Laboratory Tools

Laboratory tools are important in investigating the cause of infection, choosing appropriate therapy, and monitoring patient progress. The simplest, quickest, and most widely available and reliable tool is the Gram stain, explained earlier. Merely identifying the shape (bacillus or coccus) and the Gram stain properties (Gram-positive or Gram-negative) can be invaluable and, when combined with clinical findings, may be enough to make a provisional diagnosis and begin therapy. Occasionally other organisms (e.g., fungi) may be visible on a Gram stain. Viruses and other small nonbacterial pathogens are usually not visible by Gram stain study but may be detected by other stains and techniques in particular circumstances.

Of perhaps greater importance is microbial culture, as is illustrated in Figure 4.15. Culture is generally considered the "gold standard" for documenting an infectious organism. Obtaining a specimen for culture may be as simple as swabbing pus from a wound or collecting a urine specimen. On the other hand, obtaining a specimen may require an invasive technique such as a spinal tap to obtain cerebrospinal fluid in cases of suspected meningitis.

Cultures are performed by smearing the specimen on one or more types of special nutrient *media*, which are incubated at body temperature to encourage the growth of organisms. Typically, the specimen is smeared in a way that spreads the specimen thinly, so that it is likely that a single bacterium will be isolated and reproduce itself to form a colony apart from others. Colonies are pure cultures of a single bacterium, and can be resampled and recultured to determine other bacterial characteristics.

The type of nutrient media varies according to the type of specimen and the organism suspected. For example, stool specimens are usually cultured on media that inhibit the growth of normal intestinal bacteria and encourage the growth of intestinal pathogens such as *Shigella* or *Salmonella*. Throat swabs of suspected streptococcus infection, an important cause of pharyngitis, are inoculated onto media especially conducive to the growth of streptococci but not to other bacteria.

If a suspected pathogenic organism grows, it is subjected to other identifying tests and re-cultured (regrown) in the presence of different antibiotics, a technique known as antimicrobial susceptibility testing (Fig. 4.16). This helps clinicians determine which antibiotics inhibit growth or kill the organism and which have no effect. Modern antimicrobial susceptibility testing is automated, but the underlying principle is illustrated by the following simple manual technique:

1. Bacteria from a single colony are suspended in fluid and poured onto a culture plate in such a way as to spread organisms evenly across the entire surface.
2. Small discs soaked with various antibiotics are placed on the plate surface; antibiotic diffuses outward into the medium.
3. The plate is incubated for 24 hours and then examined.
4. Antibiotics that kill or inhibit bacterial growth are characterized by a ring of no growth around the disc.

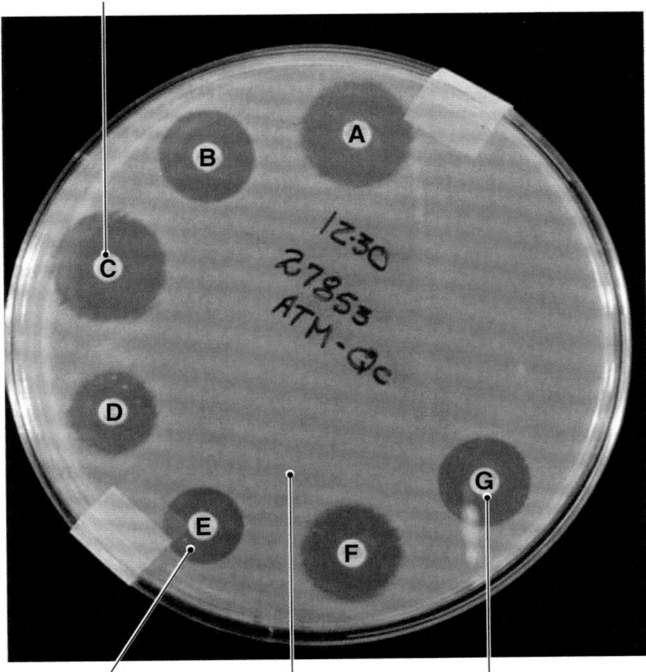

Figure 4.16 **Antibiotic sensitivity testing.** The surface of the culture plate is overgrown by bacteria that were collected from a single colony of the culture plate in Figure 4.13 and evenly spread across the surface. White paper discs soaked with different antibiotics are placed on the plate, and the plate is incubated 24 hours. Clear areas around discs are where bacterial growth has been inhibited. Bacterial sensitivity to a particular antibiotic is related to the size of the zone of inhibited: a large zone suggests the antibiotic may be effective in treating the patient's infection.

Like bacteria, fungi are relatively easy to culture and identify using similar techniques. Viruses, *Chlamydia*, *Rickettsia*, and *Mycoplasma* are difficult to culture and require more elaborate techniques, expertise, and equipment.

Detection of microbial antigens and antibodies in blood is a mainstay of diagnosis for nonbacterial infections, especially for virus infections. For example, the laboratory diagnosis of viral hepatitis (Chapter 12) depends exclusively on detection of viral antigens and antibodies in blood.

Finally, direct detection of organisms in tissue, fluids, or smears may be accomplished by a variety of immune and genetic techniques or by direct microscopic examination. For example, the *Plasmodium* parasite of malaria can be seen in RBCs on ordinary smears of peripheral blood. In the case of intestinal parasitism, the eggs or the worms themselves can be detected by direct microscopic examination of stool smears.

In addition, newer molecular techniques have been developed to detect organisms in tissues or other samples (see *Molecular Medicine*, "Polymerase Chain Reaction").

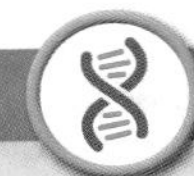

Molecular Medicine

POLYMERASE CHAIN REACTION

Culture of an organism is generally considered the "gold standard" for diagnosis of certain infections. Culturing is a time-consuming process, however, and some organisms cannot be easily cultured, if at all. To circumvent these limitations, molecular techniques, such as *polymerase chain reaction (PCR)*, can be used to detect the presence of organisms. The PCR concept is simple. A specimen is mixed with an enzyme, polymerase, which detects exceedingly small amounts of DNA or RNA and synthesizes a very large amount of identical DNA or RNA, enough to study and identify by other laboratory techniques. Incidentally, PCR is the technique used to capture DNA in crime investigations.

Pop Quiz

4.42 True or false? Molecular techniques are now considered the "gold standard" for identification of bacteria.

4.43 What are the two most important traditional techniques used to identify organisms?

Case Study Revisited

"I knew she was sick when she didn't want a cigarette." The case of Ruth R.

Ruth R.'s case illustrates that influenza can be extremely serious, even fatal, especially in elderly or debilitated persons. The most significant facts in this case were the history of cigarette smoking and the failure to obtain an influenza vaccination. When the patient first appeared, she was in the prodromal phase of influenza. Mild lymphocytosis confirmed the viral nature of her illness. Her second appearance was at the height of the acute phase of the influenza syndrome, but the marked granulocytosis (neutrophilia) and widespread pulmonary infiltrates suggested a secondary bacterial infection. Bacterial pneumonia can be a nosocomial (hospital- or clinic-acquired) infection, and she might have picked it up on her initial visit. An important question is whether or not antibiotics should have been prescribed at that point.

In light of the near-fatal course of this case of influenza, it is tempting to believe that doing so might have prevented the bacterial pneumonia. There is no guarantee, however, that the bacterium that infected her would have been susceptible to the antibiotic chosen, and there remains the possibility that killing off her normal flora might have encouraged infection by an even more dangerous bacterium.

Points to Remember

- Cigarette smoking causes lung disease and increases risks associated with other lung disease.
- Influenza vaccination is important in elderly or debilitated people, especially those with lung disease.
- Bacterial pneumonia is a common complicating illness in patients with chronic lung disease.

Chapter Challenge

CHAPTER RECALL

1. A 14-year-old Caucasian female presents to the emergency room complaining of fevers, aches, and diarrhea of several days duration. Her body is covered in a sunburn-like rash. Her mother, who has accompanied her to the hospital, states that her daughter recently started her period and has been using tampons. What is the likely pathogen?
A. *Streptococcus pneumonia*
B. *Staphylococcus aureus*
C. *Rickettsiae rickettsii*
D. *Yersinia pestis*

2. What is the likely cause of disease in a patient with a recent travel history to sub-Saharan Africa, episodes of fever and jaundice occurring every 48–72 hours, and a peripheral blood smear that reveals both anemia and the causative agent?
A. *Plasmodium*
B. *Giardia lamblia*
C. *Entamoeba histolytica*
D. *Trypanosome*

3. A 5-year-old African American boy presents to his doctor with nausea and vomiting, hoarseness, and loud rapid breathing. Physical exam reveals a swollen neck, a gray inflammatory membrane in the tonsillar area, and stridor. At 24 hours, his cultures grew anaerobic, Gram-positive bacilli. What is the pathogen?
A. *Bordetella pertussis*
B. *Listeria monocytogenes*
C. *Corynebacterium diphtheriae*
D. *Nocardia*

4. Which of the following is a corrupt form of normal brain protein, and responsible for *Creutzfeldt-Jakob* and *mad cow disease*.
A. Virus
B. Bacteria
C. Worm
D. Prion

5. What virus is responsible for invading motor neurons in the brain or spinal cord, causing paralysis?
A. Poliomyelitis
B. Measles
C. Mumps
D. Rubella

6. What is the ectoparasite responsible for the transmission of Leishmaniasis?
A. Deer ticks
B. Fleas
C. Sandflies
D. Mosquitoes

7. What is the most common cause of infection-associated death?
   A. Respiratory infection
   B. Diarrheal disease caused by infection
   C. HIV/AIDS
   D. Malaria
8. Diagnosis of which of the following worm infections is made by pressing clear acetate tape to the perianal region and examining it microscopically?
   A. Hookworm
   B. Pinworm
   C. Tapeworm
   D. Flatworm
9. A 2-year-old Hispanic male presents to his physician with blisters, some of which have ruptured and coalesced into small patches of red, "honey-crusted" lesions covered with dried exudate. Gram stain of fluid isolated from the blisters reveals Gram-positive cocci in long chains. What is the pathogen?
   A. *Candida*
   B. *Staphylococcus aureus*
   C. *Rickettsiae rickettsii*
   D. *Streptococcus pneumonia*
10. True or false? An epidemic is when a disease is found in a geographic area above normal levels.
11. True or false? A patient with gonococcus should be treated for *Chlamydia*.
12. True or false? Most exotoxins come from living Gram-negative bacteria and can cause vascular collapse.
13. True or false? Intestinal nematodes are the most common parasitic infection in the world.
14. True or false? Viruses are the only obligate intracellular pathogens.
15. True or false? Candida is the most common endemic fungal infection.
16. Match the following infective agents with the types of inflammatory cells usually associated with their infection. Some infective agents have more than one answer:
   i. Neutrophils
   ii. Lymphocyte and monocyte
   iii. Eosinophils
   iv. Granulomas
   A. Viruses
   B. Bacteria
   C. Mycobacteria
   D. Helminthes
   E. Fungi
17. Match the following sexually transmitted disease pathogens to the genitourinary lesions that are associated with them. Some lesions may have more than one answer.
   i. *Chlamydia trachomatis*
   ii. *Neisseria gonorrhea*
   iii. *Treponema pallidum*
   iv. *Haemophilus ducreyi*
   v. *Human papillomavirus*
   vi. *Herpes simplex virus*
   A. Ulcer, rash on the palms and soles, damage to aorta and CNS
   B. Crops of small, painful blisters in skin or mucosa, which fade in a week
   C. Urethritis, prostatitis, and epididymitis in men, and salpingitis in women
   D. Condyloma acuminatum or dysplasia and cancer of the cervix
   E. Chancroid, papules, ulcers, and marked inguinal lymphadenopathy, which may abscess

CONCEPTUAL UNDERSTANDING

18. What are the stages and pathological findings of *Mycobacterium tuberculosis?*
19. Name several transformative viruses and their associated cancers.
20. Put the following in order as they relate to the course of an infection and define them: recovery, acute phase, incubation, convalescence, and prodromal period.
21. What are the laboratory tools used in investigating the cause of infection?
22. Why must the influenza vaccine be given yearly?

APPLICATION

23. Discuss the methods for, and pitfalls of, diagnosing syphilis.
24. Name the organ systems most commonly affected by infections. What do they share in common?
25. Using examples from the text, discuss problems associated with the use of antibiotics.
26. An 18-year-old sexually active female goes to her doctor for a routine check-up before leaving for college. What tests do you recommend? Are there any vaccines you would recommend?

CHAPTER

5

Neoplasia

Contents

Chapter Objectives

After studying this chapter, you should be able to complete the following tasks:

CHARACTERISTICS AND DEFINITIONS OF NEOPLASIA

1. Explain how the name of a tumor provides insight into its composition and prognosis and whether there are any exceptions to this naming convention.
2. List the seven hallmarks of cancer.

THE CAUSES OF CANCER

3. Using examples from the text, explain the various etiologies responsible for carcinogenesis.

THE MOLECULAR BASIS OF NEOPLASIA

4. Name the four types of genes mutated in neoplasia.

THE BIOLOGY OF NEOPLASTIC GROWTH

5. Discuss the importance of heterogeneity, doubling time, growth fraction, angiogenesis, metastatic potential, and immunodeficiency in tumor prognosis.

CLINICAL MANIFESTATIONS

6. Describe the local and systemic (paraneoplastic) effects that might manifest secondary to tumor presence.

CLINICAL AND LABORATORY ASSESSMENT OF NEOPLASMS

7. Discuss the available methods for diagnosing malignancy, as well as their benefits and caveats.
8. Compare and contrast the gross and microscopic appearances of benign versus malignant neoplasms, and explain the difference between histologic grading and clinical staging of a malignancy.

CANCER TREATM

9. Discuss the t
to patients d

EARLY DETECTIO OF CANCER

10. Describe the
breast, prost

Case Study

"It's not my normal bleeding." The case of Brenda T.

Chief Complaint: Abnormal vaginal bleeding

Clinical History: Brenda T. was a 29-year-old Caucasian woman who saw her gynecologist for vaginal bleeding. "It's not my normal bleeding," she said. "My periods are regular as clockwork, but this bleeding tends to come between periods. It's not much, and I've noticed it sometimes occurs after I have sex." Further questioning revealed that she had her first Pap smear in college and it had been abnormal. "They told me it was a virus infection, so I didn't pay much attention." She had not had a Pap smear or seen a physician since. Sexual history revealed frequent unprotected sex with multiple male partners.

Physical Examination and Other Data: Brenda was of average height and physically fit. Vital signs were normal. Physical examination revealed that the cervix was indurated and distorted by an irregular, friable mass about 3 cm in diameter, which bled briskly when biopsied.

Clinical Course: Microscopic study of the biopsy revealed poorly differentiated squamous cell carcinoma. Further clinical evaluation concluded that the tumor may have extended beyond the cervix into parauterine tissue. There was no evidence of blood-borne metas

tissue. Radical hysterectomy was performed. Surgeons found that the tumor had extended beyond the cervix into parauterine tissue and into the upper vagina, but had not reached the pelvic wall. The peritoneum showed no tumor implants. The cervix, uterine body, fallopian tubes, ovaries and the upper one-third of the vagina were removed along with parametrial soft tissue and lymph nodes. Brenda recovered slowly and was discharged home on the ninth hospital day.

Pathologic study of the surgical specimen revealed a large tumor mass of carcinoma that invaded beyond the wall of the uterus into the upper vagina, but did not involve other parts of the specimen. A focus of carcinoma *in situ* with "HPV effect" was present in the adjacent cervical squamous epithelium. One of 17 excised lymph nodes contained metastatic carcinoma.

Brenda was treated postoperatively with chemotherapy and external pelvic radiation. Five years after diagnosis there was no evidence of local recurrence or further metastasis and she was otherwise in apparent good health.

Note: HPV infection is also an important aspect of the Chapter 17 case study, *"I can't get pregnant." The case of Susan A.*

The same people who tell us that smoking doesn't cause cancer are now telling us that advertising cigarettes doesn't cause smoking.

ELLEN GOODMAN (B. 1941), U.S. POLITICAL COLUMNIST, AS QUOTED IN NEWSWEEK (P. 17, JULY 28, 1986)

Cancer is second only to cardiovascular disease as a cause of death in the United States. Of the 300 million people living in the United States in 2011, approximately 12 million (4%) were living with cancer. This figure represents the prevalence of cancer—the fraction of a given population with a certain condition at a certain moment. Figure 5.1 shows the incidence (number of *new* cases per year) of new cancer cases and cancer deaths in the United States for 2011 (skin cancers excluded). Lung cancer is the most common cause of cancer death in both sexes. In females,

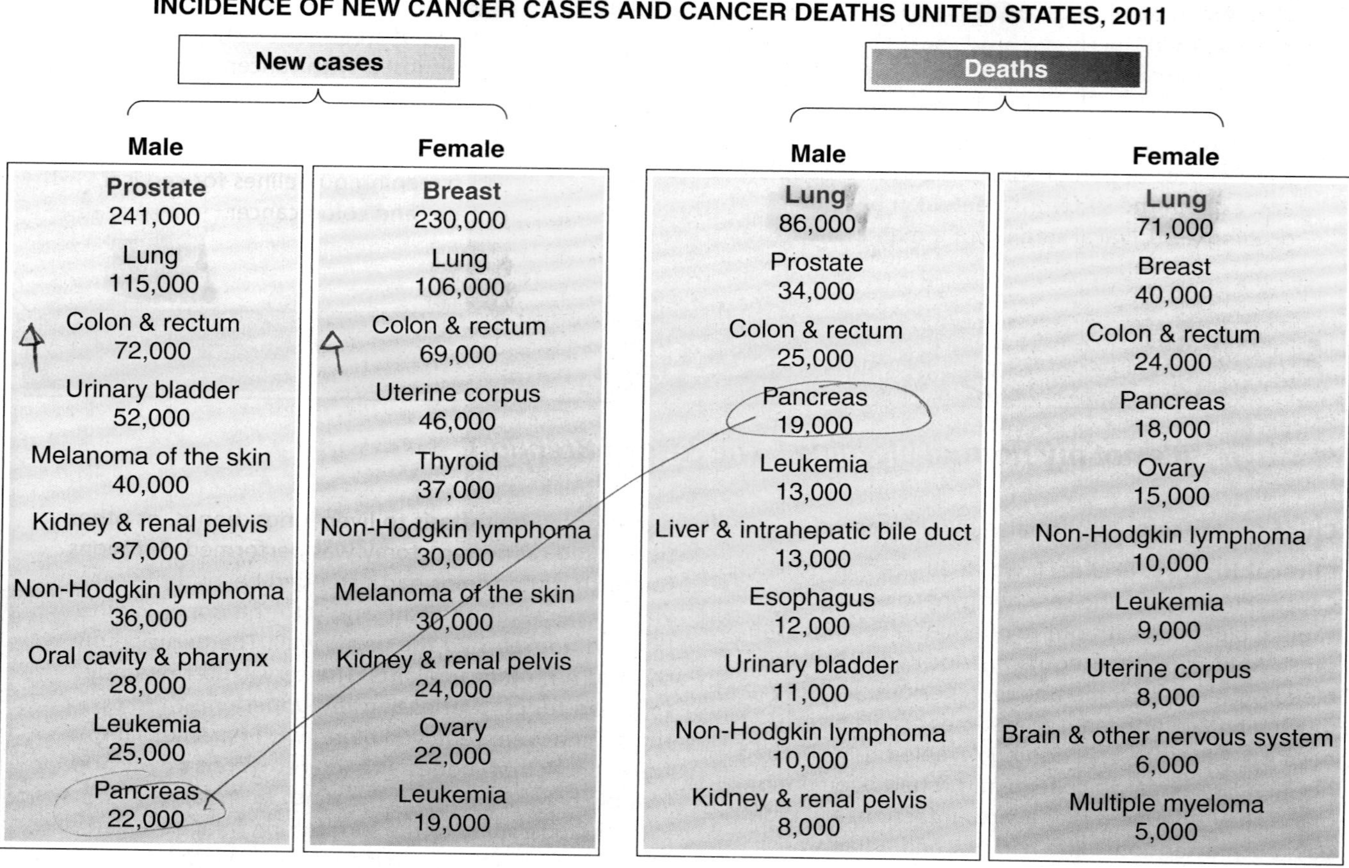

Figure 5.1 **New cancer cases and deaths, 2011.** Skin cancers are not included because they are very common but rarely fatal (the exception is malignant melanoma, which is uncommon but sometimes fatal). (Data rounded to nearest whole thousand. Modified from American Cancer Society, 2011).

breast cancer is second to lung cancer as a cause of death, while in males prostate cancer is the second most common fatal cancer. Note that prostate cancer is the most common of all cancers. Nevertheless, although 241,000 men developed prostate cancer in 2010, only 34,000 died of it because prostate cancer is not nearly as deadly as most other cancers. In contrast, the number of new cases of pancreatic cancer in both sexes and the number of deaths is roughly equal because pancreatic cancer is usually quickly lethal. Furthermore, note than *when the numbers for both sexes are summed, colon and rectal cancer rises to second place behind lung cancer as the second most common new cancer (141,000) and the second most common cause of cancer death (49,000).*

Characteristics and Definitions of Neoplasia

Neoplasias may be benign or malignant. A **benign** growth is one that usually does not have the capacity to cause death. A **malignant** growth is one that has the capacity to cause death. A **cancer** is a malignant neoplasm.

The growth process is critical in the development of neoplasms. Recall from Chapter 2 that normal cells die and are replaced regularly by new ones in an orderly growth process. Normal tissue growth is tightly regulated and occurs as a part of normal development or adaptation to the environment. This growth is governed by "go" and "stop" signals controlled by genes. If the "go" switch is stuck in the "on" position, or if the "stop" switch does not allow cells to die, *uncontrolled* growth (a neoplasm) is the result. A **neoplasm** is any *abnormal* growth of new cells. We also refer to neoplasms as *tumors*, a word meaning "mass" or "swelling." Tumors may be benign or malignant:

- A **benign** tumor is one that usually does not have the capacity to cause death. Notable exceptions are benign brain tumors, which may grow slowly but can cause death by virtue of their critical location. For example, a meningioma, a benign neoplasm of the meninges surrounding the central nervous system, can kill by compressing the brain.
- A **malignant** tumor is one that has the capacity to cause death. A **cancer** is a malignant tumor.

Oncology is the study of neoplasms. It is important to note that *benign* and *malignant* are defined primarily by behavior. Gross and microscopic appearances are important, but in the end it is behavior that matters. The following **biologic capabilities** are the seven hallmarks of neoplasia.

1. Self-sufficiency of growth ("go") signals
2. Evasion of growth suppression ("stop") signals
3. Cells divide indefinitely (unlimited reproduction)
4. Avoid apoptosis (programmed cell death)
5. Recruit nutrients via growth of new blood supply (angiogenesis)
6. Invade nearby tissue and spread to distant tissue (a feature of *malignant* neoplasms only)
7. Evade immune surveillance (the cancer detection and elimination aspect of the immune system)

It is also important to know that though most neoplasms form tumor masses, not all do. Leukemia is an example: malignant white blood cells (WBCs) are spread everywhere in the blood and bone marrow and do not form a tumor mass.

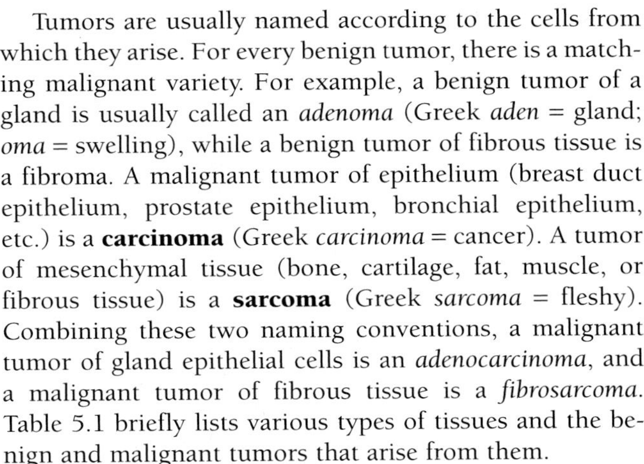
Tumors are usually named according to the cells from which they arise. For every benign tumor, there is a matching malignant variety. For example, a benign tumor of a gland is usually called an *adenoma* (Greek *aden* = gland; *oma* = swelling), while a benign tumor of fibrous tissue is a fibroma. A malignant tumor of epithelium (breast duct epithelium, prostate epithelium, bronchial epithelium, etc.) is a **carcinoma** (Greek *carcinoma* = cancer). A tumor of mesenchymal tissue (bone, cartilage, fat, muscle, or fibrous tissue) is a **sarcoma** (Greek *sarcoma* = fleshy). Combining these two naming conventions, a malignant tumor of gland epithelial cells is an *adenocarcinoma*, and a malignant tumor of fibrous tissue is a *fibrosarcoma*. Table 5.1 briefly lists various types of tissues and the benign and malignant tumors that arise from them.

Some names do not follow convention so neatly. According to the conventions above, *lymphoma* ought to be a benign neoplasm of lymphocytes. A lymphoma, however, is a malignant neoplasm of lymphocytes. Similarly, a *melanoma* is a malignant tumor of melanocytes, the pigment-producing cells in skin.

Case Notes

5.1 Brenda's tumor did not kill her. Does that mean it is not malignant?

Pop Quiz

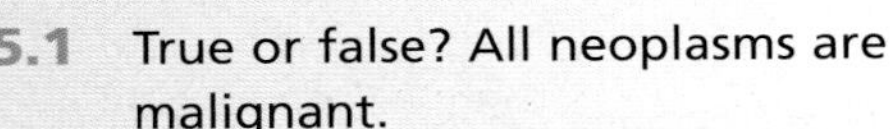
5.1 True or false? All neoplasms are malignant.

Table 5.1 The Naming of Tumors

Tissue of Origin	Benign	Malignant
Fibrous	Fibroma	Fibrosarcoma
Fat	Lipoma	Liposarcoma
Bone	Osteoma	Osteosarcoma
Cartilage	Chondroma	Chondrosarcoma
Blood vessels	Hemangioma	Hemangiosarcoma
Blood cells		
Granulocytes		Leukemia
Lymphocytes		Leukemia, if in blood
		Lymphoma, if in lymph nodes or organs
Muscle		
Skeletal	Rhabdomyoma	Rhabdomyosarcoma
Smooth	Leiomyoma	Leiomyosarcoma
Epithelium		
Epidermis, squamous mucosa	Squamous cell papilloma	Squamous cell carcinoma
Glands, other epithelium	Adenoma, papilloma	Adenocarcinoma
Melanocytes	Nevus	Malignant melanoma

5.2 True or false? Melanoma is a malignant neoplasm.

5.3 A malignant tumor composed of skeletal muscle is called ____________________.

The Causes of Cancer

The root cause of cancer is damaged DNA. A wide variety of environmental forces can cause **mutations**, permanent damage to DNA (Fig. 5.2). Mutations that lead to cancer are characterized as **carcinogenic**. As carcinogenic mutations pass down the generations of cancer cells, they not only assure their continued malignancy, but also grant the cancer cells a Darwinian growth and survival advantage over normal cells.

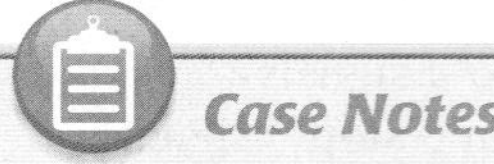

Case Notes

5.2 Will the cells in Brenda's tumor contain abnormal DNA?

Remember This! The root cause of all cancer is damaged DNA.

Sunlight
(ultraviolet radiation)
Skin cancer
Radiation
Thyroid cancer,
leukemia
Inhalation carcinogens
(cigarette smoke)
Lung cancer
Viruses
Lymphoma (thymus,
lymph nodes)
Liver carcinogens
(mildewed grain)
Liver cancer
Wild
Smoked
Salmon
Dietary carcinogens
(smoked foods)
Stomach and
intestinal cancer
Excretory carcinogens
(industrial chemicals)
Bladder cancer
Human papillomavirus
(unprotected sex)
Cervical cancer
INDUSTRIAL CLEANER
Carcinogenic
Contact
carcinogens
Skin cancer

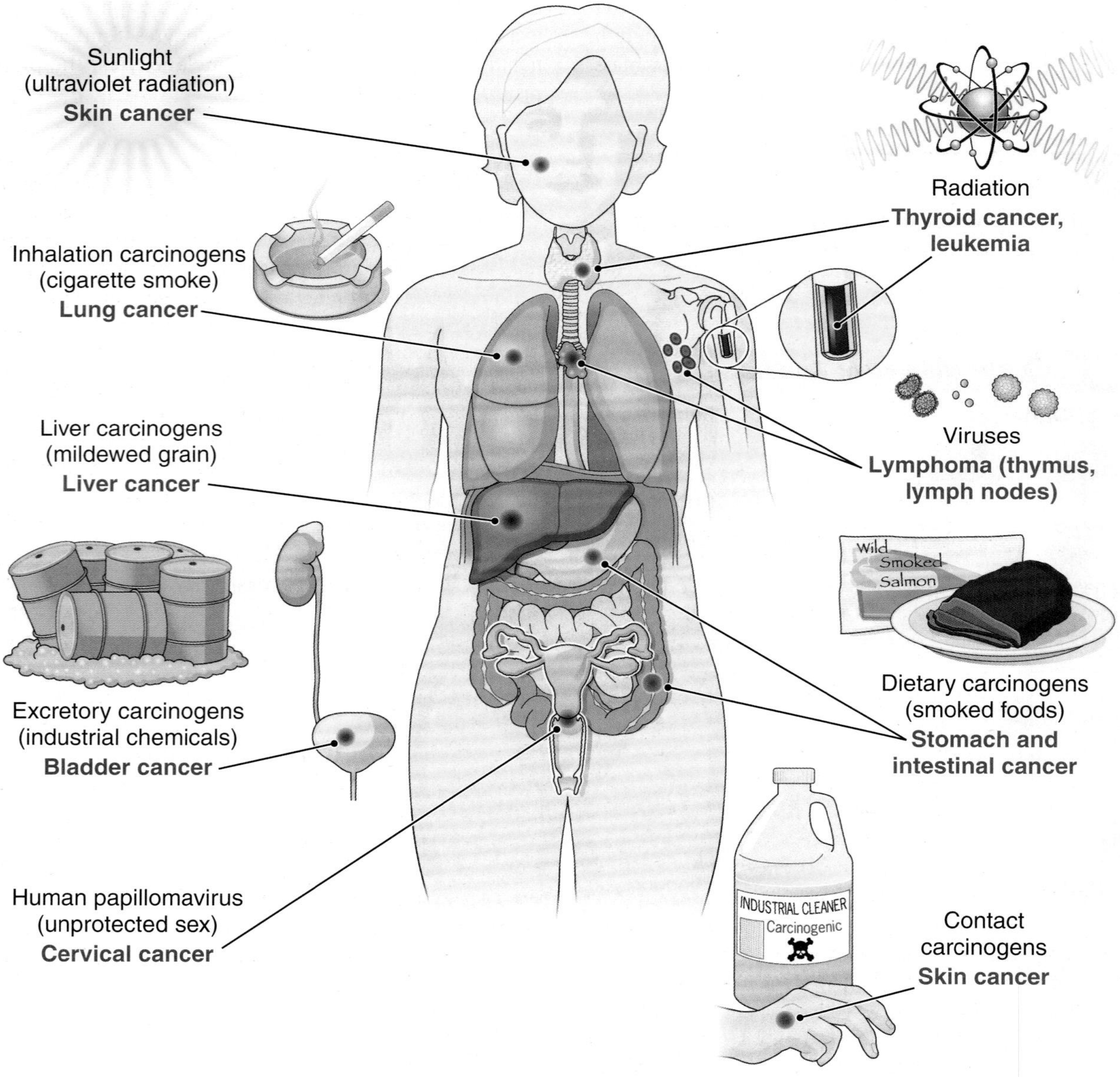

Figure 5.2 **The causes of cancer.** Cancer is caused by transformation of cells (carcinogenesis) following injuries that directly damage DNA (mutagenesis).

Neoplasms Can Be Characterized by Epidemiology

Much of what we know about neoplasms comes from epidemiology. Some links are clear—smoking and lung cancer is one example. Another is the combination of tobacco use and alcohol abuse, which is linked to cancers of the mouth and throat (see *The History of Medicine*, "The Only American President to Die of Cancer"). Long-term comparison of epidemiologic data provides valuable insights. For example, as smoking surged in popularity during and after World War II, the incidence of new lung cancer cases in men increased more than four times and in women more than eight times between 1945 and 1995. After the publication of the first U.S. Surgeon General's *Report on Smoking and Health* in 1964, which publicized the dangers of smoking, the popularity of smoking declined, and since the mid-1990s lung cancer rates have trended lower.

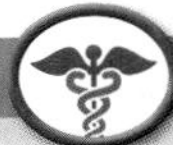

The History of Medicine

THE ONLY AMERICAN PRESIDENT TO DIE OF CANCER

The only U.S. president to die of cancer was Ulysses S. Grant (1822–1885), who gained fame during the American Civil War (1861–1865) and was appointed by Lincoln to be General-in-Chief of the Union Army in 1864. He served as President of the United States from 1869 through 1877 and succumbed to a tumor of the throat, a point worth noting because Grant loved cigars and whiskey—tobacco *use* and alcohol *abuse*, especially together, are associated with carcinomas of the mouth, tongue, pharynx, larynx, and esophagus.

Lincoln heard "Grant is a drunkard" from politicians so often and heard so little praise for the damage Grant was inflicting on the Confederates that he is said to have replied on one occasion, ". . . you just find out, to oblige me, what brand of whiskey Grant drinks, because I want to send a barrel of it to each one of my generals."

More often, however, the link between disease and behavior or environment is less obvious. Still, epidemiology can reveal subtle clues by evaluating geographic and environmental factors, personal habits, the effects of age and gender, and the role of diagnostic methods. For example, stomach cancer is much more common in Japan than in the United States. Although genetic differences play a role, most of the difference is due to *environmental* factors such as diet. Study of successive generations of Japanese immigrants to the United States shows them developing an American pattern of stomach cancer occurrence. *Personal habits* are important as well. For example, alcohol abuse is associated with cancers of the oral cavity, throat, larynx, and liver. Overeating also plays a role: among the obese, the overall cancer risk is at least 50% higher. *Age* and *gender* are also important. Older people have more malignancies than younger people do, while a few cancers occur predominantly in children. Differences in cancer rates among males and females are attributable largely to malignancies of sex organs—women have a high incidence of breast cancer, and men have a high incidence of prostate cancer. Finally, declines in the death rate for colon, breast, and prostate cancer have occurred recently due to increased public awareness and improved *diagnostic* techniques, which allow earlier diagnosis and treatment.

Environmental Factors Can Stimulate Cancer Development

Experience and research, as well as epidemiological data, show that certain environmental forces are carcinogenic. The list of *chemical* carcinogens is long. The first such example in medical history was Sir Percival Pott's linking of scrotal cancer to soot exposure in English chimney sweeps. (See *The History of Medicine*, "Where There's Smoke, There's Cancer," available online at thePoint.com, which provides details as well as additional historical context.) Modern examples include links between: 1) the chemical content of cigarette smoke and lung cancer; 2) certain dyes and bladder cancer in the dye and rubber industry; and 3) liver cancers in parts of Africa and the Far East caused by aflatoxin, a carcinogen produced by a mold in improperly stored food grain.

Ionizing radiation also can be mutagenic and carcinogenic—survivors near to the atomic bomb blasts at Hiroshima and Nagasaki, Japan, at the end of World War II have increased prevalence of leukemia and cancers of the thyroid and other organs. Very common, but not as well appreciated, is the mutagenic and carcinogenic effect of ultraviolet (UV) light in ordinary sunlight. At greatest risk are light-skinned people who receive increased sun exposure. The lower lip, the forehead, and the back of the neck and hands are particularly susceptible.

Viruses also may cause cancer. *Human papilloma virus* (HPV) is a sexually transmitted infection that after multiple reinfections is the cause of most carcinoma of the cervix (Chapters 4 and 17). *Epstein-Barr virus* (EBV) is implicated as the cause of some lymphomas, and *hepatitis B and C virus* (HBV and HCV) are important in the genesis of hepatocellular carcinoma.

Finally, chronic inflammation may cause cancer. Certain conditions are often forerunners of malignancy. The mechanism of the carcinogenesis in some of these premalignant conditions is not clear, but others are well known. One is *Barrett esophagus*, an inflammatory condition of the lower esophagus caused by gastric acid reflux, which is associated with an increased risk for development of esophageal cancer.

Case Notes

5.3 **Is HPV an environmental factor?**

Some Neoplasms Are Genetically Predisposed to Develop

A small percentage of cancer patients have an inherited mutation in their *germ cells* (ova and sperm) that predispose them to development of a certain type of cancer, which they pass to subsequent generations. Perhaps the most widely known is the *BRCA* gene, a mutated version of which encourages, but does not guarantee, the development of breast and ovarian cancer in women. In most instances, however, the genetic influence is subtler. For example, the relationship between smoking and lung cancer is indisputable. The nonsmoking relatives of lung cancer patients, however, develop lung cancer with a greater frequency than expected. Although second-hand smoke inhalation may account for a portion of this effect, the remainder is related to poorly understood genetic tendencies. On the other hand, some genetic links are specific. Children who inherit a defective copy of the retinoblastoma gene (RB gene) are almost certain to develop *retinoblastoma*, a malignant tumor of the retina.

Case Notes

5.4 Is it likely that Brenda developed cancer with her initial HPV infection?

Pop Quiz

5.4 True or false? Epidemiology is the study of the patterns and causes of diseases.

5.5 True or false? Most cancers are caused by mutations in ovarian or testicular germ cells.

5.6 Name several types of environmental carcinogenesis and give examples.

5.7 What is the root cause of cancer?

The Molecular Basis of Neoplasia

Knowledge of the molecular basis of cancer is vast, so we must confine ourselves to a short version. It is important to understand that mutant genes associated with cancer are first discovered and named because they are associated with a particular cancer; hence the name given to the gene usually is related to the abnormal (defective, cancer-causing) form of the gene, not the normal gene or its usual function. This often leads to the mistaken assumption that the abnormal gene is the only one that exists. For example, the *BRCA* gene, associated with breast cancer, is named for the cancer with which it is associated, and we know little of the normal function of the undamaged gene in healthy people.

These mutant genes fall into four categories: proto-oncogenes, tumor suppressors, genes that regulate apoptosis, and DNA repair genes. The list of identified mutations in cancers of various sorts is very long and growing daily, so we must be satisfied with a few examples.

Recall from our discussion above that all cells contain genes that function as "go" or "stop" switches, stimulating or restraining cell growth. The effect of growth-stimulating and growth-suppressing genes is in balance in normal cells. The "go" genes are **proto-oncogenes**, which promote normal cell growth, but when mutated become **oncogenes**. For example, the **HER2 gene** is a proto-oncogene that produces *human epidermal growth factor 2*, a protein that promotes normal cell growth. The mutant or over-expressed (over-active) *HER2* genes, which can be identified in breast cancer, promote uncontrolled growth. **Tumor-suppressor genes** are the opposite of oncogenes—they are "stop" switches that restrain normal cell growth by producing proteins that inhibit cell division. If a growth-suppressing gene suffers injury and loses its ability to function, it leaves cell growth uninhibited.

Case Notes

5.5 If Brenda's cancer cells were studied, is it likely that gene mutations would be found?

Some genes promote **apoptosis**, normal cell death. One such gene is the **p53 gene**, a mutant variety of which is the most common genetic defect in human cancers. About half of all cancers have a defective *p53* gene, but it is especially prevalent in cancers of the breast and colon. Without the *p53* gene to command apoptosis, cells with damaged DNA remain alive, capable of dividing indefinitely, and on the road to malignancy. Likewise, telomeres (Chapter 2) play a role in allowing some cells to divide indefinitely. Recall that telomeres are short segments of DNA at the tip of each chromosome that keep track of how many times a cell divides by shortening with each division. When a cell runs out of telomere it can no longer divide and the cell line dies. This is part of the ageing process at the cellular level, but it plays a role in carcinogenesis as well. Some cancer cells can divide indefinitely because they have developed a way to generate new telomere length. Much of the effectiveness of chemotherapeutic agents lies in their ability to induce apoptosis, and they depend upon *p53* to aid them in this task. The loss of *p53* reduces the effectiveness of chemotherapy by making cells less sensitive to chemotherapy-induced signals for apoptosis.

DNA is miscoded frequently, but the erroneous sequences are quickly repaired by **DNA repair genes**, which can be conceived of as "spell checkers" for "misspelled"

DNA. For example, if a base sequence should be AAA but is synthesized as CAA, the DNA repair mechanism corrects it back to AAA. If the DNA repair gene itself is damaged and defective, however, mutations of the DNA of other genes go uncorrected and cancer is often the result. For example, *xeroderma pigmentosa*, an inherited disease with a predisposition to development of skin cancers, is caused by a faulty DNA repair apparatus that allows defective DNA to remain mutant.

Carcinogenesis is a *multistep process*. No single mutation in any of the gene types discussed above is sufficient to produce a neoplasm, much less a malignant one. Cancers arise from an accumulation of multiple mutations: the average breast or colon cancer has 90 different mutations. Cells become cancerous due to a cycle of repeated injury and mutation. Smoking is the perfect example. One cigarette is not enough. But one pack a day for 35 years, about 250,000 cigarettes, is. Referring to our case, it seems very likely that Brenda suffered from repeated HPV infections because of her practice of unprotected sex with multiple male partners. One HPV infection is not likely to lead to cancer, but repeated infections are.

Almost all cancer-related mutations occur in *somatic* cells (e.g., lung, muscle), not the reproductive (*germ*) cells of the ovary or testis. Somatic cell DNA defects are not inheritable. They are acquired after birth and are the result of the effects of age, viruses, chemicals, or radiation. For example, smoking-related gene damage is not inheritable. However, mutations in germ cells are inherited and the defective gene is present in every cell in the body. A noncancerous example is red–green colorblindness. Though all cells in the body have the gene, it makes a difference only in certain cells, in this instance in retinal cells. Similarly, some germ cell defects increase the risk of cancer, but the risk applies only to certain cells. Such inheritable germ cell defects are called **inheritable cancer syndromes**. They increase the risk of a particular cancer to a variable degree but do not guarantee cancer development. About 20 such syndromes have been identified that link certain germ cell defects to the development of cancers of the breast, ovary, colon, skin, eye, kidney, and nerves.

Case Notes

5.6 Does Brenda's cancer arise from somatic or germ cells?

5.7 Is Brenda's cancer inheritable by her children?

Pop Quiz

5.8 True or false? Proto-oncogenes suppress cell growth.

5.9 True or false? Somatic cell mutations are inheritable.

5.10 True or false? Multiple mutations are necessary to produce a cancer.

The Biology of Neoplastic Growth

During the lengthy process of becoming malignant, the genetic molecular defects discussed above enable biologic capabilities that promote sustained cancer cell survival and growth.

Malignancies Develop through Premalignant Stages

Before becoming fully malignant, damaged DNA provokes in cells recognizable **premalignant changes**. Recall the following from Chapter 2:

- Epithelium is a membrane of cells that lines body surfaces and rests upon a basement membrane. Recall, also, from our definitions above that a carcinoma is a malignancy of epithelial cells.
- *Metaplasia* (Chapter 2, Fig. 2.10) is a reversible change of one cell type into another caused by chronic injury. It usually occurs in epithelium. Metaplastic epithelium reverts to normal when the injury stops. It is not precancerous.
- *Dysplasia* (Chapter 2, Fig. 2.11) is a *precancerous* cellular change. Most dysplasia arises in metaplastic epithelium. It may revert to normal or it may progress to malignancy.

Dysplasia is the microscopic expression of the accumulating genetic defects and special biologic capabilities described above. The degree of dysplasia varies from mild to severe according to the amount of accumulated genetic damage. It is critical to understand that *dysplasia does not always progress to malignancy*. Nevertheless, increasing degrees of dysplasia are ever more likely to progress to full malignancy. At a certain point, dysplasia becomes severe enough to become high-grade dysplasia or **carcinoma in situ**, a state that is cancer "in place" (Fig. 5.3). Carcinoma in situ is neoplasia confined to the epithelium. Since it has not penetrated the basement membrane, it cannot reach blood vessels or lymphatics (which lie beneath the basement membrane) in order to metastasize to other locations. Thus, it is not **invasive**. Nevertheless, *at some point the malignant cells acquire the ability to invade: that is, to penetrate the basement membrane, and gain access to vessels and lymphatics that can carry it to any part of the body* (Fig. 5.4). Up to this critical moment, the malignancy is 100% curable: it can be excised or obliterated and will never progress to invasion, metastasis, and death.

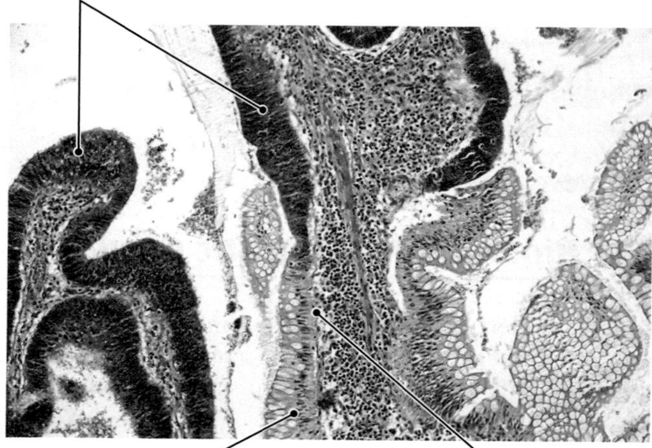

Figure 5.3 **Carcinoma in situ.** A colon polyp with an area of malignant (dark, hyperchromatic, atypical) epithelium that has not invaded the basement membrane.

Case Notes

5.8 Brenda's cancer developed in stages. Put the following stages in time sequence, first to last: 1) carcinoma in situ, 2) invasive cancer, 3) dysplasia.

Neoplasms Are Composed of Differing Populations of Cells

Neoplasms grow by forming a **clone** (Fig. 5.5), a set of identical cells descended from a single ancestor. All neoplasms are *initially* **monoclonal**, in that they arise from a single cell and grow as successive generations of that cell. As a tumor grows, however, some of the cells are altered and the tumor diverges into multiple clonal populations of cells, each with different characteristics. Some tumor cell variants have mutations of one kind, while others have mutations of a different kind, each of which produces a clone of identical descendant cells. The result is **tumor cell heterogeneity**, a tumor composed of multiple sets of cells, each differing in some respect from the others.

Among these sets of cells, a "survival of the fittest" competition ensues, and those that reproduce and grow best survive to predominate. Some cells are sturdier, more capable of defeating natural defenses, use resources more efficiently, or are more capable of surviving therapeutic anticancer drugs. These highly malignant cells generally survive, while the less malignant ones do not. For example, tumor cells that require hormone to flourish are vulnerable to therapy that reduces hormone availability. An example is prostate cancer: it thrives on testosterone and its growth is slowed if the testicles are removed or antitestosterone drugs are administered. Tumor cells that do not have such needs are less vulnerable and better able to survive. Likewise, tumor cells effective in growing their own blood supply are also more likely to survive.

Case Notes

5.9 As Brenda's tumor continues to grow, will the cells become more or less alike?

The Growth Rate of Neoplasms Depends on the Number of Dividing Cells

Cells must divide for a neoplasm to grow. A single neoplastic cell is about one-billionth of a gram. It divides into two cells, these two into four, and so on for about 30 generations—about 30 doublings—until the mass of cells is large enough to be detected. The smallest detectable mass is about the size of a grape (about one gram). This usually takes 10–20 years or more, which means that, by the time a solid malignant neoplasm becomes clinically detectible, it has already lived most of its life. If doubling continues at the same rate, the mass will reach football size in only a fraction of the time it took to reach grape size (see Fig. 5.5). This type of exponential growth explains why tumor growth seems to accelerate after detection.

Case Notes

5.10 Did it likely take Brenda's tumor months, a year, or many years to develop?

In most tumors the majority of cells are resting, only a fraction of them are dividing. This fraction, the **growth fraction**, is the main determinant of total growth rate (Fig. 5.6). For example, if 80% of cells in a tumor are dividing, it will grow much more rapidly than a tumor in which 20% of cells are dividing. How *frequently* the cells are dividing (e.g., once a day vs. once a week) is much less significant. Growth fraction is clinically important because chemotherapy drugs typically exert their effect by interrupting or slowing the growth cycle of dividing cells. Tumors with a high growth fraction—many cells that are actively dividing—are usually affected by traditional chemotherapy. Lymphomas and leukemias grow more rapidly than most other tumors because they have high growth fractions. In turn they are more sensitive than other neoplasms to drugs that inhibit cell division. By comparison, lung, breast, cervical, and colon cancer are tumors with relatively low growth fraction and are much less sensitive to chemotherapy. Some tumors grow more rapidly under certain circumstances such

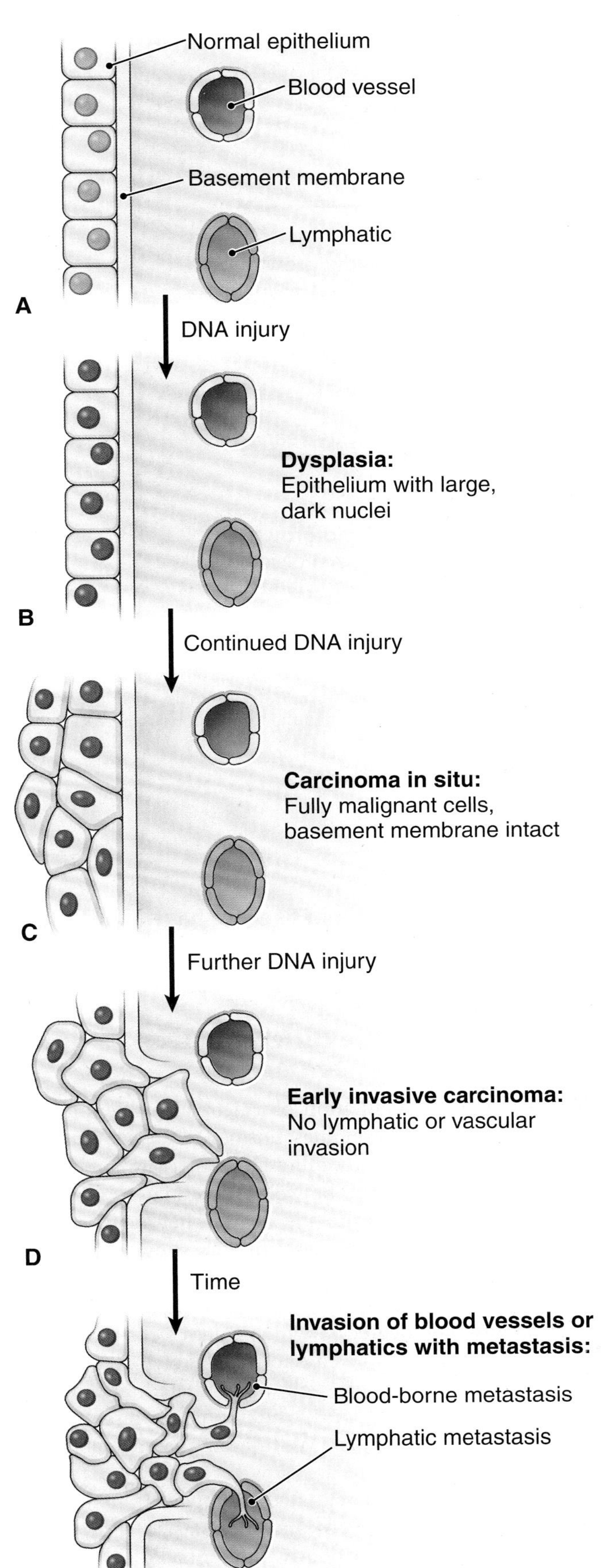

Figure 5.4 **The development of an epithelial malignancy (carcinoma). A. Normal epithelium** resting on basement membrane. Lymphatics and blood vessels are below the basement membrane. **B. Dysplasia.** Nuclei of cells with injured DNA are large and atypical but not yet malignant. **C. Carcinoma in situ.** Further DNA injury transforms the cells into a malignancy that has not crossed (invaded) the basement membrane and, therefore, cannot metastasize because it has not reached into blood vessels or lymphatics. **D. Early invasive carcinoma.** Additional injury produces malignant cells that penetrate the basement membrane. **E. Invasion of blood vessels or lymphatics** with distant metastasis.

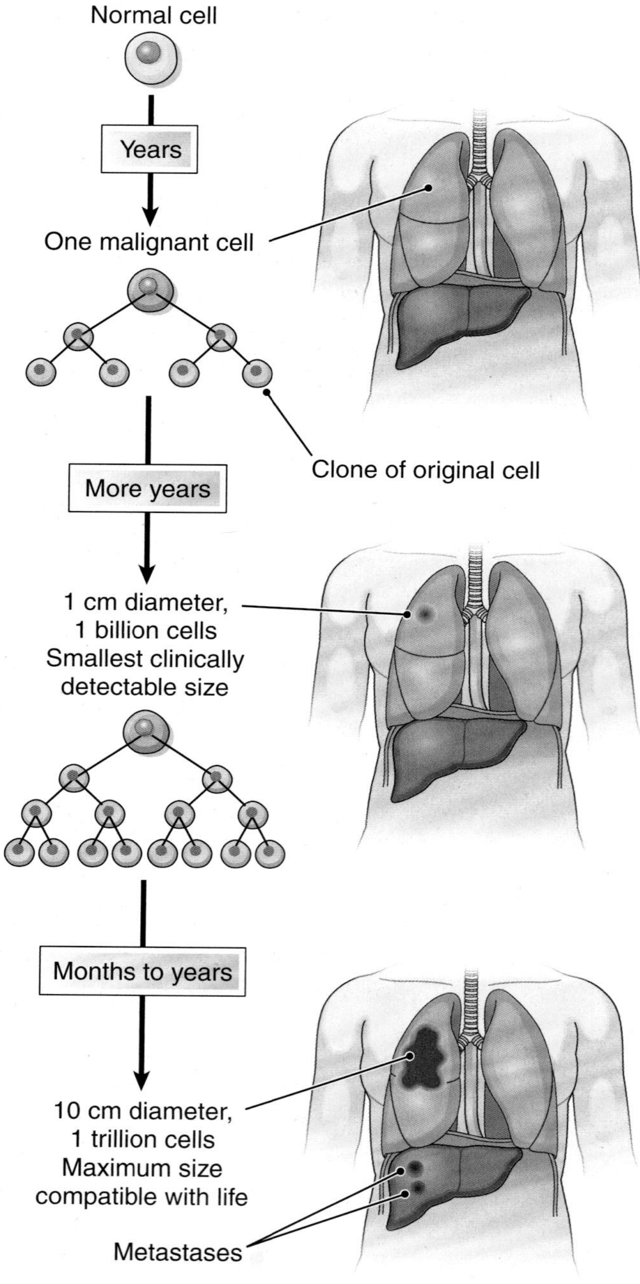

Figure 5.5 **Tumor doubling time.** Tumors arise as a single cell and are composed of cells derived from a single ancestor (a clone). One cell divides into two, two into four, four to eight, and so on, doubling in roughly the same amount of time. It takes far more time for a normal cell to become cancerous than for the tumor to grow large enough to be detectable, and it takes even less time for a tumor to grow large enough to cause death.

as changing hormone levels. For example, uterine leiomyomas (benign tumors of the uterus) may not grow for years, but with pregnancy may suddenly blossom into larger but still benign masses. Hormone-dependent breast cancers may also become more aggressive during pregnancy. Alternatively, antihormone drugs may slow the growth of such tumors in nonpregnant women.

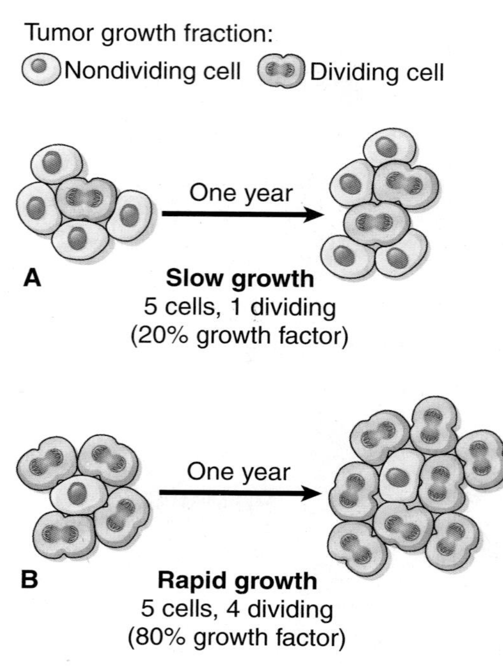

Figure 5.6 **Tumor growth fraction. A. Low (slow) growth fraction.** In this example, 20% (the growth fraction) of tumor cells are dividing at any given time, and the tumor grows relatively slowly. **B. High (rapid) growth fraction.** In this example, 80% of the cells are dividing at any given time, and the tumor grows much faster than the one shown in part A.

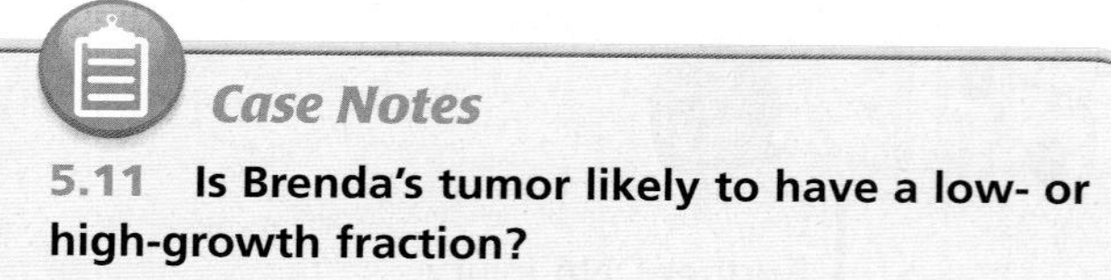

Case Notes

5.11 Is Brenda's tumor likely to have a low- or high-growth fraction?

Neoplastic Cells Are Differentiated to a Greater or Lesser Degree

The degree of differentiation of a neoplasm refers to the degree to which it resembles normal tissue in function and appearance. Perfectly differentiated tissue is normal. Neoplasms are judged to be well-differentiated or poorly differentiated according to the degree they deviate from this normal. Well-differentiated tumors show some semblance of the normal tissue from which they arose. Poorly differentiated ones (Fig. 5.7) show little or no semblance of normality. The degree to which tumor cells are differentiated is a microscopic clue to their likely behavior. As a rule, benign tumors are well differentiated, and highly malignant tumors are poorly differentiated; rarely, however, there are exceptions. Well-differentiated malignant tumors grow slowly and are slow to invade and late to metastasize. Poorly differentiated malignant tumors grow rapidly, invade aggressively, and metastasize early. Most tumors, whether well- or poorly differentiated, show little or no normal physiologic function.

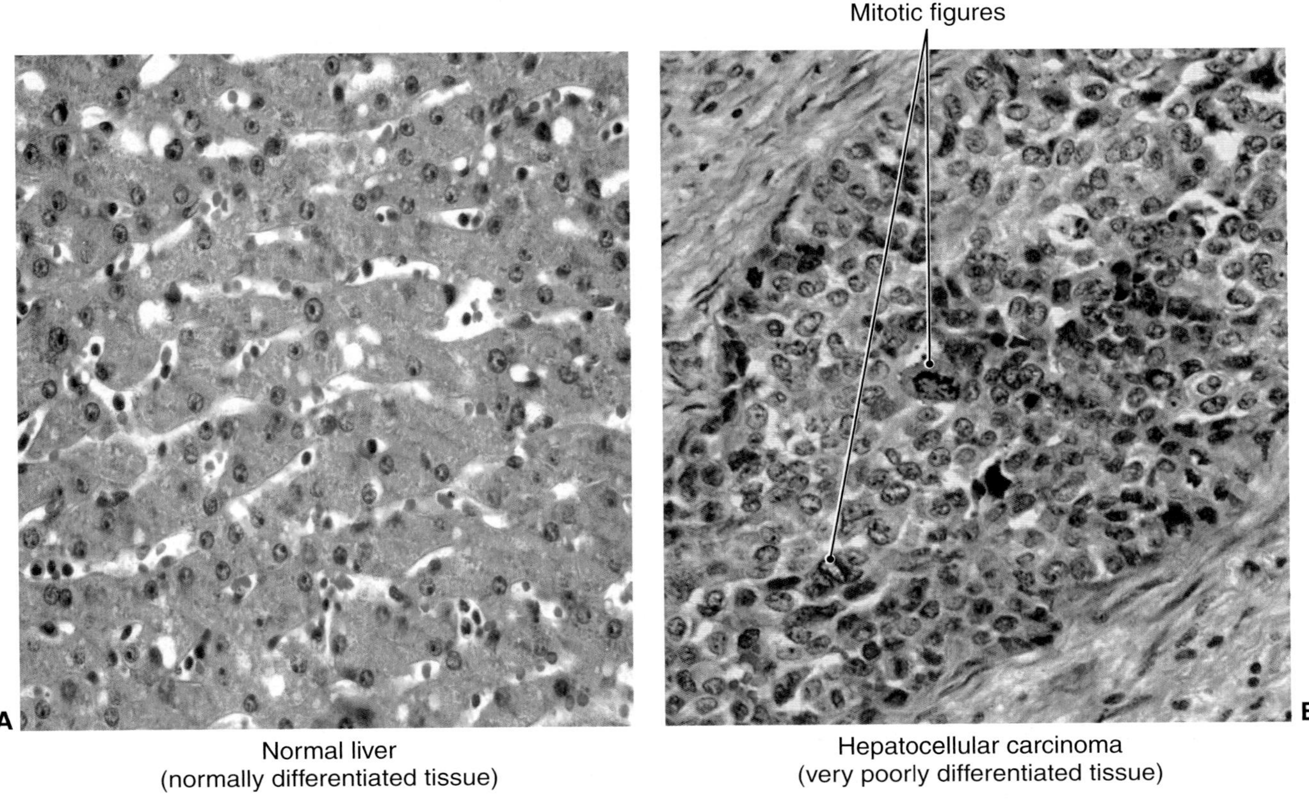

Figure 5.7 **Differentiated versus undifferentiated tissue. A. Normal liver** (microscopic view). The cells are perfectly well differentiated (normal). **B. Malignant tumor of liver.** The cells are so poorly differentiated that no hint of normal liver cells remains.

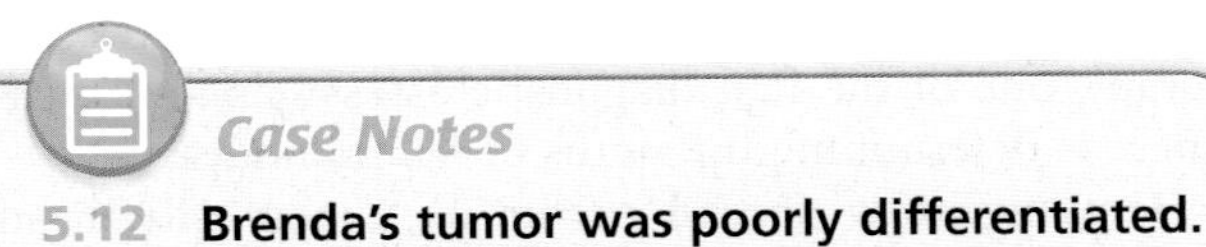

Case Notes

5.12 **Brenda's tumor was poorly differentiated. Is it likely to be indolent or aggressive?**

Neoplasms Require Nourishment

Like other tissues, neoplasms must have nourishment from the bloodstream. Because neoplasms are new growths, they must develop their own network of blood vessels—a neoplasm without a blood supply would never become larger than a few millimeters. Neoplasms develop their own blood supply by the process of angiogenesis (Chapter 2), a key element in the normal tissue repair process. Angiogenesis is as necessary for the growth of neoplasms as damaged DNA is necessary for their creation. Early in their development, most dysplastic or malignant cells do not stimulate angiogenesis; they remain dysplastic or as carcinoma in situ for years before becoming invasive and angiogenic. The degree of tumor angiogenesis affects the ability of malignant tumors to metastasize. Tumors with rich vascular networks are more prone to metastasize than are those with fewer blood vessels, because blood vessels are more abundant and accessible for invasion. Not surprisingly, cancer researchers have recently developed a number of antiangiogenesis drugs, hoping to starve cancers into submission by interfering with their blood supply. To date, the results show limited promise.

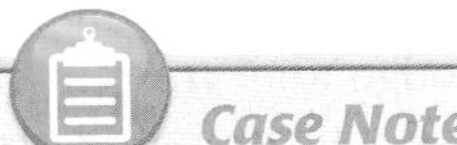

Case Notes

5.13 **Would Brenda's tumor be growing its own new blood vessels?**

Invasion and Metastasis Are Hallmarks of Malignancy

Invasion is the direct extension of tumor into adjacent tissue. *The ability to invade nearby tissues is a reliable distinction between benign and malignant neoplasms.* Benign tumors tend to grow slowly and typically are rounded masses that push aside nearby structures using blunt force. Compressed fibrous tissue usually forms a capsule around the tumor. Slow growth usually gives time for nearby tissue to adapt, so that the tumor often does not affect function. On the other hand, malignant tumors invade nearby tissue with streams of destructive cells. No capsule forms to limit the advancing army of cells. The invasive nature of malignant tumors allows them to invade blood and lymph vessels and spread discontinuously to distant tissue or organs. Some tumors may be *locally* *aggressive*, a term applied to invasive tumors that invade but do not metastasize, though they may recur after local excision or other treatment.

Case Notes

5.14 Was Brenda's tumor invasive?

Metastasis is the discontinuous spread of tumor from one site to another and is the most reliable sign of malignancy. Recall that "malignant" means capable of causing death. *Metastatic tumors are so often associated with death that the ability to metastasize is synonymous with malignancy.* About one-third of patients with malignancy have metastases at the time of diagnosis. The presence of metastases greatly reduces the chances of cure. Also recall, however, that our definition of malignancy is "usually capable of causing death." This is certainly true for metastatic tumors. Nevertheless, it is not an ironclad rule as previously mentioned—some thyroid tumors metastasize but rarely cause death.

Metastases may occur in three ways: 1) seeding across the surface of body cavities; 2) through lymphatics into lymph nodes; and 3) through blood.

Seeding (Fig. 5.8) occurs as tumor cells float from point to point in body fluid; it is most often seen in the intra-abdominal spread of ovarian cancer on the surfaces of the peritoneum. Seeding is less often seen in the meningeal, pericardial, and pleural spaces.

Lymphatic spread (Fig. 5.9) occurs as tumor cells invade lymphatic vessels and are swept up the lymphatic chain by the flow of lymph fluid. Carcinomas are especially prone to invade lymphatics. Lymph nodes filter out the carcinoma cells, which then lodge and grow in the nodes. Regional lymph nodes serve as a temporary barrier to further spread. Because there are many connections between lymphatics and blood, however, it is impossible to know if a particular tumor has spread into blood directly or through lymphatic connections. Because lymphatic spread follows the natural route of lymphatic drainage of the tumor site, nearby lymph nodes are most often the site of early metastasis. For example, breast cancer usually arises in the upper outer quadrant of the breast, which naturally drains to axillary nodes. Because the presence or absence of nodal involvement greatly alters prognosis and therapy, one of the first diagnostic assessments of breast cancer is determining the status of lymph nodes.

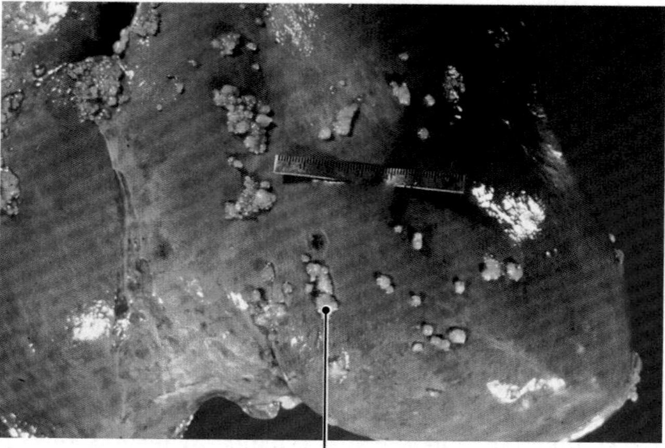

Figure 5.8 **Metastasis by seeding.** Gross study of the peritoneal surface of the liver with ovarian carcinoma implants seeded into the peritoneal space.

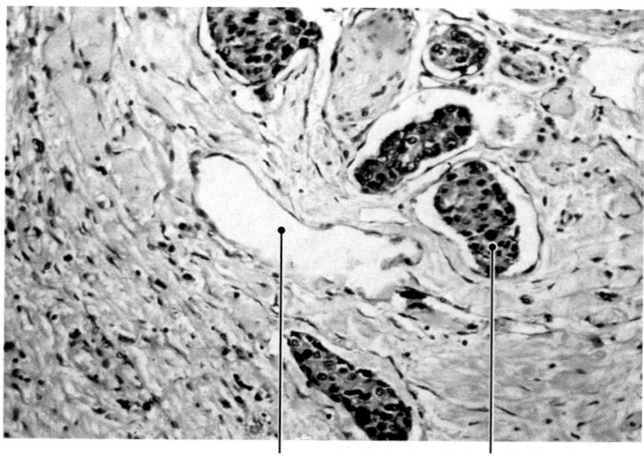

Figure 5.9 **Invasive carcinoma in lymphatics.** Shown are nests of malignant cells present in lymphatic channels. Metastases were present in lymph nodes fed by these lymphatics.

Hematogenous spread occurs as tumor cells invade blood vessels. Hematogenous spread is typical of sarcomas, less so of carcinomas. Because their walls are thin, veins are most often invaded. Tumor cells follow natural venous flow and lodge in a distant capillary bed—sometimes the first capillary bed they encounter. For intestinal malignancies, this is usually the liver (Fig. 5.10); for the remainder it is usually the lungs. Nevertheless, some of the venous drainage of the prostate and thyroid glands is through the paravertebral venous plexus, which explains the frequency of thyroid and prostate vertebral metastases. Other factors are involved as well. Some cancers find the "soil" of certain tissues more accommodating than others. For example, breast carcinoma has a proclivity to spread to bone, and lung cancer to brain and adrenals. Surprisingly, despite their great blood flow, the muscle and spleen are rarely sites of metastasis.

Case Notes

5.15 Which of the following did Brenda's tumor show: invasion, seeding, lymphatic spread, hematogenous spread?

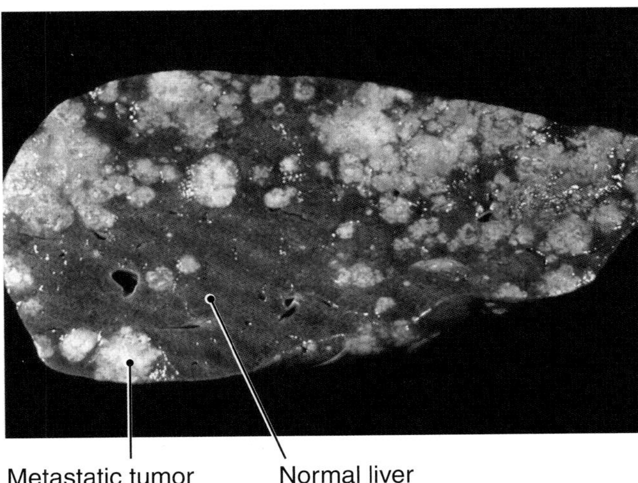

Figure 5.10 **Metastatic cancer.** This cross-section of liver shows multiple blood-borne nodules of metastatic colon cancer.

Immune Surveillance Is Immune Defense against Neoplasia

Recall from Chapter 3 that with the exception of identical twins, all of us are genetically unique: the proteins made under our DNA's control are ours alone and unlike anyone else's. Recall further a person's DNA and proteins are referred to as *self* and all other proteins as alien, or *nonself*. It is the job of the immune system to attack things that are made of nonself protein, such as an invading microbe or tissue transplanted from another person or a nonhuman species.

The concept of nonself extends to neoplasms. Once normal DNA is changed by injury (mutation), it and its proteins become nonself to a certain degree and subject to immune attack. This antineoplastic function of the immune system is referred to as **immune surveillance**. Under the watchful eye of immune surveillance, mutant cells that otherwise might develop into a neoplasm are eliminated. Sometimes, however, mutant cells escape immune attack to perpetuate themselves as neoplasms.

Logic suggests that immunodeficient patients should suffer from more neoplasms than those with normal immune systems, and they do—AIDS patients and patients on immunosuppressive therapy for organ transplants or other reasons also have a higher than expected occurrence of malignant neoplasms.

Pop Quiz

5.11 True or false? The tumor lives most of its life before it is detected.

5.12 True or false? All tumors begin as a clone of a single cell (monoclonal) and remain monoclonal.

5.13 True or false? Carcinomas tend to spread via lymphatics rather than spreading via blood vessels.

5.14 True or false? Identical twins have the identical risk for cancer.

5.15 The growth of new blood vessels into a tumor is called ______________.

5.16 The most reliable sign of malignancy is ______________.

5.17 What is the name of an epithelial malignancy that has not invaded through the basement membrane?

5.18 Why do patients with immune deficiency have more neoplasms than do normal people?

5.19 Which mainly determines the rate of tumor growth: growth fraction or rate of cell division?

Clinical Manifestations

No matter how much we may know about the usual behavior of a particular type of neoplasm, every patient and every tumor is different. The only way to understand a particular tumor in a given patient is to collect a medical history. Tumors, whether benign or malignant, may have different effects that may be local or far-reaching and systemic. Symptoms arise from the following:

- Pressure of the expanding tumor mass on nearby tissue
- Infection or bleeding from ulceration of surfaces
- Infarction or rupture
- Generalized wasting (*cachexia*)
- Production of hormones or other molecules that affect distant organs

Case Notes

5.16 Which of the effects listed above was important in Brenda's case?

Clinical History Is Supremely Important

The importance of context—*clinical history*—in pathologic, radiologic, or clinical diagnosis and treatment cannot be overstated. Clinical history is essential for bedside diagnosis; but it is just as critical for pathologic or radiologic diagnosis. For example, a microscopic slide taken from a healing bone fracture can look amazingly similar to a slide taken from some types of malignant bone tumor, so much so that even the savviest pathologist can be fooled without knowing the clinical history of a fracture. Although knowing the history of a patient changes nothing in the cells, in the X-ray images, or on the microscopic slides being read by a pathologist, clinical history can make an immense difference for the patient. The significance we attach to everything we see, be it in medicine or on the street, is determined by events (history) and context (circumstances).

The point is this: clinicians, radiologists, pathologists, nurses, and other healthcare professionals cannot fully understand what is happening to the patient without a good medical history. To act without taking clinical history into account is to risk, for example, amputating a leg for a benign bone condition that has a misleading microscopic appearance, or not doing an amputation on a malignant bone tumor that has deceptively bland microscopic features. A microscopic slide or an X-ray image is nothing more than a picture frozen in time. The circumstances—the clinical history—are extremely important if a correct conclusion is to be reached.

Most Neoplasms Are Discovered because of Their Local Effects

No matter how they grow, most neoplasms make themselves known by the effect of local pressure exerted by the expanding mass of the primary tumor or of metastatic tumor masses. Benign tumors of the pituitary may be discovered because they press on nearby optic nerves to produce disturbances of eyesight, or they may destroy the pituitary and deprive the body of pituitary hormones. Brain tumors may spark epileptic seizures. Carcinomas of the lung may irritate bronchi or obstruct airflow to cause coughing or wheezing. The advancing edge of a tumor may penetrate blood vessels or the tumor may hemorrhage from its own blood supply. Bleeding into stool or urine is a common first symptom of gastrointestinal (GI) or urinary tract tumors.

Neoplasms Can Produce Distant Effects

Neoplasms may produce far-reaching effects on the body that are distinct from the direct mass effect of the primary tumor or its metastases.

A **paraneoplastic syndrome** is a set of systemic symptoms *not* due to local or metastatic spread of tumor. About 10% of patients with malignancy will have a paraneoplastic syndrome. Some are not easily explained; others are readily explainable by known substances secreted by tumors. They are clinically important because they may be the first sign of malignancy, they may be lethal, or they may present diagnostic difficulties.

Dozens of paraneoplastic syndromes have been identified that cause mental aberration, neurologic disease, high blood calcium (*hypercalcemia*), low blood glucose (*hypoglycemia*), high blood cortisol or other hormones, and other problems. High blood calcium is perhaps the most common paraneoplastic syndrome. When appearing as a paraneoplastic syndrome and not due to some other cause, it is most often associated with cancer of the lung, breast, or kidney. Of all malignancies, *small cell carcinoma of the lung* is probably most often associated with paraneoplastic syndrome, especially *Cushing syndrome* (high blood cortisol, Chapter 14). Other tumors that commonly cause paraneoplastic syndrome include carcinomas of the kidney, pancreas, and stomach. The tendency of some patients to develop deep vein thrombi and inflammation (*thrombophlebitis*), usually in leg or pelvic veins, is another example of paraneoplastic syndromes. The cause is procoagulant proteins secreted by the tumor, and the appearance of otherwise unexplainable thrombophlebitis will prompt experienced diagnosticians to search for hidden cancer.

Some patients with malignancy suffer from **cachexia** (Fig. 5.11), a progressive loss of weight accompanied by weakness, lethargy, fatigue, and anemia that occurs to a greater or lesser degree in about half of cancer patients. Unlike starvation, in which weight loss is usually confined to fat loss, cachexia is equally fat and muscle loss. Cachectic patients usually have poor appetite (anorexia), and therefore eat less. Normally, reduced food intake reduces

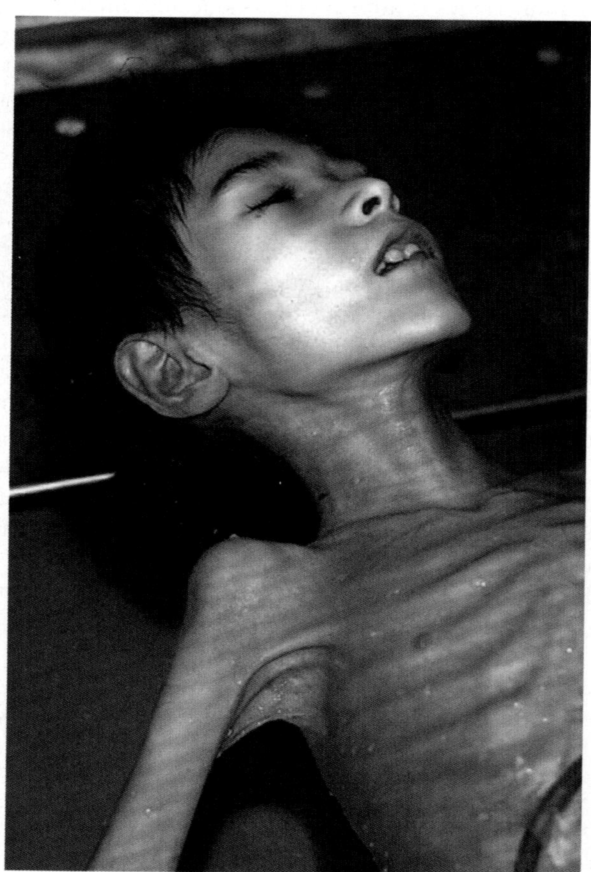

Figure 5.11 **Cachexia of malignancy.** This photo is of a patient with pancreatic carcinoma. The wasting away of body tissue is not entirely a matter of lost appetite.

metabolic rate, which in part accounts for the difficulty most people have in trying to lose weight. But in cachexia, the basal metabolic rate is increased, so the person burns calories at a faster rate than normal. This combination of reduced energy intake and increased energy output explains some of the weight loss. Other factors that prevent the breakdown of or interfere with the synthesis of protein needed to construct tissues also appear to be at work. These factors appear to be small polypeptides derived from breakdown of tumor proteins.

Case Notes

5.17 Did Brenda have a paraneoplastic syndrome?

Pop Quiz

5.20 True or false? Diagnosis of cancer is mainly a microscopic exercise in which clinical history has little importance.

5.21 Local effects of tumor masses are caused by ________.

5.22 Systemic effects of tumors are called ________.

5.23 The wasting associated with malignancy is called ________.

Clinical and Laboratory Assessment of Neoplasms

The assessment of neoplasms, especially malignant ones, is an exercise that involves obtaining a thorough clinical history, doing a complete physical examination, obtaining medical images and laboratory data, and often, undertaking microscopic study of tissues and cells. It is increasingly complex, as tumor subtypes are identified and treatments tailored for each one.

Clinically discernible masses generally require biopsy and microscopic diagnosis. There are some notable exceptions, especially in skin where the clinical look and feel of subcutaneous lipomas (benign tumors of fat) and certain skin cysts are so unmistakable that biopsy is not necessary. On the other hand, *every* breast or lung mass must be investigated thoroughly.

Study of Cells and Tissues Is Essential for Diagnosis

Cytology is the diagnostic study of individual cells for evidence of cancer or other abnormality. *The Clinical Side*, "Cytologic Diagnosis," offers more information about cytology. The best known cytology procedure for cancer diagnosis is the **Papanicolaou (Pap) smear** of the female cervix, depicted in Figure 5.12 and named after George Papanicolaou, who perfected the technique in the 1930s by study of cells scraped from the cervices of female lab rats. The technique was adopted in the 1940s and is now universally practiced. It is accepted as instrumental in a dramatic reduction of deaths from cervical cancer since its inception.

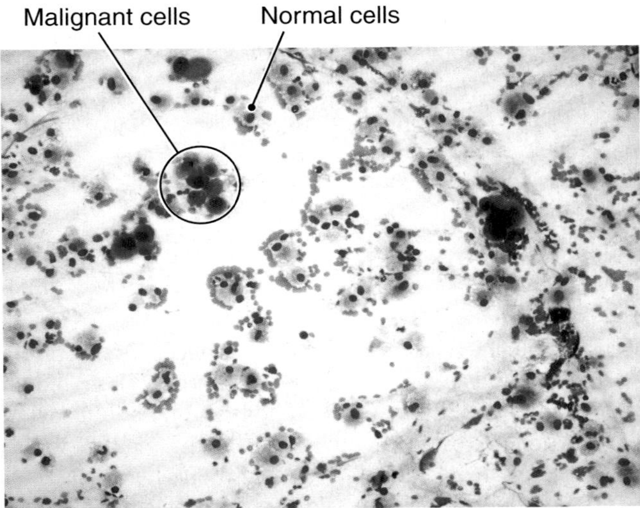

Figure 5.12 **Pap smear of the cervix.** Many normal cells are present, which have small, uniform nuclei. Also present are clumps of malignant cells, which have large, dark nuclei.

Referring to our case, it is interesting that about 10 years earlier Brenda had an abnormal Pap smear and recalls that it was related to a virus infection. Coupled with her sexual history, it seems clear that she must have had HPV infection at the time of the Pap smear and had repeated infections in the intervening years. A follow-up Pap smear and further investigation and treatment surely would have prevented her developing cancer.

The Clinical Side

CYTOLOGIC DIAGNOSIS

Cytology is the diagnostic microscopic study of collections of cells, usually with the intent to see if any of them appear to be malignant or premalignant. It is in contrast with the microscopic study of intact pieces of tissue obtained by biopsy or at autopsy. The best-known cytology study is the Pap smear, which consists of cells scraped from the female cervix and smeared on a slide for microscopic diagnosis. A new technology of liquid Pap smears offers some improvement.

Cells for cytologic exam can also be gathered by

- collecting sputum, cerebrospinal fluid, urine, joint fluid, or fluid from other body cavities, such as ascitic fluid from the peritoneal cavity;
- washing a hollow organ, such as a bronchus, with a small amount of fluid and recollecting it;
- aspirating cells and tissue juice from a solid mass (e.g., a breast tumor) or organ (e.g., the thyroid) by use of a very thin needle.

Specimens collected by scraping or needle aspiration are often spread directly on clear glass slides, which are passed through a series of chemicals and dyes to ready them for microscopic study similar to the method for biopsy specimens (Chapter 1). Cells in fluids are usually first concentrated by centrifugation or collected by filtration before being placed on a slide.

A cytology specimen found to contain malignant cells is reliable. It is very nearly 100% specific (Chapter 1). Very few false-positive results occur. On the other hand, false-negative results can occur despite the most careful and correct procedures. Most false-negative results occur because even the most carefully collected specimen may not capture malignant cells present in the patient's tissue. That false-negative results occur with regularity is one of the main reasons that regular Pap smears are recommended for most adult women. In any circumstance, a woman who has had an abnormal Pap smear must be followed carefully.

Another technique for obtaining cells for microscopic diagnosis is **fine needle aspiration**. A very thin needle is inserted into the lesion, sometimes under radiologic guidance, and clusters of cells and attendant fluid are aspirated and spread onto a slide for examination. This technique has made possible the accurate diagnosis of some lesions without the necessity of open surgical biopsy.

Flow cytometry is a method of physically separating and sorting individual cells of any kind according to certain physical characteristics, including markers expressed on the surface. This technique generally requires a small piece of fresh tissue (biopsy) and is especially useful in classifying malignancies of blood cells.

Biopsy is the collection of intact pieces of tissue for microscopic diagnosis by surgical excision or needle to obtain a thin cylinder of tissue. For example, prostate biopsies are usually obtained by needle biopsy technique. After collection, the specimen must be carefully preserved, usually in a formaldehyde solution, and properly transported. Careful attention to specimen handling is paramount: careless handling can result in dried, lost, poorly preserved, or otherwise ruined specimens.

Immunohistochemistry is a widely used method that involves bathing a biopsy specimen with antibody against specific tumor proteins to see if they attach to tumor cells, an indication tumor proteins are present. Often, the method is used in conjunction with microscopic study to identify the type of tumor or the type of differentiation of cells within a neoplasm. Some tumors present with metastases from a hidden primary site. Finding a characteristic marker can help locate the primary. In other instances, the presence or absence of certain proteins is a valuable guide to therapy. For example, finding estrogen-receptor protein in breast cancer cells indicates the tumor has a need for estrogen and that antiestrogen therapy (tamoxifen) may be beneficial.

Tumor markers are substances produced by normal or neoplastic tissue and may appear *in blood* at increased levels in the presence of a neoplasm. Dozens have been identified. Nevertheless, they are not useful for the *early detection* of cancer because they lack sensitivity and specificity. They are too often falsely positive when high and falsely negative when low. Rather than detecting cancer, these markers may be useful to confirm diagnosis or monitor therapy. For example, a falling level of blood tumor marker may validate the effectiveness of cancer therapy or surgery.

Carcinoembryonic antigen (CEA) is a protein found in the blood of patients with colon cancer and some other malignancies, but is also increased in liver disease. It may be useful as a monitor of tumor regression or progression.

Alpha-fetoprotein (AFP) is another marker that may be produced by neoplasms and appear in blood, but abnormal levels are also associated with other conditions. For example, when elevated in amniotic fluid, AFP has a positive association with fetal neural tube defects; when low, it has a correlation with Down syndrome (Chapter 22). Patients with hepatocellular cancer may have elevated AFP.

Prostate-specific antigen (PSA) is a protein made by the prostate, which has proven to have some value in screening men for prostate cancer. Nevertheless, it, too, lacks sensitivity and specificity. When compared to other markers, its greatest advantage is that it is not expressed by any tissue other than prostate. Though fraught with false positives and negatives, blood PSA measurement has become a standard screening test for prostate cancer. We discuss this issue in more detail later in this chapter.

Neoplasms Vary in Their Anatomy and Behavior

Neoplasms can be classified according to their *gross* (naked eye) and *microscopic* anatomy or their *clinical* behavior. Figure 5.13 and Table 5.2 contrast the appearance and behavior of benign and malignant neoplasms. One of the pathologist's roles in microscopic examination of a biopsy is to predict whether the microscopic appearance of the tumor suggests it will behave in a "benign" or "malignant" fashion. Usually microscopic features correlate well with clinical behavior, but not always. Some neoplasms may exhibit conflicting features that make prediction of clinical behavior very difficult. Molecular (genetic) profiling is an increasingly useful tool that further helps predict tumor behavior and serves as a guide to therapy.

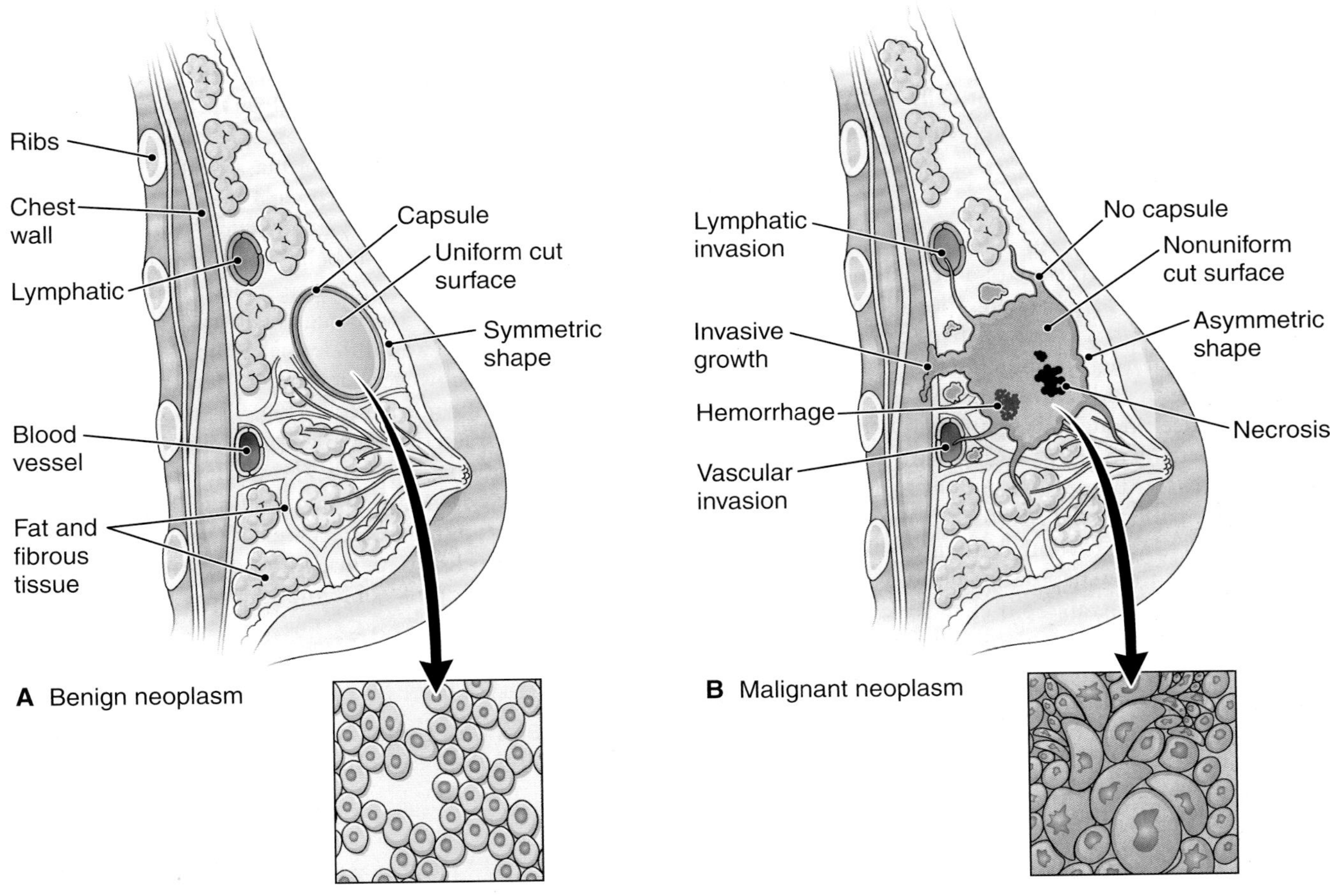

Figure 5.13 **The gross structure of neoplasms. A. Benign neoplasm B. Malignant neoplasm**

Table 5.2 ***Comparison of Clinical and Anatomic Characteristics of Benign and Malignant Neoplasms***

	Benign	Malignant
CLINICAL BEHAVIOR		
Growth	Slow	Rapid
Invasive	No	Yes
Metastasis	No	Yes
GROSS APPEARANCE		
Contour	Round, smooth	Stellate, irregular
Capsule	Present	Absent
Internal necrosis	Absent	Present
Internal hemorrhage	Absent	Present
MICROSCOPIC APPEARANCE		
Organization	Resembles normal tissue	Poor resemblance, if any
Cells	Resemble normal	Poor resemblance, if any
Nuclei	Resemble normal	Abnormal size, shape
Mitoses	Few or none, normal shape, size	Many, irregular shape, size

Case Notes

5.18 Were Brenda's tumor cells likely to resemble normal cervical epithelial cells?

Gross Anatomy

The *gross shape and structure* of a neoplasm are important diagnostic characteristics. Benign neoplasms tend to have a rounded, smooth outline with a rim of compressed fibrous tissue at the edge (a fibrous capsule). The cut surface is smooth and uniform, with a regular consistency and appearance throughout. Malignant neoplasms, on the other hand, tend to be irregular, with fingers of tumor invading adjacent tissue, and the cut surface has a varied appearance, with areas of necrosis, hemorrhage, calcification, or other. Tumors, both benign and malignant, may be described by their shape. Some grow as a **polyp**, a mass that protrudes from an epithelial surface. Others may grow as a **papilloma**, which grows in a fern- or finger-like pattern with prominent folds like a head of broccoli, and rises above the epithelial surface, like a polyp. Likewise, both benign and malignant tumors may be cystic; that is, they may have a hollow center, a feature incorporated into the name. For example, *cystadenoma* and *cystadenocarcinoma* are cystic varieties of tumors of the ovary.

Microscopic Anatomy

The *microscopic structure* of a neoplasm correlates much better with tumor behavior than does its gross appearance. Normal cells are perfectly and fully differentiated to perform their several tasks, be they neurons in the brain or skeletal muscle cells in the arm. Loss of differentiation is called **anaplasia** (Greek *ana* = without; *plassein* = shape). Benign neoplasms are well-differentiated, typical for their variety of cell, while malignant tumors are poorly differentiated (**anaplastic** or **atypical**). For example, a *lipoma* is a benign neoplasm of fat cells; the neoplastic cells so closely resemble normal fat cells that they are impossible to recognize by microscopic study alone—only their accumulation into a tumor mass offers a clue to their neoplastic nature. By contrast, *liposarcomas* are often so poorly differentiated that by microscopic study alone they may not be recognizable as being composed of fat cells.

Figure 5.14 illustrates the microscopic features of benign and malignant neoplasms. Benign neoplasms have relatively normal appearing (well-differentiated) cells (Fig. 5.14A). Malignant cells, however, lack normal differentiation and appear very unlike normal cells (Fig. 5.14B). Lack of differentiation is characterized by **pleomorphism**—great variety in the size and shape of cells and nuclei. Cells lose their orientation and do not align themselves with other cells to form normal structures. Nuclei are dark with extra genetic material (**hyperchromatism**). Mitotic figures are numerous and have abnormal configuration.

Case Notes

5.19 Brenda's tumor was poorly differentiated. Would the term "anaplastic" apply?

Treatment Depends on Tumor Grading and Staging

Malignant tumors are graded and staged (Fig. 5.15) to treat them appropriately. Later in this chapter, Table 5.3 provides an overview of treatments. *Grading* is a pathologic exercise based on microscopic characteristics. *Staging* is a clinical exercise based on tumor behavior. Benign tumors do not require grading and staging.

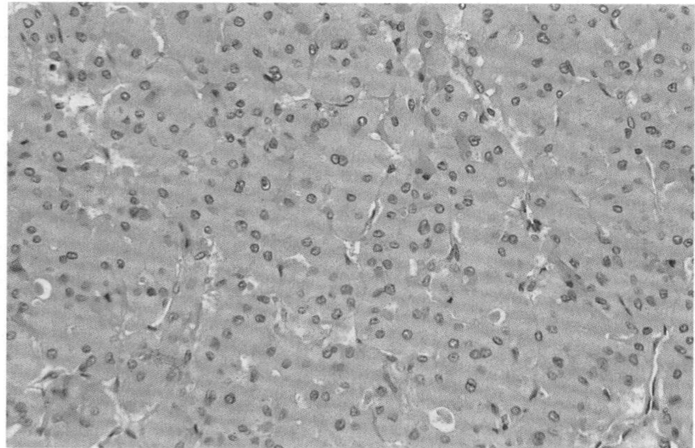

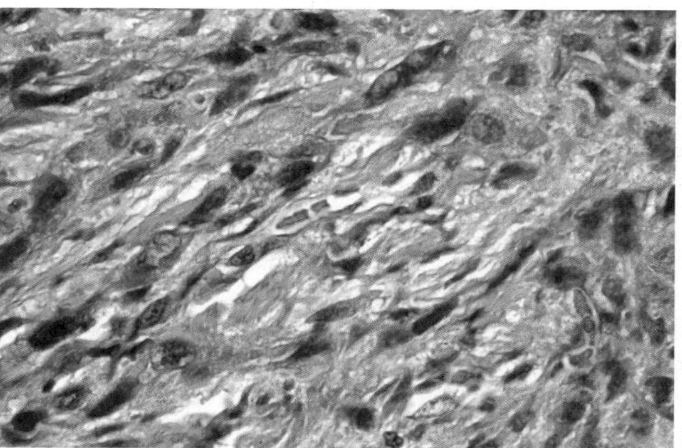

Figure 5.14 **Microscopic features of benign and malignant neoplasms. A. Benign.** This adenoma is formed of orderly small glandular acini composed of well-differentiated cells with unremarkable nuclei. No mitotic figures are present. **B. Malignant.** This adenocarcinoma originated in the same organ as A. No acini or other trace of normal gland structure is present. Growth is disorderly. Cells and nuclei vary greatly and nuclei contain an excess of chromatin. Mitotic figures are present. (**A,** Reprinted with permission from Raphael Rubin R, Strayer DS. *Rubin's Pathology: Clinicopathologic Foundations of Medicine*. 5th ed. Philadelphia, PA: Lippincott, Williams & Wilkins; 2008; **B,** Reprinted with permission from Cagle PT. *Color Atlas and Text of Pulmonary Pathology*. Philadelphia, PA: Lippincott, Williams & Wilkins; 2005).

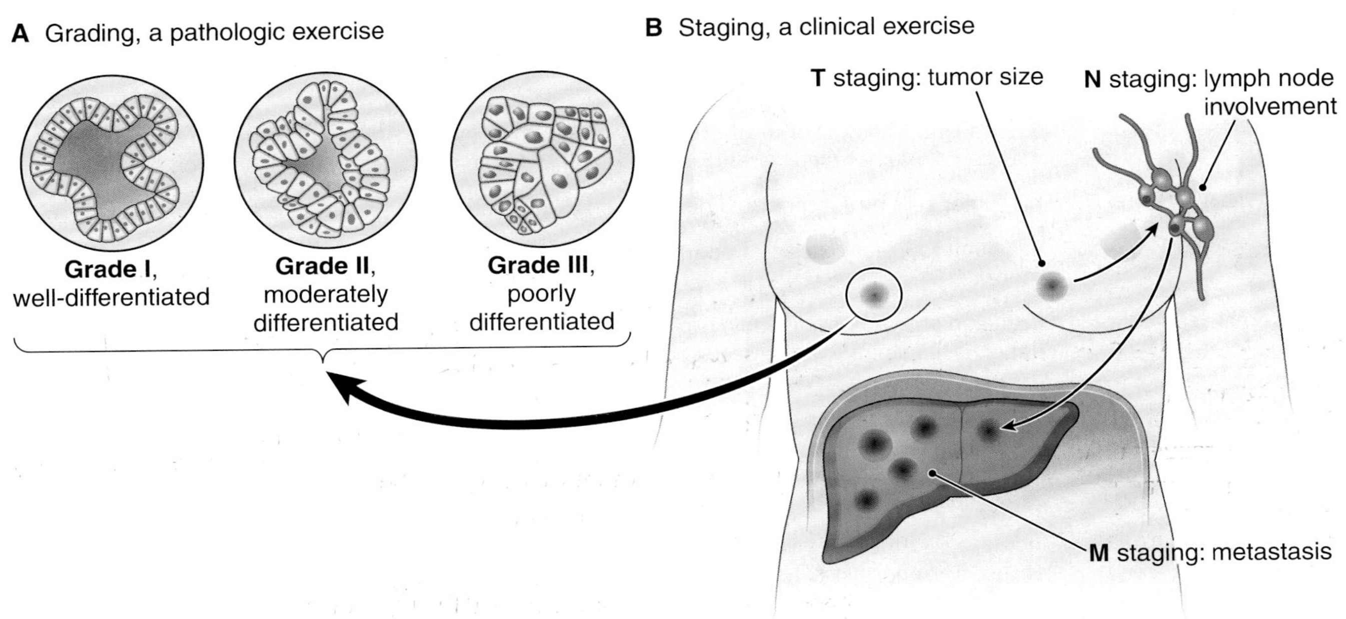

Figure 5.15 **Grading and staging of malignancies. A.** Grading is a pathologic exercise that classifies tumors according to their microscopic characteristics. **B.** Staging is a clinical exercise that classifies tumors according to their size, invasiveness, and spread. Tumors are staged according to the TNM system (T, tumor size; N, lymph node involvement; M, metastasis to distant organs). Schemes for TNM classification vary according to tumor type and organ involved.

Grading (see Fig. 5.15A) is the assessment of the degree of cell differentiation (specialization), nuclear atypia, mitotic figures, and other gross and microscopic features of malignancy listed in Table 5.3. Grading is basically an assessment of "How bad does the tumor look?" Grading practices vary somewhat from one type of malignancy to another and one pathologist to another: most tumors are graded on a scale of I to IV. Typically *grade I* (low-grade) malignancies are those with the least aggressive microscopic appearance—tumors that are well differentiated and have little nuclear atypia. *Grade II* and *Grade III* cancers are intermediate, and *grade IV* (high-grade) cancers are those that appear to be the most aggressive—poorly differentiated and highly atypical. There are exceptions. For example, the Gleason system for microscopic grading of prostate cancer grades tumors on a scale of 2–10.

Staging (see Fig. 5.15B) is an evaluation of tumor *behavior* that relies on the size of the primary tumor and its spread, either local or metastatic, as assessed by physical examination, history, and pathologic and diagnostic imaging. *Staging is a much better guide than grading for making decisions about therapy and for determining prognosis.* It's like your mother said, "It's not what you say but what you *do* that counts"—what tumors *do*, not what they look like, is most important.

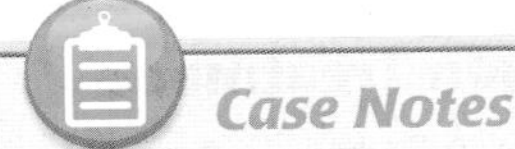

Case Notes

5.20 **Brenda's tumor was poorly differentiated. Was that assessment part of grading or staging?**

A common clinical staging convention is the **TNM system**—T for the size of the *primary* tumor; N for the extent, if any, of *regional* lymph node involvement; and M for *distant* metastases beyond local lymph nodes. TNM stages correlate closely with survival and are a valuable guide to prognosis and therapy. TNM staging criteria vary for particular types of cancer. Each feature of the malignancy—size, regional nodes, and distant metastasis—is assessed according to certain criteria. Size of the primary tumor might be graded T1 for the smallest size, T4 for the largest. No lymph node involvement is usually signified by N0, whereas N1 to N3 signifies progressively greater involvement of local lymph nodes. Likewise, M0 signifies no metastases beyond local lymph nodes, and M1 or M2 indicates progressively greater degree of distant metastasis.

Pop Quiz

5.24 True or false? Tumor markers are not a reliable method for early detection of cancer.

5.25 True or false? The gross characteristics of a neoplasm are important diagnostic characteristics.

5.26 The diagnostic study of individual cells for evidence of cancer or other abnormality is ________.

Table 5.3 Cancer Treatments

Treatment	Purpose
SURGERY	Physical removal of all or most of primary tumor; may involve removal of nearby lymph nodes that may contain tumor metastases. Example: excision of breast cancer and axillary lymph nodes.
RADIATION	Kill tumor cells by concentrated doses of ionizing radiation.
External	Radiation source is outside of body; beam of rays focused on tumor. Example: radiation of brain cancer.
Internal	Radiation source is inside body; capsules, seeds, or needles of radioactive material placed in the tumor. Example: radioactive seeds placed in prostate gland to treat prostate cancer.
Systemic	Selective tumor absorption of radioactive material. Example: radioactive iodine is selectively absorbed by some thyroid cancers.
CHEMOTHERAPY	Interferes with cancer cell reproduction. Example: oral or IV administration of drugs in leukemia and lymphoma.
TARGETED THERAPY	Individualized therapies that target the underlying pathophysiology (genes, proteins, or properties) of specific tumor types. May include immunotherapy cancer-cell hormone use, or tumor blood vessel growth (angiogenesis).
IMMUNOTHERAPY	Use of immune methods to stop or slow tumor cell growth by administering synthetic antibodies targeted at tumor antigens or by vaccinating the patient with tumor antigen to stimulate immune system production of antitumor antibodies. Example: *rituximab* is a manufactured monoclonal antibody (mab) used in the therapy of non-Hodgkin lymphomas, which targets the C20 antigen on B lymphocytes.

5.27 The collection of intact pieces of tissue for microscopic diagnosis by surgical excision or needle to obtain a thin cylinder of tissue is ________.

5.28 Great variety in the size and shape of cells and nuclei in a tumor is called ________.

5.29 Which provides the best information to guide prognosis and therapy in patients with malignancy: the stage of the tumor or its grade?

5.30 Which of the following terms describe aggressive tumors: well-differentiated, atypical nuclei, Grade I, Stage IV.

Cancer Treatment

Upon discovery of cancer, the initial hope is that it can be cured. Defining a cure is difficult, however, because some cancers may disappear with initial treatment only to recur years, even decades, later from tiny foci of tumor cells that survived treatment. For the most part, "cure" is defined as tumor-free survival for a certain period of time (usually 5 or 10 years). For every cancer there is abundant survival data for every mode of treatment, which indicate the treatment most likely to offer the best hope of cure or the longest survival. Treatments may be arduous, however, and not every patient can tolerate a given treatment or is willing to accept likely side effects, some of which are disabling. In some instances there is no reasonable hope of cure at the time of diagnosis. In such cases the aim of treatment is to prolong and improve the quality of life; in other cases the aim of treatment is *palliative*: to provide immediate comfort and relief from tumor effects.

The primary tumor mass is always the main target of treatment. Nevertheless, additional treatment may be aimed at the possibility that the tumor has spread by micrometastases that cannot be detected but that, if left untreated, would be sure to blossom into detectable metastases in the future. For example, following complete removal of a breast cancer, the patient may be offered several courses of chemotherapy and/or radiation to nearby lymph nodes in the hope that if micrometastases are present they will be eliminated. Multiple courses are offered because it is unlikely that all micrometastases will be destroyed with a single course.

Until the closing decades of the 20th century, surgery, radiation therapy, and chemotherapy were the mainstays of cancer treatment. Although all three remain important, new techniques are helping to increase options for oncologists and their patients (Table 5.3).

Surgery Is the Most Common Treatment

Surgery is typically the first choice of treatment for discrete neoplasms and involves mechanical removal of the cancer and, if possible, a rim of normal tissue to ensure complete removal. Sometimes, however, complete removal is not possible because it would require unacceptable damage to vital structures nearby. Typically, nearby lymph nodes are removed and with them any metastases they may contain.

Sometimes the aim of surgery is to destroy the tumor without removing it. **Radiofrequency ablation** involves inserting into the tumor a probe that emits high frequency radio waves, which heat tissue to the point of necrosis. **Cryotherapy** involves freezing the tumor to induce necrosis. Alternatively, liquid nitrogen can be used to destroy superficial tumors such as skin cancers. **Laser therapy** can be used to treat superficial cancers of skin or mucosa by burning the tumor away. For example, carcinoma in situ of the cervix (Chapter 17) can be easily treated with laser therapy.

Radiation Blocks Tumor Cell Reproduction

Ionizing radiation can be administered in several ways (Table 5.3). It is usually administered as external radiation in the form of X-rays, but gamma rays or other forms may also be employed. The effect is to damage DNA so that cell division stops. Therefore, for any given dose, radiation has its greatest effect on neoplasms that grow rapidly, especially lymphomas and leukemias. Adverse effects of radiation depend upon the dose and the breadth of application. Dosages are calculated carefully to avoid overexposure.

A virtue of external radiation is that it can be focused like light, but not so sharply. The result is a strong effect in the center surrounded by surrounding zones of lesser effect. Because tumors are irregularly shaped, some normal tissue is usually damaged. Much the same is true for internal radioactive implants: they provide a strong effect near the implant with surrounding zones of lesser effect.

Systemic radiation involves administration of intravenous radioactive material, which is circulated throughout the body. In most instances the material is designed to be assimilated by the tumor, so that the tumor gets a large dose and other tissues receive a much smaller one. Tissues most likely to suffer adverse effect are those that have the shortest life span and must reproduce rapidly to replace dying cells: bone marrow, epidermis, and respiratory and intestinal epithelium. Bone marrow depression is the most serious because decreased white cell and platelet production exposes patients to risk of infection and bleeding.

Case Notes

5.21 Brenda was given external pelvic radiation. Was this likely to affect her bone marrow in the spine and ribs?

Chemotherapy Is Drug Treatment of Cancer

Chemotherapy, the drug treatment of malignant neoplasms, is comparatively new and, like radiation, has its greatest effect on rapidly dividing cells. Its development can be traced to a World War II accidental spill of sulfur mustard (a chemical warfare agent), which resulted in troop fatalities. Autopsies revealed marked depletion of both bone marrow and lymph nodes. This led to successful treatment experiments in mice with bone marrow cell neoplasms, and eventually a successful trial in non-Hodgkin lymphoma (Chapter 7). Animal research gradually identified additional compounds and from the modest success of these agents came the increasingly successful use of drugs to treat malignancy. Sidney Farber, a pediatric pathologist, became the first to use chemotherapy to induce remission in childhood leukemia, which earned him fame as the "father of chemotherapy." The most notable of early drugs was *paclitaxel* (Taxol®), which was found to prevent cell division or induce natural cell death (apoptosis) in some cancers.

For the most part, chemotherapeutic agents are administered systemically by mouth or by intravenous injection. In some instances, the agent is tied to another chemical that will be assimilated by tumor cells, so that the tumor receives a much higher dose than other tissues. Typically, two or more drugs are used in combinations and sequences that have a reinforcing effect. In some instances, however, they may be injected into the arteries supplying the tumor to deliver a very high dose to the tumor and a much lower dose to the remainder of the body as the agent spreads into the general circulation. As with radiation, bone marrow cells and epithelial cells of skin, bronchial mucosa, and intestinal mucosa normally divide most rapidly and are most vulnerable to side effects. Bone marrow depression exposes the patient to the risk of infection or hemorrhage from low platelet count. Nausea, vomiting, and diarrhea are common side effects. Hair loss is common because hair cells in hair follicles grow rapidly. During chemotherapy, hair growth slows, the root of the hair becomes narrow, and hairs break off at the narrow point. Recently "cold cap" treatment has proven effective at preventing hair loss. Wearing icy caps during therapy slows normal hair growth so that chemotherapy has little effect on the dormant hair.

Case Notes

5.22 Brenda was given chemotherapy. Did it likely affect her bone marrow?

Advances in Cancer Research Have Led to New Therapies

As understanding of cancer biology and genetics has evolved, so has the treatment. Identifying the molecular abnormalities in cancer can be used to develop *targeted therapy* to treat a particular aspect of cancer. For example:

- *Hormonal manipulation*. Arguably the first molecularly targeted therapy was *tamoxifen*, a chemical that blocks the estrogen receptors present on some breast cancer cells. Tumors with estrogen receptors grow most avidly with the aid of estrogen. Depriving them of estrogen slows their growth. Women whose cancers have this receptor now receive tamoxifen in combination with surgery and/or radiation.

- *Growth factor suppression*. Aggressive breast cancers may produce an excessive amount of *human epidermal growth factor receptor 2 (HER2)*, a protein that promotes cell growth. The effect of HER2 can be reduced by administering *trastuzumab* (Herceptin®), a synthetically produced antibody (**monoclonal antibody**), which binds to HER2 and neutralizes its function.
- *Stimulating immune destruction of tumor cells*. Antibody-based drugs are engineered antibodies designed to bind to a particular tumor protein target. Monoclonal antibodies can be synthesized to attach to virtually any cell membrane protein and manipulated in a way that stimulates the body's immune system to attack the targeted cell.
- *Enzyme blockage*. Perhaps the best example of targeted therapy is *imatinib* (Gleevec®), a small molecule that has proven remarkably effective in the treatment of chronic myelogenous leukemia. Before imatinib, about 5% of patients lived two years beyond diagnosis. With imatinib, more than 90% survive five years. Imatinib blocks the action of a mutant gene that synthesizes excess, unregulated tyrosine kinase, an enzyme that promotes unregulated overproduction of myelocytes, the family of WBCs that includes neutrophils and monocytes.

As mentioned in the opening of this chapter, another relatively new therapy targets the blood vessels that feed the tumor through antiangiogenics such as *bevacizumab* (Avastin®).

Immunotherapy may prove to be the ultimate targeted therapy: the development of anticancer B and T lymphocytes that are programmed to attack tumor cells and no other. Gene therapy also holds promise. Researchers have successfully manipulated the genes of a line of T lymphocytes that specifically attacked cancer cells. The trend of current developments suggests that we are moving into an era of cancer therapy tailored to the singular molecular characteristics of each patient's cancer—personalized medicine.

Pop Quiz

5.31 The drug treatment of malignant neoplasms is called ___________.

5.32 How was cancer treated prior to the development of cancer drugs?

5.33 How has our understanding of cancer mechanisms changed cancer therapeutics?

Early Detection and Prevention of Cancer

In an ideal world, we would have a cheap, convenient, painless technique to detect all cancers early enough to cure them. The Pap smear screening for cervical cancer meets these criteria, and its widespread use has resulted in a marked decline of deaths from cancer of the cervix. But although early detection of every cancer is a worthy goal, it is not without problems. Screening can be expensive, invasive, inconvenient, and hazardous. And despite a theoretical advantage to finding cancer early, real-world experience often shows little benefit. For example, experimental, highly sensitive radiographic techniques can find lung cancer at a very early stage; however, detecting these very early cancers appears not to result in a decrease in the number of lung cancer deaths. Barnett Kramer of the National Institutes of Health, in a 2004 interview in the *Wall Street Journal*, put it this way: "Finding a cancer early is sometimes like being tied to a railroad track and given a pair of binoculars: you can see the train coming from further away, but you haven't done anything to change when the train is going to hit you."

Opinions vary, but there is general agreement that people with a positive family history of cancer benefit most from screening tests to detect cancer early. Here, slightly modified for brevity and simplicity, are some current screening guidelines from the American Cancer Society (ACS) (www.cancer.org/):

- *Cervical cancer.* The 2012 ACS guidelines recommend screening with Pap smears should begin approximately three years after the onset of vaginal intercourse, but no later than age 21, and should be done every one to two years until age 30, after which screening may continue every two to three years for those women who have had three consecutive negative results. Women over 70 may choose to cease screening if they have had three consecutive negative Pap smears and no abnormal Pap smears within the prior 10 years. In 2006, the U.S. government approved the first vaccine against the strains of HPV that cause approximately 70% of cervical cancers and 90% of genital warts. Vaccination is most efficacious when administered prior to initiation of sexual activity. Vaccination of girls is effective in reducing HPV-related cervical cancer. It is currently recommended that girls can be vaccinated at age 11 or 12. Vaccination of boys is effective in reducing the risk of HPV-related genital warts. Boys may be vaccinated as early as age 9.
- *Breast cancer*. Women age 20–40 should have a clinical breast exam once every three years, and annually thereafter. Yearly mammograms should begin at age 40 and continue for as long as the woman is in good health. Early detection has reduced the death rate

from breast cancer in the United States about 25% since 1990.

- *Prostate cancer*. Perhaps no screening program is more fraught with misunderstanding and controversy than screening men for prostate cancer. Remember that prostate cancer grows slowly and is uncommonly the cause of death in those who develop it. A widely used screening tool is blood PSA measurement. Nevertheless, after many years of routine PSA screening, practices are changing. Because of the low level of sensitivity and specificity of PSA, it is acceptable *not* to be screened. Very few men with PSA <4 ng/ml will have prostate cancer. For PSA 4–10, about 30% will. For PSA >10 ng/ml, the rate is about 60%. Deciding whom to biopsy is difficult. Favoring biopsy is younger age, higher PSA, and more rapid rise of PSA from one year to the next. Sentiment is growing that men beyond age 70–75 should not be biopsied. Those in poor health and with life expectancy <10 years should not be screened. Even more difficult is deciding whom to treat. Because prostate cancer is not usually aggressive, it is legitimate not to treat some elderly men because they are more likely to die of something other than their prostate cancer.

  The ACS notes that it is not clear that the benefit of treatment outweighs the harm. For example, it requires treating 48 men with prostate cancer to save one life. And among the 48, about one-third will lose bladder control or suffer erectile dysfunction, a heavy price. The ACS recommends that men in good health and without a family history of prostate cancer *may* want to have a blood PSA test beginning at age 50. African Americans and those with a positive family history of prostate cancer *may* want to begin as early as age 40.
- *Colorectal cancer*. Remember that colorectal cancer is the number two cancer killer in the United States. *Colonoscopy reduces the death rate from colorectal cancer more than 50%*. The ACS recommends that beginning at age 50, adults at average risk should follow one of the following two regimens.
  1. Have periodic testing that primarily detects *cancer*:
     - *Occult (unseen) blood* in stool once per year. Most colon cancers arise from pre-existing polyps, which take many years to become malignant and tend to bleed.

     OR
     - *Cancer DNA* in stool (testing interval uncertain). Cancers shed malignant cells into stool where DNA can be detected.
  2. Periodically have an annual test that detects *polyps* and *cancer*:
     - Flexible sigmoidoscopy every five years, OR
     - Colonoscopy every 10 years, OR
     - Double-contrast barium enema every five years, OR
     - CT colonography (virtual colonoscopy) every five years.

  Patients with a family history of colorectal cancer or a history of adenomas (adenomatous polyps) of the colon should begin screening at an earlier age.
- *Endometrial cancer*. Women, especially postmenopausal women, should report unexpected vaginal bleeding to their physician.

The ACS makes no recommendation about screening for *lung cancer*. Remember that lung cancer is the number one cancer killer in the United States and worldwide. Until recently, all screening methods failed for lack of sensitivity and specificity (too many false negatives and false positives). Now, specialized CT chest scans of smokers show limited promise in reducing the death rate in smokers by about 20%, but false positives are very common and lead to patient expense and anxiety.

Remember This! Regular colonoscopy reduces the death rate from colorectal carcinoma by more than 50%.

Case Notes

5.23 Which of the ACS guidelines for cancer screening did Brenda not follow?

Pop Quiz

5.34 True or false? Screening programs have no effect on the mortality rate of cancer.

5.35 True or false? Early detection of cancer guarantees cure.

5.36 True or false? Women age 20–40 should have a clinical breast exam every year.

Case Study Revisited

"It's not my normal bleeding." The case of Brenda T.

Brenda had a malignant tumor of the cervix, a carcinoma of the cervical epithelium, which proved its malignancy by invading nearby tissues and metastasizing into the lymphatic system. Of particular interest is her medical history of an abnormal Pap smear associated with a "virus infection." Given that HPV infection is known to be the cause of cancers of the cervix, the Pap smear was an early warning that went unheeded. Also, given that cancer is a multistep process of repeated injuries over time, Brenda's sexual history of unprotected sex with multiple partners strongly suggests that she was reinfected multiple times in the intervening years. It is also significant that bleeding was the sign that compelled her to seek medical attention. Bleeding is one of the hallmark signs of cancer at any site.

Chapter Challenge

CHAPTER RECALL

1. A 5-year-old Caucasian male is brought to your genetics clinic. His past medical history is significant for diffuse erythema, scaling, and freckle-like areas of increased pigmentation over areas of his body after sunlight exposure. You diagnose him with xeroderma pigmentosum and explain to the mother that it is a hereditary condition resulting in uncorrected DNA mutations that may lead to skin cancer due to what type of defective gene?
A. Apoptotic gene
B. Proto-oncogene
C. Tumor suppressor
D. DNA repair gene

2. Which of the following environmental factors plays an important role in carcinogenesis?
A. Age
B. Diet
C. Familial history
D. Gender

3. A 10-year-old Hispanic male is brought to the emergency room. His mother reports that he was sitting at the dining room table when he fell to the floor and began to twitch all over. He has no significant past medical history, but he has recently been complaining of a headache that is worse in the mornings. On MRI he is found to have a mass in the right lateral ventricle. What is the explanation of his symptoms?
A. Pressure of the expanding tumor mass on nearby tissue
B. Infection or bleeding from ulceration of surfaces
C. Infarction or rupture
D. Production of hormones or other molecules that affect distant organs (paraneoplastic syndrome)

4. A 23-year-old African American woman with a past medical history significant for cystic breast nodules undergoes a surgical biopsy of the largest nodule. Which of the following microscopic findings would be most reassuring for a benign lesion?
A. Few mitoses
B. Presence of necrosis
C. Cellular pleomorphism
D. Absence of a capsule

5. Which of the following is an ACS guideline for cancer detection and prevention?
A. Pap smears should begin no later than age 18, and be done every one to two years.
B. Women age 20–40 should have a clinical breast exam annually with mammograms starting at age 40.
C. Beginning at age 50, patients should begin periodic testing for colon cancer to detect blood/cancer DNA in stool and/or polyps via imaging.
D. Starting at age 50, all men should undergo preventative screening for prostate cancer using PSA.

6. A 55-year-old African American female with a past medical history significant for recurrent esophageal reflux presents for her scheduled upper GI endoscopy. A biopsy of the tissue surrounding the lower esophageal sphincter reveals normal intestinal epithelial cells in place of the usual squamous cells; the cells extend to the basement membrane. What type of change has occurred?
A. No change, this is normal epithelium
B. Dysplasia
C. Metaplasia
D. Carcinoma in situ

7. A 60-year-old Caucasian man with a previous history of lung cancer presents for evaluation of a nodule that is protruding from the chest wall. Which of the following is the least invasive procedure capable of providing a diagnostic sample?
A. Fine needle aspiration
B. Biopsy
C. Surgical excision
D. Tumor marker analysis

8. Which of the following statements concerning carcinogenesis is true?
A. A small percentage of cancer patients inherit somatic cell mutations from their parents, which predispose them to the development of certain types of cancer.
B. People with dark-colored skin are most prone to develop neoplasms of the lower lip, forehead, and back of the neck and hands in response to high doses of UV light.
C. Viruses such as HPV and EBV are capable of causing malignancies of the cervix and lymph nodes respectively.
D. Chronic inflammation is a rare cause of neoplasms and, due to lack of precursor lesions, is difficult to detect and prevent.

9. A 63-year-old Caucasian female presents for a routine check-up. During her physical exam, you note some unusual changes. In addition to her elevated blood pressure, she appears to have gained a significant amount of weight around her abdomen; prominent purple striae on the abdomen are also observed. You further note hirsutism, ruddy cheeks, and a pad of fat on the back of her neck and over her clavicles. Her chest X-ray reveals a centralized mass in the lower left lobe. What is the cause of her symptoms?
A. Pressure of the expanding tumor mass on nearby tissue
B. Infection or bleeding from ulceration of surfaces
C. Generalized wasting
D. Production of hormones or other molecules that affect distant organs

10. True or false? Lung cancer is the most common cancer.

11. True or false? Benign neoplasms are low grade due to their anaplastic phenotype on microscopic analysis.

12. True or false? A malignant tumor is one that has the capacity to cause death.

13. True or false? Surgery is typically the first choice in cancer treatment.

14. True or false? The smallest detectable mass is approximately 10 grams.

15. True or false? As understanding of cancer biology and genetics has evolved, so has the treatment, heralding an era of "targeted therapy."

16. True or false? Neoplasms are susceptible to immune attack secondary to acquired DNA mutations, a mechanism referred to as "immune surveillance."

17. Match the following descriptions to the appropriate tumor. Note that some choices may not be used.
i. Benign neoplasm consisting of fibrous tissue
ii. Malignant neoplasm consisting of fibrous tissue
iii. Malignant neoplasm of melanocytes
iv. Cancer of granulocytes
v. Cancer of lymphocytes
vi. Malignant neoplasm consisting of smooth muscle
vii. Benign neoplasms consisting of smooth muscle
viii. Malignant neoplasm of skeletal muscle
ix. Benign neoplasm of bone
x. Malignant neoplasm of bone
A. Leukemia
B. Fibroma
C. Osteoma
D. Melanoma
E. Leiomyosarcoma

CONCEPTUAL UNDERSTANDING

18. What are the seven hallmarks of cancer, and do all neoplasms have these features?

19. What are the types of ionizing radiation, and how do they affect cancer cells?

20. Explain why tumor stage is better than tumor grade in determining patient prognosis.

21. When should tumor markers be used in the diagnosis of cancer?

APPLICATION

22. A young man accompanies his mother to her doctor's visit, where she is scheduled to receive her first dose of chemotherapy. He is very upset about his mother's diagnosis, but is most concerned by her recent weight loss. He believes that the nursing home caring for his mother has been negligent in her care, despite his mother adamantly denying mistreatment. The patient admits to weight loss, fatigue, weakness, and a poor appetite. What advice do you give her son?

23. Citing a recent online article, one of your patients declines a mammogram, stating: "Since the implementation of screening mammograms, breast cancer has increased drastically." How do you respond?

24. Explain the "Darwinian" model (survival of the fittest) of carcinogenesis.

25. What factors affect the metastatic possibility of neoplasms?

CHAPTER

6 Disorders of Fluid, Electrolyte and Acid-Base Balance, and Blood Flow

Contents

Chapter Objectives

After studying this chapter, you should be able to complete the following tasks:

PRESSURE AND THE MOVEMENT OF BODY FLUIDS

1. Explain the difference between hydrodynamic pressure, hydrostatic pressure, and osmotic pressure.
2. Define cardiac output and what factors determines it.

FLUID FLOW IN BLOOD VESSELS AND LYMPHATICS

3. Compare and contrast arteries, arterioles, capillaries, veins, and lymphatics.

WATER AND FLUID COMPARTMENTS

4. Briefly discuss body water compartments, body water balance, and how salts regulate this balance.

FLUID IMBALANCE

5. Discuss the types of edema and separate them into exudates and transudates.
6. Using examples from the chapter, discuss the difference between hypertonic, hypotonic, and normocytic dehydration.

ELECTROLYTE IMBALANCES

7. Describe the signs and symptoms of electrolyte imbalances of sodium, potassium, calcium, phosphate, magnesium, and chloride.

ACID-BASE IMBALANCE

8. Discuss the types of acid-base imbalance, and how compensation acts to restore homeostasis.

HYPEREMIA AND CONGESTION

9. Explain the difference between congestion and hyperemia.

HEMOSTASIS

10. Name the three elements of hemostasis that act to stop bleeding.

HEMORRHAGE

11. Classify hemorrhages by size, and discuss their cause and manifestation.

THROMBOSIS

12. Compare and contrast clotting and thrombosis.

EMBOLISM

13. Discuss the different types of emboli.

INFARCTION

14. Explain why arterial occlusion is not always followed by infarction and why infarction may occur without arterial occlusion.

THE COLLAPSE OF CIRCULATION: SHOCK

15. Name the types and stages of shock.

Case Study

"I think he is having another heart attack." The case of James G.

Chief Complaint: Chest pain

Clinical History: James G. was a 49-year-old African American man whose wife brought him to the emergency room early in the morning because he was having severe substernal chest pain and shortness of breath. He was somewhat disoriented and unable to answer questions meaningfully. His wife said, "I think he's having another heart attack."

She told the ER physician he'd had a heart attack five years earlier, which was followed by successful coronary bypass surgery. He developed congestive heart failure six months ago. He was taking multiple medicines, including diuretics for his increasing tendency to retain fluids.

Physical Examination and Other Data: Vital signs included: normal temperature; heart rate 106/min (normal = 72); blood pressure 75/55 (normal = 120/80); respirations 24/min (normal = 14). He was a man of average height, obese, and clearly in respiratory distress. Breath sounds were "wet." His liver could be felt below the lower edge of his right rib cage. Severe pedal edema was present and his abdomen was swollen with fluid (ascites).

Chest X-ray revealed an enlarged heart, bilateral collections of fluid in the pleural space (pleural effusions), and pulmonary vascular congestion, findings consistent with congestive heart failure and pulmonary edema. Laboratory tests revealed low blood sodium and potassium and the presence of abnormally high troponin, a heart muscle protein, which strongly suggested heart muscle necrosis. An electrocardiogram was diagnostic of an acute myocardial infarction.

Clinical Course: The emergency room physician made a diagnosis of acute myocardial infarction, and right and left ventricular failure with congestive heart failure.

Within a few hours James went into shock. Blood pressure became unobtainable, blood oxygen content fell, blood CO_2 content rose, and he became blue (cyanotic). Respirations became deep, hard, and rapid. Blood bicarbonate fell markedly and pH fell to 7.15 (normal: 7.35–7.45). Despite heroic efforts to alleviate acidosis, stimulate cardiac output, and raise blood pressure, his heart rate slowed and he suffered cardiac arrest from which he could not be resuscitated. Immediately prior to death, blood pH was 6.96 and urine pH was 4.9.

An autopsy revealed severe coronary atherosclerosis. James had an old, healed myocardial infarct of

(continued)

"I think he is having another heart attack." The case of James G. (continued)

the posterior left ventricle. Also present was a fresh thrombus that occluded the left anterior descending coronary artery at the site of a large atheroma. This produced an infarction of the anterior apex of the left ventricle. The lungs were heavy, wet, and congested. The liver was enlarged and severely congested. Ascites and pleural effusions were noted. There was severe edema of his legs and genitals.

Of William Harvey, the most fortunate anatomist, the blood ceased to move on the third day of the Ides of June, in the year 1657, the continuous movement of which in all men, moreover he had most truly asserted . . .

FROM AN OBITUARY OF WILLIAM HARVEY (1578–1657), ENGLISH PHYSICIAN, WHO DISCOVERED THAT BLOOD CIRCULATES CIRCULARLY AND CONTINUOUSLY

Jupiter has its moons, Saturn has its rings, and Mars is "the red planet." Not for nothing is Earth called "the blue planet," for, alone among the planets, Earth has an abundance of water. Life is not possible without water: it is the major ingredient in every cell, every tissue, and every fluid in the body. Watery fluids exist in and move constantly among various *body fluid compartments*: from blood vessels into tissues, from inside cells to outside of them, and vice versa. *Fluid flow* is essential; it brings oxygen, nutrients and other essentials to cells and removes waste products.

Pressure and the Movement of Body Fluids

Fluid movement is necessary for life. The movement of fluids requires *fluid pressure* and *osmotic pressure*.

Blood Pressure Moves Large Volumes of Blood over Long Distances

Fluid pressure is the physical/mechanical pressure exerted on one object by another. **Hydrostatic pressure** is pressure caused by the weight of fluid. For example, scuba divers are subject to increasing pressure the deeper they dive due to the weight of the water above them. Municipal water towers are high so that the hydrostatic pressure of a tall column of water can force water through pipes and out of your faucet.

In most clinical circumstances, *hydrostatic* pressure has a negligible effect. Nevertheless, in some circumstances it can be clinically important.

Hydrodynamic pressure is the *increment* of pressure created by resistance to the flow of fluid in a closed system like plumbing pipes or the cardiovascular system. **Blood pressure** is the hydrodynamic pressure of moving blood. The left ventricle stuffs blood into the aorta and great vessels, which tends to raise pressure. Blood drains out of the arterial tree through tissue capillaries, which tends to lower pressure. As simple as this seems, how blood flowed was a profound mystery until William Harvey unlocked the secret nearly 400 years ago (see *The History of Medicine*, "Does Blood Ebb and Flow like the Tide?").

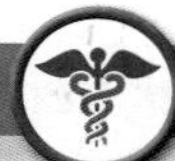

The History of Medicine

DOES BLOOD EBB AND FLOW LIKE THE TIDE?

Does blood ebb and flow like the tide? Or run one-way like a stream? The answer, we now know, is neither—it runs in a circle. In the second century CE, Greek physician Galen postulated blood was made by the liver and the heart and spread outward to tissues where it was consumed, a doctrine that survived nearly 2,000 years until it was refuted by English physician William Harvey (1578–1657). Harvey postulated that blood moved in a circle, flowing away from the heart in arteries and returning to it by veins, though he could not understand how blood passed from arteries into veins.

Harvey was an energetic anatomist, and by dissecting humans and animals he made an observation that had escaped others for centuries. He observed that the human heart could contain about 2 ounces (60 ml) of blood, and coupling this figure with the number of beats the heart makes in a day, he calculated that the volume of blood moved was many, many times the volume of the average person.

Another observation critical to his conclusion about the circular nature of blood flow was the behavior of superficial veins of the forearm after simple occlusion by finger pressure, something curious children may do.

The vein above the occlusion collapses; the vein below remains filled with blood. If occluded at two points, the vein will refill only from below. Harvey reached his conclusions in 1615 but waited until 1628 to publish his immortal paper, "On the movement of the heart and blood in animals." Why did he wait so long? He was afraid of upsetting established belief. Despite his genius, it was another 200 years before Harvey's insight was widely accepted in medicine.

Blood pressure is determined by two main variables: 1) flow into the arterial tree (determined by *cardiac output*) and 2) flow out of the arterial tree (determined by *vascular resistance* to outflow):

Blood pressure = cardiac output × vascular resistance

Cardiac output is determined by heart rate and the volume of blood ejected with each beat (*stroke volume*). Cardiac output is also influenced by *blood volume*: hemorrhage decreases the volume of blood in the arterial tree, decreases cardiac output, and decreases blood pressure. Similarly, increased blood volume is associated with increased cardiac output and increased blood pressure—the reason a blood transfusion restores blood pressure in someone who has hemorrhaged a large volume of blood. **Vascular resistance** is governed by the collective size of small peripheral arteries (arterioles), which constrict to decrease outflow and increase pressure, and vice versa.

Among the several homeostatic mechanisms for maintaining blood pressure, none is more important than the **renin-angiotensin-aldosterone system**. When blood pressure is low, the kidneys secrete **renin**, an enzyme that initiates a cascade of events to maintain blood pressure. Renin acts upon **angiotensinogen**, a protein made by the liver, and converts it into *angiotensin I*, which is in turn converted into *angiotensin II* by **acetylcholinesterase (ACE)**, an enzyme made in the lungs. **Angiotensin II** increases blood pressure by increasing both peripheral resistance and cardiac output. It is a powerful vasoconstrictor, which increases peripheral resistance. It also stimulates secretion of aldosterone from the adrenal cortex. **Aldosterone** is a steroid that acts on the kidney to retain sodium and water, which expands blood volume and, therefore, cardiac output.

Remember This! Movement of water and fluids is determined by the balance of fluid and osmotic pressures.

Blood pressure powers the flow of blood, which serves as a large-scale, bulk transfer mechanism that rapidly moves essentials over long distances, such as moving oxygen from the lungs to tissues. Blood pressure is expressed as the number of millimeters upward it can force a column of mercury (Hg) (mercury is about 13 times heavier than water). Normal *average* arterial blood pressure in the upper arm can force a column of mercury upward to about 100 mm (about 4 inches), which is expressed as 100 mm Hg. Blood pressure is highest in the aorta and great vessels and gradually falls in the circulatory path until it is near zero as it reenters the heart at the right atrium. After passing through tissues, blood in veins is assisted in its flow back to the heart by the massaging action of muscles on veins. Backward flow is prevented by one-way valves in veins.

Case Notes

6.1 James's blood pressure falls. Presuming peripheral resistance is steady, does this mean his cardiac output also falls?

6.2 What does James's low blood pressure imply about flow of blood through tissue?

Osmotic Pressure Moves Small Volumes of Fluid over Short Distances

Osmotic pressure is as important as blood pressure in the movement of body fluids. Nevertheless, it is a slower molecular process that works intimately with blood pressure in the movement of small volumes of fluid over short distances: between blood and tissues, and into and out of cells.

Understanding osmotic pressure requires an understanding of *solutions*, *solvents*, *solutes*, *osmolarity*, *semipermeable membranes*, and *osmosis*. A **solution** is a mixture of solvent and solute. The major component is the **solvent**, in which is dissolved the minor component or the **solute**. Water is the body's solvent. Solutes include carbohydrates, proteins, salts, vitamins, hormones, and many other substances that are soluble in water. Solutes do not include fats, which are not water soluble. The concentration of solute is expressed as **osmolarity**, expressed in *milliosmoles*. In most body fluids, the concentration of dissolved salts is the major determinant of osmolarity. In plasma, however, the concentration of **albumin**, a small protein made by the liver, is about 10 times that of other solutes and is the principal determinant of plasma (blood) osmolarity. Normally, albumin and other plasma proteins remain in the vascular space because they are too large to pass through the vascular wall.

A **semipermeable membrane** is one that is permeable to the *solvent* but not the *solute*. Cell membranes are semipermeable membranes. **Osmosis** is the flow of water across a semipermeable membrane from an area of high *water* concentration to an area of lower *water* concentration—water flows down its gradient, seeking to equalize water concentration across the membrane. **Osmotic pressure** is a measure of the tendency of water to move by osmosis from an area of high water (low solute) concentration across a semipermeable membrane to an area of low water

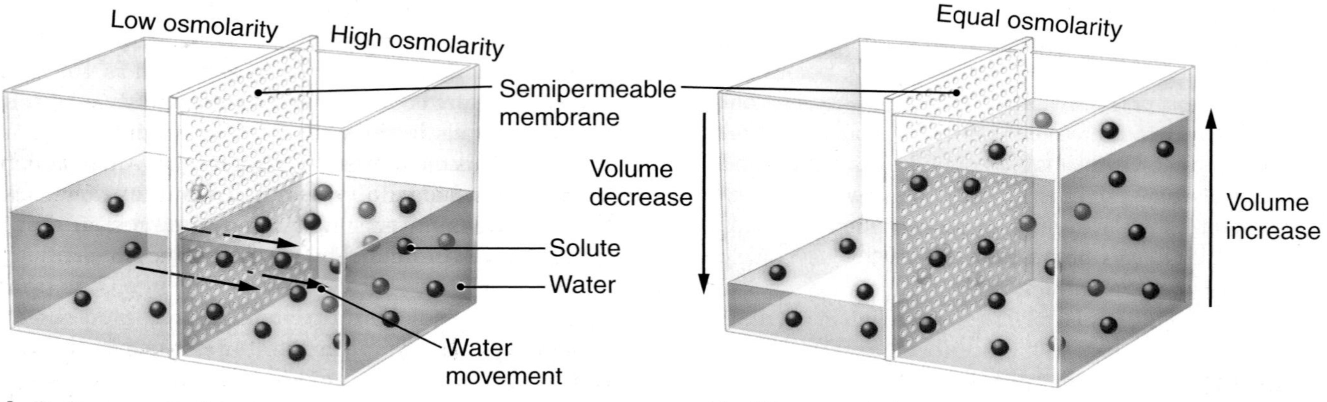

Figure 6.1 **Osmosis. A.** Two compartments in a container are separated by a semipermeable membrane, which permits water but not solute to pass. The left-hand compartment has a lower concentration of solute molecules (and correspondingly more water molecules) than the right-hand compartment. Before osmosis occurs, each compartment contains exactly 1 L of solution; that is, the volume of the two compartments is equal. **B.** After osmosis, water has moved from the left side to the right, equalizing the solute concentration but greatly changing the volume on either side. (Reprinted with permission from McConnell TH, Hull KL. *Human Form Human Function: Essentials of Anatomy & Physiology*. Baltimore, MD: Wolters Kluwer Health; 2011.)

(high solute) concentration (Fig. 6.1). Put another way, osmotic pressure is a measure of how strongly a highly concentrated solute solution "attracts" water.

Case Notes

6.3 Is the albumin in James's plasma a solvent or a solute?

6.4 If James's plasma albumin falls, will his plasma osmotic pressure rise or fall?

6.5 If his plasma albumin falls, will water move into or out of James's vascular space?

6.6 If James ate a high-salt diet, how would this affect his blood volume and blood pressure?

The average solute concentration of the body is equivalent to a 0.9% (by weight) solution of sodium chloride (NaCl) in water (commonly called *normal saline*), which accounts for the fact that such a solution is the most widely administered of intravenous fluids. For example, restoring intravascular volume and blood pressure after severe hemorrhage often depends initially on intravenous water/solute infusions while waiting for transfusion blood to arrive, as explained in *The Clinical Side*, "Emergency Salt Water Therapy."

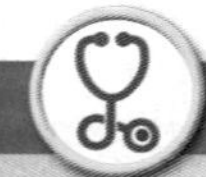

The Clinical Side

EMERGENCY SALT WATER THERAPY

Maintaining blood *volume* is physiologically critical. For example, severe hemorrhage depletes oxygen-carrying capacity because red blood cells (RBCs) are lost; but of equal importance is that blood volume (and, therefore, blood pressure) is also reduced. Merely having enough red cells to sustain life is of little value if there is not enough volume of blood to maintain the pressure necessary to force red cells to flow through the vascular tree. Only red blood cells can restore oxygen-carrying capacity, but saltwater solutions can restore blood flow quickly by increasing blood volume and blood pressure. These solutions can be life-saving because they have the same solute concentration as body fluids and remain largely in the intravascular space for some time after infusion, providing a fluid substitute for plasma. Expansion of blood volume increases cardiac output, which raises blood pressure and aids diffusion of essential substances from blood into tissues.

Under normal conditions, the osmolarity of the extracellular and intracellular fluids is equal, so cells neither swell with excess water nor shrink from loss of it. Nevertheless, a shift of solute concentration initiates water movement. If extracellular solute concentration falls, water will enter the cell, and vice versa. A specific example is *water intoxication*, which can be dangerous, or even fatal. This is well illustrated by a college hazing prank in which a student is forced to drink a very large volume of water. Recalling that water itself knows no boundaries in the body, brain cells absorb their share of the excess and enlarge. The net result is a swollen brain contained in a bony case that will not yield. Often the only adverse effect of such a prank is a bad headache, but convulsion or death can occur.

Pop Quiz

6.1 Is hydrostatic pressure higher in the arms or legs? With incompetent venous valves or functioning venous valves? Arterial or venous vasculature?

6.2 Water flows across a semipermeable membrane from compartment A to compartment B. Which compartment has higher osmotic pressure?

6.3 What are the two factors that determine cardiac output?

6.4 Define osmotic pressure.

Fluid Flow in Blood Vessels and Lymphatics

The anatomy of blood and lymphatic vessels facilitates fluid flows. Arteries and veins are tubes with walls formed of multiple layers of tissue and a central, hollow core (the lumen). Innermost are endothelial cells—the **endothelium**—which line all blood vessels and which control the exchange of substances between blood and tissue. **Arteries** have thick, rubbery walls with multiple layers and carry oxygenated blood under *high pressure* away from the heart to the body or, in the pulmonary system, to the lungs. As arteries extend further from the heart, they branch into progressively smaller channels. **Arterioles** are the smallest arterial vessel and consist only of endothelial cells and a thin wrapping of smooth muscle cells. **Capillaries** are the smallest of all vessels. They are composed only of endothelial cells and connect the arterial tree to veins. The capillary microcirculation modulates the exchange of O_2, CO_2, water, and other small molecules between blood and tissues. Large molecules, especially protein, however, cannot normally pass through the capillary wall from blood into tissue. **Veins** are pliable and relatively underfilled, much like a balloon partially filled with water. They have thin walls, and carry *low pressure*, deoxygenated blood from the body back to the heart.

Lymphatics are a low-pressure capillary-like system of vessels that collect interstitial fluid from between cells and deliver it into blood via a delicate lymph-vascular network. They originate in tissues as small arrays of blunt tubes, like the fingers of a glove. **Lymph fluid** flow is one-way, away from tissues. Lymph vessels merge to form progressively larger channels that ultimately empty into venous blood in the chest via the thoracic duct. The walls of lymph capillaries, like blood capillaries, are formed of a single layer of cells. Nevertheless, in contrast to blood capillaries, lymphatic capillaries have openings between the cells to allow entry of large molecules, especially protein, and particulate matter such as bacteria. As a result, normal lymph fluid is high in protein. In its journey, lymph fluid passes through **lymph nodes**—small nodules of immune system cells that filter lymph fluid and capture bacteria and other foreign matter.

As blood passes through the systemic microcirculation (Fig. 6.2), hydrodynamic pressure and osmotic pressure combine to cause the flow of a small amount of fluid from blood into the interstitial space, where some of it enters the lymphatic system. The remainder is reabsorbed into venous blood from interstitial tissue for return to the right ventricle. Under normal circumstances, hydrodynamic pressure in the lungs is so low that no fluid escapes into the lungs.

In a healthy person, about 5,000 ml of blood leaves and returns to the heart each minute. The movement of water and solutes into and out of blood is mainly controlled by the opposing effects of blood hydrodynamic or hydrostatic pressure and plasma osmotic pressure. Blood pressure tends to force water out of the vascular space; osmotic pressure tends to retain it within. As Figure 6.2 indicates, almost all of the fluid that flows into the interstitial tissue from blood returns to the heart through veins. Nevertheless, a small volume (2 ml/min, or 3 L/day) of fluid returns via the lymphatic system. This occurs because the balance of blood pressure and osmotic pressure forces water out of the capillary microcirculation at the arteriolar end. A small amount flows into lymph capillaries. The remainder reenters the capillary microcirculation at the venous end and is returned to the heart.

Pop Quiz

6.5 True or false? Lymphatics are a system of vessels that collect interstitial fluid rich in proteins from between cells and deliver it into blood via the thoracic duct.

Water and Fluid Compartments

The body is 45% solids such as protein, carbohydrate, and fat, and 55% fluid, virtually all of which is water. Water is the primary constituent of body cells. Total body water (100%) is divided into several compartments (Fig. 6.3). Water is by far the most plentiful element in each of these spaces and it is constantly on the move into and out of these compartments. To move water requires force: fluid pressure, mainly blood pressure, and osmotic pressure, each of which is discussed below.

On average, body water is a 0.9% (by weight) solution of dissolved solutes, mainly minerals. The most abundant are sodium and chloride, with lesser amounts of potassium, calcium, bicarbonate, and a mixture of proteins, fats, and carbohydrates. Clinically, the most important

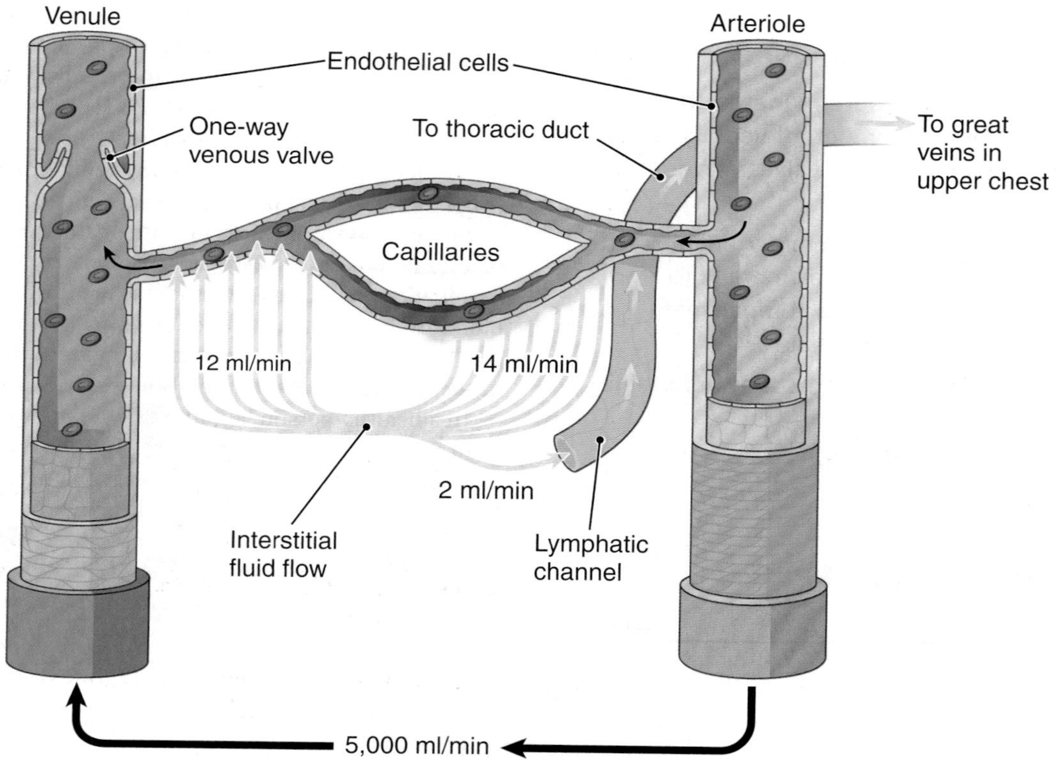

Figure 6.2 **Fluid flow in the microcirculation.** Arteries and veins are connected by capillaries, which are composed of a single layer of endothelial cells. Total normal cardiac output, about 5,000 ml/min, passes through the microcirculation. About 14 ml/min leaves capillaries and enters the interstitial space. Of this 14 ml/min, about 2 ml/min enters the lymphatic system as lymph fluid; the remaining 12 ml/min is reabsorbed into capillaries for return to the heart.

compartment is blood, the intravascular fluid. Blood is about 45% cells (mainly RBCs), and 55% plasma. More than 90% of plasma is water, which contains dissolved solutes such as sodium, potassium, bicarbonate, and other electrolytes. The remaining 10% of plasma is protein, mainly albumin. Small but important volumes of fat (cholesterol and triglyceride) and carbohydrate (glucose and other sugars) are also present in plasma.

In women water comprises about 55% of body mass (weight); the remaining 45% is solids. The proportions in males are 60% water and 40% solid. The difference is due to the relatively greater percentage of fat in women: fat contains little water.

Most water is obtained from food and drink, although a tiny amount is produced by metabolic reactions. Water is lost in stool, urine, perspiration, and respiratory air (Fig. 6.4). Water lost as vapor in breath and by sweat is called *insensible loss* because we usually are unaware of it.

Water intake is regulated by cells in the thirst center of the hypothalamus, which sense osmolarity: high osmolarity (low plasma water) sends signals to the cerebral cortex, which we sense as thirst.

Normal water loss is regulated by three mechanisms:

- *Antidiuretic hormone*, secreted by the posterior pituitary in response to osmoreceptors, influences the kidneys to retain water in blood and concentrate urine.
- *Aldosterone*, secreted by the adrenal cortex on command of renin secreted by the kidneys, influences the kidneys to retain sodium in blood rather than release it into urine.
- *Atrial natriuretic peptide*, secreted by the atrial cardiac muscle cells in response to increased blood volume, influences the kidney to release sodium and water, which lowers blood pressure by lowering blood volume.

Case Notes

6.7 James was very obese. Would his percentage of body water be higher or lower than that of a lean male?

Electrolytes Are Salts

Body fluid compartments contain many dissolved substances (*solutes*). The most important for our discussion are **electrolytes**. Electrolytes are salts. **Salts** are chemical compounds that separate into ions when dissolved in water. An **ion** is an atom or molecule with a net positive or negative electric charge. **Cations** (such as Na+ or K+) are positively charged, whereas **anions** (such as Cl^- or HCO_3^-) are negatively charged. For instance, sodium chloride (NaCl, common table salt) dissociates in water into its

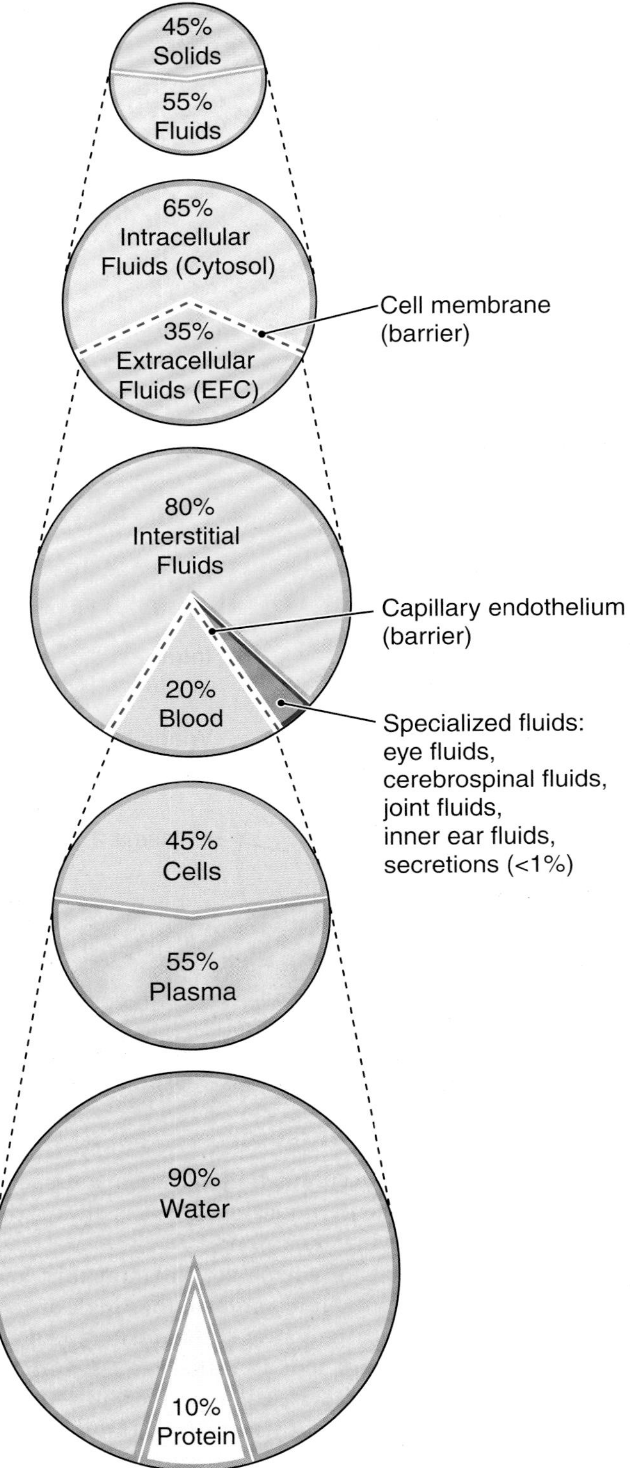

Figure 6.3 **Body fluid compartments.** Body fluids can be divided into numerous compartments. This figure shows the approximate values for a lean female.

component ions, Na^+ and Cl^-. Both the compound and its component ions are considered to be electrolytes.

We gain salts via diet. The most common dietary salt is common table salt (NaCl), even though a varied diet of unsalted foods contains more than enough NaCl for physiologic purposes. Normally, we lose a modest amount of salt (mostly sodium) in urine and sweat. Little escapes in feces.

Although we will devote most of our attention here to Na^+ and Cl^-, other important electrolytes in body fluids include potassium (K^+), bicarbonate (HCO_3^-), calcium (Ca^{++}), and magnesium (Mg^{++}). Though electrolytes have many other functions, in this chapter we will focus on their importance in determining the flow of body water among compartments.

Sodium and Water Balance Are Co-Dependent

To maintain homeostasis, body water must shift among compartments. *Sodium* (Na^+) is the major determinant of fluid shifts between one compartment and another. Blood vessel walls are lined by cells, which form a semipermeable membrane between blood and tissues. These cells are permeable to both Na^+ and water, so that Na^+ and water move easily between plasma and interstitial fluid. The same is not true for tissue cells, whose membranes strictly limit Na^+ passage into cells. Water, however, easily crosses into and out of tissue cells.

The overall body content of Na^+ is a major determinant of body water content. The rule is this: *water follows solute*. That is, Na^+ attracts and holds water. For example, think of the bloated feeling that comes with having a big bag of salty popcorn and a jumbo soft drink. Water and salt are absorbed into plasma, expanding blood volume. The salt crosses the semipermeable cell membrane lining blood vessels and water follows it into the interstitial space. Tissues swell, which produces that bloated sensation.

Remember This! Water follows solute.

But in our salty popcorn and soda example, even after losing volume into the interstitial space, blood volume will still be increased somewhat, and blood volume is a major determinant of blood pressure. It follows that sodium balance and blood pressure are codependent—increased sodium increases blood pressure and vice versa. This relationship is so absolute that body sensors use sodium concentration as a proxy indicator for blood pressure regulation.

The relationship between electrolyte balance and blood pressure has important clinical implications. Pathological alterations in electrolyte balance can alter blood pressure. Chronic abnormally high blood pressure is *hypertension* (Chapter 8), which is associated with a host of ill effects.

Pop Quiz

6.6 Name the two major extracellular fluids.

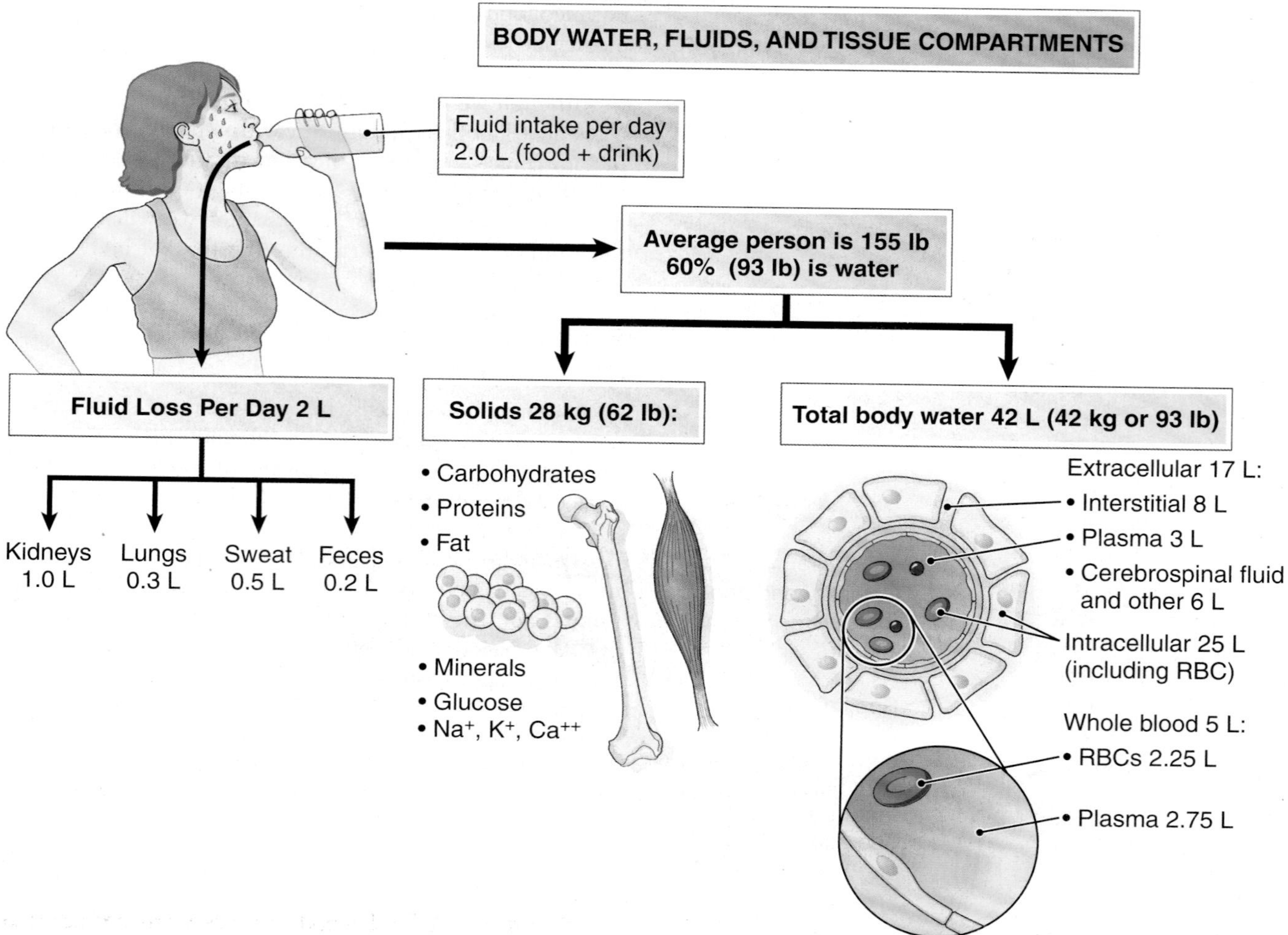

Figure 6.4 **Body water intake and loss.** In the average person weighing 70 kg (155 lb), about 60% of body weight is water. Daily average oral intake is about 2 L per day, which is lost through urine (1 L), respiratory evaporation (0.3 L), sweat (0.5 L), and feces (0.2 L). Body water resides in two main fluid compartments: intracellular and extracellular. Extracellular fluid is divided into interstitial fluid, blood, and specialized fluids.

Pop Quiz

6.7 Which fluid compartment contains the largest water volume—the intracellular compartment or the extracellular compartment?

6.8 In the absence of compensation, what effect would a high-sodium diet have on blood pressure?

Fluid Imbalance

In a healthy person, fluid moves into and out of cells and fluid compartments with quiet ease. But in some disease states the body may not be able to keep up with loss, or fluid may shift abnormally such that a compartment may have too much fluid.

Edema Is an Excess of Fluid

Edema is an abnormal accumulation of fluid in a tissue or body cavity such as the peritoneal cavity. It is always the result of some underlying condition.

The two main types of edema are inflammatory and noninflammatory. Edema fluid can be either high or low in protein according to its cause. Inflammatory edema has high protein content and is called an **exudate**. It is created by the increased vascular permeability of inflammation, which allows protein to leak through capillary walls. Low protein edema is caused by pressure imbalance and is called a **transudate** (Fig. 6.5). Either increased capillary fluid pressure or decreased plasma osmotic pressure can cause accumulation of transudate, if the net movement of water exceeds lymphatic drainage. A diagnostic feature of transudate edema is a "pitting edema"—when an area is pressed with a finger an impression—a "pit"—remains (Fig. 6.6). Inflammatory edema and lymphedema (discussed below) are high protein edemas and do not "pit."

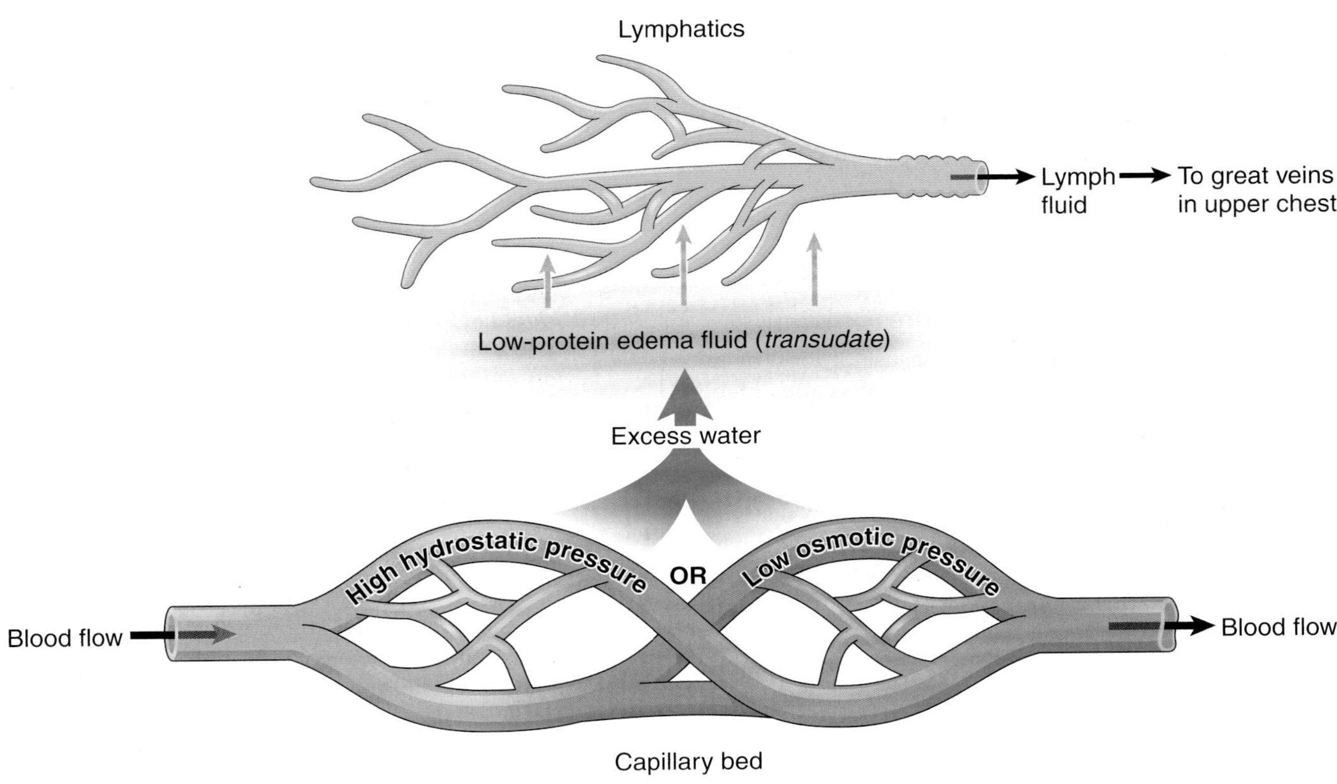

Figure 6.5 **The formation of low-protein edema (transudate).** Edema accumulates as a result of abnormally high venous hydrostatic pressure or abnormally low plasma osmotic pressure, either of which allows escape of water from blood plasma into interstitial tissue or body spaces.

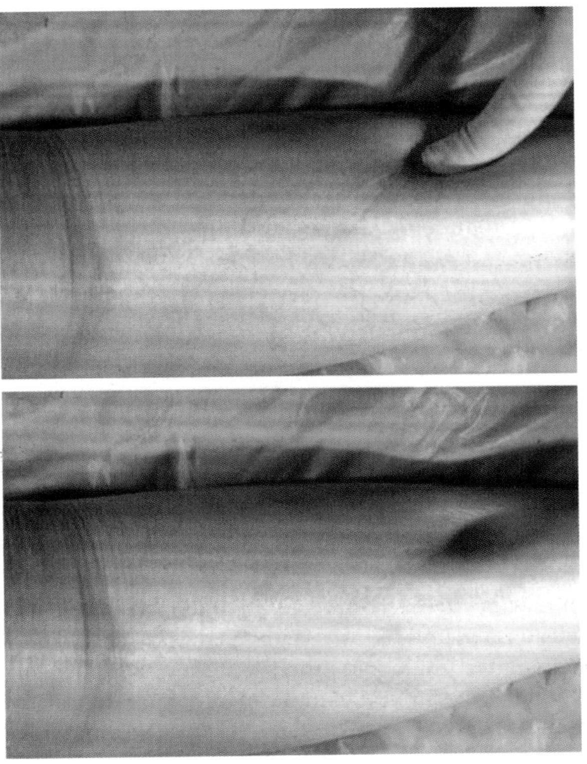

Figure 6.6 **Pitting of low-protein edema (transudate).** Gentle finger pressure leaves an impression.

Collections of fluid in body cavities are named according to the cavity: *hydrothorax*, *hydropericardium*, or *hydroperitoneum*. The latter is usually called **ascites**. Severe, generalized edema is termed **anasarca**. Clinically the word *effusion* is commonly used to describe these accumulations, as in *pericardial effusion (hydropericardium)* or *pleural effusion (hydrothorax)*.

Edema is usually mild and localized, as with the swelling associated with tissue injury and inflammation. Nevertheless, it can be generalized, as it is in heart failure and in some types of severe liver or kidney disease. Localized edema is easy to see, but generalized edema may be more difficult to appreciate. General accumulation of a few liters of edema fluid may not be visible, but can be tracked by weighing the patient daily (a liter of edema fluid weighs 2.2 lb).

The most common effect of edema is swelling, which is usually without further consequence. Nevertheless, a pleural effusion may compress the lungs enough to impair respiration. Similarly, a pericardial effusion may impair the ability of the heart to pump blood. Brain edema may prove fatal because the swollen brain has no place to expand, and the increased pressure may cause fatal injury. Chronic hydrostatic edema in the lower leg from varicose veins can impair blood flow and render skin vulnerable to skin atrophy and ulceration.

Case Notes

6.8 Assuming no inflammation is present, is the excess fluid in James's chest, abdomen, and legs a transudate or an exudate?

6.9 Is James's edema "pitting edema"?

Edema of Increased Fluid Pressure

Increased fluid pressure is often the cause of local or regional edema. The hydrostatic pressure of venous blood is greatest in the feet because the feet are normally the lowest part of the body and have a tall column of blood in veins above them. Hydrostatic pressure would be much higher in the feet except that one-way valves in the large veins of the legs prevent backflow and constrain downward hydrostatic pressure. If these valves are incompetent, however, as they are in patients with varicose veins, hydrostatic pressure increases, veins bulge, and edema results. Similarly, venous obstruction by a large thrombus (discussed below) increases resistance to venous blood flow, hydrodynamic pressure rises and edema accumulates in the affected part, usually a leg. Another important cause of increased venous fluid pressure is *right* heart failure, a condition in which the right ventricle is incapable of ejecting all of the blood delivered to it. Intravenous fluid pressure increases because resistance to flow increases as blood "dams up" as it tries to get into the right side of the heart. The result is edema in tissues below the heart, typically in the loose tissue of the genitals or the legs.

Case Notes

6.10 Does James's pedal edema argue for increased or decreased venous pressure?

Edema of Low Plasma Osmotic Pressure

Albumin is a small protein molecule made by the liver and is the major determinant of plasma osmotic pressure. Decreased plasma osmotic pressure occurs when plasma albumin falls. Low albumin occurs when synthesis is impaired by liver disease, or if albumin is lost into urine in some kidney diseases. *Cirrhosis* of the liver is a major cause of osmotic edema. The combination of osmotic edema and urinary loss due to kidney disease is called *nephrotic syndrome*. In each instance the movement of fluid out of blood into the interstitial space lowers blood volume, and with it, blood flow to organs falls. The kidneys sense this and secrete *renin*, a hormone that acts to restore blood volume and blood flow by retaining salt. The retained salt causes obligatory water retention, but cannot make up for decreased albumin, and edema increases.

Edema of Salt and Water Retention

As mentioned immediately above, salt and water retention can be a cause of edema. The most common cause of salt and water retention is *heart failure* (Chapter 9), a condition in which one or both of the ventricles is unable to pump enough blood to meet metabolic demand. One of the consequences is dilation of the ventricle and "damming up" of blood upstream of the failing ventricle: in the lungs with left ventricular failure; in the systemic circulation with right ventricular failure. Ventricular failure has a forward effect and a backward effect (Fig. 6.7).

The *forward effect* of ventricular failure is low cardiac output, low blood pressure, and low blood flow to the body, including the kidneys. Sensing this, the kidneys increase their output of *renin*, a hormone, which increases renal salt and water retention to expand blood volume and raise blood pressure. In the nonfailing heart, increased blood volume increases cardiac output and blood pressure. But in the failing heart, the opposite is true: increased blood volume increases left ventricular strain, which impairs cardiac output. The result is a vicious circle with ever-worsening failure and increasing edema.

The *backward effect* of left ventricular failure is pulmonary congestion, increased pulmonary hydrodynamic pressure, and pulmonary edema. The high pulmonary blood pressure increases the resistance to right ventricular output. This may cause the right ventricle to fail, which causes systemic venous congestion and increased venous pressure, which in turn causes further edema. The most common cause of right heart failure is left heart failure.

Case Notes

6.11 James's lungs were "wet," indicating pulmonary edema. Is this due to right or left heart failure?

6.12 James has pulmonary edema. Is it due to increased fluid or osmotic pressure?

6.13 On admission, is it likely that blood flow to James's kidneys was high or low? Why?

6.14 Does left heart failure cause the kidneys to retain or to excrete more salt and water? Why?

The Edema of Lymphatic Obstruction

Edema resulting from lymphatic obstruction is termed **lymphedema**. It is local, usually occurring in a limb. Common causes include tumor obliteration of lymph nodes, surgical interruption of lymph channels, and radiation scarring after tumor radiotherapy. Severe lymphedema of the upper arm can be a complication of surgery or irradiation of the breast or axillary lymph nodes in the treatment of breast cancer. Like inflammatory edema, lymphedema is a high protein edema and does not "pit" to finger pressure.

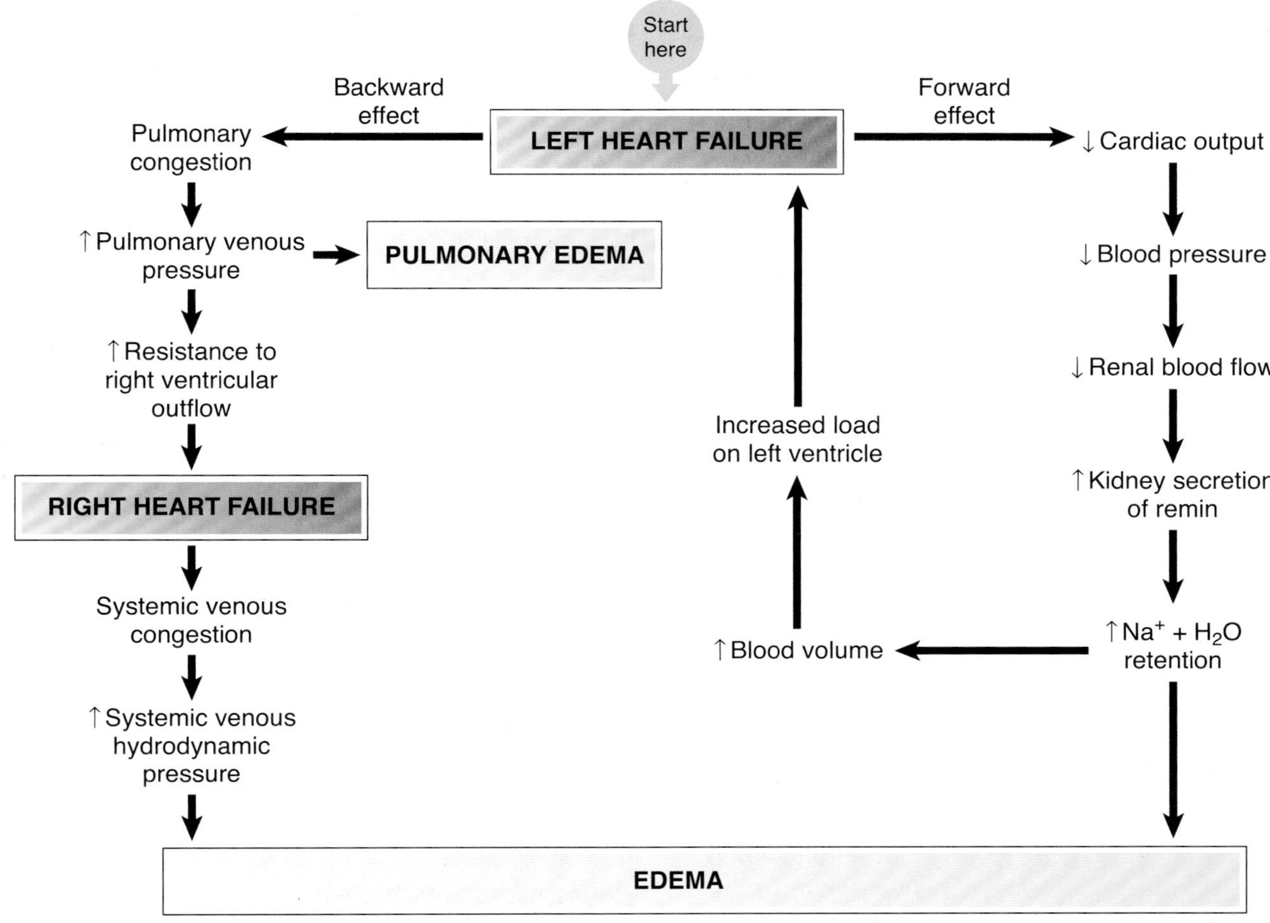

Figure 6.7 **Congestive heart failure and the formation of edema.** The forward effect of left heart failure leads to renal sodium and water retention. The backward effect of left heart failure leads to hydrostatic pulmonary edema, right heart failure and formation of peripheral hydrostatic edema, both of which are compounded by sodium and water retention.

Dehydration Is Insufficient Body Water

Dehydration is a deficiency of body water, which may be due to insufficient water intake, excess loss, or a combination of the two. Excess loss is the most common cause of dehydration. Diarrhea and heavy sweating are common causes. Because sweat and intestinal fluid are extracellular fluids, the extracellular compartment dehydrates first, but if not corrected, the intracellular compartment may be affected and cellular function may deteriorate. For example, prolonged high blood glucose in diabetes may cause brain cell dehydration and coma: high blood glucose increases osmotic pressure in blood, which draws water out of neurons, shifting it into blood (part of the extracellular space), dehydrating the neurons and causing brain malfunction. Diabetics with prolonged high blood glucose may become severely dehydrated owing to the glucose that spills into urine. Glucose is a solute that increases urine osmotic pressure, which attracts water into urine, increasing urine output and fluid loss.

The severity of dehydration is categorized by the relative amount of lost body weight. In general, 2% loss is *mild* dehydration, 5% is *moderate*, and 8% is *severe*.

Dehydration is often more severe in infants, the elderly, or those with debilitating illness. Infants have relatively larger skin surface area and higher metabolic rate than adults, and therefore have greater insensible loss. The elderly or debilitated may not drink enough fluid, and may not sense thirst or be able to communicate their need. Dehydration shifts water out of the vascular space, lowering blood pressure and blood flow, which may affect brain, heart, and kidney function.

Fluids lost carry solute, mainly electrolytes. For example, sweating causes loss of water plus sodium and chloride. Restoration of water alone is often all that is necessary in mild cases, but restoration of electrolytes is necessary when loss is severe or prolonged. A feature of many sport drinks is a small amount of electrolytes to restore electrolyte loss.

Dehydration can be according to concentration of electrolytes in the fluid lost. *Normotonic* dehydration refers to loss of a fluid roughly equivalent to normal plasma (e.g., sweat); *hypotonic* refers to loss of a fluid with low electrolyte concentration (e.g., urine); and *hypertonic* refers to loss of a fluid with high electrolyte concentration (e.g., diarrhea fluid).

Clinical signs of dehydration include dry mucus membranes; low blood pressure; weak, rapid pulse; increased relative percentage of RBCs as a fraction of blood volume (hematocrit), reflecting lost plasma water; pale, cool skin from peripheral vasoconstriction to maintain blood pressure; and low urine output. A distinctive sign is lost tissue elasticity (**tissue turgor**), which can be observed by pinching skin into a fold and releasing it. Dehydrated skin will stay pinched for a while, slowly retracting; normal skin recovers instantly.

A shift of fluid out of blood into another body space is referred to as **third-spacing**, which is associated with lost blood volume, low blood pressure, and low flow to tissues. Important causes are peritonitis, which shifts fluid out of blood into the peritoneal space, and severe skin burns, which shifts fluid out of blood into burn edema.

Pop Quiz

6.9 Edema is caused by increased ________ or decreased ________.

6.10 What type of edema will a patient with congestive heart failure have? Lymphatic obstruction?

6.11 True or false? The most common cause of right heart failure is left heart failure.

6.12 Give an example of each of the following: normocytic dehydration, hypotonic dehydration, and hypertonic dehydration.

Table 6.1 Major Electrolytes

Ions	Intracellular Fluid* (mEq/L)	Plasma and Extracellular Fluid† (mEq/L)
CATIONS		
Sodium (Na^+)	10	142
Potassium (K^+)	160	4
Calcium (Ca^{++})	Varies	5
Magnesium (Mg^{++})	35	3
ANIONS		
Bicarbonate (HCO_3^-)	8	27
Chloride (Cl^-)	2	103
Phosphate (HPO_4^{--})	140	2

*Values vary slightly from one person to another.

† Plasma, interstitial fluid, and other extracellular fluid concentrations vary slightly from one another.

Electrolyte Imbalances

Electrolytes are the ionic components of salts, which separate into their constituent positively charged (**cations**) and negatively charged (**anions**) ions in water. For example, sodium chloride dissolves in water to become Na^+ and Cl^-. Table 6.1 lists the principal electrolytes. Electrolytes have many physiologic roles. Among others, they 1) maintain the electric potential of the cell membrane, 2) propagate nerve signals, 3) enable muscle cell contraction, and 4) as solutes are very important in movement of fluids by osmosis.

Sodium and Water Balance Are Closely Interdependent

Body fluid volume and sodium concentration are normally maintained within very narrow limits. Water follows sodium wherever it goes, and vice versa. Homeostatic balance of sodium, water, and other electrolytes is modulated primarily by the kidneys.

Sodium (Na^+) passes easily and without energy consumption by simple diffusion among extracellular fluids, where concentrations are the same. For example, the Na^+ in dietary salt is absorbed into the interstitial space of gastrointestinal (GI) epithelium, and then diffuses into plasma and spreads throughout the body. Nevertheless, Na^+ concentration is much greater in extracellular fluid than in intracellular fluid, a steep gradient that requires energy to be spent by the sodium-potassium pump in the cell membrane, which pumps Na^+ out of the cell in exchange for potassium (K^+).

Sodium exists in body fluids mainly as sodium chloride (NaCl, common table salt), and sodium bicarbonate ($NaHCO_3$). Diet is the main source of sodium. Sodium is secreted into body fluids—it is lost in sweat, feces, and urine. Plasma levels are mainly maintained by aldosterone, which acts on the kidneys to reduce urine sodium excretion.

Sodium is important in the maintenance of plasma (and, therefore, blood) volume because of its osmotic power—it accounts for about 90% of electrolyte solute—and it is important in nerve signal transmission.

Hyponatremia is low plasma sodium. It is usually due to excessive loss by sweating or occurs in patients with vomiting or diarrhea. It may also be caused, however, by excessive water ingestion, or by certain diuretics that promote urinary sodium loss.

Hyponatremia impairs nerve impulses and has osmotic effects that shift water from one compartment to another. Muscle cramps are a common symptom. Low plasma sodium causes water to shift out of plasma, lowering blood volume and blood pressure. Low extracellular sodium causes water to shift into cells, causing intracellular edema and cell swelling. The effect is minimal in most cells, but swollen brain cells can cause marked increase of intracranial pressure with headaches, seizures, or death.

Treatment depends on correcting the underlying cause. For example, if loss is the cause, as in severe diarrhea, then treatment is aimed at stopping the diarrhea, supplemented by oral or intravenous replacement of sodium and water.

Hypernatremia is high plasma sodium. It is less common than hyponatremia and caused by excess salt ingestion, dehydration, or watery (low sodium) diarrhea. A rare cause is failure of the pituitary to secrete antidiuretic hormone, the absence of which causes a flood of low sodium urine output.

The major effect of hypernatremia owes to increased osmotic pressure of plasma and other extracellular fluids. Water shifts out of cells, which may cause weakness and agitation. Urine output falls to preserve water, and thirstiness is stimulated.

Treatment depends on correction of the underlying cause.

Potassium Is the Primary Intracellular Cation

Potassium (K^+), like sodium, passes by simple diffusion among extracellular fluids, where concentrations are the same. Nevertheless, K^+ concentration is much greater in intracellular fluid than in extracellular fluid, a steep gradient that requires energy to be spent by the sodium-potassium pump in the cell membrane, which actively pumps Na^+ out of the cell in exchange for K^+. Insulin shifts K^+ into cells and acidosis (low blood pH) shifts it out of cells.

Diet is the main source of K^+. It is excreted into body fluids. It is important in cardiac and skeletal muscle contraction, in nerve signal transmission, in intracellular osmotic pressure, and in many metabolic processes. Under normal circumstances, blood levels are maintained by aldosterone, which acts on the kidneys to increase urine K^+ excretion. Plasma *acid-base balance*, discussed below, also affects plasma K^+ levels. Diabetic ketoacidosis (Chapter 13) is an example. As plasma pH falls (*acidosis*, increased hydrogen [H^+] ions), H^+ moves into interstitial fluid and then into cells, where, to maintain electrical neutrality, H^+ displaces K^+ out of cells and into the interstitial fluid and then into plasma, increasing plasma K^+. The reverse occurs with increased plasma pH (*alkalosis*, low H^+).

Hypokalemia is low plasma potassium. It can be caused by fecal loss with diarrhea; by low dietary potassium with alcoholism or eating disorders; by certain antihypertensive diuretic drugs that promote urine loss; by high plasma levels of aldosterone and cortisol, which promote urine loss; and in the use of high doses of insulin in the treatment of diabetic acidosis (insulin promotes the movement of K^+ into cells).

The most important effect of hypokalemia is on the electrical activity of the heart, which is accompanied by distinctive changes in the electrocardiogram. Hypokalemia promotes electrical instability and abnormal rhythms (*arrhythmias*), which may be fatal. It also interferes with skeletal muscle contraction, causing fatigue and weakness, which begins in the legs and ascends. Hypokalemia also interferes with sensory nerve function, promoting tingling sensations (*paresthesias*). Treatment is by oral or intravenous replacement.

Hyperkalemia is high plasma potassium. It is most often caused by renal failure and by use of certain antihypertensive diuretic drugs that promote renal potassium retention. Massive tissue injury may release a large amount of intracellular potassium, which is absorbed into plasma.

Hyperkalemia impairs nerve signal transmission and skeletal muscle contraction, causing weakness, paralysis, and sensory paresthesias. Nevertheless, it is usually asymptomatic until it interferes with cardiac function, slowing heart rate or, at very high levels, causes cardiac standstill and death.

If blood K^+ is only moderately increased and the matter is not urgent, limiting dietary intake or administration of an oral K^+-binding resin may be effective. For cardiac toxicity, intravenous insulin and glucose may be effective, or dialysis may be required.

Case Notes

6.15 **James has hyponatremia and hypokalemia. What is the most likely explanation?**

Blood Calcium and Phosphate Are Inversely Related

Blood phosphate (HPO_4^{--}, $H_2PO_4^-$) and blood calcium (Ca^{++}) exist in an inverse relationship: as one goes up, the other goes down. Anything that caused blood phosphate to rise will lower blood calcium, and vice versa.

Diet is the main source of calcium. Calcium provides substance and strength to bones, is important in the propagation of nerve impulses and in cardiac muscle cell contraction, and is vital in the coagulation process. It is stored in bone and excreted in urine and feces. Calcium in blood is bound to albumin and is constantly being exchanged with calcium in bone. Calcium balance is modulated by the parathyroid glands (Chapter 14), which secrete **parathyroid hormone (PTH)**. PTH acts to raise blood calcium. It acts on bone to shift calcium into blood, it stimulates intestinal absorption of dietary calcium, and it reduces urinary calcium excretion. Low blood calcium stimulates PTH secretion, which raises blood calcium, and vice versa.

Vitamin D is important in calcium metabolism. It may be ingested, but it is also synthesized in skin by the action of sunlight. It promotes intestinal uptake of calcium and movement of calcium from bone into blood.

Hypocalcemia is low blood calcium. It is relatively uncommon. Common causes include low PTH (usually from inadvertent surgical removal of parathyroid glands during thyroidectomy), high phosphate from renal failure, vitamin D deficiency, or prolonged alkalosis (high blood pH, which limits the physiologic effect of blood calcium). There are many other uncommon causes. For example, severe pancreatitis may cause the deposition of calcium salts in pancreatic fat, which decreases blood calcium.

Hypocalcemia increases the irritability of nerve cells, which causes involuntary contractions of skeletal muscle, either fasciculations (small twitchings) or prolonged contractions (spasms, tetany), and increased skeletal muscle reflexes. Paresthesias and abdominal cramps are common. Cardiac muscle is affected differently than skeletal muscle. The effect on skeletal muscle is due to the effect on nerves, whereas low calcium directly affects heart muscle. Contractions become weaker, irregular rhythms (arrhythmias) occur, and blood pressure falls.

Hypercalcemia is increased blood calcium. It is much more common than hypocalcemia. The most common cause is slight hyperparathyroidism with increased blood PTH. It is quite common, especially in postmenopausal women, and often does little harm and needs no treatment. Also, malignant tumors metastatic to bone (often breast cancer) may dissolve bone, releasing large volumes of calcium into blood. Excess vitamin D intake is another cause, usually seen in someone who is overzealous about dietary supplements. Because healthy bones require daily activity, immobilization, such as in the bedfast, causes resorption of bone calcium into blood.

Hypercalcemia depresses neuromuscular activity and leads to weakness and fatigue. Its effect on the brain may cause lethargy and depression. The kidneys excrete the excess calcium, and increased urinary calcium is a common cause of kidney stones. Cardiac muscle becomes irritable and arrhythmias may occur. Depending on the cause, bones may be weak and fracture easily.

The main goal of treatment is correction of the underlying cause. Slight elevations usually do not need treatment. Moderate increases should respond to oral phosphates. Higher levels call for administration of Ca^{++}-lowering drugs or dialysis.

Phosphate is ubiquitous in food. It serves many physiologic functions, especially in the storing and release of energy via adenosine triphosphate (ATP). It is an integral part of bone and tooth mineralization and serves as an important acid/base buffering system in the control of blood pH.

Hypophosphatemia is low blood phosphate. It can be caused by diarrhea or any condition that raises blood calcium. *Hyperphosphatemia* is high blood phosphate. The most common cause is renal failure. There are other, uncommon, causes. For example, it may be caused by overuse of phosphate enemas in children.

Because of its tight inverse relationship with calcium, it is difficult to separate the clinical effect of change in phosphate from the related changes in calcium discussed above.

Magnesium Imbalance Is Rare

Magnesium (Mg^{++}) is plentiful in the body and in food. Maintenance of blood levels depends on dietary intake and the level of urinary and fecal loss. Because 99% of it is stored in bone and turnover is slow, blood levels are usually independent of total body content. In blood it is bound to protein. Blood levels generally fluctuate with two other blood cations, K^+ and Ca^{++}. Other than its role in the structure of bones, it is important in many enzyme reactions. Imbalances are rare.

Hypomagnesemia is low blood magnesium. The most common cause is dietary deficiency, usually in alcoholics when it is combined with use of diuretic drugs that increase urine Mg^{++} excretion. Symptoms are usually related to the accompanying hypocalcemia and hypokalemia and include lethargy, tremor, tetany, arrhythmias, and seizures. Therapy is replacement.

Hypermagnesemia is high blood magnesium. The usual cause is renal failure. Symptoms include hypotension, depressed respirations, and arrhythmias or cardiac arrest. Treatment is administration of magnesium-lowering drugs.

Chloride Tends to Follow Sodium

Chloride (Cl^-) is the main extracellular anion. Blood levels generally follow sodium levels because of the attraction of the positive (Na^+) and negative (Cl^-) ions for one another. Because both are anions, Cl^- is freely exchangeable for bicarbonate (HCO_3^-) in acid-base balance reactions (discussed below). For example, if excess acid (H^+) is present in blood (acidosis), bicarbonate ions (HCO_3^-) are consumed as they bind with excess H^+ to form H_2CO_3 to maintain normal pH. This reaction causes Cl^- ions to diffuse out of RBCs and into plasma to maintain electrical balance, which raises the Cl^- level. The opposite occurs if blood pH is high (*alkalosis*, low H^+ concentration): bicarbonate (HCO_3^-) rises as H_2CO_3 dissociates to provide more H^+. The rising bicarbonate forces plasma Cl^- into RBCs and blood Cl^- falls.

Pop Quiz

6.13 Failure of the pituitary to secrete antidiuretic hormone will cause what electrolyte imbalance?

6.14 Hypomagnesemia is often accompanied by which electrolyte imbalances?

6.15 When calcium is low, ______________ and ______________ increase, causing an increase in calcium, which then causes phosphate to ______________.

6.16 True or false? Insulin and elevated blood pH shift potassium into cells.

Acid-Base Imbalance

An **acid** is a compound that releases hydrogen ions when dissolved in water, which increases the number of free hydrogen ions in the solution. Recall that pH is a numerical expression of the degree of acidity or alkalinity of a solution—pH 7 is neutral; pH less than 7 is acidic; pH greater than 7 is alkaline. The lower the pH, the more H^+ ions are in solution. For example, HCl is a *strong* acid because it completely dissociates, releasing all of its H^+ and Cl^- when dissolved in water. A *weak* acid, such as the acetic acid (HAc; Ac = *acetate*) in vinegar, holds onto its H^+ much more avidly, and is therefore less strongly acidic. It releases only a few H^+ molecules when dissolved in water.

A **base** is a compound that decreases the number of free H^+ ions, usually by releasing OH^- ions, which combine with H^+ to form H_2O (water). The pH of a base is more than 7. As the concentration of hydroxide (OH^-) ions rises, the concentration of H^+ ions falls, and the solution becomes more basic. Normal arterial blood is slightly basic because the slight deficit of H^+ leaves more room to neutralize the byproducts of metabolic reactions, most of which are acidic. Blood pH is homeostatically controlled in a very narrow range between 7.35 and 7.45. Abnormally low blood pH is **acidosis**; abnormally high pH is **alkalosis**. *Because most metabolic processes generate excess acid, acidosis is far more common than alkalosis.*

Remember This! **Metabolism produces more acids than bases.**

Food may be acidic or basic, but the main task in regulating blood pH is to neutralize and dispose of metabolic acids. *The general principle of acid-base balance is simple—the kidneys excrete as much acid or base as we consume or generate metabolically.* Renal capacity is augmented by the ability of the respiratory system to exhale carbon dioxide, which, when dissolved in blood, is weakly acidic. But before we discuss the kidneys' role in acid-base balance, it is useful to discuss types of acid-base imbalance and the role of the lungs and of chemical buffer systems in the control of blood pH.

Case Notes

6.16 Shortly before death, James's blood pH was 6.96. Did his blood contain more free hydrogen ions than normal blood, or fewer?

There Are Four Categories of Acid-Base Imbalance

The chemical reaction above occurs in blood as well as in cerebrospinal fluid. Blood pH homeostasis is maintained by the respiratory center of the medulla, which responds to increased acidity in the cerebrospinal fluid by increasing respiration and exhaling the extra CO_2. Carbon dioxide is described as a **volatile acid** because it can be exhaled. Increased tissue CO_2 production—say, during moderate exercise—is matched with increased respiratory exhalation of CO_2, which keeps arterial pH relatively constant. But, if lung function is significantly impaired, ventilation cannot adequately rid the body of CO_2. In such cases, CO_2 accumulates in arterial blood and **respiratory acidosis** results.

Conversely, if respiration is greater than CO_2 production requires (say, during hyperventilation in a panic of anxiety), the reduction in CO_2 can raise pH and **respiratory alkalosis** results.

Acids that cannot be exhaled are **fixed acids**. They include ingested amino acids (especially from meat) and ketones produced from fatty acid metabolism. Moreover, the reactions that generate and use ATP during intense exercise also release hydrogen ions that contribute to blood acidity. Increased blood acidity resulting from fixed acids is called **metabolic acidosis**. Figure 6.8 illustrates the three systems that compensate for, and eventually correct, an increase in blood acidity: buffers, the respiratory system, and the renal system.

Metabolic alkalosis is much less common than metabolic acidosis. It results from the loss of acids, such as the loss of gastric acid following repeated vomiting, or the gain of bases, such as the ingestion of large amounts of base, often in the form of medicinal antacid compounds in the treatment of gastroesophageal conditions.

The four types of acid-base imbalance are displayed in Table 6.2. *Compensation* for acid-base imbalance is partial neutralization of excess H^+ or OH^- ions. *Correction* is return to normal blood pH.

The primary goal of treatment is correction of the underlying condition. For example, ventilatory assistance may be required to correct respiratory acidosis; intravenous infusion of bicarbonate buffer solution is indicated for metabolic acidosis, and so on.

Case Notes

6.17 What type of acid-base imbalance did James have?

Buffer Systems and the Lungs Compensate for Excess Acids

The first defense against excess acid is specialized substances called *buffers*. In physiology, a **buffer** is any substance that quickly acts to restrain a change in pH following the addition of an acid or base. Buffers bind newly introduced hydrogen ions (strong acid) and convert them into weak acids (Fig. 6.8, step 2).

Hydrogen ions in blood cells are buffered when they bind to hemoglobin, and hydrogen ions in other body cells bind to cellular proteins. But many hydrogen ions will find their way into extracellular fluid and blood

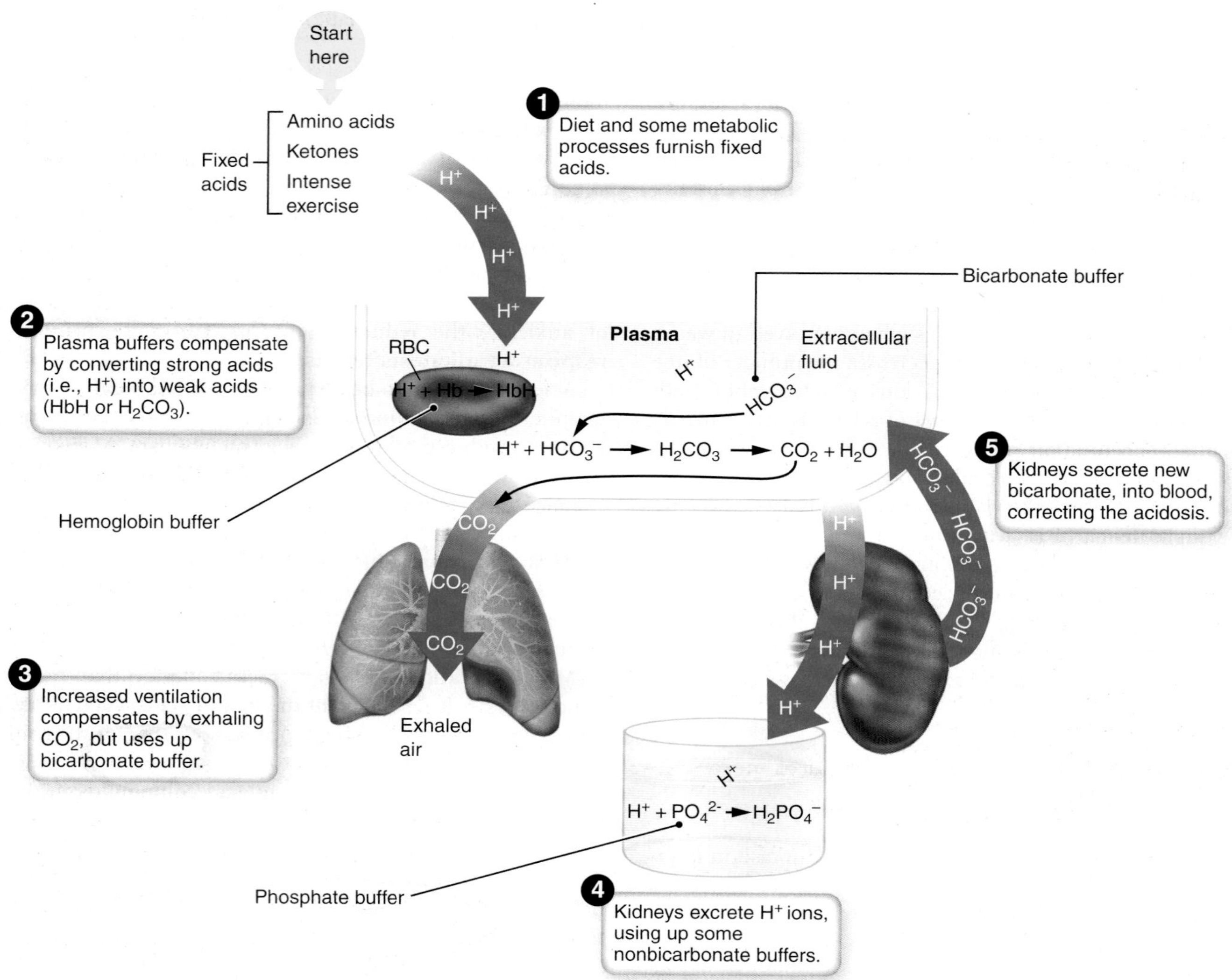

Figure 6.8 **Metabolic acidosis.** The body compensates for fixed acids using buffers and increased ventilation, but renal acid excretion is required to fully correct the pH imbalance. (Reprinted with permission from McConnell TH, Hull KL. *Human Form Human Function: Essentials of Anatomy & Physiology*. Baltimore, MD: Wolters Kluwer Health; 2011.)

Table 6.2 Acid-Base Imbalances

Origin	**Acidosis** (Common)	**Alkalosis** (Uncommon)
RESPIRATORY ORIGIN		
	Causes: Respiratory depression (e.g., drugs, coma) or chronic pulmonary disease (emphysema)	**Causes**: Hyperventilation (e.g., anxiety)
	Effect: Increased blood CO_2	**Effect**: Decreased blood CO_2
	Compensation: Increased renal acid excretion and generation of new blood bicarbonate buffer	**Compensation**: Kidneys excrete less acid and generate less new blood bicarbonate buffer
METABOLIC ORIGIN	**Causes:** Shock with poor tissue oxygenation and anaerobic metabolism, which generates fixed acids; diabetic ketoacidosis, kidney failure (less acid excretion)	**Causes:** Excess ingestion of base (e.g., antacid drugs) or severe vomiting of gastric acid
	Effect: Decreased blood bicarbonate	**Effect**: Increased blood bicarbonate
	Compensation: Rapid, deep respirations to blow of acid as CO_2; increased renal secretion of acid (in patients with good renal function)	**Compensation**: Slow, shallow respirations to retain CO_2 as acid; decreased renal secretion of acid

plasma, where they meet with the most important buffer of all: the **bicarbonate buffering system**. It combines H^+ with bicarbonate (HCO_3^-) to generate the weak acid *carbonic acid*, as shown by the equation below:

H^+	+ HCO_3^-	<=> H_2CO_3	<=> CO_2	+ H_2O
Acid (strong acid)	+ bicarbonate (weak base)	<=> carbonic acid (weak acid)	<=> carbon dioxide	+ water (neutral)
Tissues	Blood	<=> Blood	<=> Lungs	Tissues

Above, we see that acid generated in tissues can be converted into CO_2 for exhalation by the lungs (see Fig. 6.8, step 3). Note, however, that *the reaction can also run right to left*, as may occur in, for example, chronic lung disease, if normal amounts of CO_2 cannot be exhaled by the lungs. Buffer reactions are controlled by the concentration of constituents, so the addition of a buffer drives the reaction to the right and decreases blood acidity. Conversely, the loss of a buffer drives the reaction to the left, liberating a hydrogen ion and increasing blood acidity. This is a key feature of all buffers: the reaction may proceed in either direction according to the need for more or less H^+.

All of the body's buffer systems work together to limit the impact of our natural acid production. Chemical buffers, however, are only a short-term solution, because they do not actually eliminate the acid. Moreover, every buffering reaction uses up a buffer molecule, and buffer stores are not unlimited. The loss of buffers, such as the loss of bicarbonate that occurs with diarrhea, can cause metabolic acidosis as effectively as the gain of acid. Thus, buffers help *compensate* for the acid load but do not *correct* it.

As you can see in the formula above, the addition of H^+ from fixed acids increases blood CO_2. This in turn stimulates the rate and depth of breathing, which eliminates the added CO_2. The body responds to metabolic acidosis by exhaling the newly generated CO_2. While this response tends to resist acidosis, *it results in the permanent loss of a bicarbonate molecule and lessens reserve buffering capacity*. In other words, for every molecule of CO_2 lost through the lungs, a molecule of HCO_3^- is removed from the body's pool of HCO_3^- buffer. Thus, the respiratory response compensates for the acid load but cannot correct it because the fixed acids, which created the problem, have not been eliminated.

Case Notes

6.18 James's bicarbonate was low. Why?

6.19 Why was James's breathing so rapid and deep?

The Kidney Eliminates Fixed Acids

Buffers and the respiratory system essentially "hold the fort" by exhaling acid at the expense of bicarbonate buffer. This prevents big changes in blood pH while the kidney acts to excrete the bulk of acid into urine (Fig.6.8, step 4). In the process *the kidney generates new bicarbonate molecules to replenish the stock of bicarbonate buffer lost to the exhalation of* CO_2 (Fig. 6.8, step 5).

If the H^+ ions could be excreted "as is," the net result of the renal excretion of acid would be the loss of one H^+ and the gain of one blood bicarbonate buffer molecule. Nevertheless, excessively acidic urine could damage the urinary tract. So, urine H^+ itself must be buffered by consuming other blood buffers, mainly phosphate and ammonia, in a process that mimics the bicarbonate process and turns strong urine acid into weak acid. Thus, the excretion of H^+ ions into urine results in acidic, partially buffered urine and a net loss of nonbicarbonate buffers.

Case Notes

6.20 By excreting acid, are James's kidneys consuming his blood bicarbonate buffer or restoring it?

Pop Quiz

6.17 Hyperventilation causes what acid-base disturbance?

6.18 For every molecule of CO_2 lost by through the lungs, a compensatory ____________ of HCO_3 occurs.

6.19 What organ is responsible for eliminating fixed acid?

Hyperemia and Congestion

Hyperemia and *congestion* are terms that describe an increased volume of blood in an affected part of the body. **Hyperemia** is an *active* process associated with inflammation or with increased metabolic activity of the affected part (e.g., a hardworking muscle). Arterioles dilate and the site turns red (**erythema**) with bright red, oxygenated blood. Sunburn is an example of inflammatory hyperemia: arterioles dilate upon receiving chemical signals from injured cells and flood tissue with blood. **Congestion**, on the other hand, is a *passive* process associated with impaired venous outflow. The affected part is passive, has not signaled a need for blood, but is gorged with poorly oxygenated, dark blood. It can be local, as in venous obstruction in a limb, or general, as in congestive heart failure. Affected tissue turns dusky, reddish blue. *Chronic passive congestion* is a fairly common occurrence, especially in the liver. The most

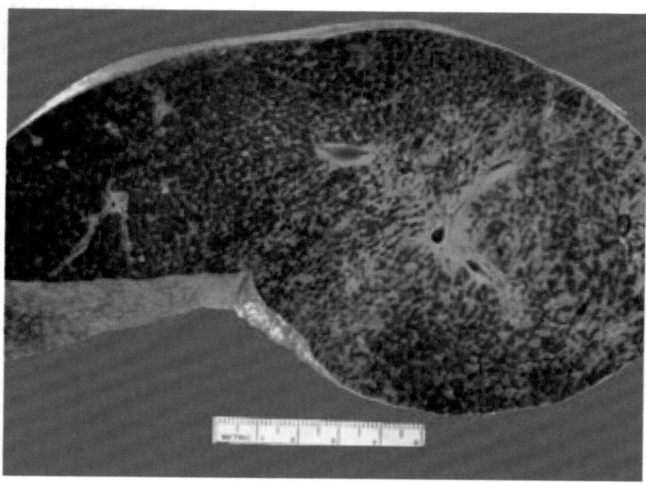

Figure 6.9 **Chronic passive congestion.** In this cross-section of liver from a patient with severe congestive heart failure, the red spots are congested central veins.

common cause of chronic passive congestion of the liver is chronic right heart failure, in which the right ventricle is unable to eject the blood delivered to it. The blood "dams up" in the vena cava, increasing venous pressure. The liver is especially affected because it is large and has a large blood supply. The result is a characteristic pattern (*centrilobular necrosis*) of liver damage depicted in Figure 6.9.

Case Notes

6.21 **Is the excess blood in James's lung vessels due to active or passive vasodilation?**

6.22 **Why is James's liver enlarged?**

Pop Quiz

6.20 Explain the difference between congestion and hyperemia.

Hemostasis

Hemostasis is the composite activity of blood vessel endothelium, platelets, and plasma *coagulation (clotting) factors* that 1) keep blood in a fluid, clot-free state and 2) form a *clot* to stop bleeding at the site of vascular injury. Hemostasis balances pro- and anti-clotting forces. If tilted too far toward anticlotting, spontaneous or excessive bleeding may occur. Tilt too far the other way and intravascular clotting occurs.

Normal hemostasis (Fig. 6.10) is evident in reaction to vascular disruption. After injury, the first reaction is temporary constriction of blood vessels (vasospasm). Injury disrupts the vascular wall and exposes blood to *tissue factors*, which cause platelets passing by to become "sticky." They adhere to the edges of the wound and form a temporary *thrombotic plug*. At the same time, escaping blood is exposed to tissue factors, which stimulate coagulation and the formation of a *permanent plug* of clotted blood. Activation of the clotting process inside of blood vessels (intravascular coagulation) without exposure to tissue factor is pathologic.

Endothelial cells are the first element of the coagulation process and play a critical role in balancing pro- and anti-clotting forces. On one hand, there is the natural tendency of platelets to adhere to endothelium. On the other hand is the antithrombotic and anticoagulant activity of endothelial cells, which prevent thrombosis and clotting unless stimulated by injury.

Platelets are the second element and are tiny, non-nucleated fragments of cytoplasm shed into blood by bone marrow **megakaryocytes**. They form the thrombotic plug that initially seals vascular defects; they attract more platelets to enlarge the plug; they initiate the clotting cascade, which forms a clot as a permanent plug; and they fuse together to form a glue-like cement to hold it all together. Platelets also secrete factors that stimulate wound healing in the repair process.

Coagulation (*clotting*) is the third element of the hemostatic process. It begins when plasma or platelets contact something they should not: extravascular tissue or a foreign surface. Clot formation is the product of a "falling dominoes" interaction among blood **coagulation factors**, most of which are proteins made by the liver and which are denoted by names and Roman numerals. In its final step, the coagulation cascade (Fig. 6.11) causes *fibrinogen (factor I)* to polymerize into strands of fibrin, which form a gel-like solid meshwork that plugs the hole.

Traditionally, the coagulation cascade is divided into two pathways. The **extrinsic coagulation pathway** is initiated when *coagulation factor VII* comes into contact with *tissue factor* in extravascular tissue. The **intrinsic coagulation pathway** is initiated when *coagulation factor XII* comes into contact with a foreign surface such as glass or plastic. This two-part division is an artifact of laboratory testing; both pathways are active in hemostasis. *The extrinsic pathway operates in most clinical circumstances.* The intrinsic pathway accounts for the clotting that occurs when blood comes into contact with labware or intravascular devices such as artificial heart valves or catheters. Table 6.3 explains the interpretation of the most important laboratory tests of coagulation and hemostasis.

Because coagulation is a self-propagating process, it must be restricted to the site of vascular injury to avoid runaway coagulation of the entire blood supply. Certain factors released by the clotting process have a negative feedback effect that self-limits coagulation. What's more, the coagulation cascade initiates the *thrombolytic cascade*, a process that slowly dissolves the clot as healing proceeds.

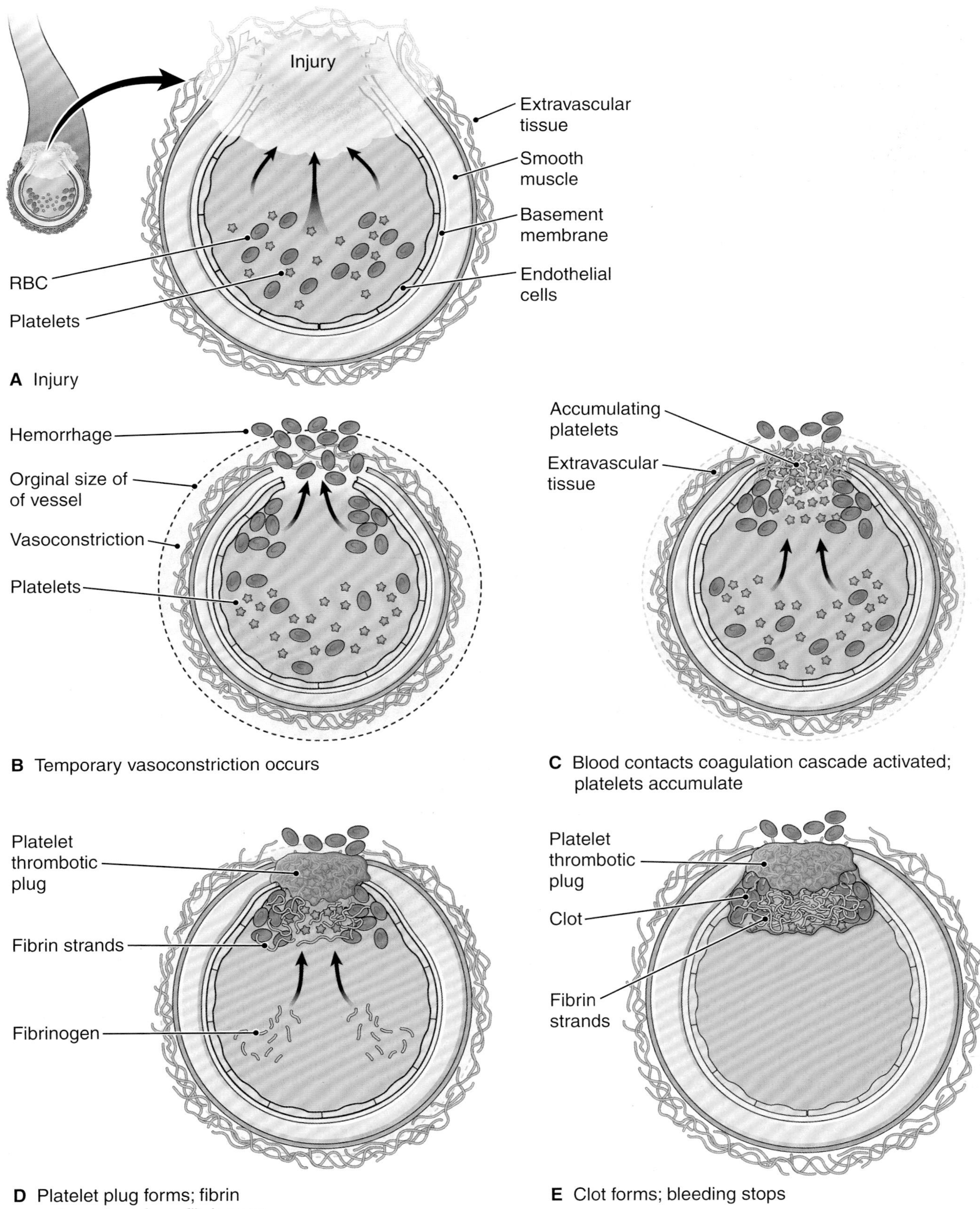

Figure 6.10 **Normal hemostasis. A.** Injury occurs. **B.** Temporary vasoconstriction occurs. **C.** Blood contacts tissue, platelets accumulate, and coagulation begins. **D.** Further platelet aggregation occurs, and coagulation produces a web of fibrin in the wound. **E.** Hemorrhage stops as fibrin traps red cells and blocks further bleeding.

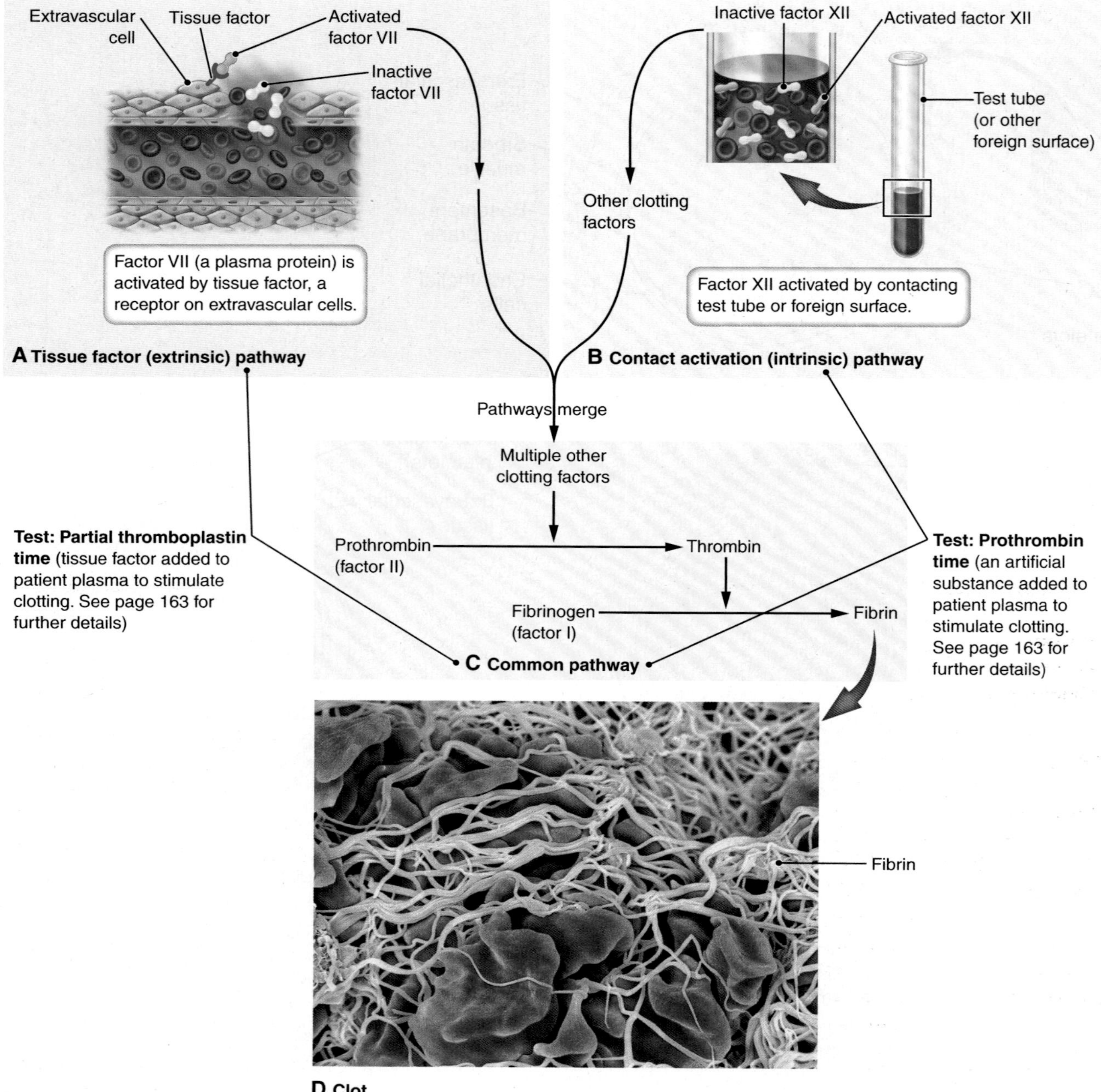

Figure 6.11 **Coagulation pathways. A.** Exposure of clotting factor VII to tissue factor on extravascular cells activates the tissue factor pathway. **B.** The contact activation pathway is activated when clotting factor XII contacts collagen or a foreign surface such as glass. Activated factor XII initiates a series of enzymatic reactions. **C.** Activated factor VII or factors activated by the contact activation pathway activate the common pathway, which terminates in the formation of a web of fibrin fibers forming a clot. **D.** Photomicrograph of a blood clot. (Reprinted with permission from McConnell TH, Hull KL. *Human Form Human Function: Essentials of Anatomy & Physiology*. Baltimore, MD: Wolters Kluwer Health; 2011.)

Pop Quiz

6.21 Define hemostasis, and name the three elements of hemostasis that act to stop bleeding.

6.22 Which coagulation factor initiates the intrinsic pathway? The extrinsic pathway?

Hemorrhage

Hemorrhage is the escape of blood from a blood vessel. Hemorrhage confined to tissue is classified according to size.

- **Petechiae** (Fig. 6.12) are the smallest hemorrhages, about one millimeter, and are often visible in skin or mucous membranes. Buccal or conjunctival mucosal petechiae are usually associated with platelet disorders,

Table 6.3 Interpretation of Tests of Hemostasis Function*

Test and Result		Conclusion
PLATELET COUNT	**BLEEDING TIME**	
Normal	Normal	**Normal.** Platelets not part of the bleeding problem; suspect coagulation factor defect
Low	Prolonged	**Low platelet count**
Normal	Prolonged	**Abnormal platelet function**
PROTHROMBIN TIME	**PARTIAL THROMBOPLASTIN TIME**	
Normal	Normal	**Normal** coagulation function. Suspect vascular or platelet factors.
Abnormal	Abnormal	**Defect** in the COMMON pathway
Normal	Abnormal	**Defect** in the INTRINSIC pathway
Abnormal	Normal	**Defect** in the EXTRINSIC pathway

* See page 163 for further details

especially bleeding caused by *thrombocytopenia* (low platelet count).

- **Purpura** is a hemorrhage <1 cm.
- **Ecchymosis** is a hemorrhage >1 cm
- **Hematoma** is a large, localized collection of blood.

There are two categories of bleeding: bleeding from *large vessels* and bleeding from *capillaries*. Bleeding from large vessels is usually caused by trauma or a coagulation factor deficiency and tends to produce the most serious hemorrhages. Because the liver makes most coagulation factors, most instances of coagulation factor defect are caused by acquired liver disease. Liver disease, however, is but one variety of coagulation defect; many coagulation defects are caused by genetic conditions, for example, factor VIII deficiency (hemophilia). Capillary bleeding most often results from a low platelet count. Sometimes capillary bleeding is due to vasculitis, usually an autoimmune disorder. Less often, it stems from poorly understood defective function of the capillaries themselves. Capillary bleeding usually presents as skin or mucosal petechiae, nosebleed, or urinary bleeding.

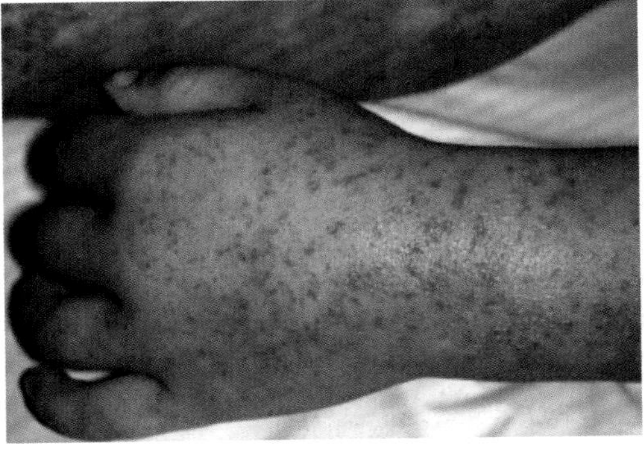

Figure 6.12 **Petechiae.** These tiny skin hemorrhages occurred in a child with low platelet count (thrombocytopenia).

Case Notes

6.23 **James developed purpura at a venipuncture site. What can you say about how large it was?**

6.24 **When the needle entered James's vein, what was the first response of the vein?**

6.25 **James's hemostasis mechanism quickly stopped the bleeding. Which occurred first, a platelet plug or a clot?**

Bleeding Disorders Are Due to Abnormal Hemostasis

Bleeding is usually the result of vascular injury. Hemostasis normally stops bleeding quickly if the injury is small. Larger injuries require intervention. **Hemorrhagic diathesis** is *excessive* bleeding beyond the expected amount for a certain injury, or bleeding without obvious injury. It is a pathologic counterpart of normal hemostasis. Excessive bleeding is caused by one of three factors:

- Fragile small blood vessels
- Decreased platelet count or ineffective platelet function
- Decreased coagulation factor activity

Case Notes

6.26 **Does James's venipuncture purpura suggest a hemorrhagic diathesis?**

Vascular or Platelet Problems

Some bleeding is related to the integrity of the vascular wall. Most hemorrhage occurs because blood vessels are disrupted by trauma. *Aneurysms*—balloon-like bulges that occur in weakened arteries—may rupture and bleed. Other causes of bleeding related to vascular integrity include autoimmune vasculitis and vitamin C deficiency (*scurvy*), which weakens the intercellular cement that holds together small blood vessels. Also, some people, especially the elderly, bruise easily for reasons that are not clear and may relate to weakening of supporting connective tissue, a condition that usually has no adverse consequences—patients usually do not bleed excessively with major trauma, surgery, or childbirth.

Low platelet count (**thrombocytopenia**) occurs in a great variety of disorders and is usually characterized by petechial bleeding in skin or mucosa. The normal range for platelet counts in most laboratories is about 130,000–400,000/mm^3. Because of this wide range, most practitioners do not grow concerned unless the platelet count falls below 100,000/mm^3. Even so, excessive bleeding after trauma rarely occurs until the count falls below 50,000/mm^3, and spontaneous hemorrhage usually does not occur until counts fall to about 20,000/mm^3. Nevertheless, with severe thrombocytopenia, hemorrhage may occur at any site. Brain hemorrhage is a particular hazard for patients with very low platelet counts. Patients with thrombocytopenia bleed longer than normal after a standardized skin puncture (see Table 6.3, abnormal bleeding time).

Thrombocytopenia may also occur when platelet production is low because of a primary bone marrow disorder (such as leukemia), toxic effect of drugs or chemicals, or with ineffective platelet production, as in the case of folate or B_{12} deficiency. Decreased platelet survival may also cause thrombocytopenia. The spleen normally filters old platelets out of the blood after about 12 days, but an overactive spleen (*hypersplenism*) may cause thrombocytopenia by removing them a few hours or days after production.

A much more common cause of low platelet count is **immune thrombocytopenic purpura (ITP)**, in which the immune system destroys its own platelets. ITP usually occurs as an isolated disease, but can be seen in association with other autoimmune disorders, or it rarely may occur as a complication of acute pediatric viral illnesses. Platelets become coated with antiplatelet autoantibodies and are quickly removed by the spleen. Thrombocytopenia usually reveals itself as easy bruisability, epistaxis (nosebleed), bleeding gums, or unusual bleeding after minor trauma. Diagnosis is clinical with laboratory detection of antiplatelet antibodies. Treatment with steroids is effective, and splenectomy is curative in most cases.

The **thrombotic microangiopathies** are disorders caused by pathologic platelet activation, which creates thrombi in small vessels. The most common underlying defect is acquired or genetic deficiency of plasma enzyme ADAMTS13. Typical symptoms include fever, thrombocytopenia, microangiopathic hemolytic anemia (Chapter 7), transient neurologic deficits, and renal failure. Two varieties are recognized.

- **Thrombotic thrombocytopenic purpura (TTP)** is more likely to occur in adults with neurologic symptoms, and renal failure is less likely.
- **Hemolytic uremic syndrome (HUS)** is more likely to occur in children who have renal failure and few neurologic symptoms. HUS is strongly associated with gastroenteritis caused by certain strains of *E. coli.*

Diagnosis is clinical and supported by typical laboratory findings and ruling out immune thrombocytopenia. Treatment includes steroids and supportive therapy, and plasma exchange in adults.

Coagulation Factor Deficiency

Liver disease is the most common cause of coagulation factor deficiency. For example, patients with *cirrhosis* (severe scarring) usually have bleeding tendencies because of underproduction of hepatic coagulation factors. Vitamin K deficiency is another example of an acquired bleeding disorder, because vitamin K is essential for the production of factors VII, IX, and X, and of prothrombin. Coagulation defects resulting from vitamin K deficiency are most often seen with lengthy antibiotic therapy that eliminates vitamin K-producing bacteria from the intestine.

On the other hand, some coagulation defects are inherited in a Mendelian fashion and involve single coagulation protein deficiencies, for example, von Willebrand disease and classic hemophilia.

von Willebrand disease stems from a deficiency of von Willebrand factor (vWF), a coagulation factor made in endothelial cells and megakaryocytes. It is one of the most common inherited coagulation disorders and is characterized by spontaneous bleeding from mouth, nose, and other mucous membranes and by excessive wound and menstrual bleeding. Bleeding time is prolonged despite normal platelet count because lack of vWF interferes with platelet adhesion to endothelium.

Classic **hemophilia** (hemophilia A or factor VIII deficiency) is the most common serious inherited coagulation disorder. It is an X-linked gene defect that occurs almost exclusively in males. It is inherited from their mothers, most of whom are unaffected carriers. Nevertheless, about one-third of cases are new mutations without positive family history. Spontaneous hemorrhage occurs only in severe deficiency (factor VIII levels about 1% of normal). Lesser deficiencies show varying amounts of post-traumatic bleeding. Intracapsular joint hemorrhage (**hemarthrosis**, especially in the knee) is a particular problem in patients with severe deficiencies. Repeated episodes may produce crippling joint strictures or frozen joints (*ankylosis*).

Patients with hemophilia characteristically have a normal bleeding time and platelet count because neither platelets nor vascular factors are at fault. Patients with hemophilia have a normal prothrombin time because the extrinsic and common pathways do not require factor VIII. Nevertheless, partial thromboplastin time is prolonged because factor VIII is in the intrinsic pathway (Table 6.3). For those with severe deficiency, periodic transfusion with factor VIII is effective. *The History of Medicine*, "The Royal Disease," available online at thePoint.com with the Chapter 7 resources, offers a glimpse into the interesting story of hemophilia.

Christmas disease (hemophilia B, factor IX deficiency) is clinically similar to classic hemophilia but is much less common. It is named for the first patient in whom the disease was identified, not for the annual holiday season. Like classic hemophilia, it is caused by an X-linked recessive gene defect, and it has test abnormalities similar to *hemophilia (factor VIII deficiency)*. Christmas disease may or may not be associated with significant bleeding problems. Diagnosis requires specialized testing specifically for factor IX deficiency.

Hemostasis Is Assessed by Laboratory Tests

Hemostasis is assessed by performing laboratory tests to assess platelet action and the clotting process. The coagulation process is assessed by *prothrombin time (PT)* and *partial thromboplastin time (PTT)*. Each is performed by adding reagent to anticoagulated plasma and timing to see how long it takes for a clot to form (see Fig. 6.11 and Table 6.3).

- **Prothrombin time (PT)** is the time it takes for a sample of patient plasma to clot after the addition of *tissue factor*. This initiates coagulation via the *extrinsic* pathway and, therefore, the result is abnormal if there are defects in the *extrinsic* or *common* pathways.
- **Partial thromboplastin time (PTT)** is the time it takes for a sample of patient plasma to clot after addition of silica powder, an *artificial surface*. This initiates coagulation via the intrinsic pathway and, therefore, the result is abnormal if there are defects in the *intrinsic* or *common* pathways.

Clotting, however, is but one of three elements important in hemostasis: clotting, platelets, and the characteristics of the vascular wall of blood vessels.

Platelets are assessed by performing a *platelet count*, a *platelet function* test, or a *bleeding time*:

- **Platelet count** measures platelet *numbers* only; it does not account for platelets that do not *function* properly.
- **Platelet function analysis** detects defective platelet function and can be performed by specialized analyzers in large laboratories.
- In the absence of these devices, a **bleeding time** can be performed to measure the length of time required for a patient to stop bleeding after skin prick with a standardized lancet. An abnormally long bleeding time is the result either of a low platelet count or of defective platelet function.

There is no test to assess factors related to the walls of blood vessels.

Table 6.3 shows how to interpret the results. With results in hand, the problem usually can be identified by process of elimination. For example, because prothrombin is made by the liver, patients with liver failure may have a prothrombin deficiency. Patients with prothrombin deficiency have a normal platelet count and bleeding time. Nevertheless, both PT and PTT are prolonged because prothrombin acts in the common pathway, which serves both intrinsic and extrinsic pathways.

Pop Quiz

6.23 Fill in the blank. ________ are small hemorrhages 1mm in size (usually caused by thrombocytopenia); ________ hemorrhages are less than 1 cm, while ____________ hemorrhages are larger than 1 cm; and _______ are large, localized collections of blood.

6.24 True or false? PT measures clotting in the intrinsic pathway, while PTT is a measure of clotting in the extrinsic pathway. For extra credit, what factors are in each of these pathways?

6.25 What is the treatment for ITP?

Thrombosis

In normal hemostasis, a small platelet plug (the hemostatic thrombus) gathers at the site of vascular disruption to fill the hole and stop bleeding. This normal, hemostatic variety of thrombosis, however, is *extravascular*. In clinical medicine, when **thrombosis** is discussed, it refers to pathologic, *intravascular* thrombosis, not the hemostatic variety. An intravascular **thrombus** is a collection of the cellular elements of blood (platelets, white blood cells [WBCs], and RBCs) that forms only under pathologic conditions. Though elements of the clotting process participate in thrombus formation, *a clot and a thrombus are not the same*. They differ in pathogenesis, structure and the time they require to form. They play very different roles and the terms are often confused.

A thrombus forms slowly and begins as aggregates of platelets and WBCs that adhere to the endothelium in a pattern that creates a *visible internal architecture*—layers of WBC and platelets that form distinct layers. An intravascular thrombus is *never normal* and is always the result of a *pathologic process*. Conversely, clotting occurs quickly is a *normal* process that normally occurs only when blood is exposed to extravascular tissue; it produces a clot, which is a featureless gel that does not have the internal architecture that characterizes an intravascular thrombus.

Formation of a thrombus requires some combination of 1) endothelial injury, 2) abnormal local blood flow (either stasis or turbulence), and 3) hypercoagulability—a tendency of blood to have more than the normal tendency to clot, as depicted in Figure 6.13. One of the most important causes of thrombosis in arteries is atherosclerosis. Inflammation, scarring, and deposits of cholesterol damage endothelial cells, prompting platelets to adhere to the vascular wall over the area of atherosclerosis (atheroma). If the thrombus grows large enough, it can completely occlude blood flow and cause death of downstream tissue (discussed below). Typically, however, thrombi form in veins, especially large veins in the legs, or on the walls of large arteries that have been damaged by atherosclerosis. Figure 6.14 illustrates the formation of a thrombus in a vein. Figure 6.15 illustrates the internal architecture of an unusual thrombus in a heart chamber.

The formation of a thrombus does not depend *initially* on the coagulation process; thrombi begin and grow initially without clot formation. Nevertheless, once a thrombus reaches a certain size, usually in a vein, it can grow by *adding* a clot. If a thrombus accumulates in a small artery narrowed by atherosclerosis it may be the final act that chokes off the blood supply, as in a heart attack or stroke (discussed below). Large thrombi usually form in veins and have three parts—*white, mixed,* and *red* (Fig. 6.14 D). The *white* part is the initial thrombus and consists of the aggregations of platelets and white cells stuck to the vascular wall. As platelets in the white part release clotting factors, the thrombus may grow by adding additional platelets and white cells mixed with clot to form the *mixed* part of the thrombus. The final, *red,* part is pure clot and may grow to be very large. However most thrombi are relatively small (a few mm or cm).

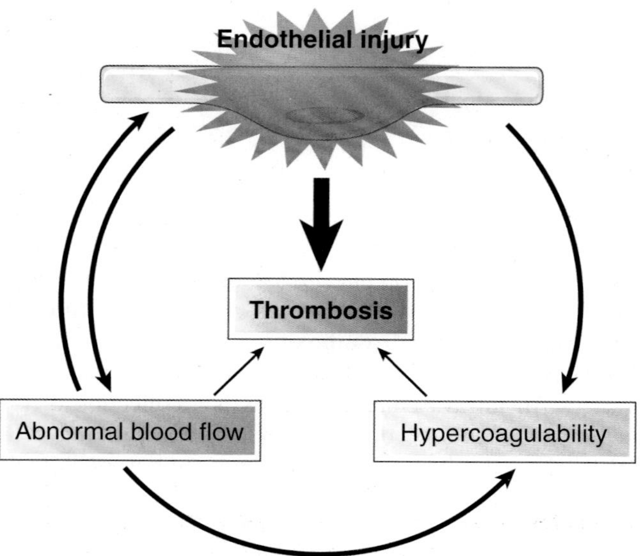

Figure 6.13 **Factors in thrombus formation.** The most important factor in thrombus formation is endothelial injury. Abnormal blood flow and hypercoagulability of blood also play a role.

Case Notes

6.27 **Will the thrombus in James's coronary artery have a visible internal architecture or will it be a featureless gel?**

6.28 **What element of blood accumulated first in the buildup of James's thrombus?**

After formation, a thrombus may evolve in one of several ways, each of which has different consequences: 1) it may grow by adding clot; 2) it may break loose into the blood stream and become an *embolus*; 3) it may dissolve; or 4) it may rechannel (recanalize), that is, it may be "bored out," and the vessel occluded by a thrombus may reopen slowly.

Venous thrombi can be relatively innocuous, or they can be life-threatening. When venous thrombi occur, the condition is usually called **thrombophlebitis** because the vein and adjacent tissue become inflamed and painful. Thrombophlebitis in a superficial arm vein is usually not a serious matter; on the other hand, thrombophlebitis in a deep vein of the leg is very dangerous because the thrombus can grow very large, break loose, and embolize to another part of the body (a phenomenon known as **thromboembolism**, discussed below). Such large thrombi can be washed through the heart and completely occlude the pulmonary artery to cause instantaneous death.

A thrombus may dissolve through normal thrombolytic activity of blood, or it may rechannel. *Rechanneling* occurs as repaired blood vessels sprout from the internal wall of the vein and work their way into the thrombus. Ultimately they connect with the lumen of the vein and enlarge enough so that normal blood flow returns.

Some diseases increase the tendency to cause thrombosis. Patients with systemic lupus erythematosus (SLE) may have in their blood an autoantibody called **lupus anticoagulant** (also called *antiphospholipid antibody*). It occurs in about 10% of patients with SLE and gets its name from the fact that it interferes with laboratory tests of blood coagulation, causing the tests to suggest that coagulation is deficient when, in fact, the opposite is true: lupus anticoagulant promotes venous thrombosis. Therefore, lupus anticoagulant is a misnomer and patients with lupus anticoagulant are at increased risk for recurrent venous thrombosis, pulmonary thromboembolism, and recurrent spontaneous

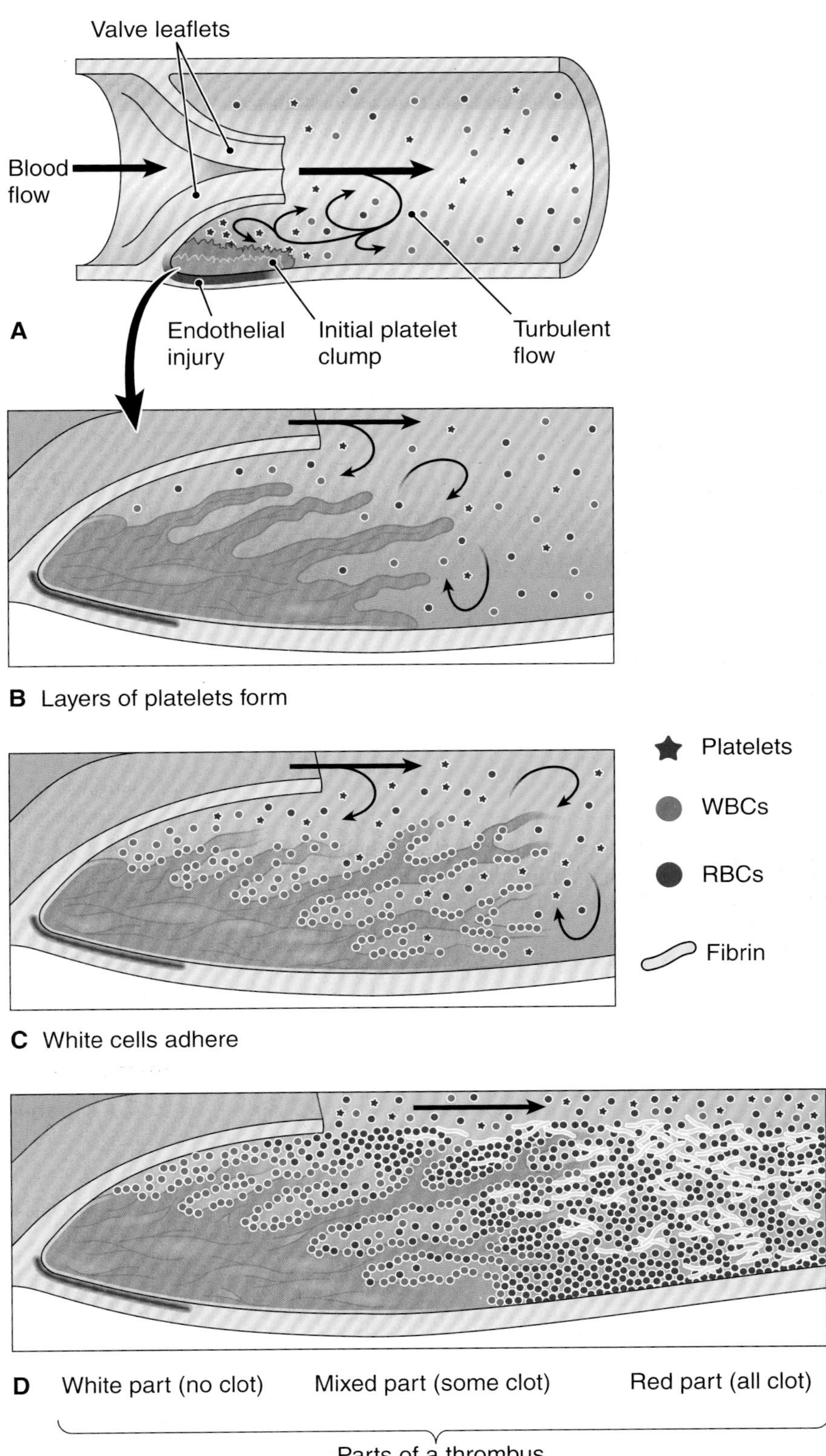

Figure 6.14 **Formation of a thrombus.** **A.** Platelets separate and agglutinate as a result of turbulent flow and endothelial injury in the valve pocket. **B.** Further platelet agglutination forms platelet layers. **C.** WBCs adhere to platelet layers. **D.** A clot adds volume as the thrombus grows.

abortions. Nevertheless, *most patients with lupus anticoagulant do not have SLE* or other clinical disease. Lupus anticoagulant should also be suspected in patients who have abnormal laboratory tests of blood coagulation (prolonged prothrombin or partial thromboplastin time, Table 6.3) but who do not have clinical evidence of a bleeding disorder.

Another condition predisposing to venous thrombosis is **Factor V Leiden**, an abnormal form of coagulation factor V produced by a defective gene. Factor V Leiden promotes a generalized tendency to form venous thrombi, thromboemboli, and spontaneous abortion. The abnormal gene is an autosomal recessive defect that is surprisingly

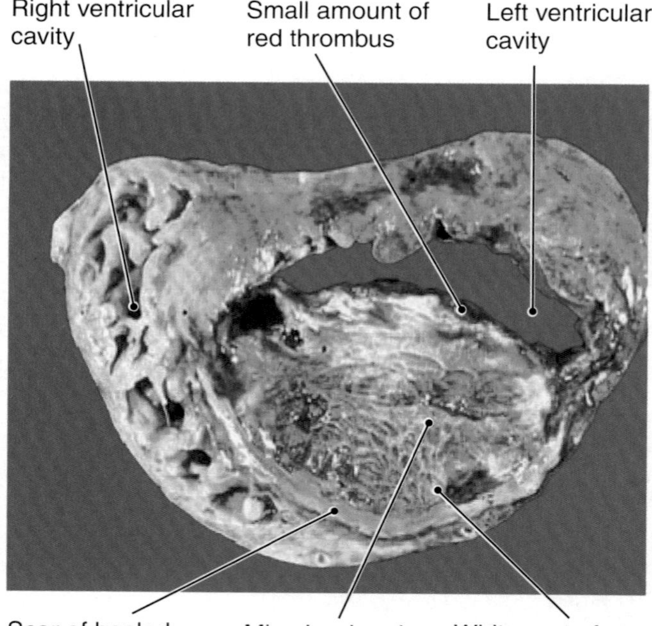

Figure 6.15 Large intracardiac thrombus. This thrombus is situated on the internal lining of the heart over muscle damaged by a myocardial infarction. It occupies most of the volume of the left ventricle.

common—it is present in about 5% of people of European ancestry and 1% of African Americans. The heterozygous state is associated with an approximate fivefold increased risk for venous thrombosis; the risk for the homozygous state is much higher. Oral contraceptive use further increases the risk, as does smoking. Factor V Leiden should be suspected in patients with venous thrombosis of any type or in those with recurrent spontaneous abortions. Laboratory tests are necessary to confirm the diagnosis.

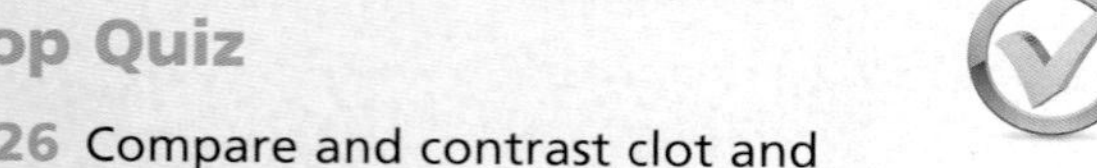

Pop Quiz

6.26 Compare and contrast clot and thrombus.

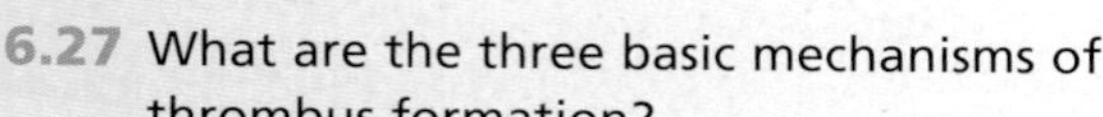

6.27 What are the three basic mechanisms of thrombus formation?

6.28 What are the possible outcomes of thrombus formation?

Disseminated Intravascular Coagulation

Just as bleeding is one pathologic counterpart of hemostasis, intravascular coagulation is another. Blood normally clots only when it comes into contact with tissues outside the vascular space. **Disseminated intravascular coagulation (DIC)** is a condition in which clotting occurs inside the vascular space without exposure to tissue. One consequence is obstruction of small vessels by clots. Surprisingly, bleeding can also be a consequence. This occurs because coagulation factors are consumed by the clotting process and no longer exist in high enough concentration in blood to prevent abnormal bleeding. Therefore, DIC is said to be a **consumptive coagulopathy**.

DIC is never a primary disease; it is always a complication of other diseases. For example, it may occur in bacterial infection of blood (*septicemia*) when bacteria release coagulogenic products that activate the coagulation cascade. DIC may be initiated by a variety of conditions, which can be grouped into several major categories:

- *Obstetrical complications*: toxemia, premature separation of the placenta (abruptio placentae), amniotic fluid embolism, retained dead fetus
- *Infections*: Gram-negative bacterial sepsis, meningococcal meningitis, malaria
- *Neoplasms*: carcinoma of stomach, pancreas, lung, and prostate, and acute promyelocytic leukemia
- *Massive tissue trauma*: crush injury, burns
- *Others*: snakebite, heat stroke, acute hemolysis, and vasculitis

Regardless of cause, DIC is usually characterized by *hemolytic anemia* (as RBCs are shredded by passing through intravascular fibrin webs), *thromboses,* and *hemorrhage* as coagulation components are consumed by the clotting process.

Pop Quiz

6.29 What types of hemostasis problems do patients with DIC present with?

6.30 What are the major categories that are capable of causing DIC?

Embolism

An **embolus** is an intravascular object that travels in the bloodstream from one place to another. The main danger of an embolus is obstruction of blood flow. Sources of emboli include:

- *Thrombi,* usually from large veins of the legs or pelvis, or from the left side of the heart
- *Marrow fat* from the yellow marrow of broken long bones
- *Air* introduced accidentally at surgery or which forms in *decompression sickness (the bends)*
- *Amniotic fluid*, which may embolize (rarely) in pregnancy

Pulmonary thromboembolism can be fatal and is a common hazard in patients hospitalized for pregnancy, surgery, or malignancy. In most instances, the thrombus forms in the deep veins of the legs or pelvis. Fragments of various sizes break free and are carried to the lungs. Most are silent, but larger ones may produce pulmonary hemorrhage, with coughed blood (*hemoptysis*) and chest pain. Very large ones may completely occlude the main pulmonary artery (saddle embolus) and produce instant death.

Systemic thromboembolism refers to arterial thromboemboli. Most arise from thrombi that cling to the inner wall of damaged left ventricular muscle from a heart attack. Others arise from the left atrium in patients with atrial fibrillation, a common form of irregular heartbeat. Emboli usually travel to the lower extremity, and sometimes the brain. Consequences vary, but tissue death (infarction, see below) is always a threat.

Fat and marrow embolism is common after long bone fracture and cardiopulmonary resuscitation, but usually does not cause clinical problems. Nevertheless, some patients may develop neurologic and pulmonary symptoms, red cell destruction and anemia, and low platelet count.

Air embolism is the introduction of air bubbles into the arterial tree, usually during cardiac or neurosurgical procedures, or the formation of gas bubbles from *decompression syndrome*. About 100 ml of gas is required to create a problem. Decompression syndrome is a hazard of scuba divers, who breathe air under pressure on a long, deep dive. If ascent to the surface occurs too suddenly, gas (nitrogen, especially) may come out of solution and form gas bubbles. The result is a painful syndrome, *the bends*, which may cause ischemia or infarction of the brain or other tissue. Treatment is recompression in a specialized pressure chamber.

Amniotic fluid embolism is a rare but usually fatal complication of pregnancy. The cause is infusion of amniotic fluid into the maternal circulation from tears in the placenta. Fetal skin debris, hair, and mucin lodge in the small vessels of the lung, which impairs gas exchange and creates general hypoxia and vascular collapse (shock). Some material passes through the lungs and into the brain to cause coma or seizures. DIC and hemorrhage is common.

Pop Quiz

6.31 Name the four types of emboli.

6.32 While scuba diving off the Great Barrier Reef, a young college student observes a shark heading in his direction. Without a second thought, he rockets to the surface, and scrambles frantically onto his boat. He immediately begins complaining of pain, especially in his joints, before collapsing. What has happened?

Infarction

Recall from Chapter 2 that **ischemia** is a lack of oxygen supply to tissue and is usually caused by obstruction of blood flow. An **infarct** is an area of ischemic necrosis. Infarcts are a very common cause of human illness. Most are caused by thrombotic occlusion of an artery. For example, most heart attacks are caused by thrombotic obstruction of a coronary artery. Nevertheless, infarction may occur with only partial or no vascular occlusion, depending on blood pressure, blood oxygen content, and other factors. For example, despite having normal cerebral arteries, survivors of near-drowning may suffer infarction of the cerebral cortex because of inadequate blood oxygen concentration. Though less common, obstruction to venous outflow may impede arterial inflow enough to produce the same effect. Most often, however, bypass channels open and adequate arterial flow resumes.

Case Notes

6.29 **An area of James's heart muscle suffered a loss of oxygen supply. What is the name for this condition?**

Sometimes venous obstruction may produce infarction if the obstruction is so severe that venous stasis prevents arterial perfusion. For example, occlusion of the hepatic vein by tumor or thrombus produces such a severe degree of liver congestion that normal arterial blood flow is insufficient and hepatic infarction occurs.

Rarely, infarcts may result from torsion (twisting) of mobile tissue around the arterial vessel supplying it. Loops of small bowel, ovaries, and testicles are most often involved. Torsion is usually sudden and painful and is a surgical emergency. Also, vasospasm (contraction of smooth muscles in the vascular wall) can narrow the lumen and cause an infarct. Cocaine is well known for its ability to induce coronary vasospasm and sudden death in drug abusers.

There Are Two Types of Infarcts: White and Red

White infarcts (bloodless infarcts) form when arterial obstruction occurs in dense, solid tissue, such as the kidney, heart, or liver, as is depicted in Figure 6.16. **Red infarcts** (hemorrhagic infarcts, Fig. 6.17) are bloody because venous or arterial obstruction occurs in loose, spongy tissue or in the lungs or liver, each of which has a dual blood supply. Interruption of one supply causes infarction while the other pumps blood into the dead tissue.

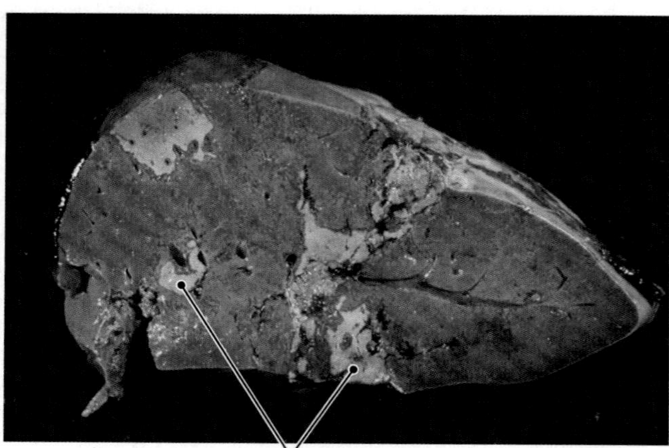

Figure 6.16 **White Infarcts.** White (bloodless) infarcts of the liver owing to arterial thromboemboli from cardiac valves.

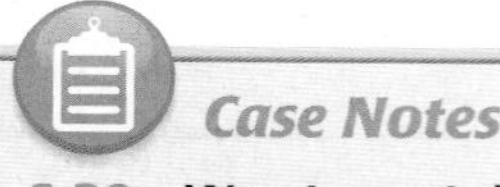

Case Notes

6.30 Was James's infarct red or white?

Infarcts Develop in Predictable Fashion

As mentioned above, *infarction does not always follow vascular occlusion*. Conversely, *infarction can occur without vascular occlusion*. Factors influencing the development of an infarct include 1) whether the organ has a single or dual vascular supply; 2) the rate at which the obstruction develops; 3) the sensitivity of downstream tissue to oxygen deprivation; and 4) the oxygen content of blood.

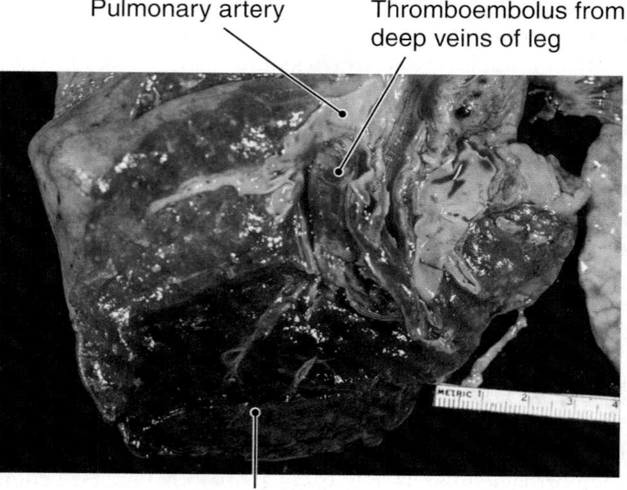

Figure 6.17 **Red infarct.** Red infarct in the lung owing to venous thromboembolus from the legs.

The dual vascular supply in the lungs and liver makes these organs resistant to infarction. Most lung infarcts are caused by pulmonary thromboemboli that occlude a pulmonary artery branch, and are red because the lungs have a dual blood supply from the pulmonary artery and bronchial artery branches from the aorta. Blood supply from bronchial arteries is not enough to prevent necrosis, but continues to pump blood into the dying tissue. A similar dual vascular supply exists in the liver. The portal vein brings venous blood from the bowel, but the liver depends on arterial supply from the hepatic artery.

At the opposite end of the spectrum, the kidney is especially sensitive to vascular insufficiency and infarction because it is metabolically very active and burns oxygen quickly, and its arteries have few interconnections with other vessels.

Occlusion of an artery can be sudden, as in occlusion from an embolus, or slow, as in the development of atherosclerotic obstruction. Slow occlusion over several years may provide enough time for alternative (collateral) circulation to develop, so that complete occlusion may not produce an infarct. For example, slow total occlusion of a carotid artery by atherosclerosis may not cause stroke, because the basilar arteries provide an alternative supply of blood (oxygen) via the circle of Willis.

Some tissues become infarcted quickly after a short period of ischemia. Brain neurons are the best example; they are exquisitely sensitive to hypoxia and die if deprived of oxygen for three or four minutes. Most other tissues are much more tolerant of ischemia: myocardial cells, for example, die after about 20 minutes of hypoxia, whereas fibroblasts may tolerate many hours of hypoxia without damage.

The oxygen content of blood is also an important determinant of infarction. All other things being equal, low blood oxygen content may facilitate transformation of ischemia into infarction. For example, a patient who is hypoxic from severe lung disease is at greater risk than usual for stroke or heart attack if coronary or cerebral blood flow is compromised.

Pop Quiz

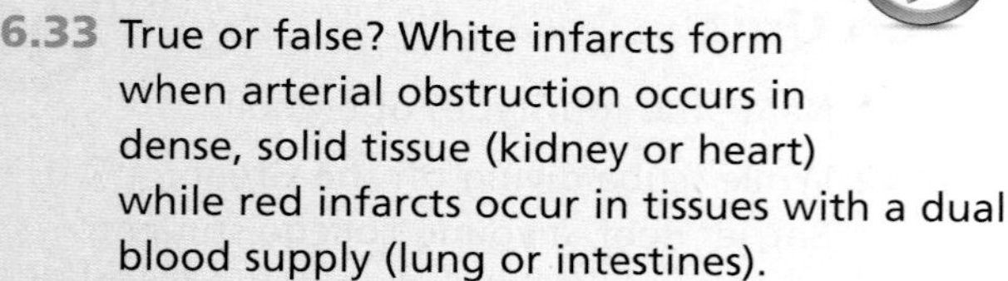

6.33 True or false? White infarcts form when arterial obstruction occurs in dense, solid tissue (kidney or heart) while red infarcts occur in tissues with a dual blood supply (lung or intestines).

6.34 Is complete occlusion necessary to cause an infarct? Does necrosis always follow arterial occlusion?

6.35 What variables affect the development of an infarct?

The Collapse of Circulation: Shock

Shock, or circulatory collapse, is a state of systemic low blood flow (hypoperfusion) when cardiac output is reduced or *effective* blood volume is decreased (i.e., either blood is lost or the vascular space dilates). Shock may be the final stage of a number of clinical conditions, including severe hemorrhage, overwhelming bacterial sepsis, catastrophic allergic reaction, burns, severe myocardial infarction, or trauma with extensive soft tissue damage. Whatever the cause, the end result of shock often is multiorgan failure and death.

There Are Several Types of Shock

Shock may be classified into four categories: *hypovolemic* shock, *cardiogenic* shock, *obstructive* shock, and *septic* shock.

Hypovolemic shock results from an underfilled vascular space, usually the result of hemorrhage. Hypovolemic shock may also be caused by fluid loss following burns or severe diarrhea. It may also occur, however, without loss of blood. In such situations, marked *vasodilation* may expand the vascular space to such a degree that the *effective* blood volume is insufficient to maintain perfusion pressure. The most common cause of marked vasodilation is acute, generalized allergic reaction (generalized *anaphylaxis*, Chapter 3). Another cause is sudden loss of autonomic function from acute, paralyzing spinal cord injury (sometimes classified as "neurogenic shock").

Cardiogenic shock (pump failure) often occurs with myocardial infarction or other myocardial disease. In such cases, cardiac muscle simply lacks the mechanical power to maintain blood pressure.

Obstructive shock is caused by mechanical interference with cardiac output. The most common cause is fluid, usually blood, accumulation in the pericardium (*cardiac tamponade*), which prevents cardiac filling.

Septic shock is associated with systemic microbial infection (*sepsis*). It ranks high as a cause of death in intensive care units—20% of affected patients die. Multiple factors are involved and have complex, self-reinforcing interactions with one another. Microbes release toxic molecules, inflammatory mediators play a role, and damaged endothelium may induce DIC and hemorrhage. Gram-positive bacteria are the usual culprits.

Case Notes

6.31 What type of shock was James in?

There Are Three Stages of Shock

Unless hemorrhage is massive and immediately fatal, as with a gunshot wound of the aorta, shock may progress through three overlapping stages: nonprogressive, progressive, and irreversible shock.

Figure 6.18 illustrates the process. The initial stage of shock is the *nonprogressive* stage, characterized by reflex actions to re-establish perfusion. Low blood pressure stimulates the sympathetic nervous system: tachycardia increases cardiac output, and systemic vasoconstriction (mainly in the skin and extremities) increases peripheral resistance, both of which act to raise blood pressure to maintain tissue perfusion. Low blood pressure and blood flow to the kidneys stimulate the renin-angiotensin-aldosterone system, which induces peripheral and renal vasoconstriction and stimulates the kidney to retain sodium and water and expand blood volume.

The second stage, the *progressive stage,* characterized by more severe hypoperfusion and metabolic imbalances, is caused by hypoxia. Insufficient oxygen shifts energy metabolism to the anaerobic cycle, producing lactic acid excess (lactic acidosis), which in turn results in vasodilation and pooling of blood in the extremities, depriving brain and abdominal viscera of blood. The result is low blood pressure, decreased tissue perfusion, further hypoxia, and more acidosis, a vicious circle that often results in the final, irreversible, stage of shock.

Without effective intervention, a final, *irreversible stage* supervenes. This is characterized by 1) progressively severe hypotension, hypoperfusion, and acidosis; 2) decreased myocardial contractility; and 3) leakage into blood of inflammatory mediators from dying cells, which spread widely and further compound the metabolic difficulties. Finally, multiorgan failure leads to death.

Case Notes

6.32 Which stage of shock was James in when he died?

Pop Quiz

6.36 True or false? Cardiogenic shock is characterized by blood loss or vasodilation.

6.37 True or false? Obstructive shock is caused by mechanical interference with cardiac output.

6.38 What stage of shock is characterized by a shift to anaerobic metabolism and is accompanied by severe hypoperfusion and hypoxia?

6.39 What are the usual culprits of septic shock?

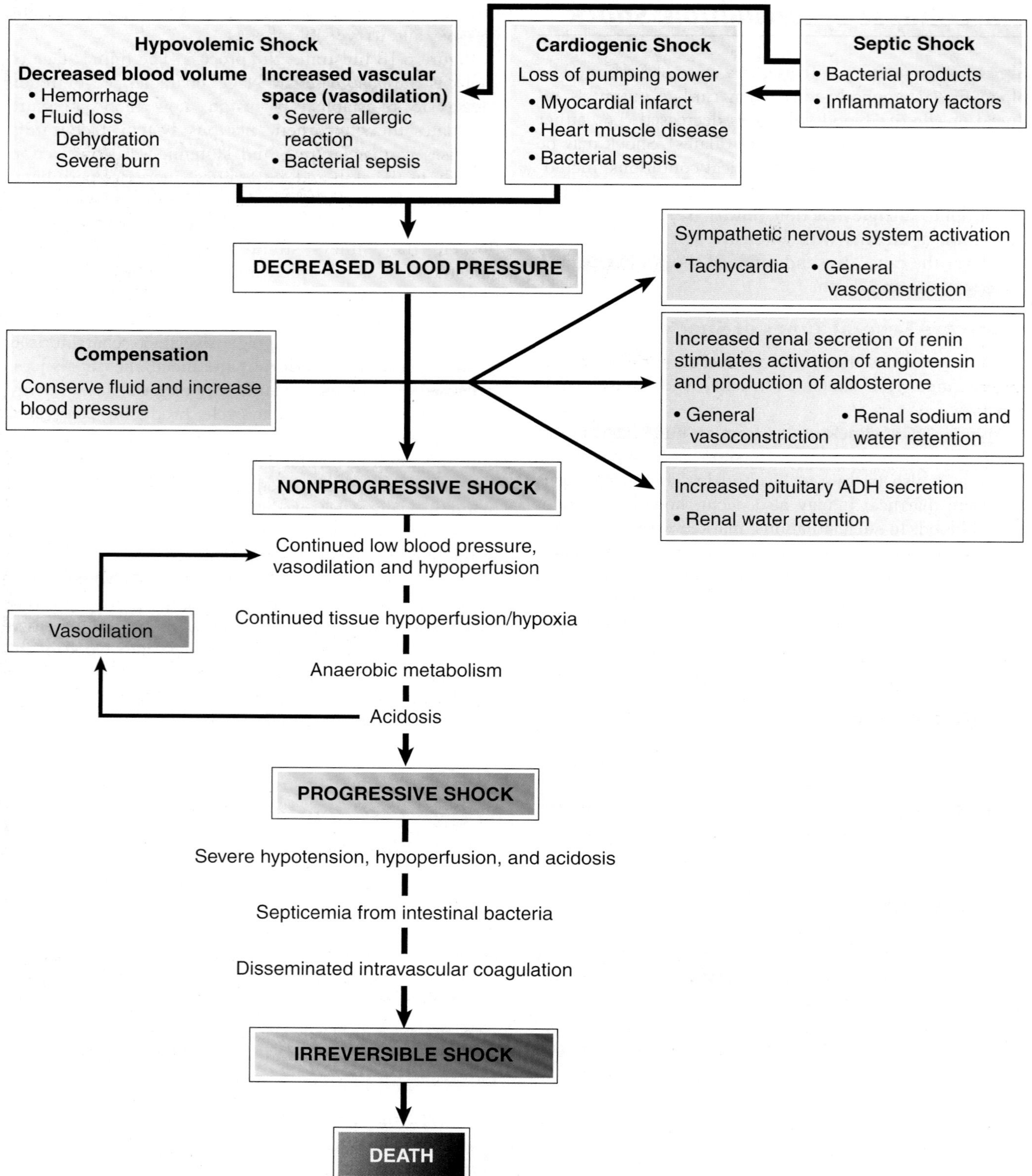

Figure 6.18 **Stages of shock.** This diagram shows the etiology, pathogenesis, and consequences of shock.

Case Study Revisited

"I think he is having another heart attack." The case of James G.

James's hospitalization was precipitated by the formation of a thrombus upon a preexisting coronary atheroma. The thrombus formed because of atherosclerotic damage to the vascular endothelium. Downstream ischemia caused death (necrosis) of the block of downstream heart muscle cells fed by the artery (an infarct). This infarct further deprived his heart of muscle power and he went into cardiogenic shock from low cardiac output. Blood acid content rose because the acidic products of metabolism could not be eliminated by lungs or kidneys, and blood oxygen fell because pulmonary edema interfered with oxygenation. Ultimately his shock became irreversible and he died.

James had severe edema of his legs and genitals and fluid accumulation in his pleural and peritoneal cavities. All of this fluid accumulated because James was retaining salt and water due to low blood pressure caused by low cardiac output, which in turn was due to muscle damage to his left ventricle from an old heart attack. With low cardiac output, less blood flowed into his kidneys, which sensed it and stimulated the secretion of renin, a hormone that promotes renal retention of salt (and water with it). This expanded blood volume, which strained the heart to an even greater degree, which further lowered cardiac output in a vicious circle of salt and water retention.

The failing left ventricle caused blood to "dam up" in the lungs, congesting them with blood and increasing capillary blood pressure. This forced water out of lung capillaries into lung air spaces, and accounted for the wet lungs sounds and X-ray findings of pulmonary edema. Congestion and fluid accumulation impaired oxygen and carbon dioxide exchange. Low blood oxygen accounted for his cyanotic (blue) appearance shortly before death.

The dammed up blood in the lungs in turn made it more difficult for the right ventricle to pump blood into the lungs and caused the right ventricle to fail. Blood dammed up in the entire venous system, congesting the viscera and accounting for James's enlarged (congested) liver; it also added to the accumulation of fluid in his chest, abdomen, and the tissues of his genitals and legs.

Low blood flow and poor oxygenation caused a buildup of tissue fixed acid. This was a major cause of his low blood pH and the fall of bicarbonate, which was being consumed by H^+ ions from fixed acids. Ordinarily, the lungs could help rid him of the excess acid, but in this instance pulmonary gas exchange was poor and carbon dioxide could not be exhaled normally. The increased carbon dioxide combined with water to cause a buildup of carbonic acid, which made him even more acidotic. His kidneys were secreting highly acidic urine (urine pH 4.96), but they were unable to handle the load and his acidosis became even worse.

His low blood sodium and potassium were surely due to diuretic therapy.

Chapter Challenge

CHAPTER RECALL

1. Which of the following is caused by an exudate?
   A. Pitting edema
   B. Ascites
   C. Lymphedema
   D. Anasarca

2. Which of the following is abnormal in a patient with von Willebrand disease?
   A. Bleeding time
   B. PTT
   C. PT
   D. Platelet count

3. Hydrostatic pressure is
   A. a measure of the tendency of water to move by osmosis from an area of high water concentration across a semipermeable membrane to an area of low water.
   B. governed by the collective size of small peripheral arteries.
   C. the increment of pressure created by resistance to the flow of fluid in a closed system like plumbing pipes or the cardiovascular system.
   D. caused by the weight of fluid in vessels.

4. Anaphylaxis causes which type of shock?
A. Cardiogenic shock
B. Obstructive shock
C. Septic shock
D. Hypovolemic shock

5. A 22-year-old African American female is being worked up for recurrent spontaneous abortions. Of interest, you note that both her PT and PTT are elevated. What is the likely cause of her spontaneous abortions?
A. Factor V Leiden mutation
B. Lupus anticoagulant
C. Idiopathic thrombocytopenic purpura
D. Hemophilia

6. Interruption of blood supply to which of the following organs will cause a white infarct?
A. Lungs
B. Kidney
C. Liver
D. GI tract

7. Which of the following has openings between the cells to allow entry of large molecules and particulate matter such as bacteria?
A. Capillaries
B. Lymphatics
C. Veins
D. Arteries

8. True or false? Albumin is the principal determinant of plasma osmolarity.

9. True or false? Excess water loss is the most common cause of dehydration.

10. True or false? In women, body water comprises 55% of mass, while in men it is only 50%.

11. True or false? Centrilobular necrosis is a result of the active accumulation of blood, or congestion, that occurs due to impaired venous outflow.

12. True or false? Activation of the clotting process without exposure to tissue factor is pathologic.

13. Put the following in order, as related to injury and coagulation:
A. Vasospasm
B. Wound healing and repair
C. Initiation of clotting cascade
D. Injury
E. Permanent plug
F. Thrombotic plug

14. Which of the following produces a transudate and which produces an exudate?
A. Nephrotic syndrome
B. Mastectomy with removal of axial lymph nodes
C. Sepsis
D. Cirrhosis
E. Tumor obstructing lymphatics
F. Congestive heart failure

15. Match the following symptoms with their cause:
i. Hyponatremia
ii. Hypernatremia
iii. Hypokalemia
iv. Hyperkalemia
v. Hypocalcemia
vi. Hypercalcemia
vii. Hypomagnesemia
viii. Hypermagnesemia
A. Weakness, thirst, and agitation
B. Slow heart rate, weakness, paralysis, and sensory paresthesias
C. Decreased blood pressure, muscle cramps, headaches, and seizures
D. Muscle fasciculations or tetany, increased reflexes, paresthesia, abdominal cramps, heart arrhythmias
E. Fatigue, lethargy, depression, kidney stones, arrhythmias, bone fractures
F. Lethargy, tremor, tetany, arrhythmias, and seizures
G. Arrhythmias, fatigue, weakness, and paresthesias
H. Hypotension, depressed respirations, and arrhythmias or cardiac arrest

CONCEPTUAL UNDERSTANDING

16. A 5-year-old male presents to the clinic for evaluation of a rash of new onset. His mother first noticed it three days ago, and complains that the affected area has continued to increase in size. On examination you notice multiple pinpoint hemorrhages on his skin. Similar findings are visible on his gums. You also note the presence of blood in his right nares. His mother denies recent illness, and reports no family history of bleeding disorders. Would you order a PTT, PT, bone marrow biopsy, or bleeding time, and why?

17. Explain why hydrostatic pressure in the feet is greater in patients with varicose veins.

18. Compare and contrast classic hemophilia and Christmas disease.

19. A 55-year-old smoker comes to the hospital complaining of painful right leg swelling. On physical exam, you note the leg is red, warm to touch, and twice the size of her left leg. What is your primary concern?

APPLICATION

20. A 60-year-old African American woman presents to the ER. Her medical history is significant for congestive heart failure. She complains of shortness of breath and swelling of her ankles. Her vitals are all within normal limits, except her blood pressure, which is extremely high. Which of the following factors could act to reduce her blood pressure by lowering blood volume?

A. Atrial natriuretic peptide
B. Aldosterone
C. Antidiuretic hormone
D. Renin

21. Fill in the following table using High, Low, or Normal:

	Respiratory Acidosis	Respiratory Alkalosis	Metabolic Acidosis	Metabolic Alkalosis
pH				
CO_2				
HCO_3				

22. Describe how the anatomy of arteries, capillaries, veins, and lymphatics contributes to circulatory flow.

23. Coumadin (warfarin) is a rat poison that blocks vitamin K action. Would this compound promote or inhibit coagulation?

24. A 16-year-old morbidly obese male is brought to the ER in an ambulance. He is comatose, with a weak, rapid heart rate, low blood pressure, dry mucous membranes, and pale cool skin. His mother reports that he has recently begun to complain of excessive thirst and increased urination. What is your diagnosis and how can you confirm it?

25. A 10-year-old male presents to the children's emergency room. He is tachycardic with decreased blood pressure. His physical exam reveals cool, clammy skin, swollen lips, and large red wheals (hives) over his entire body. A medical alert bracelet on his wrist denotes a peanut allergy. You immediately recognize this as what type of shock?

26. A young Caucasian woman presents to the clinic requesting birth control. While discussing her family history, she reports that both her mother and sister have a history of deep venous thrombosis prior to age 30. What type of birth control do you recommend to this patient and why?

27. During a follow-up physical exam 24 hours after admission for a broken leg, you notice your 65-year-old patient is breathing rapidly and seems disoriented. Pulses are palpable in both lower extremities, and no erythema, warmth, or swelling is evident. Her medications include heparin. Which is more likely—a pulmonary thromboembolism from a deep venous thrombosis or a fat embolism? Why?

PART 2

Disorders of the Organ Systems

These chapters discuss specific disorders of the organ systems.

Chapter 7 Disorders of Blood Cells
- Hemoglobin, hematocrit, red and white cell counts, red cell indices, other assessments of the formed elements of blood
- Hemorrhagic, hemolytic, and production-failure anemias; polycythemia
- Leukopenia, leukocytosis, and lymphadenopathy
- Acute and chronic leukemias; myeloproliferative syndromes; follicular and diffuse lymphomas; multiple myeloma and other plasma cell disorders
- Hypersplenism, thymic hyper- and hypoplasia

Chapter 8 Disorders of Blood Vessels
- The chemistry and optimum levels of high and low density lipoproteins and triglyceride
- Hypertension and atherosclerosis
- Aneurysms, dissections, vasculitis
- Varicose veins, thrombophlebitis

Chapter 9 Disorders of the Heart
- The cardiac conduction system and the electrocardiogram
- Right and left heart failure
- Coronary atherosclerosis, angina, coronary occlusion; valvular stenosis and insufficiency; myocarditis, cardiomyopathy, pericarditis
- Septal defects and other shunts, obstructions and other congenital disease
- Heart block, fibrillation, ectopic beats, escape rhythms, and other arrhythmias

Chapter 10 Disorders of the Respiratory Tract
- Allergic rhinitis, the common cold, sinusitis, pharyngitis, laryngitis
- Atelectasis, pulmonary edema, and acute respiratory distress syndrome
- Emphysema and chronic bronchitis, interstitial fibrosis
- Pulmonary hypertension and thromboembolism
- Lobar and bronchopneumonia
- Bronchogenic carcinoma, other tumors

Chapter 11 Disorders of the Gastrointestinal Tract
- Nausea, vomiting, diarrhea, constipation, hemorrhage, ileus, and other signs and symptoms of gastrointestinal disease
- Periodontitis, reflux esophagitis, gastritis, peptic ulcers, infectious diarrhea, hemorrhoids, and other diseases of the anatomic segments of the GI tract from mouth to anus
- Intestinal infections
- Celiac sprue and other malabsorption syndromes
- Crohn's disease and ulcerative colitis
- Tubular adenoma, carcinoma of the colon, and other neoplasms of the large and small bowel

Chapter 12 Disorders of the Liver and Biliary Tract
- Jaundice, cholestasis, cirrhosis, portal hypertension, and other liver responses to injury
- Acute and chronic viral hepatitis
- Alcoholic, toxic, and metabolic liver disease; biliary cirrhosis and other conditions of intrahepatic bile ducts
- Hepatocellular carcinoma and other tumors of the liver
- Acute and chronic cholecystitis, cholelithiasis, and other conditions of the gallbladder and extrahepatic bile ducts

Chapter 13 Disorders of the Pancreas
- Acute and chronic pancreatitis
- Diabetes and its complications: atherosclerosis, microangiopathy, glomerulopathy, peripheral neuropathy, retinopathy, infections
- Carcinoma; endocrine tumors

Chapter 14 Disorders of the Endocrine Glands
- Functioning and null pituitary adenomas, Cushing's syndrome, Addison's syndrome, goiter, thyrotoxicosis, thyroiditis, myxedema, hyperparathyroidism, diabetes insipidus, and other conditions of the pituitary-target organ axis
- Hyper- and hypoparathyroidism
- Carcinoma of the thyroid and other neoplasms of endocrine organs

Chapter 15 Disorders of the Urinary Tract
- Glycosuria, hematuria, proteinuria, ketonuria, and other urine abnormalities
- Obstruction, urolithiasis, transitional cell carcinoma, renal cell carcinoma
- Cystitis, incontinence, and voiding disorders
- Azotemia, uremia, clinical presentations of renal disease
- Acute and chronic glomerulonephritis, acute tubular injury, acute and chronic drug/toxic injury, tubulointerstitial disease
- Acute and chronic pyelonephritis, reflux nephropathy, nephrosclerosis, and other vascular disease

Chapter 16 Disorders of the Male Genitalia
- Erectile dysfunction and infertility
- Peyronie's disease, Bowen's disease, varicocele, *Taneia* infections and other conditions of the penis, scrotum, and groin
- Epididymitis, testicular tumors
- Prostatitis, prostatic hyperplasia; prostate specific antigen, prostate cancer

Chapter 17 Disorders of the Female Genitalia and Breast
- Infertility, menopause; pre-eclampsia, gestational diabetes, and disorders of pregnancy
- Vaginitis, lichen sclerosus, and other vulvovaginal conditions

These chapters discuss specific disorders of the organ systems. (continued)

- Human papillomavirus infection, dysplasia, and carcinoma of the cervix
- Endometriosis, endometrial hyperplasia, and carcinoma; uterine leiomyoma
- Ovarian cysts, carcinoma of the ovary; teratomas, fibromas, and other ovarian tumors
- Fibrocystic condition, epithelial hyperplasia, fibroadenoma, and other benign breast disease
- Ductal and lobular carcinoma of the breast

Chapter 18 Disorders of Bones, Joints, and Skeletal Muscle

- Osteoporosis, osteomalacia; osteogenesis imperfecta and other congenitial disorders of bone
- Fracture, infarction, and infection
- Osteosarcoma, chondrosarcoma, and other tumors of bone
- Osteoarthritis, rheumatoid arthritis, spondyloarthropathies, joint injuries; fibromyalgia and periarticular pain syndromes
- Fibromatoses, fibrosarcoma, and other tumors of joints and soft tissues
- Myasthenia gravis, muscular dystrophy; myopathies

Chapter 19 Disorders of the Nervous System

- Increased intracranial pressure, herniation, trauma; subdural, epidural, and subarachnoid hemorrhage
- Ischemic and hemorrhagic stroke, subarachnoid hemorrhage, laminar cortical necrosis
- Meningitis, encephalitis, brain abscess
- Multiple sclerosis and other demyelinating diseases; toxic encephalopathy
- Alzheimer disease, Parkinson disease; other degenerative conditions
- Glioma, meningioma, and other intracranial tumors

Chapter 20 Disorders of the Senses

The Eye

- Myopia, hyperopia, astigmatism; other disorders of refraction
- Conjunctivitis, uveitis; other inflammatory conditions
- Diabetic and hypertensive retinopathy, retinal detachment, macular degeneration; other conditions of the retina
- Glaucoma, optic neuritis, and other conditions of the optic nerve
- Retinoblastoma, malignant melanoma

The Ear

- Otitis media, cholesteatoma, otosclerosis; other conditions of the middle ear
- Meniere's syndrome; other conditions of the inner ear
- Deafness

Other senses

- Loss of (or distorted perception of) taste, smell, proprioception, touch, pain

Chapter 21 Disorders of the Skin

- Photoaging and other effects of sunlight; melasma and other effects of pregnancy; rheumatoid nodules and other lesions of systemic disease
- Acne, impetigo, ringworm, warts; pediculosis and other infections and infestations
- Eczema, urticaria, atopy, psoriasis; other acute and chronic dermatitis
- Vitiligo, lentigo; other conditions of abnormal pigmentation
- Nevi and malignant melanoma

CHAPTER 7

Disorders of Blood Cells

Contents

Chapter Objectives

After studying this chapter, you should be able to complete the following tasks:

THE FORMED ELEMENTS OF BLOOD

1. List the three cell lines derived from hematopoietic stem cells.

LABORATORY ASSESSMENT OF FORMED ELEMENTS

2. Explain what is meant by red cell indices, and how they are calculated.

ANEMIA

3. Compare and contrast the major types and subtypes of anemia, including those caused by hemorrhage, production defects, and destruction.

POLYCYTHEMIA

4. Explain the difference between relative and absolute erythrocytosis.

LEUKOPENIA, LEUKOCYTOSIS, AND LYMPHADENOPATHY

5. Distinguish between leukopenia, neutropenia, agranulocytosis, and leukemoid reaction, and explain the significance of a left shift.

OVERVIEW OF MALIGNANCIES OF WHITE BLOOD CELLS

6. Distinguish between leukemia and lymphoma.

MYELOID MALIGNANCIES

7. Compare and contrast acute myelogenous leukemia, myelodysplasia syndrome, and myeloproliferative diseases.

LYMPHOID MALIGNANCIES

8. Compare and contrast lymphocytic leukemias and the lymphoma subtypes.

9. Discuss plasma cell proliferations and explain why patients have abnormal blood proteins.

DISORDERS OF THE SPLEEN AND THYMUS

10. Define hypersplenism.

Case Study

"My life is running out of my nose." The case of Eleanor B.

Chief Complaint: Nosebleed

Clinical History: Eleanor B., a 52-year-old professor of anthropology, presented to the emergency room of a large metropolitan hospital with a severe nosebleed. "I never have nosebleeds. This takes the cake; it just won't stop. My life is running out of my nose!"

Questioning revealed that she had been feeling unusually tired for much of the last year. "I seem to wear out at even the smallest tasks. Last week I stopped for a rest on a park bench on my way home. That's never been necessary before."

Physical Examination and Other Data: Eleanor was pale and her skin contained numerous pinpoint hemorrhages. Her liver and spleen were easily palpable, each extending several cm beneath the rib cage. Blood analysis revealed marked deficiency in RBCs and platelets and a high WBC count containing many immature WBC forms, as shown in Table 7.1.

Table 7.1

Value	Units	Patient: High/Low	Normal Range for Females
HGB	gm/dL	9.0 **Low**	12.1–15.1
HCT	%	27 **Low**	33–43
RBC*	10^6 cells/mm^3	2.9 **Low**	3.5–5.0
MCV	fL	93	76–100
MCHC	g/dL	33	33–37
MCH	pg	31	27–33
Total WBC**	10^3 cells/ mm^3	15.8 **High**	4.5–10.5
Neutrophils	%	78 **High**	60–70
Bands**	%	8 **High**	<5
Eosinophils	%	2	2–4
Basophils	%	0	0–1
Lymphocytes	%	20	20–25
Monocytes	%	6	3–8
Platelets	10^3 cells/mm^3	18 **Low**	150–350

*Numerous misshapen RBC. Many nucleated RBC.
**Many immature myeloid cells.
Lab comment: Blood is slow to clot

Clinical Course: In the emergency room, an inflatable balloon was inserted into her nose for tamponade, and she was transfused with platelets, which stopped the nosebleed. She was admitted to the hospital and transfused with RBCs. Bone marrow biopsy showed nearly complete replacement of normal bone marrow by fibrous tissue and sparse growth of immature, malignant myeloid cells. The diagnosis was primary myelofibrosis with extramedullary hematopoiesis.

After she was discharged from the hospital, Eleanor continued to require RBC transfusions because of severe anemia. She also required antibiotic treatment on several occasions for bacterial infections—pneumonia, skin abscesses, and recurrent diarrhea. She retired from her teaching position. Nine months later she was brought to the emergency room by ambulance for severe bloody vomiting. She was pale and confused, with blood pressure 60/20 mm Hg (normal: 120/80) and heart rate 190 beats/min (normal: 70). Complete blood count (CBC) showed hemoglobin 4.8 gm/dL, WBC 6.1×10^3 cells/mm^3, and platelets 14×10^3/mm^3. Despite heroic efforts, she became pulseless and her heart could not be restarted.

"My life is running out of my nose." The case of Eleanor B. (continued)

Blood collected before her death grew *Staphylococcus aureus*. At autopsy, the bone cavities normally containing red marrow were obliterated by fibrous tissue; little normal marrow remained. The liver and spleen were massively enlarged due to marked extramedullary hematopoiesis. She was also found to have severe staphylococcal pneumonia and an extensive fungal infection in the esophagus. The latter had produced a large esophageal ulcer, which was the source of her fatal hemorrhage.

Final autopsy diagnoses were as follows:

- Primary myelofibrosis with myeloid metaplasia of liver and spleen
- Staphylococcal pneumonia and septicemia, and esophageal fungus infection due to failed leukopoiesis
- Hemorrhagic tendency due to failed thrombocytopoiesis
- Acute hemorrhagic shock due to hemorrhage from fungal ulcer of the esophagus

Blood is thicker than water.

THE SENTIMENT OF THIS PROVERB—THAT FAMILY TIES ARE THE CLOSEST OF ALL RELATIONSHIPS—IS AS OLD AS WRITING. IN ABOUT 1800 BC, THE SUMERIANS, INVENTORS OF WRITING WHO LIVED IN WHAT IS MODERN-DAY IRAQ, WROTE IT THIS WAY: "FRIENDSHIP LASTS A DAY; KINSHIP IS FOREVER."

Blood is liquid tissue, a mixture of cells and fluid. By volume, blood is about 45% cells (mainly RBCs), and 55% plasma. **Plasma** is the liquid part of blood. More than 90% of plasma is water, which contains dissolved solutes such as sodium, potassium, bicarbonate, other electrolytes, and countless numbers of hormones, cytokines, and other molecules that regulate body physiology. The remaining 10% of plasma is protein, mainly albumin. Small but important volumes of lipid (cholesterol and triglyceride) and carbohydrate (glucose and other sugars) are also present in plasma.

When referring to concentrations of substances, clinicians often use the words *blood*, *plasma*, and *serum* interchangeably, although they contain different components. **Serum** is the fluid remaining after blood clots. It is the fluid that oozes from a fresh scab formed over a bloody skin scrape and is the substance analyzed for most blood lab tests. Laboratories prefer serum because clotting consumes fibrinogen, a coagulation protein discussed later, which has a tendency to clog delicate lab instruments. The volume of fibrinogen in plasma is so small that the lost volume can be conveniently disregarded in lab testing. Nevertheless, sometimes tests are done on *anticoagulated* whole blood or plasma. Figure 7.1 details the composition of normal blood.

Case Notes

7.1 Lab tests on Eleanor were performed on fluid obtained from a tube of clotted blood. What is the name of this fluid?

7.2 What kind of sample was likely used to test Eleanor's platelets?

The Formed Elements of Blood

The **formed elements** of blood are **erythrocytes** (red blood cells, RBCs), **leukocytes** (white blood cells, WBCs), and thrombocytes (more commonly known as **platelets**). RBC and WBC are intact whole cells, whereas platelets are the fragments of the cytoplasm of a bone marrow cell, the **megakaryocyte**. These elements reside in the **bone marrow**, which is either yellow (fatty) or red (hematopoietic). Red marrow actively produces blood cells, while yellow marrow serves as a storehouse for fat, though it can become red marrow if necessary. In adults, most red marrow lies in the central cavity of bones of the spine, pelvis, ribs, cranium, and the proximal ends of long bones. Despite the fact that RBCs are 1,000 times more abundant than WBCs, only about 25% of red marrow is composed of developing red cells; the remaining 75% consists of developing white cells. This is because white cells have a much shorter life span than RBCs, so they need a bigger factory to replace them.

In addition to the blood proper and bone marrow, blood cells exist in the spleen, the lymph nodes, and the thymus (to a greater extent in the fetus and a lesser extent in adults). Like all cells, blood cells have a life cycle—they are produced, they work, and they die by apoptosis. Compared to cells in most other tissues, the life span of all blood cells is short. It is important to remember that the number of a particular type of cell in a blood sample depends upon its life span as well as its rate of production—cells with longer life spans and greater production will be present in greater numbers.

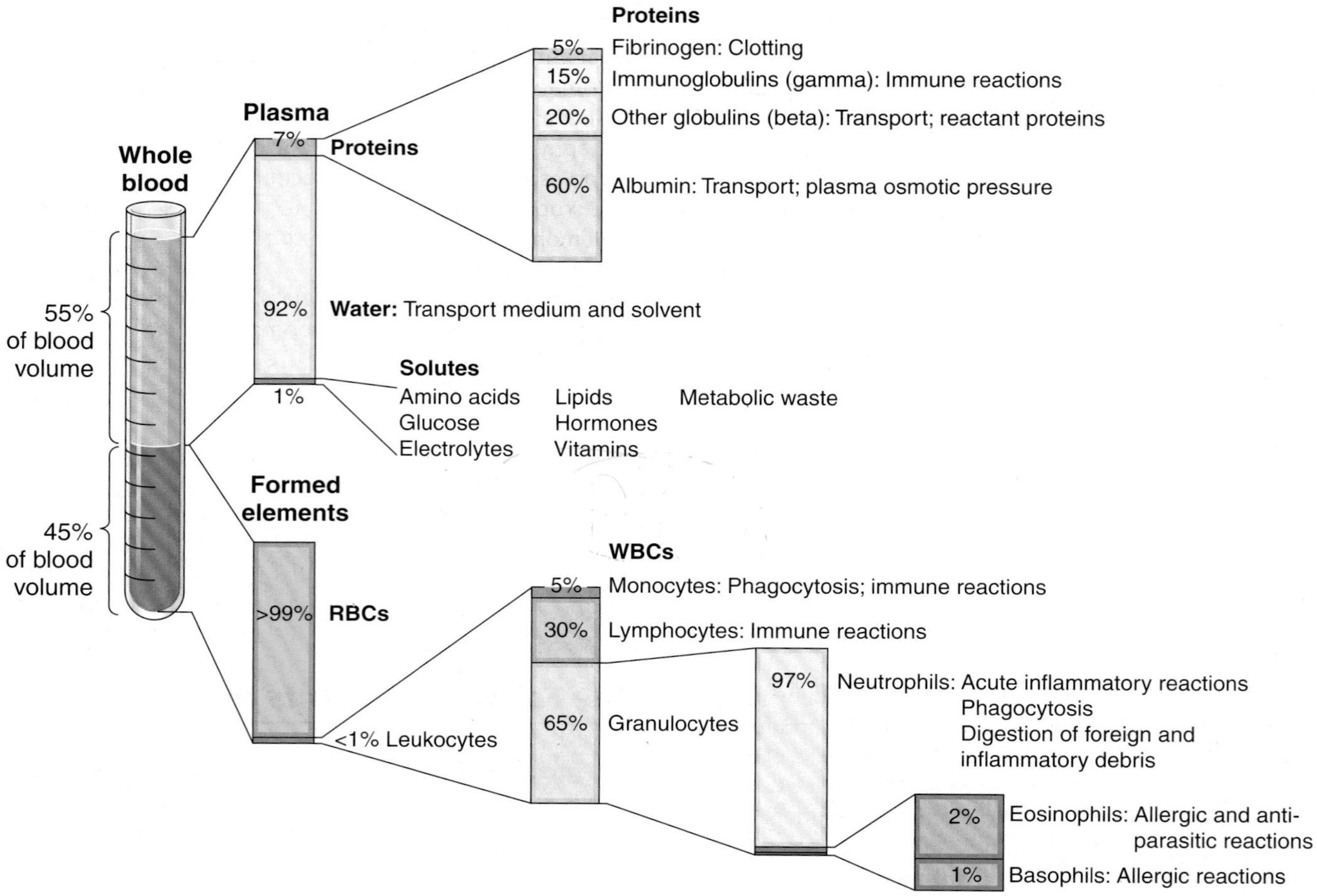

Whole blood
55% of blood volume
45% of blood volume
Plasma
7% Proteins
92% Water: Transport medium and solvent
1% Solutes
Amino acids Lipids Metabolic waste
Glucose Hormones
Electrolytes Vitamins
Proteins
5% Fibrinogen: Clotting
15% Immunoglobulins (gamma): Immune reactions
20% Other globulins (beta): Transport; reactant proteins
60% Albumin: Transport; plasma osmotic pressure
Formed elements
>99% RBCs
<1% Leukocytes
WBCs
5% Monocytes: Phagocytosis; immune reactions
30% Lymphocytes: Immune reactions
65% Granulocytes
97% Neutrophils: Acute inflammatory reactions
Phagocytosis
Digestion of foreign and inflammatory debris
2% Eosinophils: Allergic and anti-parasitic reactions
1% Basophils: Allergic reactions

Figure 7.1 **The composition of blood** (% by volume).

Hematopoiesis Is the Production of Blood Cells

The generation of blood cells is called **hematopoiesis** (Greek *haima* = blood; *poiesis* = formation). All blood cells arise from a common ancestor, a *pluripotent* hematopoietic stem cell, literally a blood cell with "many powers" (Fig. 7.2) that resides in the bone marrow. This master cell in turn gives rise to two types of specialized *multipotent* stem cells, which we will call **progenitor cells**, with several narrower powers:

- **Lymphoid progenitor cells** give rise to *lymphocytes*, a type of leukocyte or WBC.
- **Myeloid progenitor cells** give rise to all other blood cells—*granulocytes, monocytes, erythrocytes,* and *megakaryocytes.*

The production of cellular blood elements in the fetus differs from that in an adult. In the embryo and developing fetus, cellular elements of blood are produced primarily in the liver and spleen, but by the time of birth, production has gradually shifted to the red marrow. Nevertheless, the liver and spleen retain their ability to produce cellular elements throughout life and will do so, even in older adults, under some circumstances. Blood cell production by the liver and spleen in an adult is called **extramedullary hematopoiesis** (hematopoiesis away from the medullary cavity of bones). It can occur in certain conditions that wipe out the bone marrow. For example, in Eleanor's case, fibrous tissue replaced most of her red marrow, forcing the liver and spleen to take over hematopoiesis.

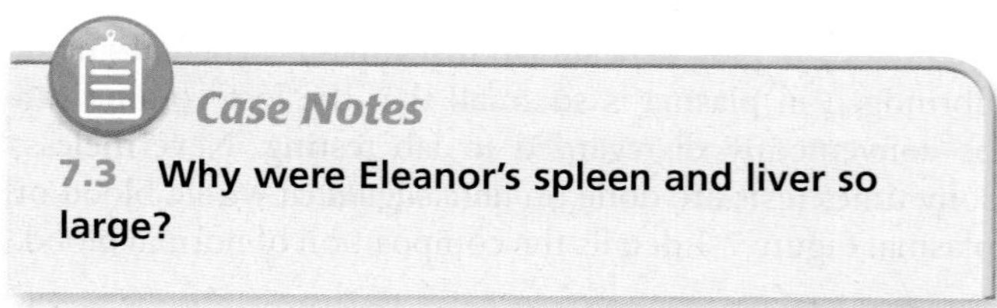

Case Notes

7.3 Why were Eleanor's spleen and liver so large?

Red Blood Cells Transport Oxygen

Red blood cells (RBCs) originate from myeloid progenitor cells in the marrow. They begin as nucleated cells, but the nucleus is ejected before the cell enters the blood stream in order to make more room for hemoglobin. **Hemoglobin** is the compound in RBCs to which oxygen attaches for transport from lungs to tissues, and its synthesis requires iron, vitamin B_{12}, vitamin B_6, and folic acid.

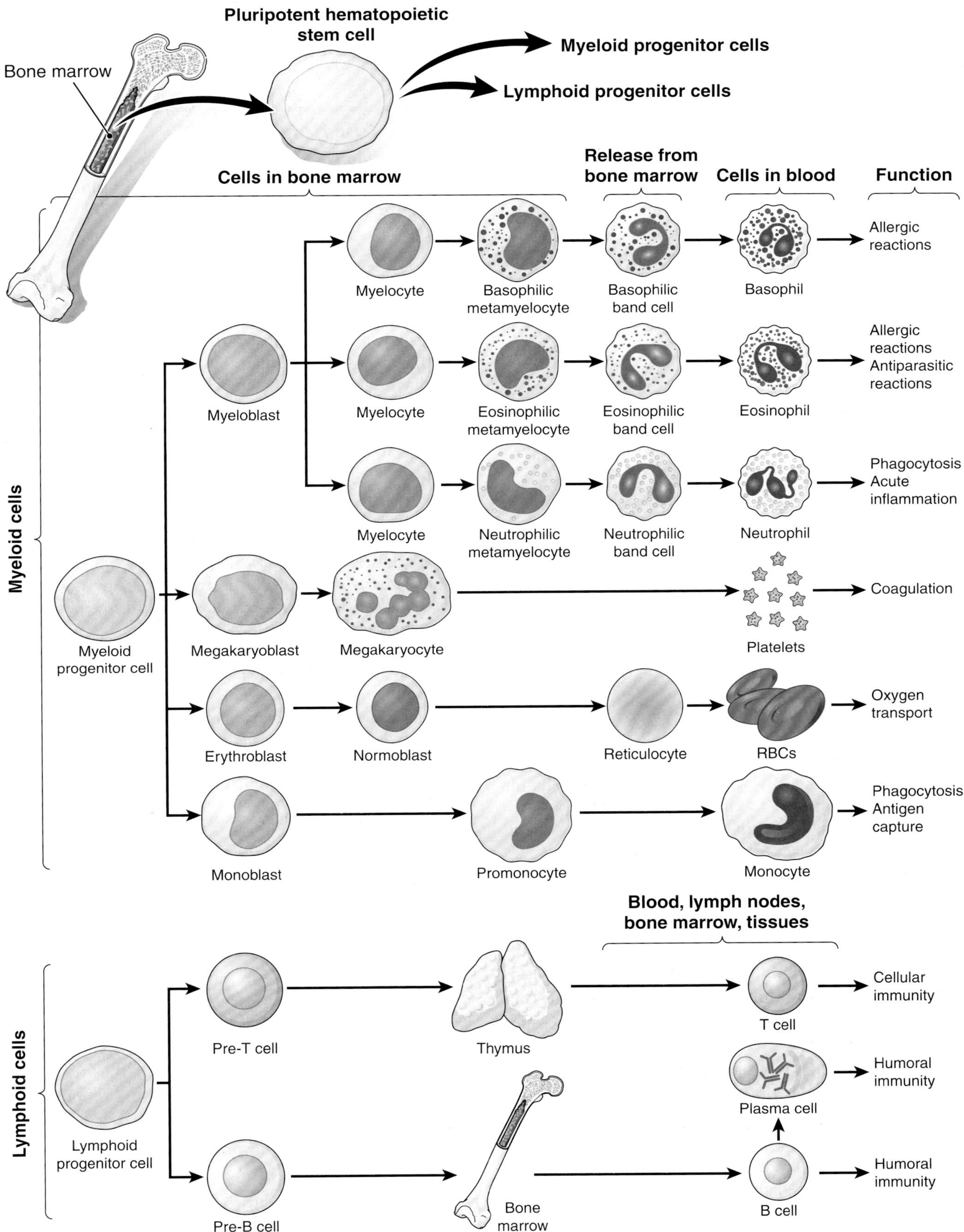

Figure 7.2 **Hematopoiesis.** There are two main groups of blood cells: myeloid and lymphoid, each derived from a primitive progenitor cell.

RBC production in the bone marrow is stimulated by **erythropoietin**, a hormone synthesized by the kidney. Erythropoietin production is stimulated by the amount of oxygen delivered to the kidney by RBCs. Low oxygen levels or abnormal hemoglobin (most of which stem from genetic defects of hemoglobin synthesis) result in increased release of erythropoietin and RBC production to make up the deficit. For example, general hypoxia occurs in people living at high altitude and their bone marrow makes extra red cells to compensate—they therefore have higher RBC counts than do people living at lower altitudes. General hypoxia also occurs in patients with chronic lung disease; they, too, have high RBC counts. Likewise, in patients who are anemic like Eleanor, erythropoietin levels increase in order to produce more RBCs.

Case Notes

7.4 On admission to the hospital, would Eleanor's erythropoietin be increased or decreased?

White Blood Cells Are Active in Inflammation and Immunity

Hormones and inflammatory and immune molecule mediators stimulate the production of WBCs and platelets. Leukocytes are nucleated phagocytic cells that fight microbes and other nonself invaders and promote the repair process.

There are three kinds of leukocytes:

- *Monocytes* are phagocytic. They migrate into tissue to become phagocytes that ingest and digest foreign antigen and present it for action to immune cells for immune response.
- *Lymphocytes* are the main cells of the immune system. Their task is to react to nonself antigen.
- *Granulocytes* have cytoplasmic granules of digestive enzymes and other substances that play an important role in inflammation. The three granulocytes are: neutrophils, eosinophils, and basophils. *Neutrophils* are the most abundant granulocyte. Their task is to react to acute injury and infection by ingesting (phagocytosis) and digesting foreign agents, especially bacteria, and by cleaning up inflammatory debris. *Basophils* and *eosinophils* are the inflammatory cells of allergic reactions and reactions to parasites.

Notice in Figure 7.2 that megakaryocytes, large bone marrow cells, produce platelets. Megakaryocytes are closely related to WBCs because they arise from the same progenitor cell. Platelets are not WBCs; in fact, they have no nucleus and aren't really cells at all. Instead, they are small fragments of megakaryocyte cytoplasm. Their task is to stop bleeding by sticking together at points of vascular injury to obstruct hemorrhage, and to initiate the clotting process at the site of bleeding.

Case Notes

7.5 Study Eleanor's lab report. Why does she have severe nosebleed and why is her blood slow to clot?

The Life Span of Blood Cells Varies Greatly

How long blood cells live (and circulate) is important. Compared to cells in most other tissues, the life span of blood cells is short; therefore, cell turnover is rapid. Red cells have the longest life span of blood cells: about 120 days. Neutrophils, basophils, and eosinophils live about four days; lymphocytes and monocytes, a week or two. Platelets live about a week. Old (senescent) blood cells and platelets are removed from circulation by the spleen. This rapid turnover means that it is critical that new cells be produced at a rate that equals the rate at which cells are dying.

Many diseases of blood cells are caused by production failure or early cell death or destruction; that is to say, by shortened cell life span. Anemia (too little hemoglobin) is usually caused by too few RBCs (anemia can also occur with normal numbers of red cells that do not contain enough hemoglobin). Some patients have a low RBC count because their bone marrow fails to produce enough RBCs. In other cases, RBC life span is short because RBCs are prematurely destroyed (*hemolysis*). The same holds true for platelets and WBCs—some conditions are attributable to failed cell or platelet production, others to early destruction or death.

Remember This! The number of WBCs, RBCs, and platelets in blood is a function of their life span and the rate of their production versus the rate of their loss.

Pop Quiz

7.1 True or false? Granulocytes are the shortest-surviving formed element in blood, surviving four days.

7.2 True or false? Leukocytes include monocytes, erythrocytes, and granulocytes.

7.3 What do myeloid progenitor cells give rise to? Lymphoid progenitor cells?

7.4 What causes erythropoietin to be released?

7.5 How long does a RBC live?

Laboratory Assessment of Formed Elements

Laboratory assessment of blood cells is usually performed on blood collected from an arm vein. Such a blood sample is typically referred to as "peripheral blood" to distinguish it from the pool of blood in large vessels and the viscera, which is slightly more dilute. Though a syringe is depicted in Figure 7.3, in modern practice blood is collected directly into vacuum tubes from which a sample is obtained for machine analysis. Formed elements typically are measured in anticoagulated whole blood; that is, blood that contains an anticoagulant to keep it clot-free. Conversely, chemical elements, such as glucose, are measured in plasma or in serum from a second tube of clotted blood. In either case, the tube is then taken to an analyzer that samples blood directly from the tube and renders a patient report within a few seconds (Fig. 7.3A). For study of features not amenable to machine analysis, a technician smears a thin film of blood on a slide, which is placed under a microscope (Fig. 7.3B).

The standard laboratory study of blood cells is referred to as a **complete blood count (CBC)**. In modern laboratories, the process is automated and at a minimum consists of a determination of the **WBC count**, the **white cell differential count** (the percentage of white cells that are neutrophils, eosinophils, or basophils), the **RBC count**, the number of grams of **hemoglobin** per unit of volume, the **hematocrit** (the percent of blood volume occupied by RBCs), and the **platelet count**.

Microscopic examination of blood cells is an important tool, but it is ordinarily not necessary unless significant abnormalities are present in the measurements obtained on a CBC. Every laboratory has criteria defining when microscopic examination is necessary. Alternatively, the clinician may know of signs and symptoms that indicate need for microscopic examination of blood cells and can order it. For example, microscopic examination may be required if the hemoglobin is below 10 gm/dL, or the WBC count is above 15,000 cells/µl. Among the important things detectable by microscopic examination are the presence of malignant white cells in leukemia, abnormally shaped RBCs, malaria parasites in RBCs, RBCs with nuclei, and giant platelets.

Also important in a CBC is determination of the **red cell indices**, which are measures of the size and hemoglobin content of the *average* RBC (Fig. 7.4):

- The average *size* of an RBC is the **mean cell volume (MCV)**.
- The average *amount* of hemoglobin in an average RBC is the **mean cell hemoglobin (MCH)**.
- The average *concentration* of hemoglobin per unit of volume in an average RBC is the **mean cell hemoglobin concentration (MCHC)**.

Red cell indices are important in the diagnosis of diseases. RBCs may be too large (**macrocytic**), normal size (**normocytic**), or too small (**microcytic**). Additionally, diseased RBCs may have a normal amount of hemoglobin per cell (**normochromic**) or too little hemoglobin (**hypochromic**). There is no such thing as a red cell with too much hemoglobin.

Case Notes

7.6 In the blood Eleanor lost from her nosebleed, did she lose a greater volume of cells or fluid?

Additionally, tests may be performed to determine the percentage of new (young) red cells (**reticulocytes**) in blood, which are elevated when red cell production increases as the bone marrow compensates for RBC shortage. Laboratories may also determine the type of hemoglobin in red cells. Normal hemoglobin is *hemoglobin A* (and consists of two alpha globin chains and two beta globin chains). Hundreds of types of abnormal hemoglobin have been described. Among the most common abnormal hemoglobin is *hemoglobin S*, the hemoglobin of sickle cell disease, which we will discuss later.

Pop Quiz

7.6 What is the equation for calculating MCV?

7.7 How would the MCHC change if hemoglobin production were decreased?

7.8 What is the best measurement of erythrocyte size?

Anemia

Anemia is abnormally low hemoglobin in blood. It may be caused by decreased numbers of RBCs, decreased amounts of hemoglobin in red cells, or both. Laboratory measures of hemoglobin, red cell count, and hematocrit usually move up and down together. Anemia demands thorough investigation because it is always a sign of some underlying condition. Some patients present with signs or symptoms of the primary disease and are found upon investigation to be anemic. For example, a slowly bleeding intestinal cancer may not be detected until it produces intestinal obstruction; and the patient is then found to

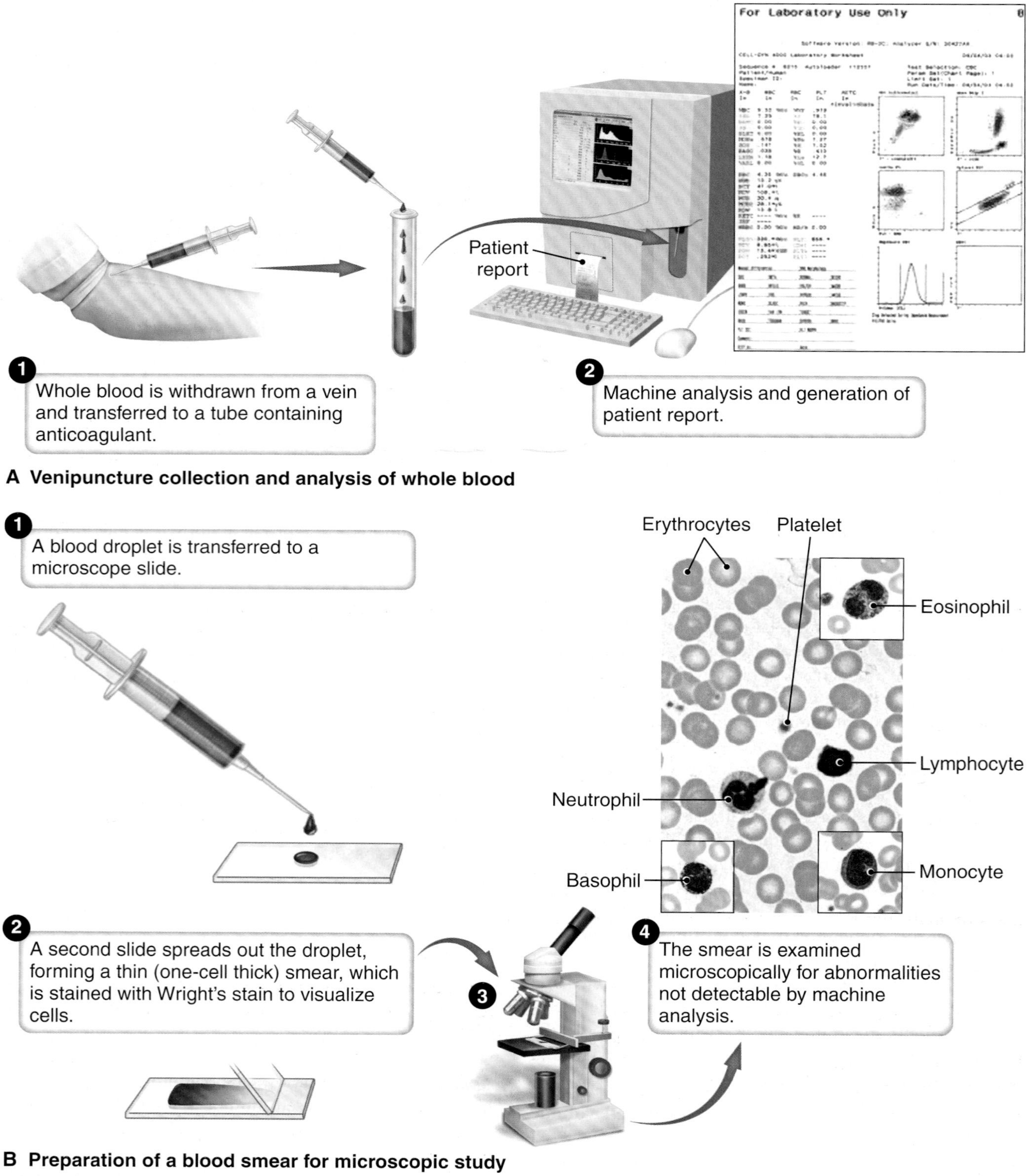

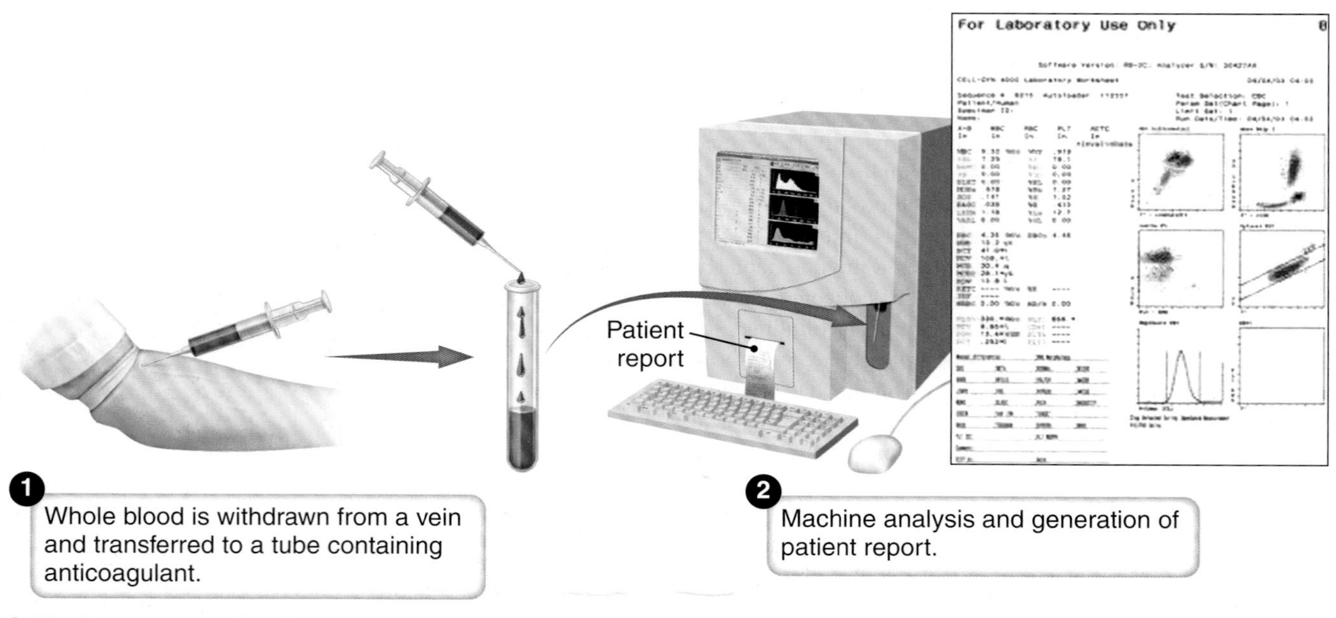

For Laboratory Use Only
Patient report
1
Whole blood is withdrawn from a vein and transferred to a tube containing anticoagulant.
2
Machine analysis and generation of patient report.
A Venipuncture collection and analysis of whole blood
1
A blood droplet is transferred to a microscope slide.
Erythrocytes
Platelet
Eosinophil
Lymphocyte
Neutrophil
Basophil
Monocyte
2
A second slide spreads out the droplet, forming a thin (one-cell thick) smear, which is stained with Wright's stain to visualize cells.
3
4
The smear is examined microscopically for abnormalities not detectable by machine analysis.
B Preparation of a blood smear for microscopic study

Figure 7.3 **Laboratory assessment of the formed elements of blood. A.** Machine determination of hemoglobin, hematocrit, red and white blood cell counts, platelet count, and red cell indices. **B.** Microscopic study of formed elements. (Adapted with permission from McConnell TH, Hull KL. *Human Form Human Function: Essentials of Anatomy & Physiology*. Baltimore, MD: Wolters Kluwer Health; 2011.)

be anemic from chronic blood loss. Other patients present with symptoms that are almost universal and caused directly by the anemia owing to less than normal capacity to deliver oxygen to tissues: chronic fatigue, shortness of breath (because of lack of oxygen), or pale appearance (pallor). Skin is pale. Anemia in people with dark skin can be detected by pallor of the oral and conjunctival mucosae, as well as the bed of fingernails. Resting heart rate and

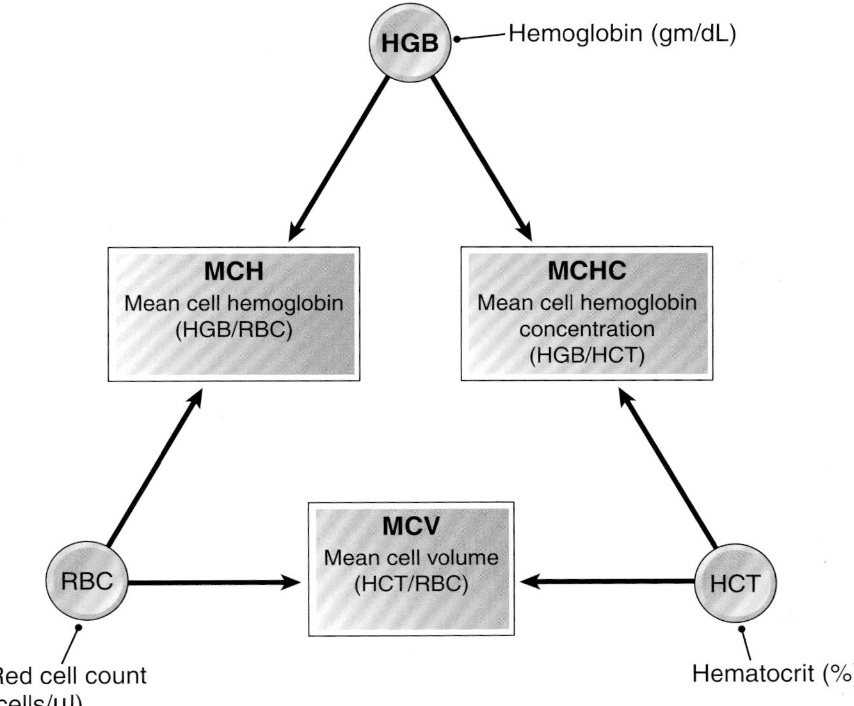

Figure 7.4 **Red blood cell indices.** Measurement of red cell size (MCV), hemoglobin content (MCH) and concentration (MCHC) are calculated from blood hemoglobin (HGB), red cell count (RBC), and hematocrit (HCT).

respiratory rate are increased. Severely anemic patients may faint or become comatose.

The first step in the diagnosis of anemia is a CBC and determination of red cell indices, because the different types of anemia are typically characterized by red cells of a certain size (MCV) and hemoglobin content (MCHC). For example, iron deficiency impairs hemoglobin synthesis, so iron-deficient RBCs contain less hemoglobin than normal. The RBCs are pale (hypochromic, low MCHC) and small (microcytic, low MCV). Few diseases other than iron deficiency produce small, pale RBCs. Conversely, other types of anemia are characterized by macrocytic cells (large MCV). Knowing the red cell indices dramatically narrows the number of diseases to be considered in the differential diagnosis.

The second step in the diagnostic routine for anemia is to determine if the anemia is associated with 1) *failed bone marrow production* of RBCs (not enough cells or hemoglobin), versus 2) RBC loss either by a) *hemorrhage* or b) *destruction*. A reticulocyte count should be near 0% in failed production, and greater than 2.5% in red cell destruction. Every anemia fits into at least one of these categories.

It helps to think of the intravascular space as a tank into which RBCs are pumped from the bone marrow. They enter the intravascular space and survive an average of 120 days before they die a natural death by apoptosis and are filtered out of circulation by the spleen. Figure 7.5 illustrates the production, circulation, and destruction of RBCs.

Treatment is twofold. One aspect is to replenish RBCs, either rapidly by transfusion, or more slowly by supplying iron or other nutrients necessary for bone marrow generation of new blood cells. The other aspect is to identify the cause and reverse it: stop bleeding or intravascular red cell destruction, or eliminate the cause of marrow suppression.

Despite their similarities, the various types of anemia differ to some degree in their signs, symptoms, and treatment.

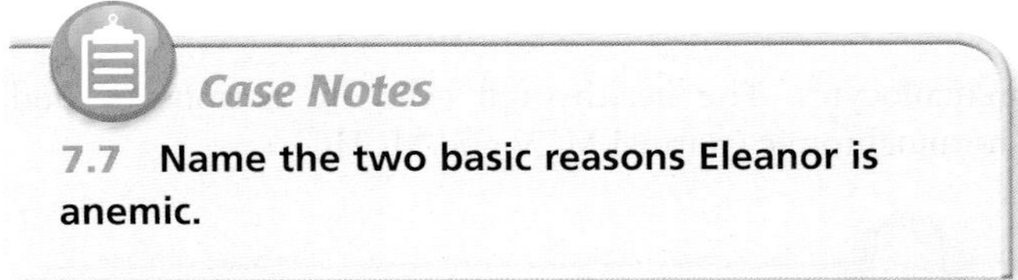

Anemias of Hemorrhage Are Due to Blood Loss

Hemorrhage creates two problems: 1) loss of oxygen-carrying capacity; and 2) loss of iron (80% of body iron is in the hemoglobin in RBCs). If bleeding is limited, lost red cells can be replaced in a few weeks or months by normal bone marrow; however, lost iron is not easily or quickly replaced. If bleeding continues for a long time (e.g., from an undetected colon cancer), the patient may become iron deficient (discussed below).

The main threat of **acute blood loss** is not anemia, but shock or death from lost blood volume. If the patient survives an acute hemorrhage, the volume of lost red cells is initially replaced by water and albumin synthesis by the liver, and the patient develops a temporary **dilutional anemia** until the marrow can replace the lost RBCs. Dilutional anemia features healthy red cells, which have normal size and hemoglobin content, and increased numbers of

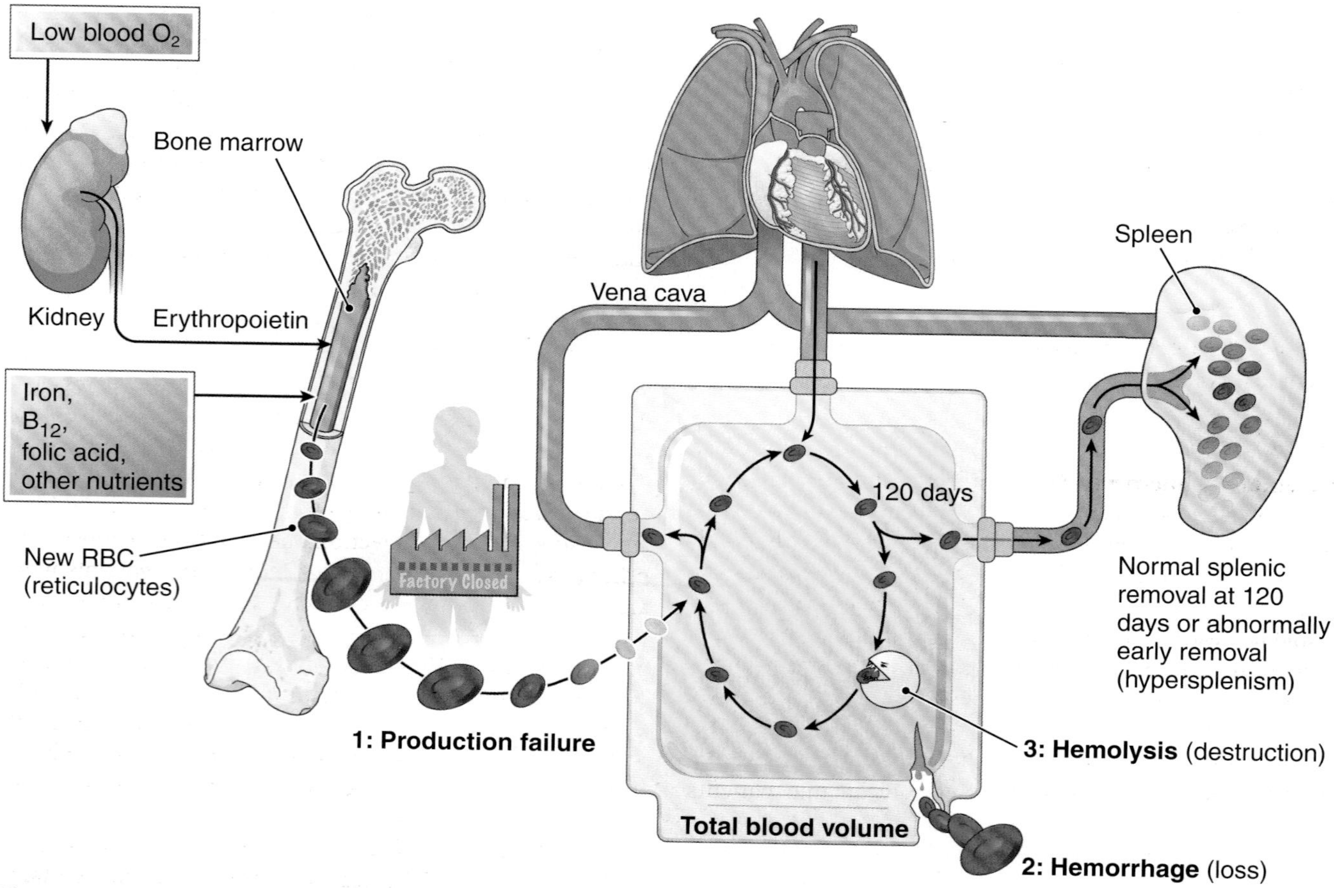

Low blood O_2
Bone marrow
Kidney
Erythropoietin
Iron,
B_{12},
folic acid,
other nutrients
New RBC
(reticulocytes)
Factory Closed
1: Production failure
Vena cava
Spleen
120 days
Normal splenic removal at 120 days or abnormally early removal (hypersplenism)
3: **Hemolysis** (destruction)
Total blood volume
2: **Hemorrhage** (loss)

Figure 7.5 **Production, circulation, and death of RBCs.** Every anemia is caused by at least one of three mechanisms: 1) decreased red cell production, 2) loss of red cells by hemorrhage, or 3) early death (destruction) of RBCs.

reticulocytes. The healthy red cells are normocytic and normochromic (normal MCV and MCHC).

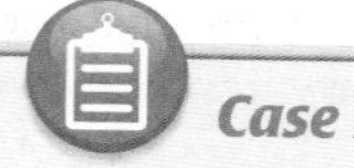

Case Notes

7.8 Did Eleanor have dilutional anemia on her final admission?

Chronic blood loss usually occurs with one of two conditions: 1) abnormal menstrual bleeding in women during their reproductive years; or 2) intestinal bleeding in either sex, especially from undetected colon cancer. Intestinal bleeding is often very slow, new cells from the bone marrow replace lost red cells, and the patient does not become anemic. If, however, the rate of red cell loss is greater than the marrow can produce, the lack of red cells in the vascular space is made up by fluid and the patient *initially* develops a *dilutional anemia* until the bleeding stops. In chronic bleeding, however, the intestinal absorption of dietary iron usually cannot make up for iron lost in the hemorrhaged RBCs, and the patient eventually becomes *iron deficient* and develops iron deficiency anemia (discussed below).

Case Notes

7.9 Did Eleanor die of acute or chronic blood loss?

Hemolytic Anemias Are Due to Red Cell Destruction

Premature destruction of RBCs is called **hemolysis**, which shortens red cell life span below the normal 120 days. Hemolytic anemias feature

- *anemia and short RBC life span*;
- *active, hypercellular bone marrow*, as the marrow works overtime to replace dying cells;
- *increased blood erythropoietin*, as the kidney secretes more to stimulate RBC production;
- *blood that contains a high count of new RBCs (reticulocytes)*. These new red cells are easy for

laboratory technicians to identify on conventional microscopic examination because they have a bluish cast; they can be revealed even more clearly by special stains.

Depending on the cause, hemolytic anemia may also result in the following signs: an enlarged spleen (*splenomegaly*), increased free hemoglobin in plasma (*hemoglobinemia*), dark urine due to hemoglobin in the urine (*hemoglobinuria*), or *jaundice*, a yellow discoloration of skin caused by increased bilirubin (a metabolic product of hemoglobin breakdown).

Many hemolytic diseases are caused by genetic defects. The most common of these are discussed next.

Hereditary Spherocytosis

Hereditary spherocytosis is a genetic disorder of structural protein (spectrin) in the red cell membrane that renders cells stiff and spherical rather than flexible and biconcave. The cells are therefore less able to deform themselves to successfully pass through the spleen. The result is a splenic destruction (hemolysis). Signs and symptoms are variable degrees of anemia, jaundice, and splenomegaly. Diagnosis is by microscopic study of RBCs and by laboratory demonstration of the increased susceptibility of RBCs to hemolysis by hypotonic saline solutions. Treatment is supportive. Splenectomy is effective, but it does not, of course, remedy the genetic defect.

Glucose-6-Phosphate Dehydrogenase Deficiency

Glucose-6-phosphate dehydrogenase (G6PD) deficiency is an X-linked recessive genetic disorder that causes deficiency of G6PD in red cells. G6PD is important in the supply of energy to stabilize the red cell membrane. Deficiency destabilizes the membrane, rendering RBCs fragile and susceptible to destruction. The mutant gene is present in 10% of African American men, rendering them subject to acute hemolytic episodes upon exposure to certain oxidizing drugs, toxins, or infections. Signs and symptoms are typical of hemolytic anemia. Diagnosis is by laboratory assay for G6PD. Treatment is supportive.

Sickle Cell Disease

Sickle cell disease is one of more than 300 **hemoglobinopathies**, a family of autosomal recessive genetic disorders of hemoglobin synthesis. The hemoglobin is *molecularly defective*, unstable, and causes early red cell death (hemolysis) The most notable among these is *hemoglobin S*, the cause of **sickle cell disease**. About 10% of African Americans are carriers (heterozygotes, genotype SA); about 0.3% of African Americans are homozygotes (genotype SS) and have sickle cell anemia.

Pathophysiology

In Hb S valine is substituted for glutamic acid in the sixth amino acid of the beta globin chain of hemoglobin (Chapter 22). Oxygenated Hb S is less soluble than oxygenated Hb A, so that at sites with low oxygen levels it tends to form a gel that causes RBCs to deform in a sickle shape. This process, called "sickling," subjects cells to premature death (hemolysis) as they pass through the spleen. These misshaped, inflexible RBCs also plug small arterioles and capillaries, which can lead to infartion of any tissue. Venous plugging predisposes to thrombosis, and chronic compensatory marrow hyperactivity deforms bones, especially in children.

Signs and Symptoms

Sickle cell disease (hemoglobin SS) usually becomes evident shortly after birth, presenting as a severe anemia with chronic hemolysis. The clinical course of sickle cell disease is punctuated by periodic sickle "crises," episodes of acute severe abdominal or bone pain caused by vascular occlusions stimulated by infection, dehydration, acidosis, or other physiologic stress. On the other hand, patients who are carriers of the sickle cell trait tend to remain asymptomatic unless their blood oxygen content falls, as happens in ascents to high altitudes, severe lung disease, or other conditions associated with low blood oxygen. Children with sickle cell disease tend to be poorly developed and have skeletal abnormalities. Hepatosplenomegaly is common in children, but later the spleen shrinks to a nubbin from repeated infarcts.

The clinical and pathologic findings in sickle cell disease are those of hemolytic anemia, but with certain unique features (Fig. 7.6A). These findings result from the following:

- *Obstruction of small blood vessels*, which causes ischemia and infarction of various tissues, including gangrene of fingers and toes
- *Anemia*, which can be severe enough to cause high-output heart failure and cardiomegaly, bone marrow hyperplasia, and bone deformities induced by the overactive bone marrow
- *Hemolysis*, which produces many of the clinical features of hemolysis mentioned above, but may also cause pigment gallstones owing to bilirubin secretory overload on the liver and biliary system
- *Infections*, caused by loss of splenic immune function (*hyposplenism*) as accumulated infarcts destroy the spleen; or by pathogens that find their way into necrotic bone, lung, and other tissues. Only about half of patients with sickle cell disease reach midlife, but others succumb to a variety of infections—such as *Salmonella* bone infections or pneumococcal sepsis—or to bone marrow failure triggered by *parvovirus* infection of red cell precursors in the bone marrow.

Diagnosis and Treatment

Diagnosis is by laboratory demonstration of S hemoglobin by one of two methods. The simplest technique involves

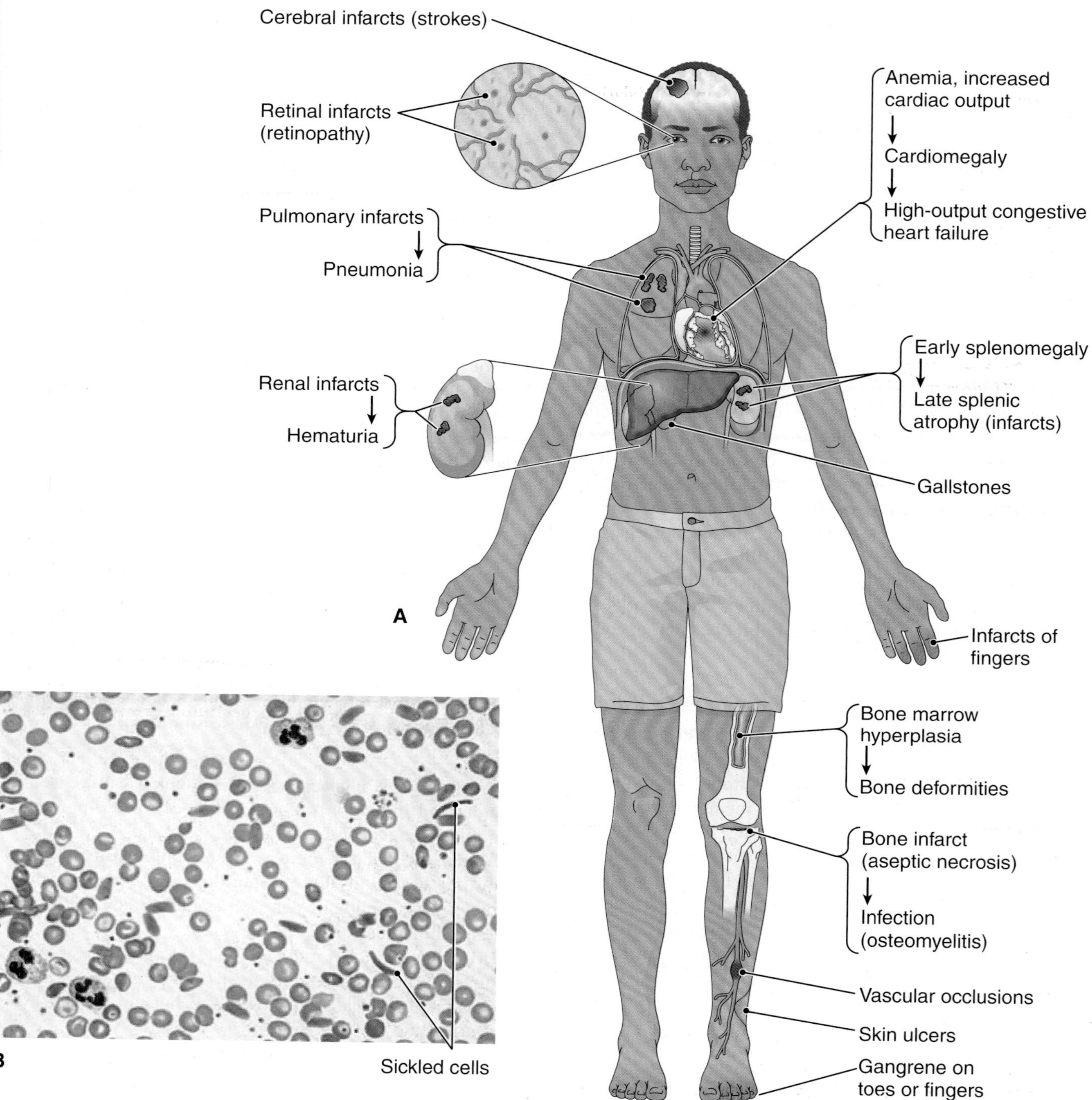

Figure 7.6 **Sickle cell anemia. A.** Clinical and pathologic findings. **B.** Sickled RBCs. Sickled red cells appear in peripheral blood specimens only in patients with sickle cell *disease* because all of their hemoglobin is hemoglobin S. Sickled cells do not normally appear in the blood of patients with sickle cell *trait* because their red cells contain roughly equal amounts of hemoglobin S and normal hemoglobin. Red cells with any amount of hemoglobin S, however, can be induced to sickle as part of a laboratory test for the presence of hemoglobin S.

adding a chemical to bind all oxygen in a drop of blood and then inspecting the specimen for sickled cells. The microscopic appearance of sickled red cells in smears of untreated patient blood is also diagnostic (Fig. 7.6B). Electrophoresis can directly demonstrate hemoglobin S, hemoglobin A, or both. Prenatal diagnosis can be made by DNA testing for the sickle gene.

Treatment is generally supportive. An occasional transfusion may be necessary. Prophylactic daily penicillin may be useful to ward off infections to which these patients are vulnerable because of hyposplenism. Because crises are often initiated by infection, vaccinations are important.

For an interesting and unexpected aspect of sickle cell trait, see *The Clinical Side*, "Sickle Cell Hemoglobin and Malaria."

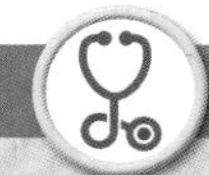

The Clinical Side

SICKLE CELL HEMOGLOBIN AND MALARIA

About 10% of African Americans are carriers of the **hemoglobin** *S* genetic mutation. The prevalence is as high as 30% in some populations of African Americans. The higher rate in Africa appears to be Darwinian: hemoglobin S appears to render carriers resistant to the deadly *falciparum* strain of malaria, which is endemic in the region. The sickle cell defect is a mutation in the gene that codes for beta globin chain, a protein molecule of hemoglobin, which is inherited according to the Mendelian model (the genetic defect and its inheritance is discussed in Chapter 22). Since this is a recessive trait, people who inherit the defective beta globin (causing hemoglobin S) from only one parent and a normal gene from the other parent are healthy carriers of *sickle trait* (genotype *SA*, phenotype *healthy*). But in people who inherit a defective beta globin from both parents, *sickle cell disease* is the result (genotype *SS*, phenotype *sickle cell disease*).

Thalassemias

The **thalassemias** are a group of inherited microcytic (low MCV), hemolytic diseases that tend to occur most commonly in people of Mediterranean and Southeast Asian origin. They are inherited in Mendelian fashion. Prevalence is 0.1% in northern Europe, 1% in Thailand, 3%–8% in India and China, and 16% in Cyprus.

Pathophysiology

The genetic defect impairs synthesis of the alpha or the beta polypeptide chains of the globin protein of hemoglobin. The hemoglobins are molecularly normal fetal (F) or adult (A) hemoglobin—the genetic defect affects the *amount* of hemoglobin synthesized. The defective globin renders RBC membrane fragile and susceptible to hemolysis. RBCs are pale and small because they lack normal amounts of hemoglobin cytoplasm.

Decreased production of beta globin is the cause of **beta thalassemia**. Beta globin synthesis is governed by a single gene and is inherited in Mendelian fashion—heterozygous cases (**beta thalassemia minor**) are mild. Homozygous cases (**beta thalassemia major**) are severe.

In **alpha thalassemia**, the alpha chain of hemoglobin is affected. Two different genes govern alpha synthesis, so the inheritance patterns and disease presentation are more variable and complex than for beta thalassemia.

Signs and Symptoms

Clinical features of alpha and beta thalassemias are similar but vary in severity. The most severe clinical form is *beta thalassemia major*. Many patients die before age 20. It features severe microcytic, hypochromic hemolytic anemia. Red cells have a striking appearance: they look like shooting targets and are called "target cells." Other features include jaundice, massive splenomegaly, hyperactive bone marrow, and bony deformities. The liver and spleen may enlarge as they revert to their fetal capacity to produce blood cells (*myeloid metaplasia* of spleen and liver). Iron overload (*hemochromatosis*) is a major hazard caused by repeated transfusions and increased iron absorption by the gastrointestinal (GI) tract as it accumulates raw material for RBC production. More common and much less severe is *beta thalassemia minor*. Most patients are mildly anemic and asymptomatic.

Alpha thalassemia is less common, but has multiple presentations, which vary from mild, asymptomatic anemia to severe fetal anemia and intrauterine death.

Diagnosis and Treatment

Diagnosis is by detection of hemolytic anemia followed by laboratory study of blood for microcytic, hypochromic RBC and quantitative assay of Hb A and F levels.

Patients with mild thalassemia may need no treatment. Patients with severe disease may need transfusions, but they should be kept to a minimum because chronic iron toxicity (hemochromatosis) is a risk. Iron chelation therapy may be necessary. Splenectomy may be required to mitigate splenic hemolysis. Bone marrow transplant may be effective, but use is limited by clinical difficulties.

Non-Genetic Hemolytic Anemias

Antibodies directed against antigens on the red cell membrane cause **immune hemolytic anemia**. When RBCs become coated by antibodies, they are susceptible to premature removal by the spleen.

The two types of immune hemolytic anemia reflect the two different types of antibodies that may be involved. Antibody activity varies by temperature. **Warm antibodies** (IgG) are most active at normal body temperature. Symptoms of warm antibody hemolysis tend to be due to anemia; mild splenomegaly is common. **Cold antibodies** (IgM) are most active at lower temperatures and are precipitated by exposure to cold air, drinking cold fluid, handwashing with cold water, and so on. Accordingly, symptoms of hemolysis are usually sudden and may be severe: back or leg pain, fever, vomiting and diarrhea, and passage of dark brown urine (hemoglobinuria).

Immune hemolytic anemia often occurs in association with autoimmune disease (especially systemic lupus erythematosus), malignancies of WBCs (lymphoma and leukemia), infectious mononucleosis and *Mycoplasma pneumoniae* pneumonia, and as a reaction to certain drugs that act as haptens, which turn normal red cell protein into nonself antigen that renders red cells subject to immune attack.

Diagnosis is by demonstration of antibody on the surface of RBC or in plasma. Treatment depends on the type of antibody. For warm antibodies: withdrawal of the drug, if drug induced, and corticosteroids. For cold antibodies: avoid cold and provide supportive care.

Mechanical hemolytic anemia is caused by physical shredding of red cells as they pass through mechanical devices, such as artificial heart valves. A similar mechanical effect may occur as red cells squeeze through swollen, inflamed small blood vessels affected by autoimmune disease (*autoimmune vasculitis*) or as red cells pass through blood vessels partially blocked by intravascular blood clotting (*disseminated intravascular coagulation*).

Hemolysis is also a feature of **malaria** (Chapter 4), a parasitic disease that infects red cells. It is caused by four varieties of tiny amoebae smaller than a RBC, the *Plasmodium* species, which are transmitted by mosquitoes from infected to noninfected persons.

Some Anemias Are Due to Insufficient Red Cell Production

Inadequate bone marrow red cell production is another cause of anemia. Most cases are due to nutritional deficiency of essential substances necessary for red cell production—iron, folic acid, or vitamin B_{12}. Low marrow output is also a common complication of severe chronic infections and of kidney failure, which is associated with low erythropoietin production. Other causes include adverse effects of drugs or toxins or destruction and/or replacement of the marrow by scar tissue or malignancy.

Iron Deficiency Anemia

Iron deficiency is the most common nutritional deficiency in the world. Without iron, hemoglobin cannot be synthesized and anemia occurs. Worldwide, iron deficiency anemia is by far the most common anemia.

Etiology

Think of iron deficiency anemia as a symptom, not a disease; there is always some underlying condition. In developed nations, most iron deficiency is due to blood loss. Other less common causes include poor intestinal absorption owing to intestinal disease, or increased need for iron caused by normal growth and development. For example, after about six months of age, infants are at risk for iron deficiency because breast milk contains little iron, and the iron stores built up during fetal life become depleted because growth of new tissue requires iron. Thus, iron-fortified rice cereal is often recommended as a first infant food. Toddlers and older children can also develop iron deficiency, as their rapid growth demands iron for expansion of blood volume and other tissues.

In the United States by far the most common cause is chronic blood loss, though low dietary intake of iron or low intestinal absorption is rarely responsible. The most common causes of chronic blood loss are menstrual abnormalities and GI bleeding. The diagnosis of menstrual loss is usually easy to establish; however, loss from GI bleeding is much more sinister, difficult to document, and often associated with intestinal malignancy, especially carcinoma of the colon. Therefore, it is a good rule to assume that, *until proven otherwise, the cause of iron deficiency anemia in adult men or postmenopausal women is occult (undetected) bleeding from the GI tract*. Often it is an intestinal neoplasm.

In developing nations, the most important cause of iron-deficiency anemia is chronic intestinal bleeding caused by parasitic intestinal worms. Growing children are most affected because they are most often infected and need iron to fuel tissue growth.

Pathophysiology

Iron deficiency hinders the ability of the bone marrow to make hemoglobin. The body is stingy with iron—in males and nonmenstruating females natural losses from shedding skin and cells of the GI tract are on the order of just 0.1% of total body iron per day. Iron balance is maintained largely by intestinal absorption of dietary iron from animal hemoglobin in meat, poultry, and fish. Plant foods provide iron, but it is not as bioavailable. The average Western diet contains more than enough iron for men, but barely enough for menstruating women, who normally have low iron reserves due to iron loss from menstrual bleeding. During pregnancy, iron reserves can fall even further because of the extra demand of providing iron for the fetus.

About 80% of total body iron is in the hemoglobin of red cells; the remaining 20% is stored as **ferritin**, an iron-protein complex found in the bone marrow, liver, spleen, and skeletal muscle. Plasma ferritin levels vary directly with the amount of ferritin stored in bone marrow; therefore, the level of plasma ferritin is a good indicator of the amount of body iron stores. Iron is transported from one place to another bound to a special blood protein, **transferrin**, made by the liver. Total transferrin is measured by testing the ability of transferrin to bind to iron and is expressed as **total iron binding capacity (TIBC)**. The degree to which this *potential* transporting capacity is occupied by *actual* plasma iron is referred to as the "percent *saturation* of TIBC."

In any case, when patients lose or require more iron than they absorb intestinally, iron stores gradually become depleted. Iron stores must be completely exhausted, however, before red cell production is affected. Therefore, patients must become *iron deficient* before they become *anemic*, and they become anemic only if iron deficiency persists. This preanemic stage is characterized by normal levels of plasma iron and transferrin (expressed as total iron binding capacity, TIBC), but low levels of plasma ferritin, reflecting low marrow iron stores. If negative iron balance persists, plasma iron levels fall and the liver increases transferrin (TIBC) levels in an effort to deliver more iron to the bone marrow. Finally, **iron deficiency anemia** develops as red cell production becomes impaired owing to lack of iron. TIBC is high while plasma iron, ferritin, and percent saturation of transferrin by iron are low. The bone marrow, lacking sufficient iron to make hemoglobin, produces RBCs that are small (microcytic, low MCV) and pale (hypochromic, low MCHC), as illustrated in Figure 7.7.

Diagnosis and Treatment

Symptoms are those of any anemia: fatigue, shortness of breath, weakness, dizziness, and pallor. Diagnosis is by finding microcytic, hypochromic anemia and the characteristic iron, ferritin, and transferrin changes described above. Thalassemia also causes microcytic, hypochromic RBC, but in thalassemia the bone marrow pours out fresh RBCs, which can be documented by high reticulocyte count. In contrast, the marrow in iron deficiency anemia makes few new RBCs and the reticulocyte count is low. Oral iron supplementation can rebuild iron stores, but the underlying cause of the iron deficiency must be found and treated.

Remember This! Iron deficiency anemia in a man or in a postmenopausal woman should be considered GI bleeding, most likely from cancer, until proven otherwise.

Megaloblastic Anemia

Anemia associated with deficiency of either vitamin B_{12} (cobalamin) or folic acid is characterized by enlarged (macrocytic) red cells, depicted in Figure 7.8. Together these are known as the **megaloblastic** or **macrocytic anemias**. *Megalo* and *macro* mean large, and in these anemias the red cells and their bone marrow precursors (blasts) are unusually large. Clinically, the two deficiencies are very similar, except for the neurological symptoms that occur in B_{12} deficiency.

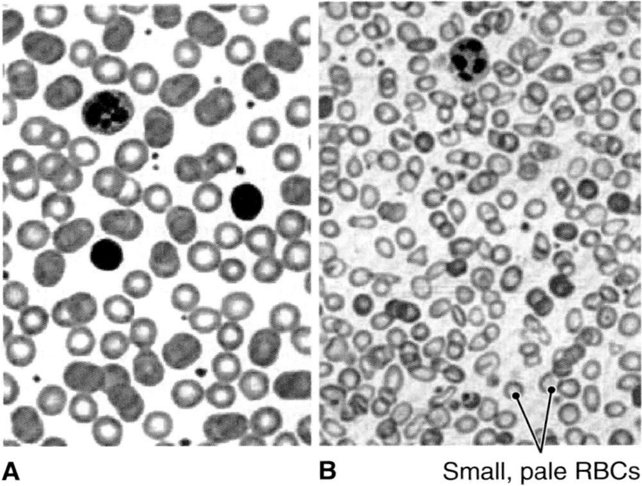

Figure 7.7 **The blood in iron deficiency anemia. A.** Normal blood smear. **B.** Blood smear in iron deficiency anemia. The red cells are small (microcytic) and pale (hypochromic).

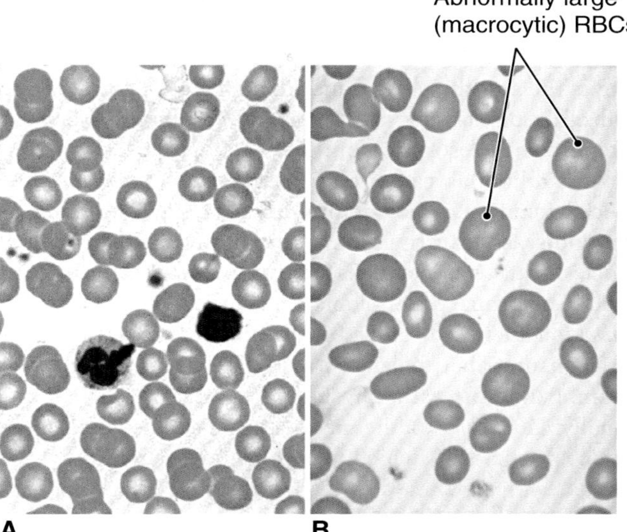

Figure 7.8 **The blood in vitamin B_{12} deficiency. A.** Normal blood smear. **B.** Macrocytic RBCs in a patient with vitamin B_{12} deficiency. Folic acid deficiency also causes red cell macrocytosis.

Pathophysiology

Vitamin B_{12} and folic acid are necessary for DNA synthesis. If DNA cannot be produced, cells cannot be made, hence a deficiency of either B_{12} or folic acid results in decreased production of cells. It is especially notable in bone marrow cells, which have a short lifespan. Though DNA synthesis is impaired, RNA synthesis continues, which results in fewer cells but cells with a large nucleus and abundant cytoplasm. The result is *macrocytic* red cells (high MCV), low WBC count (leukopenia), and low platelet count (thrombocytopenia).

Inadequate diet or deficient intestinal absorption may cause deficiency of either B_{12} or folic acid. Megaloblastic anemia associated with folic acid (folate) deficiency is uncommon because folate is abundant in raw vegetables (it is largely destroyed by cooking) and in folate-supplemented breads and cereals. Nevertheless, depressed folic acid levels may be found in anyone with a poor diet—chronic alcoholics are especially prone to folic acid deficiency. Dietary vitamin B_{12} deficiency is also rare—B_{12} is abundant in meat, poultry, fish, eggs, and dairy products, and multiyear reserves are stored in the liver. It is almost impossible to devise a diet deficient in B_{12} except by observing a strict vegan diet for many years.

The most common cause of B_{12} deficiency is defective intestinal absorption. B_{12} absorption requires **intrinsic factor (IF)**, a protein secreted by the gastric mucosa. IF binds to dietary B_{12} and travels to the lower end of the small bowel (ileum), where absorption occurs. B_{12} cannot be absorbed by the ileum unless it is bound to IF. Causes of insufficient B_{12} absorption include gastrectomy (which limits IF production), surgical resection of the ileum (which removes the absorbing site), and inflammatory bowel disease and other diseases affecting the distal ileum, all of which interfere with absorption of the B_{12}-IF complex.

An additional cause of B_{12} deficiency that deserves special mention is **pernicious anemia (PA)**, an autoimmune disease featuring autoantibodies against the gastric mucosal cells (parietal cells) that produce IF, or against IF itself. The primary pathologic abnormality in PA is *chronic atrophic gastritis*, discussed in detail in Chapter 11. Lack of IF ensures that dietary B_{12} will not be absorbed by the ileum. Before the pathophysiology was discovered, PA was usually fatal due to the neurological effects, hence the name "pernicious," which means evil or deadly.

Signs and Symptoms

Both folate and B_{12} deficiency anemia usually develop very slowly, so slowly that patients may physically and mentally adapt to their condition and not complain (become symptomatic) until the anemia is quite severe.

B_{12} deficiency can lead to neurological damage, which is manifest by peripheral neuropathy, dementia, and a severe neurological syndrome—*subacute combined degeneration*, which includes decreased position sense (proprioception) and vibratory sensation in the extremities accompanied by mild-to-moderate weakness. In later stages, spasticity and ataxia may occur. Touch, pain, and temperature sensations are usually spared.

Clinical features of folate deficiency are those of any anemia and do not affect the nervous system.

Diagnosis and Treatment

In macrocytic anemia, it is especially important to be certain of the cause before beginning treatment. If the patient has B_{12} deficiency but is treated with folate, red cell production will improve, and may leave the impression that the proper diagnosis is folate deficiency. Folate does nothing for the neurological problems, however, which can be managed only with B_{12} therapy.

Diagnostic features of folate or B_{12} deficiency include megaloblastic RBCs, low reticulocyte count, low WBC and platelet count, and low plasma folate or B_{12}. Bone marrow studies in each reveal a hypercellular, active bone marrow filled with enlarged (megaloblastic) red and white cell precursors. The marrow is overly cellular because it is striving ineffectively to produce red and white cells.

Therapy is folate or B_{12} supplementation, sometimes by injection, and treatment of the underlying cause of the deficiency.

Anemia of Chronic Disease

Low output of RBCs by the bone marrow in patients with chronic disease is perhaps the most common of all anemias in the United States. Worldwide, it is second to iron deficiency anemia.

The major issue is that bone marrow mass does not expand appropriately to the anemia. Three pathologic mechanisms appear to be at work.

- RBC survival is shortened.
- Erythropoiesis is impaired.
- Iron reutilization is impaired.

The chronic diseases usually involved are malignant neoplasms, chronic infections, and chronic autoimmune disorders. It appears that inflammatory mediators interfere with the mechanism that transports iron from iron storage into red cell production. Iron stores (ferritin) increase even as red cells starve for iron. These same mediators interfere with erythropoietin production by the kidney.

Symptoms are those of anemia and the underlying disease (cancer, infection, inflammation). Red cells may be normocytic and normochromic or microcytic and hypochromic. Increased bone marrow iron stores and low transferrin are important diagnostic clues that it is not iron deficiency anemia. Treatment of the underlying disorder is supplement by erythropoietin to boost marrow output and iron supplementation to improve iron utilization.

Aplastic Anemia

Primary bone marrow failure is called **aplastic anemia**. The name, however, is a misnomer: the disease is not just a failure to produce RBCs, it is a primary failure of *all* marrow elements—red cells, white cells, and megakaryocytes. Nevertheless, anemia is usually the presenting problem. In fatal cases, the cause of death is usually *hemorrhage*, because of a low platelet count, or *infection,* secondary to a low WBC count. In about half of cases the cause is unclear, although autoimmunity is suspected. When the cause is known, drugs and chemicals are usually responsible because they exert a toxic effect on bone marrow cells. In some cases the toxic effect is dose related, as is the case with chemotherapy drugs given to patients with a malignancy. In others, the reaction is termed *idiosyncratic*; that is, the toxic effect is far out of proportion to the dose. Some cases owe to rare genetic defects, others to disorders of the thymus. **Pure red cell aplasia** is a variant affecting only RBCs and is usually caused by viral infection, especially in children.

In addition to the fatigue and pallor of anemia, most patients have low platelet count (thrombocytopenia) resulting in hemorrhages (skin petechiae and ecchymoses, or internal bleeding) and low WBC counts (granulocytopenia) resulting in bacterial infections. Peripheral blood studies show anemia, low white count, and low platelet count. Bone marrow biopsy reveals a hypocellular bone marrow that is mostly fat, with few hematopoietic cells

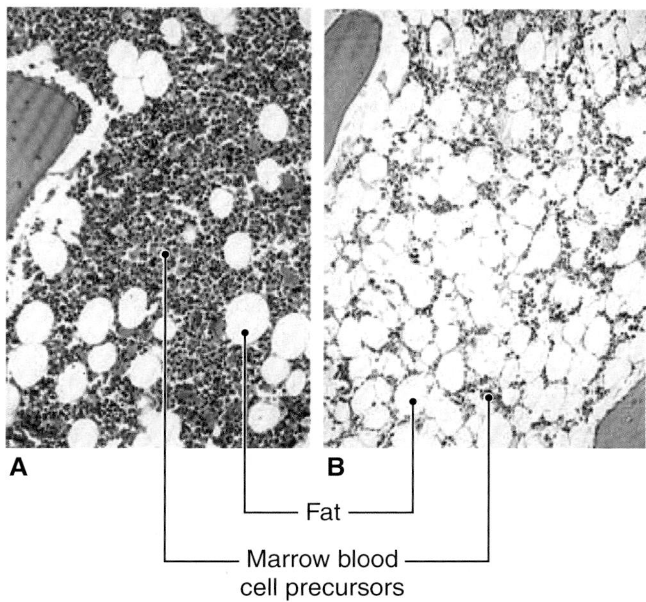

Figure 7.9 **Bone marrow in aplastic anemia. A.** Normal bone marrow. **B.** Bone marrow in aplastic anemia. Few bone marrow cells are present. Most of the tissue is fat.

(Fig. 7.9). Treatment depends on the cause. For most patients the treatment of choice is equine (horse) antithymocyte globulin, which is effective in more than half of patients. Bone marrow transplant, steroids, and other therapies may also be useful.

Case Notes

7.10 How does Eleanor's case differ from aplastic anemia?

Myelophthisic Anemia

Myelophthisis (Latin *phthinein* = to decay) is replacement of the marrow by malignancy or fibrosis. *Primary* myelophthisic anemia is marrow fibrosis of unknown cause and is rare. Marrow fibrosis may be a feature of sarcoidosis, tuberculosis, or other inflammatory or infectious diseases. The marrow may be displaced in some genetic lipid-storage diseases such as Gaucher disease. The most common cause, however, is marrow displacement by metastatic cancer, most commonly breast and prostate. Radiation, lymphoma, leukemia, and multiple myeloma may have a similar displacement effect. Bone marrow fibrosis is also the end stage of some bone marrow malignancies, especially those that comprise the *chronic myeloproliferative syndromes* discussed later in this chapter.

As the marrow fails, the spleen and liver enlarge as they revert to their fetal capacity to produce blood cells (*extramedullary hematopoiesis* or *myeloid metaplasia*). Red cells produced by extramedullary hematopoiesis are misshapen, and many of them still contain their nuclei. White cells are not deformed but are often released early in their life cycle, so that immature forms may outnumber mature cells.

Signs and symptoms are those of anemia, often accompanied by hepatosplenomegaly. Diagnosis is suggested by CBC showing normochromic, normocytic anemia; nucleated RBCs and immature WBCs. Other findings depend on the underlying cause. Confirmation requires bone marrow biopsy. Treatment begins with attention to the underlying disorder. Transfusions and corticosteroids may also be employed. For primary myelofibrosis no effective treatment exists.

Case Notes

7.11 In microscopic examination of her peripheral blood what are clues in Eleanor's red and white cells that her marrow is failing?

Pop Quiz

7.9 True or false? In sickle cell anemia, defective hemoglobin causes cells to sickle, clogging capillaries and impairing blood flow.

7.10 True or false? IF is secreted by the gastric mucosa.

7.11 True or false? Aplastic anemia causes death by hemorrhage or infection.

7.12 In iron deficiency anemia, what happens to *ferritin, iron, transferrin, and iron binding capacity?*

7.13 Defective hemoglobin synthesis is a characteristic of what type of disease?

7.14 A patient's RBCs are seen to lyse when placed in hypotonic saline. What hereditary deficiency might you diagnose him with?

7.15 Iron deficiency anemia in older adults indicates what disease process until proven otherwise?

7.16 A patient has surgical removal of part of his colon because of ulcerative colitis. Is he expected to have PA after the surgery?

Polycythemia

Polycythemia (**erythrocytosis**) is an excess number of red cells in blood. The most common cause of *apparent* polycythemia is **relative polycythemia**, which is caused by low plasma volume. For example, in dehydration, loss of fluid causes concentration of RBCs, but the *absolute* number of red cells is unaffected. Among the most common causes of relative polycythemia is a poorly understood condition called *stress polycythemia*, which is usually seen in overweight, anxious (stressed), or hypertensive patients. For reasons that are not well understood, these patients have low plasma volume. There are no pathologic consequences that owe to mere low plasma volume, though patients may suffer directly from the associated stress and hypertension.

Other patients have an increased red cell count because there is an *actual* increase in the total number of RBCs in the body; these patients have **absolute polycythemia**. Absolute polycythemia can be primary or secondary.

Secondary absolute polycythemia is caused by conditions outside the bone marrow that stimulate the marrow to produce red cells. For example, chronic hypoxia, as in chronic lung disease, stimulates the kidney to produce erythropoietin, which increases red cell production. For the same reason, people living at high altitudes have secondary polycythemia as compared to those living at lower altitudes. Secondary polycythemia can also be caused by renal tumors that secrete erythropoietin, or as a paraneoplastic syndrome caused by tumors of other organs. Other causes are congenital heart diseases with right-to-left shunting of blood so that it does not pass through the lungs and vascular malformations with venoarterial shunting.

Primary absolute polycythemia occurs with a bone marrow malignancy called **polycythemia vera (PV)** (literally, true polycythemia), a proliferation of primitive bone marrow red cell precursors that is related to certain leukemias and related neoplasms collectively discussed below as one of the *myeloproliferative syndromes*.

Most of the time an abnormally high red cell count is accompanied by increased hematocrit and hemoglobin and can be explained by conditions other than PV. For example, patients who smoke more than just an occasional cigarette damage their lungs enough to reduce oxygen uptake, which stimulates red cell production and a secondary increase of RBCs.

Apart from PV, which has distinctive signs and symptoms, symptoms are those of the underlying disorder. The main sign is plethora—a florid, red face. Laboratory RBC count, hematocrit, and hemoglobin are correspondingly increased. Determining whether or not patients have an absolute or relative increase of red cells can be very difficult because red cell count in *peripheral* blood is significantly higher than the relatively dilute *central* pool of blood in viscera and large blood vessels. Laboratory determination of total body RBC mass is required to make the distinction. Treatment is for the underlying disorder.

Pop Quiz

7.17 True or false? Dehydration causes a relative polycythemia.

7.18 True or false? Patients with stress polycythemia have an increase in the absolute red cell mass.

7.19 Low erythropoietin in a setting of elevated RBC count is consistent with a diagnosis of ______________.

Leukopenia, Leukocytosis, and Lymphadenopathy

Increase or decrease in the number of leukocytes in blood and lymph nodes can be due to infection, immune reaction, or malignancy. Here we discuss nonmalignant changes.

Leukopenia Is Low White Cell Count

Leukopenia is a WBC count of <4,000/μl. It is usually caused by decreased numbers of granulocytes, especially neutrophils, a condition called **granulocytopenia** or **neutropenia**. Low numbers of lymphocytes (**lymphopenia**) is uncommon and is usually associated with steroid therapy or immunodeficiencies such as AIDS.

Neutropenia may result from accelerated destruction of neutrophils or from a failure of production. Among the causes of increased destruction are increased filtering of neutrophils from blood by an enlarged spleen (hypersplenism), autoimmune disease, and overwhelming sepsis, which uses up the supply of neutrophils faster than they can be produced. Bone marrow white cell production failure can be caused by cancer chemotherapy, radiation, or environmental toxins; by replacement of marrow by tumor or fibrosis; by B_{12} or folate deficiency; or by adverse reaction to therapeutic drugs.

When neutropenia is severe (<500/μl) it is called **agranulocytosis**. Most agranulocytosis is caused by therapeutic drug toxicity. In most instances the degree of white cell decline is *dose related*, and the drugs are those administered as cancer chemotherapy. Many drugs, however, are known to cause a rare, *idiosyncratic* (not dose related) agranulocytosis. The major clinical problem resulting from agranulocytosis is bacterial or fungal infection. Treatment depends on cause. The underlying condition should be treated if it can be identified. For example, splenectomy may be necessary if the cause is hypersplenism.

Antibiotic prophylaxis may be necessary to prevent infection and existing infection should be treated vigorously. In some cases, myeloid growth factors may be administered.

Leukocytosis Is High White Cell Count

Leukocytosis is an increase in WBCs. It may be benign (reactive) or malignant (leukemia). Most leukocytosis is secondary (reactive), and is the result of bacterial infection or inflammation associated with tissue necrosis.

The most common form of leukocytosis is **granulocytosis**—increased numbers of granulocytes (neutrophils, eosinophils, basophils). In virtually every case it is due to increased numbers of neutrophils (**neutrophilia**). The normal WBC count is usually <10,000/µl. In most instances of infection, the WBC count does not rise above 20,000/µl. Sometimes, however, very high reactive white counts occur that may appear alarming, especially in uncommon cases when the count rises to over 50,000/µl. Such a high reactive WBC count is termed **leukemoid reaction** (literally, "like leukemia"). Sometimes bacterial infection or other injury causes such demand for neutrophils from the bone marrow that an excess number of immature granulocytes are released into blood. Normally, the least mature WBC found in the peripheral blood is the **band neutrophil** (Fig. 7.2), a WBC with a banana-shaped nucleus that normally accounts for <5% of WBC count. An increased number of band neutrophils is referred to clinically as a "left shift." This owes to the fact that the maturation sequence of WBC is typically depicted in left to right fashion (Fig. 7.2) and band cells are one step to the left of mature neutrophils. Increased numbers of bands usually indicate bacterial infection, but sometimes it occurs in conjunction with blood cell malignancies, which typically release increased numbers of immature cells into blood.

Viral infection usually causes **lymphocytosis**, an increase in the number of lymphocytes in blood. *Eosinophilic* leukocytosis is uncommon and when present is almost always associated with *allergic* reactions or *parasitic* infection.

Case Notes

7.12 Study Eleanor's initial lab report. Which of the boldfaced terms above are present?

Lymphadenopathy and Lymphadenitis Are Conditions of Lymph Nodes

Lymph nodes are involved in the most common diseases: infection, malignancy, immune reactions, and autoimmune disease. The lymphatic system (Chapter 3) filters bacteria, cancer cells, and other alien substances from tissues. Lymph node lymphocytes are involved in immune reactions, and most lymphomas arise in lymph nodes. Therefore, most lymph nodes involved in a disease process are enlarged, a condition termed **lymphadenopathy**. In the absence of apparent infection or injury, enlarged lymph nodes are worrisome and deserve investigation, primarily because they may contain malignant cells. *Chronic nonspecific lymphadenopathy* is usually caused by prolonged antigenic stimulation. The nodes enlarge slowly and are usually not tender. Inguinal nodes are most often involved because the genitalia are often the site of infection and inflammation.

Lymphadenitis is a benign inflammatory change in lymph nodes. It may be due to infection of the node, but much more often is a reactive change caused by antigens and inflammatory mediators draining into the node from a nearby infection. *Acute nonspecific lymphadenitis* is characterized by enlarged, *tender* nodes and is usually seen in cervical (neck) nodes in association with dental infections or sore throat. When occurring in the axillae or inguinal regions, the culprit is usually genital infection or infections of the distal arm or leg. Systemic viral infections in children may produce generalized acute nonspecific lymphadenitis. Painful acute lymphadenitis may also occur in the intestinal mesentery and mimic acute appendicitis.

Pop Quiz

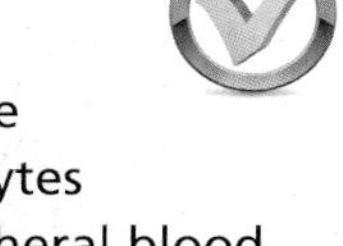

7.20 True or false? A left shift is the release of immature granulocytes from bone marrow into peripheral blood, and occurs only during an acute infection.

7.21 What are the two types of agranulocytosis?

7.22 If there is no infection, enlarged lymph nodes are worrisome for ________________.

Overview of Malignancies of White Blood Cells

Some general themes underlie the etiology and pathogenesis of WBC malignancies:

- Various types of acquired mutations cause most of them.
- Some are caused by inherited genetic defects.
- Normal cell maturation (Fig. 7.2) is blocked and immature cells accumulate.
- Chronic immune stimulation plays a role in the mutations occurring in some neoplasms of lymphocytes.
- Viruses play a role in the pathogenesis of some lymphocyte neoplasms.

- Cancer radiation and chemotherapy can, paradoxically, increase the risk of developing one of these malignancies.

The key to understanding any malignancy is to know the progenitor cell from which it arose. For WBC malignancies, the malignant cell represents the transformation of a normal, benign cell from a particular stage in the maturation of the cell line: some malignant cells arise from progenitor cells, others from various stages of more mature cells (Fig. 7.2).

- **Myeloid malignancies** arise from myeloid cells: the precursors of granulocytes, RBCs, and megakaryocytes.
- **Lymphoid malignancies** arise from lymphoid cells: B lymphocytes (including plasma cells), T lymphocytes, or natural killer (NK) lymphocytes.

Remember This! There are only two varieties of WBC malignancies: lymphoid and myeloid.

Apart from this basic distinction, WBC malignancies traditionally have been divided into two large groups, leukemia and lymphoma, based on their clinical and pathologic presentation and behavior. **Leukemia** is a malignancy of myeloid or lymphoid cells in which malignant cells are widespread in blood and bone marrow. It is characterized by the following:

- Widespread infiltration of the bone marrow by malignant cells (Fig. 7.10).
- Malignant cells in blood. Usually many malignant cells are present, but sometimes the total WBC count is normal or low.
- Proliferation of a clone of malignant cells with a characteristic genetic defect for each type of leukemia.

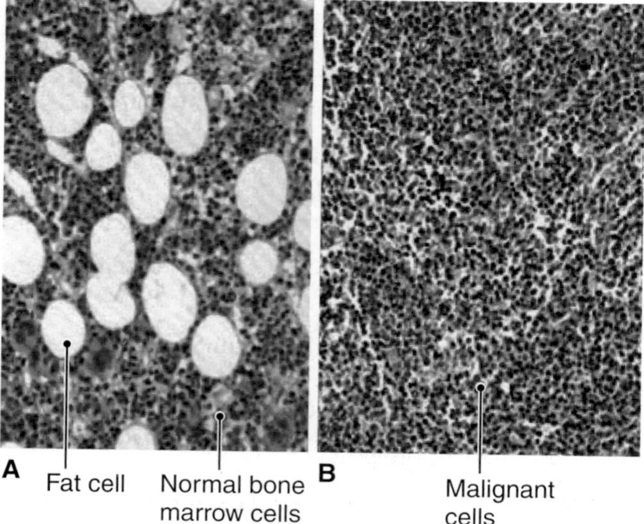

Figure 7.10 **The bone marrow in leukemia. A.** Normal bone marrow. **B.** The marrow in leukemia. The marrow is packed with cells of a single type. No fat remains.

- Complications that include anemia, infection, and hemorrhage owing to the fact that dysfunctional malignant cells replace normal red cells, white cells, and megakaryocytes. Overwhelming infection is the usual cause of death.

Acute leukemia features abrupt onset—it often presents as acute infection or hemorrhage. Symptoms are related to a decrease in the numbers and functionality of normal marrow cells, such as might be seen in anemia, infection, or bleeding from thrombocytopenia. Bone pain and tenderness occur as bone marrow becomes packed with malignant cells. Lymph nodes, spleen, and liver enlarge as malignant cells infiltrate them. Nervous system symptoms such as headache, vomiting, or nerve palsies occur if malignant cells infiltrate the meninges. WBC counts often are very high—sometimes >100,000 cells/µl—but about half the cases have total WBC counts near normal. It is the microscopic appearance of the cells in bone marrow and peripheral blood that is diagnostic—both contain many immature WBCs (blasts).

Chronic leukemia is insidious—patients present with fatigue or pallor from anemia, night sweats, low-grade fever, secondary infection, or enlarged spleen or liver. The clinical course is less rocky and the prognosis is better than for acute leukemia, although ultimately the cause of death is similar in both acute and chronic leukemia: hemorrhage as a result of low platelet count, or infection because leukemic WBCs are not effective at fighting infection.

By contrast, **lymphoma** is a malignancy of *lymphoid* cells that grows as discrete masses in lymph nodes or organs and is not easily described as acute or chronic. Myeloid proliferative malignancies that grow as masses are rare and are termed "myeloid sarcomas" or "chloromas."

Case Notes

7.13 Does Eleanor have a lymphoid cell or a myeloid cell disease?

It is critical to realize, however, that these distinctions are often not as sharp as this scheme suggests. For example, some myeloid malignancies do not neatly fit into the leukemia category, and some lymphomas may spread in a leukemic manner. This simple way of classification has been greatly complicated by modern science. Malignancies are now classified based on cell type as determined by various antigenic markers (CD antigens and others) on the cell membrane and on the genetic or chromosomal defects responsible. More than 20 types of malignant WBCs can be identified based on their CD antigen type, and there are at least 15 major types of chromosomal defect. These categories and others are combined to characterize each type of malignancy. The World Health Organization (WHO) recognizes 31 varieties of neoplasms of lymphoid cells and nearly as many myeloid ones. In the interest of simplicity, we will follow the simpler, traditional path, which offers a sound basis for further learning.

Pop Quiz

7.23 True or false? Acute leukemia often presents as infection or hemorrhage.

7.24 True or false? Plasma cell proliferations are a myeloid neoplasm.

7.25 True or false? Lymphomas and leukemias are categorized by the WHO based on cell types and not on genetic defects.

7.26 What are the two major groups of bone marrow malignancy?

7.27 What is the difference between leukemia and lymphoma?

Myeloid Malignancies

Myeloid malignancies (Fig. 7.11) are leukemias and related disorders that arise from myeloid progenitor cells, which in normal hematopoiesis develop into normal bone marrow and blood cells. The myeloid malignancies are **acute** and **chronic myeloid leukemia (CML)**, the **myelodysplastic syndromes**, and the **myeloproliferative syndromes**. The latter two groups of myeloid malignancies have distinctive characteristics and may evolve into leukemia or bone marrow fibrosis.

Acute Myeloid Leukemia Is Rapidly Progressive

Acute myeloid (myelogenous) leukemia (AML) (Fig. 7.12) is a variable family (16 WHO varieties) of acute leukemias characterized by increased numbers of myeloblasts in bone marrow and blood. Malignant cells crowd out normal bone marrow, and granulocytes, red cells, and megakaryocytes fail to develop. It may arise *de novo* or may evolve from one of the myelodysplastic or myeloproliferative syndromes discussed below. AML accounts for 70% of acute leukemias. It occurs at all ages, but is most common in adults over 50 years of age. Cigarette smoking is a risk factor.

Onset is typically sudden, and symptoms of marrow failure appear rapidly as the bone marrow becomes packed with malignant cells. Red cell, granulocyte, and platelet counts fall, and anemia, infection, and hemorrhage occur. Symptoms include bone pain, lymphadenopathy, enlarged spleen and liver, and neurologic defects from leukemic infiltrates in the brain and peripheral nerves.

Diagnosis requires that >20% of bone marrow cells must be myeloblasts. Chemotherapy induces remission in a majority of patients, but only about 25% remain disease free for five years. Nevertheless, AML arising from myelodysplasia or myeloproliferative syndrome is usually a final and quickly lethal development. Without treatment most patients die within six months.

Chronic Myeloid Leukemia Is Slowly Progressive

Chronic myeloid (myelogenous) leukemia (CML) is the chronic counterpart of AML. It is rare in children, but prevalence increases with each decade. It is often classified as one of the chronic myeloproliferative syndromes discussed below. A very important aspect of CML is its molecular pathogenesis, which features a unique acquired reciprocal translocation of genes between chromosomes 9 and 22, a combination that produces an abnormally small chromosome 22 and a very large chromosome 9. The small 22 is called the **Philadelphia chromosome** after the city of its discovery. It is present in 95% of cases. Demonstration of its presence is diagnostic. It renders CML especially vulnerable to chemotherapy. One of the genes is a proto-oncogene that produces *tyrosine kinase*, which when fused to the other gene becomes permanently active, initiating the production of excess numbers of immature granulocytes. Chemotherapy blocks the activity of tyrosine kinase.

Disease progression is slower than AML and tends to evolve through three phases. First is an indolent period that may last about three years even in untreated patients. Incidental discovery of leukocytosis, anemia, or an enlarged spleen may be the first diagnostic clue. Second is an accelerated phase in which it becomes resistant to treatment, and anemia and thrombocytopenia become worse. The third and terminal phase is quick evolution into AML or an acute variant of lymphoid leukemia. Infection and hemorrhage are the most dangerous threats.

In contrast to AML, many of the malignant cells are mature neutrophils, but some eosinophils and basophils are usually present. WBC counts tend to be very high, sometimes >100,000 cells/μl. RBC precursors and megakaryocytes proliferate to a lesser degree—*nucleated* RBCs may be found in the peripheral blood, and platelet counts may be high (*thrombocytosis*). Therapy with imatinib (Gleevec®) is very effective: >90% of treated patients survive five years. Therapy greatly reduces the number of malignant cells, and reduces the risk of transformation into acute leukemia, though it is not yet clear if a permanent cure occurs, and patients must continue taking the medication for the duration of their lives.

Myelodysplasia Is a Preleukemia Syndrome

Myelodysplasia syndrome (MDS) is a group of hematopoietic progenitor cell disorders that feature ineffective myeloid cell maturation, defective hematopoiesis, and

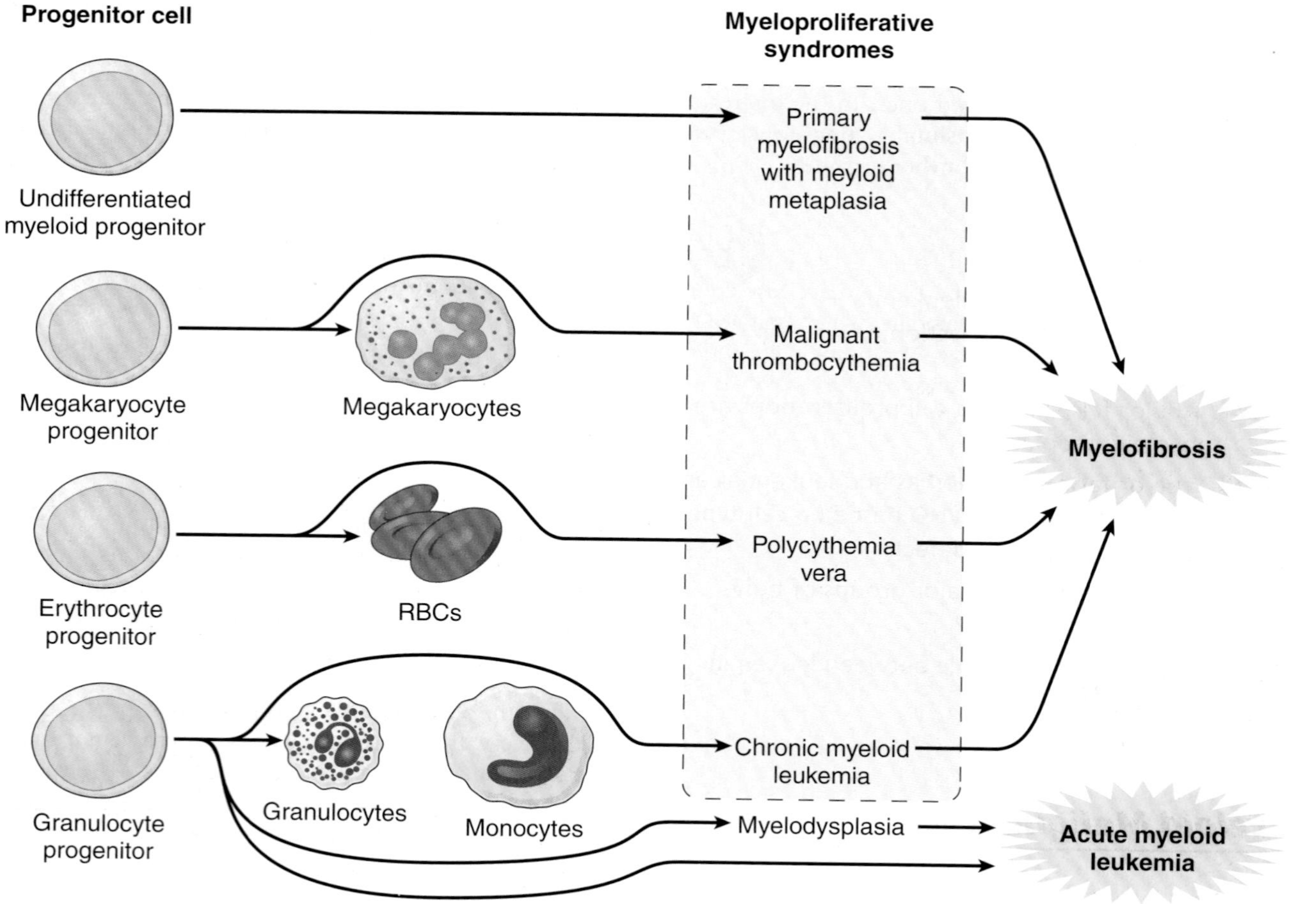

Progenitor cell
Myeloproliferative syndromes
Undifferentiated myeloid progenitor
Primary myelofibrosis with meyloid metaplasia
Megakaryocyte progenitor
Megakaryocytes
Malignant thrombocythemia
Myelofibrosis
Erythrocyte progenitor
RBCs
Polycythemia vera
Granulocyte progenitor
Granulocytes
Monocytes
Chronic myeloid leukemia
Myelodysplasia
Acute myeloid leukemia

Figure 7.11 **The origin of bone myeloid malignancies.** Each malignancy derives from a particular type of myeloid progenitor cell.

A
B
Neutrophil
Lymphocyte
Malignant myeloblasts

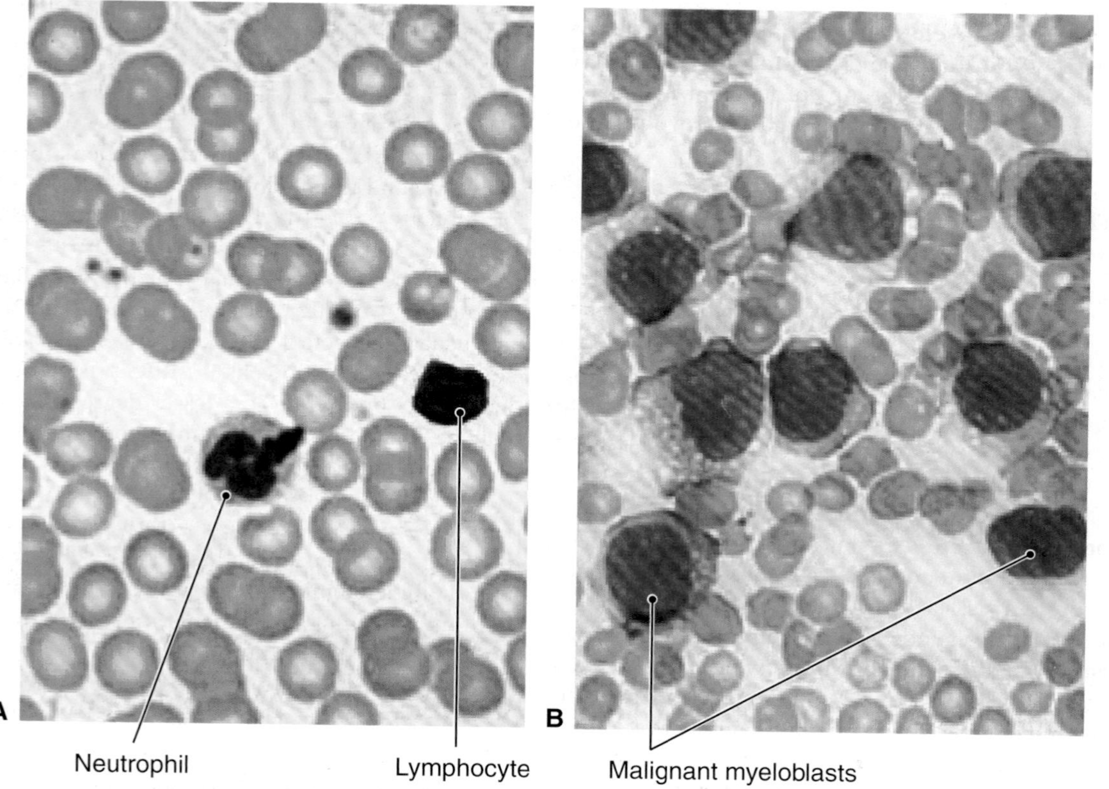

Figure 7.12 **Acute myeloid (myelogenous) leukemia. A.** Normal blood showing neutrophil and lymphocyte. **B.** AML showing immature myeloid cells (malignant myeloblasts).

increased risk for development of AML. MDS is also referred to as *preleukemia* or *smoldering leukemia*; both terms convey a correct sense of the disease. Some cases occur spontaneously, others six to eight years after chemotherapy or radiation. The bone marrow is partly occupied by dysplastic progenitor cells that can multiply but do not develop into mature, functional cells. Patients tend to have low counts of one or more of the formed elements, which may lead to infection, anemia, or hemorrhage. Microscopic changes in the bone marrow can be subtle and diagnosis may depend on genetic analysis. Chemotherapy may be helpful.

Myeloproliferative Syndromes Are Related Myeloid Malignancies

As is illustrated in Figure 7.10, the **chronic myeloproliferative syndromes** are related neoplastic diseases. All arise from myeloid progenitor cells and can be considered one condition with various expressions. Several mutations are responsible, and all activate a related set of enzymes that circumvent cell growth control mechanisms. They share the following common tendencies:

- *Neoplasia* of marrow cells
- *Extramedullary hematopoiesis* in the liver and spleen due to spread of primitive myeloid cells. (Clinical features of extramedullary hematopoiesis include deformed, nucleated red cells in peripheral blood and hepatosplenomegaly. The spleen is sometimes gigantic.)
- *Progression* into a final, fatal phase featuring either marrow fibrosis (myelofibrosis, myelophthisis) or acute leukemia

Four disorders are recognized according to the manner in which the progenitor cells differentiate. There is considerable overlap among them.

- *Chronic myeloid (myelogenous) leukemia*—malignant granulocytes predominate
- *Polycythemia vera*—malignant red cells predominate
- *Malignant (essential) thrombocythemia*—malignant megakaryocytes predominate
- *Primary myelofibrosis with extramedullary hematopoiesis*—marrow cells are displaced by nonmalignant fibrous tissue; neoplastic myelocytes populate the liver and spleen

Polycythemia Vera

Polycythemia vera (PV) is a rare condition, but the most common of the myeloproliferative disorders. It occurs almost exclusively in adults. Incidence increases with age. It owes to malignant transformation of red cell progenitor cells caused by a specific mutation (in another kinase) in a majority of cases. Rarely, some cases may evolve into acute leukemia or myelofibrosis. There is an absolute increase of total red cell mass, and hematocrit is usually above 60% with corresponding increased RBC counts and hemoglobin levels. The WBC and platelet counts are often high as well. Clinical features include a tendency to develop deep vein thrombophlebitis and stroke, hepatosplenomegaly, gout caused by uric acid metabolized from the DNA of malignant cells, hypertension because of expanded intravascular volume, intense pruritus (itching) of unknown cause, and a flushed complexion. Blood erythropoietin is low. Conclusive diagnosis requires determination of total red cell mass and sequencing for the mutation. Treatment is phlebotomy and aspirin to prevent thromboses. Chemotherapy tends to promote PV into AML and is usually avoided. Median survival is about 10 years.

Malignant Thrombocythemia

Malignant thrombocythemia (*essential thrombocythemia*) is a rare myeloproliferative syndrome that occurs when malignant progenitor cells develop toward megakaryocytes. Platelet count is high, but high platelet counts are common in all chronic myeloproliferative syndromes, so the diagnosis is one of exclusion of leukemia, polycythemia, and myelofibrosis. This myeloproliferative disorder often shares the same mutation as PV. Thrombosis and hemorrhage are the most common clinical problems. It is a sluggish disorder with periods of quiet; average survival is about 10–15 years. Low-level chemotherapy is helpful.

Primary Myelofibrosis

Primary myelofibrosis (Fig. 7.13) is a malignant disease of myeloid cells that stimulates *nonmalignant* obliteration of normal bone marrow by fibrous tissue (*myelophthisis*). This type of marrow fibrosis may also occur as a final, fatal phase of one of the other myeloproliferative syndromes. The bone marrow contains a few immature, malignant myeloid cells,

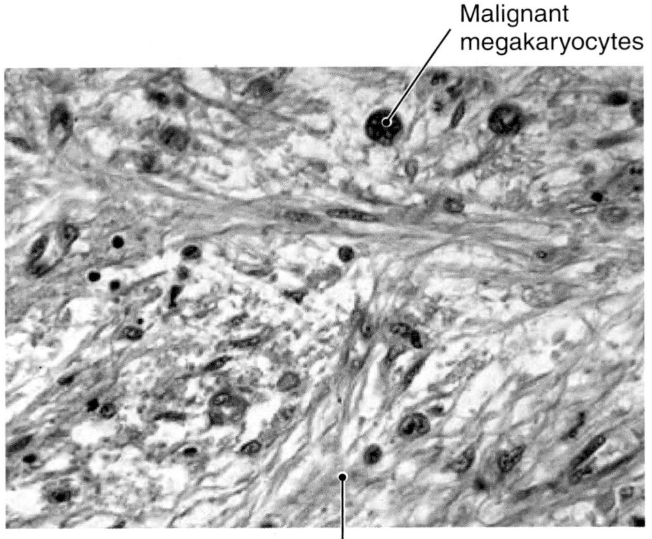

Figure 7.13 **Myelofibrosis.** This high-power microscopic view reveals that the marrow is completely replaced by malignant fibrous tissue. No normal marrow elements remain.

which stimulate scar-like proliferation of fibrous tissue that replaces normal marrow. Some malignant cells are present in blood though not nearly so many as in myeloid leukemia. Most of the malignant cells are in the liver and spleen, which rekindle their fetal capacity as hematopoietic organs (*neoplastic extramedullary hematopoiesis*; or *myeloid metaplasia*). Hepatosplenomegaly and nucleated red cells are the result. As extramedullary hematopoiesis is not nearly as effective as normal hematopoiesis, however, patients present with severe anemia, thrombocytopenia, and leukopenia. Chemotherapy is not effective, and median survival is about five years.

Case Notes

7.14 Does Eleanor have a chronic myeloproliferative disease?

7.15 Why are Eleanor's liver and spleen enlarged?

Pop Quiz

7.28 True or false? More than 90% of CML patients survive after treatment.

7.29 True or false? Extramedullary hematopoiesis causes deformation of RBCs.

7.30 A patient presents to the clinic complaining of shortness of breath, nosebleeds, and recurrent sinus infections. His WBC count is >100,000 and a genetic study reveals the 9;22 translocation. What is the treatment of choice?

7.31 Name the myeloproliferative disorders and the cell precursor they affect.

7.32 AML accounts for ______________% of acute leukemias.

7.33 What symptoms commonly characterize leukemias and myelodysplastic syndromes?

7.34 Which malignancy leads to too many RBCs? Platelets?

Lymphoid Malignancies

Recall from the overview above that we said that lymphoid malignancies could be divided into leukemias and lymphomas. Generally, "leukemia" is used for neoplasms that present with widespread involvement of the bone marrow and peripheral blood and usually present with symptoms of bone marrow suppression: anemia, infection, or bleeding. "Lymphoma" is used for neoplasms that arise as discrete masses in lymph nodes, organs, or tissues. Nevertheless, molecular diagnosis and cell typing—B cells, T cells, and subtypes—is blurring these simple distinctions. Most cell types usually behave in a predictable fashion: this one usually behaves as a lymphoma, that one as leukemia. Sometimes, however, tumor behavior does not follow the rules—a cell type that usually behaves as leukemia will behave as a lymphoma, and some tumors that present initially as lymphomas will later evolve into leukemia.

Figure 7.14 presents a simplified scheme of the development of lymphoid neoplasms. Recall from Chapter 3 that B cells mature in the bone marrow and T cells mature in the thymus. From there, B and T cells populate lymph nodes and other lymphoid organs. Mutations may transform B or T cells into malignancy at any stage of their development. Malignant transformation of bone marrow B or T cells usually behaves as leukemia. Malignant transformation of B or T cells in lymph nodes or other organs usually behaves as lymphoma. Plasma cell neoplasms are a distinctive subset of B cell neoplasia. Most arise as bone marrow masses and present with bone pain or pathologic fracture.

About 90% of lymphoid neoplasms are of B cells. Despite cell typing and other diagnostic advances, pathologic study of biopsy material is mandatory for diagnosis of lymphoid neoplasms.

Case Notes

7.16 Why is Eleanor's disease not classified as a lymphoma?

Lymphoid Leukemia Features Malignant Lymphocytes in Blood

As we did with myeloid leukemia, we divide lymphoid leukemia into acute and chronic types.

Acute Lymphoid Leukemia

Acute lymphoid (lymphoblastic) leukemia (ALL) is a malignant proliferation of immature lymphocyte precursors, usually B cells, and is the most common malignancy of children (though uncommon among all leukemias). Although ALL differs greatly from AML in cell type and genetic defects, clinically the two are similar. Both feature accumulation of immature blasts in bone marrow that crowd out normal hematopoiesis. Onset is typically near age three to four years and is abrupt. It is accompanied by widespread malignant cell infiltration of bones, lymph nodes, liver, spleen, and meninges, resulting in bone

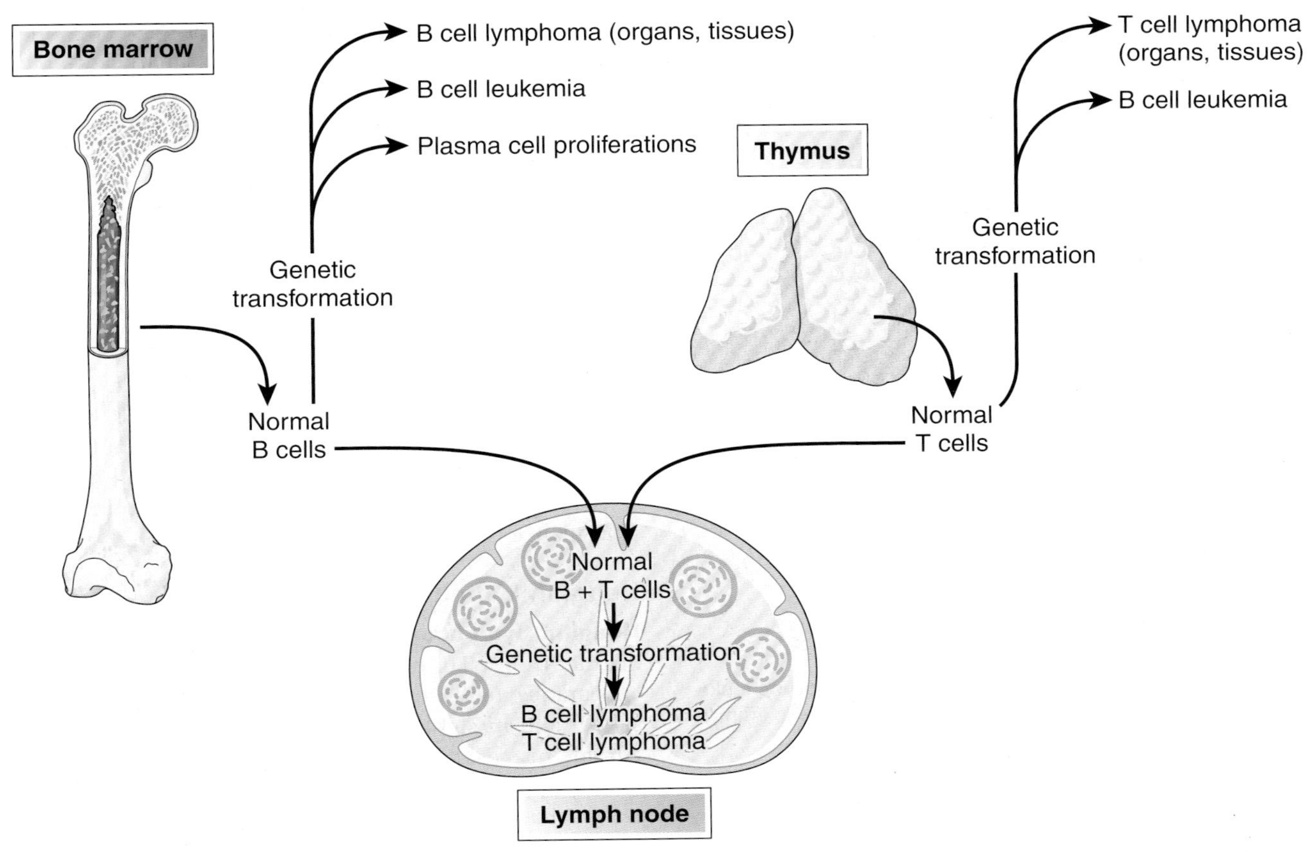

Figure 7.14 **The development of lymphoid malignancies.**

pain, lymphadenopathy, hepatosplenomegaly, headache, nerve paralysis, and pain. Malignant cells overrun blood and bone marrow; red cell, granulocyte, and platelet counts fall; and anemia, infection, and hemorrhage follow. Among children, chemotherapy induces remission in 95% of patients, and about 75% are ultimately cured. Nevertheless, ALL remains the leading cause of cancer death in children. Among adults younger than 60, chemotherapy allows about one in three to survive five years. Among older patients only about 10% survive five years.

Chronic Lymphoid Leukemia

Chronic lymphoid (lymphocytic) leukemia (CLL) and **small-cell lymphocytic lymphoma (SLL)** are different expressions of the same disease and are often referred to as CLL/SLL. The only difference is the number of lymphocytes in blood: few in SLL (an uncommon lymphoma discussed below) and many in CLL. CLL is a malignant proliferation of mature B cells that accounts for about one-third of all leukemias, and is therefore the most common leukemia in the Western world.

The onset of CLL is slow; most patients are asymptomatic and the disease is discovered incidentally in the course of a medical visit for another condition. When symptoms appear, they are constitutional: malaise, mild fever, minimal lymphadenopathy, weight loss, and loss of appetite. As malignant B cells proliferate, normal B cells are in short supply. Because B cells produce immunoglobulins (antibodies) to fight infection, patients are predisposed to developing infections.

For a diagnosis of CLL, the blood lymphocyte count must be >4000/μl. The total WBC count is highly variable, from > 20,000/μl to leukopenia if malignant cells have overrun the bone marrow. As malignant cells multiply in the blood (Fig. 7.15), lymph nodes, and spleen, they cause lymphocytosis, lymphadenopathy, and splenomegaly. Diagnosis is by examination of peripheral smear and bone marrow aspirate.

Though CLL is a progressive disease, patients discovered early may live for 20 years without treatment. Overall survival, however, is about 10 years. Approximately 25% of patients progress to ALL or an aggressive lymphoma. Treatment should be delayed until symptoms appear. Chemotherapy, steroids, immune therapy, and radiation are effective depending on disease presentation and progression.

Lymphomas Do Not Feature Malignant Lymphocytes in Blood

Recall that lymphomas are malignant neoplasms of lymphocytes that grow as nodular masses, usually in lymph nodes (Fig. 7.16) but sometimes in organs. In contrast

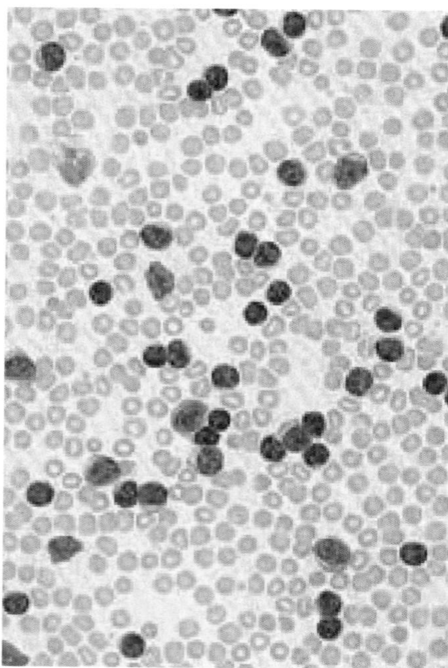

Figure 7.15 **The peripheral blood in chronic lymphocytic leukemia.** In this smear, all of the white cells are lymphocytes. No granulocytes are present.

to leukemia, in most lymphomas malignant cells are not detectable in blood.

There are two broad types of lymphoma: Hodgkin lymphoma (HL), and all others, which are designated non-Hodgkin lymphomas (NHL). HL is separated from all others because of its distinctive features and behavior. Another distinctive group of lymphoid tumors is the plasma cell neoplasms, which arise in bone marrow and rarely involve lymph nodes or peripheral blood.

Modern classification of lymphomas is exceedingly complex because of the use of molecular markers to identify cell types and subtypes, and is beyond the scope of this textbook. Nevertheless, certain simple principles are worth noting:

- According to cell type there are three basic groups: tumors of B cells, tumors of T cells, and tumors of Reed-Sternberg cells, the malignant cell of HL.
- Despite clinical and molecular features, biopsy is required for diagnosis.
- About 90% of NHL are of B cell origin.
- Malignant lymphocytes proliferate at the expense of normal lymphocytes and normal immune function: lymphomas are often associated with immune problems including infection, autoimmunity, and increased risk for other malignancies due to loss of immune surveillance (Chapter 3).

Hodgkin Lymphoma

Hodgkin lymphoma (HL) is a group of lymphomas distinct from NHL because it has distinctive microscopic appearance, tends to arise in a single lymph node, spreads slowly and in steplike fashion to adjacent nodes, and is curable in most instances. It is the most common malignant neoplasm of Americans between ages 10 and 30. It often originates in the lymph nodes of the chest or neck and usually presents as cervical lymphadenopathy (Fig. 7.17). HL rarely involves structures other than lymph nodes but it may spread to the spleen, liver, and bone marrow. It is associated with defective cell-mediated (T-cell) immunity and associated infections; other symptoms include fever,

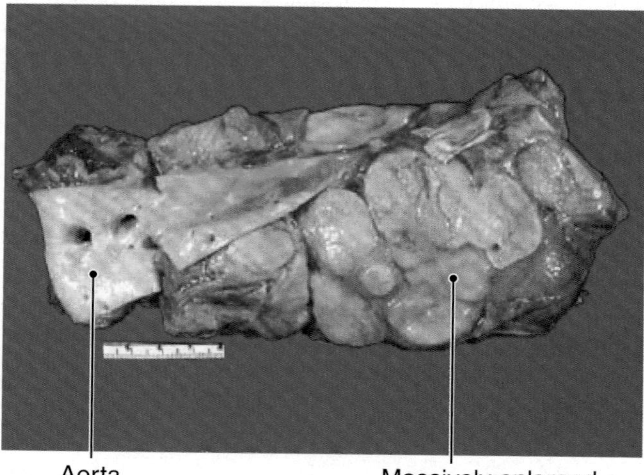

Figure 7.16 **Malignant lymphoma in lymph nodes.** Shown here is a gross autopsy study of lymphoma in paraaortic, retroperitoneal lymph nodes.

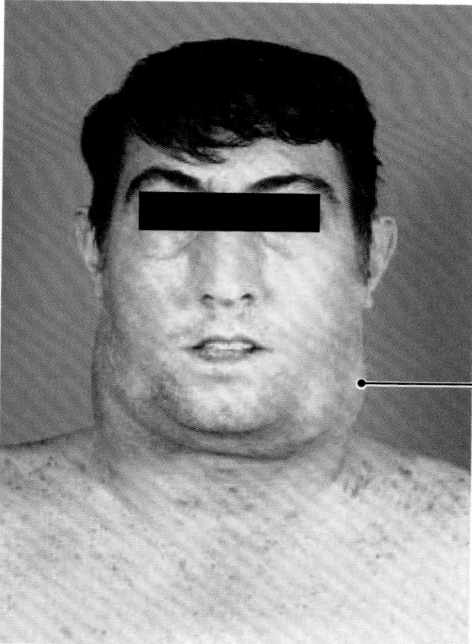

Figure 7.17 **Hodgkin disease.** This photo shows a patient with nodular sclerosis Hodgkin disease and marked enlargement of the cervical lymph nodes.

night sweats, weight loss, pruritus, splenomegaly, and hepatomegaly.

The malignant cell of HL is the **Reed-Sternberg (RS) cell**, a B lymphocyte with a distinctive appearance. There is evidence that it becomes malignant because of infection by the *Epstein-Barr virus (EBV)*. Microscopic study defines five variants, each of which has somewhat differing anatomic presentation and prognosis. **Nodular sclerosing Hodgkin lymphoma (NSHL)** is the variant that accounts for about 70% of cases. It is the only variety of HL that is more common in women than men; it has a conspicuous tendency to involve neck, upper chest, and mediastinal lymph nodes, and it is the least aggressive.

Diagnosis is based on lymph node biopsy. Because of its local origin and tendency to spread in stepwise fashion, clinical staging is more important for HL than NHL. Treatment consists of chemotherapy with or without radiation therapy. Survival beyond five years is considered curative. The overall cure rate is about 75%, but exceeds 90% for patients diagnosed with early stage disease.

Remember This! Hodgkin disease differs in important ways from all other lymphoid malignancies.

Non-Hodgkin Lymphomas

About 80% of **non-Hodgkin lymphomas (NHL)** are malignant tumors of B lymphocytes. These lymphomas are similar to HL: both are tumors of lymphocytes, both usually present as a painless enlargement of lymph nodes, and both are associated with immune deficiency and infections.

Nevertheless, NHL differs from HL in important ways. On average, NHL is more aggressive and is in a more advanced clinical stage at time of diagnosis. Its microscopic appearance and behavior vary greatly from one type to the next. In sharp contrast to HL, one-third of NHLs arise not in lymph nodes but in other organs, such as brain, bone, or bowel. NHL tends to spread widely from the original site into other lymph nodes, spleen, liver, and bone marrow, and at time of diagnosis, most patients are presumed to have widespread disease; therefore, clinical staging is not as important as in HL.

The pathologic classification of NHL is complex—the WHO classification lists dozens of types. A simpler but useful method classifies NHL into two main groups: those with a follicular microscopic appearance are called **follicular lymphoma**; the remainder lack follicles and are called **diffuse lymphoma**. Follicular lymphoma (Fig. 7.18A) is so-named because its growth pattern is similar to the lymphoid follicles of normal lymph nodes (Fig. 7.18B). Of all NHL, about half have a follicular microscopic appearance and half diffuse.

Follicular lymphomas arise, mainly in adults, as painless, enlarged lymph nodes. They have a microscopic architecture that roughly approximates the anatomy of normal lymph nodes by having lymphoid follicles. Follicular lymphomas are less aggressive and have a better prognosis than diffuse lymphomas, and median survival is nearly 10 years. Nevertheless, despite this sluggish behavior, they do not respond well to chemotherapy.

Diffuse lymphomas (Fig. 7.18C) grow in a uniform microscopic pattern without follicles. They occur mainly in people over 60 years old, but there are two notable age exceptions: childhood lymphomas and the lymphomas associated with AIDS. Most appear quickly, grow rapidly, and are quickly lethal unless treated. After chemotherapy, about 30% of patients experience a permanent remission and can be considered cured. Most of the others undergo temporary complete remissions, but the disease recurs in a few years. *Small cell lymphocytic lymphoma (SLL)*, the low-grade NHL discussed above, is essentially the same disease as *chronic lymphocytic leukemia (CLL)*, and has a good prognosis despite having a diffuse microscopic pattern.

The clinical features of NHL include 1) enlarged, nontender lymph nodes; 2) an increased metabolic rate that is responsible for constitutional symptoms such as fever, weight loss, malaise, and sweating; and 3) autoimmune phenomena or immunodeficiency problems such as infection. Prognosis and therapy of NHLs of any kind are guided by the microscopic pattern (follicular or diffuse pattern and other microscopic features), cell type (B cell or T cell, other protein markers), and clinical stage (extranodal or organ involvement).

Most Plasma Cell Proliferations Are Malignant

Recall from Chapter 3 that a plasma cell is an active B lymphocyte that is making antibodies (immunoglobulins IgG, A, M, D, and E, each of which is composed of two *heavy chain* and two *light chain* proteins). **Plasma cell proliferations** are overgrowths of a single clone of plasma cells. Most are malignant. They are often referred to as **plasma cell dyscrasias**. *Dyscrasia* is an old term that essentially means *disease*. It is useful in plasma cell proliferations because their behavior varies widely from nearly innocuous to lethal.

Pathophysiology

The proliferating clone of plasma cells makes excess whole immunoglobulin molecules, or, less commonly, excess pure heavy or light chains. These immunoglobulins are functionally useless and are made at the expense of normal immunoglobulin production. Heavy and light chains can also appear as a metabolic product of the breakdown of whole immunoglobulin molecules. Whole immunoglobulin molecules and heavy chains are confined to blood because they are too large to pass through vessel walls. Free light chains, however, are small enough to pass out of the renal glomerulus (a vascular structure), and into urine, where they are known as **Bence-Jones protein**. These free light chains have a toxic effect on the kidney.

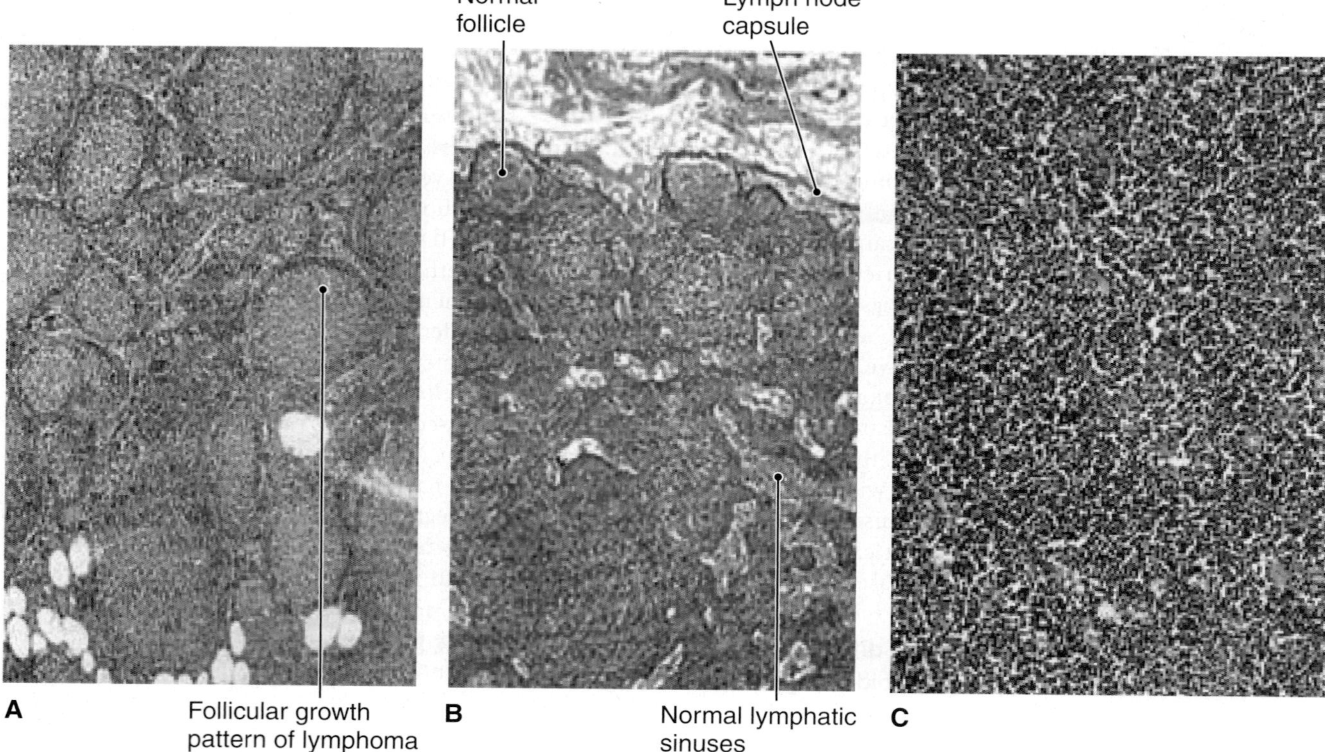

Figure 7.18 **Follicular lymphoma. A.** Lymph node involved by malignant lymphoma with nodular pattern. **B.** Normal lymph node demonstrating follicular pattern. **C.** Lymph node involved by malignant lymphoma with diffuse pattern.

Whether a whole immunoglobulin molecule, heavy chain fragment, or light chain fragment, these proteins are the product of a single clone of plasma cells and are referred to as **monoclonal proteins**, or **M-proteins**. In blood or urine they can be separated, identified, and studied by **protein electrophoresis** (Fig. 7.19). Monoclonal protein appears as a dense band in the *gamma globulin* region along with normal immunoglobulins, and when the strip is scanned to make a graph, it produces a tall peak or **monoclonal spike**. That the abnormal protein appears with normal gamma globulins accounts for the name **monoclonal gammopathy**, which is applied to any plasma cell proliferation with monoclonal protein in blood or urine.

The most common plasma cell proliferation is **monoclonal gammopathy of undetermined significance (MGUS)**, which affects about 1% of the U.S. population over age 25 and 5% over age 70. MGUS is usually asymptomatic. No treatment is necessary. Each year about 1% of MGUS patients will develop an overt plasma cell dyscrasia.

Multiple Myeloma

Multiple myeloma is a malignant neoplasm of plasma cells that features multiple bone lesions. A more limited form known as **solitary myeloma** (or *plasmacytoma*) may precede multiple myeloma for many years, but it always progresses. The peak incidence of multiple myeloma is about age 65. Men are affected more than women, and blacks more than whites. The malignant plasma cells do not circulate in blood but appear as nodular masses in bone marrow (Fig. 7.20). These nodules destroy bone and produce solitary, "punched out" bone defects, especially in the spine and skull (Fig. 7.21), which are so distinctive radiographically that the appearance is diagnostic.

As the clone of malignant plasma cells grows, it replaces normal plasma cells, causing a decline in the production of normal antibodies. The result is low levels of gamma globulin (*hypogammaglobulinemia*) and subsequent susceptibility to infections due to impaired humoral immunity. Bone pain, hypercalcemia (as a result of bone destruction), anemia (because of bone marrow replacement), and recurrent infections are common complaints. The most common cause of death is infection, followed by renal failure due to the toxic effect of Bence-Jones protein on renal tubules.

The diagnosis of multiple myeloma can be made by finding characteristic "punched out" bone lesions on radiographs or by finding monoclonal proteins in plasma or urine. Therapy includes conventional chemotherapy and steroids. Radiation may be effective for painful bone lesions. Survival is usually three to five years.

Lymphoplasmacytic Lymphoma and Waldenström Macroglobulinemia

Lymphoplasmacytic lymphoma is a B cell neoplasm of older adults that is related to chronic lymphocytic

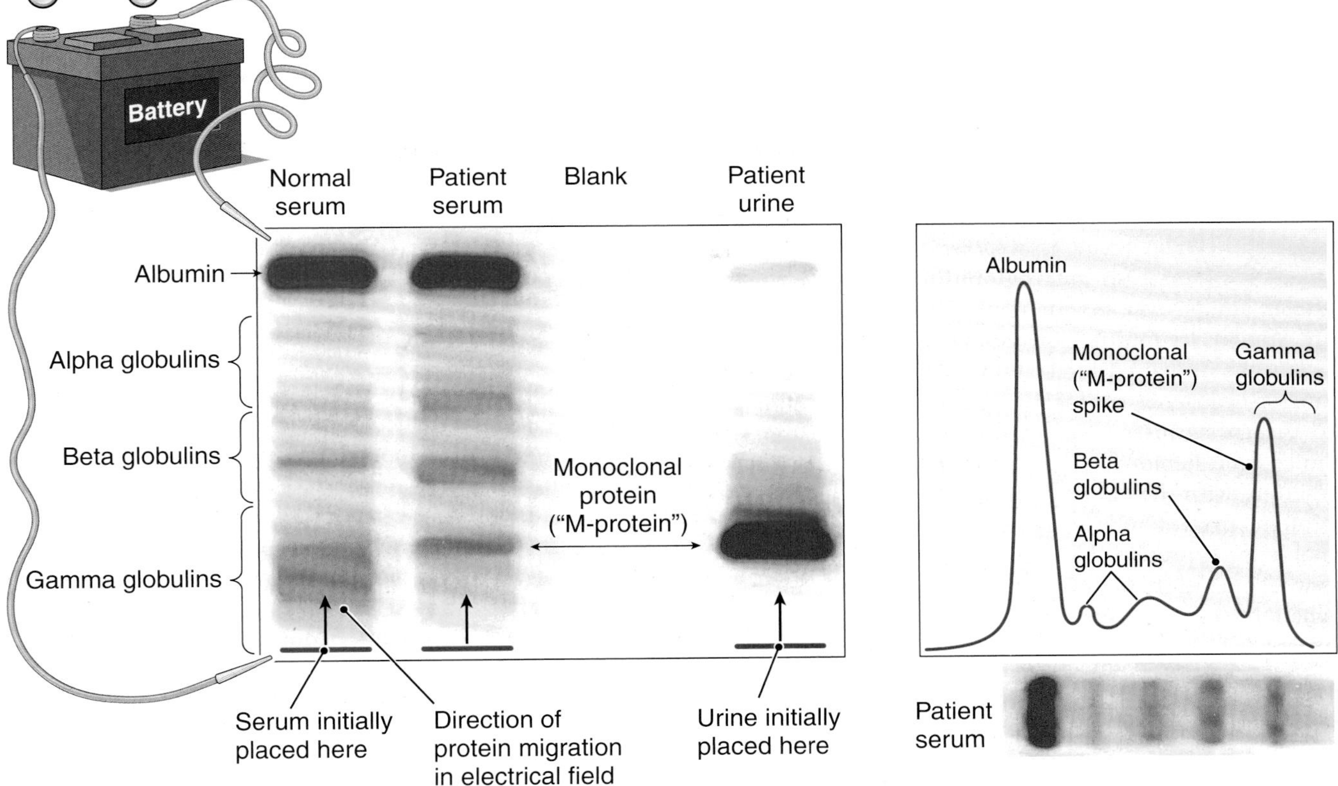

Figure 7.19 **Protein electrophoresis in plasma cell disease.** Serum or urine is placed at one end of a strip of gel, across which a direct electrical current is applied. Most proteins have a negative charge and migrate toward the positive pole at various speeds according to their molecular weight and charge. The serum on the left shows a narrow band in the gamma globulin region. Serum protein has spilled into urine, which demonstrates a matching band. In the scan of patient serum on the right, the height of the tracing is proportional to the amount of protein stained in each band. Monoclonal protein appears as a tall, narrow (monoclonal) "M-protein."

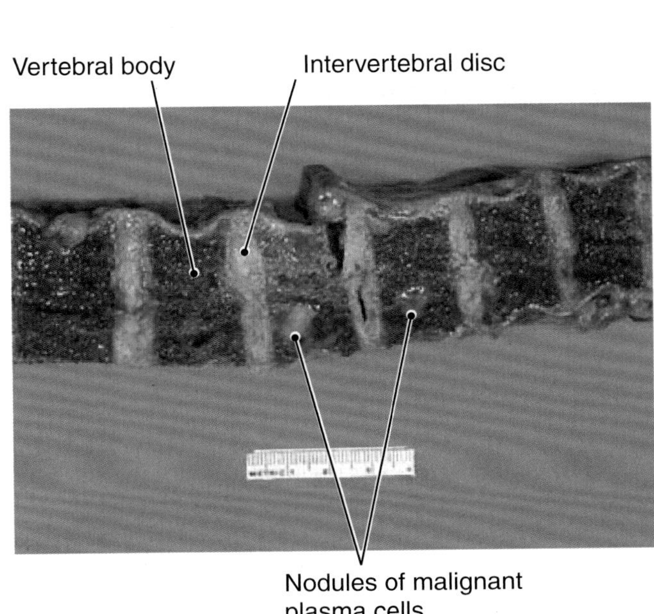

Figure 7.20 **Multiple myeloma.** In this autopsy photo of vertebrae, nodules of malignant plasma cells are visible.

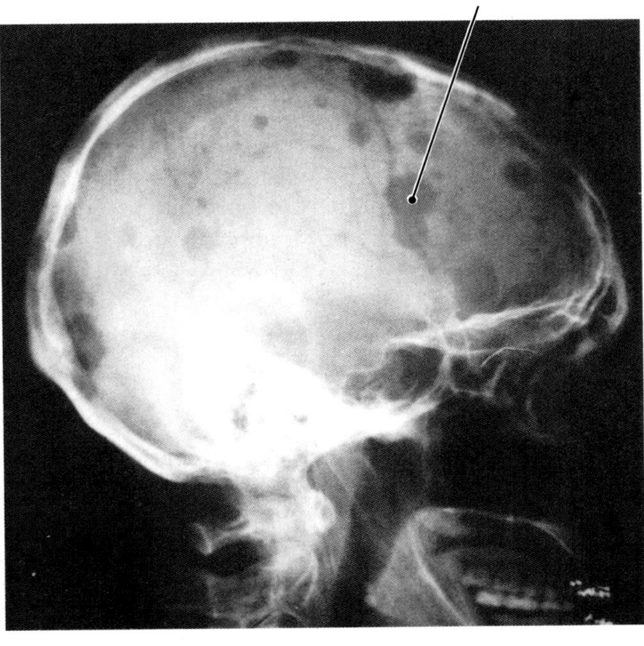

Figure 7.21 **Multiple myeloma.** In this radiograph of the skull in multiple myeloma, the "punched out" radiolucent lesions are the result of destruction by nodules of plasma cells. (Reprinted with permission from Rubin E. *Pathology*. 4th ed. Philadelphia, PA: Lippincott Williams and Wilkins; 2005.)

leukemia and small cell lymphocytic lymphoma (CLL/SLL, discussed above). In this instance the malignant cells differentiate into plasma cells, which usually secrete IgM immunoglobulin. IgM is the largest of all immunoglobulin molecules. When present in excess, it thickens plasma into a syrupy, viscous fluid, which causes sluggish blood flow. The result is *hyperviscosity syndrome*, also called **Waldenström macroglobulinemia**, which mainly affects adults over 60. In most patients, the symptoms are similar to multiple myeloma, but bone lesions do not occur. Impaired blood flow to the brain causes dizziness, headache, confusion, and stroke, and poor flow to the eyes causes visual symptoms. Patients may also suffer from hemorrhages because increased levels of IgM interfere with the clotting process. Diagnosis is by serum protein electrophoresis, determination that IgM is the monoclonal protein, blood viscosity test, and bone marrow examination. Many patients require no treatment, but when hyperviscosity occurs, plasmapheresis to harvest excess IgM is usually effective. Some patients require chemotherapy. Average survival is a few years, similar to multiple myeloma.

Pop Quiz

7.35 True or false? SLL is very aggressive.

7.36 True or false? Nodular sclerosis type is the most common type of HL.

7.37 True or false? Bence-Jones proteins can be detected in a sample of blood.

7.38 A microscopic pattern on a lymph node biopsy resembling normal lymphoid follicles is characteristic of which lymphoma?

7.39 A patient is found to have an elevated WBC count, Bence-Jones proteins in her urine, and "punched" out lesions on an X-ray of the spine. What will protein electrophoresis reveal?

7.40 The major groups of lymphomas are ______________________ and ______________________.

7.41 What do blood samples from patients with multiple myeloma and Waldenstrom macroglobulinemia have in common?

7.42 Which lymphoma has a better prognosis, follicular or diffuse?

7.43 For which lymphoma is chemotherapy more effective at killing tumor cells, follicular or diffuse?

Disorders of the Spleen and Thymus

The **spleen** is the largest organ of the immune system and home to the largest collection of macrophages in the body. It nests under the lower edge of the left rib cage and weighs about 150 gm, but may enlarge to 5,000 gm in pathologic states, and can very nearly fill the abdomen. It is highly vascular and filters blood, ridding it of microbes, old or damaged RBCs, WBCs, platelets, and particulate matter. It is particularly active in removing cellular elements in autoimmune disease in which antibody is attached. For example, in immune hemolytic anemia, RBCs coated with antibody are avidly trapped and hemolyzed early in their life span. The spleen also houses macrophages that trap and present alien antigens to splenic B and T cells, which respond by producing antibodies (B cells) or directly attacking the antigen (T cells). Finally, the spleen retains a latent capacity to revert to fetal status and produce RBCs, WBCs, and platelets (extramedullary hematopoiesis).

Loss of the splenic function, as with surgical removal after trauma or repeated infarction in sickle cell disease ("autoinfarction"), is characterized by increased risk for fatal septicemia by pneumococcus, meningococcus, and *H. influenza*. Patients without a functioning spleen should be immunized against this risk.

Splenomegaly is an enlarged spleen. Because it is an immune organ, it may enlarge reactively as its component cells proliferate in immune disease or infection, especially blood infection. The catalog of conditions that enlarge the spleen is too long to list, but among the most common are viral infections such as infectious mononucleosis, chronic autoimmune disease, malaria, lymphoma, and leukemia. And because it is highly vascular, it may enlarge as it congests with venous blood (**congestive splenomegaly**), as in right heart failure, cirrhosis of the liver, and other conditions. Regardless of cause, an enlarged spleen may become overactive and remove more than the normal number of red cells, white cells, and platelets, a condition called **hypersplenism**. The result can be hemolytic anemia, leukopenia, and thrombocytopenia, each of which has consequences discussed above.

Case Notes

7.17 **Does Eleanor have splenomegaly?**

The **thymus** sits behind the upper end of the sternum and is critical to the development of the T lymphocytes of the immune system. It features a cortex of lymphocytes and a medulla of thymocytes (thymic epithelial cells). Relative to body size, it is largest at birth, but in absolute terms it becomes largest at puberty and shrinks to a few grams in adults.

Underdevelopment of the thymus causes serious immune deficiency. **Thymic hyperplasia** is a term applied to hyperplasia of thymic lymphocytes. It is associated with a variety of endocrine and autoimmune diseases but is most commonly found in association with **myasthenia gravis** (Chapter 3), a rare, acquired autoimmune disease in which antibodies block transmission of nerve signals across the neuromuscular synapse. About half of cases have thymic hyperplasia or thymoma. **Thymoma** is a tumor of thymic epithelial cells. It is very rare and may be either benign or malignant ("thymic carcinoma"). Most cases are discovered in association with myasthenia gravis.

Pop Quiz

7.44 Define hypersplenism.

7.45 Thymic hyperplasia and thymoma are associated with what autoimmune disease?

7.46 After removal of the spleen (or autoinfarction in sickle cell anemia), the patient is susceptible to what infections?

7.47 How can these infections be prevented?

Case Study Revisited

"My life is running out of my nose." The case of Eleanor B.

Eleanor died of bone marrow failure caused by one of the myeloproliferative syndromes: primary myelofibrosis. Malignant myeloid cells stimulated scar-like proliferation of fibrous tissue that replaced her bone marrow, forcing her spleen and liver to take over blood cell production (extramedullary hematopoiesis). This type of blood cell production, however, is not efficient. As a result, she was anemic and had a very low platelet count. On the initial visit, her WBC count was slightly elevated due to the presence of malignant cells. At the time of her death, however, each of her major cell lines was affected: platelet and leukocyte cell counts were very low, and she was severely anemic, even before her final, fatal hemorrhage. Let's discuss each of these elements.

- *Leukocytes:* When she first appeared in the emergency room, Eleanor's total white cell count was moderately increased. From the time of her initial emergency room visit until the time of her death, she required antibiotic treatment for pneumonia, skin infections, and recurrent diarrhea. The medical record does not indicate WBC counts during the interim between diagnosis and death, but recurrent infections strongly suggest that WBC function was inadequate, whether due to poorly functioning malignant cells, low numbers of WBCs, or both. Autopsy findings were confirmatory: bacterial infection of blood and lungs and fungus infection in her esophagus.
- *Platelets:* Note that on her initial hospitalization the platelet count was very low and she had a severe nosebleed and tiny skin hemorrhages (*petechiae*, which are characteristic of platelet-induced bleeding). Physicians transfused her with platelets, which stopped the bleeding. On her final admission with massive GI hemorrhage, the platelet count was again very low. The thrombocytopenia and bleeding esophageal ulcer combined to produce uncontrollable acute esophageal hemorrhage, shock, and death.
- *Erythrocytes:* When she initially appeared with a nosebleed, Eleanor was severely anemic, reflecting the dual effect of marrow production failure and hemorrhage. Though her final blood hemoglobin level was extremely low, some patients with very low hemoglobin levels can survive if their blood volume is adequate; that is, if their bleeding is slow enough (or therapy quick enough) for their plasma volume to expand to make up for the lost blood volume. But Eleanor's blood volume was not adequate—she bled so rapidly that both blood volume and blood pressure fell to undetectable levels and she expired from lack of oxygen (hypoxia).

Chapter Challenge

CHAPTER RECALL

1. What is the lifespan of a neutrophil?
   A. 4 days
   B. 120 days
   C. 1–2 days
   D. 7 days

2. A 42 year-old African American male comes to your office for a checkup. His CBC shows a mild microcytic hypochromic anemia, and hemoglobin electrophoresis shows elevated hemoglobin F and decreased hemoglobin A. Target cells are also visible on a peripheral smear. Which of the following diseases does the patient suffer from?
   A. Sickle cell disease
   B. Iron deficiency anemia
   C. Alpha-thalassemia
   D. Beta-thalassemia minor

3. Warm antibody hemolytic anemia is characterized by which of the following?
   A. Room temperature antibodies that cause anemia and splenomegaly
   B. Autoimmune antibodies that form after exposure to drugs or an infectious etiology
   C. Sudden severe back/leg pain, vomiting, diarrhea, and hemoglobinuria
   D. Antibodies that are produced after exposure to a cold shower

4. A 54-year-old Japanese female presents to the clinic complaining of numbness and tingling in her hands and fingers. Physical exam is positive for plethora, and a CBC demonstrates a hematocrit greater than 60% and thrombocytosis. Which of the following is true about her disease?
   A. It is caused by an autoimmune disease resulting in low B_{12}.
   B. Erythropoietin is increased.
   C. The treatment of choice is a therapeutic phlebotomy.
   D. A bone marrow biopsy will demonstrate fibrosis.

5. Which cell digests foreign antigens for presentation to immune cells?
   A. Lymphocytes
   B. Monocytes
   C. Neutrophils
   D. Granulocytes

6. An eight-year-old Hispanic female is brought to the clinic because she has been increasingly tired over the last month. Her mother reports that in addition to pallor, she also has increased bruising and complaints of bone pain. What do you expect to see on her CBC?
   A. Elevated WBC count, with greater than 20% blasts
   B. Anemia
   C. Thrombocytopenia
   D. All of the above

7. NHL and HL can be differentiated based on the presence of which of the following?
   A. Reed-Sternberg cells
   B. Blasts in peripheral blood
   C. Malignant cells in lymph nodes
   D. Malignant cells in bone marrow

8. A 65-year-old African American male comes to the clinic complaining of bone pain and fatigue. Incidentally, he notes a recent change in urination. A urinalysis reveals Bence-Jones proteins and a skull X-ray shows punched out lesions. What is your diagnosis?
   A. Waldenström macroglobulinemia
   B. Multiple myeloma
   C. Monoclonal gammopathy of undetermined significance
   D. Lymphoplasmacytic lymphoma

9. A 22-year-old Hispanic male presents to the ER for evaluation of a fever of 103°F, abdominal pain, and diarrhea of three days' duration. His CBC is concerning for a WBC count greater than 50,000/µl, with a marked increase in band cells, while his platelet and RBC counts are within normal limits. What is the most likely explanation of his elevated WBC count?
   A. Leukemoid reaction
   B. Acute myelogenous leukemia
   C. Neutropenia
   D. Acute lymphocytic leukemia

10. A 65-year-old Caucasian female with a past medical history significant for rheumatoid arthritis presents for evaluation of shortness of breath, fatigue, and pallor. Her peripheral smear demonstrates microcytic hypochromic anemia, and blood work reveals low transferrin and elevated ferritin. Which of the following anemias is responsible for her symptoms?

A. Iron deficiency anemia
B. Megaloblastic anemia
C. Hereditary spherocytosis
D. Anemia of chronic disease

11. True or false? An anemia of production deficiency can be differentiated from an anemia of blood loss/destruction using a reticulocyte threshold count of 2.5%.

12. True or false? The most common cause of B_{12} deficiency is defective intestinal absorption.

13. True or false? Acute nonspecific lymphadenitis is caused by prolonged antigenic stimulation, and is characterized by slowly enlarging nontender nodes.

14. True or false? Primary myelofibrosis is a malignant disease of myeloid cells that stimulates myelophthisis.

15. True or false? Loss of the splenic function places the patients at risk for infection by pneumococcus, meningococcus, and *H. influenza*.

CONCEPTUAL UNDERSTANDING

16. What are red cell indices?

17. Compare and contrast the megaloblastic anemias. How can they be differentiated from one another?

18. Explain extramedullary hematopoiesis.

APPLICATION

19. Discuss how a massive hemorrhage might result in two different types of anemia.

20. A 55-year-old Caucasian male comes to your office complaining of fatigue. You perform a routine blood draw and note a microcytic anemia. What tests should you run, and what is your concern?

21. Explain why the hemoglobin S mutation remains in the population when it causes severe disease in homozygous patients.

CHAPTER 8

Disorders of Blood Vessels

Contents

Chapter Objectives

After studying this chapter, you should be able to complete the following tasks:

OVERVIEW OF VASCULAR STRUCTURE AND FUNCTIONING

1. Discuss how vessel structure varies with its function.
2. Classify the plasma lipids.

HYPERTENSIVE VASCULAR DISEASE

3. Discuss the risk factors, clinical manifestations, and pathological findings associated with hypertension.

ATHEROSCLEROSIS

4. List the predisposing factors, indicators of risk, pathologic processes, clinical complications, and treatment of atherosclerosis.

ANEURYSMS AND DISSECTIONS

5. Name the most common causes of aneurysms and dissections.

VASCULITIS

6. Describe the pathological findings associated with the affected vessel and the clinical manifestations of the following vasculitides:
   - Temporal arteritis
   - Takayasu arteritis
   - Polyarteritis nodosa
   - Kawasaki disease
   - Microscopic polyangiitis
   - Wegener granulomatosis
   - Thromboangiitis obliterans

RAYNAUD

7. Compare and contrast primary and secondary Raynaud syndrome.

DISEASES OF VEINS

8. Describe the pathogenesis of varicose veins and thrombophlebitis.

TUMORS OF BLOOD AND LYMPHATIC VESSEL

9. Know whether the following are benign or malignant: hemangioma, lymphangioma, vascular ectasia, Kaposi sarcoma, and angiosarcoma.

Case Study

"A man found dead in his office." The case of Leon F.

Chief Complaint: Sudden, unexpected death

Clinical History: Sixty-two-year-old African American real estate executive Leon F. was found dead in his office late at night by the cleaning crew. The police report said he was found on the floor beside his desk with a small amount of dried blood around a superficial scalp laceration. There was no sign of forced entry, altercation, or theft.

The Office of the Medical Examiner obtained his medical record from his doctor. The physician said she had been seeing Leon for five years for hypertension that was difficult to control. Leon's first visit to the physician's office had been for a minor ailment during which a routine check of his blood pressure revealed it to be 145/90. Her notes said he was "overweight" but his weight was not recorded. He admitted to smoking a half a pack of cigarettes a day. His mother had died of diabetes and his father of a heart attack. The physician ordered laboratory tests and X-rays and asked him to return in two weeks. Laboratory data and imaging studies revealed no evidence of underlying disease that would explain the hypertension. Blood tests revealed total cholesterol 265 mg/dL, LDL cholesterol 200 mg/dL, and HDL cholesterol 45 mg/dL. Increased plasma levels of creatinine and blood urea nitrogen (BUN) suggested impairment of kidney function. A diagnosis of primary hypertension was made.

The physician said when Leon returned for follow-up she told him his cholesterol and blood pressure were dangerously high, that it was affecting his heart and kidneys, and that he needed to lose weight and quit smoking. She gave him prescriptions for a statin drug to lower his cholesterol and a drug for blood pressure control. On the next office visit, his blood pressure was even higher—150/95—but his cholesterol numbers were "much improved."

The medical record showed irregular office visits over the next few years and apparent failure to have his prescriptions refilled despite documented notices that he should return to the office regularly for monitoring and medication adjustment. One entry indicates Leon cut down on cigarettes but was never able to quit except for brief intervals. The last note in the physician's records was two years earlier. The record from that visit included an electrocardiogram indicating left ventricular enlargement, beside which was scribbled "Hypertension!" On that last visit the physician refilled Leon's hypertension prescriptions and referred him to a hypertension specialist at the local medical center, but their records found no evidence of him as a patient.

Investigators concluded that Leon probably died of a heart attack or stroke, but the circumstances warranted a medicolegal autopsy. Major findings were confined to the cardiovascular system, kidneys, and brain. The adrenals and other endocrine glands were unremarkable, and no tumors were found in any organ. The left ventricle was very hypertrophic. A $3 \times 3 \times 1$ cm fibrous scar was present in the anterior wall of the left ventricle in tissue fed by the anterior coronary artery, which was severely atherosclerotic (90% narrowing of the lumen). The kidneys were small and granular. The renal arteries were mildly atherosclerotic and showed no evidence of significant obstruction. No renal hemorrhages were present. The abdominal aorta was especially atherosclerotic and aneurysmally dilated. The scalp laceration was superficial and associated with mild superficial hemorrhage. The skull was not fractured. In the midbrain and basal ganglia was a 6 cm hematoma that ruptured into the left lateral ventricle, filling it with blood. Microscopic studies were unremarkable except in the kidney, where there was severe nephrosclerosis.

(*continued*)

"A man found dead in his office." The case of Leon F. (continued)

Final autopsy diagnoses were the following:

- Acute intracerebral hemorrhage (clinical history of severe hypertension)
- Marked left ventricular hypertrophy (clinical history of severe hypertension)
- Severe coronary atherosclerosis (clinical history of severe hypertension and hypercholesterolemia)
- Old, healed myocardial infarction (clinical history of severe hypertension and hypercholesterolemia)
- Severe arteriolar nephrosclerosis (clinical history of severe hypertension)
- Moderate fusiform aneurysm of the abdominal aorta (clinical history of severe hypertension and hypercholesterolemia)

Humorous health definitions:

- *Artery: the study of fine paintings*
- *Varicose: nearby*
- *Vein: conceited*
- *Capillary: a boy's hat*

ANONYMOUS, 2005

Unlike an amoeba, which can wander about to find life's necessities, the cells of our body are fixed in place and must have oxygen, food, and other requirements brought to them and waste carried away by a transport vehicle—blood. In transporting these materials, blood travels through a network of about 50,000 miles of arteries and veins.

Overview of Vascular Structure and Functioning

In historical terms, that blood moves within vessels is a relatively recent discovery. Greek physician Hippocrates (~400 BCE) knew of blood vessels but believed they contained air and foodstuffs. About 600 years later, Roman physician Galen (131–201 CE) theorized that blood surged and ebbed like the ocean's tide. Galen's idea persisted until English physician William Harvey (1578–1657), in a series of very careful animal experiments and human observations, concluded that blood flowed circularly in a closed system and inferred that arteries and veins were connected.

There Are Three Types of Blood Vessels

There are three basic types of blood vessels (Fig. 8.1). **Arteries** carry high-pressure, pulsating blood away from the heart. **Veins** carry low-pressure, nonpulsating blood toward the heart. **Capillaries**, the smallest vessels, lie in tissues and join the arterial network to the venous network. Both arteries and veins are composed of similar layers of cells, but layer thickness varies according to local functional requirements.

Large vessels are composed of three concentric layers. From outside to in they are the **adventitia**, **media**, and **intima**. The adventitia is composed of supporting fibrous tissue. The media is composed mainly of smooth muscle. The intima in most vessels is composed of a single layer of **endothelial cells** that rest on a basement membrane; larger vessels also have a thin subendothelial layer of connective tissue. Endothelial cells serve two important functions: 1) they control diffusion of substances across the wall into adjacent tissues and 2) they are in constant contact with blood and keep it in a smooth, unclotted state by preventing coagulation.

As Figure 8.1 illustrates, the anatomy of arteries and veins varies as the vessels branch into smaller-diameter tubes. As vessels become smaller, the outer layers fall away until the tiniest vessels, capillaries, are composed only of endothelial cells.

To withstand the higher pressure and pulsing flow, artery walls are usually thicker than the walls of veins. Based on their size and structural features, arteries are divided into four types:

- **Elastic arteries** are large and include the aorta and its initial branches, and the main pulmonary arteries. The smooth muscle of their media is rich with elastic fibers, which imparts to them a springy resiliency.
- **Muscular arteries** are middle-size, and include the renal and coronary arteries. In muscular arteries (Fig. 8.2) the media is composed predominantly of encircling smooth muscle cells. In the muscular arteries and arterioles, regional flow and pressure are regulated by the change in lumen size as smooth muscle cells contract to narrow the lumen (**vasoconstriction**) and decrease blood flow, or relax to enlarge it (**vasodilation**) and increase blood flow. Vasoconstriction and vasodilation are controlled by the autonomic nervous system, by hormones, and by local metabolic factors.

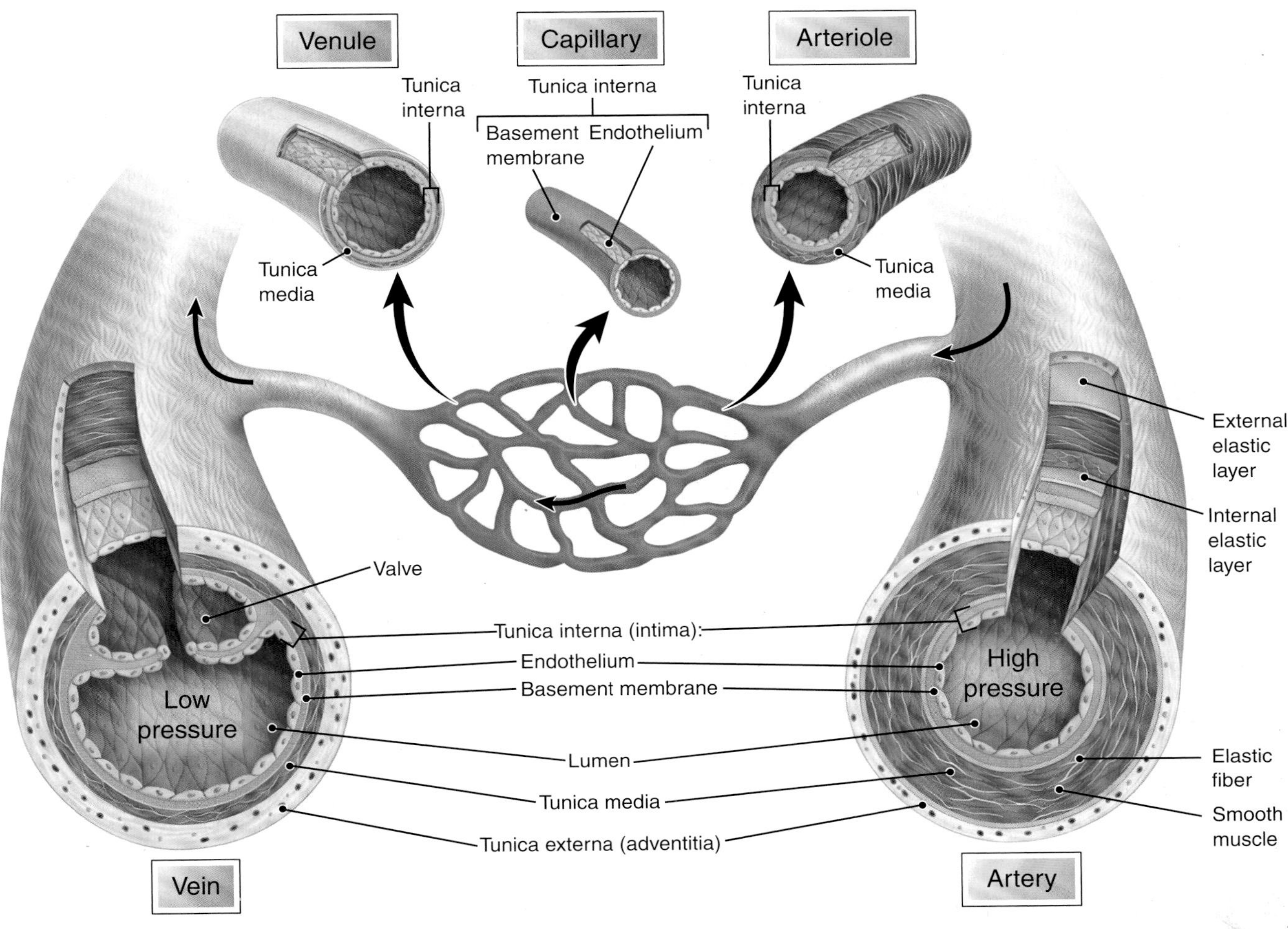

Figure 8.1 **The structure of the vascular tree.** The basic structure of blood vessels is uniform, but the thickness of layers varies according to local pressure and tissue demand. (Adapted with permission from McConnell TH, Hull KL. *Human Form Human Function: Essentials of Anatomy & Physiology*. Baltimore, MD: Wolters Kluwer Health; 2011.)

- **Small arteries** are less than about 2 mm in diameter, and include the retinal arteries.
- **Arterioles** are tiny precapillary arteries less than 0.1 mm, which are wrapped by a thin layer of smooth muscle.

Capillaries are about the diameter of a red blood cell (7 to 8 μm) and are composed only of endothelial cells resting on a basement membrane, which promotes free exchange of gases and fluids. As blood flows out the arterial tree, the cross-sectional area of each vessel becomes smaller, but the number of vessels increases such that total cross-sectional area increases rapidly. Though they are the tiniest of vessels, they are by far the most numerous, so the collective cross-sectional area of capillaries is many, many times larger than the aorta. As total cross-sectional area increases, the speed of blood flow falls. Within capillaries, flow rate is very slow, a pace nicely suited to the need for exchange of gases, nutrients, and wastes between blood and tissues.

Blood from capillaries flows into **venules** and then sequentially through small, medium, and large **veins**. Compared to arteries, veins have a larger diameter, larger lumen, and thinner wall. Veins are pliable and expand easily, much like a rubber balloon partially filled with water, which expands and contracts to accommodate more or less volume with little pressure change. At any given moment about two-thirds of all blood is in veins. In the standing position, venous blood from most of the body must flow against gravity to return to the heart. Flow is assisted by one-way venous valves in the extremities. When skeletal muscles contract and relax, the massaging action squeezes blood toward the heart and the valves prevent reverse flow.

Blood Pressure Causes Blood to Flow

Blood flow is required for life. Blood will not flow without pressure. Blood pressure is, therefore, required for life. Blood, like any fluid, flows from high pressure to low.

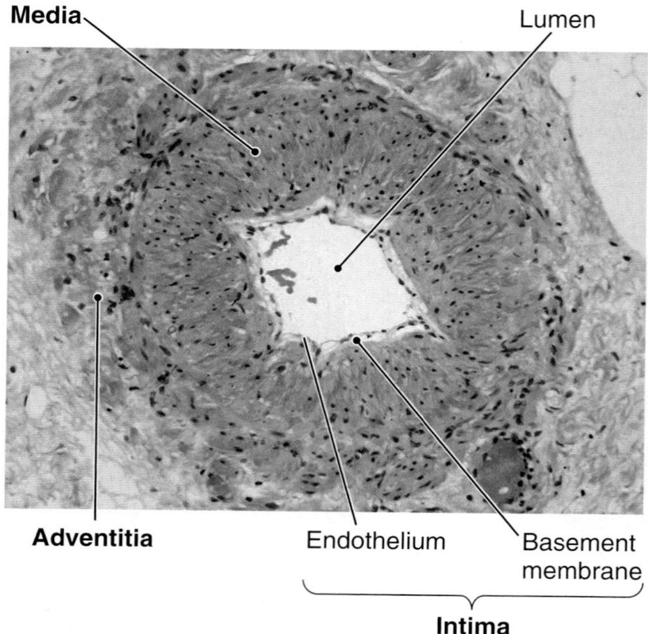

Figure 8.2 **Normal small muscular artery (arteriole).** Arterioles like this are a key point in blood pressure control because their muscular wall can contract or relax to change lumen diameter.

Pressure is highest in the aorta and falls steadily until it is near zero in the vena cava before entering the right ventricle. With each left ventricular contraction, blood is forced under high pressure into the aorta and other large elastic arteries, stretching them tense. As the left ventricle relaxes and refills (diastole), blood pressure and flow are maintained until the next beat by the elastic squeeze of the wall aorta and large arteries.

In 1733, an English clergyman, Stephen Hales, became the first person to demonstrate blood pressure. His subject was a horse, and his equipment consisted of a small brass pipe connected to a 12-foot long glass tube. The intrepid cleric bound the struggling horse and, stabbing the sharpened brass pipe into a carotid artery, was astonished to see blood rise 9 feet in the glass tube. Fortunately, we can now measure blood pressure more gently by use of a **sphygmomanometer**, a jawbreaker name derived from Greek *sphugmos* for pulse (Fig. 8.3). Conventional sphygmomanometers rely on a pressure gauge attached to an inflatable cuff, which is placed around the upper arm at heart level. The cuff is inflated to a pressure certain to cut off all blood flow by squeezing shut the brachial artery. The cuff is then deflated gradually as the examiner listens with a stethoscope placed over the artery at the lower end of the cuff just above the crook of the elbow. As cuff pressure falls below systolic blood pressure, blood begins to squirt through and makes a sound (the *Korotkoff sound*). The Korotkoff sound continues with each pulse wave until it is silenced as cuff pressure falls below diastolic blood pressure. The range between the pressure at the time of first appearance of the sound and the pressure at its disappearance is the blood pressure. High-tech devices that do not require a listener are also available. Despite its apparent simplicity, *accurate* sphygmomanometer readings are difficult to obtain as they are influenced by posture, breathing, girth of the upper arm, clothing, anxiety, drugs, whether taken before or after a meal or exercise, and many other variables. For more about measuring blood pressure, see *The Clinical Side*, "Measuring Blood Pressure."

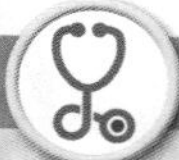

The Clinical Side

MEASURING BLOOD PRESSURE

Blood pressure is often—perhaps usually—measured incorrectly. Blood pressure varies with body position: it is lower when a person is lying down than when that person is sitting or standing. Blood pressure also varies with physical activity and emotion: it is higher with physical activity or emotional stress. Blood pressure is also increased by other activities such as smoking and consumption of caffeinated beverages.

For a correct measurement, the patient should be rested, not recovering from climbing a flight of stairs or walking a long way to get to an appointment. For several hours before the measurement, the patient should not smoke and should ingest nothing but water. Seat the patient in a chair with back and armrests, the absence of which increases blood pressure. The arm to be used for the measurement should be supported by an armrest; an unsupported arm causes higher readings. If the patient is wearing long-sleeved clothing, ask for it to be removed rather than having the patient roll up the sleeve, which interferes with the measurement. Wrap the cuff around the arm at heart level. Use special large- or small-size cuffs for obese or pediatric patients. Cuffs too large for the patient produce erroneously low readings; cuffs too small produce erroneously high readings.

Role of Cardiac Output and Vascular Resistance

Blood pressure is the product of *cardiac output* and *vascular resistance* (Fig. 8.4). **Cardiac output** is the volume of blood per unit of time (L/min) ejected by the left ventricle into the aorta. **Vascular resistance** is the resistance to flow that must be overcome for blood to flow through the circulatory system.

It is important to keep in mind when considering cardiac output that increased *total* blood volume causes increased cardiac output. The reason is simple. Increased blood volume usually owes to increased plasma, in which case the oxygen-carrying capacity of blood is unchanged. In this circumstance, more volume must be pushed through the system to maintain the same level of oxygen

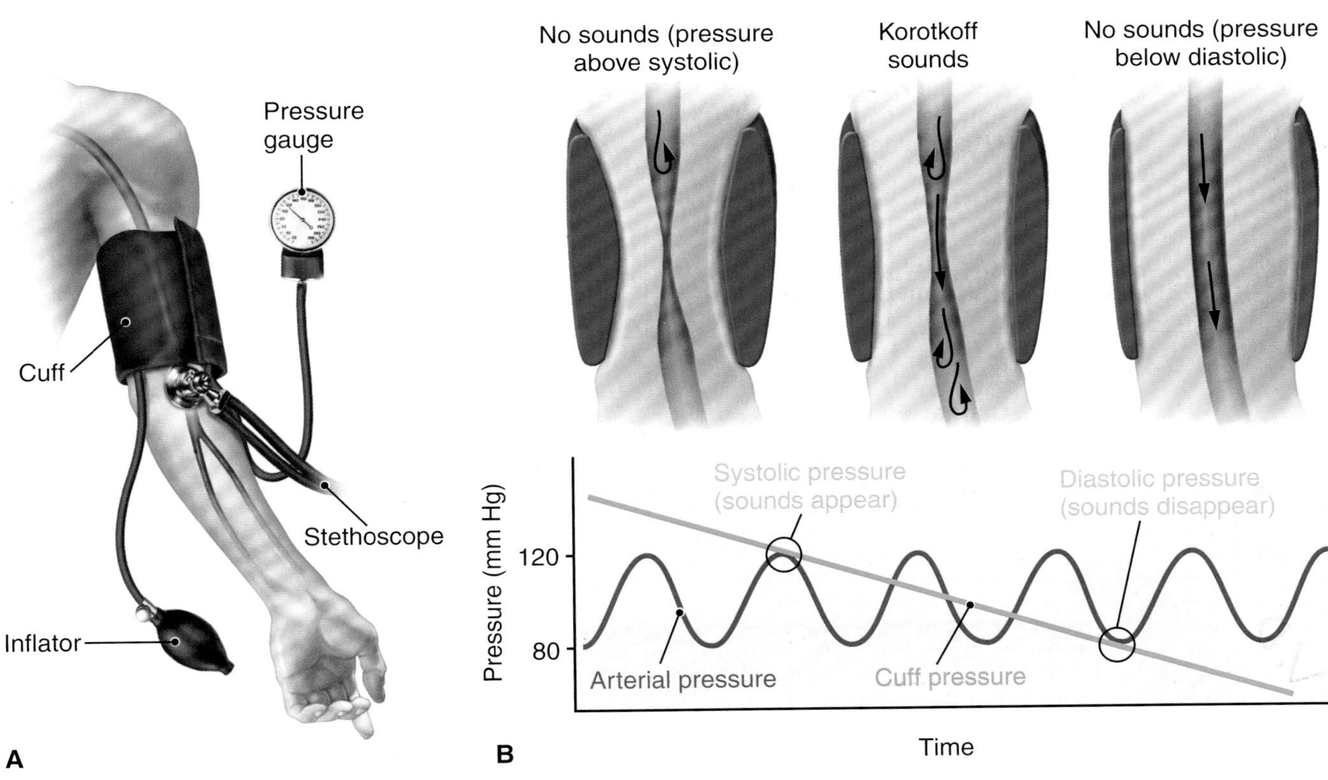

Figure 8.3 **The measurement of blood pressure. A.** Blood pressure can be measured by a using a sphygmomanometer. **B.** As cuff pressure lowers, Korotkoff sounds begin at the systolic pressure and disappear at the diastolic pressure.

supply, and blood pressure rises along with increased total blood volume.

Fluid dynamics are important in blood flow. The resistance to fluid flow in a tube is inversely proportional to the fourth power of the diameter. As resistance increases, flow must slow or pressure must increase, and vice versa. For example, halving vessel diameter increases resistance 16-fold (inverse of ½ is 2; $2^4 = 16$). It follows that small changes in the lumen diameter of small arteries has a marked effect on vascular resistance and resistance has a marked effect on pressure and flow. Peripheral arterioles are the principal point at which resistance is regulated. Peripheral arterioles constrict to narrow the arteriolar lumen and increase resistance to flow, or relax with opposite effect. If peripheral vascular resistance increases, flow must decrease or pressure must rise to maintain flow. The opposite is also true.

The autonomic nervous system innervates small arterioles and stimulates smooth muscle contraction to maintain a normal level of tension (sympathetic tone) in the vascular wall. Increased or decreased sympathetic tone has an immediate effect to increase or decrease peripheral vascular resistance. The autonomic nervous system also stimulates secretion from the adrenal medulla of the vasoconstrictors epinephrine and norepinephrine (collectively called *catecholamines*), which have a longer lasting effect on arteriolar resistance. Arteriolar resistance is also influenced by local factors such as blood pH, anoxia, inflammatory mediators, and certain hormones.

Role of the Kidneys in Blood Pressure Regulation

The kidneys play a major role in blood pressure regulation by their influence on total blood volume (and with it cardiac output) and peripheral vascular resistance. The kidney senses blood pressure and acts to increase or decrease peripheral resistance and increase or decrease blood volume as pressure rises or falls. For example, if blood pressure falls, arterioles constrict, including those leading to the kidney.

Renal vasoconstriction has two effects. First, constriction decreases the amount of blood passing through the kidney, which limits urine output and preserves water, increasing blood volume. Second, as blood pressure falls, the kidney receives less blood and is stimulated to secrete *renin*. Renin acts in concert with *angiotensin-converting enzyme*, to produce *angiotensin*, which in turn causes peripheral and renal vasoconstriction. The actions of renin and angiotensin-converting enzyme also stimulate the adrenal cortex to release *aldosterone*, a hormone that acts on the kidney to cause retention of sodium, thereby attracting water to expand blood volume, which increases cardiac output and blood pressure.

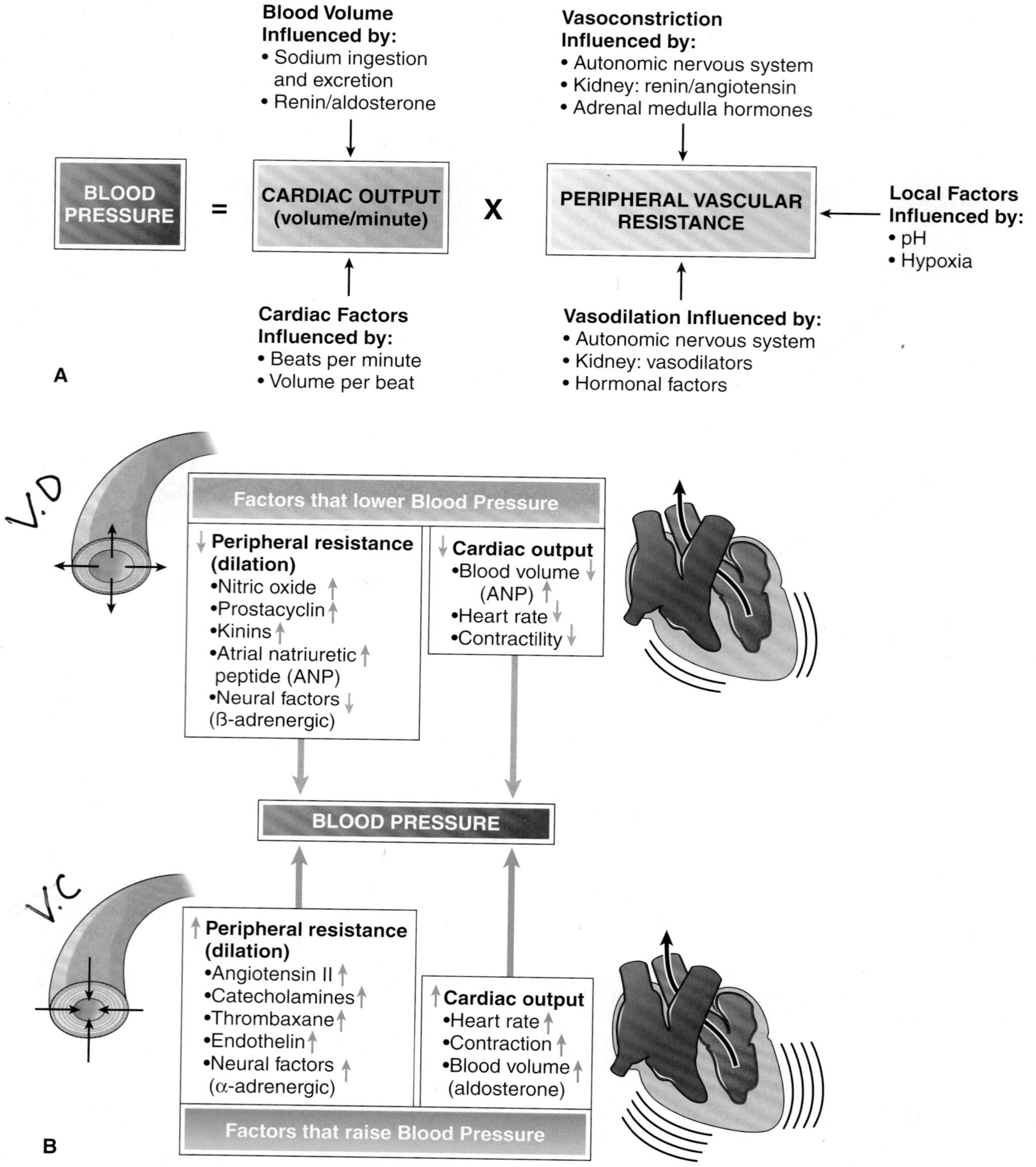

Figure 8.4 **The regulation of blood pressure. A.** Blood pressure is a product of cardiac output (volume of blood flow) and peripheral vascular resistance. **B.** Multiple factors influence blood pressure.

Plasma Lipids Influence Vascular Health and Disease

A **lipid** is a slick, greasy organic substance not soluble in water. A lipid that is solid at room temperature is a **fat**. A lipid that is not solid at room temperature is an **oil**. In the human diet, most fats are of animal origin and most oils are of vegetable origin. Lipids are very important in human physiology and disease. Free lipid is oily and not soluble in plasma, which is composed mainly of water. To be soluble in plasma, lipids must be attached to specialized plasma proteins (**apoproteins**). The combination of an apoprotein and a lipid is a **lipoprotein**. The several types of lipoproteins are classified according to their molecular density. Because protein is denser than lipid, high-density lipoproteins contain more protein than lower-density lipoproteins:

- **High-density lipoproteins (HDL)** are about half protein and half lipid, and most of their lipid is phospholipid and cholesterol.
- **Low-density lipoproteins (LDL)** are only about 22% protein, and most of their lipid is cholesterol, with smaller amounts of phospholipid and triglycerides.
- **Very-low-density lipoproteins (VLDL)** are only about 10% protein, and most of their lipid is triglycerides, with smaller amounts of phospholipid and cholesterol.

The *cholesterol portion* of each lipoprotein type is referred to as *HDL cholesterol* (HDL-C), *LDL cholesterol* (LDL-C), and *VLDL cholesterol* (VLDL-C). *Total cholesterol* is the sum of LDL, HDL, and VLDL cholesterol. For example, a blood sample from a patient with total blood cholesterol of 240 mg/dL might be composed of the following: LDL-C 160 mg/dL, HDL-C 50 mg/dL, and VLDL-C about 30 mg/dL.

After ingesting a meal containing fat or oil, most of the lipid is absorbed by the intestinal epithelium and repackaged into **chylomicrons**, exceedingly small lipid droplets that pass from bowel mucosa into intestinal lymphatics, which dump them into the bloodstream. Chylomicrons are about 85% triglyceride and are cleared from plasma by the liver, where they are attached to apoproteins to form blood HDL, LDL, and VLDL.

High levels of LDL cholesterol promote vascular disease, and so we will call it "Lousy cholesterol." High LDL is causative, that is, it actually *causes* atherosclerosis. *High* levels of HDL cholesterol, on the other hand, are *associated* with lower risk of vascular disease. We will call it "Helpful" cholesterol, a convenient name but one that may be misleading. Until recently, this relationship was thought to be *causative*; now it appears that it may only be a *marker*, much like a red flag may mark a road hazard but is not the *hazard itself*. It's a good thing to have high HDL, but why this is so is unclear.

VLDL is nearly all triglyceride. High triglyceride alone may not promote vascular disease; however, high triglyceride amplifies the vascular risk of *high* LDL cholesterol or *low* HDL cholesterol. Eating a diet high in saturated fat and cholesterol is dangerous, for reasons discussed shortly. Researchers are finding that the total percentage of fat in the diet is not all that important; rather, it is the type of fat that matters: saturated fats (most animal fats) promote vascular disease and monounsaturated and polyunsaturated fats are protective against vascular disease. A rule of thumb is this: If it's solid at room temperature, it's probably saturated and bad for you; if it's liquid at room temperature, it's probably unsaturated and good for you. The new nutrition message is: Don't focus on reducing your fat consumption, but rather on changing the type of fat you consume from animal fats to plant and fish oils.

Regarding plasma lipids, the concept of *normal* is misleading because it relies on calculations to determine the *average* cholesterol of presumably healthy people. Nevertheless, the average cholesterol of presumably healthy Americans is unhealthfully high. *Desirable* is a better concept. *The Clinical Side*, "Plasma Lipids," contains additional information about plasma lipids.

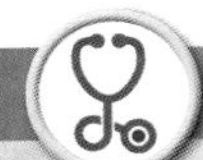

The Clinical Side

PLASMA LIPIDS

Patient plasma lipids can be assessed by direct measurement of total plasma cholesterol, HDL cholesterol, and triglyceride. LDL cholesterol is more difficult and expensive to measure than are the others and is usually calculated according to the following formula:

LDL cholesterol = total cholesterol – (HDL cholesterol + [triglyceride/5])

Calculated LDL, however, is not valid for triglyceride levels >400 mg/dL, and a direct LDL assay must be performed.

After a 12-hour fast, generally accepted desirable ranges for plasma lipids are:

Component*	Desirable (mg/dL)	Increased Risk (mg/dL)	High Risk (mg/dL)
Total cholesterol	<200	200–240	>240
HDL cholesterol (HDL-C)	>60	40–60	<40
LDL cholesterol (LDL-C)	<100	100–160	>160
Triglyceride	<150	High level increases risks of high LDL or low HDL	

*Results obtained with less than a 12-hour fast are not reliable.

Case Notes

8.1 Leon's LDL-C falls into which risk category?

Total cholesterol below 200 mg/dL is considered desirable for good health, and the lower the better: lowering total cholesterol has benefits at almost any initial cholesterol level (any starting point). That is to say, people

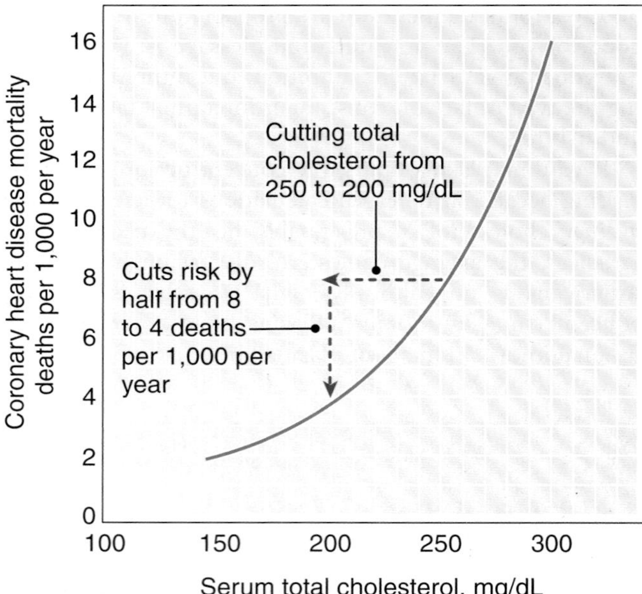

Figure 8.5 **Total plasma cholesterol and relative cardiovascular risk.** Reducing total plasma cholesterol 50 mg/dL from any given initial point cuts relative cardiovascular risk in half.

benefit by lowering their total cholesterol, whether they start with total cholesterol of 300 mg/dL or 200 mg/dL. As shown in Figure 8.5, decreasing total cholesterol by 50 mg/dL cuts in half the risk of dying from a heart attack, whether it's a drop from 300 mg/dL to 250 mg/dL or from 250 mg/dL to 200 mg dL. And the result compounds: lowering it by another 50 mg/dL cuts the risk by half again. Evidence suggests that atherosclerosis may not develop with total cholesterol levels below 150 mg/dL, a level unreachable without a strict, low saturated fat diet, usually a vegetarian diet, something few people in industrialized nations are willing to do. Indeed, when various countries are compared, the countries with the lowest blood levels of cholesterol have the lowest rates of cardiovascular disease.

Remember This! Lowering total plasma cholesterol by 50 mg/dL reduces cardiovascular risk by half; each additional 50 mg/dL decrease cuts the rate in half again.

Case Notes

8.2 What would be the atherosclerosis risk reduction if statin drug therapy had succeeded in lowering Leon's total cholesterol from 265 mg/dL to 165 mg/dL?

Pop Quiz

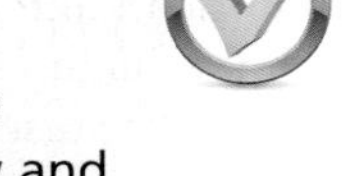

8.1 True or false? Vasoconstriction generally increases blood flow and vasodilation generally decreases blood flow.

8.2 True or false? Two-thirds of blood volume is found in the veins.

8.3 True or false? Populations with the lowest average total blood cholesterol have the highest rates of cardiovascular disease.

8.4 True or false? Total cholesterol <200 mg/dL and LDL-cholesterol <100 is desirable.

8.5 Fill in the blanks. The endothelium functions to maintain ________ blood flow and modulate ________ of substances across the wall into tissues.

8.6 What are the three layers of large vessels?

8.7 HDL and LDL are composed of what four molecular components?

8.8 What is the name of the droplet that carries lipid from the intestines to the bloodstream?

Hypertensive Vascular Disease

Good health requires that homeostatic mechanisms maintain blood pressure within a narrow range. Low pressure (*hypotension*) results in low tissue blood flow and can cause organ dysfunction or tissue necrosis. On the other hand, chronic high pressure (*hypertension*) causes endothelial injury, which evolves into vascular damage. Aside from stepping on a scale, blood pressure measurement is the most common and widely used measure of cardiovascular health, and one of the most important. In the United States, normal and abnormal blood pressures have been defined by the Seventh Report of the Joint National Committee on Prevention, Detection, Evaluation, and Treatment of High Blood Pressure (JNC7) (Tab. 8.1).

Case Notes

8.3 When Leon first appeared in the doctor's office, what was his JNC blood pressure classification?

Hypertensive vascular disease begins with injury to the endothelium. Other causes of endothelial injury include turbulent blood flow, high blood cholesterol, high blood glucose, cigarette smoke, acidosis, hypoxia, viruses,

Table 8.1 JNC7 Classification of Blood Pressure in Adults

Classification	BP (mm Hg)
Normal	<120 (systolic) *and* 80 (diastolic)
Prehypertension	120–139 (systolic) *or* 80–89 (diastolic)
Stage 1	140–159 (systolic) *or* 90–99 (diastolic)
Stage 2	≥160 (systolic) *or* ≥100 (diastolic)

JNC, Joint National Committee on Prevention, Detection, Evaluation, and Treatment of High Blood Pressure.

bacterial products, and inflammatory mediators. The reaction of the endothelium initiates and drives the vascular lesions of hypertension, atherosclerosis (discussed below), and thrombosis (Chapter 6).

Case Notes

8.4 Name some factors injuring Leon's endothelium.

Endothelial cells are metabolically active. They modulate the flow of gases, nutrients, waste, and other soluble products between blood and tissues and play an important role in vasoconstriction and vasodilation. Injury can critically affect these functions and can loosen the normally tight seams that bind the cells to one another, allowing harmful leaking of blood proteins and fats into tissues or leaking of tissue substances into blood. More important, injured endothelial cells become activated and synthesize biological products that have an important effect on the smooth muscle cells of the media.

The hallmark change of hypertensive injury is *intimal thickening* (Fig. 8.6). Endothelial chemical mediators stimulate the proliferation and migration of media smooth muscle cells, which accumulate in the subendothelial space and lose their ability to contract. They also synthesize scar-like accumulations of collagen, elastin, and other extracellular substances.

The Cause of Most Hypertension Is Unknown

The specific cause of about 95% of hypertension is unknown; that is, no underlying disease or condition can be blamed. These patients are classified as having **primary hypertension**. Nevertheless, much is known about its characteristics.

Case Notes

8.5 Other than stroke, name two other conditions from which a patient like Leon might have died.

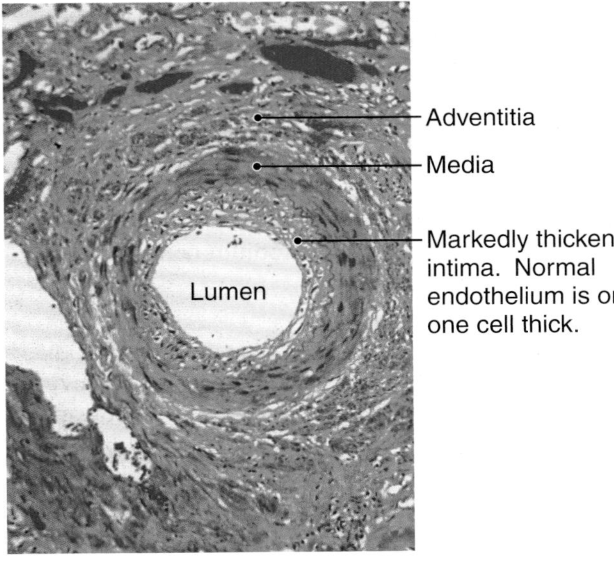

Figure 8.6 **Intimal thickening.** Intimal thickening is the hallmark indicator of hypertensive endothelial injury.

Genetic factors are important. The concordance rate in identical twins is high, and some ethnic groups are at greater risk. African Americans are twice as affected as Caucasians, and at any given level of blood pressure, are more vulnerable than Caucasians to complications such as stroke, heart attack, and kidney damage.

We also know that *the kidney plays a starring role*. For example, animal renal transplant experiments show that if a kidney from a hypertensive animal is transplanted into a normotensive animal, the normotensive animal will become hypertensive; that is, "Hypertension travels with the kidney."

High dietary sodium intake is especially associated with increased prevalence of hypertension, and dietary sodium restriction is effective in reducing hypertension of any type. Sodium balance is a function of the kidney and is important because of sodium's role as a solute. Retained sodium expands total blood volume because water follows solute. In excess of 99% of sodium passes from plasma into the glomerular filtrate and is returned to plasma as renal tubules reabsorb it. In 24 hours, this amounts to more than a pound of sodium. Even a small aberration of sodium balance can result in significant sodium retention. It appears that the final common pathway linking sodium to primary hypertension is reduced renal sodium excretion (increased sodium retention). This appears to increase blood volume and cardiac output and to cause peripheral vasoconstriction, all of which increase blood pressure. The body's internal blood pressure "thermostat" then appears to reset and higher pressure becomes "normal."

Case Notes

8.6 Is Leon's primary hypertension associated with increased or decreased total blood volume?

Stress, obesity, smoking, and lack of exercise are environmental factors that also have been implicated in the development of primary hypertension.

Case Notes

8.7 We know nothing of Leon's diet. Was it likely to have high or low sodium content?

In summary, primary hypertension is a complex disorder that features interplay between genetic and environmental factors. Patients with primary hypertension appear to have increased blood volume and increased peripheral resistance. Normally, if short-term dietary sodium intake increases and blood pressure rises, renal homeostatic mechanisms excrete sodium to lower blood pressure. In patients with primary hypertension, however, genetic mechanisms diminish this adaptive response and leaves them hypertensive.

Case Notes

8.8 Name several of Leon's known hypertension risk factors.

A Few Cases of Hypertension Can Be Linked to Specific Causes

Of the 5% of patients who are hypertensive due to an underlying disease (**secondary hypertension**), most have renal disease. One cause is stenosis of a renal artery, usually due to atherosclerosis. Blood pressure falls downstream of the stenosis, so that renal blood pressure is lower than systemic. The lower renal pressure stimulates release of renin, which raises blood pressure throughout the body. Other causes of secondary hypertension include chronic renal failure and renal tumors that secrete renin. Secondary hypertension can also be induced by steroid hormone excess (*Cushing syndrome*, Chapter 14) because steroids promote sodium and water retention and expanded blood volume. The most common cause of Cushing syndrome is medical steroid therapy; other causes include adrenocortical hyperplasia or tumor. Adrenal medullary tumors may secrete epinephrine or norepinephrine, which increase blood pressure because of increased peripheral resistance due to systemic vasoconstriction.

Hypertension Damages Arteries and Organs

The ill effect of hypertension is directly related to blood pressure. Even slight long-term increases have an adverse effect on vascular and organ health and can lead to increases in illness and death. About 25% of people in the general population are hypertensive. By age 60, about 60% of the U.S. population is hypertensive.

Hypertension is a key risk factor for atherosclerosis and plays a role in many other conditions—particularly cardiac hypertrophy, heart failure, and renal failure. Perhaps the most sinister aspect of hypertension is that it is asymptomatic until organ dysfunction is severe, after which full recovery may not be possible. Without treatment, about half of patients with hypertension will die of coronary artery disease (CAD) or congestive heart failure, and another third will die of stroke.

Early hypertension remains silent even as pathologic changes develop. Hypertension initiates and accelerates atherosclerosis (discussed below) and increases the risk of stroke, renal failure, CAD, heart attack, aortic aneurysm, and aortic dissection (discussed shortly). Severe hypertension may cause retinal hemorrhages and exudates (**hypertensive retinopathy**), which can impair vision. Because of increased ventricular strain, the left ventricle gradually hypertrophies and dilates. Heart failure and dilated cardiomyopathy (Chapter 9) may supervene.

Remember This! Hypertension is silent until complications occur.

Hypertension also causes distinctive arteriolar degenerative lesions, called *arteriolosclerosis*, in the walls of small blood vessels in the kidney. **Hyaline arteriolosclerosis** is the fingerprint of hypertension. It features narrowing of the arteriolar lumen and waxy (*hyaline*) degenerative changes of the arteriolar wall (Fig. 8.7). The accumulation of these lesions is the cause of *nephrosclerosis*, ordinarily an

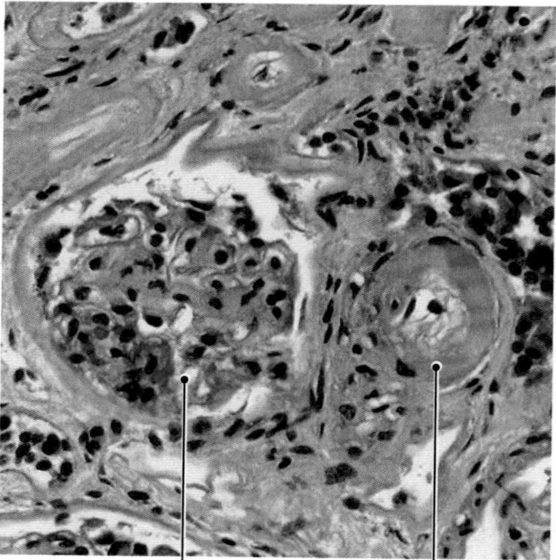

Figure 8.7 **Hyaline arteriolosclerosis.** In this lesion of benign nephrosclerosis, the waxy, red change in the afferent arteriole (hyaline arteriolosclerosis) and atrophy of the nearby glomerulus are characteristic.

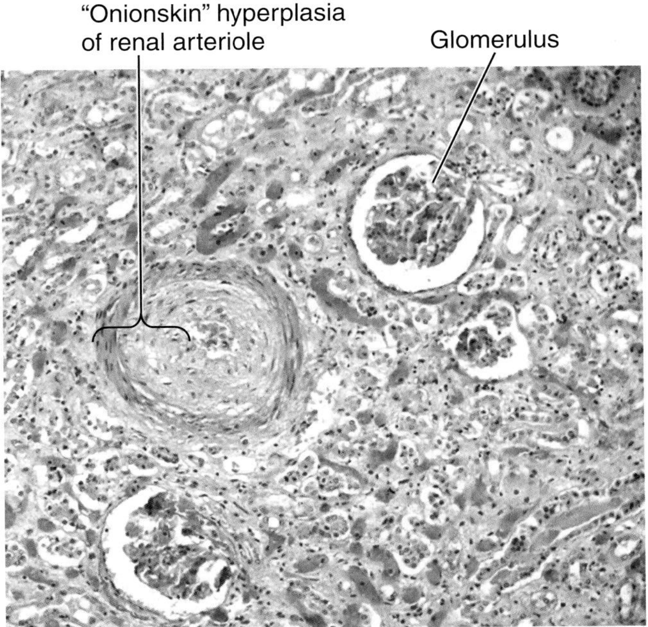

Figure 8.8 **Hyperplastic arteriolosclerosis.** Renal arteriole in severe chronic hypertension.

age-related degenerative kidney disease of the elderly, but one that may occur much earlier in hypertension. Identical changes may occur in the kidneys of the elderly or in the small vessels in multiple organs of patients with diabetes (*diabetic microangiopathy*, Chapter 13). **Hyperplastic arteriolosclerosis** occurs in severe hypertension. It is characterized by concentric layers of hyperplastic cells in the arteriolar wall (onionskin hyperplasia, Fig. 8.8). It is most often seen in the kidney in severe systemic hypertension.

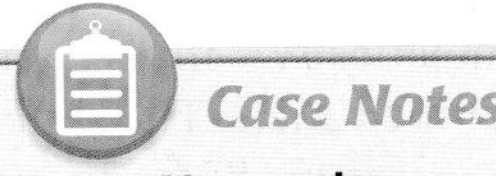
Case Notes

8.9 **Name the renal lesion in Leon's kidneys.**

Diet and Drug Treatment is Usually Effective

It is worth saying once more: hypertension is asymptomatic—symptoms appear only when vascular or organ damage is severe enough to become symptomatic. Diagnosis of hypertension is by sphygmomanometry. Multiple measurements are required to confirm the diagnosis. After the diagnosis is confirmed, causes of secondary hypertension must be ruled out before settling on a diagnosis of primary hypertension. Renal function in particular must be evaluated carefully by urinalysis and standard blood tests. If renal function is impaired, further investigation is mandatory. If blood pressure is exceptionally high or labile, the patient should be investigated for *pheochromocytoma*, an adrenal medullary tumor that secretes epinephrine and norepinephrine. Cardiac evaluation begins with a standard electrocardiogram. If left ventricular hypertrophy is present, echocardiographic imaging may be indicated. Ophthalmoscopy should be performed to check for hypertensive changes to the retina.

Laboratory findings in hypertension vary according to the cause and degree of renal involvement. Patients with early primary hypertension usually have no laboratory abnormalities. Study of blood renin levels is not helpful in most cases. Patients with significant renal disease may have blood or protein in the urine and increased levels of blood urea nitrogen (BUN) and creatinine, waste products eliminated by the kidneys.

General treatment includes weight loss, exercise, cessation of smoking, reduction of alcohol intake if excessive, and dietary salt restriction. Findings by the National Heart, Lung, and Blood Institute (NHLBI) showed that blood pressure was reduced with a diet that is low in saturated fat, cholesterol, and total fat and that is rich in fruits, vegetables, fat-free or low-fat milk and milk products, whole grain products, fish, poultry, and nuts. Such a diet is reduced in lean red meat, sweets, added sugars, and sugary beverages compared to the typical American diet. If these methods fail—and they frequently do because they are a lifestyle change—drug therapy is required.

Drug treatment should be initiated immediately for Stage 2 hypertension. Thiazide-type diuretics are a mainstay of treatment. They are safe, cheap, and effective, especially in people under age 60 and in African Americans. If thiazides fail to achieve control, many other drug options, too numerous to discuss here, are available. Multiple drugs may be required.

Blood pressure control is effective in limiting adverse consequences. Control may be difficult to achieve, however, and may require subspecialist supervision. Treatment should aim to reduce BP to <140/90 mm Hg. If systolic BP remains >140 mm Hg or diastolic BP remains >90 mm Hg after six months of lifestyle modifications, drugs are required.

Case Notes

8.10 **When the physician measured Leon's blood pressure, did the first Korotkoff sound signal systolic or diastolic pressure?**

Pop Quiz

8.9 True or false? Intimal thickening is a hallmark of vascular injury that occurs as a response to chronic injury of the endothelium.

8.10 True or false? Hyperplastic arteriolosclerosis occurs in long-term low-level hypertension.

8.11 Why do you suppose it is often challenging to maintain patients on hypertension medications?

8.12 Many patients are anxious when waiting to see the doctor and find it a stressful experience. Will this influence the patient's blood pressure?

8.13 What percent of people with hypertension have an unknown cause (primary hypertension)?

8.14 What ancillary findings on blood or urine analyses might support a diagnosis of hypertension?

8.15 A patient has a blood pressure of 135/80 on multiple visits to the doctor. Does she have hypertension?

Atherosclerosis

The terms *atherosclerosis* and *arteriosclerosis* are related and often confused. **Arteriosclerosis** literally means "hardening of the arteries." It is not widely used in daily medical practice, but is useful in an academic sense to classify certain diseases of arteries and arterioles. The three varieties of arteriosclerosis are the following:

- *Arteriolosclerosis*, discussed above as a consequence of hypertension, is a disease of *small* arteries and arterioles caused by hypertension and a few other conditions.
- *Mönckeberg medial sclerosis* features marked calcification of the media in the large arteries of patients over age 50. It is seldom the cause of clinical problems.
- *Atherosclerosis* is discussed next.

Atherosclerosis is a lifestyle disease associated with an unhealthful diet, obesity, smoking, and lack of exercise; it is characterized by fatty deposits in the arterial wall. The term derives from the Greek *athero* (gruel or thick soup) for the fatty, soft character of the fatty portion of the deposits; and *scleros* (hard), for the dense scar tissue that develops in and around the fatty deposits. The basic lesion of atherosclerosis is the **atheroma**, a fatty deposit in the arterial wall. Atheromas tend to obstruct arterial blood flow and cause hypoxia and death of downstream tissue (*ischemia* and *infarction*, Chapter 2) by hampering the swift, smooth flow of blood. Atheromas also weaken the arterial wall, causing dilation (aneurysm) and increasing the risk of arterial rupture and hemorrhage. Atherosclerosis accounts for about one-third of deaths in the industrialized world.

Atherosclerosis Is Associated with Risk Factors

The main risk of atherosclerosis is *coronary artery disease (CAD)*, which develops as a consequence of coronary atherosclerosis (Chapter 9). CAD is omnipresent in the industrialized West, but rare in Asia, Africa, and South America. Cultural influence is strong: immigrants from nations with low CAD risk soon assume the local risk when they move to a country with high CAD risk. The presence of multiple factors in a single person has a multiplier effect: two risk factors increases risk fourfold; three factors increase risk sevenfold.

Non-Controllable Risk Factors

There are some major risk factors over which the patient has no control.

- *Age*. Atherosclerosis begins in the crib. Autopsy evidence of people in their 20s who die of violence demonstrates that the majority have atherosclerosis. About one in five has more than 50% narrowing of one coronary artery. Atherosclerosis risk increases fivefold between ages 40 and 60, and continues to rise with each decade thereafter. As age-related risk increases, the risks from hypertension, smoking, high cholesterol, and other risk factors discussed below become relatively less important. Nevertheless, it remains important to pay attention to these and other risk factors regardless of patient age.
- *Gender*. Premenopausal women have fewer atherosclerosis events than men of comparable age. Nevertheless, after menopause the prevalence of atherosclerosis in women rises dramatically—in the very elderly, women have more CAD than men. The difference is presumed to be due to estrogen, but estrogen replacement therapy in postmenopausal women has not shown consistent risk reduction.
- *Genetics*. Family history is the strongest uncontrollable factor. Families with clear multigenerational risk usually display other risk factors as well, such as diabetes and hypertension.
- *Vascular inflammation*. Inflammation is a key element in the pathogenesis of atherosclerosis. In the absence of known inflammation anywhere else—an infection or arthritis, for example—it can be safely assumed that laboratory evidence of inflammation is due to vascular inflammation. The most valuable marker of systemic inflammation is **C-reactive protein (CRP)**, a substance made by the liver in response to inflammation anywhere in the body. The relationship between the development of atherosclerosis and increased levels of plasma CRP is striking. Studies show that an increased level of CRP is an independent risk factor for

atherosclerosis; that is to say, patients with an increased CRP level have an increased risk for heart attack, stroke, and other atherosclerosis complications even if all other risk factors (e.g., blood pressure, cholesterol) are normal. Studies are ongoing to determine whether or not CRP is causally related or just a marker for atherosclerosis.

Remember This! Atherosclerosis begins in the crib and progresses with age.

Case Notes

8.11 **Which were the particular noncontrollable risk factors in Leon's case?**

Controllable Risk Factors

By modifying behavior, the patient can exert substantial influence on the factors listed below. Nevertheless, roughly 20% of atherosclerotic complications occur in patients who have none of the following risk factors.

- *High blood lipids (hyperlipidemia).* LDL-cholesterol is especially important because high levels promote atherosclerosis. Diet has a major influence on LDL-C, which is increased by consumption of foods high in **saturated fats** (e.g., butter, cheese, beef, bacon, and other animal fats). A second source of LDL-C is ingested cholesterol from cholesterol-rich foods (e.g., egg yolks, shellfish), but it is minor compared to dietary animal fat. A third dietary source of saturated fat is **trans fats** (transformed fats), which are saturated fats produced by artificially *trans*forming unsaturated oils into animal-like saturated fats. Until recently, trans fats were widely used in the food industry (e.g., in baked goods, margarines, and deep-fried fast or frozen foods). Public objection has resulted in a great decline in trans fat usage. Plant oils (e.g., canola oil, olive oil) and fish oils (e.g., omega-3)are low in saturated fat and much healthier. Diets rich in plant and fish oils are associated with a lower atherosclerotic risk. *Statin drugs* are very effective in lowering LDL-C.

  On the other hand, a *high* level of HDL-cholesterol (HDL-C) is associated with *less* risk of atherosclerosis. HDL-C is not as easily influenced as LDL-C. Moderate alcohol consumption and exercise increase it; smoking and obesity reduce it. With new evidence that high HDL may only be a marker, not a cause, it is now questionable if effort should be made to raise HDL. People should exercise, lose weight, stop smoking and change destructive lifestyle habits, but not because it will raise HDL.
- *Hypertension.* Both systolic and diastolic pressures are important. Hypertension independently increases atherosclerotic risk about 50%.
- *Cigarette smoking.* Smoking one pack a day doubles the risk of CAD death. The younger the person, the more dangerous smoking is—smoking accounts for about 50% of coronary risk in people under 65, but only 15% of the coronary risk for people over 65. Cessation of smoking cuts smoking-related cardiovascular risk by 50% in one year.
- *Metabolic syndrome.* The metabolic syndrome (Chapter 23) features a number of characteristics linked to *insulin-resistance*: abnormal glucose metabolism, abdominal obesity, abnormal blood lipids, and hypertension.
- *Diabetic hyperglycemia.* As is discussed in Chapter 13, diabetes accelerates atherosclerosis. Ninety percent of diabetes is type 2, the variety that occurs in overweight or obese people. So, to the extent that these patients could have controlled their weight, they might have been able to avoid diabetes. And inasmuch as the vascular pathology of diabetes is directly related to the degree of hyperglycemia, diabetics who are fastidious about controlling their blood glucose suffer less vascular disease than those who are less diligent.
- *Additional factors.* Atherosclerotic risk is increased by *lack of exercise*, *obesity*, and *stress*.

Case Notes

8.12 **Name the particular controllable risk factors in Leon's case.**

8.13 **We do not know Leon's CRP. But was it likely low or high?**

Remember This! Atherosclerosis is accelerated by lifestyle: diet, obesity, smoking, and lack of exercise are key factors.

The Pathogenesis of Atherosclerosis Is Clear

Atherosclerosis begins with subtle, nonlethal damage to endothelial cells (Fig. 8.9). The major culprit is abnormal blood lipid concentration, especially increased LDL-C. Cigarette smoke, high blood glucose, and hypertension are also damaging. Other factors may also play a role. For example, abnormally high blood uric acid or blood homocysteine (an amino acid) and intravenous drug use are known to injure endothelium, but these factors are not important in most instances.

There is some evidence that infection of the vascular wall may be an early cause of endothelial damage. Various viruses and *Chlamydia* have been detected in atheromas, but not in normal vessels.

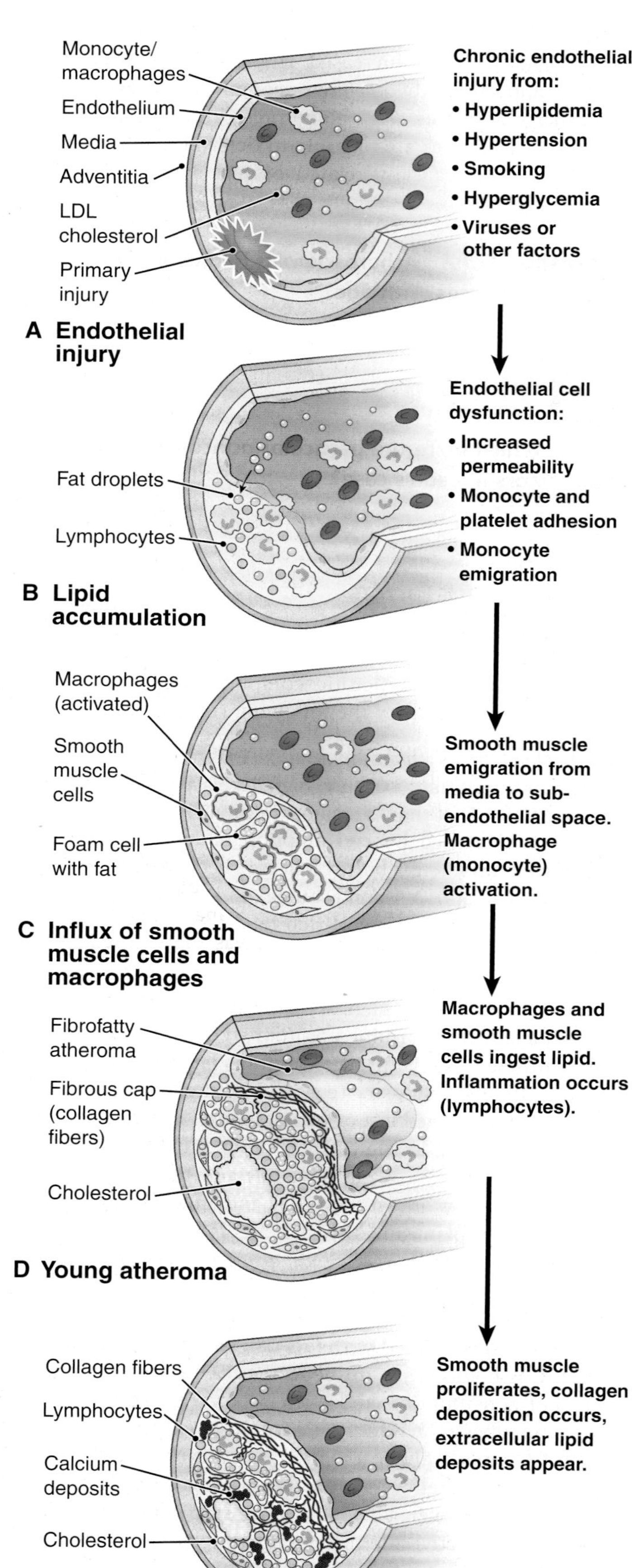

Figure 8.9 **Formation of an atheroma. A.** Subtle injury to intact endothelium. **B.** LDL cholesterol and other lipids "leak" into the site across damaged endothelium. Macrophages invade and phagocytize the lipids. **C.** The atheroma grows as smooth muscle cells invade and evolve into fibroblasts and phagocytes. Lymphocytes and other inflammatory cells appear. Cells with phagocytized fat appear as foam cells. **D.** Further accumulation of fat, foam cells, inflammatory cells, and migrating, evolving smooth muscle cells form an unstable, soft, young atheroma prone to ulceration, hemorrhage, thrombosis, and sudden vascular occlusion. **E.** Fibrosis (scarring) and chronic inflammation produce a hard, sometimes calcified, old, stable atheroma.

Atherosclerosis Has Distinct Vascular Pathology

Normal endothelium is smooth and pink (Fig. 8.10A). The earliest visible change of atherosclerosis is microscopic accumulation of lipid (mainly cholesterol) deposits in the arterial wall immediately beneath endothelial cells, evidence that damaged endothelium has become "leaky" and has lost its ability to prevent passage of cholesterol into the arterial wall. With time, grossly visible, flat, yellow fatty streaks appear. Damaged endothelial cells become "sticky" due to release of inflammatory mediators. Neutrophils, macrophages, and platelets attach to them and invade the wall of the vessel. Macrophages engulf (phagocytize) the lipid to become foam cells. Later, local factors stimulate proliferation and migration of media smooth muscle cells, which invade the site and produce collagen and other extracellular matrix, and the atheroma grows. These early, soft atheromas are obstructive and induce turbulent blood flow. Turbulence in turn causes further endothelial damage and acceleration of atheroma development.

These initial lesions evolve into advanced atherosclerosis (Fig. 8.10B), which are microscopically a mixture of fat, fibrous tissue, macrophages, and a sprinkling of lymphocytes. The result is a rough, stiff, caked appearance to the endothelial lining. Atheromas may occur anywhere, but they are most common in (in descending order) the lower abdominal aorta, coronary arteries, popliteal arteries in the back of the knee, descending thoracic aorta, internal carotid arteries in the neck, and the circle of Willis at the base of the brain. Atheromas grow slowly, gradually choking blood flow; but they can crack or ulcerate, initiating instant thrombosis or intra-atheroma hemorrhage, either of which can produce sudden vascular occlusion and infarction of downstream myocardial muscle.

Atheromas change with time. Young atheromas are soft, with a mealy, semisolid consistency, and are the most dangerous because they are prone to cause sudden thrombosis and occlusion, and the infarction of downstream tissue. On the other hand, old lesions contain much less fat and have an abundance of hard scar tissue and calcium, hence the common practice of calling atherosclerosis "hardening of the arteries."

Weakening of the arterial wall can allow bulges (*aneurysms*), which are less common than are complications from blocked blood flow. Aneurysms occur most commonly in the abdominal aorta and may become caked with thick layers of old thrombus material (Chapter 6).

Case Notes

8.14 **Name some factors that damaged Leon's endothelial cells.**

Obstructed Blood Flow Is the Cause of Most Atherosclerotic Complications

For most of their existence, atheromas are silent and subclinical. Figure 8.11 illustrates that atheromas enlarge over the decades until they become symptomatic, usually by acute or chronic obstruction of blood flow, which usually causes ischemia or infarction of downstream tissue. Less commonly, the weakened wall of a diseased vessel balloons into an aneurysm. The most common clinical consequences of atherosclerosis are (in descending order) heart attack (*myocardial infarction*, Chapter 9) due to CAD, *stroke (cerebral infarction)* from carotid or intracranial disease, *aortic aneurysm*, and *peripheral vascular disease*.

Case Notes

8.15 **Leon had an old scar from a prior myocardial infarct in the distribution of the anterior descending coronary artery, which was severely atherosclerotic. How did the atherosclerosis cause the infarct?**

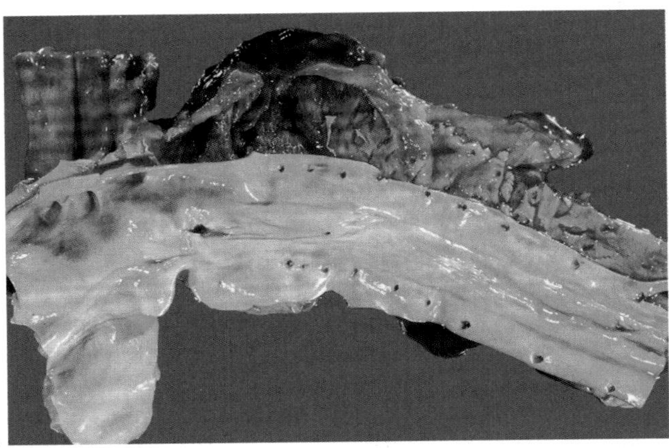

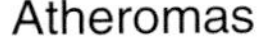

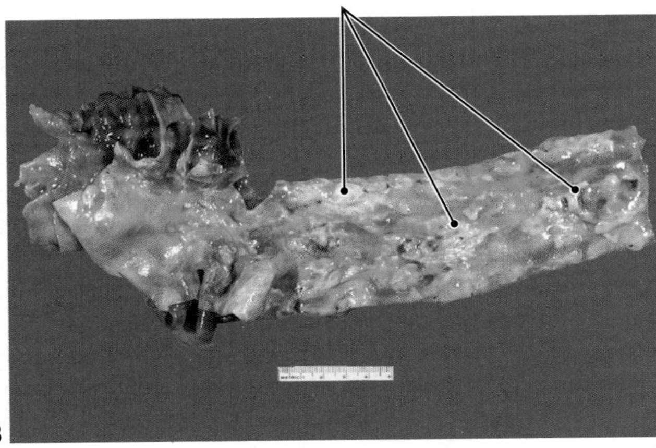

Figure 8.10 **Atherosclerosis of the aorta. A.** The normal aorta. **B.** Severe atherosclerosis.

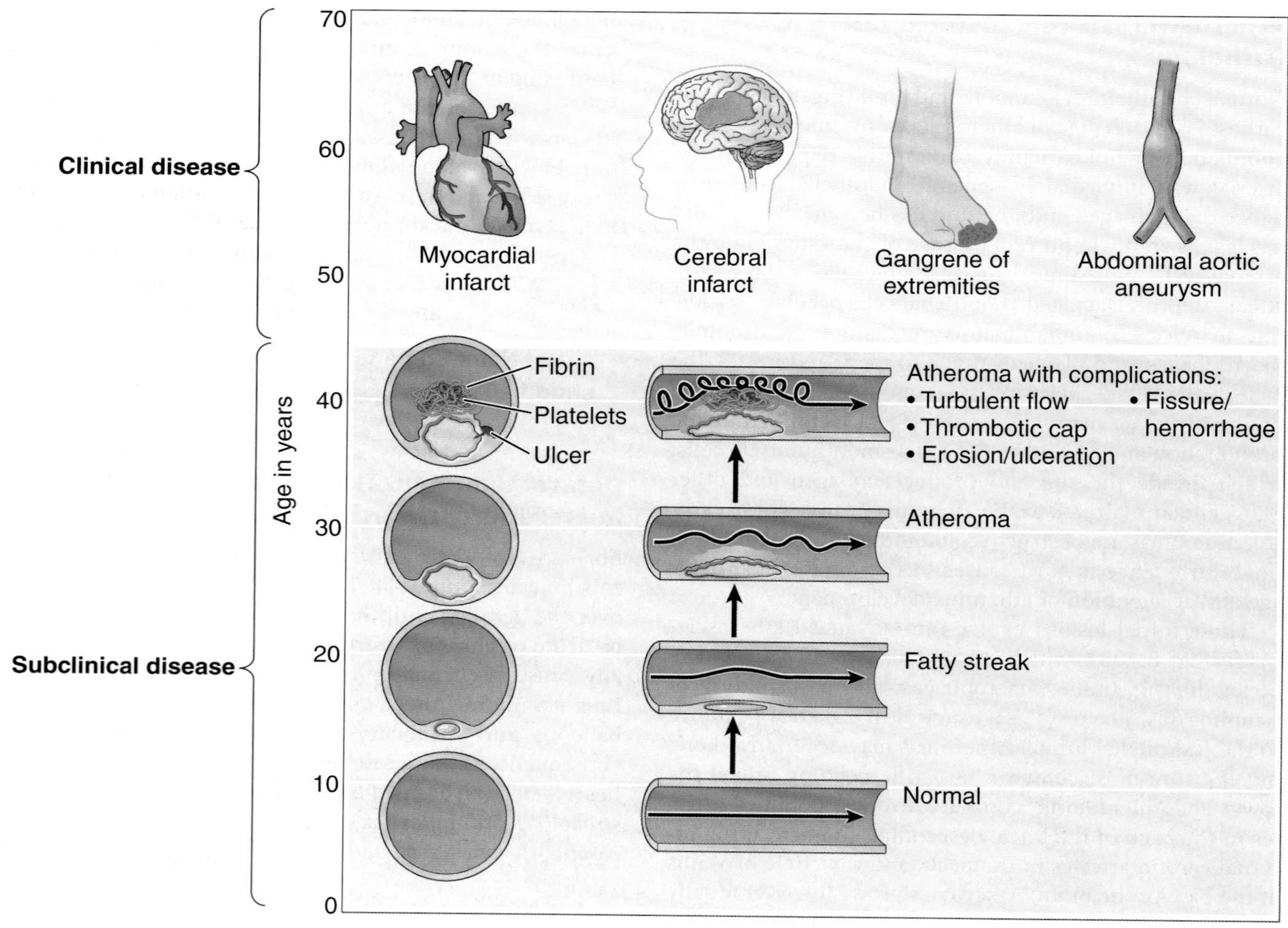

Figure 8.11 **Blood flow and the progression of atherosclerosis.**

Gradual **stenosis** is the result of slow atheroma growth. An atheroma must grow to obstruct about 70% of vessel cross-sectional area before causing clinical symptoms as a result of impaired flow. Downstream ischemia in coronary disease produces a signature type of cardiac pain and chest discomfort called *angina*. Brain ischemia may produce temporary neurologic problems (*temporary ischemic attack, TIA*), and ischemia in the legs produces cramps with exercise (*intermittent claudication*). Chronic ischemia takes its toll and may produce gradual atrophy and dysfunction. In the heart, this usually appears as heart failure; in the brain, it may cause dementia or other chronic brain disease.

Early atheromas are unstable and especially dangerous because plaque erosion, ulceration, fissuring, or rupture exposes blood to tissue factors (Chapter 6), which can cause thrombosis and complete vessel occlusion and infarction of downstream tissue. Acute occlusion can also be caused by hemorrhage into a plaque, which expands its volume. By contrast, old atherosclerosis lesions tend to be hard, scarred, calcified, and sealed with a fibrous cap. They impede blood flow gradually, producing progressive downstream ischemia, but they are usually stable and not commonly the cause of acute thrombosis and infarction. If rupture of the fibrous cap occurs, however, the contents of the atheroma can spill into the vessel and cause thrombosis.

The Best Treatment Is Prevention

Atherosclerosis is epidemic in the United States and other developed nations. Despite public health campaigns, many people are unwilling to stop smoking, lose weight, eat less animal and saturated fat, increase their intake of healthy plant and fish oils, control their blood pressure by reducing dietary salt, and exercise regularly. But these preventive behaviors do work, lowering plasma LDL-C, which in turn reduces the incidence of atherosclerosis and its complications. The effect is incremental—a 10% reduction of LDL-C is not as effective as 20%, and so on.

Until now, most treatment efforts have been reparative—surgery to bypass or reopen clogged arteries, and drugs to aid failing hearts. Nevertheless, emphasis on maintaining desirable plasma lipid levels shows promise of preventing atherosclerosis.

A desirable LDL-C level is <100 mg/dL, but as with total cholesterol, lower is better: evidence suggests that people are likely to benefit further by lowering LDL-C levels below 80 mg/dL, and studies suggest that atherosclerosis does not occur in people with LDL-C levels about 50-60 mg/dL. Remembering that HDL-C may only be a marker, not a cause of atherosclerosis, HDL-C above 60 mg/dL is not associated with increased cardiovascular risk. Values less than 40 mg/dL are associated with high atherosclerosis risk. Until further evidence accumulates, however, it is doubtful if it is worthwhile to try to raise low HDL. (For further information, see *Molecular Medicine*, "A Tale of Two Sources of Cholesterol.")

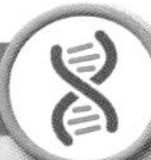

Molecular Medicine

A TALE OF TWO SOURCES OF CHOLESTEROL

Traditionally, the two major influences on the cholesterol in your body are said to be "food and family." It is true that genetics and the environment do determine your blood levels of cholesterol, but more accurately, your body acquires cholesterol either from the diet (by absorbing it from the intestine) or by synthesizing it (in the liver). These two sources of cholesterol require different drugs to treat high cholesterol. Statin drugs target liver synthesis of cholesterol by inhibiting an enzyme (HMG-CoA-reductase) in the cholesterol synthesis pathway. A newer drug, ezetimibe, blocks the molecular transporter in the small intestine that is responsible for absorbing dietary cholesterol.

Case Notes

8.16 Which should Leon have done, try to lower LDL-C or raise HDL-C?

Statin drugs block a liver enzyme important in cholesterol synthesis and have proven very effective in lowering levels of LDL-C, total cholesterol, and the incidence of atherosclerotic vascular disease and death. Nevertheless, good as they are, statins cannot lower cholesterol to optimal levels in all treated people. Other drugs are proving effective by inhibiting cholesterol absorption in the bowel.

If prevention fails and atherosclerosis becomes too advanced or causes symptoms, then surgical or "intraluminal" intervention may be necessary to repair, unblock, or bypass damaged arteries or the thrombi. Cardiac artery bypass grafting (Fig. 8.12) involves surgery to graft veins or arteries between the aorta and coronary arteries beyond the point of obstruction. Cardiac catheterization (Fig. 8.13) involves threading a catheter into the coronary artery, usually with the aim of inserting an expandable mesh tube (stent) to enlarge the narrowed area and keep it open.

For acute ischemia due to partial obstruction, aspirin or other antithrombotics may be helpful to forestall thrombosis. For acute, complete thrombotic obstruction, thrombolytic drugs may dissolve the thrombus and avoid infarction or at least reduce the size of the infarct by reestablishing perfusion. Cardiac catheterization may be employed to extract or break up the thrombus or deliver thrombolytic therapy to the site of occlusion.

Case Notes

8.17 On a follow-up visit, Leon's cholesterol was said to be "much improved." What is the most likely explanation?

Pop Quiz

8.16 True or false? Noncontrollable risk factors are more likely to change with lifestyle modifications.

8.17 True or false? Atherosclerosis is one of the three varieties of arteriosclerosis.

8.18 List controllable risk factors for atherosclerosis.

8.19 List noncontrollable risk factors for atherosclerosis.

8.20 What are some of the complications of atherosclerotic disease?

Aneurysms and Dissections

An **aneurysm** is a localized dilation of an artery or heart chamber, usually owing to a weakness of the wall. Aneurysms may be congenital or acquired. Atherosclerosis and hypertension are the most common causes. Rarely, an aneurysm may be the result of local infection (mycotic aneurysm), late stage syphilis (syphilitic aneurysm, Chapter 4), or congenital defect, or it may occur consequent to aortic injury from frontal chest trauma, as in a steering wheel injury in an auto accident. Left ventricular aneurysms may occur at the site of an old, healed myocardial infarction. These conditions weaken the wall, which balloons outward because of intravascular pressure; most are elongated swellings (fusiform aneurysms), but some are saccular, especially those of intracranial arteries (*berry aneurysms*, Chapter 19).

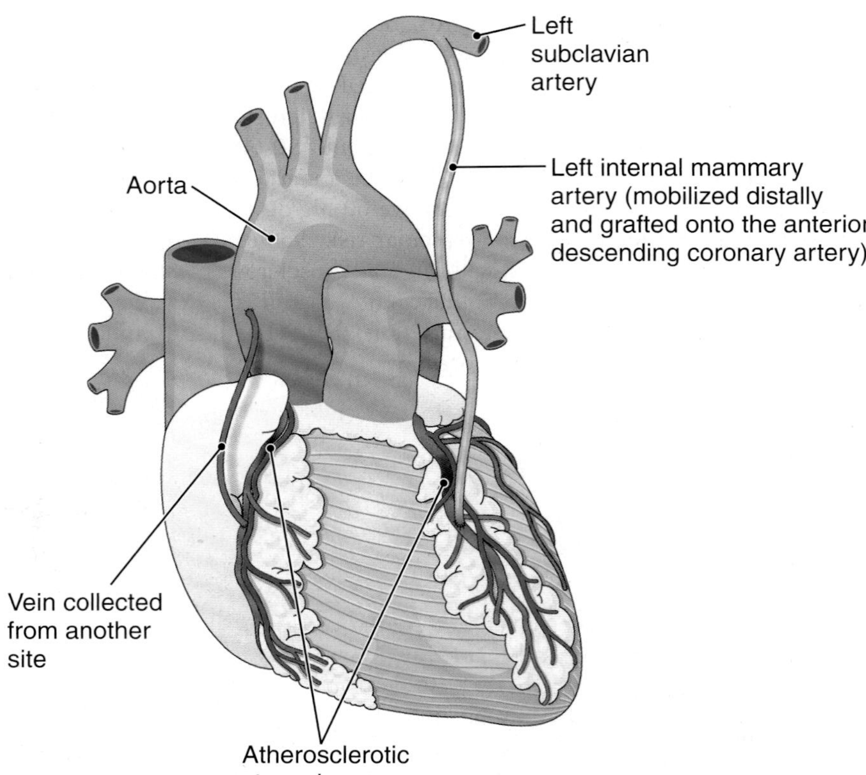

Figure 8.12 **Coronary Bypass Grafting.**

The abdominal aorta is the most common site of an atherosclerotic aneurysm (Fig. 8.14). *Abdominal aortic aneurysms (AAA)* usually occur below the renal arteries in male smokers over age 50 who have severe aortic atherosclerosis. Most AAAs grow slowly, a few millimeters each year, and become more dangerous as they enlarge. They are usually asymptomatic until complication occurs. The most feared complication is rupture, because it is often fatal. More commonly, however, AAAs develop thrombi on the internal wall (*mural thrombi*, Fig. 8.15), which may embolize into the arteries of the legs or intestines, where they can produce ischemia or gangrene.

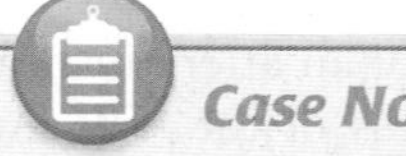

Case Notes

8.18 Name the risk factors for Leon's abdominal aortic aneurysm.

Thoracic aortic aneurysms are more often associated with hypertension and late syphilis (Chapter 4), though hereditary connective tissue defects are being increasingly recognized. Surgical replacement of the aneurysm by prosthesis is an effective treatment, but operative mortality is near 5%. Patients with small aneurysms can be safely followed by regular imaging to gauge size or detect the development of a thrombus.

Vascular dissection (dissecting hematoma) is a longitudinal tearing within the wall of an artery, most often the aorta, caused by blood that enters the wall through a defect in the lining, usually a tear or ulceration in an atheroma. Blood pulses into the wall and progresses (dissects) along tissue planes in the wall until it re-enters the main channel (rare) or exits externally (ruptures) with catastrophic hemorrhage. It usually affects older men with hypertension. In younger men the cause is often a hereditary connective tissue defect such as Marfan syndrome or Ehlers-Danlos syndrome. These and other such defects have a widespread effect on connective tissues, including the elastin and collagen in the aortic wall, which weaken the wall and allow blood to break in. Dissections produce severe, tearing chest and back pain. Some cause partial or complete occlusion of one of the great vessels, which may cause neurological symptoms or a difference in blood pressure between the right and left arms. Emergency surgery is necessary. The cause of death is usually rupture into the pericardium, pleural space, or abdominal cavity.

Pop Quiz

8.21 What are the two most common causes of an aneurysm?

8.22 What two genetic conditions can cause vascular dissection?

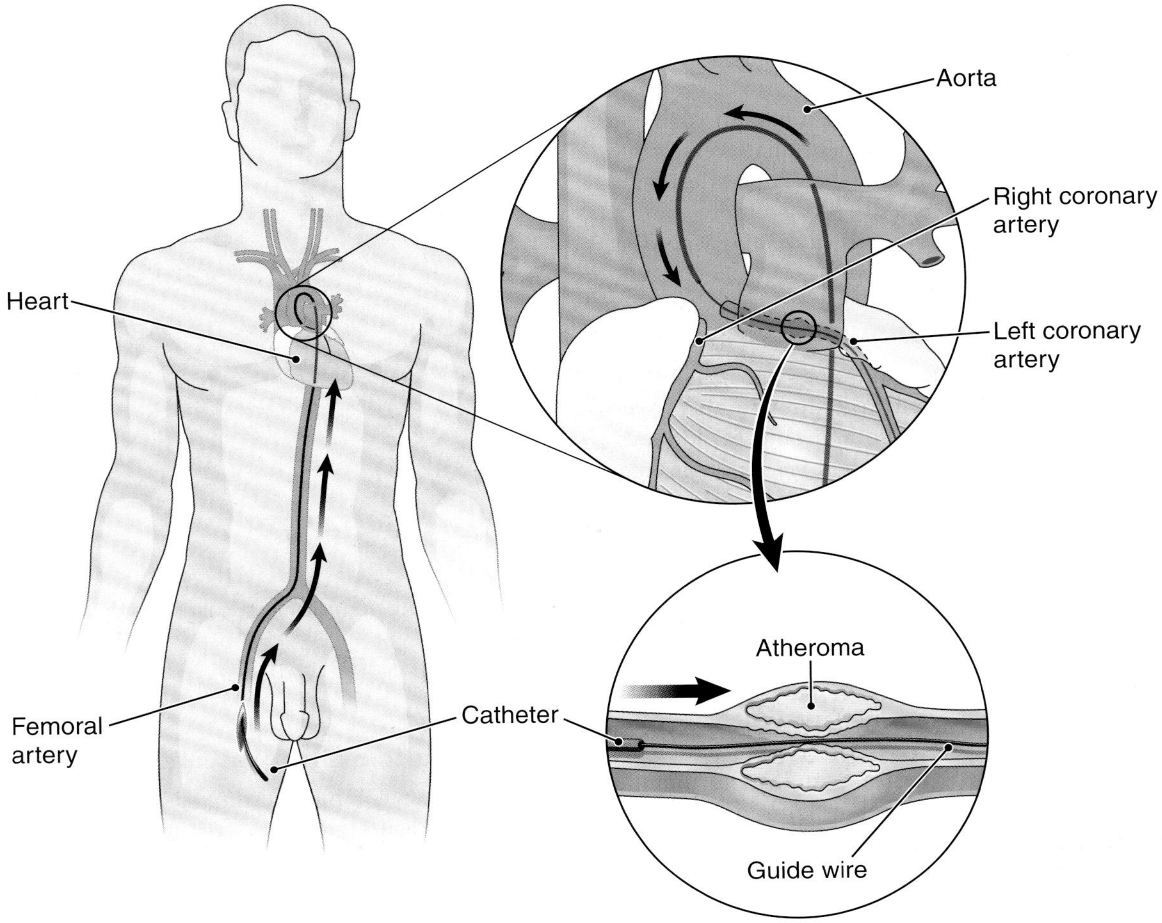

Figure 8.13 **Coronary catheterization.** Catheters are used for injecting radiographic contrast media to visualize lumen size, to establish improved flow removing atheromatous or thrombus material, or to force and hold open the lumen by insertion of a stent.

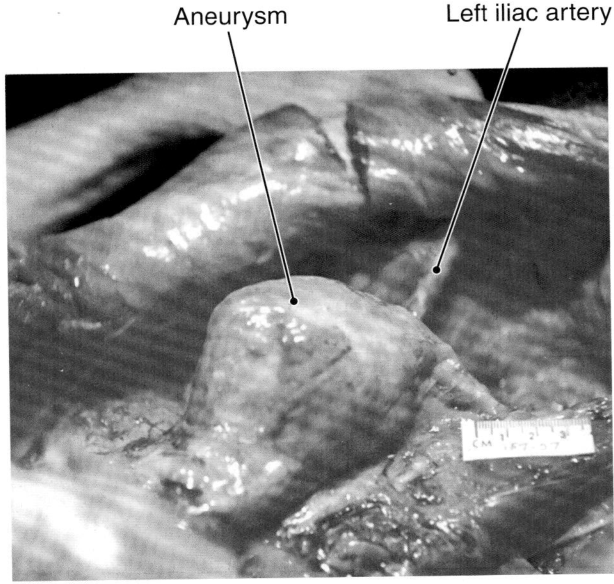

Figure 8.14 **Abdominal aortic aneurysm.** This photo was taken from above the right shoulder of the supine corpse.

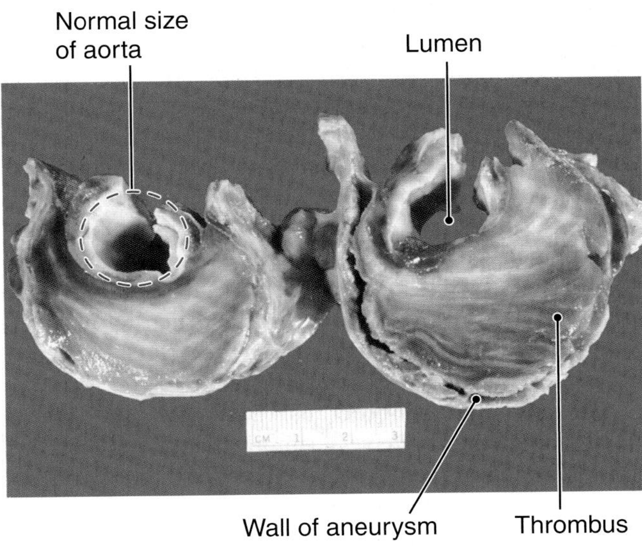

Figure 8.15 **Thrombus in an aortic aneurysm.** Layers of thrombus material fill most of the aneurysm.

Vasculitis

Vasculitis is a general term that applies to a group of uncommon diseases that feature inflammation of blood vessels, almost always arteries. When small vessels are involved, it may be called *angiitis*; when large arteries are involved, it may be called *arteritis*. Vasculitides can be classified as *autoimmune* or *infectious* (rare) and according to the size of vessel typically involved.

Most Vasculitis Is Autoimmune

Many autoimmune vasculitis syndromes are recognized, each characterized and named according to the tissue most severely affected (e.g., nose and sinuses, kidneys, aorta), and the size and type of blood vessel (large, medium, or small artery or vein).

Local Autoimmune Vasculitis

Although most autoimmune vasculitides are systemic, the most common one is a local vasculitis—**temporal arteritis** (*giant cell arteritis*). It is characterized by chronic granulomatous inflammation of large and medium-size arteries: the temporal and cranial arteries, including the carotids and ophthalmic arteries. The typical patient is a woman about age 70. Symptoms and signs include headaches, scalp tenderness, visual or neurological problems, and pain in jaw muscles during chewing. Fever is common. Erythrocyte sedimentation rate (ESR) and CRP are usually elevated. About 25% of cases occur in conjunction with a *polymyalgia rheumatica* (Chapter 18). Temporal arteritis is a medical emergency because of the risk of stroke and permanent blindness. Diagnosis is clinical and confirmed by temporal artery biopsy, which will show lymphocytes infiltrating the blood vessel wall. Treatment with high-dose steroids and aspirin is usually effective.

An example of large vessel vasculitis is **Takayasu arteritis**, which is characterized by granulomatous inflammation in the aorta and its main branches. It occurs mainly in women under 40. Pathologic features are similar to temporal arteritis. It is convenient to think of Takayasu as a different expression of temporal arteritis. The result is scarring of the aortic arch and fibrous obliteration of the main branches, which impairs blood flow to the head and arms. Diagnosis is clinical and by imaging studies of the great vessels. Drug therapy includes corticosteroids, immunosuppressives, and antihypertensives. Surgical vascular bypass of obstructed vessels may be required.

Thromboangiitis obliterans (*Buerger disease*) affects small- and medium-size vessels in the hands and feet. It is most common in young, heavy cigarette smokers and frequently leads to painful ulcers or gangrene of the fingers and toes. Prompt cessation of smoking usually results in dramatic improvement. Treatment may include amputation of the affected extremity.

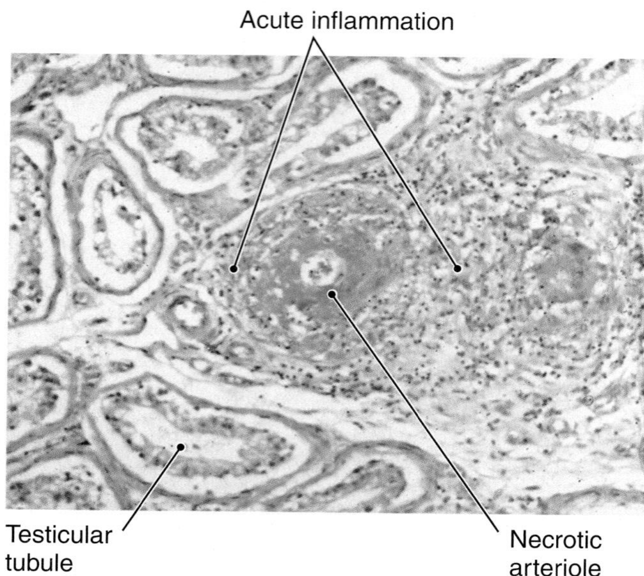

Figure 8.16 **Acute necrotizing vasculitis in a patient with polyarteritis nodosa.** This specimen is from a testicular biopsy in a patient with polyarteritis nodosa. The biopsy was performed to confirm a provisional clinical diagnosis.

Systemic Autoimmune Vasculitis

The four most common forms of systemic autoimmune vasculitis are as follows:

- **Polyarteritis nodosa** (Fig. 8.16) is a generalized autoimmune disease of small- and medium-size muscular arteries, which tends to affect the kidneys and abdominal viscera. It is typically a disease of young adults, but may occur in children or the elderly. Occasionally, it mainly affects skin. Some cases are etiologically linked to hepatitis B infection.
- **Kawasaki disease** is an important cause of acquired heart disease in children because of its predilection to affect coronary arteries. It is also known as *mucocutaneous lymph node syndrome* because it typically presents with fevers, conjunctivitis, oral ulcers, redness of palms and soles, rash, and lymphadenopathy. Treatment is high-dose aspirin and intravenous immunoglobulin, whereas other systemic autoimmune vasculitides may be treated with steroids (see below).
- **Microscopic polyangiitis** (*hypersensitivity vasculitis*) affects arterioles, capillaries, and venules. It can affect any tissue, but most cases feature involvement of renal glomeruli (glomerulonephritis) and pulmonary capillaries. It usually can be traced to reaction to a drug such as penicillin or to a bacterium such as streptococcus.
- **Wegener granulomatosis** is a vasculitis affecting small- to medium-size arteries in the nose, throat, sinuses, lungs, and kidneys of middle-aged men.

Apart from specific signs and symptoms related to the particular tissues involved, clinical manifestations of systemic autoimmune vasculitis are constitutional: malaise, fever, muscle aches, and joint pain. Standard treatment includes steroids and cyclophosphamide (an immunosuppressant- antineoplastic drug).

Remember This! Three of the most common diseases of humankind—atherosclerosis, hypertension, and diabetes—have their primary effect on arteries.

Infectious Vasculitis Is Rare

Infectious vasculitis is local and usually due to bacterial or fungal infection. It may represent the spread of nearby tissue infection to vessels, or it may represent hematogenous seeding of a vessel from infection elsewhere. Infection can weaken the vascular wall to create an aneurysm or it can induce thrombosis and infarction. For example, a major risk of *meningococcal meningitis* (Chapter 4) is inflammation and thrombosis of cerebral venous sinuses with infarction of the nearby brain tissue.

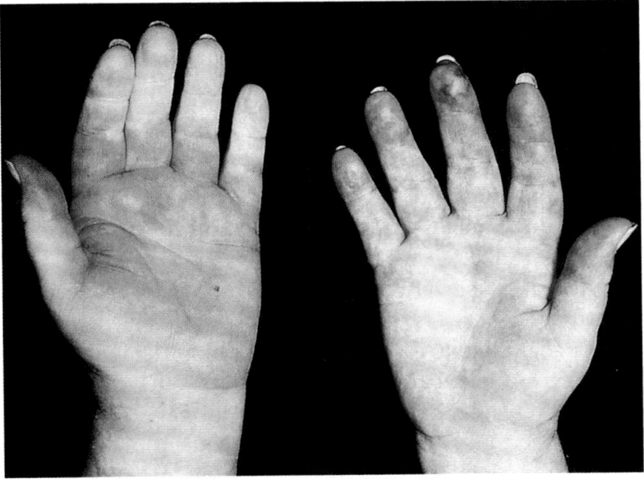

Figure 8.17 **Raynaud syndrome.** Red, white, or blue discoloration is the hallmark of Raynaud syndrome. (Reproduced with permission from Effeney, DJ, Stoney, RJ. *Wylie's Atlas of Vascular Surgery: Disorders of the Extremities.* Philadelphia, PA: Lippincott Williams & Wilkins; 1993.)

Pop Quiz

8.23 True or false? Most vasculitis is infectious in origin.

8.24 Which systemic autoimmune vasculitis is treated differently from the others?

8.25 Which vasculitis affects the small- to medium-size arteries in the nose, throat, sinuses, lungs, and kidneys of middle age men?

8.26 Which vasculitis is responsible for painful ulcers of the fingers and toes in a smoker?

Raynaud Syndrome

Raynaud syndrome is a common condition that results from exaggerated vasomotor reactivity in the small arteries and arterioles in the hands and fingers (Fig. 8.17). Occasionally, the nose, earlobe, or lips may be affected. The trigger is usually cold or emotional stress. Nicotine use may be a factor. No pathologic lesion is present; that is, the condition is purely functional. Women are affected far more often than men. Typically one or more fingers blanch at the tip when exposed to cold, after which the fingers may then turn blue (cyanotic). The part may become numb, but pain is uncommon. When rewarmed, the part becomes flushed with blood (hyperemic).

When no underlying disease can be found, the condition is called *primary* Raynaud syndrome, which accounts for over 80% of patients. When an underlying cause is found, the condition is *secondary* Raynaud syndrome, most of which occurs in conjunction with autoimmune diseases. For example, 80% of patients with systemic sclerosis and 20% with systemic lupus erythematosus (SLE) have secondary Raynaud syndrome.

Diagnosis is clinical. Autoimmune disease should be ruled out by ESR to detect hidden inflammation, plus rheumatoid factor, and antinuclear antibody test for SLE.

Treatment is to avoid triggers, especially smoking. Vasodilator drugs may be helpful.

Pop Quiz

8.27 True or false? Raynaud syndrome is usually associated with autoimmune disease.

Diseases of Veins

Among diseases of the veins, varicose veins and thrombophlebitis are the most common.

Varicose veins are abnormally dilated veins due to incompetent venous valves that owe to age-related relaxation of supporting tissues. With time, the internal valves of veins, which ordinarily prevent downward backflow and backpressure, become incompetent. As dilation progresses, the column of blood above the varicosity puts more hydrostatic pressure on the vein wall. Superficial veins are more often affected than deep ones because they are surrounded by less supporting tissue. Leg veins are most susceptible—hydrostatic pressure is greatest there because the column of blood is tallest between the lower leg and the heart. Most patients are over 50, obese, or have a career that requires them to stand for long periods of time. About 15% of men and 30% of women are affected. Because, however, the weight of the pregnant uterus increases pressure in the pelvic veins, reducing venous return, pregnant women—especially those who have had several pregnancies—are the population most commonly affected.

Ordinarily, leg varicosities are nothing more than an unsightly nuisance. The most common result is edema of the feet (pedal edema). In severe cases, blood stagnates and flow is insufficient to maintain proper tissue oxygen supply, which results in skin atrophy, inflammation (*stasis dermatitis*), and poor wound healing. In exceptionally severe cases, skin ulcers may occur. Thrombosis may occur, but, in contrast to deep vein thrombosis, embolization is rare.

Diagnosis is clinical. Compression stockings are helpful, but surgical excision may be necessary. Injection of sclerosing drugs into local lesions is useful to remove unsightly superficial skin varicosities. Treatment offers short-term relief, but varicosities usually reappear and require further treatment.

Hemorrhoids are varicose veins of the anus and deserve mention because they are common and painful. Topical, soothing creams may offer temporary relief, but sclerotherapy or surgery is required for cure. The veins of the esophageal mucosa can also develop varicosities. These *esophageal varices* occur with cirrhosis of the liver (Chapter 12), because portal venous blood flow through the liver is obstructed. Obstruction raises pressure and forces blood to seek alternate routes back to the heart—esophageal veins are one route. Esophageal varices can rupture and cause fatal gastrointestinal bleeding.

Thrombophlebitis is the formation of venous thrombi (Chapter 6). Venous thrombus formation and inflammation tend to occur together and it is usually difficult to know which came first. The deep veins of the legs account for 90% of thrombophlebitis. This form is commonly referred to as *deep venous thrombosis (DVT)*. Any condition that causes increased venous pressure or sluggish blood flow can cause DVT, including pregnancy, heart failure, obesity, and prolonged bed rest. *Prolonged immobilization is the most common predisposing factor*, as in bed rest following surgery or injury, or a very long air flight. Sometimes thrombophlebitis results from a paraneoplastic syndrome (Chapter 5), and is the first clue to an undiagnosed internal malignancy.

Venous thrombi in the legs usually arise silently and can grow up to two feet long without producing clinical signs or symptoms. Not infrequently, thrombi break loose and embolize to the lungs, where they may cause infarcts or, if very large, instantaneous death by complete occlusion of the pulmonary artery. Treatment includes thrombolytic drugs, anticoagulants, or surgery to ligate the vein or remove the thrombus.

Pop Quiz

8.28 True or false? Thrombophlebitis is simply inflammation of the veins.

8.29 What anatomic abnormality causes varicose veins?

Tumors of Blood and Lymphatic Vessels

Tumors of blood vessels (*hemangiomas*) or lymphatics (*lymphangiomas*) are benign neoplasms that may occur anywhere in the body, usually in soft tissue.

Hemangiomas are common and usually are found in skin as small, red, blood-filled lesions composed of capillary-size blood vessels (*capillary hemangioma*). They become malignant only very rarely. They usually occur in the skin of children and are called *infantile hemangiomas*. According to location and appearance, some have special names (*port wine stain; nevus flammeus*, Fig. 8.18). Most resolve without therapy. Oral corticosteroids may hasten involution of large lesions that interfere with vision or airway. Surgery is usually not recommended.

Spider angiomas are acquired, bright red, pulsatile vascular growths with a central arteriole from which small vessels radiate outward, in some cases like spider legs. They are most common on the face and upper anterior chest. They owe their development to high blood estrogen levels and are usually found in pregnant women or in patients

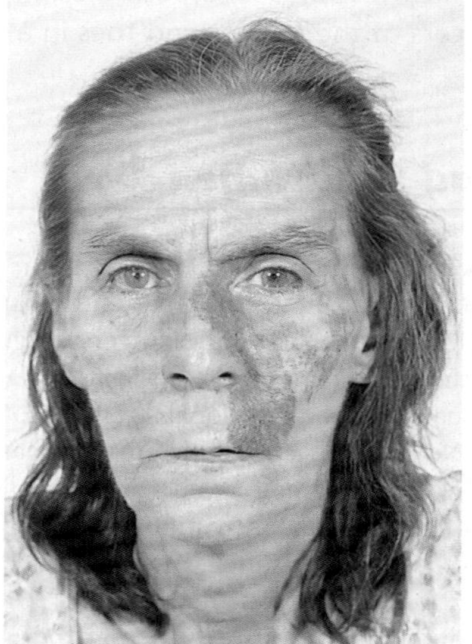

Figure 8.18 **Nevus flammeus.** One type of vascular malformation. (Reproduced with permission from Tasman W, Jaeger E. *The Wills Eye Hospital Atlas of Clinical Ophthalmology*. 2nd ed. Baltimore, MD: Lippincott Williams & Wilkins; 2001.)

with liver cirrhosis (who are unable to metabolize and excrete estrogen). They regress if estrogen levels decline, as they do at the end of pregnancy.

Less commonly, some hemangiomas are composed of larger vessels. These *cavernous hemangiomas* tend to occur in deeper tissue, such as the brain and liver. They usually remain silent, but may bleed spontaneously.

Hemangiomas should not be confused with similar-appearing *pyogenic granuloma*, a small nodular collection of inflamed capillaries that forms as a result of pathological wound healing (Chapter 2).

Lymphangiomas are collections of lymphatic capillaries. These are less common than hemangiomas. They are benign and usually are found in the subcutaneous tissues of the head and neck.

Kaposi sarcoma (KS) is an intermediate-grade malignant vascular tumor that is most often seen in patients with AIDS, but can also occur in other circumstances in which immunity is impaired. It was first described in 1872 by Dr. Moritz Kaposi as an affliction mainly affecting older men of Mediterranean descent. That variety, *chronic KS*, is not associated with AIDS or immunodeficiency. *African KS* is seen most often in Africans with lymphoma. It is more aggressive and may spread widely. In conjunction with *AIDS-related KS*, it is the most common neoplasm of men in central Africa. In the early stages of the AIDS epidemic, *AIDS-related KS* was common, but drug therapy has sharply reduced prevalence to about 1%, though it remains the most common tumor in AIDS patients in the United States. KS is caused by *human herpesvirus-8* (HHV-8, also termed *KS-associated herpesvirus*, KSHV). In most patients, KS presents as a sluggish skin tumor composed of small purple plaques or nodules. Aggressive varieties, however, may balloon into fleshy, bloody masses in lymph nodes or other organs. Treatment is a combination of antiretroviral therapy, chemotherapy, radiation, and cryotherapy.

Angiosarcoma is a rare malignant tumor of vascular endothelial cells that occurs most frequently in skin, breast tissue, soft tissue, and liver. Some angiosarcomas occur after irradiation or prolonged exposure to certain chemicals. Others arise in areas of chronic lymphedema (Chapter 6). Treatment is with a combination of surgery, chemotherapy, and radiation.

Pop Quiz

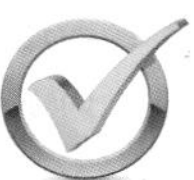

8.30 True or false? All KS is caused by infection with HIV and HHV8.

8.31 True or false? Tumors of blood vessels can be benign or malignant.

8.32 What hormone is responsible for causing spider angiomas?

8.33 In what cells of the blood vessel do angiosarcomas commonly occur?

Case Study Revisited

"A man found dead in his office." The case of Leon F.

Recall that Leon was found dead in his office with a bloody head wound. He died unobserved and the medical examiner's office investigated. His medical record revealed longstanding, poorly treated hypertension and hypercholesterolemia. He was overweight, a chronic smoker, and showed lab evidence of an enlarged heart and poor kidney function.

A medico-legal autopsy was performed by the medical examiner's office. The scalp wound was superficial, and no skull fracture was present; the examiner concluded it arose when Leon hit his head on the desk or floor as he collapsed from intracranial bleeding. No lesions were found that could explain the hypertension, which validated his physician's diagnosis of primary hypertension.

Acute bleeding into the brain is a common hazard of hypertension and is often fatal. Leon suffered other consequences of hypertension. He had an enlarged left ventricle that resulted from the strain of pumping blood into a hypertensive arterial tree. Leon had high LDL-cholesterol, which formed the basis of his atherosclerosis. Hypertension and smoking accelerated the effect of cholesterol. Together these three forces gave him unusually severe general and coronary atherosclerosis, which compromised coronary arterial flow and accounted for the scar in his heart from an old, silent myocardial infarct and

(continued)

"A man found dead in his office." The case of Leon F. (continued)

for his abdominal aortic aneurysm. Hypertension accounted for his severe arteriolar nephrosclerosis, which explained his abnormally high blood BUN and creatinine: his kidneys were not excreting waste products as well as they should.

This case is a lesson in the pathogenesis of hypertension and the consequences associated with it, proving that mild or moderate hypertension is a serious disease. First, Leon was clearly hypertensive—his diastolic pressure was consistently over 90 mm Hg. Second, he was African American and male, which put him especially at risk—men are more often hypertensive than women, and African Americans are more often hypertensive than other Americans and suffer more serious consequences from it. Third, he was a smoker, which added to his vascular risk. Fourth, he did not take his medicine regularly and did not return for regular follow-up care as recommended, nor did he apparently keep his appointment with the hypertension specialist, which illustrates the problem of patient noncompliance. Patients who do not take their medicine regularly, or at all, are a major problem in healthcare. Most problematic are those patients who are on drugs that have no immediate, detectable effect on the way the patient feels, which is often the case for antihypertensive and cholesterol-lowering drugs. For example, before he had a heart attack in 2004, former President Clinton had stopped taking the statin drug prescribed for him.

Chapter Challenge

CHAPTER RECALL

1. Which of the following regarding cholesterol is true?
   A. Decreasing total cholesterol by 50 mg/dL cuts cardiovascular risk by half.
   B. For every 5 mg/dL LDL is increased, coronary risk declines by 2–3%.
   C. Smoking raises HDL-C.
   D. Exercise and consumption of moderate amounts of alcohol raise LDL-C.

2. A seven-year-old Hispanic male presents to his pediatrician's office with five days of unexplained fever. On physical exam, conjunctivitis, oral ulcers, and desquamation of the palms and soles of his feet are noted. He also has bilateral lymphadenopathy of his cervical lymph nodes. From what vasculitis does he suffer?
   A. Microscopic polyangiitis
   B. Takayasu arteritis
   C. Temporal arteritis
   D. Kawasaki disease

3. Which one of the following is the site of the initial arterial injury in atherosclerosis?
   A. Endothelial cell
   B. Basement membrane
   C. Muscular wall (media)
   D. Adventitia

4. With regards to vascular injury, which of the following is true?
   A. Neutrophils are responsible for synthesizing the biological products that effect on smooth muscle cells of the media.
   B. The causative agents of endothelial damage are purely genetic in nature.
   C. Endothelial chemical mediators stimulate the proliferation and migration of media smooth muscle cells, which accumulate in the subendothelial space.
   D. Injured endothelial cells retain their ability to contract and synthesize scar-like accumulations of collagen and elastin.

5. A 70-year-old Caucasian woman presents to your office complaining of headaches, vision changes, and pain in her jaw muscles during chewing. Her labs reveal an elevated ESR and CRP, and a biopsy reveals lymphocytes infiltrating the affected blood vessel wall. What is your diagnosis?
   A. Polyarteritis nodosa
   B. Takayasu arteritis

C. Temporal arteritis
D. Kawasaki disease

6. Which of the following is a modifiable risk factor in atherosclerosis?
   A. Inflammation
   B. High blood homocysteine
   C. Hypertension
   D. Gender

7. Which of the following statements about varicose veins is true?
   A. The population most commonly affected by varicose veins is women who have had several pregnancies.
   B. Deep veins are more often affected than superficial ones.
   C. Skin ulcers are a common result of varicose veins.
   D. Varicose veins are found only in the extremities, most commonly the legs.

8. Which one of the following explains most aneurysms?
   A. Cystic medial necrosis of the wall of the aorta
   B. Atherosclerotic weakening of the vascular wall
   C. Anatomic weakness in the wall of arteries at a branching point
   D. Vasculitis of large arteries

9. Which one of the following is a marker for increased risk of atherosclerosis?
   A. HDL cholesterol <40 mg/dL
   B. LDL cholesterol <100 mg/dL
   C. VLDL cholesterol <30 mg/dL
   D. Triglyceride <150 mg/dL

10. True or false? Blood pressure is the result of cardiac output and vascular resistance.

11. True or false? Most aneurysms occur in the thoracic aorta and are a result of atherosclerosis.

12. True or false? Atherosclerosis begins around age 30.

13. True or false? Autoimmunity is the most common basic mechanism of vasculitis.

14. True or false? Halving vessel diameter increases resistance 16-fold.

15. True or false? Elevated triglyceride levels have no effect on atherosclerosis.

16. Match the following. Each will be used only once:
   i. Hemangioma
   ii. Lymphangioma
   iii. Pyogenic granuloma
   iv. Angiosarcoma
   v. Spider angioma
   vi. Hemorrhoids
   vii. Kaposi sarcoma
   A. Malignant tumor often found in AIDS patients, caused by HHV8
   B. Benign, small, red, blood-filled lesions composed of capillary-size blood vessels
   C. Small nodular collection of inflamed capillaries usually found on skin (e.g., the healing umbilical stump of a newborn) or in the oral cavity
   D. Benign tumor of lymphatic capillaries, found in subcutaneous tissue of head and neck
   E. Malignant tumor of vascular endothelial cells that occur most frequently in skin, breast, soft tissue, and liver
   F. Acquired skin lesions, usually on the upper chest or face that resemble a spider

CONCEPTUAL UNDERSTANDING

17. Classify each of the following blood pressure readings as prehypertension, stage 1, stage 2, or stage 3. Answers may be used more than once.
   A. 135/90
   B. 135/80
   C. 150/105
   D. 160/105
   E. 140/95

18. Briefly explain Raynaud syndrome.

19. What is the function of the vascular endothelium?

20. Which has a worse prognosis, a young atheroma or an old atheroma?

21. In what populations does vascular dissection occur?

22. What is your primary concern in a patient presenting with thrombophlebitis?

APPLICATION

23. Explain why "normal" is not a useful concept in study of plasma lipid levels.

24. A patient is reluctant to take medication to control his blood pressure. What lifestyle modifications can you recommend, and when are lifestyle modifications not an acceptable alternative to medication?

25. A 35-year-old African American male presents to your office complaining of headaches. This is his fourth visit in three months. You note that, despite aggressive lifestyle modification, his blood pressure has continued to increase. What must you consider prior to prescribing antihypertensive agents?

26. A 40-year-old Caucasian male presents to your office for a physical before starting his new job. He discloses that his father died of a stroke at age 53, and that his grandfather died of a ruptured abdominal aneurysm at age 60. What recommendations would you make?

CHAPTER 9

Disorders of the Heart

Contents

Chapter Objectives

After studying this chapter, you should be able to complete the following tasks:

THE UNIQUENESS OF THE HEART

1. The anatomy of the heart is a reflection of its function; describe its manifestation in muscle contraction, one-way valves, blood supply, and conduction.
2. List the three waves of an electrocardiogram (EKG or ECG) and give their source.
3. Name the five principles of healthy cardiac function.

HEART FAILURE

4. Compare and contrast the different types of heart failure, discussing their etiology, clinical

signs/symptoms, and the lifestyle changes and medications indicated for treatment.

CORONARY ARTERY DISEASE

5. Discuss the etiology of coronary artery disease, distinguishing angina pectoris from a true myocardial infarct, and identify the signs/symptoms, diagnosis, treatment, and complications of each.

VALVULAR HEART DISEASE

6. Discuss the etiology, signs/symptoms, diagnosis, treatment, and complications of valvular degeneration, rheumatic heart disease, and endocarditis.

DISEASES OF THE MYOCARDIUM

7. List the causes of myocarditis, and describe disease presentation and diagnosis.
8. Compare and contrast dilated, hypertrophic, and restrictive cardiomyopathy.

PERICARDIAL DISEASE

9. Discuss the etiology, presentation, diagnosis, and treatment of pericardial effusions and pericarditis.

CONGENITAL HEART DISEASE

10. Compare and contrast acyanotic, cyanotic, and obstructive heart disease, and give examples of each.

TUMORS OF THE HEART

11. List the tumors that can arise in the heart.

CARDIAC ARRHYTHMIAS

12. Explain the causes of arrhythmia, the locations from which they can arise, and their diagnostic findings on ECGs.

Case Study

"I only fainted." The case of Willard S.

Chief Complaint: Syncope.

Clinical History: Willard S. was an eight-year-old child living in a rural community when the family's general practitioner detected a heart murmur on a routine physical examination. The doctor told Willard's mother and said it was nothing to worry about. When Willard was 23, the murmur was noticed on a military physical examination. An echocardiogram revealed that he had a congenital bicuspid aortic valve, but he was accepted for service and told again it was not a matter of consequence. For the next 40 years, he lived a vigorous life and became a marathon runner. At 63, he began to have exertional dyspnea and chest pain, which was relieved by rest. Being exceptionally fit, he dismissed the pain as inconsequential. He told friends in the gym about being short of breath but they joked that he was just getting old.

"I told myself I couldn't have heart trouble because I run marathons," he said. One day, however, he fainted at the gym during a treadmill session and paramedics were called. As he was being loaded into the ambulance, he protested, "I just fainted. No reason to be so excited." At the hospital, a physician examined him for the first time in many years.

Physical Examination and Other Data: Willard was 5′9″ and weighed 158 lbs. Blood pressure was 100/40 (normal: 120/80); heart rate was normal, but the beats were especially forceful, and his head shook with each beat. Other vital signs were normal. Auscultation revealed a loud crescendo-decrescendo systolic murmur and a faint diastolic murmur. Chest X-ray showed an enlarged heart. ECG showed no evidence of recent or old myocardial infarction. Twenty-four hour ECG monitoring revealed periodic short episodes of ventricular tachycardia. Echocardiography confirmed the earlier diagnosis of bicuspid aortic valve and severe left ventricular hypertrophy (LVH), and also confirmed the clinical suspicion of severe aortic stenosis (AS): the aortic valve area was 0.9 cm^3 (normal: 3–4 cm^3). Studies of cardiac motion showed the left ventricular wall to be stiff and noncompliant, with poor diastolic filling. Catheter studies revealed high left ventricular end-diastolic pressure. The pressure gradient across the aortic valve was markedly increased. A limited degree of aortic insufficiency was also found. His ejection fraction was normal. Coronary angiography revealed very little coronary atherosclerosis.

Echocardiography of the heart of Willard's son revealed that he, too, had a bicuspid aortic valve.

Clinical Course: While awaiting surgery, Willard developed uncompensated left-heart failure, which responded slowly to salt restriction and drug therapy. After some delay, he had open-heart surgery and was on cardiac bypass for three hours. His aortic valve was

"I only fainted." The case of Willard S. (continued)

replaced with a pig valve. Postoperatively, he had periodic episodes of ventricular tachycardia, which responded to drug therapy. He was discharged home on the seventh hospital day. He recovered slowly at home, gradually regaining strength. "Physically he was fine," his son said, "but mentally he wasn't quite himself for about six months." Follow-up one year later found that his LVH had regressed somewhat and he was exercising regularly.

"... another supper from a sack, a ninety-nine cent heart attack."

TIM MCGRAW (B. 1967), AMERICAN MUSICIAN, SINGER, AND ACTOR. FROM "WHERE THE GREEN GRASS GROWS".

The heart propels blood through the vascular tree. It is a tireless bundle of muscle and a complex mechanical and electrical pump whose normal function depends on flawless, perfectly timed, interlocked movement of its various parts. Daily it beats about 100,000 times, pumping about 6,000 liters of blood, an activity it normally sustains quietly for a lifetime. It follows, therefore, that heart disease is a serious matter. In the United States, heart disease alone accounted for nearly one out of four deaths in 2011, more than all types of cancer combined.

The Uniqueness of the Heart

Much about the heart is unique. Of particular note are the myocardium, which never fatigues; the valves, which act in perfect mechanical harmony; the coronary arteries, which supply oxygen and other necessities; and the conduction system, a self-stimulating network of specialized muscle cells that performs like a miniature nervous system to carry beat signals.

Myocardial Cells Function Together like a Single Large Cell

Heart muscle is the **myocardium**. It is composed of specialized muscle cells, **cardiac myocytes**, which contract to eject blood during **systole** and relax during **diastole** so that the chambers can refill. Cardiac muscle and skeletal muscle are very different. Skeletal muscle cells lie next to one another but are not electrically connected: each one is connected separately to the nervous system and each responds individually to neural commands. The brain can command a few cells to contract to lift a small load, or it can command many to lift a heavy load. On the other hand, cardiac myocytes are intimately fused to one another and contract as a single entity—all cardiac muscle cells must contract together in an "all or nothing" manner.

This does not mean, however, that cardiac muscle cannot contract with extra *force* under some circumstances. Like skeletal muscle, cardiac myocytes contain overlapping bundles of actin and myosin fibrils joined by "teeth," which ratchet across one another, causing them to slide to and fro in the cycle of contraction and relaxation. During systole, the fibrils ratchet their bundles shorter, contracting the cell. During diastole, the teeth relax their grip and fibrils slide back as the bundles stretch. The *distance* each bundle shortens during contraction determines the amount of *force* generated. As the ventricle dilates, the fibrils slide further, stretching the bundle. This increases the distance the fibrils must contract during systole, which increases the force of the beat. A slightly dilated ventricle, therefore, generates more pumping force with each beat. Beyond a certain point, however, the opposite occurs and further ventricular dilation causes less forceful contractions. Heart failure, discussed below, is an example of this principle in action.

A further difference is that some atrial myocytes contain granules containing **atrial natriuretic peptide**, which acts to produce a number of effects, including vasodilation and increased sodium and water excretion by the kidney, actions beneficial in conditions such as hypertension and heart failure.

Cardiac Valves Ensure One-Way Blood Flow

The cardiac valves ensure one-way flow into and out of each chamber (Fig. 9.1). They are composed of tough, thin, pliable fibrous flaps, called *leaflets* in the tricuspid and mitral valves, and *cusps* in the pulmonary and aortic valves. They must open fully and close tightly with every beat, otherwise blood flow is not optimal. Failure to open (**stenosis**) or to close fully (**incompetence**, or **regurgitation**) is a feature of some cardiac disease.

The atria are separated from the ventricles by a nonconductive, electrically insulating fibrous collar to which the valves are hinged (Fig. 9.2). The free ends of the tricuspid and mitral valve leaflets are tethered by thin ligaments (**chordae tendineae**) to small mounds of muscle (**papillary muscles**) projecting from the interior of the heart wall, which ensure the leaflets do not invert. Rupture of either muscle or ligament can cause leaflet inversion and regurgitation.

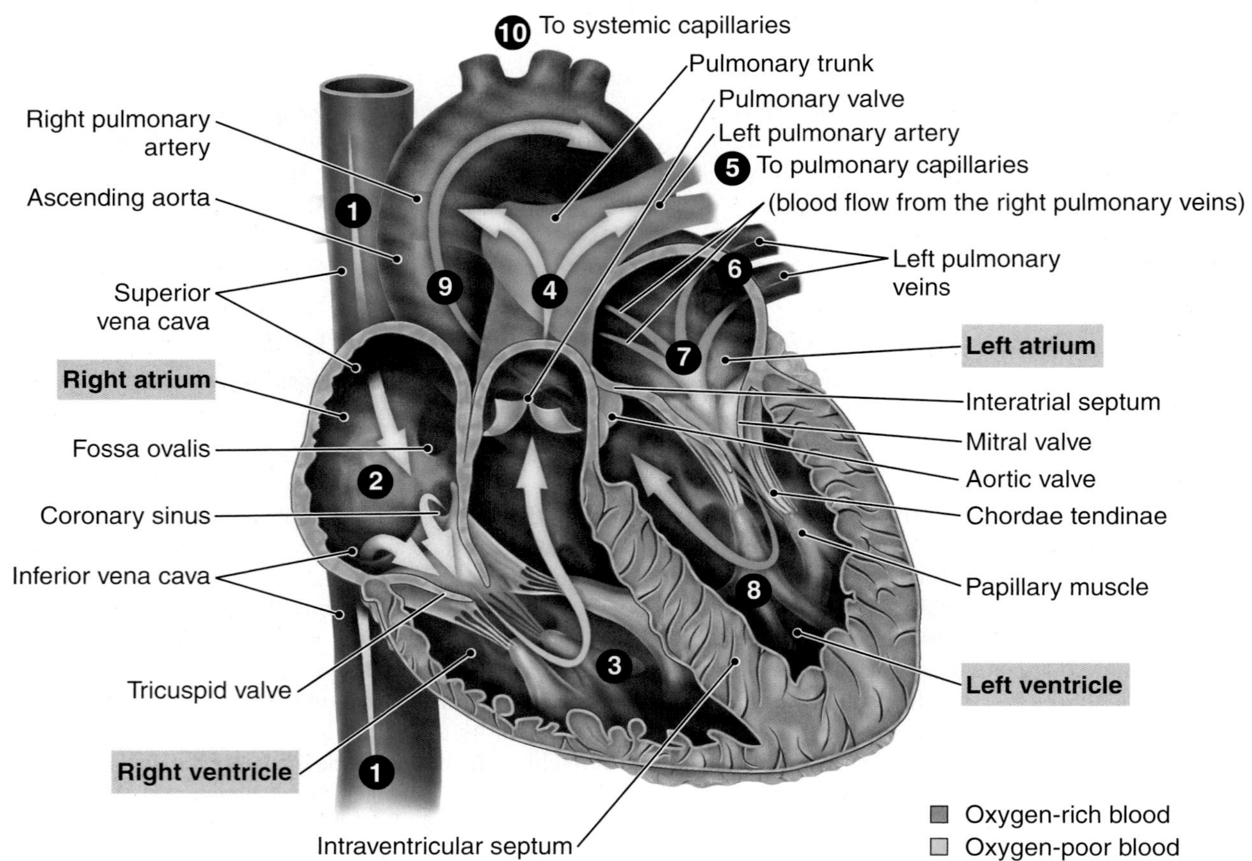

Figure 9.1 **Blood flow through the heart.** The numbered steps begin with return of blood from the systemic circulation and end with ejection of blood into the systemic circulation. (Adapted with permission from McConnell TH, Hull KL. *Human Form Human Function: Essentials of Anatomy & Physiology*. Baltimore, MD: Wolters Kluwer Health; 2011.)

The aortic and pulmonary cusps are anchored, respectively, within the base of the aorta and pulmonary artery. Dilation of the root of either vessel can cause regurgitation.

Apart from mechanical problems of the type discussed above, heart valves are subject to three types of pathological processes. First, valve collagen may stretch to create lose or "floppy" valve leaflets, as in *mitral valve prolapse* (inversion). Regurgitation is the result. Second, calcification may make the valve leaflets or cusps board-stiff, as in *calcific aortic valve disease*. Stenosis and/or regurgitation are the result. Third, the leaflets or cusps may thicken and stiffen with scar tissue due to an inflammatory process, as in *rheumatic fever (RF)*. Stenosis and/or regurgitation are the result.

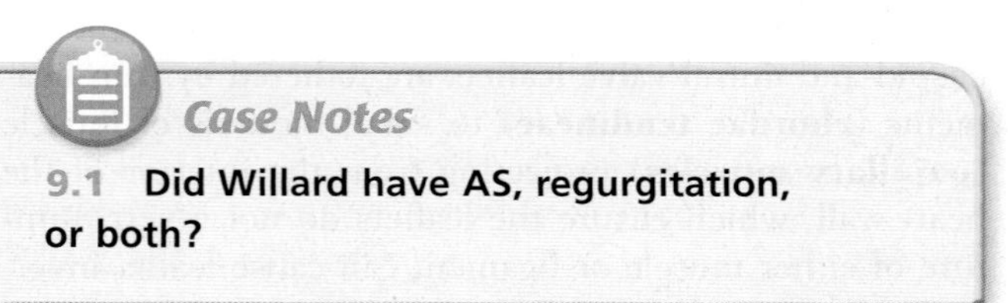

Case Notes

9.1 Did Willard have AS, regurgitation, or both?

Coronary Arteries Supply Blood to the Heart

The myocardium's high metabolic rate and ceaseless beating cause it to consume a lot of energy, which must be provided abundantly and quickly from mitochondria, the energy producing organelles of cells. Cardiac myocytes are packed with mitochondria, which derive energy from fatty acids and glucose by oxidative phosphorylation, an aerobic (requiring oxygen) process that is the body's most efficient mechanism for claiming energy from glucose. Some organs can derive energy from nonaerobic metabolism, but the heart cannot. The myocardium is, therefore, absolutely dependent on an abundant supply of oxygen.

Oxygen and other essentials are supplied to myocardium by blood from the two main **coronary arteries** (Fig. 9.3), the left main coronary artery and the right coronary artery. Both originate from the root of the aorta behind the aortic valve cusps, the first possible point of origin and the point of highest pressure in the arterial tree. The coronary arteries and their major branches travel on the outer surface (epicardium) of the heart, sending *penetrating branches* downward into the myocardium.

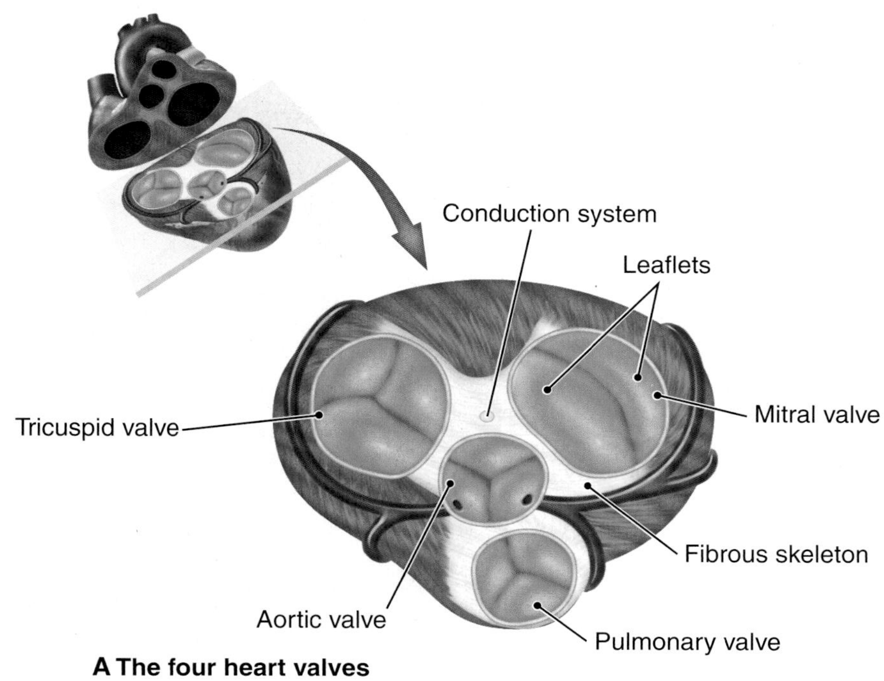

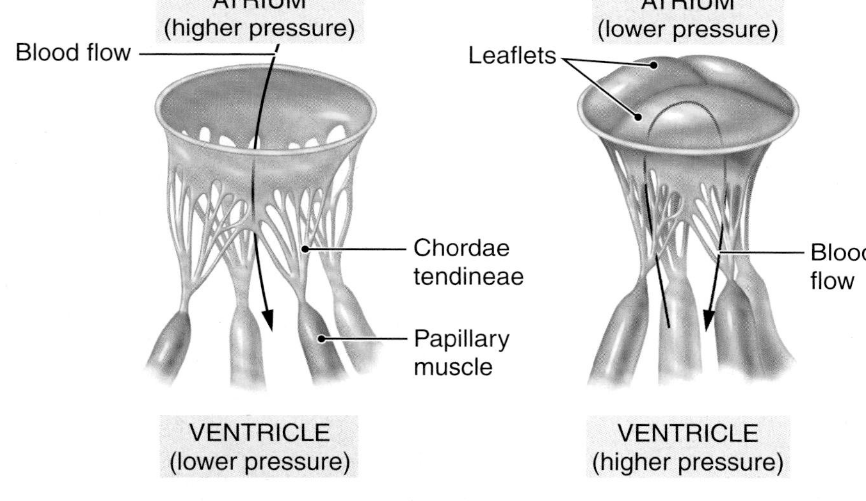

Figure 9.2 **Valves and the fibrous skeleton. A.** The fibrous skeleton physically and electrically separates the atria from the ventricles and supports the heart valves. **B.** In response to higher pressure in the atrium than in the ventricle, the right atrioventricular (AV) valve opens, enabling blood to flow from the atrium to the ventricle. **C.** The right AV valve closes, preventing blood flow from the ventricle to the atrium. (Reprinted with permission from McConnell TH, Hull KL. *Human Form Human Function: Essentials of Anatomy & Physiology*. Baltimore, MD: Wolters Kluwer Health; 2011.)

In most people, the *right coronary artery* wraps around the right side of the heart along the upper edge of the right ventricle before turning downward along the posterior side of the interventricular septum. As it descends, it is called the *posterior descending coronary artery,* and it supplies the right ventricle and the posterior aspect of the left ventricle. The *left main coronary artery* branches immediately after leaving the aorta, sending the *anterior descending artery* down the anterior aspect of the interventricular septum to supply the anterior septum and left ventricle. The main left coronary continues as the *left circumflex coronary artery*, which wraps around the upper edge of the left ventricle to supply its anterior and lateral aspects. There are many variations of this general configuration. Coronary blood returns via *coronary veins*, which gather on the posterior aspect of the heart in the *coronary sinus* before flowing into the right atrium.

The Electrocardiogram Is an Electric Record of the Heartbeat

Voltage is the difference in electrical potential between two points. An **electrocardiogram** (**ECG**, or EKG from the original German) is a graphical tracing of the voltage *changes*—greater or lesser than the moment before—caused by each heartbeat (Fig. 9.4). It depicts the sum of all of the electrical changes of cardiac muscle fibers as they polarize and

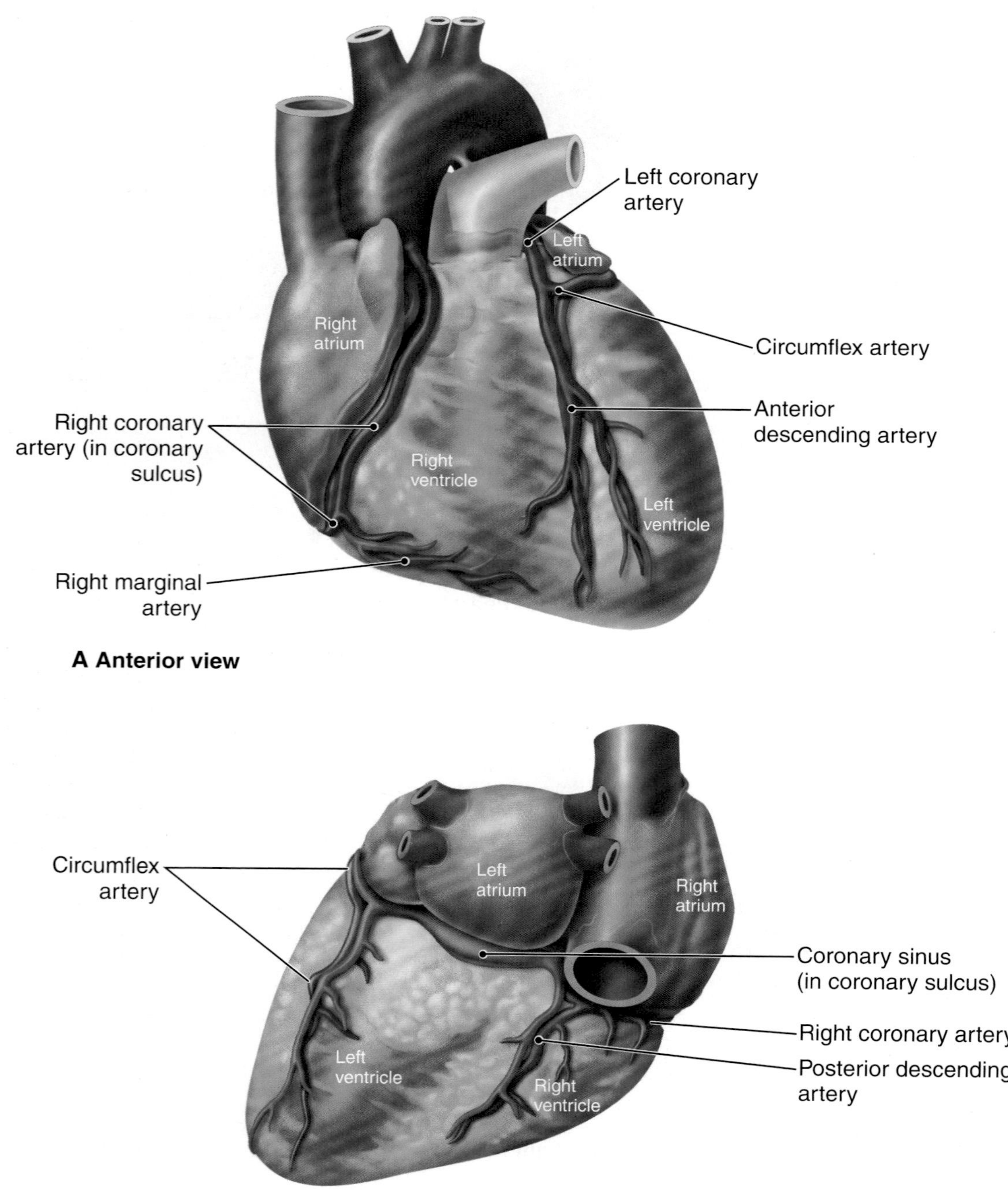

Figure 9.3 **External heart features and the coronary circulation.** The coronary circulation supplies the heart muscle. **A.** Anterior view. **B.** Posterior view. (Adapted with permission from McConnell TH, Hull KL. *Human Form Human Function: Essentials of Anatomy & Physiology*. Baltimore, MD: Wolters Kluwer Health; 2011.)

depolarize in the beating heart. If the voltage is not *changing*, the EKG shows a flat line.

Four major voltage changes are associated with each heartbeat: 1) atrial depolarization with atrial systole; 2) atrial repolarization during atrial diastole; 3) ventricular depolarization with ventricular systole; and 4) ventricular repolarization during ventricular diastole. Each generates a waveform signal. Only three corresponding waves are detectable in a normal ECG, however, because the small wave of atrial repolarization is masked by the large wave of ventricular depolarization. The three waves are referred to as follows:

- The **P wave** is first. It is small and represents atrial depolarization.

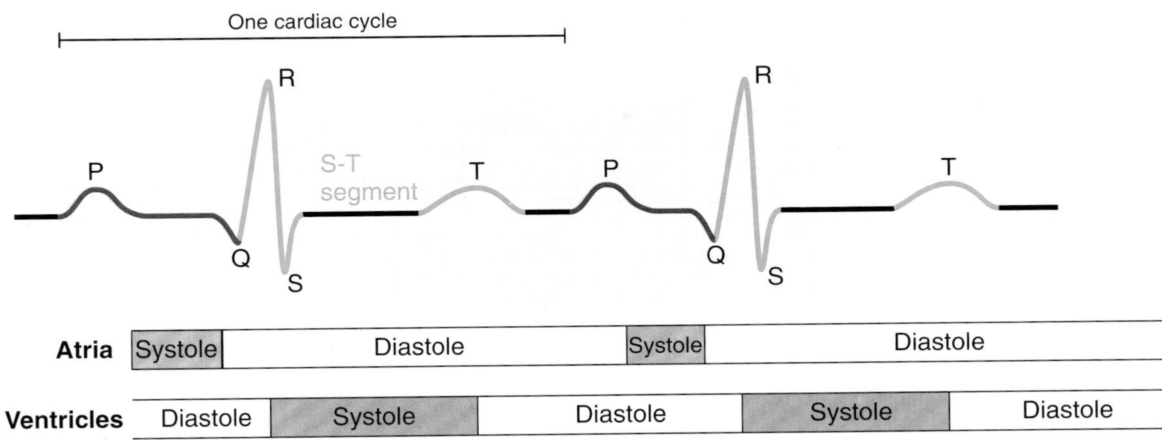

Figure 9.4 **Electrocardiogram.** The electrical changes in the heart over two heartbeats. (Reprinted with permission from McConnell TH, Hull KL. *Human Form Human Function: Essentials of Anatomy & Physiology*. Baltimore, MD: Wolters Kluwer Health; 2011.)

- The **QRS complex** is next. It is a rapid series of three waves that represent ventricular depolarization. The repolarization of the atria is hidden in this large wave.
- Finally, the **T wave** comes. It is a mid-size wave that represents ventricular repolarization.

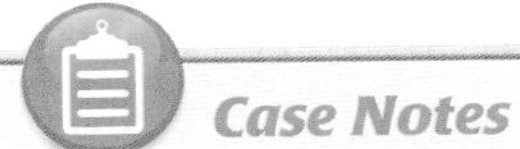

Case Notes

9.2 During his episodes of ventricular tachycardia, Willard's ventricle contracted very rapidly. Which of the three main ECG waves would these contractions generate?

The time period between the beginnings of successive P-waves is one complete cardiac cycle. This period can be used to calculate the heart rate (e.g., a P-P interval of one second indicates a heart rate of 60 beats/min).

ECGs are invaluable aids in the diagnosis of heart conditions. For example, an enlarged P-wave suggests enlarged atria, because there are more cells contributing to the voltage changes. For the same reason, an enlarged T-wave suggests an enlarged left ventricle. A prolonged P-R segment indicates some degree of pathological delay of the signal (heart block, discussed below) as it travels from atria to ventricles.

The Cardiac Conduction System Transmits the Signal for Each Heartbeat

Each normal beat of the heart is initiated by a self-excited, automatic discharge of an electrical signal from the heart's natural pacemaker in the right atrium, the **sinoatrial (SA) node** (Fig. 9.5). This signal is carried throughout the heart as a wave of electrical stimulation by the **cardiac conduction system (CCS)**, composed of specialized myocardial muscle fibers. The fibrous collar mentioned above serves to electrically insulate the atria from the ventricles, and is penetrated only by the CCS.

After the signal leaves the SA node, it sweeps over the atria and passes into a second node, the **atrioventricular (AV) node**, which sits at the peak of the interventricular septum. The AV node serves as a gatekeeper, stalling the signal slightly. This ensures that only one signal passes through to the ventricles. Extra signals occur in some diseases. Beneath the AV node the signal passes through a thick bundle of conductive fibers, the **bundle of His**, which penetrates the insulating fibrous collar and branches into two main bundles of CCS fibers, the **right and left bundle branches**. The AV node, bundle of His, and bundle branches are capable of self-excitation at a progressively slower rate than the SA node. If an SA signal fails to arrive at the AV node, the highest active part of the CCS discharges a new, slower signal automatically to prevent cardiac standstill.

The right and left branches continue down either side of the interventricular system to the apex of the heart, where fibers first connect to cardiac muscle cells. This guarantees that ventricular contraction begins at the apex of the heart, ensuring efficient emptying of the ventricle, like squeezing toothpaste from the bottom of the tube. From the apex, the remaining fibers turn upward and spread through the ventricular walls.

The SA node has a native discharge rate of about 70 beats/min. The CCS is innervated by the autonomic nervous system, however, which can increase or decrease the rate of discharge to increase or decrease heart rate.

Heart Disease Affects Cardiac Output and/or Effort

Heart disease arises from a failure of one or more of the five principal mechanisms of healthy cardiac function. In each instance, the result is decreased cardiac output and/or increased cardiac work to maintain normal output.

- *Pump failure.* Weak contraction results in poor cardiac output. For example, infarcted (dead), diseased, or stiff muscle cannot contract with normal force.

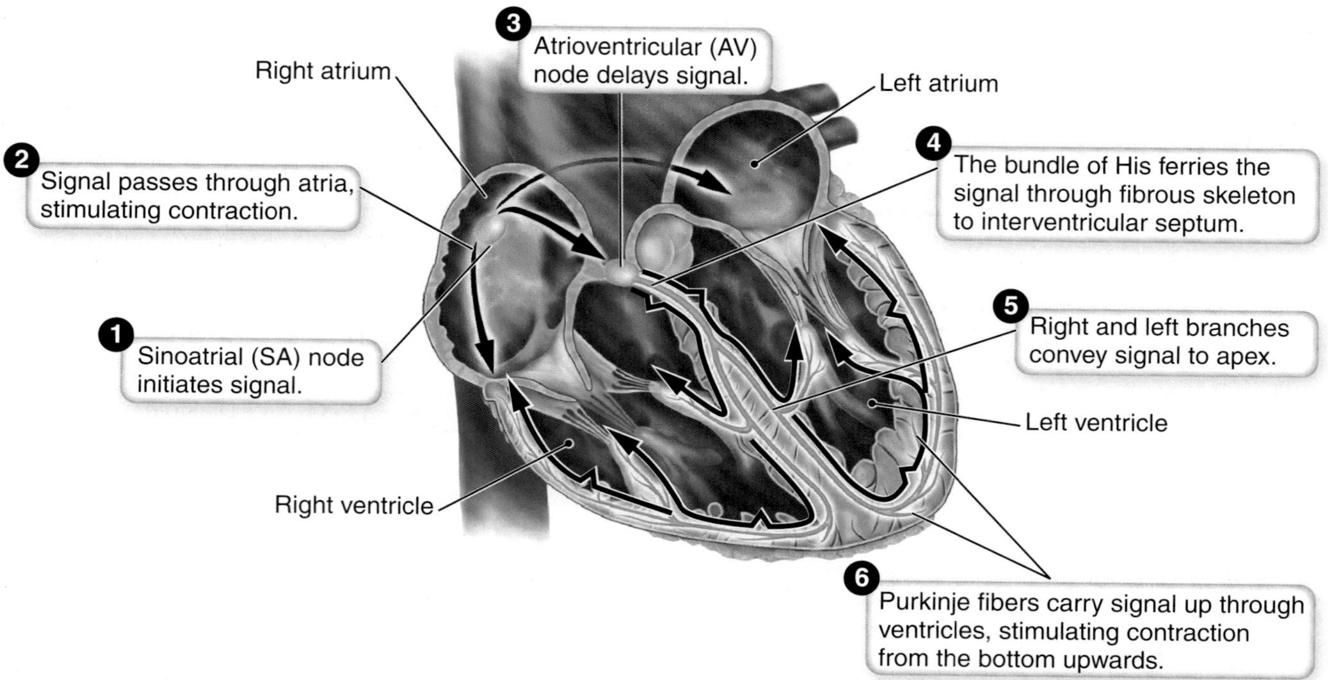

Figure 9.5 **The cardiac conduction system.** The anatomical components of the CCS and the steps involved in one heartbeat. The black arrows indicate the spread of electrical impulses through the conducting system. (Adapted with permission from McConnell TH, Hull KL. *Human Form Human Function: Essentials of Anatomy & Physiology*. Baltimore, MD: Wolters Kluwer Health; 2011.)

- *Obstructed flow.* Atherosclerosis may impair coronary blood flow to heart muscle, causing pump failure. Any of the four valves may become stiff or the leaflets may fuse, causing the heart to work harder to force blood past the obstruction.
- *Regurgitant flow.* Backward flow across a valve subtracts from normal output and the heart must repump the loss with the next beat. This is mechanically inefficient and causes extra cardiac effort.
- *Shunted flow.* Blood is diverted, usually by congenital defect. This is mechanically inefficient. For example, a hole in the interventricular septum may allow blood that should flow into the aorta to flow into the right ventricle, from which it flows into the lungs and back to the left ventricle in an endless loop. This, too, is mechanically inefficient and causes extra cardiac effort.
- *Abnormal conduction.* Conduction defects result in ill-timed, premature or late, mechanically inefficient beats in which the ventricle is under- or overfilled at the beginning of systole. The result is low cardiac output.

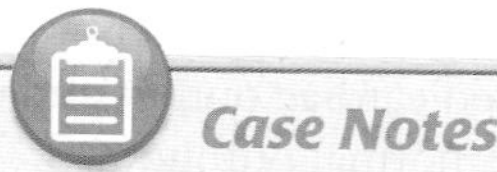

Case Notes

9.3 **Which of the five principal mechanisms of heart disease did Willard have?**

Pop Quiz

9.1 True or false? Cardiac myocytes contract during diastole to eject blood from the ventricle, and relax during systole to allow the ventricle to fill.

9.2 True or false? The tricuspid and mitral valve leaflets are tethered by chordae tendineae to papillary muscles.

9.3 Put the following in order from superior to inferior: Right and left bundle branches, AV node, SA node, bundle of His.

9.4 What causes stenosis? Regurgitation?

9.5 Which of the four major waveforms is not visible on an ECG?

9.6 What are the five principal mechanisms of cardiac dysfunction?

Heart Failure

Heart failure (HF, or *congestive* heart failure) is a syndrome of ventricular dysfunction in which the heart cannot pump blood at a rate sufficient to meet metabolic demand or can do so only if the ventricle is dilated. The **Frank-Starling Law**

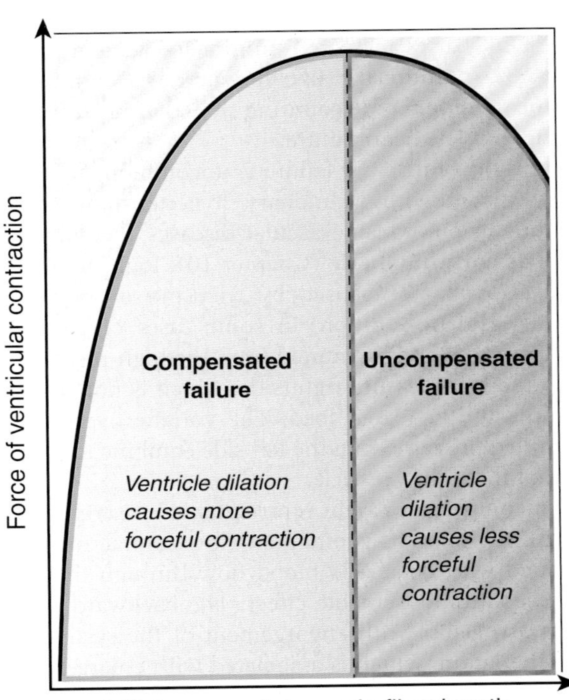

Figure 9.6 **The Frank-Starling curve.** Up to a point (the apex of the curve), cardiac myocytes contract with more force when stretched. Beyond that point, the fibers contract less forcefully.

(Fig. 9.6) describes the relationship between ventricular dilation and cardiac performance as indicated by *cardiac output* (Chapter 8) or **stroke volume**, the volume of blood ejected with each ventricular beat. Ventricular dilation is an adaptive response to certain myocardial conditions. Dilation stretches myocardial muscle fibers, which react by contracting more forcefully, somewhat like a stretched spring or rubber band pulls ever harder as it lengthens. The result is increased cardiac contractile power and improved stroke volume and cardiac output. Nevertheless, this adaptation works only up to a certain point of stretch. Like a spring that deforms and loses its pull or a rubber band that snaps, beyond this point further stretching causes contractile force to decline.

HF is the endpoint for most serious heart disease: coronary atherosclerosis, hypertension, valve disease, cardiomyopathy, and congenital cardiac malformation. It is a common and serious condition affecting 1–2% of Americans.

Causes of failure fall into two broad groups: increased workload and muscle failure, the details of which will be discussed as this chapter progresses. Causes of increased *left* ventricular workload include hypertension, mitral or aortic valvular regurgitation (incompetency), aortic valvular stenosis, and some congenital heart diseases. Causes of left ventricular muscle failure include ischemic coronary artery disease (CAD) (with or without myocardial infarction) and cardiac muscle disease (cardiomyopathy).

The most common cause of *right* ventricular failure is increased workload due to left ventricular failure, which increases pulmonary venous pressure and results in pulmonary arterial hypertension and right heart failure, if the process is not reversed. Additional causes of increased right ventricular workload include other causes of pulmonary hypertension and right heart failure, if the process is not reversed. (especially chronic lung disease), tricuspid and pulmonary valve disease, and some congenital heart diseases. Causes of right ventricular muscle failure include right ventricular infarction and cardiomyopathy.

There Are Several Modes of Heart Failure

Before failing, the heart compensates for muscle weakness or valve inefficiency in two ways: 1) sympathetic nervous stimulation and release of adrenal hormones (e.g., epinephrine) to increase heart rate and the force of contraction; and 2) cardiac muscle hypertrophy. If these adaptations are unable to maintain cardiac output, then congestive failure occurs.

In **systolic failure** the ventricle contracts poorly and empties incompletely. The ventricle fills properly, but the **ejection fraction**, the fraction of total ventricular volume ejected with each stroke, is abnormally low. Systolic dysfunction is caused by myocardial muscle damage due to ischemia, infarction, inflammation or intrinsic myocardial muscle disease (cardiomyopathy, discussed below).

In **diastolic failure** ventricular relaxation and filling are impaired. Contractile power and ejection fraction remain normal but cardiac output falls. Diastolic dysfunction is caused by ventricular stiffness that can be the result of cardiac hypertrophy (usually secondary to hypertension or valvular disease), cardiomyopathy, or infiltration of the myocardium by amyloid, an abnormal protein (*amyloidosis*, Chapter 3).

As the failing ventricle dilates, the ventricular wall stretches and the ventricle maintains cardiac output according to the Frank-Starling Law. This state is known as **compensated heart failure**.

As Figure 9.6 illustrates, however, if pathologic forces continue to damage heart muscle, further stretching muscle fibers results in weaker, not stronger, contractions. Like a spring that loses its power or a rubber band that snaps, if myocardial fibers are stretched too far the heart goes into **uncompensated failure**. Cardiac output falls and blood "backs up" like water behind a dam. The right and left ventricles can fail independently, but usually they fail together. There are two components of uncompensated failure. The **forward failure** component is low cardiac output; the **backward failure** component is upstream venous congestion.

The *renin-angiotensin-aldosterone system* (Chapter 6) is important in the pathogenesis of heart failure. In normal circumstances, this system is designed to regulate blood pressure by influencing peripheral resistance and blood volume. Angiotensin II is a powerful vasoconstrictor. It also stimulates secretion of aldosterone, which acts on the kidney to retain sodium and water, which expands blood volume. In left-heart failure, low cardiac output and low blood pressure are associated with decreased renal blood flow, causing an outpouring of renin and aldosterone, which creates a vicious circle: increased fluid retention and expanded blood volume further burden the failing chamber.

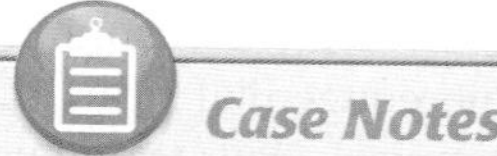

Case Notes

9.4 Did Willard have diastolic or systolic heart failure?

Remember This! Low cardiac output is the forward component of heart failure, while congestion is the backward component of heart failure.

One or Both Ventricles May Fail

Left-heart failure is much more common than right. The most common cause is cardiac muscle damage, usually caused by CAD. Less common causes are valve defects that result in stenosis or regurgitation and an inefficient pumping stroke. Left-heart failure can also be caused by the excess strain of high blood pressure or aortic or mitral valve disease. Much less commonly, primary disease of cardiac muscle (cardiomyopathy) is the culprit.

In uncompensated left ventricular failure (**left-heart failure**) (Fig. 9.7), the forward component (low cardiac output) is associated with decreased blood flow to vital organs. The backward component is associated with engorgement of the left atrium, pulmonary veins, and lungs. This causes increased pulmonary venous pressure and forces fluid into the alveoli, where it accumulates as **pulmonary edema**, accounting for the breathlessness (dyspnea) of left-heart failure.

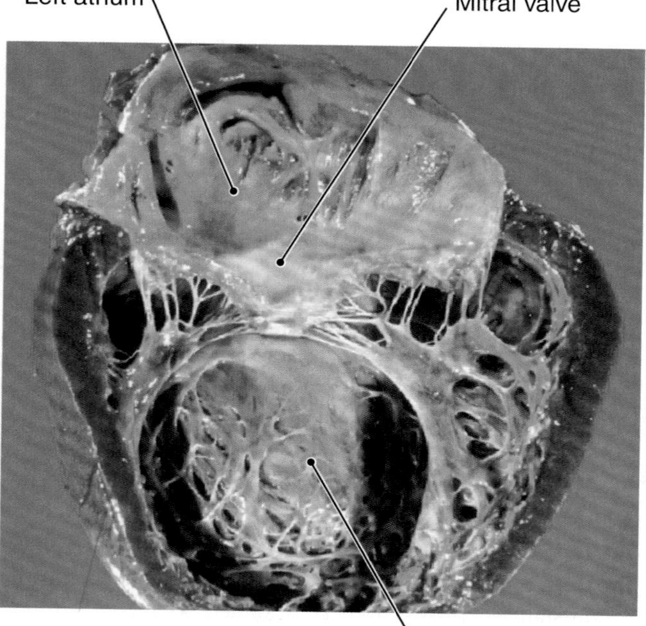

Figure 9.7 **Left-heart failure.** The left ventricle is markedly dilated.

Pure right ventricular failure is uncommon and is usually associated with pulmonary hypertension resulting from lung or pulmonary vascular diseases, a combination known as **cor pulmonale** (Chapter 10). Right ventricular failure also may be caused by tricuspid or pulmonary valve disease. In addition, in some cases of congenital heart disease, blood is shunted from the high-pressure left side to the low-pressure right side, which is not equipped to handle the increased load. The volume overload and transmitted pressure from the left side combine to produce failure of the right ventricle.

In uncompensated right ventricular failure (**right-heart failure**), the forward component (low cardiac output) is associated with decreased blood flow through the lungs, which has little observable effect. The backward component is associated with engorgement of the systemic venous circulation, which is associated with enlargement of the liver and spleen as they become overfilled with blood. Increased venous hydrostatic pressure forces fluid into tissues and body spaces, where it accumulates as edema of the feet and legs, ascites, and pleural effusion. *The most common cause of right-heart failure is left-heart failure*—the failing left ventricle so gorges pulmonary blood vessels that the right ventricle must work extra hard to force more blood through them and the ventricle fails as a result.

Case Notes

9.5 What are the forward and backward components of Willard's left-heart failure?

Heart Failure Has Widespread Signs and Symptoms

Heart failure has a widespread ill effect on the body (Fig. 9.8), but signs and symptoms differ according to the cause of heart failure.

One of the most prominent clinical features of left-heart failure is breathlessness (**dyspnea**). Typically accompanied by tachypnea and fatigue, it is most noticeable when the patient is physically active (exertional dyspnea) or lying down (**orthopnea**), and it is relieved by rest in a sitting position. As failure worsens, dyspnea can occur even at rest. Chest X-ray typically reveals prominent pulmonary veins (owing to congestion) and an enlarged cardiac silhouette (owing to ventricular dilation). Patients also typically have rapid heart rate, because of sympathetic impulses. On physical exam, murmurs and exaggerated heart sounds are common, and the apical impulse

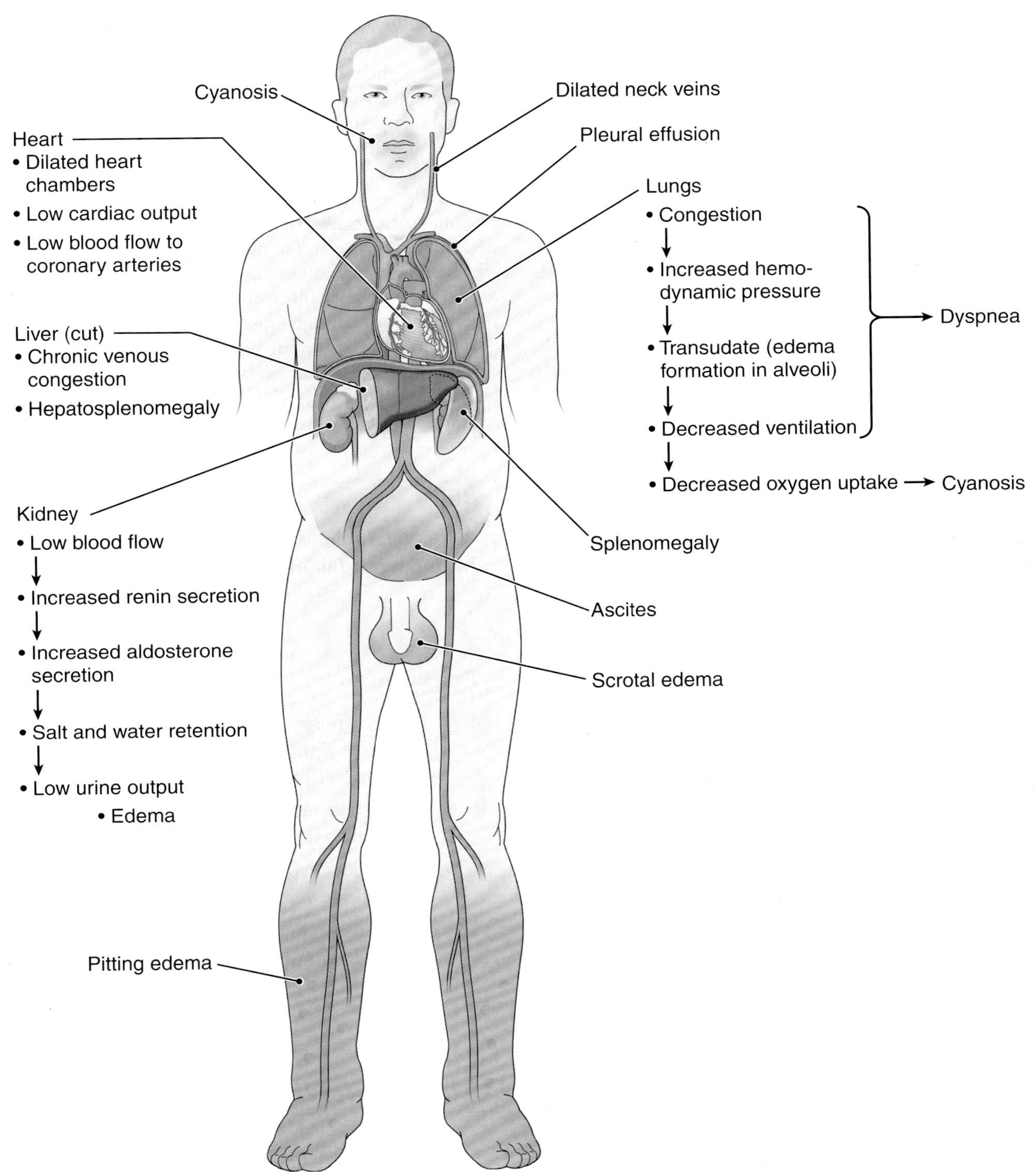

Figure 9.8 **Clinical findings in heart failure.** Left heart failure is associated with salt and water retention, general edema, ascites and other effusions, pulmonary congestion and edema, dyspnea, poor ventilation, poor oxygen uptake, and cyanosis. Right heart failure is associated with systemic venous congestion, peripheral edema, and hepatosplenomegaly.

is displaced to the left. Pulmonary edema, when present, can be detected by hearing in the lung bases fine *rales* (wet, tissue-paper, crinkling sounds) that do not clear with coughing.

With severe left-heart failure, the left ventricle becomes so dilated (the cardiac wall is pushed so far outward) that the mitral valve cannot close completely during systole, and mitral regurgitation (insufficiency) occurs, adding a burden of valvular inefficiency and increased workload that further exacerbates the failure. In addition, the left atrium dilates and may lose its ability to maintain a regular beat, causing *atrial fibrillation*, an irregular rhythm pattern discussed below. Severe failure may also be associated with low blood pressure, confusion or agitation, and **cyanosis** (blue–gray skin color owing to **hypoxia**, low blood oxygen), all due to low cardiac output. The sluggish blood flow and bed rest associated with heart failure can also cause deep venous thrombi and pulmonary embolism (Chapter 6).

Left-heart failure is often fatal because it produces hypoxia, acidosis, and cardiac *arrhythmias* (disturbed patterns of heartbeat, discussed later). Hypoxia arises because cardiac output is not sufficient to meet the demands of tissues, and because pulmonary edema interferes with oxygenation of blood in the lungs. Acidosis occurs secondary to impairment of CO_2 discharge by pulmonary edema (retained CO_2 is acidic); low cardiac output is also associated with reduced renal blood flow, which deprives the kidney of some of its opportunity to purge acid from blood. Fatal arrhythmias occur when the myocardium becomes irritable following sympathetic nervous system stimulation, the purpose of which is to increase cardiac output by increasing heart rate and contractile force.

The clinical features of right-heart failure are different from those of left-heart failure but derive from the same cause—engorgement with blood and increased venous pressure. In pure right failure, dyspnea is usually not present unless related to coexisting pulmonary disease. Signs of systemic venous congestion include distended neck veins, edema in the feet and genitals; and in severe cases, pitting edema extending to the thighs or hips. Other signs include congestive enlargement of the liver and spleen, which may become so engorged with blood that they become palpable below the rib cage, and accumulations of fluid (*effusions*) in the peritoneal and pleural spaces.

Diagnosis sometimes requires only clinical evaluation. Chest X-ray, echocardiography, and ECG may be required to confirm the clinical impression.

Treatment Includes Diet and Drug Therapy

The primary goal of treatment is to correct or ameliorate the underlying cause. Acute heart failure caused by acute myocardial infarction or arrhythmia may require hospitalization. Chronic CHF can be treated at home. The short-term goal is to relieve symptoms and improve cardiac output. Long-term goals include correcting hypertension, preventing myocardial infarction, and avoiding hospitalization by controlling symptoms.

Weight loss and a low-salt diet are important. Weight loss reduces the demand for cardiac output. Reducing salt intake retards the accumulation of fluid and edema and avoids expanding blood volume, which adds to cardiac stress. Stopping smoking is also important.

A broad menu of drug therapies is available. Among the most commonly used are diuretics for control of fluid accumulations. Angiotensin-converting enzyme (ACE) inhibitors and aldosterone-receptor blockers are used to counteract the effect of the renin-angiotensin-aldosterone mechanism. Digoxin and other digitalis preparations enhance myocardial contractility. Beta-blockers improve ejection fraction and cardiac output and lower myocardial work by lowering heart rate. Other categories of drugs are also available.

Some patients may benefit from surgery to correct valve disease or a congenital defect. Mechanical ventricular-assist devices may offer temporary help for those awaiting a heart transplant. Intracoronary stem cell infusion for regeneration of cardiac muscle remains experimental.

The prognosis is poor unless the underlying cause is correctible. Low blood pressure, CAD, and low ejection fraction are key markers of poor outlook. Annual mortality varies from 10% to 40%.

Case Notes

9.6 Willard did well postoperatively despite having heart failure. Why?

Pop Quiz

9.7 True or false? The most common cause of right-sided heart failure is left-sided heart failure.

9.8 What happens to the ejection fraction in systolic heart failure?

9.9 Is pulmonary edema associated with right-sided or left-sided heart failure?

9.10 What lifestyle changes are important in the treatment/prevention of heart failure?

Coronary Artery Disease

Coronary artery disease (CAD) arises because of atherosclerotic narrowing or complete occlusion of one or more coronary arteries, which deprives cardiac muscle of blood and results in ischemia or infarction of cardiac muscle. Risk factors are the same as for atherosclerosis. CAD is the leading cause of death in the United States in both sexes, accounting for about one-third of all deaths.

CAD begins surprisingly early in life. Autopsy studies of American soldiers killed in the early 1950s during the Korean War revealed an astonishing degree of coronary atherosclerosis in these otherwise healthy young men, most of whom were in their late teens or twenties. More recent studies show that cholesterol deposits literally begin in the crib; however, most CAD does not become clinically apparent until after age 60 in men and age 70 in women. CAD is more common in males, but women tend to catch up after menopause, when they lose the protective effect of estrogen. The difference narrows and by age 75 women are affected as much as or more than men. For unknown reasons, the sex difference is less in nonwhites.

In both sexes, age is one of the most important risk factors—the older you become, the more at risk you are. There is some familial influence, but it is much less than lifestyle. It is worth [illegible] that *half of acute myocardial infarction*[illegible] *or no risk factors and no prior s*[illegible]

Remember This! [illegible] **occur in previously asympt**[illegible]

Obstructed Co[illegible] uses Myocardial Isc[illegible]

Recall from Chapt[illegible] e basic lesion of atherosclerosis[illegible] struction becomes progressiv[illegible] f downstream myocardium occ[illegible] partial or complete, and tempo[illegible] gree of stenosis required to prod[illegible] oxygen demand (e.g., increased [illegible] emotion). Some cell necrosis oc[illegible] mia, so that the consequences va[illegible] myocardial dysfunction to irreversible myocardial infarction—75% fixed reduction of the coronary lumen may be enough to cause infarction if oxygen demand is high. In such cases, the partial obstruction is usually attributable to an old, stable atheromatous plaque. Partial, reversible obstruction may also occur when aggregates of platelets temporarily accumulate on the surface of an atheroma (early thrombus formation, Chapter 6), further narrowing the lumen without proceeding to complete thrombotic occlusion and infarction.

Although atherosclerosis is the underlying cause of CAD, vascular spasm may be a contributing or precipitating factor in some instances. The cause of vasospasm is not clear in most instances, but smoking and cocaine abuse are well-known culprits. Obstruction due to vasculitis and embolism are rare.

Ischemia can occur without CAD in patients with massive cardiac hypertrophy because even normal coronary arteries may not be able to meet the metabolic demand of the large amount of muscle mass, especially if blood pressure is relatively low.

Acute complete occlusion (Fig. 9.9) is usually caused by events occurring in a soft, unstable, young atheroma. The atheroma may fissure, rupture, or hemorrhage, exposing blood to tissue factors that initiate thrombosis and cause acute ischemia due to further narrowing or complete occlusion. Prior to occlusion, these atheromas usually are not large enough to cause symptoms, which make them very difficult to detect in asymptomatic persons. Alternatively, slow complete occlusion by old, fibrotic (often calcified) atheromas may not cause infarction because alternative (collateral) vessels develop to supply the affected area. These older atheromas, while likely to produce ischemia and angina, are not so prone to sudden occlusion and infarction and are easier to identify by diagnostic imaging.

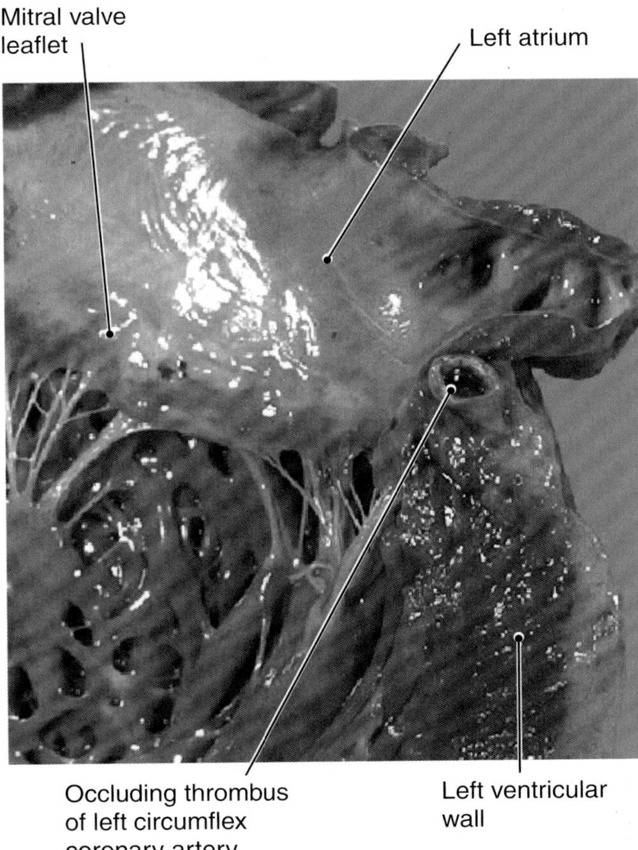

Figure 9.9 **Acute thrombosis of a coronary artery.** This thrombosis caused infarction of part of the posterior wall of the left ventricle (not visible).

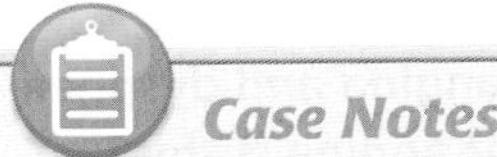

Case Notes

9.7 **Willard had ischemia and angina but had negligible coronary atherosclerosis. Explain.**

Acute Ischemia Produces a Spectrum of Effects

Acute ischemia produces a spectrum of effects that vary depending on the size of the ischemic area and the duration of the obstruction. They range from temporary chest pain (*angina*) to survivable myocardial infarction to instant death from arrhythmia. Myocardial infarction is not necessary to produce dire effects.

Angina Pectoris

Angina pectoris is a distinctive sensation caused by myocardial ischemia with or without infarction. Usually the patient seeks care for a frightening feeling of chest discomfort, described as smothering, pressing, aching, choking, or heaviness. They may not describe the feeling as painful. The sensation occurs beneath the sternum and may radiate to the left jaw, shoulder, elbow, or wrist or even to the back, neck, both arms, or upper abdomen.

It is clinically difficult to determine whether a patient is experiencing ischemia without infarction or is having a myocardial infarct. Angina without infarction typically rises or fluctuates and then disappears, or is relieved by coronary vasodilators, especially nitroglycerin.

Stable angina rises and falls smoothly over a period of a few minutes and is relieved by rest or medication. It may be precipitated by exertion and emotion or by a heavy meal or sudden exposure to cold. It rarely arises spontaneously.

Unstable angina is caused by aggregates of platelets accumulating on an atherosclerotic plaque. It is a very serious condition that may herald impending myocardial infarction. It is characterized by intensification of existing angina, new onset of angina at rest, nocturnal angina, or onset of prolonged angina. Patients with unstable angina, especially angina at rest accompanied by temporary electrocardiographic abnormalities, are at high risk for impending myocardial infarction and need vigorous intervention. About 30% of patients with unstable angina will have an MI within three months of onset.

Unremitting angina is angina that does not fluctuate and cannot be relieved by therapy. It is caused by myocardial infarction. The angina is a steady, crushing substernal chest discomfort or pain with radiation to the neck, jaw, epigastrium, shoulder, or left arm. Patients usually have dyspnea, nausea and vomiting, and sweat profusely.

To learn something of the history of angina, see *The History of Medicine*, "... a disorder of the breast, marked with strong and peculiar symptoms."

Case Notes

9.8 Willard had exertional angina and dyspnea relieved by rest. What type of angina is this?

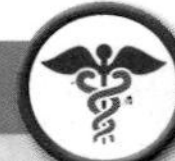

The History of Medicine

"... A DISORDER OF THE BREAST, MARKED WITH STRONG AND PECULIAR SYMPTOMS"

Coronary artery ischemia is the most common potentially fatal disease of people living in the United States and other developed Western nations. Whereas infectious diseases, diabetes, and many other illnesses were described in antiquity, CAD is a relatively recent discovery.

The typical chest pain of myocardial ischemia was first clearly described by English physician William Heberden (1710–1801). In 1768 he wrote: "There is a disorder of the breast, marked with strong and peculiar symptoms, considerable for the kind of danger belonging to it, and not extremely rare . . . [which causes a] sense of strangling and anxiety . . . [called] angina pectoris." Heberden studied a series of patients and noted that the malady came over them when walking and disappeared with rest, that most patients were overweight, stocky men, and that the malady sometimes killed them quickly, observations that remain valid today.

Nevertheless, the syndrome was not clearly identified as being caused by coronary obstruction until 1912, when American physician James B. Herrick published his landmark paper, "Clinical Features of Sudden Obstruction of the Coronary Arteries."

Myocardial Infarction

A **myocardial infarct (MI)** is a circumscribed area of myocardial necrosis caused by ischemia. MI is the most important consequence of CAD and is the single, most common cause of death in industrialized nations. In the United States, about 1.5 million persons suffer a MI each year; about one-third die of it. The usual infarction is accompanied by *angina*, the signature severe chest discomfort or pain discussed above. Infarction may be asymptomatic, however, and discovered incidentally by routine ECG. About 20% of MIs are silent, especially in people with diabetes or hypertension, or in the very elderly.

As described above, most MIs are initiated by atherosclerotic plaque rupture, ulceration, or hemorrhage, precipitating the formation of an obstructing thrombus (**coronary thrombosis**) (Fig. 9.9). The size of an infarct is largely determined by the anatomy of the coronary artery tree and the location of the occlusion. For example, proximal occlusion of an artery is more likely to produce a larger infarct than is distal occlusion of a smaller branch. The coronary distribution varies—the right or left coronaries and their branches supply varying amounts of myocardium from one person to the next; occlusion of a branch supplying a large amount of myocardium produces a correspondingly larger infarct.

The left ventricle is most affected, though large infarcts may involve the muscular interventricular septum and right ventricle. Anterior infarcts tend to be larger and have a worse prognosis than posterior infarcts. Occlusion of the anterior descending branch of the left coronary artery, which usually supplies the anterior wall and apex of the left ventricle, is the cause of nearly half of all infarcts. The right coronary artery, which usually supplies the posterior left ventricular wall, is the culprit in about one-third of the cases. The left circumflex artery, which usually supplies the left lateral ventricular wall, accounts for the remainder.

Coronary arteries run on the surface of the heart and send penetrating arteries inward to supply the myocardium. The last muscle to be supplied is that deepest in the wall—the subendocardial muscle, which is the first to die when an infarct develops. Decreased flow through a particular segment of a coronary artery or occlusion of small coronary branches may cause infarction only of subendocardial muscle—a *subendocardial infarct*. As Figure 9.10 shows, an infarct associated with the occlusion of a larger (more proximate) coronary branch may begin as an area of subendocardial infarction and continue to enlarge for three to six hours, until it involves the full thickness of the ventricular wall—a *transmural infarct*.

The age of a MI can be determined by the gross and microscopic findings at autopsy (Fig. 9.11). Coagulative necrosis (Chapter 2), characterized by blocks of yellow tissue, appears early and gradually heals. By eight weeks a mature scar is present.

CAD Should be Suspected in Adult with Chest Pain

CAD should be suspected in men over 30 and women over 40 whose main complaint is chest pain or discomfort (Fig. 9.12). The first task in diagnosis of a patient with chest pain or discomfort is to rule out conditions other than angina: pneumonia, pulmonary embolism, pericarditis, rib fracture, inflammation of costochondral joints, esophageal spasm, aortic dissection, gallstones, gastric ulcer, and many others.

If CAD is suspected, diagnosis requires serial ECGs and highly sensitive blood tests for the presence of cardiac

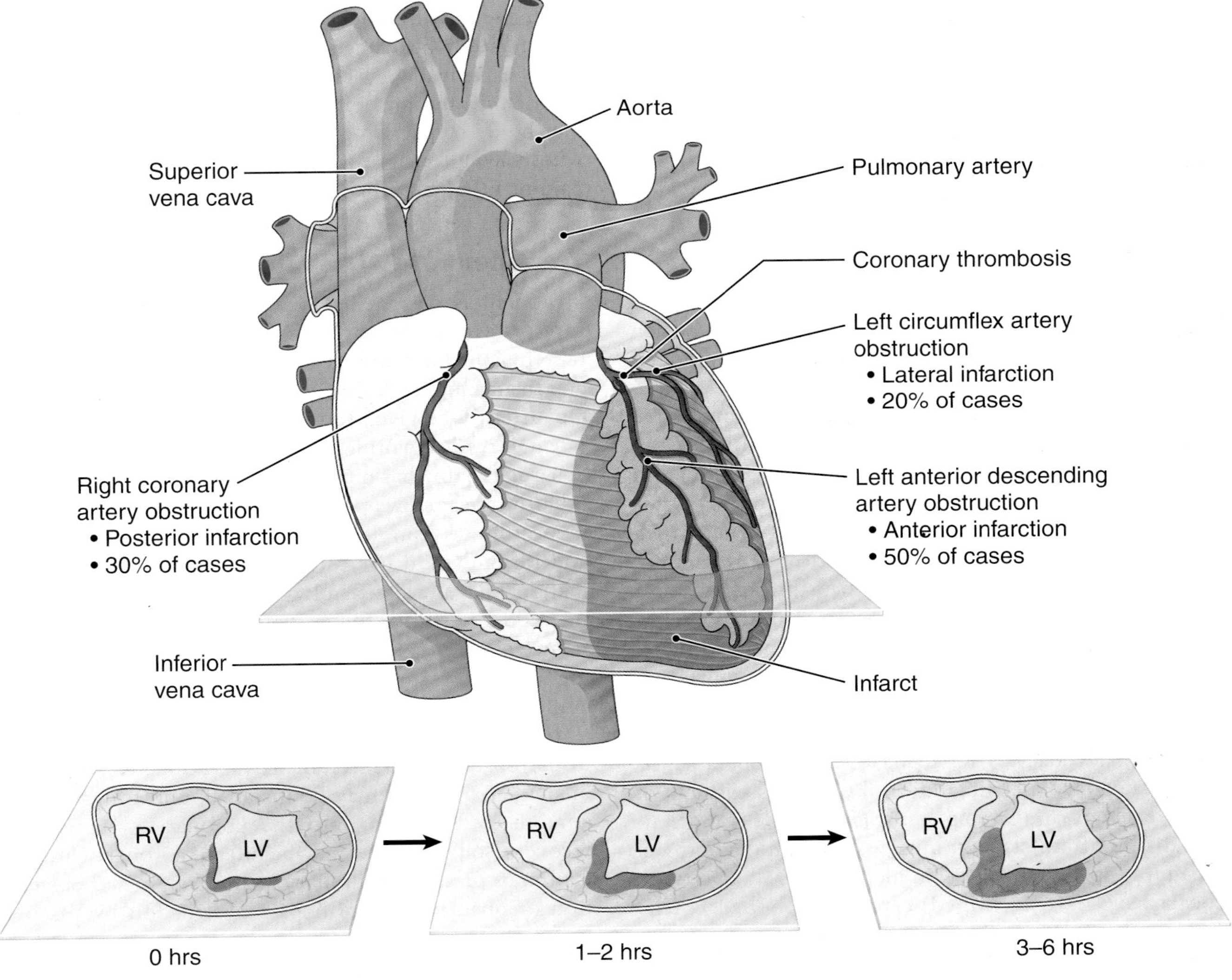

Figure 9.10 Evolution of an acute myocardial infarct. The area of infarcted muscle is small at the onset and larger three to six hours later.

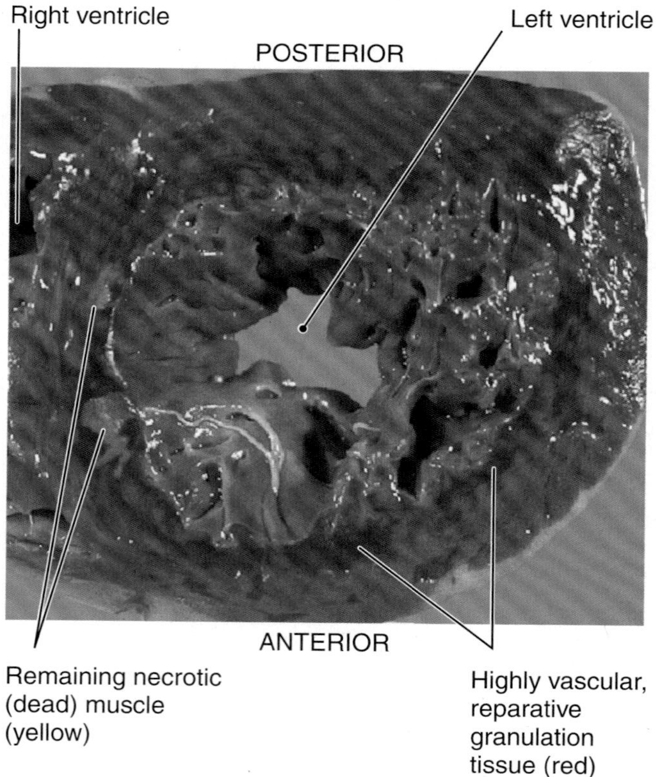

Figure 9.11 **Myocardial infarct.** Two-week-old infarct of the left ventricle. The infarct completely encircles the ventricle. Note sunken, red granulation (repair) tissue with a few remaining islands of yellow, necrotic cardiac muscle not yet removed by the repair process.

markers. ECG is most important and should be done immediately. ECG findings are used to distinguish which patients need immediate catheterization, angiography, and administration of thrombus-dissolving fibrinolytic drugs.

Blood assays for cardiac markers are also imperative in the differential diagnosis of chest pain, in the follow-up assessment of the size of a MI, and in the evaluation of recovery and treatment. Dead cardiac muscle cells release enzymes and proteins into blood where they can be measured. Even in patients without infarction, temporary electrocardiographic abnormalities may occur and some cardiac markers may be present in blood. The degree of increase of these enzymes in blood is roughly proportional to the size of the infarct. One enzyme is *creatine kinase (CK)*, which is found in high concentration in cardiac and skeletal muscle, and in the brain. *CK-MB* is the cardiac variety. CK-MB has proven to be a sensitive, but not very specific, indicator of MI. Assessment of blood levels of *cardiac troponin (cTn)*, which is molecularly distinct from skeletal muscle troponin, has proven to be more specific than CK in identifying MI. Two types of cTn have been identified, cardiac troponin I (cTnI) and cardiac troponin T (cTnT). Neither type is present in significant amounts in the blood of healthy people; therefore, detection of even small amounts offers a sensitive and specific indicator of myocardial infarction. The time period for these markers to rise and fall is also different—CK-MB falls back to normal in two to three days, while troponin takes seven to ten days.

Remember This! The measurement of blood cTn is the most specific test for detection of a myocardial infarction.

Although enzymes can confirm damage is present, recognizing the full extent of obstruction and the size of affected muscle is difficult without angiography. *Coronary angiography* is used to visualize both the location and the extent of coronary obstruction and often combines diagnosis with therapy (discussed below). Immediate angiography is indicated in patients with certain ECG findings, persistent pain despite maximal medical therapy, unstable arrhythmias, cardiogenic shock, and some other conditions. Angiography can be delayed a day or two in patients with small infarcts or whose pain has resolved with medical therapy. In addition, echocardiographic imaging can be used to study heart mechanical action for defects such as mitral valve leaflet eversion and ventricular wall inertia or paradoxical motion. Finally, cardiac exercise stress imaging should be performed in patients with noninfarct CAD whose symptoms resolve to check for exercise-related pain or ECG abnormalities.

Treatment of CAD Is Multimodal

Treatment is designed to comfort the individual, interrupt or reverse coronary thrombosis, reverse ischemia by reperfusion, limit infarct size, reduce cardiac workload, and treat complications. Oxygen and bed rest are required. Opiates may be given to relieve anxiety and reduce heart rate and cardiac workload.

Drug therapy has multiple objectives. Nitroglycerine or other nitrates relieve pain and aid in reperfusing ischemic myocardium. Antiplatelet, thrombolytic, anticoagulant, and fibrinolytic drugs can halt or reverse thrombus formation and reestablish blood flow, which may prevent infarction or reduce the size of the infarct. Beta-blockers reduce cardiac workload by slowing heart rate and lowering blood pressure. Antiarrhythmics regularize rhythm and control heart rate.

If immediate coronary angiography is warranted after initial observation, thrombi may be directly broken up or extracted, stents may be installed, and drugs may be administered directly into the coronary system. After recovery, some patients may be offered coronary catheterization to place intracoronary stents at points of obstruction or open surgery to bypass obstruction by vascular grafts.

For additional insight into the treatment of CAD, see *The Clinical Side*, "Lifestyle and Coronary Artery Disease."

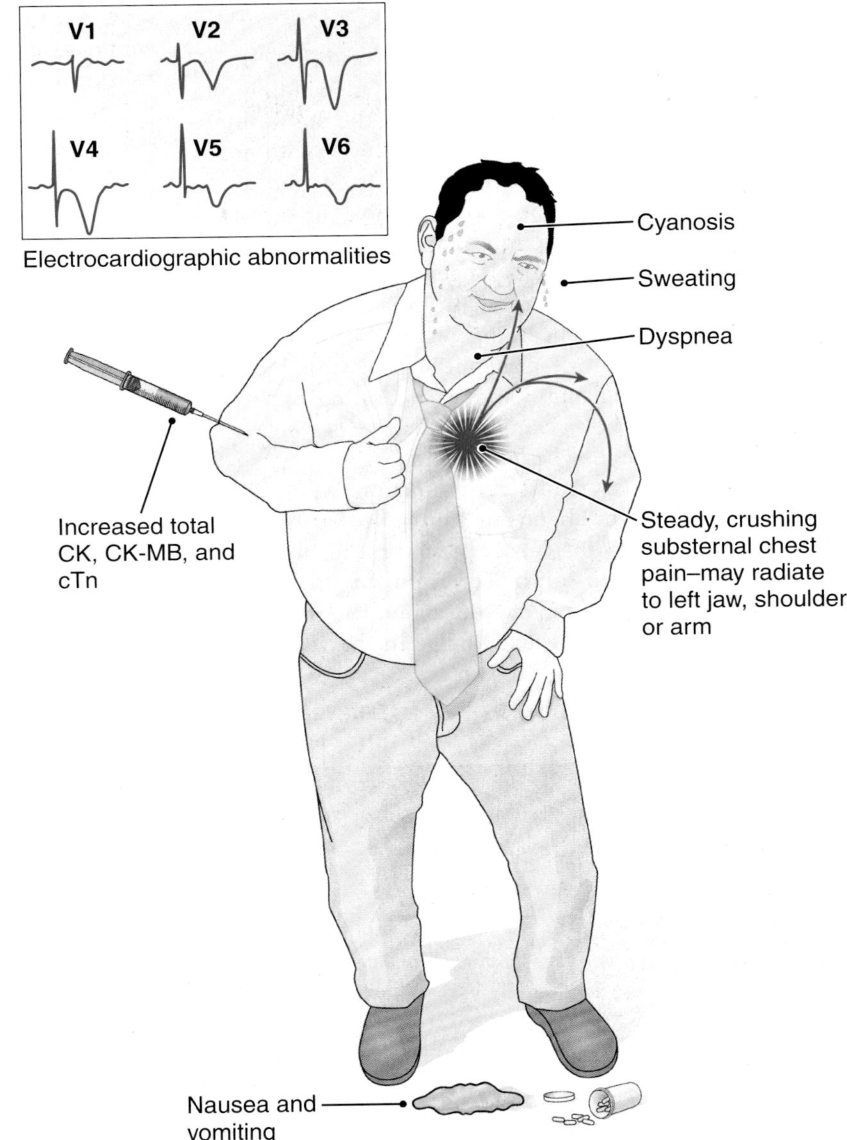

Figure 9.12 **Clinical picture of acute myocardial infarction.** ECG abnormalities are characteristic. In blood, total creatine kinase (CK), cardiac creatine kinase (CK-MB), and cTn are increased.

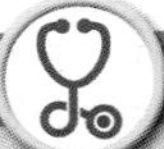

The Clinical Side

LIFESTYLE AND CORONARY ARTERY DISEASE

What can the average Joe or Jane do to pevent a heart attack?

- Giving up cigarettes is at the top of the list—nothing else comes close.
- Regular exercise, even a small amount, helps.
- Maintain a healthful weight.
- Reduce intake of foods high in saturated fat, such as burgers, full-fat cheeses, butter, and ice cream, as well as foods high in *trans* fats.

Evidence suggests that moderate consumption of alcohol can lessen the risk of cardiovascular disease. The equivalent of one to two alcoholic drinks a day (beers, glasses of wine, cocktails) reduces the risk of cardiovascular disease. Too much alcohol, however, eliminates the benefit and leads to other health problems, and no one recommends that nondrinkers take up the habit for cardiovascular benefit. Recent studies indicate that the number of drinking days per week is more important than the amount of alcohol consumed; persons drinking in moderation nearly every day appear to have a greater benefit than those drinking episodically. The benefit is only slightly reduced by the adverse effects of alcohol (such as obesity, liver disease, and accidents). But it is folly to think that moderate alcohol intake, exercise, weight loss, or a healthful diet will trump the devastating effect of smoking—it won't.

Complications Are Common

Ischemic (even though not infarcted) myocardium does not contract normally. Consequences vary depending on the size of the area of affected muscle and the duration of the obstruction. Some cell necrosis occurs even with mild ischemia, so that the consequences vary from transient, mild myocardial dysfunction to irreversible myocardial infarction. Transient obstruction of a small vessel may be asymptomatic, but larger and longer-lasting obstruction may not be able to support normal cardiac output. Mild-to-severe heart failure or cardiogenic shock may result. The electrical function of ischemic cells is not normal and may cause *arrhythmias* (abnormal beating patterns, discussed below). They occur in 90% of MIs. Most are temporary, but some may be fatal.

Temporary papillary muscle dysfunction with mitral regurgitation occurs in about one-third of MI patients in the first few days. Scarring causes permanent regurgitation in some patients, which can be corrected surgically. Myocardial rupture and death occurs in about 1% of infarcts. Ventricular aneurysm, a localized bulge in the ventricular wall, develops in some transmural infarcts. It is associated with reduced mechanical efficiency, low cardiac output, and risk for formation of a mural thrombus (Fig. 9.13). Mural thrombus occurs in about 20% of MIs and is associated with risk of thromboembolism to the brain and other organs.

Prognosis varies depending upon the location and size of the infarct; the presence or absence of arrhythmia, heart failure, or shock; and many other variables. Overall mortality in the first 30 days is about 25%, with half of those dying, usually of an arrhythmia, before reaching the hospital. Of those who survive, annual mortality is about 10%.

Chronic myocardial ischemia, from recurrent acute attacks or due to decreased blood supply, may lead to **ischemic cardiomyopathy**, a condition in which heart failure develops as the mass of healthy ventricular muscle deteriorates following infarcts both large and small, clinical or subclinical (asymptomatic), or with the accumulated withering effect of chronic ischemia. The ventricles become dilated, thin-walled, and flabby, similar to *dilated cardiomyopathy (DC)* (discussed below), a type of cardiomyopathy with the same features but usually of unknown

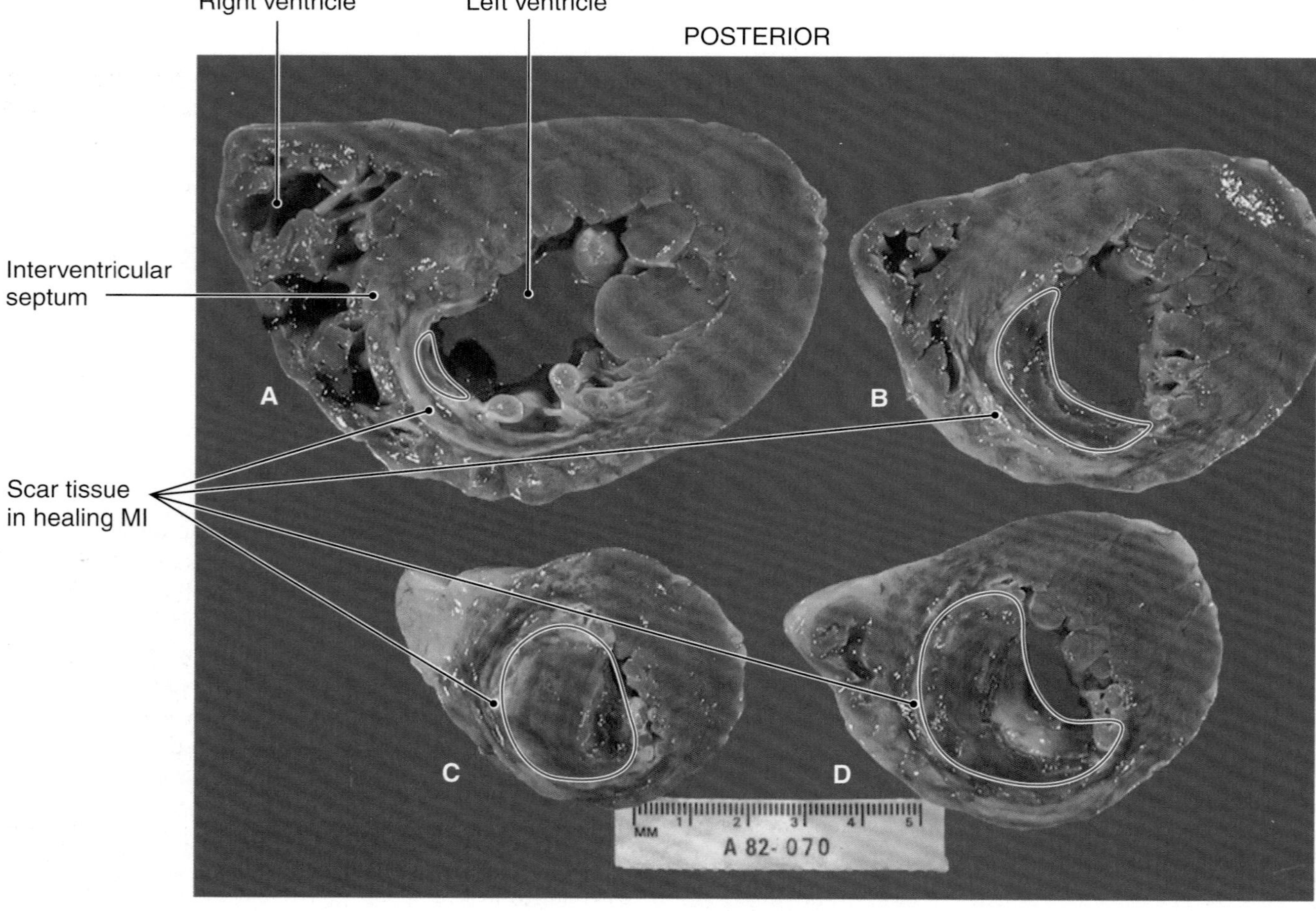

Figure 9.13 **Intracardiac mural thrombus (encircled).** Superior view of serial cross-sections. **A.** Section high, near the mitral valve. **B** and **C.** Middle sections. **D.** Section near the apex, where the thrombus fills most of the ventricular cavity.

cause. Most patients with ischemic cardiomyopathy are elderly and present with heart failure.

Pop Quiz

9.11 True or false? A blood test for troponins is more specific in detecting a MI than a blood test for CK.

9.12 True or false? Ischemia can occur without CAD.

9.13 True or false? ECG abnormalities mean a MI has occurred.

9.14 What is the difference between stable and unstable angina?

9.15 What are the main elements of the treatment of an MI?

Valvular Heart Disease

Normal cardiac valves function like one-way gates. Valve malfunctions include the following:

- **Valvular stenosis** is failure of the valve to open fully. It is usually due to stiff or fused valve leaflets caused by chronic inflammation and scarring.
- **Valvular insufficiency** (regurgitation, backflow, incompetence) is failure of the valve to close fully. Sometimes referred to as a "leaky valve," it is usually due to a structural defect. Valves are usually stiff or deformed by inflammation, or eaten away by bacterial or fungal infection. *Functional* insufficiency is valve incompetence owing to abnormality of valve support structures. For example, the aortic root may dilate and prevent complete closure of aortic valve cusps or mitral valve leaflets may invert secondary to papillary muscle infarction or rupture.

Stenosis and insufficiency are mechanically inefficient. In some severe cases, valves may be both stenotic and insufficient, usually when the valve is stiff and locked into a midway point between being open and closed (Fig. 9.14). Regardless of cause, diseased, damaged, or deformed valves are susceptible to bacterial infection (*infective endocarditis*).

Degeneration Is the Most Common Cause of Valve Disease

Valves are delicate structures subject to great stress: they flex at hinge points and snap closed about 40 million times

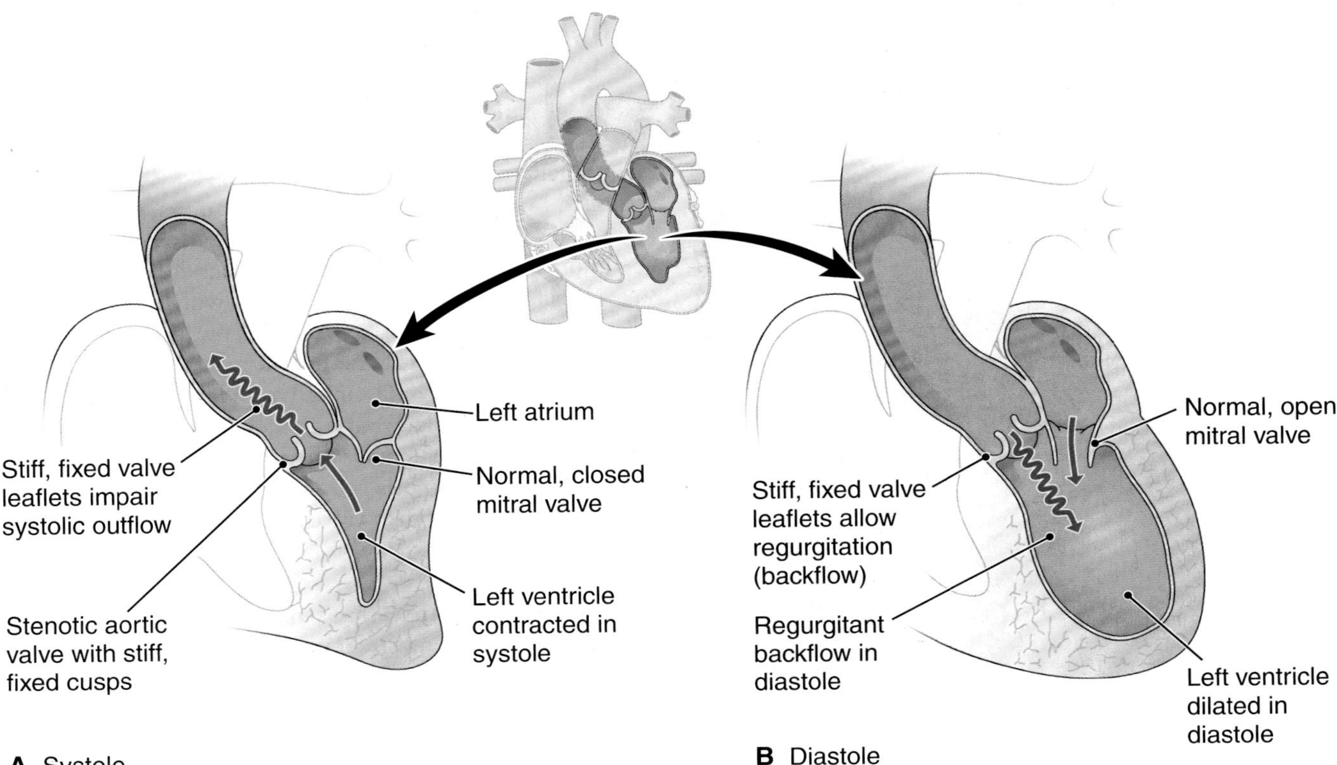

Figure 9.14 **Aortic stenosis and insufficiency.** Severe aortic valve disease can immobilize aortic valve cusps, so that both obstruction to outflow (stenosis) and regurgitant backflow (insufficiency) occur. **A.** Systole: flow across the aortic valve is obstructed. **B.** Diastole: incomplete closure of aortic valve allows backflow.

per year. When closed, they are strained by high-pressure gradients—especially the mitral and aortic valves, which are most often affected by degenerative valve disease. Aortic stenosis (AS) and mitral valve prolapse are the two most common valvular abnormalities.

Aortic Stenosis

Most cases of AS are age-related, wear-and-tear disease, most commonly in patients over 60. AS can also be caused, however, by congenital bicuspid aortic valves and by rheumatic fever, an autoimmune disorder discussed below, in which valve cusps fuse together. In each instance the valves are stiff and laden with lumps of rock-hard calcific nodules (**calcific aortic stenosis**) (Fig. 9.15). The valve orifice gradually narrows, putting strain on the left ventricle. The ventricle compensates by becoming hypertrophic, but ultimately cannot maintain sufficient cardiac output when demand is high.

Congenital bicuspid aortic valve (Fig. 9.15) occurs in 1% of the population. The normal valve consists of three equal leaflets. A congenitally bicuspid valve has two functional leaflets, one larger than the other, reflecting failure of two of the three embryologic precursor leaflets to separate normally. It is associated with increased valve leaflet wear and tear because the valve leaflets are stretched with each beat. (In a normal valve the three leaflets are designed so that they are merely pushed out of the way.) Most cases are associated with early-onset AS.

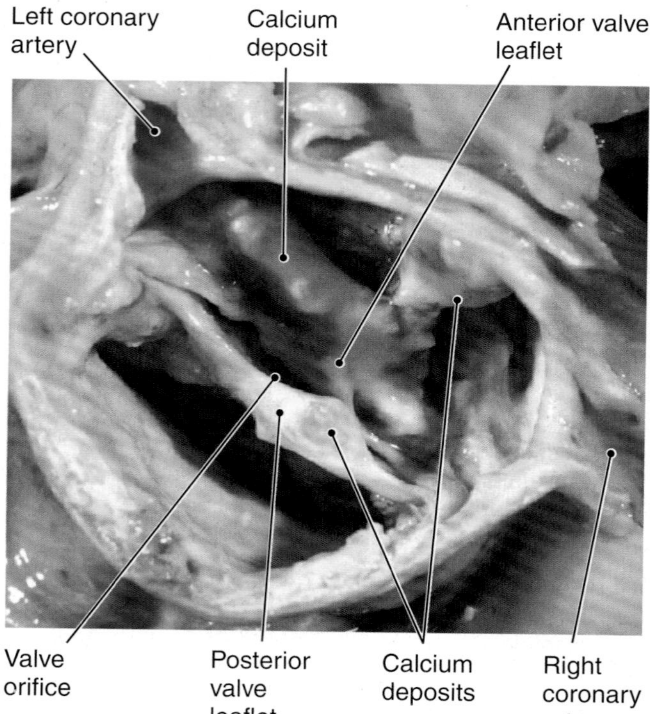

Figure 9.15 **Calcific aortic stenosis of a congenital bicuspid aortic valve.** Valve leaflets are thick and crusted with calcium and frozen in position. This valve is both stenotic and insufficient.

The classic clinical diagnostic triad of AS is exertional dyspnea, syncope, and angina pectoris. With exertion, cardiac output becomes insufficient. Right ventricular output cannot be greater than left, so low pulmonary blood flow causes dyspnea. Low systemic flow causes syncope, and low coronary flow to a laboring left ventricle causes angina pectoris. A systolic crescendo-decrescendo murmur is characteristic. Diagnosis is by echocardiographic imaging of the valve. Average survival for untreated symptomatic patients is two to three years. Valve replacement or balloon valvotomy is effective: it relieves symptoms and extends survival. Surgery is delayed until symptoms develop because, in asymptomatic patients, the risk of surgery outweighs the benefit and because grafts have an effective lifespan of about 10 years and may have to be repeated.

Case Notes

9.9 **Willard had known of his valve defect for 40 years before having surgery to correct it. Why the long wait?**

Calcification of the Mitral Annulus

Calcific deposits can develop in the ring of fibrous tissue (annulus) that supports the mitral valve (**annular calcification**). Risk factors are the same as for atherosclerosis and CAD. The deposits are similar to those of calcific AS: rough, rock-hard calcific nodules that can form an unyieldingly stiff collar around the base of the valve. Valvular function is usually not affected. In some cases, however, regurgitation may occur because the valve leaflets are restrained from full closure. In other instances, the ring may cause stenosis. Sometimes the ring may cause arrhythmia by impinging on the CCS near the AV node. The ring may also precipitate thrombus formation with increased risk of embolization and stroke. Additionally, the rough edges and crevasses of the calcific nodules can be the nidus for implantation of bacteria (*infective endocarditis*, discussed below). Annular calcification is most common in women over age 60 and patients with *mitral valve prolapse* (discussed below). Diagnosis is by chest X-ray. There is no specific treatment other than valve replacement in some cases.

Mitral Valve Prolapse

Mitral valve prolapse (*myxomatous degeneration of the mitral valve*) is the most common valve disease, affecting about 3% of the U.S. adult population between ages 20 and 40. Two-thirds of patients are women. It is a common problem in patients with inheritable connective tissue disorders such as *Marfan syndrome* (Chapter 22). It is characterized by an accumulation of interstitial myxoid material in the valve leaflets. The cause is usually unknown. The result is regurgitant, "floppy" mitral valve leaflets attached to elongated chordae tendineae. The great majority of patients are asymptomatic and suffer no ill effect, but some may develop severe regurgitation.

Initial presentation may be subtle and erroneously attributed to psychological problems. Anxiety, fatigue, palpitations, odd chest pain, and syncope are common. Chest X-ray, ECG, blood tests, and other data are usually normal. Chest auscultation may reveal the late systolic murmur and mid-systolic click that is characteristic of affected patients (the click occurs as elongated chordae tendineae snap tight). Diagnosis is by echocardiography. Treatment is surgical valve repair or replacement.

Rheumatic Fever Is a Cause of Valve Disease

Acute rheumatic fever (RF) is an acute autoimmune disease that occurs in children 5–15 years old about two to six weeks after group A streptococcal pharyngitis (Fig. 9.16). It is a syndrome of various combinations of *arthritis, valvulitis, myocarditis, pericarditis, subcutaneous nodules, skin rash,* and *chorea (see below)*. It is a transient disease but may recur in some patients. For unknown reasons, it does not occur with group A streptococcal infections at other sites. RF owes to autoimmune attack on self-tissues by antistrep antibodies. Recall from our discussion of immune disease that molecular mimicry is one way in which the immune system can be tricked into attacking self-tissues—a foreign antigen (streptococcus antigen in this case) is similar to self-antigens found in the heart and joints, and antibodies produced against strep antigens also attack these similar self-antigens.

Fever and migratory polyarthritis are the most common symptoms. Acute carditis and pericarditis occur in about half of cases, but if chronic valve disease appears, it presents much later. Cardiac murmurs are common. Subcutaneous inflammatory nodules and a distinctive serpiginous skin rash (*erythema marginatum*) usually occur together. A few patients develop *Sydenham chorea*, a slowly developing movement disorder of rapid, irregular, jerky movements, and speech abnormalities. Diagnosis is clinical and supported by increased markers of inflammation such as increased WBC and elevated erythrocyte sedimentation rate (ESR) and C-reactive protein (CRP).

RF is usually self-limiting and often not recognized for what it is. Most patients recover completely without long-term ill effect. Prognosis depends on the severity of the initial carditis—severe carditis is more likely to recur and may progress to chronic myocardial or valve disease. In about 5% of acute cases, severe carditis with heart failure occurs. Sydenham chorea usually lasts several months, but may recur.

Acute rheumatic carditis may progress to *chronic rheumatic heart disease* (RHD), the main manifestation of which is valvular disease. RHD is virtually the sole cause of mitral stenosis. RF and RHD are uncommon today in developed nations because of the effective use of antibiotics in the treatment of streptococcal pharyngitis, but RHD remains a serious problem in developing nations.

Alternatively, streptococcal infection and immune attack may be chronic and subclinical (silent), and the first clinical sign may be **chronic rheumatic valvulitis (RV)** (Fig. 9.17). Patients with RV rarely have a history of RF and the diagnosis is made in retrospect as a diagnosis of exclusion in the workup of patients with chronic valve disease, especially mitral stenosis. A history of streptococcal pharyngitis is rarely obtained.

Treatment is supportive and includes aspirin and other nonsteroidal anti-inflammatory drugs (NSAIDs). Corticosteroids may be required if NSAIDs do not quell the inflammation. Antistreptococcal antibiotics should be administered prophylactically. How long to continue prophylaxis is uncertain. The American Academy of Pediatrics recommends 10 years for patients with carditis.

Endocarditis Is Usually a Disease of Valves

The growth of vegetations on cardiac valves (or, rarely, other endocardial sites) is called "endocarditis." Two types are recognized: *noninfective thrombotic endocarditis* and *infective endocarditis*. Both can cause valve malfunction and carry increased risk for embolization and stroke.

Noninfective Thrombotic Endocarditis

Noninfective thrombotic endocarditis (Fig. 9.18) is characterized by 1–5 mm valvular vegetations composed of platelets and fibrinous material. The mitral and aortic valves are most often affected. If valve malfunction occurs, it is most likely to be mitral regurgitation. The lesions contain no microorganisms, and affected valves are otherwise normal. The pathogenesis is obscure; however, the lesions are found most often in patients with severe lupus erythematosus (SLE) or in severely debilitated patients such as those with terminal cancer or sepsis. The lesions are almost always asymptomatic and are discovered incidentally at autopsy. Rarely, they may embolize and cause infarction, most notably in the brain. It is also important to note that the lesions are susceptible to microbiologic colonization and the added development of infective endocarditis. Diagnosis is clinical. There is no specific treatment.

Infective Endocarditis

Infective endocarditis is infection of the endocardium, usually in the endothelium lining the aortic or mitral valve. It is almost always caused by bacterial infection (**bacterial endocarditis**), usually by staphylococci or streptococci, which appear as ragged masses (vegetations) (Fig. 9.19). The most common associated conditions are congenital heart defects, rheumatic valvular disease, bicuspid or calcific aortic valves, and prolapsed mitral valves. Artificial valves are at special risk. Rarely, a previously normal valve may be affected, especially in IV drug abusers. Anything that causes bacteremia (transient or otherwise) can seed an abnormal cardiac valve and

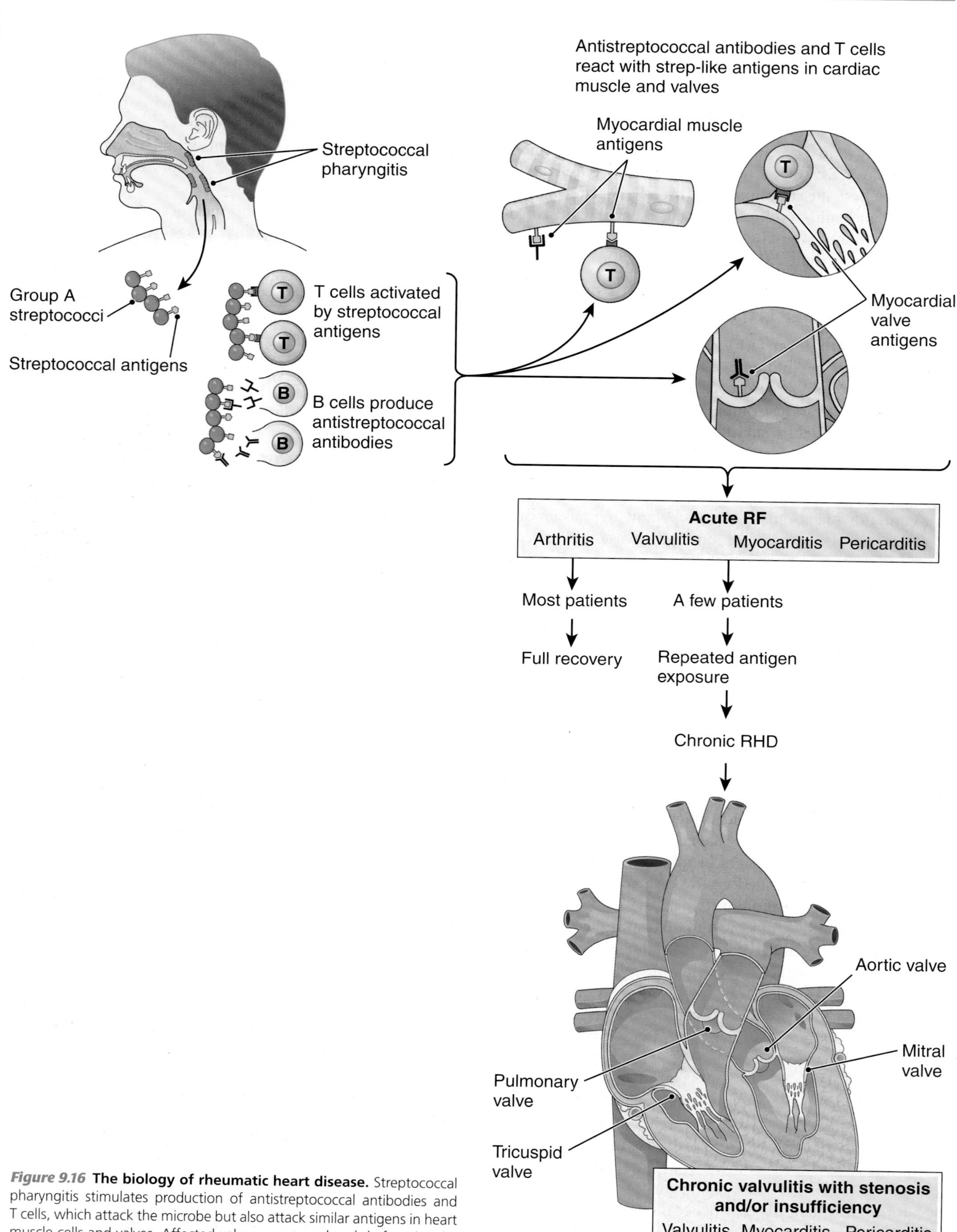

Figure 9.16 **The biology of rheumatic heart disease.** Streptococcal pharyngitis stimulates production of antistreptococcal antibodies and T cells, which attack the microbe but also attack similar antigens in heart muscle cells and valves. Affected valves are scarred and dysfunctional.

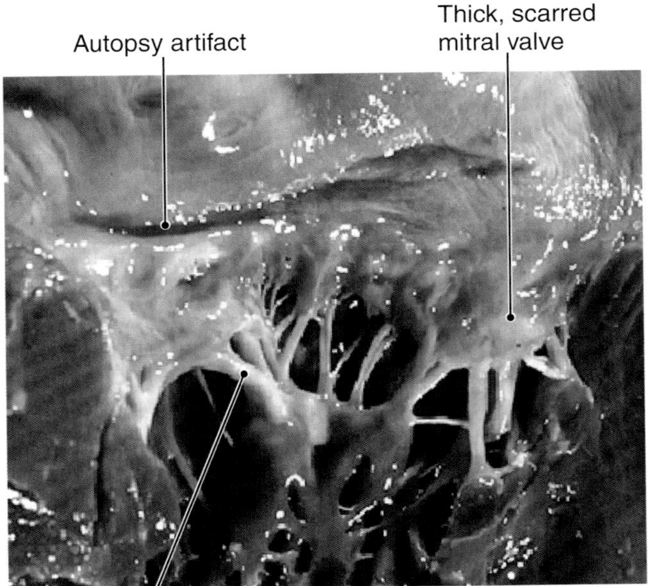

Figure 9.17 **Chronic rheumatic mitral valvulitis.** Inflammation and scarring produce a stiff, thick valve and short, thick chordae tendineae. Such valves may be stenotic or regurgitant.

establish infection—inflamed gums, abscesses, shooting intravenous drugs with dirty needles, cardiac catheterization, and endoscopic examinations of the lungs, joints, intestine, or urinary tract.

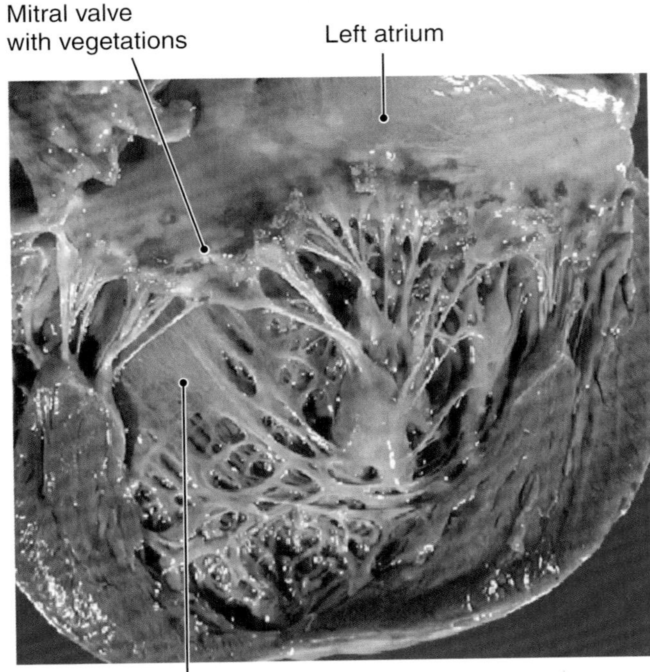

Figure 9.18 **Nonbacterial thrombotic endocarditis.** Valve vegetations are composed of platelets and fibrin. They are subject to bacterial infection (bacterial endocarditis) and may break away and embolize to distant organs. The cause is unknown.

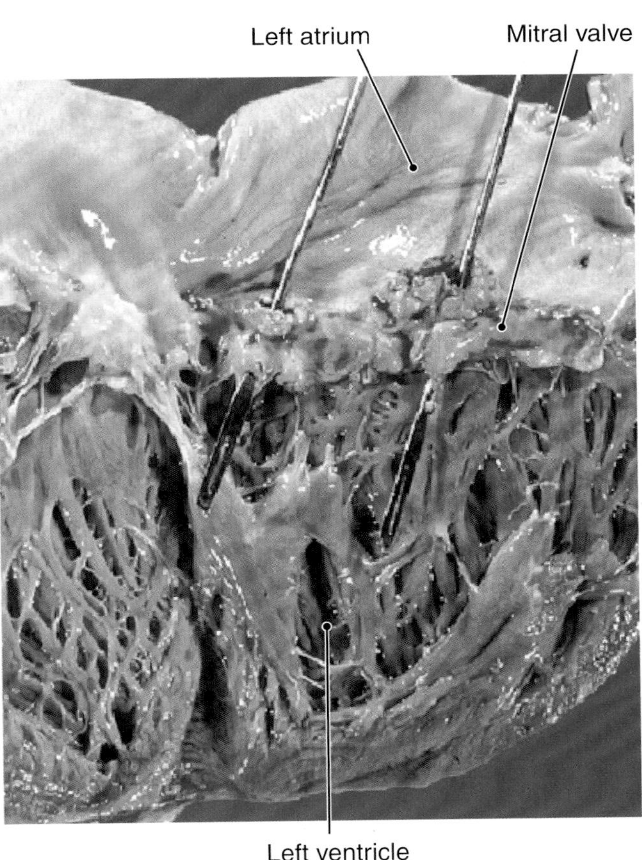

Figure 9.19 **Bacterial endocarditis of the mitral valve.** Probes demonstrate valve perforations caused by bacterial destruction of valve tissue. This case was associated with severe valvular insufficiency (regurgitation).

Valve infections may be acute or chronic, depending on the infective organism. For instance, staphylococcal infection may cause rapidly progressive valve destruction with devastating regurgitation and is referred to as *acute bacterial endocarditis*. It is uncommon and is usually a consequence of IV drug abuse. Infections by less virulent organisms such as *streptococcus* or *enterococcus* are much more common and usually referred to as *subacute bacterial endocarditis (SBE)* because of their slow course. Infection usually occurs in previously diseased valves.

The clinical onset of infective endocarditis may be gradual or explosive, depending on the infective agent. Acute infections feature high fever and shaking chills, but subacute infection may present with innocuous-appearing low-grade fever, weight loss, and malaise. Cardiac murmurs are usually present, and the spleen may be enlarged if hyperplasia develops associated with chronic bloodstream infection. A valuable clue sometimes is oral, conjunctival, retinal, or subungual (beneath the nails) tiny hemorrhages (*petechiae*) caused by bacterial microemboli. Larger emboli may cause abscesses or infarcts, with specific symptoms, such as brain abscess or stroke, or visual impairment from retinal emboli.

Diagnosis is clinical. Infective endocarditis should always be suspected in a patient with fever of unknown origin (FUO). Echocardiographic imaging and repeated and carefully collected blood cultures may be necessary to confirm the diagnosis. Compounding the difficulty of diagnosis is that patients may have been treated with antibiotics for malaise and fever before a diagnosis of endocarditis is considered. Such prediagnosis administration of antibiotics can render blood cultures negative when they otherwise would have been positive.

Infection has local and systemic consequences. The most serious local consequence is erosion or perforation of the valve with valvular insufficiency. Less often myocardial abscess may occur with involvement of the CCS. Systemic consequences mainly owe to embolization with infarction or abscess formation. Right-heart infection seeds the lungs and causes lung infarction, pneumonia, or pulmonary abscess. Emboli from left-heart infection most often infarct the brain, retina, or kidney.

Untreated infective endocarditis is uniformly fatal. Prognosis is poor for patients with drug-resistant organisms, delayed treatment, aortic valve infection, and embolization of clumps of bacteria. In general, mortality is about 10%, but approaches 100% in patients with fungal infection of an artificial valve. Treatment usually requires large doses of intravenous antibiotics over a prolonged period. Rarely, surgical debridement and valve repair may be necessary.

Remember This! Untreated infective endocarditis is uniformly fatal.

Pop Quiz

9.16 True or false? Streptococcal bacterial endocarditis is less virulent than staphylococcal.

9.17 True or false? Noninfective thrombotic endocarditis is most commonly found in people with lupus or in severely debilitated patients.

9.18 What causes RHD?

9.19 What are the two most common valvular diseases?

Diseases of the Myocardium

Disease of cardiac muscle is caused either by inflammation (*myocarditis*) or by intrinsic cardiac muscle disease (*cardiomyopathy*). The usual manifestation is heart failure. Several types are recognized according to anatomic and functional characteristics, each of which may result from inflammation, metabolic disorder, autoimmune disease, or muscular dystrophy or another genetic condition. The cause is often unknown.

Myocarditis Is Inflammation of the Myocardium

Myocarditis is inflammation of the myocardium. It is usually caused by viral infection, especially *Coxsackie A or B* viruses. Some cases are autoimmune (e.g., RF). The list of other causes is long and includes other infectious agents, drugs, chemicals, and pregnancy. Disease usually presents as heart failure or arrhythmia in a patient in otherwise good health with few cardiovascular risk factors. There is no age, ethnic, or sex predilection. Most cases are mild and resolve without therapy, but some proceed to chronic heart failure and the syndrome of dilated cardiomyopathy (see below). The diagnosis is clinical and by exclusion of other causes. Cardiac markers are often present in blood. The prognosis is guarded. Most of those with mild disease recover completely, but about one-third develop dilated cardiomyopathy (see below). Mortality is high for those with severe disease.

Cardiomyopathies Are Non-Inflammatory Diseases of Myocardium

Primary cardiomyopathy refers to intrinsic disease of cardiac muscle. Often the cause is unknown; however, genetic defects are increasingly being identified as a cause of each of the varieties described below. **Secondary cardiomyopathy** may be associated with ischemic heart disease, cardiac hypertrophy due to hypertension or valve disease, infections, acquired metabolic disturbance, congenital heart abnormalities, nutritional deficiency, and immune dysfunction. No matter the cause, cardiomyopathies are classified into one of three categories according to the shape, size, and function of the heart.

Dilated Cardiomyopathy

Dilated cardiomyopathy (DC), or *congestive cardiomyopathy* (Fig. 9.20), is characterized by progressive heart failure with cardiac hypertrophy, dilation, and low ejection fraction. DC occurs most commonly between ages 20 and 60. Usually the cause is not known, but genetic influence is present in about 25% of cases. Viral infection is often suspected. Some cases are clearly associated with chemotherapy. There is a strong association with alcohol abuse. Men are more frequently affected than women, perhaps because more men than women abuse alcohol. Chronic ischemia of the myocardium caused by CAD (*ischemic cardiomyopathy*) can also produce a clinical syndrome indistinguishable from that stemming from other causes of DC. Peripartum and postpartum cardiomyopathy has been described as well.

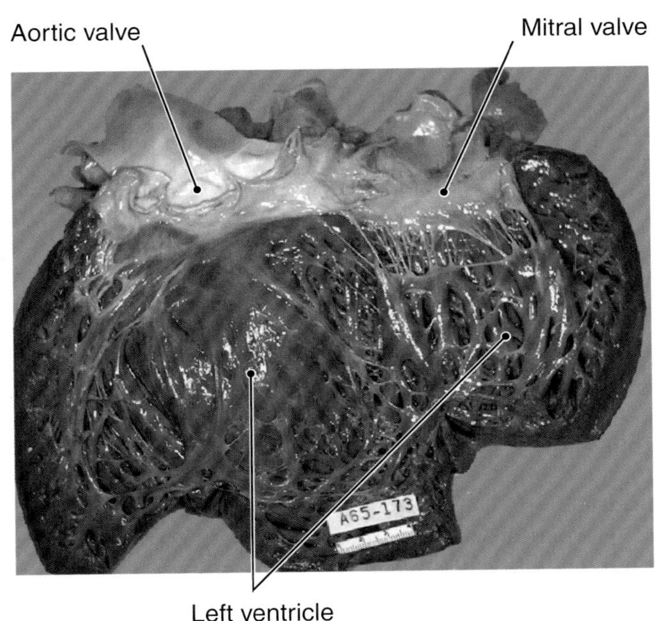

Figure 9.20 **Dilated cardiomyopathy.** The markedly dilated left ventricle is so flabby that it lies flat on the examining table.

The pathology of DC is characterized by dilation and hypertrophy of all chambers. The affected heart features weak, ineffectual contractions. Arrhythmias are frequent. The signs and symptoms are those of heart failure. Diagnosis is clinical by exclusion of other categories of heart failure.

Treatment is symptomatic and aimed at the cause, if one can by found. Prognosis is poor. About 20% die in the first year and 10% annually afterward. Half of deaths are sudden.

Hypertrophic Cardiomyopathy

Hypertrophic cardiomyopathy (HC) can be congenital or acquired. It features marked myocardial hypertrophy. About half of the cases result from an autosomal dominant gene defect. Most of the remaining cases are idiopathic.

In HC, the heart is shaped like, and about as stiff as, one end of a football. The myocardium resists filling, which increases end diastolic and pulmonary venous pressure and causes lung congestion and dyspnea. The muscular hypertrophy is deforming, so much so that diastolic filling may be chaotic and incomplete, and systolic ejection forceful but ineffective. The upper ventricular septum may be especially thick, sometimes to the point of obstructing left ventricular outflow. Because tachycardia allows less time for filling, symptoms usually appear with exercise because cardiac output cannot meet demand. In striking contrast to the weak contractions of DC, systolic contractions are powerful and hyperactive. Arrhythmias are common. Heart failure is uncommon.

Clinical features include systolic murmur, myocardial ischemia, and angina without CAD because the thick, stiff muscle is difficult to perfuse with blood. HC usually comes to attention in the 30- to 50-year-old age group because of dyspnea, angina, fainting spells (syncope), or irregular heartbeat. The first clue that something is wrong, however, may be sudden death, especially in children or young adults, often during or immediately after exertion: sudden death of young athletes is a well-known manifestation of HC. In Europe, trial programs to screen youngsters involved in sports or other exertions have reported as much as a 90% drop in sudden cardiac deaths. Diagnosis is clinical. Echocardiography is confirmatory.

Beta-blockers, ACE inhibitors, nitrates, and other drugs may be useful in decreasing myocardial contractility and improving diastolic filling. Surgical excision of the upper ventricular septum may improve outflow. Annual mortality is 1–3%. Most deaths are sudden and due to arrhythmia.

Remember This! HC is a life-threatening condition in young athletes.

Restrictive Cardiomyopathy

Restrictive cardiomyopathy (RC) is the rarest cardiomyopathy and is characterized by a stiff, noncompliant ventricle that fills incompletely in diastole. There are two varieties. Worldwide, the most common cause is *endomyocardial fibrosis*, a mysterious condition of uncertain cause that occurs most commonly in children and is characterized by markedly thickened, stiff endocardium. The other variety is characterized by infiltration of the myocardium by some substance, such as amyloid protein (*amyloidosis*), iron (*hemochromatosis*), or scar tissue. Poor ventricular compliance increases end diastolic and pulmonary venous pressure, which causes lung congestion and pulmonary hypertension. CHF is the usual outcome. Other complications and symptoms are similar to those of DC and HC. Diagnosis is clinical. Echocardiography is confirmatory. Treatment is symptomatic. Transplantation is not recommended because RC may recur in the transplant.

Hypertension Is a Cause of Ventricular Hypertrophy and Dysfunction

The strain imposed by pumping against high blood pressure or through a stenotic tricuspid or aortic valve can cause right or left ventricular hypertrophy and malfunction.

Systemic hypertension with left ventricular hypertrophy (LVH) is the most common form (Fig. 9.21). Prolonged mild systemic hypertension can induce mild LVH that has few adverse myocardial consequences. Severe and prolonged hypertension, however, can cause massive LVH. In such cases the myocardium becomes stiff and has higher-than-normal metabolic requirements, which render the muscle more susceptible to infarction and arrhythmia. Stiffness reduces ventricular compliance and diastolic

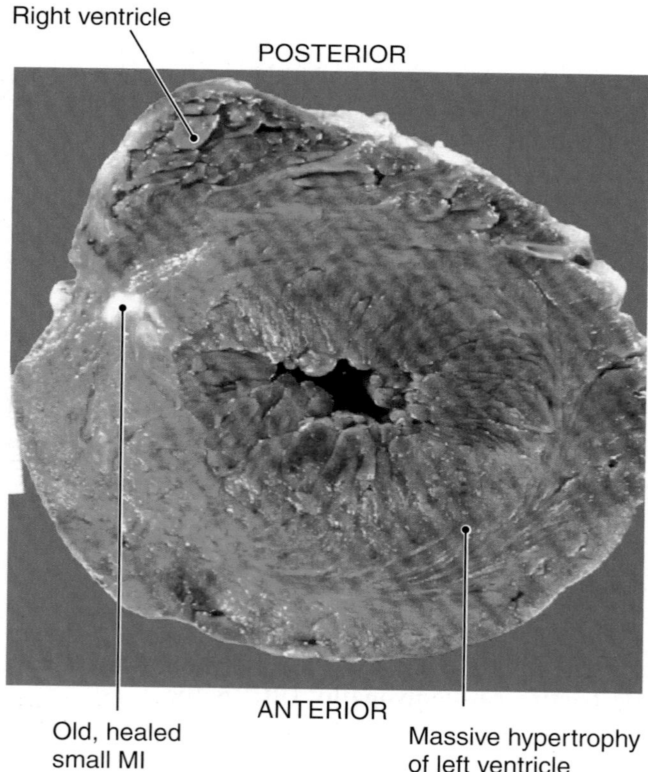

Figure 9.21 **Left ventricular hypertrophy.** The left ventricle is thickened because of the strain of chronic hypertension. Also present is scar from small, old MI.

filling and increases the distance over which oxygen and nutrients must diffuse through the ventricular wall. The end result often is heart failure, myocardial infarction, and cardiac arrhythmia. Effective control of hypertension can prevent or reverse LVH. Diagnosis is clinical. Treatment is aimed at the cause and complications, such as arrhythmia or heart failure.

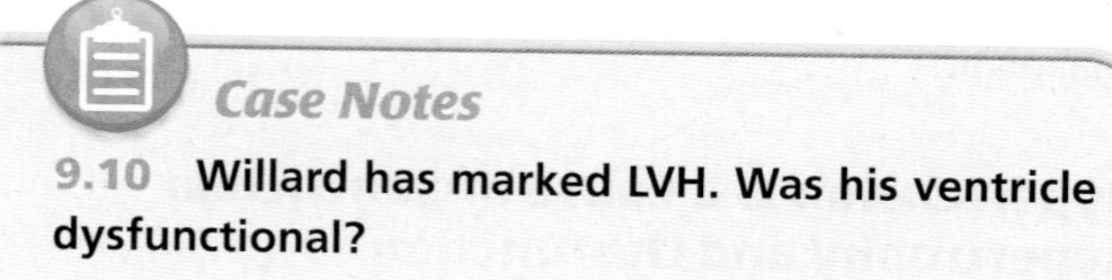

Case Notes

9.10 **Willard has marked LVH. Was his ventricle dysfunctional?**

Pulmonary hypertension with right ventricular hypertrophy (*cor pulmonale*) is usually the result of chronic obstructive pulmonary disease (COPD), discussed in detail in Chapter 10. Acute cor pulmonale also can be caused by large or repeated pulmonary emboli, or by any other cause of pulmonary hypertension, which is much more difficult to treat than systemic hypertension. Irrespective of cause, right-heart failure is a common complication. Treatment is aimed at the cause. Prognosis is poor.

Pop Quiz

9.20 True or false? Half of the cases of HC are the result of an autosomal dominant gene defect.

9.21 What is the most common cause of myocarditis?

Pericardial Disease

Almost all diseases of the pericardium are secondary to some other condition. Primary pericardial disease is unusual.

The pericardial sac normally contains a small amount of fluid that lubricates the motion of the heart within the sac. **Pericardial effusion** is an increased amount of pericardial fluid. If it accumulates slowly, the pericardial sac expands, but rapid accumulations can so increase pressure that the heart cannot fill (cardiac tamponade) and cardiac output falls, sometimes fatally. Among the causes of effusion are inflammation, metastatic malignancy, heart failure, and blunt anterior chest trauma. **Hemopericardium** refers to undiluted blood in the pericardial sac and is to be distinguished from bloody effusion and bloody exudate. Hemopericardium may be caused, for instance, by retrograde extension of an aortic dissection or rupture of the myocardium. Treatment is needle or open surgical drainage.

Pericarditis is inflammation of the pericardium. The most frequent cause is MI. The pericardial inflammation results from inflammatory mediators released from infarcted muscle into the pericardial fluid. It may also occur after an MI as an autoimmune triad of fever, pericardial effusion, and chest pain (*Dressler syndrome*). It may also as a complication of noninfectious inflammatory disease such as RF, lupus, or uremia (renal failure). Infectious pericarditis is most often caused by viral infection, which also may cause an associated myocarditis. Most cases are characterized by atypical chest pain and a loud friction rub. Treatment is aimed at the cause.

Some cases may progress to chronic scarring and obliteration of the sac, which usually has no adverse consequences. A few cases, however, may progress to **restrictive pericarditis**, which impairs diastolic filling and may be difficult to distinguish from cardiomyopathy. Treatment is surgical excision of the fibrous casing.

Pop Quiz

9.22 True or false? The most frequent cause of pericarditis is a MI.

Congenital Heart Disease

Congenital heart malformations occur in about 1% of live births, making such malformations among the most common congenital abnormalities. Most arise from faulty embryogenesis in fetal weeks three to eight. The abnormalities may be innocuous and not detected until late adult life, or they may be fatal in utero. The cause of many cases is unknown. The main known causes are specific genetic defects, of which *Down syndrome* (Chapter 22) is most common. Environmental causes include viral infections (especially first trimester maternal rubella), fetal alcohol syndrome, and maternal diabetes.

The embryologic heart begins as a tube and becomes an anatomically complete heart by the 10th week of pregnancy. Development has two important characteristics: 1) the primitive heart expands and twists in a complicated way that results in the chambers and vessels being the right size and in the correct place, and 2) the septum that divides the heart into right and left sides grows internally from one end to the other. Anatomically, there are three types of defects: 1) *malrotation defects*, which result in misplacement of a vessel—for example, transposition of the great vessels; 2) *expansion defects*, which result in hypoplastic chambers or vessels—for example, coarctation of the aorta; and 3) *septal defects*, which result in direct connections between atria or ventricles—for example, interatrial or interventricular septal defects. Combinations of defects may occur.

Normal fetal circulation is depicted in Figure 9.22A. Understanding cardiac malformations and shunts requires study of the path of fetal blood flow in utero. The major differences from adult circulation are that in the fetus: 1) oxygenated blood flows in veins (not arteries) from the placenta to the fetal heart; 2) oxygenated and deoxygenated blood is mixed in most of the circulation; and 3) little blood flows through the lungs because blood is shunted from the right atrium to the left atrium through the foramen ovale, and from the pulmonary artery to the aorta through the ductus arteriosus. At birth, these bypasses close, and the lungs become suffused with blood.

Clinically, congenital heart disease falls into two major categories: *shunts* and *obstructions*. A **cardiac shunt** is a defect that diverts blood from one side of the heart or great vessels to the opposite side (e.g., from aorta to pulmonary artery). Blood always flows, of course, from an area of high pressure to one of low pressure. If the low-pressure right side (right atrium, right ventricle, pulmonary artery) is open to the high-pressure left side (left atrium, ventricle, and aorta), oxygenated blood will naturally flow from the left side to the right, producing a *left-to-right shunt*. Other defects or conditions may cause the normally low pressure, unoxygenated right side to have greater pressure than the left, which produces a *right-to-left shunt*.

Right-to-Left Shunts Are Cyanotic

Right-to-left shunts are less common than left-to-right and result from malrotation of the embryonic chambers, which creates a defect that allows poorly oxygenated venous (right side) blood to flow into the oxygenated left side of the circulation. The result is poor oxygenation of arterial blood, leading to **cyanosis**, a bluish discoloration of skin due to the poor oxygenation.

Tetralogy of Fallot

The most common right-to-left shunt is **tetralogy of Fallot (TOF)** (Fig. 9.23), which consists of four (*tetra-*) anatomical abnormalities:

- *Ventricular septal defect (VSD)*
- *Small pulmonary artery or pulmonary valve stenosis*, which obstructs flow out of the right ventricle and raises right ventricular pressure, which pushes blood through the VSD
- *Misplaced aorta* that overrides (sits low on) the VSD and catches venous blood passing through the septal defect
- *Right ventricular hypertrophy*, which is a consequence of increased RV workload: the RV is straining against an obstructed outflow tract and is pumping extra blood lost through the shunt

Clinical presentation depends on the degree of pulmonary outflow obstruction. If mild, R to L shunting may be negligible and the infant will not be cyanotic at birth ("pink TOF"). Nevertheless, obstruction may progress so that cyanosis appears later, usually in the first few months or years. Sudden and severe cyanosis may occur with crying or defecating, each of which increases intrathoracic pressure enough to force more R to L shunting. Most patients have a loud systolic murmur. Diagnosis is clinical and confirmed by echocardiography. Surgical correction is effective if diagnosis is made early.

Transposition of the Great Arteries

Transposition of the great arteries is the second most common cause of early cyanotic heart disease. In this condition, the aorta rises from the right ventricle and the pulmonary artery from the left, a condition that isolates the arterial and venous systems into nonconnected circuits, a condition not compatible with life. Newborns who survive birth do so only because they have an atrial or ventricular septal defect that allows shunting of oxygenated blood from the left side to the right ventricle (which supplies the aorta), or to the aorta itself. Diagnosis is clinical and confirmed by echocardiography. Treatment is surgical correction.

Persistent Truncus Arteriosus

A related anomaly is **persistent truncus arteriosus**, a condition in which the roots of the pulmonary artery and

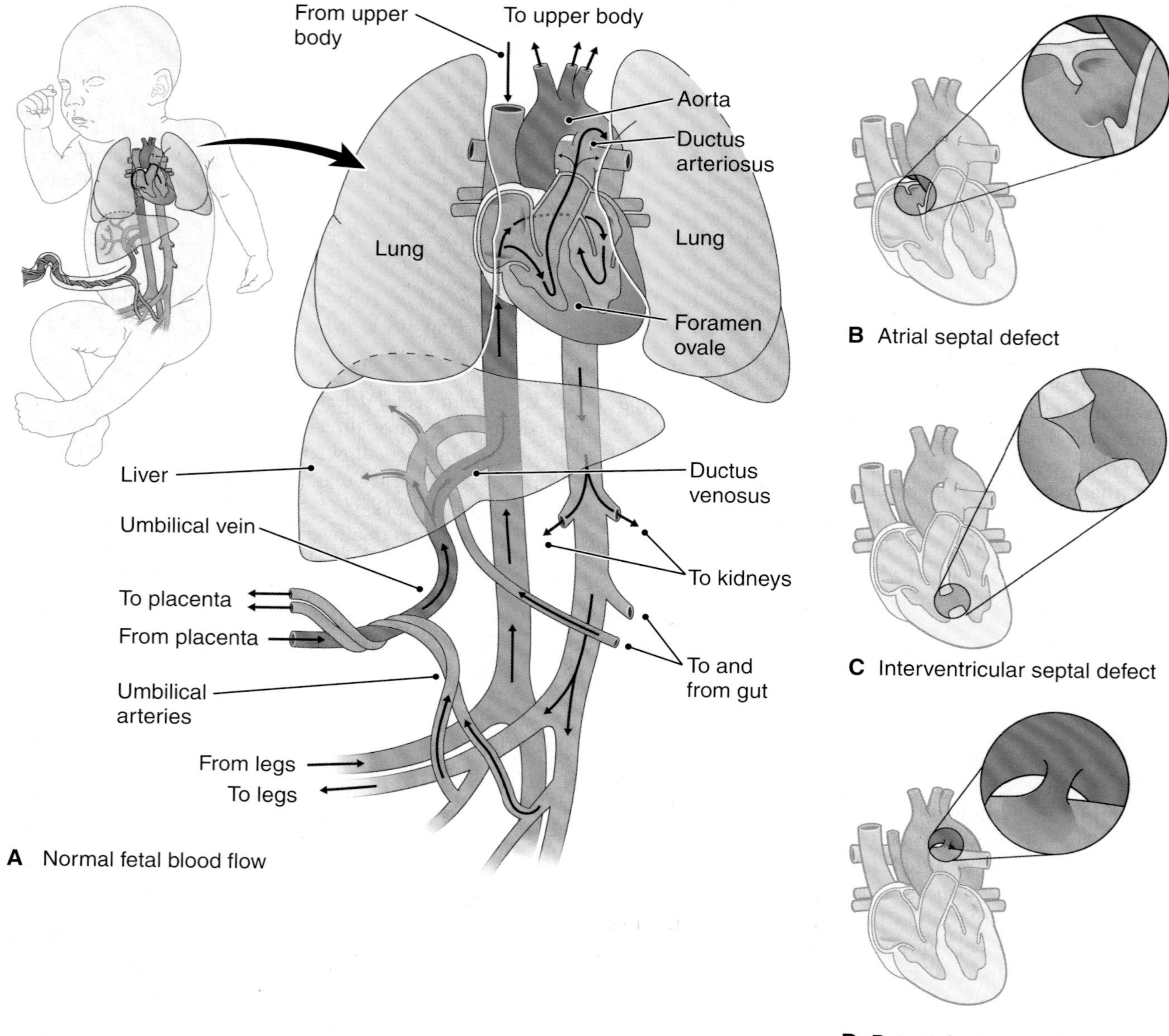

Figure 9.22 **Left-to-right congenital cardiac shunts.** Blood travels from the high-pressure left side (left atrium, ventricle, or aorta) to the low-pressure right side (right atrium, ventricle, and pulmonary artery). These shunts "short circuit" blood flow by recirculating it through the right heart and lungs, which causes right-side volume overload and abnormally high pressure in the pulmonary blood vessels. Pulmonary hypertension and right side heart failure may result. **A.** In the normal fetal blood flow, blood is oxygenated in the placenta and bypasses the lungs. **B.** In an atrial septal defect, instead of flowing from the left atrium into the left ventricle and then into the aorta, some blood flows from the left atrium to the right atrium and back through the lungs. **C.** In a ventricular septal defect, instead of flowing from the left ventricle into the aorta, some blood flows from the left ventricle into the right ventricle and back through the lungs. **D.** In patent ductus arteriosus, some blood flows from the aorta into the pulmonary artery and back through the lungs.

aorta are fused into a single vessel that receives blood from both ventricles. A VSD is always present, which allows enough mixing of blood to sustain life for a while. Diagnosis is clinical and confirmed by echocardiography. Treatment is surgical correction.

Left to Right Shunts Are Acyanotic

Blood normally reaches the right side of the heart only after flowing from the left side through tissues. **Left-to-right shunts** (Fig. 9.22 B, C, and D) are those in which high-pressure, oxygenated blood flows from the arterial (left) side of the heart or one of the great vessels directly into the low-pressure, unoxygenated venous (right) side of the circulation. L-R shunts are the most common type of congenital heart defect. Left-to-right shunts are troublesome because the additional volume of flow adds to right ventricular workload and increased pulmonary artery pressure, which, if not corrected, can cause right-heart

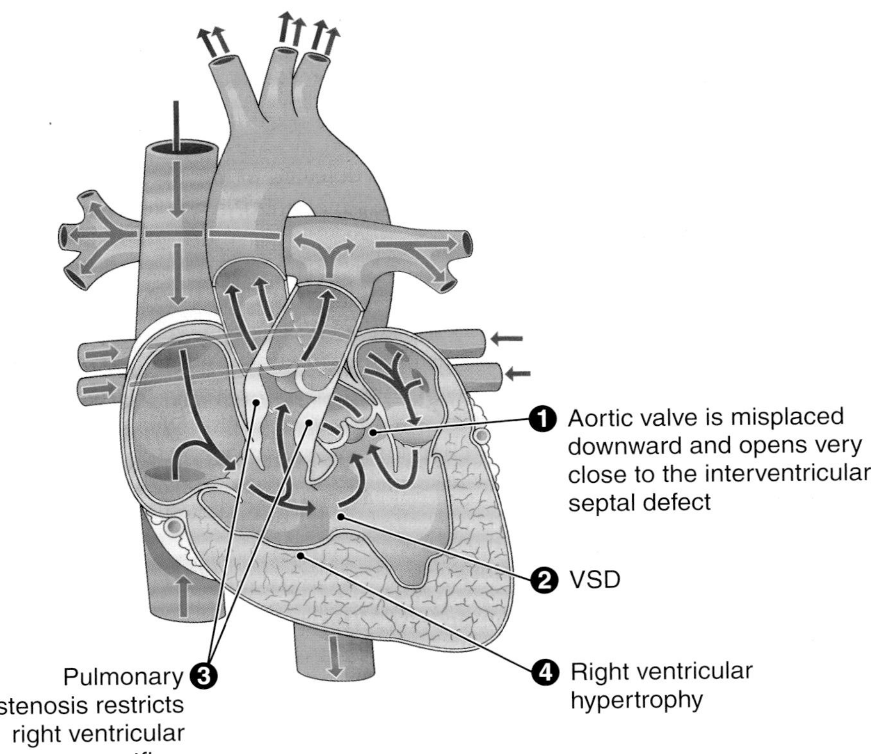

Figure 9.23 **Tetralogy of Fallot: a right-to-left cardiac shunt.** The defects are: **1)** misplacement (rightward shift) of the aortic valve so that the aortic orifice catches unoxygenated blood coming through the **2)** VSD in a right-to-left shunt because **3)** pulmonary stenosis restricts pulmonary outflow, which increases right ventricular pressure, causing **4)** right ventricular hypertrophy.

failure and irreversible (and usually fatal) pulmonary hypertension.

The three main types of left-to-right shunts are the following:

- **Atrial septal defect**: Atrial septal defect (Fig. 9.22 B) occurs when there is incomplete closure of the embryonic atrial septum. It presents as a congenital hole in the septum that separates the atria. Even though pulmonary blood flow may be several times normal, the majority of patients with atrial septal defect do not develop irreversible pulmonary hypertension. Atrial septal defect is not to be confused with **patent foramen ovale**, in which the foramen ovale, which usually closes in the first year of life, remains at least partially patent. Patent foramen ovale occurs in about one-fifth of healthy people without ill effect. Some shunting occurs but it usually remains asymptomatic. Nevertheless, with either defect, pulmonary hypertension is an increasing hazard with passing time. A mild systolic murmur may be present. Diagnosis is by echocardiography. Catheter or open surgical correction is the treatment of choice.
- **Ventricular septal defect (VSD)**: VSD (Figs. 9.22C and 9.24) is incomplete closure of the embryonic ventricular septum. It is the most common congenital cardiac anomaly; about three-quarters are associated with other congenital cardiac defects. Small VSDs may close spontaneously after a few years, or they may exist a lifetime without creating significant problems.

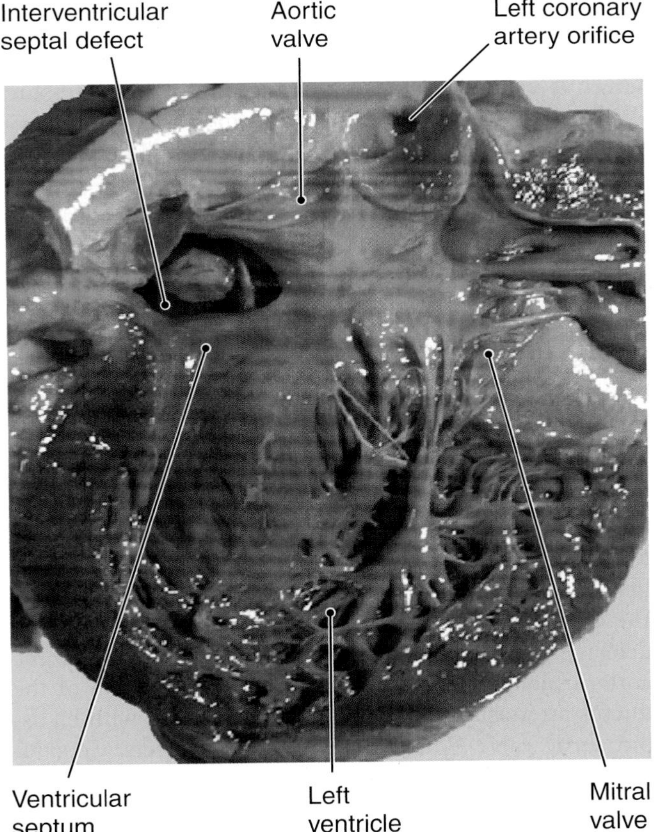

Figure 9.24 **Ventricular septal defect.** This defect is at the upper end of the interventricular septum.

When discovered, small defects may be followed while waiting for spontaneous closure. Large defects require surgery because, left untreated, they can prompt pulmonary hypertension by allowing increased flow of blood through the lungs. Diagnosis is by echocardiography. Catheter or open surgical correction is the treatment of choice.

- **Patent (persistent) ductus arteriosus**: In utero the ductus arteriosus serves to allow blood to bypass the lungs. If it fails to close at birth, blood is shunted from the aorta to the pulmonary artery (Fig. 9.22D). About 90% of patent ductus arteriosus occurrences are a solitary abnormality, but some are associated with other congenital cardiac defects. Patent ductus arteriosus is characterized by a continuous, "machinery-like" murmur. Diagnosis is by echocardiography. Some close following drug treatment; catheter or open surgical closure is effective in the remainder. Closure should be achieved as early in life as is practicable. Unclosed shunts may cause pulmonary hypertension because they allow increased flow of blood through the lungs.

Timely correction of left-to-right shunts is critical. Uncorrected shunts lead to pulmonary hypertension, right-heart failure, and death. Heart-lung transplant is the only hope after a certain point because surgical repair of the defect after development of severe pulmonary hypertension would deprive the pulmonary tree of the high pressure necessary to force blood through the lungs. A vicious circle is operating: high blood pressure damages pulmonary arterioles and increases pulmonary resistance, which in turn requires even higher pressure to sustain adequate blood flow. In some L-R shunts, right-side pressure can rise high enough to exceed left-side pressure, causing a reversal of shunt flow and *late cyanosis* as the shunt conveys unoxygenated blood into the systemic circulation.

Remember This! Uncorrected left-to-right shunts may lead to irreversible pulmonary hypertension requiring heart and/or lung transplant.

Some Malformations Obstruct Flow

Malformations with obstruction to flow occur when embryonic vessels fail to expand properly. **Coarctation of the aorta**, one of the most common congenital cardiac defects, consists of a ring-like fibrous narrowing of the aorta, usually in the aortic arch near the location of the ductus arteriosus. Half of cases are associated with bicuspid aortic valve. Some also have septal defects. Coarctation is associated with high blood pressure in the upper extremities and low blood pressure in the legs. Some have a patent ductus arteriosus distal to the lesion, which allows low-oxygen blood from the pulmonary artery to flow into the aorta because aortic pressure is low distal to the narrowing. The result is cyanosis of the lower half of the body. Low blood flow to the kidneys (below the obstruction) stimulates renin and aldosterone output, which expands blood volume and elevates blood pressure even further. Hypertension is detected in most patients because blood pressure is always measured in the arm, above the obstruction. Most patients have a murmur. Diagnosis is clinical, aided by echocardiography. Treatment is surgical.

Segments of vessels other than the aorta may also not expand properly during fetal development. Failure of expansion is responsible for congenital pulmonary and aortic valve stenosis or hypoplasia of the root of the aorta or pulmonary artery. An example is mild *pulmonary atresia*, which is fairly common and may be compatible with long life. Treatment is surgical.

Pop Quiz

9.23 True or false? The most common right-to-left shunt is a VSD.

9.24 True or false? Coarctation is associated with high blood pressure in the upper extremities and low blood pressure in the legs.

9.25 A continuous machinery-like murmur characterizes what shunt?

9.26 During what fetal weeks do most congenital heart malformations arise?

9.27 What are the major differences between adult and fetal circulation?

Tumors of the Heart

Primary tumors of the heart are rare. Cancer metastases occur more often—about 5% of patients dying of metastatic cancer will have a cardiac metastasis, most of which are silent.

About 90% of primary tumors are benign. Diagnosis is by echocardiography. Surgical excision is curative. The most common is a **myxoma**, 90% of which occur in the atria, most commonly in the left atrium. They are caused by a genetic defect and become symptomatic by obstructing flow, usually at the mitral valve, or by fragmenting and embolic phenomena.

Papillary fibroelastomas are benign papillary growths with hair-like appendages located most commonly on the aortic valve. They may cause thromboemboli or foster bacterial endocarditis.

Lipomas are benign fatty tumors in the myocardium that are similar to their counterparts elsewhere in the body. They are usually small and asymptomatic but may obstruct flow.

Rhabdomyomas are benign tumors of cardiac muscle that usually come to attention in children because they obstruct flow.

Pop Quiz

9.28 True or false? The most common primary cardiac tumor is a myxoma.

Cardiac Arrhythmias

Every beat of the heart is a symphony of coordination—valves open and close at just the right moment, electrical signals race through with perfect timing, and chambers contract when they are filled with the optimum amount of blood. The timing of every activity is critical to produce the right rhythm. When timing is not right, the diagnosis is an **arrhythmia** (also called **dysrhythmia**). A **heartbeat** is defined as a ventricular contraction; in an arrhythmia, the heartbeat may occur too soon or too late, or in an abnormal pattern. **Tachycardia** is rapid ventricular beating, and **bradycardia** is slow ventricular beating. In any case, *arrhythmias are mechanically inefficient* because they cause the ventricles to be under- or overfilled with blood as systole begins.

Minor arrhythmias are fairly common. Strictly speaking, a single premature beat (see premature ventricular contractions, below) is an arrhythmia and is quite common and usually innocent. Several such beats are usually perceived by the patient as "palpitations," but most go unnoticed. Arrhythmias become more frequent and less innocent, however, with advancing age and the onset of coronary atherosclerosis and other heart disease.

The consequence of some arrhythmias is death from **cardiac arrest**. Cardiac arrest is an imprecise term that is widely used to describe sudden cardiovascular collapse and unconsciousness. It can be caused by many cardiac diseases and preceded by other arrhythmias. Whatever the cause (e.g., MI or methamphetamine abuse) the outcome is usually *ventricular fibrillation* (discussed below), an uncoordinated contraction of the ventricles that produces no cardiac output—the cardiac fibers are writhing like a pile of worms.

Normal Cardiac Rhythm Depends on Unique Anatomy and Electrophysiology

Orderly and efficient cardiac rhythm depends on the following characteristics:

1. *The heartbeat is a muscular contraction in response to an electrical signal,* which is a wave of heart cell membrane depolarization that sweeps through the heart in a fraction of a second.
2. *Heartbeats are paced according to the need for more or less blood flow (cardiac output),* rapid for certain occasions, slow for others. Mistimed beats, either too early or too late, are inefficient. The normal "resting" heart rate is about 60–90 beats/min, less in conditioned athletes.
3. *The electrical activity of the heart is a cascading series of separate events. Each heartbeat has an electrical beginning and end. Signals do not run in a loop.* Recirculating loops may occur, however—the result is an arrhythmia.
4. *The heart contains a network (the conduction system) of specialized muscle cells (Purkinje fibers) that conduct electrical signals through the heart* like nerves conduct impulses through the remainder of the body.
5. *The electrical signal begins at a focus (the sinoatrial, or SA, node) in the right atrium,* which is self-stimulated due to spontaneous triggering of an "internal pacemaker" in the node. A heart beating at a smooth, normal rate in response to normally initiated SA signals is said to have a **normal sinus rhythm** (Fig. 9.25).
6. *The electrical signals normally follow the same anatomic pathway with every beat.* If signals get off track, they can be detoured and arrive too late, or they can take a short cut and arrive too early. In both cases the result is bad timing—an arrhythmia.
7. *The atria and ventricles are electrically insulated from one another and connected only at a single point,* through which the electrical signal passes.
8. *Every part of the conduction network is capable of self-stimulation* (initiating a beat), but at progressively slower rates from the SA node downward into the ventricles; that is, if the SA node does not initiate a signal when it should, then a lower part of the conduction system will assume the pacemaker function, albeit at a slower rate.

   Such rhythms are called **escape rhythms**. Those originating near the AV node are about 40–60 beats/min, whereas those originating from ventricular Purkinje fibers are about 15–40 beats/min.
9. *Cardiac muscle cells are interconnected in a special way to allow uninterrupted flow of electrical stimulation from cell to cell.*
10. *Cardiac fibers stay contracted (electrically depolarized) for a few tenths of a second before relaxation*

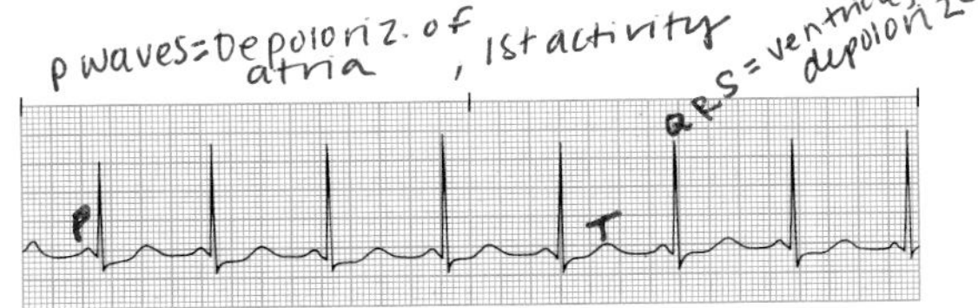

Figure 9.25 **Normal sinus rhythm.** Normal rate with evenly spaced P, QRS, and T waves. (Reproduced with permission from Springhouse. *ECG Facts Made Incredibly Easy.* 2nd ed. Ambler, PA: Wolters Kluwer Health; 2010.)

and repolarization, an effect that promotes electrical orderliness by preventing the muscle from being restimulated too early by a rogue signal. This is an electrically quiet period in the heart, represented on the ECG by the S-T segment.

The list of conditions that can cause arrhythmias is long, and includes certain genetic defects, myocardial ischemia or infarction, inflammation, drugs, and blood electrolyte disturbances, especially low magnesium or potassium.

Case Notes

9.11 When Willard is resting and is not having arrhythmias, what kind of rhythm does he have?

Arrhythmias Are Caused by Faulty Electrophysiology

Arrhythmias are caused by one or more faulty electrical mechanisms.

Faulty automaticity is the spontaneous discharge of a signal from a focus of heart cells that is ordinarily incapable of initiating a signal. The signal sweeps through the heart, conflicting with the normally generated signal and causing an abnormal, mistimed beat (see characteristic 2, above).

A **reentry loop** is a signal that runs along the normal conduction pathway but somehow loops back into the conduction network and recirculates before a newly generated SA signal can arrive (see characteristics 3 and 6, above).

Electrically unstable cell membrane can also cause arrhythmia. Recall that each heartbeat is caused by a wave of cell membrane depolarization that sweeps down the conduction system and through heart muscle, and that the membrane must repolarize before the heart can beat again. Sometimes, however, membrane polarity does not return to its normal state, but fluctuates somewhat like a flickering light bulb. Some of these fluctuations can become large enough to initiate an early new signal, which conflicts with normal signals (see characteristic 10, above).

Clinically and functionally, however, arrhythmias are classified anatomically into three broad categories according to the site of impulse origination, or how the impulse is conducted through the conduction system:

- Those associated with impulses arising from the SA node
- Those associated with impulses arising at a site other than the SA node
- Those in which the signal is delayed, interrupted, or misdirected in its travel through the conduction pathway

Any beat that originates at a site other than the SA node is said to be an **ectopic beat**. Ectopic beats occur for two main reasons. First, the SA node may be slow to discharge, which allows origination of beats to occur low in the conduction system (*escape rhythm*). Second, a focus of heart muscle away from the SA node may begin to fire because it is irritable or unstable or a reentry loop develops.

Abnormal Sinus Rhythms Originate from the SA Node

Recall from above that a normal sinus rhythm is an evenly spaced series of normally initiated and developed beats occurring at a rate of about 60–90 beats/min. Sinus rhythms can be normal, fast, or slow according to healthy physiologic demand, or they can be pathologically slow or fast. Other than more or less frequent beats, the ECG shows normal P, QRS, and T waves.

Sinus tachycardia (Fig. 9.26) is an otherwise normal sinus rhythm in which the ventricle is beating faster than the normal "resting" rate. Some instances of sinus tachycardia are normal responses to certain physiologic conditions, such as exercise, emotional stress or excitement, or ascent to high altitude (where oxygen is less abundant and higher cardiac output is required). On the other hand, sinus tachycardia can be an adaptive, homeostatic response to certain pathologic conditions, such as fever, low blood pressure, low blood oxygen (e.g., from lung disease), or hyperthyroidism (Chapter 14). Most sinus tachycardia is efficient and smoothly meets the body's demand for more cardiac output, but at extreme rates (near 200 beats/min) the ventricle beats before it fills with an optimum amount of blood and cardiac output suffers. Absent the above conditions, tachycardia may be one manifestation of a condition called *sick sinus syndrome* in which the SA node discharges too rapidly for reasons unknown. Rate control treatment with drugs may be necessary.

Case Notes

9.12 When Willard is exercising and not having arrhythmias, what kind of rhythm does he have?

Sinus bradycardia is the opposite—a ventricular rate less than about 60 beats/min in a person with otherwise

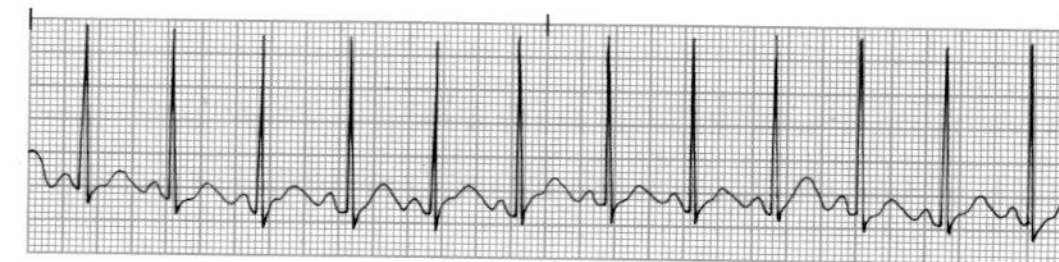

Figure 9.26 **Sinus tachycardia.** Rapid rate with evenly spaced P, QRS, and T waves. (Reproduced with permission from Springhouse. *ECG Facts Made Incredibly Easy*. 2nd ed. Ambler, PA: Wolters Kluwer Health; 2010.)

normal sinus rhythm. Conditioned athletes normally have sinus bradycardia when at rest, however, because their bodies are trained to superior efficiency. In people other than conditioned athletes, sinus bradycardia can be caused by parasympathetic vagus nerve signals produced, for example, by the Valsalva maneuver (straining at stool or similar lung pressure against a closed glottis), or by massage of the carotid body (in the neck at the separation of the external and internal carotid arteries). Other causes include medications such as beta-blockers and digitalis. Absent the above conditions, sinus bradycardia is often part of *sick sinus syndrome* in which the SA node discharges too slowly for reasons unknown. Drug therapy or an implanted pacemaker may be required for severe cases.

Remember This! Sinus bradycardia is normal in well-conditioned athletes.

Sinus arrhythmia is a condition in which the heart sometimes beats slow or fast in response to otherwise normal signals from the SA node. The most common form of sinus arrhythmia is the normal slight increase of rate with inspiration and a corresponding lower rate with expiration. In children, fluctuating autonomic activity is the usual cause and needs no therapy.

Sinus arrest (Fig. 9.27) is absence of electrical discharge from the SA node. Cardiac arrest may occur and is usually followed after a few seconds by initiation of new but slower-paced signals originating from a point lower in the conduction system. Sinus arrest is associated with lack of cardiac output and syncope (fainting) with or without grand mal epileptic seizures and may be called *Stokes-Adams syndrome*.

Ectopic Signals Originate Away from the SA Node

An ectopic beat is one that originates from a site other than the SA node. They may occur at any site in the atrial or ventricular musculature or in the cardiac conduction system.

Ectopic Atrial Arrhythmias

Ectopic beats originating in the atria are called **premature atrial beats** (or premature atrial complexes, or **PACs**, in reference to the electrocardiographic tracings). They are common and in most people have no association with underlying cardiac or systemic disease. They may, however, occur with greater frequency—several a minute—and be quite disconcerting if the patient can feel them in the chest. Emotional stress, excitement, and/or too much caffeine are the usual culprits. Runs of PACs may occur for short periods of time at rates of 120–200 beats/min. In most such patients, no underlying disease is present; however, some patients have underlying CAD. No treatment is necessary.

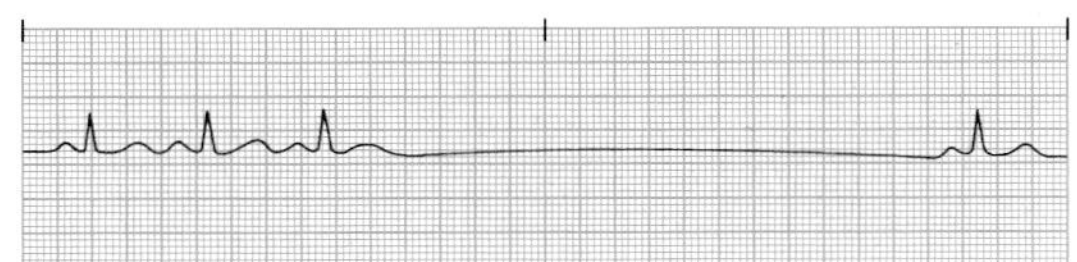

Figure 9.27 **Sinus arrest.** An interval with no sinus activity and no beats. Normal rate and sinus activity before and after. (Reproduced with permission from Springhouse. *ECG Facts Made Incredibly Easy*. 2nd ed. Ambler, PA: Wolters Kluwer Health; 2010.)

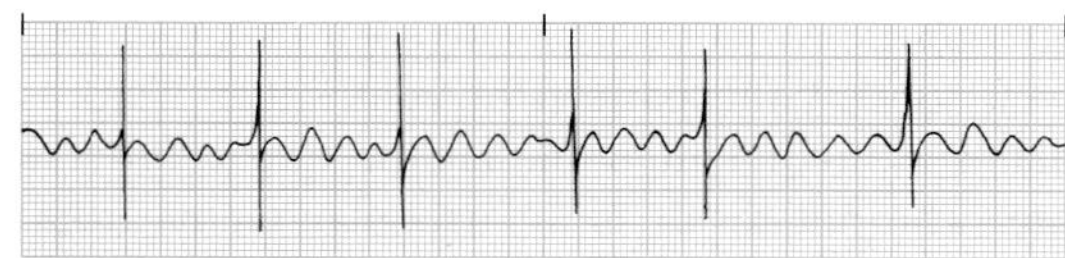

Figure 9.28 **Atrial flutter.** Very rapid atrial beats. Ventricular rate is slower because most atrial signals cannot get through the AV node because it is depolarized from the prior ventricular beat. (Reproduced with permission from Springhouse. *ECG Facts Made Incredibly Easy*. 2nd ed. Ambler, PA: Wolters Kluwer Health; 2010.)

Atrial flutter (Fig. 9.28) is an unusually rapid but *regular*, evenly spaced beating of the atrium (and ventricle) at rates from 120–350 beats/min. The underlying electrical mechanism is a reentry loop. At very high atrial rates, not all signals may get through the AV node to the ventricle, so that the ventricular rate may be, for example, half the atrial rate if half of the atrial signals do not get through. QRS complexes are normal and there may be more P waves than QRS complexes. Extremely high ventricular rates may be life threatening because the under-filled ventricle cannot produce effective cardiac output. Some patients may have underlying cardiac disease or high blood pressure; others have no underlying disease. Chronic or recurrent atrial flutter predisposes to formation of atrial thrombi, which can break away and embolize to the brain to cause ischemic infarction (white stroke, Chapter 19). Breathlessness and palpitations are common complaints. Diagnosis is by ECG. Treatment is by electroconversion or rate-slowing drugs to achieve ventricular rate control. Anticoagulants are necessary to retard thrombus formation.

Atrial fibrillation (Fig. 9.29) is an unusually rapid and *irregular*, unevenly spaced beating of the atria, commonly referred to as "irregularly irregular." Reentry loops are the underlying mechanism in most cases, but in some instances there is a focus of ectopic discharge. In a certain sense, the atria are not even beating: they are just squirming ineffectively as electrical chaos reigns. In this state, some signals

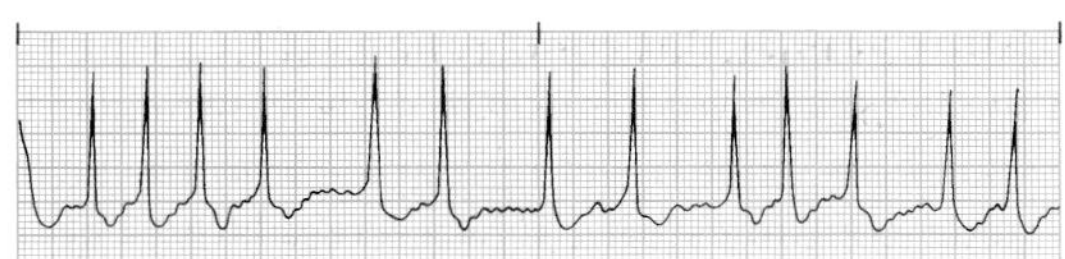

Figure 9.29 **Atrial fibrillation.** Chaotic atrial activity with no P waves. Some signals get through to ventricle but others do not because of AV node depolarization from the prior ventricular beat. Ventricular rhythm is irregular. (Reproduced with permission from Springhouse. *ECG Facts Made Incredibly Easy*. 2nd ed. Ambler, PA: Wolters Kluwer Health; 2010.)

get through the AV node. They do so at irregular intervals, however, so that the pattern of ventricular beats is very irregular and inefficient: some far too quick, others much too late. The net result is an irregular tachycardia. QRS complexes are normal, but normal P waves are replaced by small and highly irregular baseline fluctuations.

The most common causes are hypertension, ischemic heart disease, mitral or tricuspid valvular disease, hyperthyroidism, and binge drinking.

Atrial fibrillation is quite common, especially in older patients with underlying CAD. Patients with atrial fibrillation fall into two broad groups. Those with *paroxysmal atrial fibrillation* have unpredictable episodes of atrial fibrillation that may last a few hours or a few days. Others develop *chronic atrial fibrillation*, which is present at all times. Breathlessness and palpitations are common complaints. Diagnosis is by ECG. Treatment is rate-slowing drugs to achieve ventricular rate control. If an ectopic focus can be identified, it can be treated by catheter-delivered *radiofrequency ablation*, in which the focus is obliterated by heat. Anticoagulants are necessary to retard thrombus formation.

Ectopic Junctional Arrhythmias

In a **junctional arrhythmia**, the ectopic beats originate near the atrioventricular (AV) node, which is located where the atria and ventricles join together. It is sometimes called *supraventricular tachycardia* because it arises above the ventricle but is not of atrial origin. The mechanism is a reentry pathway near the AV node. Junctional dysrhythmias typically cause moderate tachycardia in the range of 80–120 beats/min. QRS complexes are normal but P waves may be inverted, due to retrograde flow of the signal across the atrium, or P waves may be lost in the QRS complex or occur after the QRS complex.

Breathlessness and palpitations are common complaints. Diagnosis is by ECG. Many episodes stop spontaneously. Vagotonic maneuvers such as coughing or the Valsalva maneuver (straining to exhale against a closed glottis) may be effective. Chronic cases require drug rate control or radiofrequency ablation of the alternate pathway.

Ectopic Ventricular Arrhythmias

Ventricular dysrhythmias are those in which the ectopic electrical impulse originates in one of the ventricles.

Premature ventricular contractions (PVC) (Fig. 9.30) arise in the ventricles and cause an early ventricular beat, but the signal does not travel retrograde into the atria, so the SA node continues to discharge regularly. The next SA signal is ineffective, however, because the ventricle is electrically refractory following the PVC and cannot be stimulated. The result is a missed normal sinus beat and a pause that is twice the usual time between beats. QRS complexes are wide and often inverted, and the T wave is often inverted as well. Occasional PVCs are common in

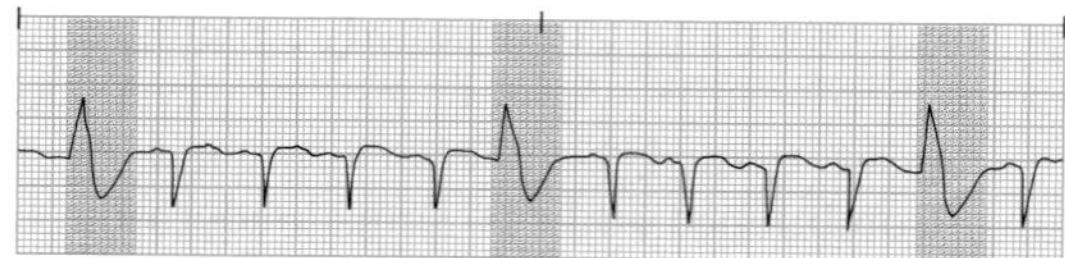

Figure 9.30 **Premature ventricular contractions.** Periodic malformed QRS complexes. Remainder of QRS complexes are normal but appear different from prior figures because they are recorded from a different ECG lead. (Reproduced with permission from Springhouse. *ECG Facts Made Incredibly Easy*. 2nd ed. Ambler, PA: Wolters Kluwer Health; 2010.)

healthy people and have no pathologic significance unless they are associated with known underlying heart disease. Other causes include stimulant drugs, caffeine, and electrolyte disturbances, especially low blood potassium or magnesium. Other than avoiding triggers, healthy patients require no treatment.

Ventricular tachycardia (Fig. 9.31) is defined as three or more consecutive ectopic ventricular beats at a rate that exceeds 120 beats/min. The sinus node continues its activity but is ineffective because the ventricle is electrically refractory when the signal arrives. Most ventricular tachycardia is thought to be due to reentry of the previous signal (see characteristic 3, above). QRS complexes are wide, often inverted, and T and P waves are often not identifiable. A common cause of ventricular tachycardia is myocardial ischemia or infarction—compromised myocardium can change conduction times and pathways, which sets the stage for reentry loops caused by misrouted or mistimed signals. Ventricular tachycardia is a serious dysrhythmia that always indicates serious heart disease and merits aggressive drug therapy or electroconversion. Breathlessness and palpitations are common, but syncope or sudden cardiac death may occur. Diagnosis is by ECG. Acute episodes are treated with electroconversion or intravenous drugs. Longer term, the goal is to prevent sudden death by use of an implantable cardioversion device.

Case Notes

9.13 Willard has episodes of ventricular tachycardia. What is the most likely mechanism?

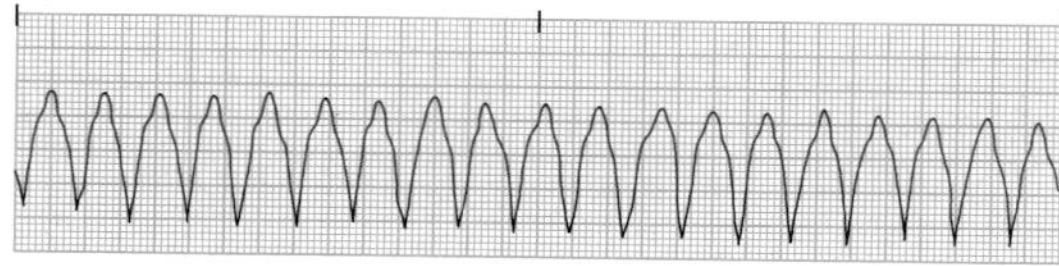

Figure 9.31 **Ventricular tachycardia.** Rapid, malformed QRS complexes. P and T waves are not visible. (Reproduced with permission from Springhouse. *ECG Facts Made Incredibly Easy*. 2nd ed. Ambler, PA: Wolters Kluwer Health; 2010.)

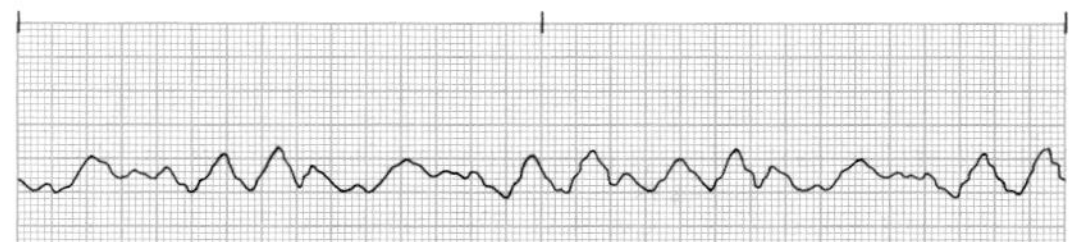

Figure 9.32 **Ventricular fibrillation.** Chaotic ventricular activity. (Reproduced with permission from Springhouse. *ECG Facts Made Incredibly Easy*. 2nd ed. Ambler, PA: Wolters Kluwer Health; 2010.)

Ventricular fibrillation (Fig. 9.32) is uncoordinated contraction of myocardium—the ventricles more or less quiver ineffectively, and cardiac output is zero. The patient collapses with sudden syncope, usually as a consequence of acute myocardial ischemia or infarction—in about one-quarter of people with acute myocardial infarction the initial symptom is sudden death from ventricular fibrillation. Normal P, QRS, and T waves are absent and replaced by irregular wiggles along the baseline. The mechanism is thought to be multiple reentry loops. Diagnosis is by ECG. Ventricular fibrillation is fatal unless corrected within two or three minutes. Electroconversion is the most effective treatment (>90% survival for those treated within three minutes). Those who have one episode are at high risk for another.

Abnormal Conduction Can Cause Arrhythmia

Recall that under normal circumstances an impulse originates from the SA node and races down the Purkinje fibers of the conduction system in a fraction of a second. If the signal goes off track, however, or is slowed or blocked, an arrhythmia occurs.

Atrioventricular Block

Recall that the sinus signal passes through the atrial musculature, causing atrial contraction as it goes, and enters the conduction system through the AV node. From the AV node, the signal passes through the bundle of His as it penetrates the ring of fibrous tissue that separates the atria from the ventricles. Then it is conducted throughout the ventricles by the branches of the conduction system. Slowing or complete obstruction of a sinus impulse in its course through the conduction system is called **atrioventricular block**. Three degrees of AV block are recognized.

First-degree block is retardation of the sinus signal, but every signal causes a ventricular beat. The P-QRS interval is prolonged. It is a common finding that may occur in otherwise healthy people, but also may be a consequence of myocardial ischemia or infarction of tissue in the region of the AV node, bundle of His, or the upper parts of the bundle branches. First-degree block does not cause functional problems and does not warrant therapy independently, though it may resolve with treatment of the underlying condition.

Second-degree block is diagnosed when some of the sinus signals are not conducted into the ventricles. Myocardial ischemia or infarction is the usual cause. The result is dropped ventricular beats. The P-QRS interval is longer than in first-degree block and a QRS complex does not follow some P waves. In some instances only a few beats are missed, but it usually causes little impairment of cardiac output. In some cases, however, bradycardia may occur and warrant drug or pacemaker therapy.

Third-degree block (Fig. 9.33) is complete obstruction of the sinus signal in the region of the AV node or bundle of His with the development of a junctional or ventricular escape rhythm. QRS complexes are wide and may be inverted, and there are fewer QRS complexes than P waves; moreover, the two bear no relationship to one another. Myocardial ischemia or infarction is the usual cause. Bradycardia occurs and may require drug or pacemaker treatment.

Accessory Conduction Pathways

Some people have congenital abnormalities of the conduction system called **accessory pathways**, which provide an alternate route for the sinus signal. The best known of these is *Wolff-Parkinson-White syndrome*, a congenital anomaly of the conduction system that features a pathway that bypasses the AV node and enters the ventricle directly. The P-QRS interval is short and the QRS complex is wide and sometimes merges with the P wave. This produces a slurred stroke in the initial movement of the QRS called a "delta wave." The result is tachycardia. The accessory pathway sometimes serves as a reentry point in the creation of a reentry loop that produces a supraventricular tachycardia. Sometimes atrial or ventricular fibrillation may supervene. Rate control by drug therapy may be necessary.

Intraventricular Conduction Defects

Below the bundle of His the conduction system branches into two main bundles of fibers: the right bundle, which supplies the right ventricle; and the left bundle, which supplies the left ventricle. Either of these bundles may be blocked, producing **right bundle branch block (RBBB)** or **left bundle branch block (LBBB)**. Either may be caused by myocardial infarction or other heart disease, and either may occur as an isolated abnormality in otherwise healthy people. Neither RBBB nor LBBB impairs cardiac function. No therapy is indicated. In both cases,

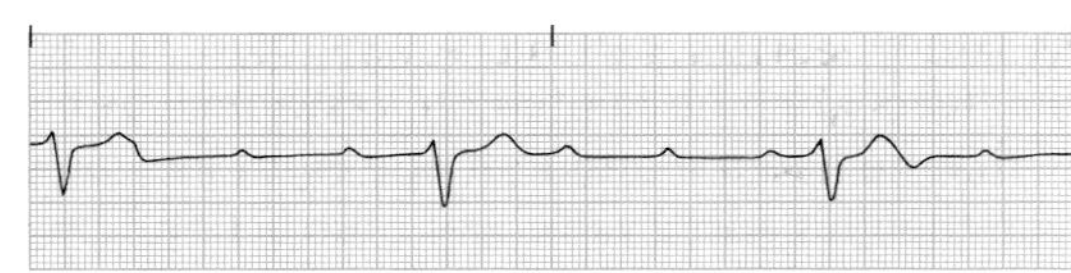

Figure 9.33 **Third-degree block.** Multiple atrial P waves without corresponding ventricular QRS. No atrial P wave signals can pass into the ventricles because signal is blocked near AV node or bundle of His. Atrial and ventricular contractions are independent of one another. (Reproduced with permission from Springhouse. *ECG Facts Made Incredibly Easy*. 2nd ed. Ambler, PA: Wolters Kluwer Health; 2010.)

LBBB especially, ECGs can be so distorted as to preclude other electrocardiographic diagnoses.

Arrhythmias Require Specialized Diagnosis and Treatment

Patients with tachycardia due to any of the conditions above often have similar symptoms: a disturbance under the breastbone ("flip flops" or palpitations), chest pain (e.g., in patients with CAD), shortness of breath, dizziness, or fainting. In many patients, however, the dysrhythmia is clinically silent and may be detected or analyzed only by ECGs, especially a 24-hour continuous recording that is analyzed by computer. Bradycardia is usually less evident to the patient and may become evident as fatigue due to lack of adequate cardiac output.

In any event, the main aim of therapy is rate control—increase the rate in bradycardia, slow it in tachycardia—and decrease the irritability of the myocardium to avoid more serious dysrhythmias. Drug therapy is usually effective, but electroconversion by pacemaker or defibrillator may be required.

Formation of atrial thrombi is a distinctive threat of chronic atrial dysrhythmias, especially chronic atrial fibrillation. If a left atrial thrombus forms, pieces can break away and embolize anywhere in the body, usually with minimal effect, but on occasion the embolus lodges in a cerebral artery and causes a stroke. Most patients with chronic atrial fibrillation are treated with anticoagulants to lessen the likelihood of atrial thrombus formation.

Treatment of arrhythmias is usually by drugs, though some cases require **electroconversion** (or *defibrillation*), in which a strong electrical current is passed through the heart to terminate the irregular pattern and allow a sinus rhythm to begin again. Some arrhythmias may require implantation of an electrical device into the body. These devices are commonly called **pacemakers**, but they can perform a wide variety of functions, including continuous monitoring and recording of cardiac beats for later study. A pacemaker can be programmed to set a lower limit on heart rate, to reestablish normal rhythm when an arrhythmia occurs, and a variety of other functions.

Pop Quiz

9.29 True or false? When resting, conditioned athletes may have sinus bradycardia.

9.30 True or false? Any beat that originates at a site other than the SA node is said to be an ectopic beat.

9.31 True or false? In a junctional dysrhythmia, the ectopic beats originate near the SA node.

9.32 What arrhythmia is characterized by the phrase "irregularly irregular"?

9.33 Which electrolyte disturbances are capable of causing arrhythmias?

9.34 Which variety of AV block is characterized by a complete dissociation of P waves and QRS complexes?

Case Study Revisited

"I only fainted." The case of Willard S.

Recall that Willard was discovered to have a heart murmur at age eight. At age 23 the cause was found to be a bicuspid aortic valve. He led a vigorous, asymptomatic life for many more years but in his early 60s began to have exertional chest pain. Matters came to a head when he fainted on a treadmill at his gym.

That he had a murmur at age eight indicates that even then his aortic valve was obstructing flow to some degree. Because the leaflets had to be stretched apart to allow blood to pass, they began to scar and calcify, finally becoming much like the bicuspid valve in Figure 9.15.

When Willard fainted while exercising, he fulfilled the classic triad for AS: exertional angina, dyspnea, and syncope. Echocardiography demonstrated marked narrowing of the valve orifice. Catheter studies demonstrated a marked pressure gradient across the valve and some aortic insufficiency as well.

Willard's chest pain was angina. He could not develop enough aortic flow to feed his coronary arteries, which needed more blood than normal because his left ventricular muscle mass was so large, a consequence of decades of hypertrophy in response

"I only fainted." The case of Willard S. (continued)

to the extra workload imposed by his aortic valve disease. It could have looked like the left ventricle in Figure 9.21. Syncope occurred because he could not develop enough cardiac output to meet the brain's need for oxygen. Myocardial ischemia also accounts for his episodes of ventricular tachycardia. Ventricular tachycardia also could have been responsible for his syncope: at high rates ventricular filling is incomplete and cardiac output falls.

Open surgical replacement with a pig valve was successful and his physiology returned to normal. His LVH began to regress after the excess workload was removed.

His son's remark that "mentally he wasn't quite himself for about six months" can probably be traced to *postperfusion syndrome*, a constellation of neurocognitive impairments that occurs in a small percentage of individuals undergoing cardiac bypass. The deficit is most noticeable early in the postoperative period. Symptoms are subtle and include defects associated with attention, concentration, short-term memory, fine motor function, and speed of mental and motor responses. Most cases resolve spontaneously, as in Willard's case. The cause is speculative, but increasing time on bypass is associated with increasing prevalence and severity.

Chapter Challenge

CHAPTER RECALL

1. A 63-year-old Caucasian male presents to the clinic for evaluation of recurrent chest discomfort that he describes as pressure and pain in his left jaw and shoulder. Previously, the sensation occurred only after walking up a few flights of stairs, but now the sensation occurs at rest. You warn him that he has a 30% chance of having a MI in the next three months. What is his diagnosis?
   A. Stable angina
   B. Unstable angina
   C. Unremitting angina
   D. Myocardial infarct

2. A 55-year-old African American male presents for episodes of breathlessness, coughing, and rapid breathing that have gotten progressively worse over the last month. A chest X-ray shows a remarkably enlarged heart while his ECHO reveals a normal ejection fraction but decreased cardiac output. What is the cause of his symptoms?
   A. Left-heart failure
   B. Right-heart failure
   C. Diastolic failure
   D. Uncompensated heart failure

3. A 44-year-old Caucasian woman presents to the emergency room complaining of breathlessness and heart palpitations. Her past medical history is significant for breast cancer treated with several chemotherapies including Adriamycin. Her ECG strip reveals an elevated (350 bpm) heart rate; it is regular with more P waves than QRS complexes; and her QRS complexes are normal. What arrhythmia do you suspect?
   A. Ventricular fibrillation
   B. Ventricular tachycardia
   C. Atrial fibrillation
   D. Atrial flutter

4. Which of the following is true concerning the drug therapies used to treat heart failure?
   A. Beta-blockers improve ejection fraction by lowering heart rate.
   B. Aldosterone blockers are the mainstay of therapy.
   C. Digoxin effects the renin-aldosterone mechanism.
   D. Angiotensin converting enzyme inhibitors improve myocardial contractility.

5. A young athlete presents to your clinic for a physical prior to trying out for his high school basketball team. He denies any complaints or significant past medical history. His family history is positive for the sudden death of his father, at age 35, while playing tennis. On physical exam, you identify a systolic murmur. What are you most concerned about in this patient?
   A. Myocarditis
   B. Restrictive cardiomyopathy
   C. Hypertrophic cardiomyopathy
   D. Dilated cardiomyopathy

6. A 29-year-old Caucasian female presents to the cardiologist for evaluation of syncope. Her symptoms are precipitated by long periods of standing and are characterized by a prodrome of light-headedness, loss of vision, and diaphoresis (excessive sweating). Her ECG strip shows a prolonged P-QRS interval, which is characteristic of which of the following?
   A. Normal ECG
   B. First degree AV block
   C. Second degree AV block
   D. Third degree AV block
7. A mother brings her six-month-old infant son to the pediatrician's office. She is concerned because every time her son cries, he turns blue. He was born term, without complications. He has no significant medical history. On physical exam, he is found to have a loud systolic murmur. An ECHO confirms your diagnosis. You tell his mother that surgery is necessary to correct what cardiac defect?
   A. Patent ductus arteriosus
   B. Transposition of the great arteries
   C. Tetralogy of Fallot
   D. Persistent truncus arteriosus
8. A 10-year-old Hispanic female is brought to the clinic by her mother for evaluation of a skin rash and some recent unusual behavior. Over the last several weeks, her daughter has developed rapid, irregular, jerky movement of her extremities. She also notes that her daughter has been walking more slowly recently, and seems to be favoring her right knee. On physical exam, the patient has a new-onset murmur. Her findings are classic. You forgo the confirmatory tests and explain to her mother that the patient has what valvular abnormality?
   A. Atrial stenosis
   B. Atrial regurgitation
   C. Mitral valve prolapse
   D. Rheumatic valvular disease
9. What type of arrhythmia is characterized by a heart rate of greater than 120 beats/min with a wide (often inverted) QRS, and absence of T and P waves?
   A. Ventricular tachycardia
   B. Supraventricular tachycardia
   C. Ventricular fibrillation
   D. Atrial fibrillation
10. A 65-year-old Caucasian male who was recently admitted to the hospital for a MI presents to the ER several weeks later complaining of chest pain. He says this pain is different from before, and on physical exam a loud friction rub is present. What is his diagnosis?
    A. Stable angina pectoris
    B. Unstable angina pectoris
    C. Myocardial infarct
    D. Pericarditis
11. A 23-year-old Caucasian woman presents to the clinic with odd chest pain and palpitations. Her past medical history is significant for Marfan syndrome. On physical exam, you note her marfanoid body habitus (tall thin stature, with slender long fingers) and chest auscultation reveals a late systolic murmur and mid-systolic click. What valvular defect do you suspect?
    A. Aortic stenosis
    B. Mitral insufficiency
    C. Mitral valve prolapse
    D. Infective endocarditis
12. True or false? Atrial natriuretic peptide serves as a vasodilator in addition to increasing sodium and water excretion by the kidney.
13. True or false? Heart disease is the second leading cause of death worldwide (cancer is the first).
14. True or false? The vasoconstrictor angiotensin II stimulates secretion of aldosterone, which stimulates the kidney to conserve sodium and water.
15. True or false? Though 90% of primary cardiac tumors are benign, they are problematic due to their propensity to obstruct blood flow in the heart.
16. True or false? About 75% of MIs are heralded by CAD symptoms.

CONCEPTUAL UNDERSTANDING

17. What are the three waveforms of an echocardiogram, and what causes them? Which waveform is hidden?
18. Left-sided heart failure can cause hypoxia and acidosis. What is the difference between the two?
19. What are the four cardiac defects that make up the tetralogy of Fallot?
20. Explain the Frank-Starling law.

APPLICATION

21. A 45-year-old man presents to the clinic with fatigue. He is concerned about occasional chest palpitation and the blue tinge of his skin, as well as recent onset episodes of fainting. On physical exam, you note cyanosis, clubbing of his fingertips, and a loud heart murmur. You suspect a left-to-right shunt that went undiagnosed in his childhood. What are the possible etiologies? What has occurred? What treatment is available?

22. Your patient presents to the clinic and tells you that in light of your conversation several months ago he has made a drastic lifestyle change to decrease his risk for a heart attack. He has stopped drinking alcohol, is now eating a diet low in saturated fat, smokes less, and even started exercising. What words of encouragement do you have to offer, and what should accompany them?

23. An 18-year-old Hispanic female is brought to the ER by her boyfriend for a fever of 104.5°F and shaking chills. Your questioning reveals that she drinks socially and uses IV drugs. On physical exam, crackles are evident throughout her lungs. The attending physician suspects pneumonia, admits the patient to the hospital, and starts treatment with antibiotics. The next day, during your morning rounds, you note additional physical findings: Your patient now has tiny oral, conjunctival, and subungual hemorrhages. A new-onset cardiac murmur is also apparent. The patient is taken for an ECHO, but the images are inconclusive. Blood cultures are also negative. How should this patient be treated?

24. You discharge your patient from the hospital following resolution of his MI symptoms. What possible complications should you warn him about?

CHAPTER

10

Disorders of the Respiratory Tract

Contents

Chapter Objectives

After studying this chapter, you should be able to complete the following tasks:

THE NORMAL RESPIRATORY TRACT

1. Discuss the organization of the respiratory tract, and explain how its varying morphology reflects its function.

LUNG VOLUME, AIR FLOW, AND GAS EXCHANGE

2. Using spirometry patterns, distinguish between obstructive and restrictive airway disease.

DISEASES OF THE UPPER RESPIRATORY TRACT

3. List the diseases affecting the upper respiratory tract and describe their etiology.

ATELECTASIS

4. Identify the three types of atelectasis and their respective causes.

PULMONARY EDEMA

5. Discuss the pathophysiology, signs and symptoms, and treatment of pulmonary edema.

ACUTE RESPIRATORY DISTRESS SYNDROME

6. Describe the etiology, clinical presentation and findings, prognosis, and treatment of acute respiratory distress syndrome.

OBSTRUCTIVE LUNG DISEASES

7. Compare and contrast the symptoms and associated pathological findings of obstructive apnea, asthma, bronchiectasis, and chronic obstructive pulmonary disease.

RESTRICTIVE LUNG DISEASES (DIFFUSE INTERSTITIAL DISEASE)

8. Discuss the clinical presentation and diagnostic findings of restrictive lung disease.

VASCULAR AND CIRCULATORY LUNG DISEASE

9. Summarize the etiology, presentation, findings, and potential complications of pulmonary thromboemboli, including pulmonary hypertension; and explain alternative causes of pulmonary hypertension.

PNEUMONIA

10. Characterize, where applicable, the etiologies of pneumonia as: lobar or interstitial, and/or nosocomial, community acquired, aspiration, chronic, or occurring in an immunodeficient host.

LUNG NEOPLASMS

11. Compare and contrast small-cell and nonsmall-cell carcinomas of the lung.

DISEASES OF THE PLEURA

12. Identify the potential substances that might be found in the pleural space, and the consequences of their accumulation.

Case Study

"She has cigarette asthma." The case of Myrtle M.

Chief Complaint: Difficulty breathing, drowsiness.

Clinical History: Myrtle M. was a 51-year-old woman who was accompanied to the emergency room (ER) by her son, who had been taking care of her for several years. She was wheezing and struggling to breathe and so drowsy that she could not give a medical history. He said, "She has cigarette asthma." He revealed that she began smoking as a teenager and had been smoking two packs a day since she was 20. Her original visit to the hospital was 12 years ago, when she was seen in the pulmonary clinic for coughing, wheezing, and shortness of breath. Many similar, more severe episodes followed, and she was diagnosed with chronic asthmatic bronchitis. A spirogram at the time revealed low FEV1 and normal FVC. Two notations were present on the graph: "obstructive" and "chronic asthmatic bronchitis." "Still smoking" was a regular chart entry for subsequent visits. In the last few years, she had visited her physician with increasing frequency. Her son brought her to the emergency room because he became alarmed by her constant sleepiness.

Physical Examination and Other Data: Myrtle was cyanotic, dyspneic, somnolent, and quite obese—estimated in the ER about 5′4″ and 225 lb. She had marked expiratory obstruction and wheezing, and coughed a lot, hacking up yellow sputum. Her temperature was 100.5°F, respirations 36, blood pressure 115/75, heart rate 105. Breath sounds were distant, with rales and expiratory wheezes.

Her chest X-ray showed evidence of moderate emphysema and shadows that suggested bronchopneumonia in both lower lobes. The blood gas study showed low pH, high CO_2, and low oxygen. The total WBC count was moderately elevated (16,500/mm^3) with an increased percentage of neutrophils and a few immature "band" neutrophils. Hemoglobin (18.1 gm/dL) and hematocrit (52%) were high. Red cell indices and blood chemistries were unremarkable.

Clinical Course: Myrtle was admitted to the hospital for antibiotic and bronchodilator therapy, oxygen supplementation, and ventilation assistance. With antibiotics, bronchodilators, and ventilation assistance she became more alert, her fever disappeared, and she found it easier to breathe. The admission sputum culture grew mixed flora, probably oral contaminants. An echocardiogram showed moderate right ventricular dilation and hypertrophy; the left ventricle and valves appeared to be normal.

(continued)

"She has cigarette asthma." The case of Myrtle M. (continued)

On the fifth hospital day she became feverish again, respirations become labored, and she became difficult to arouse. A chest X-ray revealed widespread changes in both lungs that suggested severe pneumonia. An emergency bronchoscopy revealed abundant purulent mucus in the airways, which on culture grew methicillin-resistant *Staphylococcus aureus* (MRSA). Despite intense antibiotic and respiratory therapy, the pneumonia grew more severe, she become progressively unresponsive and eventually comatose, and she died on the tenth hospital day.

It is better to have bad breath than to have no breath at all.

PROVERB, ORIGIN UNKNOWN

Respiration is more than breathing. It includes three separate but related functions:

1. *Ventilation* (breathing) is a function of the lungs. It is also called *external respiration*.
2. *Gas exchange* is the movement of oxygen and carbon dioxide between lungs and tissues via blood.
3. *Oxygen utilization* is the use of oxygen by cells to release energy. Gas exchange and oxygen utilization are together referred to as *internal respiration*.

The single greatest cause of respiratory-related death in the United States is lung cancer, which in 2012 claimed nearly 160,000 lives. A close second is chronic lower respiratory disease, which in 2011 killed another 137,000 Americans, and respiratory infections—mainly pneumonia—caused another 50,000 deaths. The main risk factor in mortality due to respiratory disease is, of course, smoking.

The Normal Respiratory Tract

The **upper respiratory tract** consists of the nose, sinuses, pharynx, epiglottis, and larynx. The nose and sinuses are lined by mucus-secreting, ciliated columnar **respiratory epithelium**. Hairs in the nose, the cilia of the respiratory epithelium, and a coat of mucus trap bacteria and particulate matter as air is warmed, moistened, and channeled to the lower respiratory tract. The pharynx, epiglottis, and larynx are lined by squamous epithelium, which facilitates phonation and the passage of food.

The **lower respiratory tract** (Fig. 10.1) consists of the trachea, bronchi, lungs, and pleurae. The trachea and bronchi are lined by respiratory epithelium, which further trap bacteria and particulate matter. The main function of the lower respiratory tract is to oxygenate blood and collect and discharge the carbon dioxide (CO_2) produced by energy metabolism. Air enters through the **trachea**, which divides into right and left main **bronchi**, one for each lung. The main bronchi divide into smaller tubes, one for each lung lobe: two on the left, three on the right. The right main bronchus is more vertical and more directly in line with the trachea. As a result, aspirated foreign materials, such as vomitus or foreign bodies, are more likely to enter the right lung rather than the left. The lobar bronchi continue to divide into progressively smaller airways, the smallest bronchial division of which is the **bronchiole**. Distal to the bronchioles are the **alveoli** (*acini*), the blind-end sacs of the lung and smallest division of the airway, where gas exchange occurs in blood vessels (capillaries) in the alveolar walls.

Case Notes

10.1 Does Myrtle's lung disease involve her upper respiratory tract or lower?

The Airway Channels Air to the Lungs

The pharynx and epiglottis are lined by smooth squamous epithelium to facilitate the slide of food. Except for the vocal cords, which are covered by stratified squamous epithelium, the entire respiratory tree, including the larynx, trachea, and bronchioles, is lined by epithelium composed of columnar ciliated epithelial cells. Numerous mucus-secreting *goblet cells* and *submucosal glands* are spread throughout the trachea and bronchi. The respiratory mucosa is also populated by neuroendocrine cells that release a variety of hormonal factors.

As shown in Figure 10.2, the trachea and bronchi are held open by an outer ring of stiff cartilage, encircled by bands of smooth muscle and lined by mucosa. As bronchi branch into smaller tubes, cartilage and mucous glands gradually disappear until they are no longer present in bronchioles; only epithelium and smooth muscle remain, allowing the bronchioles to dilate or constrict easily.

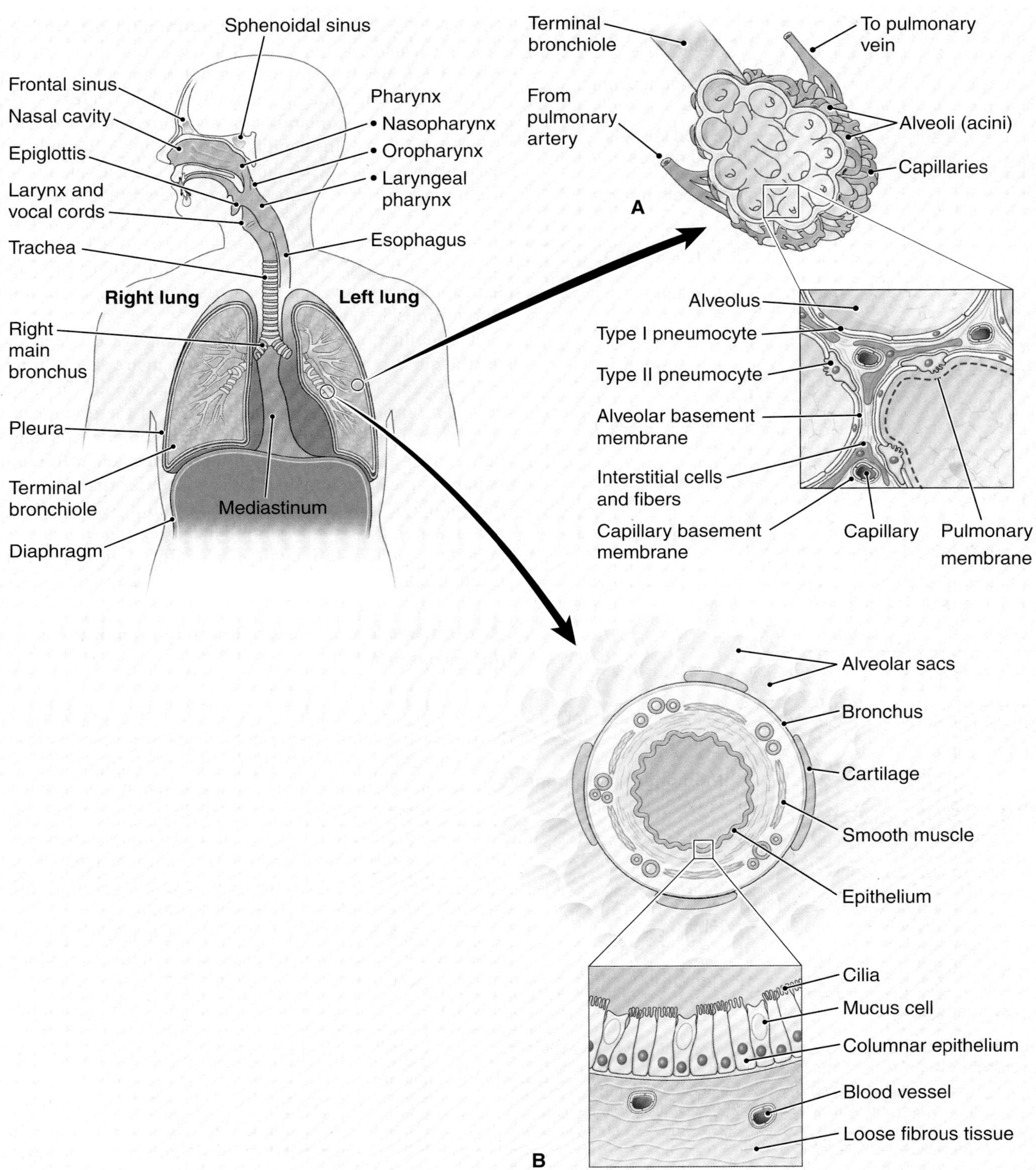

Figure 10.1 **The respiratory system. A.** Alveolar detail. **B.** Bronchial detail.

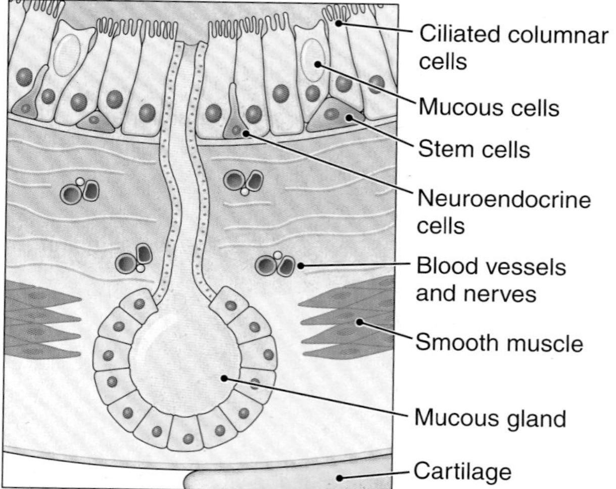

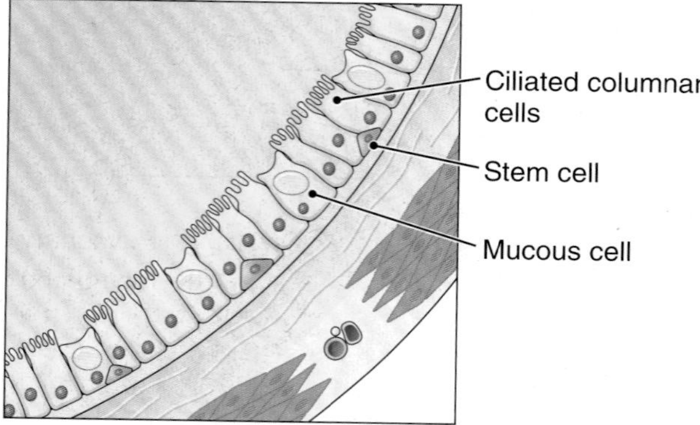

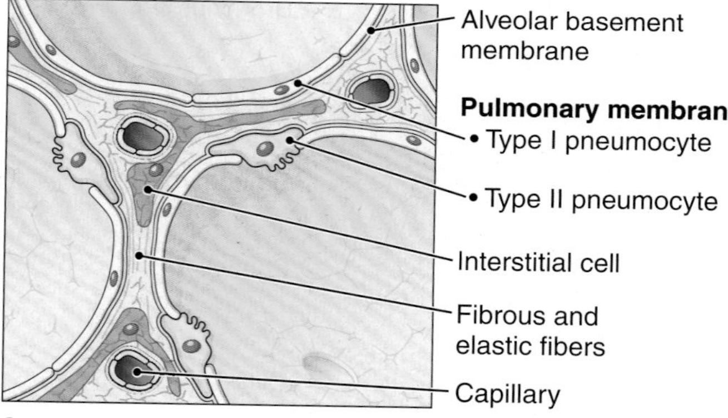

Figure 10.2 **Microscopic anatomy of bronchi and alveoli. A.** Bronchi are stiff tubes composed of linked rings of cartilage and lined by mucosa that is itself lined by ciliated epithelial cells, mucus cells, neuroendocrine cells, and stem cells. Beneath the epithelial cells are mucous glands, bundles of smooth muscle, blood vessels, and autonomic nerves. **B.** Bronchioles are smaller, have thinner walls, and are composed of epithelium and smooth muscle; no cartilage or mucous glands are present. **C.** Alveoli are lined by Type I and Type II (surfactant-secreting) pneumocytes and supported by a basement membrane, beneath which are interstitial cells, fibrous and elastic fibers, and pulmonary capillaries. Collectively, the pneumocytes form the pulmonary membrane.

Gas Exchange Occurs in the Alveoli

Alveoli are lined by Type I and Type II **pneumocytes** (see Figs. 10.1 and 10.2). The exposed surface of pneumocytes (the gas exchange surface) is the **pulmonary membrane**. *Type I pneumocytes* are flat, thin cells that form about 90% of the alveolar surface. *Type II pneumocytes* secrete pulmonary surfactant, a soapy fluid that decreases alveolar surface tension and helps alveoli remain open. The alveolar wall contains capillaries that connect the pulmonary artery, carrying incoming unoxygenated blood, to the pulmonary veins, carrying oxygenated blood back to the heart. Beneath the pneumocytes that line the alveoli is the pulmonary interstitium, which is formed of a lacy network of fibrous and elastic tissue, pulmonary capillaries, capillary and alveolar basement membranes, and a few smooth muscle cells and fibrocytes.

The ability of the lungs to exchange gases depends on the surface area of the pulmonary membrane—in an average adult it is about 750 square feet (about the floor area of a four-car garage). The capacity of the pulmonary membrane to allow oxygen and carbon dioxide exchange between air and blood is called the **pulmonary diffusion capacity**; it can be impaired by any disorder that destroys membrane or limits the ability of oxygen or carbon dioxide to diffuse across it. *Destroyed pulmonary membrane can never be recovered*—not by time, exercise, medications, not by anything short of a lung transplant. Smokers, take note.

Remember This! Lost pulmonary membrane is not recoverable.

Normal gas exchange keeps blood richly oxygenated. Normally, oxygenated arterial and capillary blood is brilliant red and accounts for the healthy pink appearance of skin in light skinned people. After gas exchange in tissues, venous blood is deoxygenated and dark blue–red. If gas exchange is impaired, arterial blood becomes darker and bluish like venous blood and the skin takes on a gray–blue color, a condition called **cyanosis**. Cyanosis is more difficult to detect in dark-skinned individuals.

The lung is served by two vascular systems: the pulmonary and the bronchial. The pulmonary circulation, which consists of the pulmonary artery and veins and their connecting capillaries in the alveolar wall, provides nourishment to the alveoli only. The trachea and bronchi are nourished by the bronchial arteries, which are branches of the thoracic aorta.

The respiratory system, like the skin, is in direct contact with the environment. Therefore, it has a special defense system. The first line of defense is the respiratory epithelium, the mucous and ciliated cells of which trap bacteria and other microbes, pollen grains, soot, and other particles. A coordinated sweeping motion of the cilia moves mucus upward to be swallowed, spit out, or blown from the nose. Also present in the respiratory mucosa are nodules of mucosa-associated lymphoid tissue (MALT, Chapter 3), which includes the tonsils, adenoids, and numerous small collections of lymphocytes in the trachea and bronchi. MALT secretes high concentrations of immunoglobulin A into the respiratory mucus to form the "immune paint" of the respiratory tree. Finally, the alveoli contain macrophages that scavenge inhaled particulate material.

Case Notes

10.2 Over the years, Myrtle's smoking began destroying her pulmonary membrane. Were more Type I or Type II pneumocytes destroyed?

Pop Quiz

10.1 True or false? The pulmonary membrane is capable of regenerating after injury.

10.2 What is the smallest division of the lung?

10.3 Define pulmonary diffusion capacity.

10.4 Which immunoglobulin paints the respiratory epithelium?

Lung Volume, Air Flow, and Gas Exchange

For normal ventilation, the lungs must freely exchange oxygen and carbon dioxide, a function that requires the following:

- *The alveoli must be open*. Disease example: *atelectasis*, in which alveoli are collapsed.
- *Air must move freely*. Disease example: *asthma*, in which spasm of bronchiolar smooth muscle narrows the airway and restricts airflow.
- *There must be sufficient pulmonary membrane*. Disease example: *emphysema*, in which smoking has destroyed the pulmonary membrane.
- *The interstitium must be thin and delicate*. Disease example: *interstitial fibrosis*, in which an accumulation of fibrous tissue interferes with gas diffusion between blood and alveoli.

The total volume of the lungs is about six liters. As illustrated in Figure 10.3, total lung volume is subdivided into smaller *volumes*. A combination of volumes is a "*capacity*." Lung diseases alter volumes and capacities.

Normal lung function requires that the lungs draw in and expel air at a certain rate and that the lungs expand normally. **Spirometry** is a diagnostic procedure that measures lung *volumes* (capacity) and the *flow rate* (liters per second) of air going into and out of the lungs. The technique is simple: the patient is given a mouthpiece and tube connected to a measuring device and instructed to breathe normally. Then the patient is asked to take the deepest possible breath and exhale as rapidly as possible. The results are recorded on a graph similar to the one shown in Figure 10.3A. The major categories of lung disease have signature spirometry patterns.

Using lung volumes and flow rate, clinicians can classify respiratory disease into two categories: obstructive and restrictive. *Obstructive disease* (Fig. 10.3B) is characterized by limitation of airflow, *restrictive disease* (Fig. 10.3C) by limitation of lung expansion.

- **Forced vital capacity (FVC)** is a *volume* measurement—the amount of air expelled from maximum inspiration to maximum expiration, regardless of the time taken to expel it. FVC is measured by asking the patient to take the deepest possible breath and blow out as much air as possible; no timing is involved.
- **Forced expiratory volume (FEV1)** is a *rate* measurement—the amount of air expelled from maximum inspiration in the first second of effort. The patient is instructed to take the deepest possible breath and breathe out as hard as possible. The amount of air expelled in the first second is recorded.
- The **FEV1/FVC ratio** is critical in separating obstructive and restrictive lung disease.

Case Notes

10.3 From reading Myrtle's physical examination, which one of the requirements for normal ventilation can you be sure is not normal?

10.4 On her clinic visit 12 years earlier, was Myrtle's FEV1/FVC ratio high, normal, or low?

In *obstructive disease* the rate of air flowing out of the lungs is slowed; therefore the amount the patient can expel is low. What's more, in obstructive disease, lung volumes are usually normal or expanded, so the ratio of airflow to lung volume is quite low; that is, the FEV1/FVC ratio is low. In *restrictive disease*, the ratio of airflow to lung volume is usually near normal because restrictive disorders limit both volume and flow rate proportionally, and the FEV1/FVC ratio remains near the normal range. The ratio may vary slightly up or down, but it is

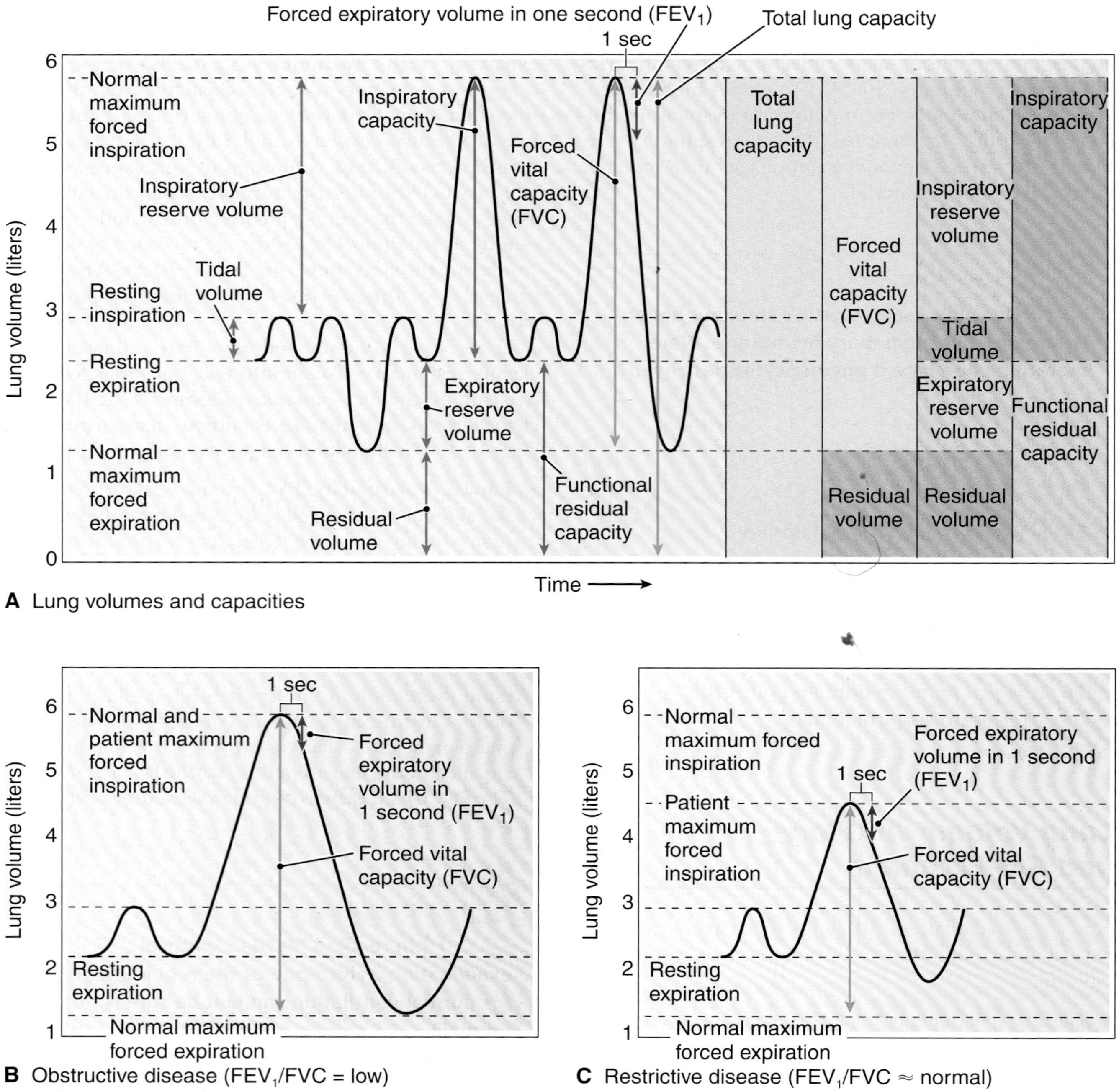

Figure 10.3 **Spirography. A.** Normal spirogram tracings with lung volumes and capacities. **B.** Spirogram in obstructive disease: One-second forced expiratory volume (FEV1) is low; forced vital capacity (FVC) is normal. **C.** Spirogram in restrictive disease: Both one-second forced expiratory volume (FEV1) and forced vital capacity (FVC) are low.

not markedly decreased, as it is in obstructive disease. Both obstructive and restrictive disease limit CO_2 and O_2 exchange: patients get less O_2 and retain more CO_2 than healthy people. Laboratory study of arterial blood O_2 and CO_2 ("arterial blood gases") is critical in assessing lung function.

Classic signs and symptoms associated with impaired ventilation include wheezing, **hypoxia** (low arterial blood oxygen), **dyspnea** (shortness of breath), and cyanosis.

Pop Quiz

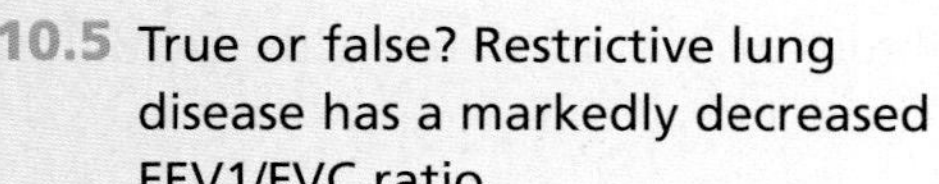

10.5 True or false? Restrictive lung disease has a markedly decreased FEV1/FVC ratio.

10.6 List the two broad categories of lung disease.

Diseases of the Upper Respiratory Tract

Among the most common of respiratory ailments are acute upper respiratory infections, most of which occur in children (Chapter 22).

Infectious rhinitis, synonymous with "common cold" or upper respiratory infection (URI), is caused by virus infection in almost every instance. Infection evokes mild fever, mucosal congestion, and watery, clear nasal discharge. Treated or untreated, symptoms usually disappear in about a week. Because uncomplicated URIs are purely viral, antibiotics are useless; indeed, widespread use of antibiotics to treat colds has promoted the development of strains of antibiotic-resistant bacteria. Nevertheless, the appearance of yellow, purulent nasal discharge or ear or sinus pain usually signifies secondary bacterial infection, which warrants antibiotic therapy.

Allergic rhinitis (*hay fever*), which affects about 20% of the U.S. population, is an exaggerated immune reaction to plant pollens, fungi, animal dander, or dust mites. Clinical manifestations include nasal mucosal edema, nasal discharge, and sneezing. Allergic conjunctivitis (itchy, red eyes) may also occur. Oral antihistamines are the mainstay of treatment, though intranasal corticosteroid sprays may also be useful.

Recurrent rhinitis of any type may lead to development of **nasal polyps**, which are exaggerated folds of edematous mucosa with inflammation and epithelial hyperplasia. They are not neoplastic. They may be 4–5 cm long and obstruct the airway or cause sinusitis by impairing sinus drainage. Treatment is surgical excision.

Impaired sinus drainage is usually due to mucosal edema or polyp. Accumulation of sinus mucus is the cause of **mucocele**, which is usually associated with an uncomfortable sense of fullness in the affected sinus. Tenderness may be present; no fever occurs unless infection arises. Diagnosis is clinical plus radiologic imaging. Treatment consists of nasal decongestants and nasal lavage or needle drainage for severe cases.

Impaired drainage and retained sinus fluid is an invitation to infection and **acute sinusitis**. The offending bacteria are usually streptococci, pneumococci, or *Haemophilus influenza*. Signs and symptoms are pain, nasal drainage, congestion, fullness, and fever. Diagnosis is clinical plus imaging studies. Treatment is decongestants, lavage, and a two-week course of antibiotics. Needle drainage may be necessary in some cases.

Continued sinus obstruction may also cause **chronic sinusitis**. Chronic sinusitis due to fungus infection is especially severe and is usually seen in diabetics. Severe or persistent infection may penetrate into the cranial cavity. Signs and symptoms are similar to acute sinusitis but less intense and longer lasting. Diagnosis and treatment are similar to acute sinusitis, but may require extended antibiotic therapy or surgical drainage and removal of hyperplastic sinus mucosal membrane.

Sinonasal papillomas are benign neoplasms that arise from nasal or sinus mucosa. Their cause is unknown, but human papillomavirus (HPV) is suspected. They usually cause symptoms of nasal obstruction or nosebleeds. Most are exophytic, cauliflower-like growths that can be easily removed, but may regrow; however, the inverted variety grows downward and can sometimes transform to squamous cell carcinoma.

Pharyngitis and **tonsillitis** (each called "sore throat") are inflammations of the throat that are usually viral and respond to supportive therapy. The usual case has its origins in a virus infection and is mild, with fever, slight mucosal reddening, painful swallowing, and swelling of the tonsils and neck lymph nodes. These symptoms usually resolve in about a week and don't require antibiotic treatment. Bacterial infection, however, is more serious. Fever, local pain, and other symptoms are more severe. The mucosal membranes may be involved by a yellow, purulent exudate. Treatment consists of antibiotics. In some cases, inflammation and edema, or the formation of an abscess, can cause airway obstruction (see *The History of Medicine*, "The Strangulation of George Washington"). What's more, if infection is caused by Group A streptococcus (**acute streptococcal pharyngitis**), autoimmune reactions may result in either acute rheumatic fever (Chapter 9) or acute glomerulonephritis (Chapter 15).

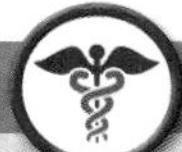

The History of Medicine

THE STRANGULATION OF GEORGE WASHINGTON

On December 12, 1799, still physically robust at age 68, General Washington rode his horse around his beloved Mt. Vernon most of the day in a heavy snowfall and near freezing temperatures. The following day he complained of a sore throat and hoarseness, but again rode most of the day in the snow and cold. In the early hours of the next day, December 14, he woke suddenly with difficulty breathing. His assistant, Colonel Lear, was summoned and prepared a medicinal mixture of molasses, vinegar, and butter, which the general tried to drink but which caused a convulsion of coughing and suffocation. Washington was a strong believer in bloodletting as a cure-all, so his estate manager was summoned and drained about a pint of blood from his forearm.

Later, physicians arrived and more blood was drained. Seeing the great man struggling so hard to breathe, a junior physician argued for cutting into the trachea (tracheostomy) to allow air to enter through the neck, a procedure known for centuries but never performed by any of those in attendance. The senior physician ruled against it, arguing that such a surgical "experiment" could not be tried on a man who was not just the foremost Founding Father but, for many years, the most famous man on the planet.

Finally, late in the afternoon, Washington realized he was dying and called his assistant to receive his deathbed instructions. "I feel myself going. I thank you for your attentions but I pray you take no more troubles about me. Let me go off quietly. I cannot last long." At 10:10 that night, after raising his arm to check his pulse, he died.

Several weeks later, his physician published an account of Washington's death, citing a fatal inflammation of the epiglottis, larynx, and upper trachea. The exact nature of the infection remains a matter of speculation.

The total quantity of blood removed from Washington has been estimated by various authorities to be 5–7 pints. General Washington was a physically impressive man, 6 feet 3 inches tall and weighing about 230 pounds, from which it is easy to calculate that his blood volume was about 14 pints. That he was drained of nearly half his blood volume surely played some role in his demise. The fact that Washington stopped struggling and appeared calm shortly before his death may have been due to weakness from excessive bloodletting.

Laryngitis is usually a part of a URI or upper airway irritation by cigarette smoke or other irritant. Most infections resolve spontaneously as the URI fades. Nevertheless, in infants and children, mucosal swelling may threaten airway closure. Respiratory syncytial virus, *Haemophilus influenza*, and beta-hemolytic streptococcus can cause severe laryngeo-epiglottitis. Children are much more likely to have airway problems than adults because their anatomic structures are smaller. *Croup* (Chapter 22) is the name of the syndrome of airway obstruction in children. Treatment is supportive. Antibiotics are necessary if bacterial infection is suspected.

Vocal cord nodules (or polyps) are benign, small (2–3 mm), smooth fibrous nodules or polyps caused by smoking or chronic vocal stress. More men are affected than women. Those in singers are usually bilateral and called *singer's nodes*. Symptoms are hoarseness and painful vocalization. Treatment is to stop the irritation by cessation of smoking and voice rest.

Laryngeal papillomas are small, benign, raspberry-like growths that may cause hoarseness or bleeding. Lesions are usually single in adults. In children they may be multiple (*juvenile papillomatosis*) and recur after removal owing to human papillomavirus (HPV) infection. Recurrences fade after puberty. Treatment is surgical.

Carcinoma of the larynx is common; most cases occur in male smokers over age 40. Chronic alcohol abuse is also a risk factor. The lesion begins as hyperplasia of the laryngeal squamous mucosa and develops through progressive stages of dysplasia, carcinoma in situ, and invasive carcinoma. The patient typically presents with hoarseness, pain, cough, painful swallowing, or coughing blood. Most tumors are confined to the larynx at time of diagnosis. If the neoplasm has metastasized, the metastases are most likely to be found in neck lymph nodes; distant metastases are uncommon and occur late. Many patients can be cured by radiation and surgery, but about one-third die of the disease.

Pop Quiz

10.7 True or false? Uncomplicated URIs are typically bacterial.

10.8 True or false? Fungal infection of the sinuses is a severe infection usually seen in diabetics.

10.9 What are the two most important risk factors in laryngeal cancer?

Atelectasis

Atelectasis is collapse of part of the lung. Collapsed lung tissue does not exchange gases properly, causes hypoxia, and invites infection. The three types of atelectasis are the following:

- *Resorption* atelectasis occurs when a bronchial obstruction prevents air from reaching part of the lung, and the air in the alveoli beyond the obstruction is completely absorbed by blood circulating through the alveoli. Causes include mucus plugs that accumulate during general anesthesia, asthma, bronchitis, and obstructing tumors. A cause in children is aspiration of foreign objects.

  A particular variety of resorption atelectasis is right middle lobe syndrome. The right lung has three lobes, the smallest of which is the right middle lobe, which is sandwiched anteriorly between the much larger upper and lower lobes. The right middle lobe is served by an unusually long, thin bronchus that is particularly prone to obstruction from bronchial mucus or inflammatory debris. Recurrent episodes of atelectasis may evolve into right middle lobe pneumonia or abscess.
- *Compression* atelectasis (Fig. 10.4) occurs when external pressure is exerted on the lung from pleural blood, fluid, or air (*pneumothorax*) or from abdominal upward pressure on the diaphragm. For example, in heart failure, fluid accumulates in the pleural space (*pleural effusion*, discussed below). Another common cause is compression of the posterior lower lobes by upward pressure on the diaphragm. This occurs, for example, in patients who have had chest or abdominal surgery and are not breathing normally because of pain associated with each breath.

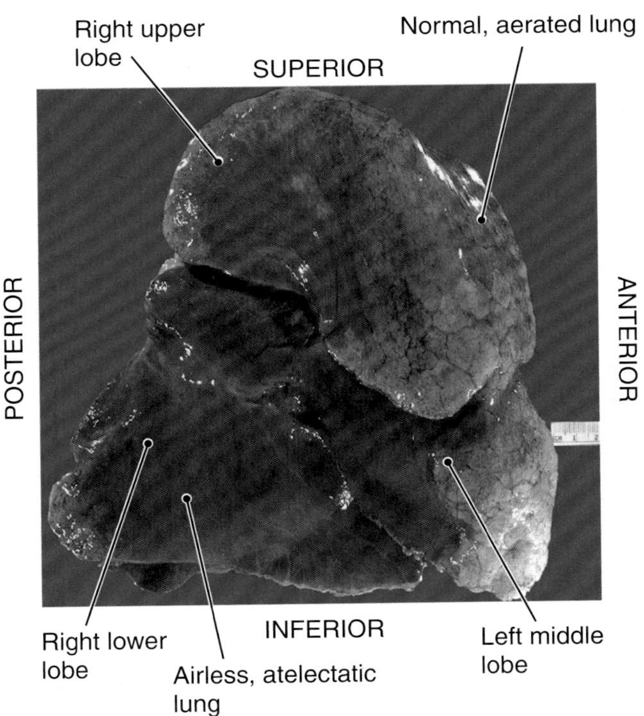

Figure 10.4 **Compression atelectasis.** Lateral view of right lung. In this reclining patient, pleural fluid compressed the lower and posterior aspects of the right lung, which are dark and airless.

- *Contraction* atelectasis occurs when scars in the lung or pleura constrict, collapsing the lung. Examples include tuberculous lung scars and pleural scars from chronic pleural inflammation.

Compression and resorption atelectases are reversible; contraction atelectasis is not. Severe atelectasis can cause hypoxia, and chronic or recurrent atelectasis invites infection.

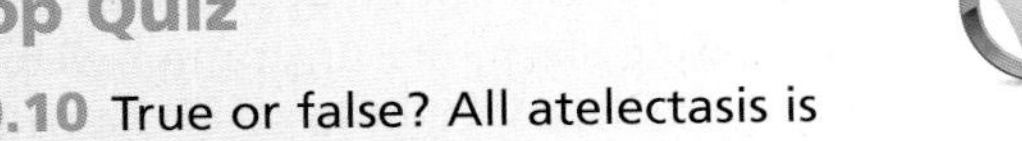

Pop Quiz

10.10 True or false? All atelectasis is reversible.

Pulmonary Edema

Normal alveoli contain only a thin film of surfactant that coats the alveolar walls.

Pulmonary edema is an abnormal accumulation of fluid in the alveoli, which resolves slowly and interferes with gas exchange. The two varieties are the following:

- *Hemodynamic* edema accumulates when there is increased hemodynamic pressure (blood pressure) in the lung vascular bed, most often as a result of left-heart failure. Increased left ventricular end diastolic pressure is associated with increased pulmonary venous pressure and pulmonary congestion. The increased hemodynamic pressure causes fluid to seep from blood into the alveolar air space.
- *Microvascular* injury edema occurs when capillaries in the alveolar walls are injured and leak protein-rich inflammatory fluid into the alveolar space. Causes from the alveolar side include inhaled toxic fumes or hot gases from a fire. Causes from the vascular side include septicemia with release of bacterial endotoxin, intravenous drug abuse, and many other conditions. Diffuse pulmonary edema from microvascular edema may evolve into *acute respiratory distress syndrome*, a very dangerous condition discussed below.

The main symptom of pulmonary edema is shortness of breath. Sweating, wheezing, and blood-tinged sputum may also be present. Breath sounds are distant, crackling rales are heard in the lung bases, and chest X-ray usually reveals widespread, splotchy infiltrates. Treatment is elimination of the cause (usually heart failure), oxygen, and respiratory support. In patients who do not survive, the lungs at autopsy are heavy and wet, and they exude a frothy, slightly bloody fluid.

Pop Quiz

10.11 What are the two varieties of pulmonary edema?

Acute Respiratory Distress Syndrome

Acute respiratory distress syndrome (ARDS) is a medical emergency associated with alveolar or pulmonary capillary injury. Causes are varied: sepsis (bacterial endotoxic shock), smoke inhalation, near drowning, oxygen toxicity, burns, heroin overdose, disseminated intravascular coagulation, pancreatitis, uremia, and large bone fracture with bone marrow fat embolism.

The pathogenesis may be roughly summarized as follows. The offending condition injures vascular endothelium and/or alveoli. For poorly understood reasons, an exceptionally severe acute inflammatory reaction ensues. Pneumocytes die and microthrombi form in capillaries. Neutrophils infiltrate the alveolar wall and a protein-rich fluid exudes into the alveolar space. Gas transfer falters and there is an abrupt onset of hypoxia. Both dyspnea and tachypnea ensue, drying the fluid into a thick membrane that coats the alveolar wall like glue. This stiffens the lung and limits airflow, which further interferes with gas diffusion.

The clinical course of ARDS is often dreadful—the fatality rate is about 40%, and even higher if it is associated with bacterial sepsis. Clinical deterioration is rapid, usually within 24 hours of the initial problem. Blood oxygen is low and often cannot be increased by oxygen supplementation. Chest X-rays often show a "white lung" of nearly complete airlessness. The protein-rich alveolar exudate invites growth of microorganisms, and secondary pneumonia is a frequent complication.

Treatment is mechanical ventilation with oxygen supplementation, steroids, and elimination of the underlying cause. In those fortunate to survive the acute phase, after about a week, fibrous repair begins in the interstitium. This may proceed, however, to interstitial fibrosis. Some patients do regain normal pulmonary function in a few months; some, however, are permanently crippled by diffuse interstitial fibrosis.

In those who do not survive, autopsy reveals striking pathologic findings. Grossly, the lungs look like liver—heavy, dark, airless, and wet, their alveoli filled with edema fluid. Microscopically, as shown in Figure 10.5, inflammatory edema condenses into a thick protein membrane that lines the alveolar walls.

Pop Quiz

10.12 True or false? In ARDS, a thick protein membrane lining the alveoli is responsible for faulty gas exchange.

10.13 True or false? In ARDS, blood oxygen content usually rises with supplemental oxygen therapy.

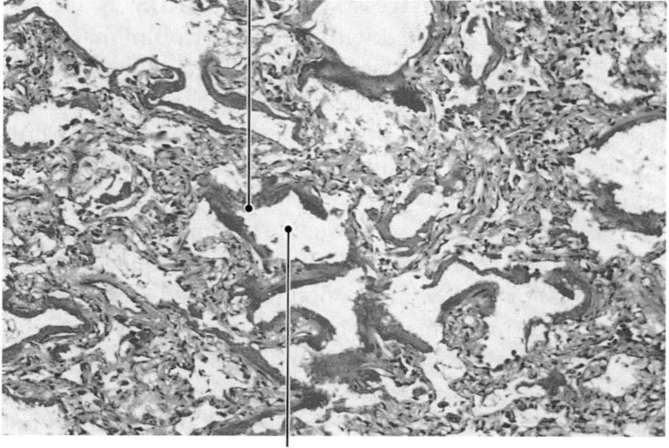

Figure 10.5 **Alveoli in acute respiratory distress syndrome (ARDS).** Edema accumulates in the alveoli as a result of alveolar and pulmonary capillary damage and condenses into a thick protein membrane, which coats alveolar walls and impairs gas exchange. (Reproduced with permission from Rubin E. *Pathology*. 4th ed. Philadelphia, PA. Lippincott Williams and Wilkins; 2005.)

Obstructive Lung Diseases

In **obstructive lung disease**, there is some general barrier to the smooth flow of air, usually at the level of the small branches of the bronchial tree. Lung volume is not affected. The problem is getting air out, not getting it in. The patient can draw a quick and deep breath, but exhalation is difficult and slow because bronchioles are constricted, and the patient must breathe in again before the previous breath has been completely exhaled. The result is slow, labored breathing with an audible expiratory wheeze as air whistles through tight bronchi. Obstructive apnea, discussed below, is an exception to these generalities.

Recall from the discussion above and Figure 10.3 that, in obstructive disease, the one-second forced expiratory volume (FEV1) is low, and volume (forced vital capacity, FVC) is normal. Therefore, the ratio FEV1/FVC is low.

Upper Airway Obstruction Causes Sleep Apnea

Obstructive sleep apnea (OSA) consists of sleep-related episodes of partial or complete closing of the upper airway that lead to breathing cessation (a breathless period of >10 seconds). About 5% of the population is affected. OSA results when relaxed pharyngeal tissues collapse, usually while the patient is recumbent. Obesity is a common risk factor. Men are much more vulnerable than women. The result is chronic hypoxemia, insomnia, daytime somnolence, and fatigue. Signs and symptoms include loud snoring and gasping followed by periods of apnea as the patient tries to inhale but cannot. Diagnosis is based on sleep history and sleep lab studies. Spirometry is normal. Treatment is with continuous positive airway pressure (CPAP), which is a stream of air, delivered via a mask that keeps the airways open while the patient sleeps. Other treatments include a variety of oral appliances that hold the jaw forward during sleep, or surgery in severe cases when other treatments fail. Weight loss—if the patient is obese—is strongly advised. With treatment, prognosis is good. Most cases remain undiagnosed and untreated and are associated with hypertension, heart failure, and injury or death due to auto and other accidents caused by severe drowsiness.

Asthma Is Characterized by Bronchospasm

Asthma is a chronic inflammatory disease of bronchioles that is characterized by recurring episodes of bronchospasm and excessive production of mucus. In normal breathing, bronchioles expand slightly with inhalation and constrict slightly on exhalation. In asthma, the constriction on exhalation is exaggerated and obstructs air outflow. The rates of asthma have been increasing every year in the United States since at least 2001. In the United States in 2012, about 7 million children and 18 million adults had asthma.

Pathophysiology

Asthma can be classified according to the irritant involved.

- *Atopic (allergic) asthma*: In some patients the irritant is an allergen that stimulates a Type I hypersensitivity (anaphylaxis) reaction. Some of the most common culprits are dust mites, cockroach allergen, mold, and pet dander. Allergic asthma occurs most often in children who have a genetic tendency toward other atopic allergies, usually "hay fever" (allergic rhinitis) and skin allergies. Many patients may have positive skin tests for particular allergens and a family history of asthma.
- *Nonatopic asthma*: Other factors that may precipitate an acute attack include URI, strenuous exercise, a drug reaction (most commonly to aspirin), and severe air pollution—*especially exposure to secondhand smoke*. Usually there is no family history of asthma and allergen skin tests are negative. Sometimes severe emotional distress may precipitate hyperventilation and an attack.
- *Occupational asthma*: Wood, grain, or textile dust; industrial chemicals, and dozens of other workplace substances can cause asthma or precipitate an acute episode.

Regardless of the initial irritant, with repeated exposure bronchioles become progressively inflamed and irritated. In many patients with chronic asthma, bronchospasm and chronic inflammation become interlocked and evolve into simple airway hyperreactivity. Similar airway overreactivity can also be seen in some patients, usually smokers, who have chronic bronchitis or related chronic obstructive pulmonary disease (discussed below). As depicted in Figure 10.6, recurrent episodes induce permanent remodeling of the airway, characterized by hyperplastic mucus glands, mucus plugs, hypertrophied bronchial smooth muscles, edema, and marked eosinophilic inflammation.

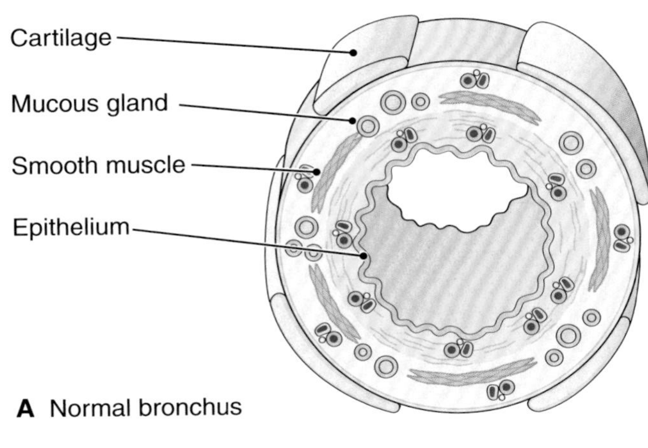

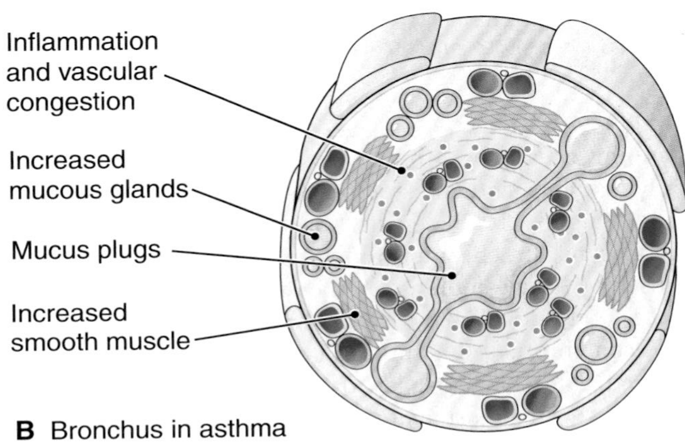

Figure 10.6 **The bronchi in asthma. A.** The normal bronchial lumen is wide; normal numbers of smooth muscle cells and mucous glands are present. **B.** In asthma, the lumen is narrow and contains a large amount of mucus; inflammatory cells are present; the mucus glands are larger and more numerous; and there are increased numbers of smooth muscle cells.

Diagnosis and Treatment

Most asthma begins in childhood; females are slightly more often affected than males. A typical asthmatic attack begins suddenly, most commonly at night or in the early morning, and if not treated can last several hours or longer. It features dyspnea, wheezing, tightness in the chest, and spasms of coughing that produce abundant mucus. In especially severe cases (*status asthmaticus*, see below) airflow may be so restricted that wheezing stops. Diagnosis depends on clinical history and spirometry.

Avoidance of triggers is key to prevention. Once exposure has occurred, however, drug therapy has two aims: to reduce chronic inflammation and relieve bronchospasm. Inhaled or oral steroids are used to reduce chronic inflammation. Bronchospasm is relieved by injectable or inhalant drugs (bronchodilators) that block bronchial smooth muscle contractions.

Prognosis is usually good. Asthma usually resolves in children but episodes may continue into adulthood. Adults with asthma may suffer episodes the whole of their lives if they are unable to avoid triggers. Nevertheless, asthma can be fatal: In 2009, it was responsible for more than 3,300 deaths in the United States. *Status asthmaticus*, a severe, prolonged state of asthmatic bronchospasm, is the usual cause of these deaths. Bronchioles become plugged with thick, sticky mucus that obstructs airflow into and out of the alveoli, and gas exchange falls dangerously. Patients become cyanotic from hypoxia and acidotic from retained carbon dioxide. *Status asthmaticus* is a life-threatening emergency that requires vigorous treatment.

Remember This! Acute asthma can be fatal.

Chronic Obstructive Pulmonary Disease (COPD) Features Bronchial Airtrapping

Chronic obstructive pulmonary disease (COPD) is the name applied to two related diseases—*emphysema* and *chronic bronchitis*, which have in common chronic air

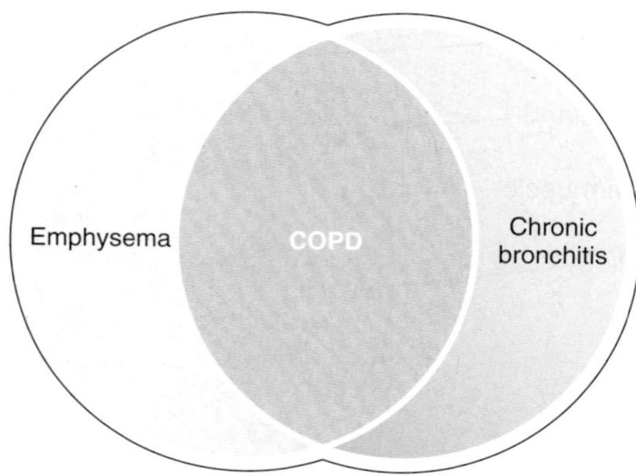

Figure 10.7 **Chronic obstructive pulmonary disease (COPD).** The relationship between emphysema, chronic bronchitis, and COPD. Most patients have a mix of emphysema and chronic bronchitis.

trapping caused by bronchial outflow obstruction. Typically, patients with these diseases have overlapping features. Figure 10.7 depicts the relationship. Whether emphysema or chronic bronchitis, almost every case is caused by heavy smoking. By the time patients finally seek medical attention after years of smoking, the distinction between chronic bronchitis and emphysema has typically blurred, and the physician diagnoses COPD. Asthmatic episodes (*chronic asthmatic bronchitis*) are also common. No matter the expression, the fundamental pathophysiologic problem is slow flow of air into and out of the lungs, which impairs uptake of oxygen and discharge of carbon dioxide. In 2011, COPD was diagnosed in about 14 million Americans, and killed about 120,000.

Emphysema

Emphysema is characterized by irreversible destruction of alveolar walls and merging of alveoli to form large air spaces. The destruction causes marked decrease of pulmonary membrane surface area and diffusion capacity. Emphysema is a common condition, present in about half of patients coming to autopsy, most of whom had no symptoms. Women and African Americans are at greater risk. There is a clear relationship to smoking—90% of cases, especially severe emphysema, occur in smokers. Nevertheless, only about 10% of smokers develop emphysema; the other 90% do not, for reasons not yet understood.

Pathogenesis

The pathogenesis of emphysema relates to an imbalance of inflammatory versus anti-inflammatory forces, and oxidant versus antioxidant forces. Cigarette smoke irritates lung tissue and causes inflammation. Inflammatory cells release digestive enzymes as part of their normal activity. These digestive enzymes are normally inhibited by alpha-1 antitrypsin, a protein made by the liver, whose purpose is to neutralize these enzymes to prevent overactivity and digestion of normal tissue. Tobacco smoke not only inflames the lung, it inhibits alpha-1 antitrypsin, which leaves the enzymes free to digest (dissolve) lung tissue. Pulmonary membrane is destroyed, alveoli merge into larger spaces and diffusion capacity is reduced (Figs. 10.8 and 10.9). Of interest is that, not only do patients with congenital alpha-1 antitrypsin deficiency (Chapter 22) have a marked tendency to develop early emphysema, it is also more severe.

Tobacco smoke also contains abundant oxidants that destroy the natural elasticity of the lungs that keeps

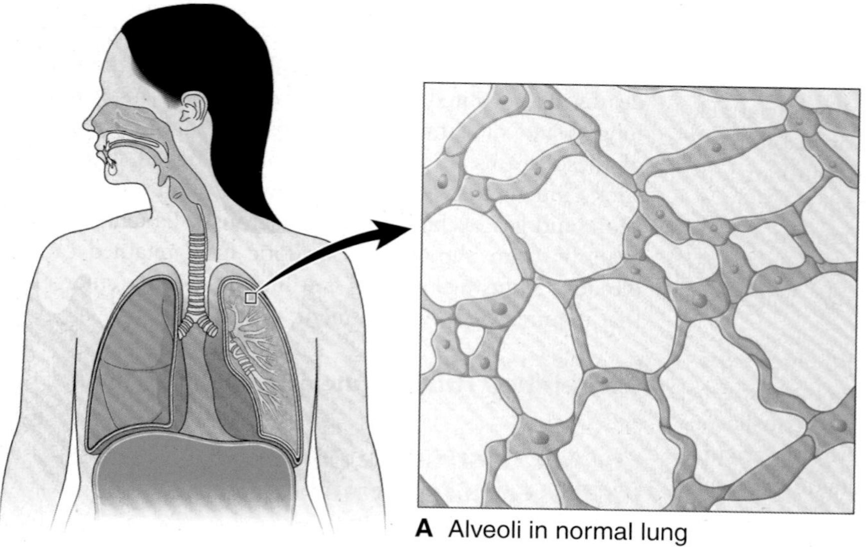

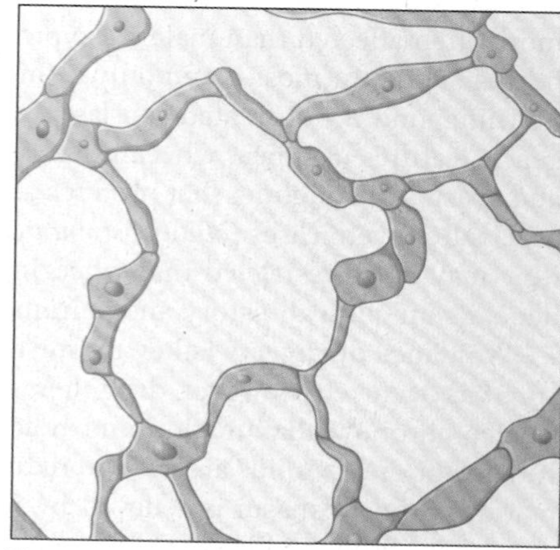

Figure 10.8 **Emphysema, microscopic development. A.** Normal alveoli. **B.** In emphysema, destruction of alveolar walls results in large air spaces with decreased pulmonary surface area for gas diffusion.

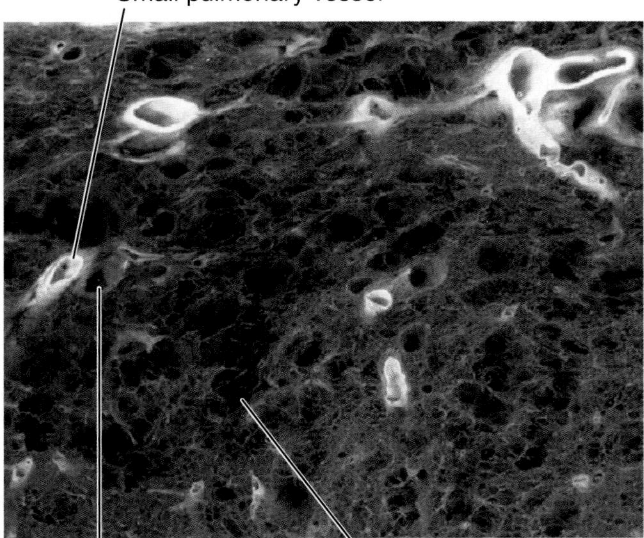

Figure 10.9 **Emphysema.** Close-up view. Normal alveoli are too small to be visible to the unaided eye. Merger of alveoli into larger air spaces makes them plainly visible in this specimen.

small airways open. Ordinarily, the lung contains great quantities of antioxidants, but those antioxidants are not plentiful enough to counter the flood of oxidants in tobacco smoke. Oxidants damage the elastic tissue to which bronchiolar walls are attached, allowing them to collapse.

Signs and Symptoms

Dyspnea is usually the first symptom of patients suffering primarily from emphysema; however, wheezing and coughing may be the first symptoms in patients whose initial disease is primarily chronic bronchitis (see below). Weight loss in patients with emphysema can be dramatic: the body sheds muscle the lungs cannot support. The typical emphysema patient is an emaciated smoker with severe dyspnea—the chest is barrel-shaped from strained overexpansion, neck muscles bulge with each breath, and the patient sits hunched forward, hands on knees, elbows spread out, breathing out through pursed lips. Nevertheless, patients remain well oxygenated and pink, an appearance sometimes uncharitably described as "pink puffers." Development of pulmonary hypertension (PH) and cor pulmonale may lead to right heart failure.

Diagnosis and Treatment

Clinical diagnosis is confirmed by spirometry, which shows low one-second forced expiratory volume (FEV1) and relatively normal forced vital capacity (FVC). The FEV1/FVC ratio is markedly decreased. Chest X-ray shows fully inflated lungs with poor markings, which indicate a loss of lung substance.

The gross and microscopic anatomy of emphysema features large air spaces throughout the lungs, especially in the apex of each lung. Large air spaces are clearly visible to the naked eye. An unusually large air space is a *bulla* or *bleb*.

Treatment options include bronchodilators and steroids for short-term relief, or bullectomy or lung transplant for longer-term relief. Long-term outlook is poor. The best policy is prevention: do not smoke cigarettes, cigars, or any other form of tobacco. Death is usually due to respiratory acidosis from retained CO_2, right heart failure, pneumonia, or rupture of a bulla into the pleural space with lung collapse (pneumothorax).

Chronic Bronchitis

Chronic bronchitis is a clinical diagnosis that can be made in any patient who has had a chronic cough that produces sputum for three consecutive months two years in a row. Chronic bronchitis, no matter the cause, may lead to emphysema or right heart failure and is implicated as an added factor in the development of lung cancer.

Tobacco smoke is the main irritant, but industrial gases, fibers, or grain dust may also irritate the bronchi and stimulate chronic inflammation and marked bronchial mucus gland hyperplasia and mucus secretion. Infection is usually secondary and adds to the insult. In contrast to emphysema—where the initial lesion is in the alveoli—in chronic bronchitis, the initial lesion is in the bronchi and bronchioles.

Signs and Symptoms

Patients with pure chronic bronchitis (a rarity) have a cough productive of abundant sputum but do not have airway obstruction. Some patients with chronic bronchitis have sudden episodes of asthma-like wheezing and are said to have **chronic asthmatic bronchitis**. Others have consistent wheezing and obstruction and are said to have *obstructive chronic bronchitis*. Nevertheless, as depicted in Figure 10.10, virtually all patients with chronic bronchitis also have significant emphysema, the reason why chronic bronchitis and emphysema are lumped together as COPD.

When obstructive chronic bronchitis is the main problem, patients have airflow obstruction and airtrapping with wheezing, coughing, infection, and sputum production. They do not move air well enough for good oxygenation or CO_2 elimination, so they are hypoxic and cyanotic, as well as acidotic from retained CO_2. These patients do not lose weight like emphysema patients because they have not lost much pulmonary membrane. Because they are bulkier and cyanotic, they are sometimes uncharitably called "blue bloaters" to contrast them with emphysematous "pink puffers." Most patients, however, fall somewhere between these extremes.

At autopsy, the bronchi and bronchioles are chronically inflamed. The mucosa is thickened due to marked hyperplasia of mucus glands. The lumen is filled with mucus and inflammatory cells.

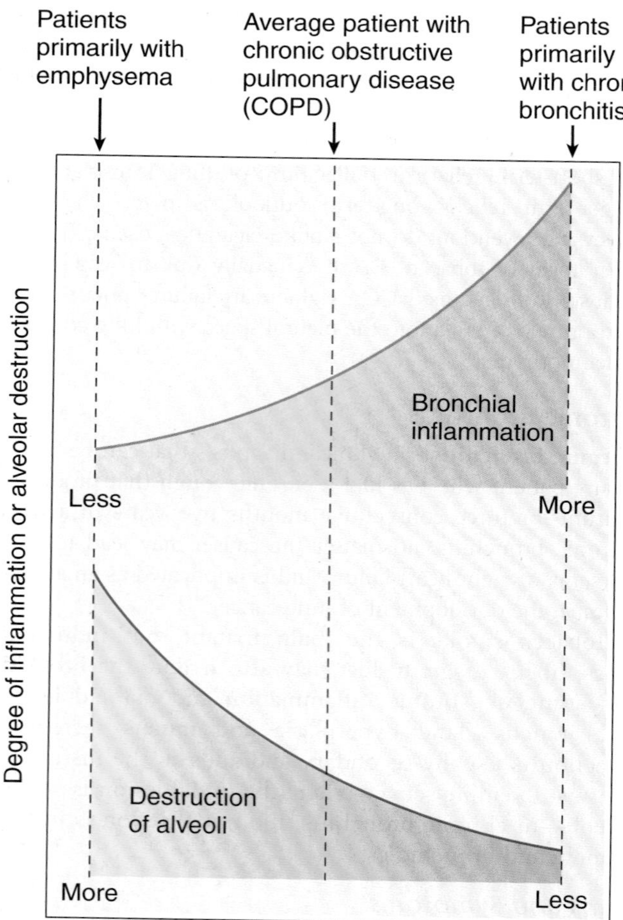

Figure 10.10 **The relationship between emphysema and chronic bronchitis.** Most patients with chronic obstructive pulmonary disease (COPD) have a mixture of bronchial inflammation and alveolar destruction.

Diagnosis and Treatment

Clinical diagnosis is confirmed by spirometry.

Prognosis and treatment are similar to emphysema, excepting that in pure bronchitis surgery is not an option. Complications are also similar to emphysema, and all patients with chronic bronchitis or other COPD are at risk for chronic hypoxia, which can lead to pulmonary vasospasm, PH, cor pulmonale, and right heart failure.

Case Notes

10.5 Would Myrtle be informally called a "pink puffer" or a "blue bloater"?

10.6 Which is more likely: A) that Myrtle has more chronic bronchitis than emphysema, or B) the opposite?

Remember This! Most patients with COPD have a mixture of chronic bronchitis and emphysema.

Bronchiectasis

Bronchiectasis (from Greek *ektasis*, for dilated) is caused by chronic, necrotizing bronchial infection. It is characterized by marked, permanent dilation of small bronchi owing to destruction of smooth muscle and elastic-supporting tissue of the airway, leaving a dilated, flaccid, pus-filled tube (Fig. 10.11). The lower lobes are most seriously involved because they are dependent. Both obstruction and infection are required; either may come first. Obstruction can cause mucous retention, which offers a breeding ground for infection; or chronic infection may damage bronchial walls, leading to excess mucous production and mucous retention. In either instance, a vicious circle ensues.

Bronchiectasis is not a primary condition; it is always secondary to other, underlying disorders, including

- immunodeficiency states, which encourage infection;
- chronic infections such as tuberculosis (TB), which damage bronchial walls;
- retained bronchial foreign body, which causes mucous retention and infection;
- genetic conditions, such as cystic fibrosis (Chapter 22), that cause generation of thick mucus, which obstructs bronchi. In cystic fibrosis, the gene defect causes accumulation of thick mucus, which encourages infection that feeds a vicious circle of destruction.

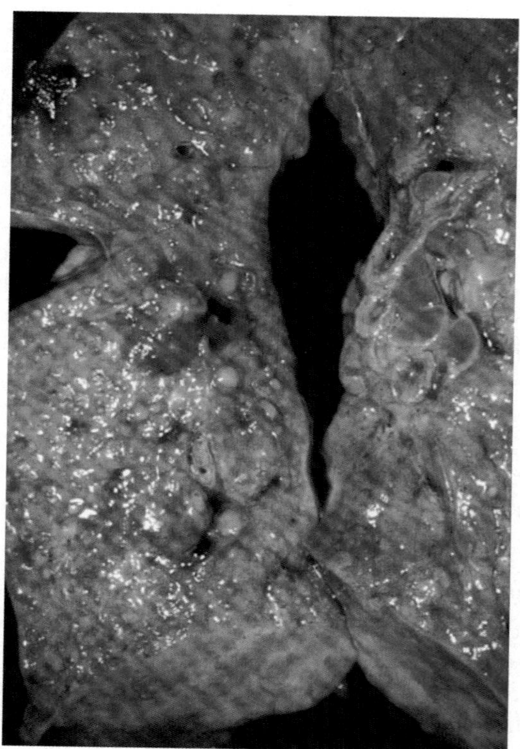

Figure 10.11 **Bronchiectasis.** The lungs of a patient with bronchiectasis due to cystic fibrosis.

The clinical picture in bronchiectasis is dominated by chronic infection and a persistent cough productive of copious amounts of infected, foul-smelling, yellow sputum. Dyspnea and cyanosis may be severe, and life-threatening pulmonary hemorrhage can occur. The severe chronic inflammation can also cause complications such as amyloidosis (Chapter 3), brain abscesses from hematogenous spread of infectious organisms, and cor pulmonale.

Clinical diagnosis is confirmed by chest imaging that demonstrates bronchial dilation. Specialized laboratory tests are necessary to rule out immunodeficiency and cystic fibrosis or other genetic condition.

The general prognosis is fairly good, especially with vigorous treatment (pulmonary toilet, antibiotics). Patients with cystic fibrosis have an average survival of nearly 40 years. Lung transplant is an option in some patients.

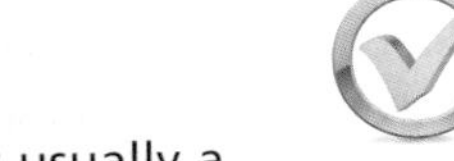

Pop Quiz

10.14 True or false? COPD is usually a blend of emphysema and chronic bronchitis.

10.15 True or false? Unlike other obstructive lung diseases, FEV1 and FVC are normal in obstructive sleep apnea.

10.16 True or false? The diagnosis of chronic bronchitis is made after three consecutive months of a cough productive of sputum.

10.17 What is the etiology of bronchiectasis?

Restrictive Lung Diseases (Diffuse Interstitial Disease)

Restrictive lung disease is a disease of stiff lungs, which limits the volume of lung expansion and the rate of expansion and contraction. Restrictive diseases are characterized by chronic inflammation, fibrosis, and stiffening of the delicate interstitium of the alveolar walls. Most of the time, the cause is unknown. The normal interstitium—alveolar walls, capillaries, and supporting tissue—is pliable and very thin, a condition necessary for easy lung expansion and gas diffusion. Of equal or greater importance, less air is moved in and out of the lungs because of the stiffness. The result is that blood oxygen saturation falls and blood carbon dioxide rises.

Spirometry in restrictive disease shows roughly equal declines of one-second forced expiratory volume (FEV1) and forced vital capacity (FVC). Therefore, the FEV1/FVC ratio is often near normal.

Patients have dyspnea, tachypnea, and end-inspiratory crackles without wheezing or other evidence of obstruction. Chest X-rays show small nodules, streaks, and ground-glass haziness. PH and cor pulmonale with right heart failure follow. Though many of these cases begin as a particular disease entity (discussed below), with time they evolve into a similar end-stage clinical picture of severe scarring, lung destruction, hypoxemia, right heart failure and death.

Interstitial lung diseases can be classified using several criteria—acute or chronic, granulomatous or nongranulomatous, known cause or unknown cause, primary lung disease or secondary to some systemic disease. Below we classify them using a mixture of these characteristics.

Case Notes

10.7 **Is there any evidence that Myrtle had restrictive lung disease?**

Simple Fibrosis Is the Only Element of Most Interstitial Disease

Most interstitial disease is characterized by simple fibrosis (Fig. 10.12). **Idiopathic pulmonary fibrosis** is known

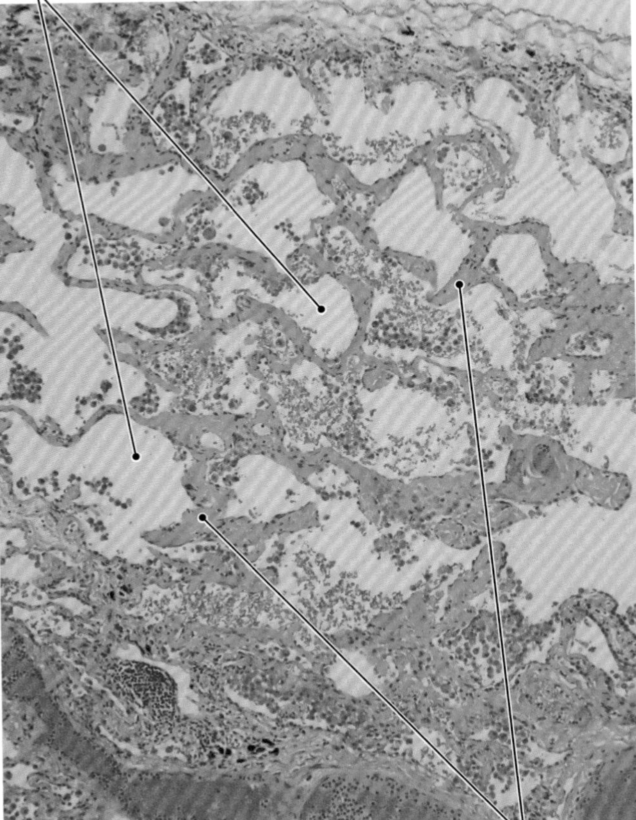

Figure 10.12 **Interstitial fibrosis.** Marked thickening of many alveolar walls by dense, scar-like fibrous tissue.

by a dozen or more names, a clue that its cause often is a mystery. At time of diagnosis, most patients are middle-aged adults, but the process presumably has been under way for many years. Men are affected more often than women. By definition (idiopathic) the cause is unknown. In these cases, the fibrosis seems to be abnormally exuberant fibrous repair (scarring) reaction to an unknown insult. Recent research finds, however, that about 15% of interstitial fibrosis is due to a genetic defect in the maintenance of telomeres (Chapter 24), a region of DNA that retards cell aging. In idiopathic and genetic cases, steroid therapy is ineffective, suggesting that inflammation is not an important pathophysiologic factor.

Immune reactions are strongly suspected of playing an important role in those cases in which some cause is found that may be related. For example, some patients will be found to have connective tissue disease (Chapter 3) as the underlying cause. Some degree of pulmonary involvement is present in about one-third of patients with rheumatoid arthritis (RA). Less commonly, patients with systemic lupus or systemic sclerosis may have pulmonary lesions. Other known causes of interstitial fibrosis include a few drugs and radiation injury.

Fibrosis begins insidiously and usually presents as shortness of breath in patients 40–70 years old. Nevertheless, in most the prognosis is bleak—median survival is about five years. Lung transplant is the only effective therapy.

Pneumoconiosis is a term applied to lung disease caused by inhaled dusts and fumes. Coal dust causes coal worker's lung (*black lung disease, anthracosis*), and rock or stone dust causes *silicosis*, the most common chronic occupational disease in the world.

Asbestosis is a chronic interstitial lung disease caused by inhalation of asbestos particles, tiny silicate fibers formerly used in industry, especially for fireproofing and insulation. When inhaled in quantity, asbestos causes interstitial pulmonary fibrosis, pleural fibrosis, pleural effusion, or pleural *mesothelioma*, a neoplasm of the pleura that can be either benign or malignant. Symptoms may not appear for 10–20 years after first exposure. Asbestosis is associated with a fivefold increased risk of lung cancer. Adding cigarette smoking increases the lung cancer risk 55-fold, perhaps because asbestos traps and retains the carcinogens in cigarette smoke. This is not the case in mesothelioma, where smoking is not a contributing factor. Prognosis is guarded. Development of lung cancer or mesothelioma is an especially grim prospect.

Most exposure to asbestos occurs in industrial settings; however, improved industrial hygiene has nearly eliminated the risk. In nonindustrial settings, asbestos is found as old spray-on insulation on ceilings, walls, and pipes. The risk from undisturbed asbestos in these settings, even in densely occupied public spaces, is virtually zero. Removal is expensive and experts conclude asbestos can be left safely in place if not disturbed.

Some Interstitial Disease Features Granulomatous Inflammation

Granulomatous inflammation (Chapter 2) is a special variety of chronic inflammation, which characterizes some interstitial disease.

Sarcoidosis

Sarcoidosis is a systemic granulomatous disease of unknown cause that affects many tissues. Sarcoidosis occurs worldwide, but is most common in northern Europeans, especially Scandinavians. It occurs 10 times more frequently in African Americans than in Caucasian Americans. Evidence suggests that the cause is a combination of immune dysfunction and genetic susceptibility, perhaps in response to exposure to a microbe. Nevertheless, despite highly distinctive pathology and decades of research, the cause is unknown.

Sarcoid granulomas may develop in any organ, but chiefly appear in the lungs and mediastinal lymph nodes. Ninety percent of patients present with chest X-ray findings of bilateral hilar lymph node enlargement and lung infiltrates. Eye (iritis, glaucoma, and retinitis, Chapter 20) and skin lesions are next most common. Other common sites include mucous membranes of the nose and mouth, and the spleen and liver.

Signs and Symptoms

The clinical picture of sarcoidosis is especially varied because so many anatomic sites may be involved. Many cases are asymptomatic and are initially diagnosed on chest X-ray taken for some other purpose. In other cases, the first clue may be skin lesions, or enlargement of lymph nodes, spleen, or liver. Nevertheless, most patients seek medical attention for pulmonary symptoms: shortness of breath, cough, chest pain, or hemoptysis.

Diagnosis and Treatment

Diagnosis is by the distinctive pattern on chest imaging and a biopsy that demonstrates distinctive sarcoid granulomas. Two-thirds of patients recover completely, some spontaneously, others after steroid therapy. Patients with mild disease should be closely followed without treatment. Prognosis is generally good for those with mild symptoms, but is poor with cardiac, brain, or extensive lung involvement.

Hypersensitivity Pneumonitis

Hypersensitivity pneumonitis is a T-cell–mediated, delayed hypersensitivity immune reaction. Also called *allergic alveolitis*, it occurs as a response to inhaled antigens, such as moldy hay and other organic dusts found in occupational settings. The acute form may present as a "flu" syndrome of cough, fever, and leukocytosis after exposure to the offending dust. One-time, acute exposure has no lasting consequences; however, chronic exposure can cause interstitial fibrosis with clinical feature like other forms of interstitial fibrosis. Diagnosis requires a high index of suspicion and rests on typical clinical history supported by chest imaging. Lung biopsy, which reveals widespread interstitial granulomatous inflammation, may be necessary. Early diagnosis is critical: elimination of the offending agent can halt the process and prevent chronic lung disease.

Pop Quiz

10.18 True or false? In patients with asbestosis, smoking increases the risk of mesothelioma.

10.19 True or false? Patients with idiopathic pulmonary fibrosis should begin steroid therapy at time of diagnosis.

10.20 What are two examples of granulomatous lung disease?

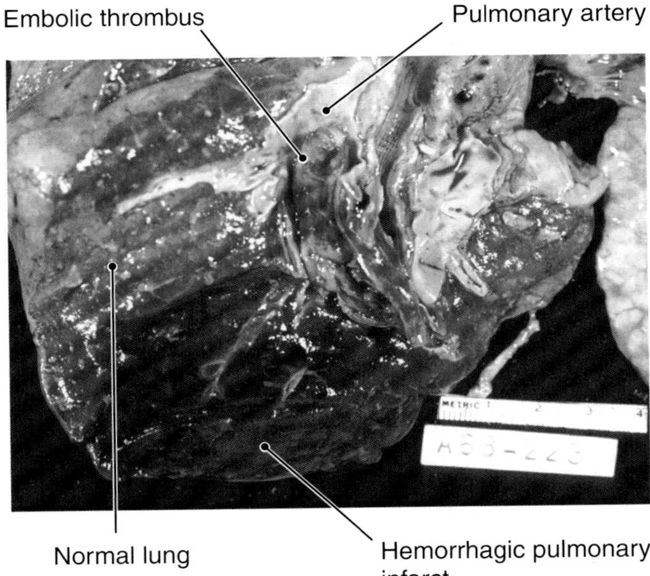

Figure 10.13 **Pulmonary thromboembolus with infarct.** A thrombus has embolized from one of the great veins of the thigh to the lung and fills a branch of the pulmonary artery. The dark, hemorrhagic tissue is infarcted lung.

Vascular and Circulatory Lung Disease

The pulmonary arterial tree is fed by venous blood returning to the heart through the great veins. Compared to the arterial tree, veins are thin-walled, pressure is low, and flow is relatively sluggish—physical factors that make it easier for thrombi to form and grow in veins. Thrombi are usually small and flexible, regardless of size, which enables them to pass easily up the ever-enlarging highway of veins and then into the right heart and into the pulmonary arterial tree. There the network becomes smaller with each branch until the thromboembolus can go no further and it occludes the lumen.

Another factor important in pulmonary vascular disease is that the pulmonary circulation is a low-pressure system—about 25/8 mm Hg (the average is about 15 mm Hg). Resistance in the pulmonary vascular bed is low, too, as it must be for blood to flow normally under such little pressure. Small increases in pulmonary vascular resistance increase pulmonary pressure, which irreversibly damages the pulmonary vascular bed, further raising pressure in a vicious circle.

Pulmonary Thromboembolism Can Be Fatal

Pulmonary thromboembolism (Fig. 10.13) is movement (embolization) of a thrombus from its origin in a vein, through the venous system into the pulmonary arterial system. Pulmonary thromboemboli are common: they cause more deaths annually than traffic accidents, and they are frequently an asymptomatic incidental finding at autopsy.

Almost all thromboemboli arise from the deep veins of the knee, upper leg, or pelvis. Local predisposing conditions include inflammation associated with major surgery, trauma, or infection. General predisposing conditions include patients with heart disease or cancer, or who are immobilized for a lengthy period, especially those with a hip fracture. Hypercoagulable states also predispose to thromboembolism (Chapter 6). Acquired hypercoagulable conditions include obesity, cancer, oral contraceptive use, lupus anticoagulant, and pregnancy; factor V Leiden is a genetic hypercoagulable state.

The pathophysiologic response to thromboembolism depends on the number and size of the emboli and the size of the occluded vessel(s). The hemodynamic consequence is increased resistance to pulmonary blood flow and a rise of pulmonary blood pressure as diverted blood flows through the remaining patent vasculature. The respiratory consequence is that segments of lung are no longer perfused, which prevents gas exchange even though they are aerated.

Signs and Symptoms

Although small emboli may cause only fleeting chest pain and cough, and sometimes hemoptysis, most do not cause symptoms. A large pulmonary thromboembolus, on the other hand, is one of the few nontraumatic causes of instantaneous death. If not fatal, the symptoms mimic those of myocardial infarction: chest pain, dyspnea, and shock.

Diagnosis and Treatment

Detection of small emboli is important, as a small embolus may herald a larger one and recurrent small thromboemboli can cause PH. Diagnosis depends on finding wedge-shaped lung defects by imaging techniques, or by sonography of deep veins that reveals a thrombus.

Treatment is anticoagulant and thrombolytic drugs. Occasionally an umbrella sieve must be inserted into the inferior vena cava to prevent emboli from reaching the lungs. Prevention is important and includes early ambulation after surgery and in postpartum patients. Mechanical compression stockings and anticoagulation may also be necessary in high-risk patients.

Pulmonary Hypertension Is Often Irreversible and Fatal

Pulmonary hypertension (PH) is abnormally high blood pressure (mean pressure ≥25 mm Hg at rest) in the pulmonary vascular tree. It is a very serious condition that feeds on itself in a vicious circle: high pressure damages the pulmonary vascular bed, increasing vascular resistance; increased resistance increases pressure.

The various types of PH share similar pathophysiology, clinical presentation, and treatment. The most common underlying cause is COPD, but other causes include genetic defects, left-to-right congenital cardiovascular shunts (Chapter 9), recurrent pulmonary thromboemboli, systemic connective tissue disease, or obstructive sleep apnea. Rarely, PH may occur as a primary disease of unknown cause (*primary PH*). The most common mechanism is increased pulmonary vascular resistance traceable to vasospasm and endothelial cell proliferation, which accounts for the distinctive onionskin endothelial hyperplasia (Fig. 10.14) so characteristic of the pathology of PH. About 5% of cases are idiopathic PH, which usually occurs in young women, less commonly in children.

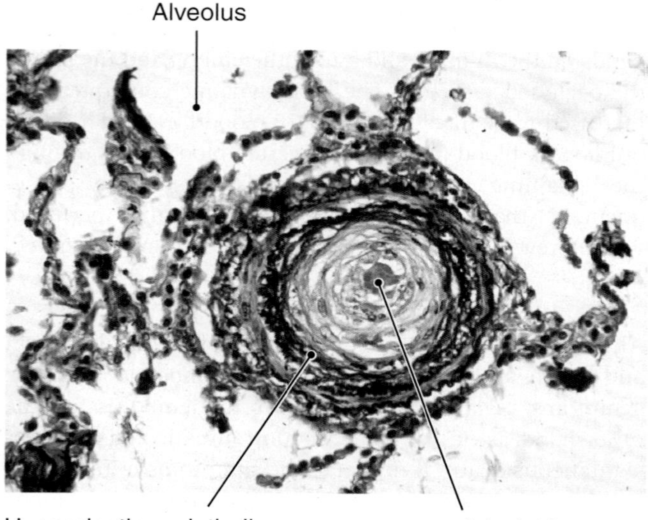

Figure 10.14 **Pulmonary arteriole in pulmonary hypertension.** High pulmonary vascular pressure injures the arterial wall and causes endothelial cell hyperplasia.

Case Notes

10.8 Is it likely that Myrtle had pulmonary hypertension (PH)?

No matter the cause, presentation is similar and does not appear until disease is advanced. Apart from signs and symptoms of an underlying disease, PH presents as dyspnea and fatigue, sometimes with angina-like chest pain. With time, severe respiratory distress, cyanosis, and right ventricular hypertrophy appear. Until recently, the only available treatment was lung transplantation. Progress is being made with new drugs, however, to arrest endothelial hyperplasia and to dilate the pulmonary vascular bed. Death usually occurs from heart failure, pneumonia, and cor pulmonale. Most patients die within two to five years of diagnosis.

Pop Quiz

10.21 True or false? The most common mechanism of PH is increased pulmonary vascular resistance.

10.22 True or false? The symptoms of a pulmonary embolism may be very similar to those of a heart attack.

Pneumonia

The respiratory tract is more often infected than any other organ system. Most infections are viral and confined to the upper respiratory tract. The local defenses, consisting of mucociliary apparatus and MALT antibody production (both described above), can be impaired by the following:

- Tobacco smoke, alcohol, toxic gas, or genetic defect
- Accumulation of bronchial mucus as with cystic fibrosis, bronchial obstruction, or suppression or loss of the cough reflex as a result of coma, anesthesia, or drugs
- Accumulation of alveolar fluid with pulmonary edema

What's more, the lungs are especially vulnerable to infection in immunodeficiency. Also, pneumonia caused by one microbe, often a virus, renders the lungs vulnerable to superinfection by another microbe, bacteria, for example. Finally, patients with chronic diseases are vulnerable to infection and are often hospitalized. The result is that many pneumonias are hospital acquired, which is especially dangerous because many bacteria found in hospitals are antibiotic-resistant.

Case Notes

10.9 Which of Myrtle's local respiratory defenses were impaired?

Strictly speaking, **pneumonia** is inflammation of the lungs. Though pneumonia may be caused by inhaled irritants, in this section we will confine our discussion to pneumonia caused by infection. It is surprisingly common, killing more Americans (50,000+) each year than die in auto accidents (30,000+).

Clinically, pneumonia is classified according to the etiologic agent, which determines treatment. (See Chapter 4 for more information about particular infective agents.) If the culprit cannot be identified, the pneumonia is classified into **pneumonia syndromes** according to the setting in which it occurs, which narrows the list of possible culprits enough to allow empiric antimicrobial therapy:

- Community-acquired pneumonia
  - Bacterial: staphylococci, streptococci, *H. influenza*, others
  - Other: viruses, *Chlamydia*, *Mycoplasma*, others
- Hospital-acquired (nosocomial) pneumonia: Gram-negative rods, penicillin resistant staphylococci
- Aspiration pneumonia: anaerobic oral flora, others
- Chronic pneumonia: TB; histoplasmosis, and other deep mycoses
- Pneumonia in the immunodeficient host: *Pneumocystis* and other opportunistic pathogens

Case Notes

10.10 Did Myrtle have a pneumonia syndrome?

Most Treated Pneumonia Is Bacterial

Of patients *treated* for pneumonia, about 75% have acute bacterial infection. About half of these have lobar pneumonia caused by S. *pneumoniae*. These statistics are misleading, however, because patients with milder pneumonia (*primary atypical pneumonia*, discussed below) do not seek medical care and are thus underrepresented in the data.

Most bacterial pneumonia is caused by organisms that normally reside in the upper respiratory tract in equilibrium with local tissues. Nevertheless, if organisms are aspirated deep into the lungs, pneumonia may occur. Organisms vary according to the setting (*pneumonia syndromes*).

Microbes find their way into the lungs by 1) inhalation of droplets that originate from the nose or that are in the air; 2) aspiration of gastric contents, food, or drink; or 3) blood-borne spread from infection elsewhere, such as the urinary tract or gastrointestinal (GI) tract.

There Are Two Anatomic Forms of Pneumonia

Pneumonia occurs in two anatomic forms: *alveolar* and *interstitial*.

Alveolar pneumonia is characterized by an acute inflammation that completely fills alveoli with neutrophils (Fig. 10.15). Alveolar pneumonia is usually bacterial and much more common than pneumonia of the pulmonary interstitium (*interstitial pneumonia*). As is illustrated in Figure 10.16, alveolar pneumonia also occurs in two anatomic forms.

- **Bronchopneumonia** (Fig. 10.16A) is characterized by patchy, noncontiguous inflammation, usually involves the alveoli of more than one lobe, and is most likely to occur in the inferior (basilar) parts of the lower lobes.
- **Lobar pneumonia** (Fig. 10.16B) is characterized by intense, consolidated acute inflammation of the alveoli in an entire lobe and is the form that is much more

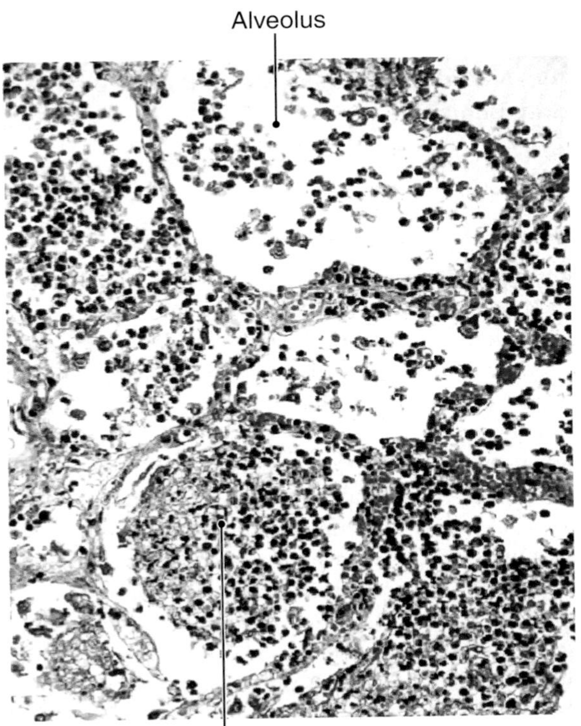

Figure 10.15 **Alveolar pneumonia.** Bacterial infection has stimulated an intense acute inflammatory reaction that fills alveoli with neutrophils and strands of fibrin (inflammatory exudate).

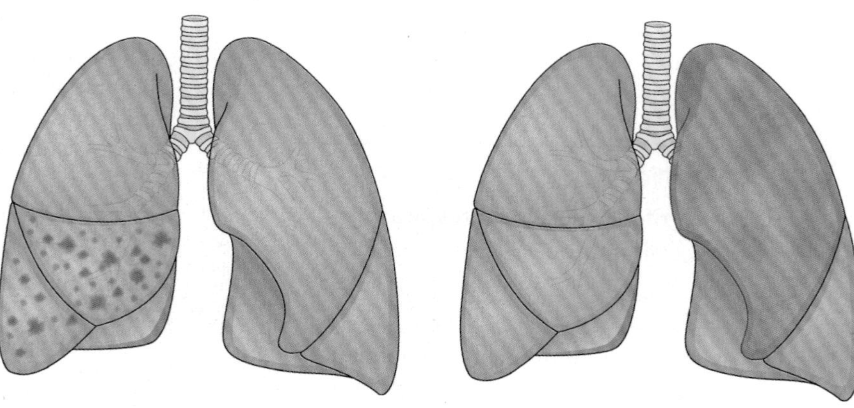

Figure 10.16 **Patterns of acute bacterial pneumonia. A.** In bronchopneumonia, alveolar inflammation is widespread and patchy, leaving some alveoli unaffected. **B.** In lobar pneumonia, all alveoli in the lobe are involved by intense acute inflammation.

likely to occur in patients with congestive heart failure, COPD, diabetes, or alcoholism. Virtually all lobar pneumonia is caused by *Streptococcus pneumoniae* (also called *pneumococcus*). Lobar pneumonia is usually confined to a single lobe that is an airless, solidified gel.

Interstitial pneumonia is inflammation confined to the alveolar septa; it does not fill the alveoli with inflammatory exudate. The inflammation is diffuse and bilateral and is usually caused by virus infection.

Case Notes

10.11 Did Myrtle have alveolar or interstitial pneumonia?

Most Pneumonias Are Community Acquired

Community-acquired pneumonia (CAP) is acute pneumonia not acquired in some special circumstance, such as in a hospital or via aspiration. The most common bacterial CAP is caused by *S. pneumoniae*. Risk factors include advanced age, diabetes, heart failure, COPD, and other chronic diseases.

The usual CAP infection is characterized by sudden onset with high fever, shaking chills, and cough productive of copious yellow sputum. Pleural inflammation is often present and features breathing-related chest wall pain and friction rub. Chest X-ray shows patchy, dense infiltrates or complete consolidation of a lobe according to whether the pattern is bronchopneumonia or lobar pneumonia. Neutrophilic leukocytosis is present in blood. Diagnosis is clinical and radiologic. Paramount for effective antibiotic therapy is identification of the infective organism by sputum or blood culture. Microscopic examination of sputum is critical—Gram stain can reveal the organism quickly and narrow the possibilities for choice of antibiotics. Most patients recover at home. Complications include pleural empyema, meningitis, endocarditis, or pericarditis. Death may occur in patients debilitated by alcoholism or other chronic illness.

Some CAP is caused by viruses, *Mycoplasma pneumoniae*, and other nonbacterial microbes, infections that may be dismissed as a "chest cold." Such infections are often called **primary atypical pneumonia (PAP)** because they are atypical in that 1) they cause interstitial rather than alveolar inflammation; 2) in most cases the agent cannot be proven; and 3) when an agent is identified, it is usually *Mycoplasma*, *Chlamydia*, or *Rickettsia*.

Patients are atypical in that symptoms are less severe. Coughing may be minimal or absent and the only other symptoms are moderate fever, myalgia, achiness, and headache. Blood leukocytosis is mild and may be lymphocytic instead of neutrophilic. Diagnosis is clinical. Minimal chest X-ray findings are confirmatory. Most patients recover spontaneously. Antibiotics are usually not necessary. Death is rare and usually due to bacterial superinfection in a debilitated patient.

Nosocomial Pneumonia Is Acquired in a Hospital

Nosocomial pneumonia is pneumonia acquired in a hospital. It is common in patients who have other severe disease, are on prolonged antibiotic therapy, or have internal medical devices such as intravascular catheters. Especially at risk are patients on mechanical ventilation. *S. aureus*, *E. coli*, and *Pseudomonas* are the most common pathogens. The most dangerous, however, are methicillin-resistant *S. aureus* (MRSA) and vancomycin-resistant enterococcus (VRE).

Case Notes

10.12 Myrtle's sputum grew MRSA. Is this evidence for or against hospital-acquired pneumonia?

Aspiration of Gastric Contents Causes Aspiration Pneumonia

Aspiration pneumonia is caused by aspiration of gastric contents in debilitated patients, especially in patients who are comatose or nearly so, as with stroke or alcoholic stupor. The inflammatory reaction is partially the result of the corrosive effects of gastric acid and partially the result of infection by a mixed flora of bacteria from the mouth. Aspiration pneumonia is serious and carries a relatively high mortality rate. Lung abscess is often a complication.

A **lung abscess** is anatomically like any other abscess—a localized area of purulent inflammation with tissue necrosis and liquefaction. Nevertheless, lung abscesses are different from other abscesses in that the bacterial population differs greatly from those of other lung infections:

- Lungs abscesses often contain several types of bacteria.
- Almost all lung abscesses contain anaerobic bacteria.
- Two-thirds of lung abscesses contain bacteria normally found in the mouth that do not usually infect other body sites.

Less commonly, lung abscess is caused by bronchial obstruction or as a complication of bacterial pneumonia.

Lung abscesses may be solitary or multiple. In addition to the usual symptoms of lung infection, they usually cause production of copious amounts of foul-smelling sputum. Lung abscesses constantly seed bacteria into the bloodstream, and patients are at risk for encephalitis or meningitis. Lung abscesses occur with some regularity with bronchogenic carcinoma, so it is wise to suspect bronchogenic carcinoma as the underlying cause in older persons with a lung abscess. Treatment includes antibiotics and surgical drainage.

Chronic Pneumonia Is Usually Due to Tuberculosis or Deep Mycosis

Chronic pneumonia is usually localized to a single lobe. Hilar lymph nodes draining the lobe also may be involved. The tissue reaction is usually granulomatous inflammation (Chapter 2). The most common etiologic agents are *M. tuberculosis* and deep mycoses (both Chapter 4) such as *Histoplasma*, *Blastomyces*, or *Coccidioides*. Chronic pneumonias often occur in immunocompromised patients.

Two kinds of fungi cause deep infection. Yeast fungi, such as *Candida* species and *Cryptococcus neoformans*, are opportunistic pathogens that primarily infect patients with diminished immunity. Dimorphic fungi, such as *Histoplasma capsulatum* and *Coccidioides immitis*, may exist as yeast or as branching, filamentous forms. They are ordinary pathogens that produce disease in patients with a normal immune system.

Candidiasis is caused by *C. albicans* and is found normally in the mouth of healthy people. Apart from dermatophytes, which infect only skin, candida is the most common cause of fungus infection. It most often causes superficial mucosal infections but may cause chronic pneumonia in debilitated or immunocompromised hosts. Antifungal drugs are available but eradication can be difficult.

Cryptococcosis is a disseminated or pulmonary infection acquired by inhalation of soil contaminated with the yeast *Cryptococcus neoformans*. It is often seen in immunocompromised patients. Symptoms depend on the site of infection: lungs, meninges, bone, skin, or abdominal viscera. Diagnosis is clinical and confirmed by culture or biopsy. Treatment, when necessary, is with specialized antifungal drugs.

Histoplasmosis, caused by *H. capsulatum*, is one of the most common systemic fungal infections in the United States, and is endemic in the general region of the Ohio River, the central Mississippi River, and along the Appalachian Mountains. It is spread by inhalation of dried bird droppings. Clinically, histoplasmosis mimics TB: Even the pathologic lesions are similar to TB, except that fungi rather than mycobacteria are the cause. Disseminated disease may occur in patients who are severely debilitated by other conditions, or who have immune deficiency. The Mantoux skin test is usually negative and is helpful in differentiating histoplasmosis from TB in the clinical workup. Positive diagnosis is made by culture, biopsy, or finding high levels of *Histoplasma* antigen or anti-Histoplasma antibody in blood. Treatment may not be necessary if the disease arrests, as it often does. Antifungal therapy is usually effective.

Coccidioidomycosis is caused by *C. immitis*, a fungus endemic in the western United States, particularly the San Joaquin Valley of central California, where infection is known as *valley fever*. As with TB, many people are infected by *Coccidioides*, but few become diseased—in the San Joaquin Valley about 80% of the population have a positive skin test. Also as with TB, most infected people remain asymptomatic, but disseminated disease can develop. Most cases do not require treatment, but some will require antifungal therapy.

Pneumonia Is Common in the Immunocompromised

Pneumonia is one of the most serious and most common complications of immunodeficiency. The usual causes are HIV/AIDS infection, immunosuppression therapy for transplants, chemotherapy for malignancy, or genetic defect. The usual agents are *Pneumocystis* (Fig. 10.17), mycobacteria, cytomegalovirus, *Candida*, gram-negative rods, and *S. aureus*. Mortality is high.

Pneumonia is the leading cause of morbidity and death in HIV infection. Opportunistic pathogens are important, but "usual" organisms are at least equally so. Patients with CD4+ counts <200 cells/mm^3 tend to develop opportunistic infection; "usual" infections tend to occur in those with higher counts.

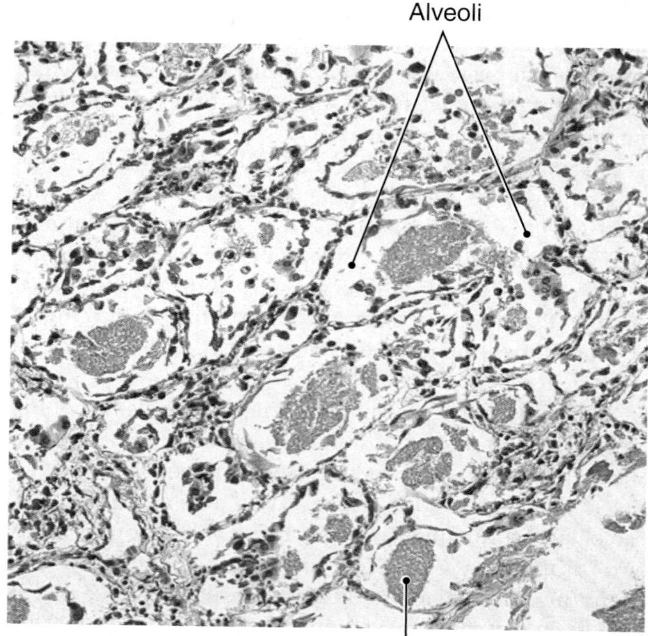

Figure 10.17 *Pneumocystis jiroveci* **pneumonia.** Microscopic study of the lungs in a patient with AIDS. Clouds of organisms fill the alveoli. Tellingly, little inflammatory reaction is present because of the patient's impaired immune system.

Pop Quiz

10.23 True or false? Nosocomial pneumonia is pneumonia acquired in a hospital.

10.24 True or false? Most bronchopneumonia is viral.

10.25 True or false? Staphylococcus, streptococcus, and pneumococcus are the most common bacteria found in lung abscesses.

10.26 Explain the terms *community-acquired pneumonia* and *nosocomial pneumonia*.

10.27 Patients with a CD 4 count less than ____________ tend to develop opportunistic infections.

Lung Neoplasms

The most common neoplasm *in* the lung is a metastasis from a cancer somewhere else in the body. The most common tumor *of* the lung is bronchogenic carcinoma ("lung cancer"), almost all of which arise from the epithelium lining the bronchi. Benign neoplasms of the lung are rare.

Bronchogenic Carcinoma Is the Most Common Fatal Malignancy in the World

Bronchogenic carcinoma is a malignancy of the bronchial epithelium. Apart from skin cancers (Chapter 21), which are largely innocuous, bronchogenic carcinoma is the most common of all human cancers worldwide and is the number one cause of cancer death for men and for women in the United States. In the United States in 2012, there were 225,000 new cases and 160,000 deaths (double the *combined* deaths for breast and prostate cancer). Another way of looking at the numbers is this: over 70% of people who develop lung cancer will die of it.

Remember This! Bronchogenic carcinoma is the most common fatal malignancy in the world.

Role of Smoking

Smoking—primarily cigarette smoking—is the main cause of bronchogenic carcinoma. The evidence is utterly convincing.

- Cigarette smoking grew exponentially beginning with World War II (1939–1945) and, in time, lung cancer rates grew in parallel. In the United States in 1950, there were only about 20,000 cases of lung cancer, one-tenth the current figure.
- Current and former cigarette smokers account for 85–90% of all lung cancer patients.
- There is a direct relationship between the number of cigarettes smoked and the likelihood of developing lung cancer (Chapter 23, Fig. 23.8). A common clinical estimate of lifetime cigarette consumption is pack-years: the average number of packs smoked per day multiplied by the number of years smoking. Higher numbers of pack years are associated with increased risk of developing lung cancer.
- Pathologic evidence shows a direct relationship between the number of cigarettes smoked and precancerous changes in bronchial mucosa: from normal to metaplasia, dysplasia, carcinoma in situ, and finally to invasive malignancy.
- Experimental evidence is compelling. Cigarette smoke is a cocktail of chemicals capable of inducing cancers in experimental animals.

Publication of this evidence, mainly in a series of reports from the U.S. Surgeon General beginning in 1964, has had a positive effect in reducing cigarette smoking: in 1955 nearly 60% of men in the United States were smokers; in 2010, 21% smoked. Lung cancer rates have declined as a result: the number of new lung cancer cases occurring each year in the United States peaked in the early 1990s and has been declining since.

It is important to note, however, that each year about 20,000–30,000 cases of lung cancer occur in nonsmokers. Factors include secondhand smoke, asbestos and other industrial exposures, and genetic predisposition.

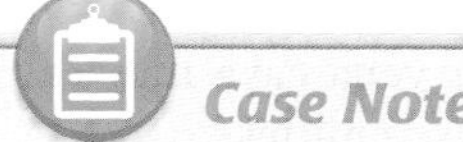

Case Notes

10.13 **How many pack-years of cigarettes had Myrtle accumulated since age 20?**

Remember This! Smoking is the cause of 85–90% of lung cancer.

Types of Lung Cancer

Based on the likelihood of metastasis and response to therapy, for clinical purposes lung cancers are grouped into two main pathologic types: *small cell* and *nonsmall cell* (Tab. 10.1).

Small cell carcinoma (Fig. 10.18) is distinctive on several counts. Most important, small cell carcinoma is the most lethal and resistant to therapy. It differs also in that it is derived from neuroendocrine cells of the bronchial mucosa, has a distinctive microscopic appearance, and occurs only in smokers. The other types vary microscopically from one another, look nothing like small cell carcinoma, and some of them arise in nonsmokers. They are lumped together as **nonsmall cell carcinomas**.

Small cell carcinomas are composed of distinctive small, dark cells that look much like large lymphocytes. They are aggressively malignant—most patients have metastases at time of diagnosis, and surgery is ineffective even in patients without demonstrable metastases.

There are three main subtypes of *nonsmall cell carcinoma*. Frequently they show a mixture of the types below.

- **Adenocarcinomas** are formed into glandular acini. They are the most well-differentiated lung cancers, and they have a slightly better prognosis than other nonsmall cell cancers. They comprise about one-third of lung cancers in men and nearly one-half in women. They tend to arise peripherally in small bronchi and therefore are easier to remove surgically because they are away from critical mediastinal structures. They are the most common type in nonsmokers.
- **Squamous cell carcinoma** is composed of malignant cells that differentiate toward flat (squamous) cells like

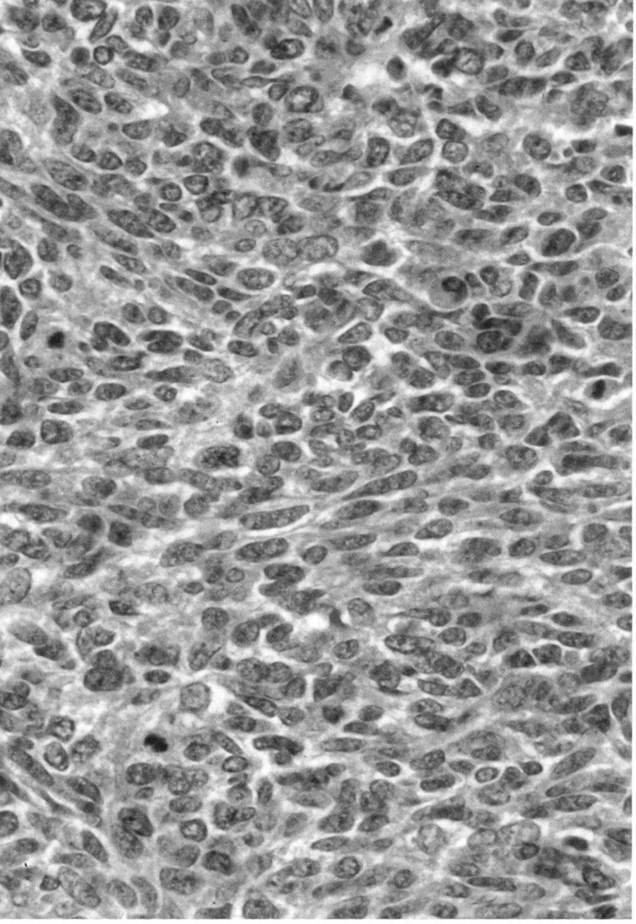

Figure 10.18 **Small cell carcinoma of the lung.** (Reproduced with permission from Cagle PT. *Color Atlas and Text of Pulmonary Pathology*. Philadelphia, PA: Lippincott Williams & Wilkins; 2005.)

Table 10.1 ***Carcinomas of the Lung: Prevalence and Survival***

Type	Small Cell	Nonsmall Cell		
		Adenocarcinoma	Squamous cell carcinoma	Large cell carcinoma
PREVALENCE	~15%	~42%	~28%	~15%
	Stages:*	Stages:†		
SURVIVAL AT FIVE YEARS	Limited ~20 Extensive <1%	Stage I ~62% Stage II ~47% Stage III ~15% Stage IV <1%		

Note: Survival figures for adenocarcinoma are slightly better than the group average figures above.
*Small cell carcinoma staging: Limited = confined to one side of the chest; Extensive = spread beyond one side of the chest
†American Joint Committee on Cancer staging : Stage 0 = carcinoma in situ; Stage I = local invasion only; Stage II = metastasis to nearby bronchial or hilar nodes; Stage III = metastasis to contralateral or extrathoracic lymph nodes; Stage IV = metastasis to any organ other than a lymph node

the epithelium of the epidermis, mouth and esophagus, and vagina. They are more common in men. Invasive cancer is preceded for years by progressive changes—first squamous metaplasia, then dysplasia, then carcinoma in situ, and finally invasive carcinoma (Chapter 5). They tend to arise centrally in the main bronchi near critical mediastinal structures and therefore may not be as easy to remove surgically as other types.

- **Large cell carcinomas** (Fig. 10.19) are composed of large, fleshy, rounded or elongated cells that lack differentiation toward any particular type of tissue and probably represent squamous carcinomas or adenocarcinomas that are too undifferentiated to permit specific classification.

Case Notes

10.14 Myrtle had a bronchogenic carcinoma in situ. Is this a small cell or nonsmall cell carcinoma?

Signs and Symptoms

About 25% of bronchogenic carcinomas are detected incidentally on chest X-ray. Local growth usually causes persistent coughing, but may cause wheezing or dyspnea from local airway obstruction. Vague chest pain is common. Lung cancer is always a suspect in investigation of unexplained weight loss. Extension of the growth may cause pleuritic chest pain or hoarseness from involvement of the recurrent branch of the laryngeal nerve. Broad extension may invade the chest wall, esophagus, or pericardium with predictable symptomatology. Invasion of the great arteries of the chest may produce severe hemorrhage. Compression of the superior vena cava may cause congestion of the head and upper extremities.

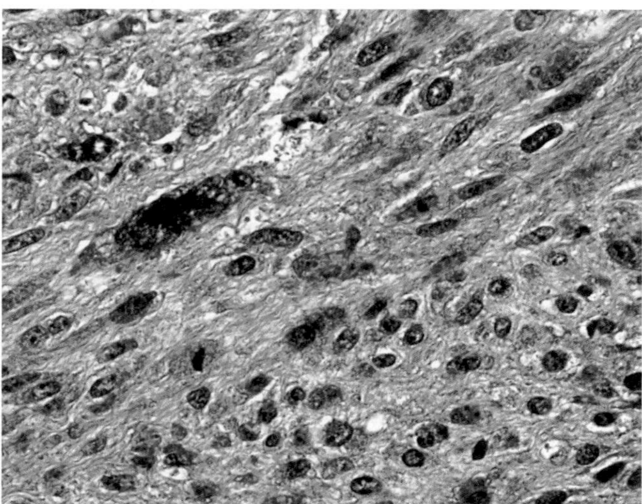

Figure 10.19 **Large cell carcinoma of the lung.** (Reproduced with permission from Cagle PT. *Color Atlas and Text of Pulmonary Pathology*. Philadelphia, PA: Lippincott Williams & Wilkins; 2005.)

Metastases cause symptoms according to the location. Brain metastases cause mental or motor symptoms, nausea and vomiting from increased intracranial pressure, or seizures. Liver metastases cause upper abdominal pain and GI symptoms. Bone metastases usually cause localized pain.

Paraneoplastic syndromes (Chapter 5) are systemic symptoms owing to tumor secretion of hormones or other substances. Small cell carcinoma is particularly likely to produce a paraneoplastic syndrome. Common syndromes include hypercalcemia, migratory thrombophlebitis, hypercortisolism (*Cushing syndrome*, Chapter 14), and neurologic syndromes such as encephalopathy, peripheral neuropathy, and *myasthenia gravis* (Chapter 18).

Diagnosis and Treatment

Diagnosis is by chest X-ray and other imaging, cytologic detection of abnormal cells in sputum, endobronchial biopsy, or fine-needle biopsy. Open biopsy is usually not required.

Screening apparently healthy smokers is usually fruitless and leads to many false positives. Many methods have been tried but all have failed. Nevertheless, the search goes on. Clinical staging (Chapter 5) is essential for prognosis and therapy. Survival closely parallels staging (Tab. 10.1). Clinical stage is determined by tumor size, local invasion, and metastasis. The American Joint Committee on Cancer (AJCC) sponsors the currently accepted system for classifying the stages of lung cancer. The system for nonsmall cell cancers is elaborate, but roughly as follows:

- Stage 0 Carcinoma in situ
- Stage I Local invasion only
- Stage II Metastasis to nearby bronchial or hilar nodes
- Stage III Metastasis to contralateral or extrathoracic lymph nodes
- Stage IV Metastasis to any organ other than a lymph node

Staging for small cell carcinomas is simple:

- Limited Confined to one side of the chest
- Extensive Spread beyond one side of the chest

The median survival for untreated small cell tumors is six months; with treatment, it is nine months.

Case Notes

10.15 In what stage was Myrtle's bronchogenic carcinoma?

Treatment for carcinomas is surgery (depending on cell type and stage), chemotherapy, and radiation. (For recent developments in lung cancer treatment, see *Molecular Medicine*, "Lung Cancer Treatment Goes Molecular: Epidermal Growth Factor.") Surgery rarely plays a role in treatment of small cell carcinoma, most of which respond initially to radiation or chemotherapy but soon relapse. Patients with nonsmall cell carcinoma in Stage I or II are eligible for surgery, which is curative in about two-thirds of those with Stage I tumors and nearly half of those with Stage II. Beyond this group, surgery is usually palliative and the mainstay of treatment is chemotherapy and radiation.

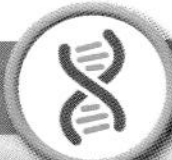

Molecular Medicine

LUNG CANCER TREATMENT GOES MOLECULAR: EPIDERMAL GROWTH FACTOR

Epidermal growth factor (EGF) is a protein that normally binds to epidermal growth factor receptor (EGFR) to promote cell growth and migration. DNA mutations can cause increased activity of EGFR—the mutation turns on the gene and leaves it on, which promotes excessive cell growth. Overactive EGFR has been discovered to be an important feature in many lung cancers. Now it is possible to test lung cancers for EGFR mutation. This is important in lung cancer treatment because specific antibody-based drugs have been developed that target and block EGFR. These drugs can be used to better treat patients whose cancers have EGFR overactivity.

Bronchial Carcinoid Is a Neuroendocrine Tumor

About 1%–5% of lung neoplasms are *carcinoid tumors*, which, like small cell carcinomas, arise from bronchial neuroendocrine cells. About one-third occur in nonsmokers. They are low-grade malignancies and are related to similar carcinoid tumors that occur in other organs. They grow slowly and protrude into the bronchial lumen, which accounts for their clinical behavior. Coughing is common. They tend to bleed and cause hemoptysis, and they tend to obstruct bronchial secretions and cause localized infection, atelectasis, bronchiectasis, and emphysema. Rarely, they secrete vasoactive amines that cause systemic flushing, tachycardia, diarrhea, and cyanosis (**carcinoid syndrome**). They rarely metastasize. Most are candidates for surgery. After surgical resection, 90% of patients survive tumor-free for five years. A carcinoid tumor may be part of the multiple endocrine neoplasia (MEN) syndrome, which features neoplasms of the parathyroid, pancreas, thyroid, and pituitary (Chapter 14).

Pop Quiz

10.28 True or false? Most lung adenocarcinomas arise in the lung periphery.

10.29 What causes carcinoid syndrome?

10.30 What is the single most common risk factor for lung cancer?

Diseases of the Pleura

The pleural space is a potential space between the parietal pleura of the chest wall and the visceral pleura covering the lung. The lungs are held to the chest wall and the diaphragm by the capillary attraction force of a thin film of fluid between the two pleural surfaces. With each breath the lungs are filled by the outward pull of the chest wall and the downward pull of the diaphragm.

If air enters the pleural space (**pneumothorax**), it breaks the capillary fluid bond and causes collapse (atelectasis) of the lung, roughly equal to the volume of air introduced. Pneumothorax may occur spontaneously in young adult smokers, but it more often occurs in patients with emphysema who have unusually large air sacs (blebs) near the pleura—a bleb that ruptures into the pleural space is a common cause of pneumothorax. Traumatic penetration of the pleura, by a foreign object or the edge of a broken rib, is another common cause. A small pneumothorax may be asymptomatic. Dyspnea and chest pain are the cardinal symptoms. Breath sounds are diminished. Pain may be in the chest wall or may mimic angina. Chest X-ray is usually diagnostic. Treatment is needle aspiration or tube thoracotomy suction.

Pneumothorax is potentially fatal. Some cases resolve spontaneously as the air is slowly resorbed by blood. An especially dangerous variant of pneumothorax is *tension pneumothorax*—the opening allows air to come in but not to escape, so that air can enter the pleural space but cannot exit, creating an increasingly high pressure that may fatally smother cardiorespiratory function.

Accumulation of fluid in the pleural space is a **pleural effusion**. There are two varieties: inflammatory and noninflammatory. Inflammatory exudates (Chapter 2) arise from pleural inflammation (**pleuritis**), which causes sharp, localized pain (*pleurisy*) with each breath. Pleuritic inflammatory exudate can accumulate because lung infection spreads to the pleura. Pleuritis may also occur with RA and other connective tissue diseases, pulmonary infarcts, or uremia (Chapter 15), or the pleura may be infected by bacteria or other microbes. Diagnosis is by finding great numbers of neutrophils in fluid from needle aspiration. Treatment depends on the cause.

Alternatively, the fluid may be noninflammatory (**hydrothorax**). Fluid accumulates due to hemodynamic forces (as with the high venous pressure of heart failure) or osmotic forces (low plasma protein in nephrosis, Chapters 6 and 15). The most common cause is a transudate formed in congestive heart failure.

Blood in pleural fluid (bloody effusion) should prompt a search for tumor cells in the fluid and an evaluation of the patient for chest malignancy. The escape of whole blood into the pleural space is a **hemothorax**. It is identifiable by clots in the blood. It is usually the fatal result of a ruptured aortic aneurysm or trauma.

Mesothelioma, as discussed above, is a rare malignancy of the pleura that is a late (20–40 years) complication of chronic inhalation of asbestos fibers (*chronic pulmonary asbestosis*).

Pop Quiz

10.31 True or false? Bloody pleural effusion is usually a sign of a ruptured aneurysm.

Case Study Revisited

"She has cigarette asthma." The case of Myrtle M.

At autopsy, major abnormalities were confined to the lungs and heart. The right ventricle was moderately dilated and hypertrophic. Grossly, in the lungs the lower lobes were heavy, boggy, and showed multiple areas of yellowish firmness from which a cloudy yellow fluid could be expressed. The upper lobes were pale and airy, with moderate emphysematous enlargement of the air spaces. Microscopic examination confirmed moderate emphysema. Marked mucous gland hyperplasia and chronic inflammation were present in the walls of small bronchi, and intense acute inflammatory exudate in the alveoli of both lower lobes. A Gram stain revealed gram-positive cocci in the inflammatory exudate. Multiple samples of bronchial mucosa revealed squamous metaplasia and carcinoma in situ in the left main bronchus.

This case is a classic example of the ill effects of cigarette smoking—Myrtle smoked a lot of cigarettes over a long time and acquired severe COPD and bronchial carcinoma from it. Her initial condition was chronic bronchitis with a severe obstructive component (chronic asthmatic bronchitis), which was confirmed by autopsy findings of marked bronchial chronic inflammation and mucous gland hyperplasia. The chronic bronchitis produced obstructive lung disease, which resulted in poor pulmonary gas exchange, hypoxia, and retained CO_2 with acidosis. The high CO_2 levels caused somnolence to such an extent that it alarmed her son, who brought her to the hospital. Her chronic hypoxia stimulated bone marrow production of RBCs, which raised her hemoglobin and hematocrit levels.

Her bronchogenic carcinoma was in situ and therefore asymptomatic, but had she not died from COPD and pneumonia, it would have invaded and become clinically apparent sooner or later.

Like most smokers with chronic asthmatic bronchitis, she also had emphysema. On admission, she was found to have CAP. The increased WBC count with neutrophilia and band neutrophils (left shift) suggested that the pneumonia was bacterial, although the initial sputum culture was inconclusive. The reappearance of fever and pneumonia on the fifth hospital day, and sputum culture positive for *Staphylococcus aureus*, strongly suggested that she had developed a nosocomial secondary infection after admission. The dense acute inflammatory reaction and gram-positive cocci found in her lungs at autopsy strongly suggested staphylococcal pneumonia, which was confirmed by postmortem culture of the lungs. The clinical diagnosis of emphysema was confirmed by the large air spaces, especially in the apex of each lung. Mild right ventricular hypertrophy and dilation indicated early PH and cor pulmonale secondary to COPD.

There are lessons in every case. In this one they are the following:

- Cigarette smoking can cause severe pulmonary disease and lung cancer.
- Fatal pneumonia is a common final event in patients with severe cardiorespiratory disease.
- Nosocomial infections are a hazard to every hospitalized patient.

Chapter Challenge

CHAPTER RECALL

1. A 25-year-old Caucasian female presents to the clinic for evaluation of a "chest cold." Her symptoms began one week ago and include: moderate fever, muscle aches, headaches, and chest heaviness. Her CBC demonstrates mild lymphocytic leukocytosis. There are minimal findings on chest X-ray consistent with diffuse inflammation of the alveolar septa bilaterally without evidence of consolidation. What disease is responsible for her symptoms?
   A. Lobar pneumonia
   B. Interstitial pneumonia
   C. Pulmonary edema
   D. Pleural effusion

2. A 65-year-old African American male with a shortness of breath and tachypnea presents to your ER. On exam he is febrile (103.5°F) and his mental status is altered. A chest X-ray demonstrates "white out" lung. Which of the following statements is true regarding his disease etiology?
   A. Chronic course leading to pulmonary failure in nearly 100% of cases
   B. Characterized by injury to bronchi and bronchioles
   C. Can be caused by many different underlying conditions
   D. Caused by *Mycoplasma pneumonia*

3. Which of the following diseases is characterized by hyperplastic mucus glands, mucus plugs, hypertrophied bronchial smooth muscles, edema, and marked eosinophilic inflammation secondary to long-term exposure to severe air pollution?
   A. Hypersensitivity pneumonitis
   B. Occupational asthma
   C. Atopic asthma
   D. Nonatopic asthma

4. A 50-year-old African American female presents to your clinic for shortness of breath, chest pain, chills, cough, and fever. She recently moved to the area after being diagnosed with AIDs, and is presenting to your clinic to establish care. On further questioning, she confirms exposure to bird droppings. As suspected, her Mantoux skin test is negative. An elevated antibody titer in the blood confirms your suspicion. What organism is responsible for her symptoms?
   A. Histoplasmosis
   B. Coccidiomycosis
   C. Candida
   D. Cryptococcus

5. A five-year-old Hispanic male is brought to the children's ER for evaluation following smoke exposure. On exam, crackling rales are heard at the lung bases. Which of the following etiologies are you concerned about?
   A. Hemodynamic edema
   B. Microvascular injury edema
   C. Pneumothorax
   D. Pleural effusion

6. Which of the following statements is true regarding the respiratory tract?
   A. Lacking both glands and cartilage, the smallest airway division is the bronchiole.
   B. Due to lung anatomy, aspirated items are more likely to end in the right lung than the left lung.
   C. The lung is served by the pulmonary vasculature system alone.
   D. The first line of defense in the lung is mucosal associated lymphoid tissue (i.e., MALT), which is responsible for secreting IgA.

7. A 24-year-old Caucasian male presents to the clinic complaining of hoarseness and pain when he speaks or sings. He is concerned about the upcoming opening night of his troupe's newest production, which has been practicing for "night and day." An upper endoscopy confirms your suspicions and you prescribe vocal rest. What is his diagnosis?
   A. Vocal cord nodules
   B. Laryngeal papillomas
   C. Laryngitis
   D. Carcinoma of the larynx

8. A 54-year-old man with a pack-a-day history of smoking complains to you of a chronic cough. The cough has lingered for greater than four months this year, and he reports a similar episode last year. On exam, he appears cyanotic, in particular at the tips of his fingers, which are also club shaped, indicating chronic hypoxia. His FEV1 is markedly decreased, while his FVC remains near normal. What is your diagnosis?
   A. Asthma
   B. Chronic bronchitis
   C. Bronchogenic carcinoma
   D. Emphysema

9. A 55-year-old Caucasian female with a history significant for RA presents to your office complaining of sharp localized pain under her right breast with each breath. On exam, her breath sounds are muffled at the right base and percussion is dull at the right base as well. The presence of neutrophils

on fine needle aspiration confirms your diagnosis of which of the following?
A. Lobar pneumonia
B. Interstitial pneumonia
C. Pneumothorax
D. Pleural effusion

10. A child who has inhaled a foreign object is at risk for what type of atelectasis?
A. Contraction atelectasis
B. Compression atelectasis
C. Resorption atelectasis
D. Obstructive atelectasis

11. A 45-year-old African American female complains of shortness of breath and hemoptysis. Her exam is positive for tachypnea and end-inspiratory crackles without wheezing or other evidence of obstruction, and her chest X-ray shows small nodules, streaks and ground-glass haziness, and bilateral hilar lymph node enlargement. You explain to her that her symptoms may resolve spontaneously, but she may require treatment with steroids for what disease?
A. Hypersensitivity pneumonitis
B. Pneumoconiosis
C. Idiopathic pulmonary fibrosis
D. Sarcoidosis

12. A 60-year-old Indian female presents to the clinic for a checkup. She complains of dyspnea and a chronic nonproductive cough. Her history is positive for smoking. On exam, she is thin, with a barrel-shaped chest, and you note that she breathes through pursed lips. On spirometry, her FEV1/FVC ratio is markedly decreased. Which of the following is true regarding her disease?
A. The surface area of the pulmonary membrane (gas exchange surface) is decreased.
B. Expiratory airflow is normal or near normal.
C. Sputum production is a key diagnostic point.
D. CO_2 retention is prominent.

13. Small cell carcinomas are ________.
A. composed of distinctive large cells formed into glandular acini.
B. aggressively malignant, but fortunately do not often present with metastasis.
C. particularly likely to produce a paraneoplastic syndrome such as hypercalcemia and Cushing syndrome.
D. the most common lung carcinoma.

14. True or false? Type II pneumocytes secrete pulmonary surfactant.

15. True or false? Anthracosis and silicosis are classified as pneumoconiosis, a restrictive lung disease with a normal/near normal FEV1/FVC ratio.

16. True or false? Obstruction of incoming air is the main problem in obstructive lung disease.

17. True or false? Approximately half of bronchogenic carcinomas are caused by cigarette smoking.

18. True or false? Repeated small pulmonary thromboemboli may result in chronic PH.

CONCEPTUAL UNDERSTANDING

19. What preventative measures can be taken for patients at risk of thromboembolism?

20. Briefly discuss spirometry and why FEV1/FVC is the best indicator of restrictive versus obstructive disease.

21. What etiologies should be included in the differential diagnosis of idiopathic pulmonary fibrosis?

APPLICATION

22. A mother brings her daughter to the clinic for a runny nose and fever of less than one week's duration. You diagnose an uncomplicated upper respiratory infection (URI) and explain that antibiotics are unnecessary. Why is this the case? If the mother calls back after another week and reports that symptoms have gotten worse, would this change your mind?

23. Explain why small cell carcinoma is placed in a separate category from other lung malignancies.

24. While renovating an old house, you determine that the attic insulation contains asbestos. What diseases does asbestos place you at risk for? What precautions should be taken?

CHAPTER

11

Disorders of the Gastrointestinal Tract

Contents

Chapter Objectives

After studying this chapter, you should be able to complete the following tasks:

NORMAL ANATOMY AND PHYSIOLOGY

1. Explain how the organs of the gastrointestinal (GI) system perform their six functions.

SIGNS AND SYMPTOMS OF GI DISORDER

2. Describe the various signs and symptoms of GI disorder including: anorexia, nausea, emesis, diarrhea, dysentery, steatorrhea, belching, flatulence, constipation, bleeding, and obstruction.

DISEASES OF THE ORAL CAVITY

3. Name and describe the lesions that can affect the oral cavity including: malformations, tooth loss, ulcers, autoimmune disease, and cancer.

DISEASES OF THE ESOPHAGUS

4. Compare and contrast esophageal adenocarcinoma with squamous cell carcinoma.

DISEASES OF THE STOMACH

5. Discuss the manifestations and treatment options for the following diseases: pyloric stenosis, bleeding gastric erosions, autoimmune gastritis, chronic peptic ulceration, Helicobacter pylori infection, and stomach cancer including lymphoma.

CONGENITAL ANOMALIES OF THE SMALL AND LARGE BOWEL

6. Define the following congenital anomalies of the small and large intestines: Meckel diverticulum, omphalocele, gastroschisis, Hirschsprung megacolon.

VASCULAR DISEASES OF THE SMALL AND LARGE BOWEL

7. Define ischemic vascular disease and hemorrhoids.

INFECTIOUS DISEASES AFFECTING THE SMALL AND LARGE BOWEL

8. Discuss the pathogenesis and manifestations of the viruses, bacteria, and protozoa responsible for causing infections of the bowel.

MALABSORPTION SYNDROMES

9. Among patients with malabsorption syndrome, distinguish between luminal and intestinal malabsorption.

INFLAMMATORY BOWEL DISEASE

10. Compare and contrast ulcerative colitis and Crohn disease, including the extraintestinal manifestations.

DISEASES OF THE APPENDIX AND PERITONEUM

11. Discuss the pathogenesis and manifestations of appendicitis.

NEOPLASMS OF THE LARGE AND SMALL BOWEL/ CARCINOMA OF THE COLON

12. Explain the importance of non-neoplastic polyps of the colon, and their relationship to colonic carcinoma.

COLONIC DIVERTICULOSIS AND ANORECTAL CONDITIONS

13. Define diverticulosis, anal fissure, anorectal abscess, and anal fistula.

Case Study

"Her intestines are acting much worse this time." The case of Melanie K.

Chief Complaint: Abdominal cramps; vomiting

Clinical History: Melanie K. was a 26-year-old woman brought to the hospital by her mother, who told the triage nurse: "Her intestines are acting much worse this time." The nurse called her doctor's office and obtained the following history.

Melanie first went to the doctor five years earlier complaining of intermittent episodes of fever, diarrhea, weight loss, crampy abdominal pain and tenderness, and bloody stools. Some flare-ups were associated with joint pain. An aunt was known to have long-standing "colon trouble" that required surgery. Melanie had not traveled internationally, and no pathogens had been found in stool culture. X-rays had revealed abnormalities of several segments of the ileum and the proximal colon. The physician had diagnosed Crohn inflammatory bowel disease (IBD). Melanie was initially treated with antibiotics and a variety of other oral medicines with good results, but recurrent and more severe episodes of similar symptoms eventually required intermittent use of oral steroids to control symptoms.

"Her intestines are acting much worse this time." The case of Melanie K. (continued)

Her mother explained that in the last year Melanie had experienced a few flare-ups requiring steroids, but in the last few months she had been relatively well. In the last few weeks, however, symptoms recurred and she had higher fevers and more than the usual amount of bright red blood mixed into her stools. A day earlier, she developed severe abdominal cramps, but, unlike previous episodes that usually abated, this time the pain grew steadily worse and she began to vomit. "She can't even keep down clear liquids, and she's very thirsty," her mother added.

Physical Examination and Other Data: Her mother said Melanie was 5′ 6″ and weighed about 100 lb, indicating her body mass index was 16 (normal: 18–25). Heart rate was 88 (normal 72), blood pressure was 96/68 (normal 120/80), and oral temperature was 99.8°F (normal 98.7). Pertinent blood values included hemoglobin 10.4 gm/dL (normal female 12–15.5), hematocrit 34% (normal female 35–44), red cell count 4.72×10^6 (normal 4.2–5.4), white blood cell count 14,600 cells/mm^3 (normal 3,500–10,500), and total blood protein 5.5 gm/dL (normal 6–8.3). Red cell indices were: MCV 72 (normal 80–100) and MCHC 30.5 (normal 32–36). Serum iron was 44 ncg/ml (normal 60–170).

Melanie was a pale, anxious young woman complaining of severe abdominal pain. Her abdomen was rigid and during the exam she vomited a small amount of thin, yellow fluid. Imaging studies revealed a mass in the right lower abdominal quadrant.

Clinical Course: Melanie was taken to surgery for abdominal exploration. Multiple segments of small bowel showed gross evidence of Crohn disease: firm, thickened walls with inflammatory exudate and peritoneal adhesions. The cecum, appendix, and right fallopian tube and ovary were involved by an inflammatory mass. Biopsy and quick microscopic examination of a cecal mass and nearby lymph node revealed metastatic adenocarcinoma of the cecum. Surgeons removed the mass intact with 60 cm of distal ileum and the entire ascending colon. During surgery, Melanie was given two 500 ml units of whole blood. During recovery, she began taking an oral iron supplement.

Pathological study of the specimen revealed Crohn disease of the ileum and colon with a fistulous tract into the right ovary and fallopian tube; a 6 cm adenocarcinoma of the cecum that extended through the muscular wall of the bowel and into the right fallopian tube; and metastatic adenocarcinoma in 3 of 13 lymph nodes. The cecum, appendix, ovary and fallopian tube were bound together into an inflammatory mass around the fistula.

Her discharge diagnoses were: adenocarcinoma of the cecum, Crohn disease, malnutrition, and iron deficiency anemia.

I would like to be a figment of my own imagination, but belly and bowels will not permit.

MASON COOLEY (1927–2002), AMERICAN WRITER

The *digestive system* includes the GI system plus the liver and pancreas, which will be discussed in the following chapter. The **gastrointestinal (GI) tract** digests and absorbs food. It consists of the mouth, teeth, and tongue; the pharynx; the esophagus; the stomach; and the small and large bowel (Fig. 11.1). Accessory organs in the digestive process are the salivary glands, liver, gallbladder, and pancreas.

Important in understanding GI pathology and pathophysiology is the fact that the GI tract is open to the environment at both ends and is occupied at every point by material from the environment. In an important sense, the lining of the GI tract is exposed to the environment every much as the skin or the lining of the bronchial tree.

The Normal Gastrointestinal Tract

The functions of the GI tract are the following:

1. **Ingestion** (eating) brings food into the oral cavity.
2. **Secretion** is the release of fluids—mainly water with acids, buffers, and enzymes—into the lumen by epithelial cells and accessory digestive organs. These secretions provide the chemical tools for digestion and help protect the digestive tract wall.
3. **Digestion.** *Mechanical digestion* is the tearing and cutting of food into small pieces by the teeth, and the churning action of the stomach. *Chemical digestion* is the cleaving of large food molecules into smaller ones by the secretions mentioned above.

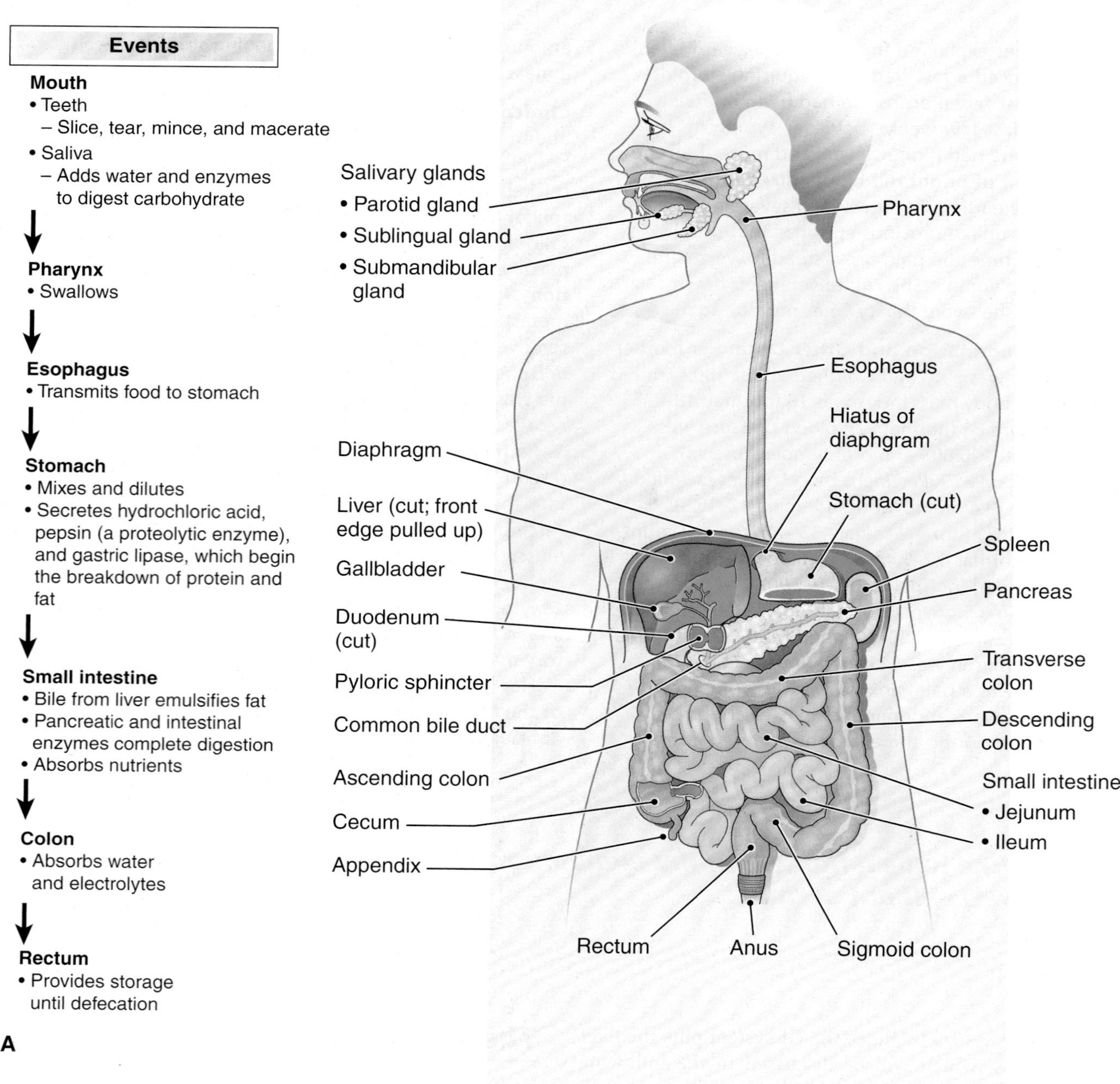

Figure 11.1 **gastrointestinal tract and accessory organs. A.** Overview. Accessory organs and structures include the salivary glands, liver, and pancreas. **B.** Close anatomy of the small intestine. **C.** Microanatomy of an intestinal villus. **D.** Microanatomy of intestinal epithelium.

4. **Motility.** Muscular contractions of the GI tract propel foodstuffs forward and mix them with digestive secretions.
5. **Absorption** is the uptake of small nutrient molecules from the GI tract into the blood or lymph.
6. **Defecation** is the passage of feces—compacted indigestible food material, bacteria, and shed epithelial cells—through the anus.

The salivary glands, liver, gallbladder, and pancreas are important in the digestive process. Saliva contains enzymes, which begin the digestive process, and mucus, which lubricates food for its slide down the esophagus. The liver secretes bile, which is stored in the gallbladder and released into the intestine through bile ducts, where it disperses fat into tiny globules so that it can be acted upon by lipase secreted by the pancreas. The *pancreas* secretes digestive enzymes into the small bowel through the pancreatic duct. These enzymes (amylase, lipase, and protease) break large molecules of carbohydrate, fat, and protein, respectively, into their constituent molecules, which are much smaller and therefore absorbable.

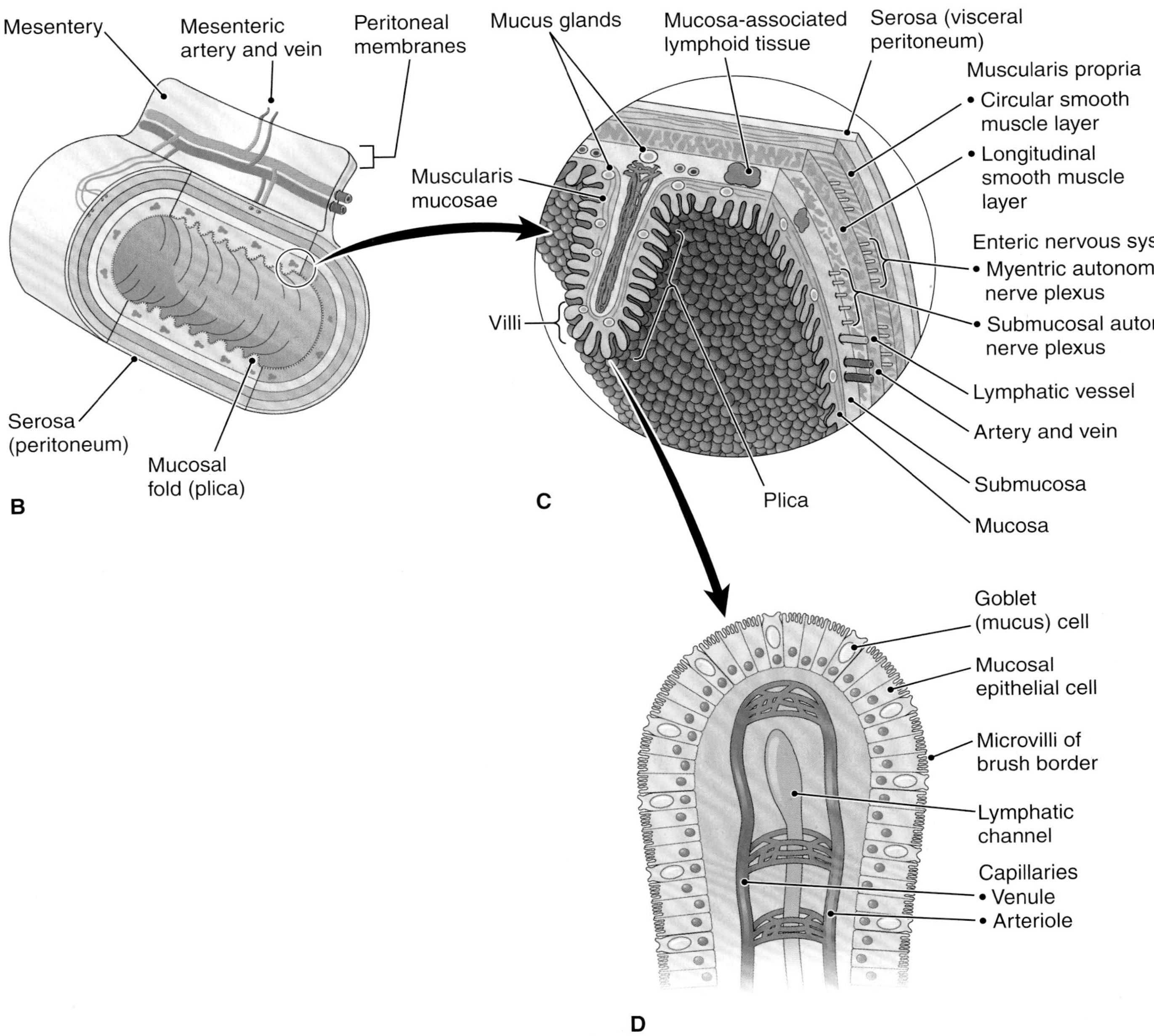

Figure 11.1 (continued)

The Gastrointestinal Tract Is a Multilayered Tube

The GI tract is a long, convoluted tube that starts at the mouth and ends at the anus. It is composed of concentric layers (Fig. 11.1, B, C, and D), which from inside to out are the following:

- *Mucosa*: the innermost layer of the mucosa is epithelium, which rests upon a basement membrane. In the mouth, the esophagus, and the last centimeter of the anus, the epithelium is composed of layers of flat (squamous) cells. Their smooth surface and many layers of cells ease the slide and resist the harsh effect of rough food and feces. In the stomach, small bowel, and colon, the epithelium is composed of tall, columnar cells conducive to digestion and absorption. Beneath the basement membrane are blood vessels, lymphatics, and interstitial tissue (called the "lamina propria"), and a thin layer of smooth muscle, the muscularis mucosa.
- *Submucosa*: In the submucosa are accessory glands, specialized lymphoid tissue known as MALT (mucosa-associated lymphoid tissue, Chapter 3), lymphatics, blood vessels, loose fibrous tissue, and the submucosal nerve plexus.
- *Muscularis propria*: The main muscular layer of the bowel is called *propria* (or sometimes *externa*) to distinguish it from the innermost muscular layer, the thin

layer of muscle in the mucosa (the *muscularis mucosae*). The muscularis propria is formed of two layers of smooth muscle: an outer longitudinal layer and inner circular layer. Between the layers of the muscularis propria is the *myenteric nerve plexus*, which along with the *submucosal nerve plexus*, makes up the **enteric nervous system**. The plexus consists of a network of autonomic ganglia that innervates the muscularis and propagates peristaltic waves of contraction and relaxation of the gut wall. The enteric nervous system also regulates the secretions of various digestive glands.

- *Serosa*: The outermost layer is composed of flat peritoneal cells. The relationship of the peritoneum to the intestines is discussed later in this chapter.

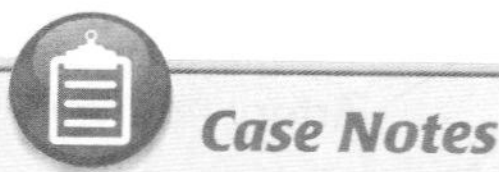

Case Notes

11.1 Which of these bowel wall layers were penetrated by Melanie's cancer?

The Gastrointestinal Tract Is Regulated by Chemical and Neural Signals

Endocrine and neural signals regulate these functions (Tab. 11.1). Endocrine control is mediated by hormones secreted by gastric and intestinal epithelial cells. Nervous control is mediated by the autonomic nervous system, which relays signals to the myenteric plexus (Fig. 11.1B). Parasympathetic signals, the "rest and digest" half of the autonomic nervous system, stimulate gland secretions and intestinal motility. Sympathetic signals, the "fight or flight" half, suppress secretions and motility.

Even before we take a first bite of food, parasympathetic signals aroused by the thought, sight, and/or smell of food stimulate salivary gland secretion of saliva to begin the digestive process. Neural signals also prepare the stomach to receive food, in part by triggering the release of digestive hormones and fluids. In the stomach, food and secretions mix to form **chyme**, a term applied to the digestive "soup" until it enters the colon, where water is absorbed from it, and it becomes **feces**. The presence of chyme itself stimulates neural and hormonal activity (Tab. 11.1), which in turn stimulates peristalsis, the release of additional hormones, secretion of bile by the liver, and secretion of intestinal and pancreatic enzymes.

The Gastrointestinal Tract Bears an Important Relationship to the Peritoneum

The **peritoneum** is a translucent membrane composed of flat (squamous) epithelial cells. The portion of the peritoneum that lines the interior abdominal wall is the **parietal**

Table 11.1 Hormonal and Neural Signals Involved in Digestion

Hormone Signal	Origin	Stimulus	Action
GASTRIN	Gastric enteroendocrine cells (G cells)	Proteins/peptides in stomach	Stimulates secretion of *hydrochloric acid*
GASTRIC INHIBITORY PEPTIDE	Small intestine enteroendocrine cells (K cells)	Glucose in small intestine	Stimulates release of *insulin* by pancreatic islands of Langerhans, inhibits secretion of *hydrochloric acid*
PEPSINOGEN	Gastric epithelial cells (chief cells)	Hydrochloric acid	Becomes *pepsin*, which digests protein
CHOLECYSTOKININ	Small intestine enteroendocrine cells (I cells)	Fat and protein in duodenum	Slows gastric motility; stimulates release of *bile* from gallbladder; stimulates secretion of *pancreatic enzymes*
SECRETIN	Small intestine enteroendocrine cells (S cells)	Acidic chyme in duodenum	Stimulates release of *bicarbonate* from pancreas to neutralize acidic chyme
Neural Signal	Route	Stimulus	Action
PARASYMPATHETIC	Vagus nerve	Sight, smell, taste or thought of food	Stimulates secretions and peristalsis
SYMPATHETIC	Multiple routes	Stress	Inhibits secretions and peristalsis
ENTERIC NERVOUS SYSTEM	Local, within bowel wall	Multiple	Modulates secretions and peristalsis

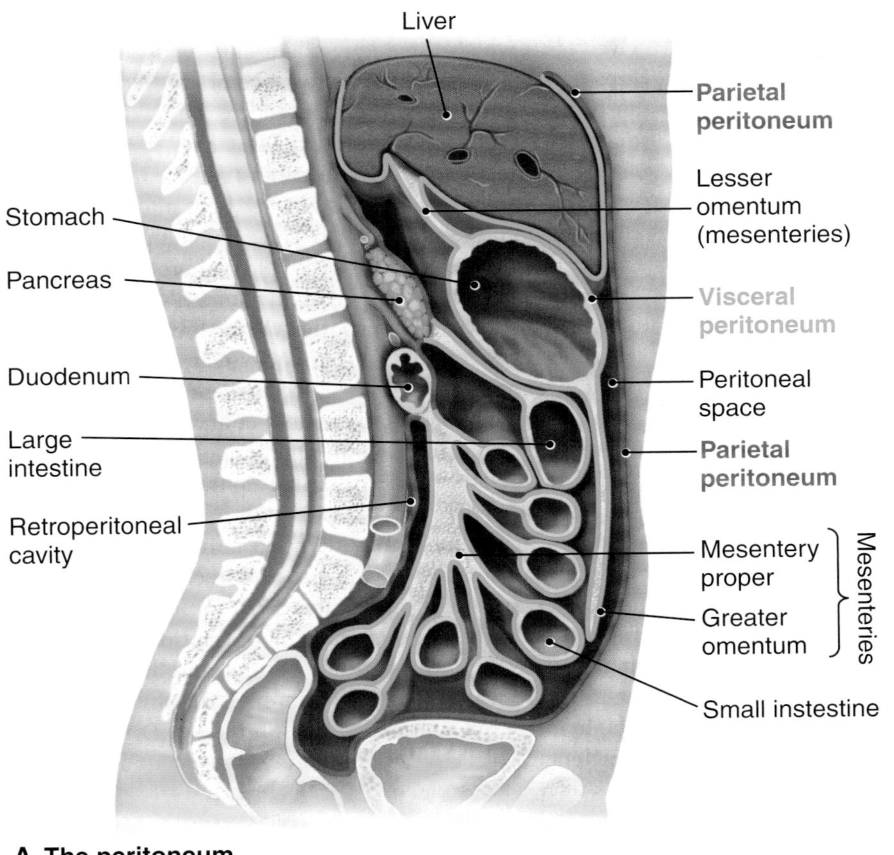

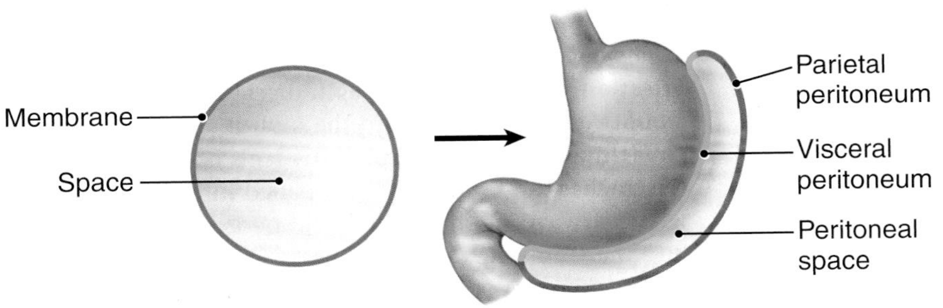

Figure 11.2 **The peritoneum and mesenteries. A.** The visceral peritoneum (green) covers organs and forms mesenteries. The parietal peritoneum (orange) lines the walls of the abdominal cavity. **B.** Peritoneal membranes form around a cavity in the embryonic abdomen. The stomach and other intestinal structures, the liver, spleen, and other organs push in the sides of the cavity as they grow and the peritoneal membrane covers them as they advance. The peritoneal space is the thin space between the peritoneal membranes. A distinction is to be made between the peritoneal space and the abdominal cavity. The abdominal cavity is bounded by the parietal peritoneum and contains the organs and the peritoneal space. (Reproduced with permission from McConnell TH, Hull KL. *Human Form Human Function: Essentials of Anatomy & Physiology*. Baltimore (MD): Wolters Kluwer Health; 2011.)

peritoneum. The rest of the membrane, described as the **visceral peritoneum**, folds over all or part of the abdominal organs (Fig. 11.2). Between the parietal and visceral peritoneum is the **peritoneal space**, a thin space between loops of bowel and other viscera. The peritoneal space is filled with a small amount of slippery **peritoneal fluid**. This fluid enables bowel loops to slide over each other, and enables the liver and other abdominal organs to move smoothly relative to movements of the chest wall and trunk. A distinction is to be made between the peritoneal space and the abdominal cavity. The **abdominal cavity** is bounded by the parietal peritoneum and contains the organs and the peritoneal space.

During fetal development, the stomach, intestines, and liver advance from the posterior part of the abdomen near the vertebral column and push their way into the peritoneal space (Fig. 11.2B) like a fist pushing into the side of a balloon. As they advance, they carry with them their blood vessels, lymphatic vessels, and nerves, which lengthen and trail behind and remain attached to the aorta, vena cava, and lymph ducts. Peritoneal membrane covers the advancing organs as the visceral peritoneum and envelops the bundles of vessels and nerves to form a **mesentery**, a broad, thick membrane formed of two layers of peritoneum that envelop vessels, nerves, and adipose tissue and forms the stabilizing *pedicle* that anchors them. The pancreas, the proximal part of the small intestine (called the *duodenum*), and parts of the large intestine do not advance, but remain near the spine in the **retroperitoneal space** (*retro* = behind).

The major mesenteries are the following:

- The *greater omentum* is a double fold of peritoneum that hangs from the large intestine and stomach like an apron. The amount of fat stored between the layers of the greater omentum is related to nutritional status. An overweight (and overnourished) person will have a larger omentum than a malnourished one.
- The *mesentery proper* arises in a thick vertical strip anterior to the lumbar vertebrae and attaches to the small intestine. This mesentery provides a stable base (pedicle) for the intestines, acting somewhat like a tree trunk that stabilizes the motion of its limbs.
- The *lesser omentum* suspends the stomach from the undersurface of the liver. Just as the mesentery proper stabilizes the bowel, the lesser omentum stabilizes the stomach.

Case Notes

11.2 Which mesentery attaches to Melanie's ileum?

Digestion Breaks Food into Its Building Blocks

Unlike plants, humans cannot make most of the nutrients they need and must obtain them from food. The organic molecules in food serve two purposes: they are burned for energy, and they provide the basic building blocks to synthesize physiologic compounds and grow new tissues.

Digestion begins in the mouth and is completed as residue enters the colon. **Mechanical digestion** begins as teeth slice, tear, and crush food into small pieces. It continues in the stomach and intestines as food particles are tossed, turned, and mixed with intestinal juices.

The three basic foodstuffs are carbohydrate, protein, and fat. Chemical digestion breaks these molecules—which are too big to be absorbed directly—into their building blocks. With the aid of enzymes from the salivary glands, pancreas, and the stomach and intestinal mucosa, these large molecules interact with water and by the process of **hydrolysis** are broken down into smaller molecules, which are absorbed by the mucosal epithelial cells lining the small intestine.

Carbohydrates (sugars and starches) are composed of one or more *monosaccharide* molecules (glucose, fructose, and galactose). A variety of enzymes (amylases, saccharidases, and others) break carbohydrates into monosaccharides for absorption.

Proteins are composed of *peptides*, which in turn are composed of *amino acids*. Protein-digesting enzymes (proteases) break proteins and peptides into amino acids for absorption.

Most dietary *fat* (lipid) is **triglyceride**, a molecule of glycerol to which three long-chain fatty acids are attached. Lipases break triglycerides into glycerol and fatty acids for absorption. But unlike the monosaccharides from carbohydrate and amino acids from protein, digested fats are not absorbed directly into blood because they are not soluble in water. Instead, epithelial cells cluster them into lipoproteins called **chylomicrons**, which are spherical compounds with a triglyceride center and a phospholipid and protein coat. Chylomicrons are picked up by lymph channels (lacteals) in the intestinal mucosa and transported via the thoracic duct to the left subclavian vein. From the bloodstream, they can travel to the liver, muscle, or fatty tissues, where they are metabolized for energy, used to make lipid-containing compounds, or stored. **Cholesterol** is another important lipid that is absorbed directly by the intestinal epithelium. Cholesterol is chemically different from triglyceride: a sterol, it is closely related to steroid molecules like testosterone and estrogen.

Some substances are absorbed directly. Like cholesterol, they are small molecules. They include water, vitamins, trace minerals such as iron and iodine, electrolytes such as sodium and potassium, drugs, and alcohol. Some vitamins are water-soluble (vitamin C, the B vitamins and folic acid), while others are fat-soluble (A, D, E, and K). Deficiencies of fat-soluble vitamins can occur in diseases that affect fat absorption.

The Role of the Mouth and Esophagus

Chewing macerates food into manageable, small pieces. Salivary glands—*parotid*, *sublingual*, *submaxillary* and *submandibular*—add saliva, which contains mucus for lubrication and enzymes to begin digestion. In swallowing, a bolus of food moves from the mouth and into the *pharynx* (throat). There, the epiglottis seals off the entrance to the trachea, and the food is propelled into the esophagus, where a wave of smooth muscle peristalsis transports it into the stomach.

Near the stomach, the distal esophagus passes through an opening in the diaphragm, the *esophageal hiatus*. The esophagus terminates at the *lower esophageal sphincter (LES)*, through which food passes into the stomach. These anatomical features of the terminal esophagus are important in gastroesophageal reflux disease (GERD), discussed later in this chapter.

The Role of the Stomach

The upper (proximal) part of the stomach is the *cardia*, the mid-part is the *body* (or *fundus*), and the distal part is the *pylorus*. The stomach produces lubricating mucus and holds food temporarily, mixing it with fluids to form chyme. It also begins the digestion of protein and fats. The presence of protein in the stomach stimulates gastric epithelium to secrete **gastrin**, a hormone that stimulates gastric peristalsis and the release of hydrochloric acid. Glucose in the small intestine stimulates enteroendocrine cells to release **gastric inhibitory peptide**, which in turn stimulates the pancreas to secrete insulin. In response to the presence of hydrochloric acid, the chief cells of the gastric epithelium secrete **pepsinogen**, which gastric acid converts into **pepsin**, a protein-digesting enzyme. Chief cells also secrete gastric lipase, which initiates lipid digestion.

Chyme is released gradually into the duodenum by relaxation of the *pyloric sphincter*, which encircles the distal pylorus. The opening and closing of the sphincter is regulated by the **enterogastric reflex**, a parasympathetic reflex activated by the arrival of chyme in the duodenum. This reflex stimulates intestinal peristalsis but inhibits release of chyme through the pyloric sphincter, ensuring a gradual release of chyme that doesn't overwhelm the small intestine.

The Role of the Small Intestine

The small intestine extends from the stomach to the colon. The first 10–12 inches is the *duodenum*, into which the pancreatic and bile ducts empty through an opening in a small mound of tissue, the *ampulla of Vater*. Most digestion occurs in the duodenum, with assistance from intestinal and pancreatic enzymes and bile.

The remaining small bowel is divided into two roughly equal parts: the proximal *jejunum* and the distal *ileum*. The transition from one to another is gradual. The jejunum absorbs most nutrients, including most vitamins, and iron, calcium, and some other minerals. The ileum absorbs water, bile salts, and electrolytes, as well as vitamin B_{12}.

Case Notes

11.3 Presume that the yellow in Melanie's vomitus was duodenal bile. Starting in the first centimeter of the duodenum and proceeding superiorly, name several important anatomic structures the vomitus passed on its way to the mouth.

As depicted in Figure 11.1 B, C, and D, the absorptive surface of the small intestine is multiplied by its anatomy. First, the mucosa is pleated into large inward folds (plica) of mucosa that provide about two feet of mucosa for every foot of bowel. Second, the mucosa is composed of millions of tiny *villi*, which multiply the absorptive surface many more times. Third, the surface of each villus is covered by intestinal epithelial cells, each of which has dozens of *microvilli*, referred to collectively as the *brush border*. In addition to increasing absorption of nutrients, the brush border contains digestive enzymes that act on nutrients as they are absorbed.

Spread among the absorptive epithelial cells are *goblet* cells that produce mucus that lubricates the intestinal contents. Waves of peristaltic contraction—much weaker than those of the esophagus and stomach—move intestinal contents forward. Also present throughout the small (and large) bowel are patches of lymphoid tissue (*Peyer patches, mucosal associated lymphoid tissue [MALT]*) that are immunologically active—that is, they secrete high concentrations of immunoglobulin A, the "immune paint" of the GI tract, which protects against invasion of the intestinal wall by bacteria in the GI lumen.

Like the stomach, the small intestine is subject to neural and hormonal control (Tab. 11.1). Secretions and peristalsis are stimulated by neural signals, one of which is the enterogastric reflex mentioned earlier. The presence of fat and protein in the duodenum stimulates intestinal epithelial cells to secrete **cholecystokinin**, a hormone that stimulates the gallbladder to release bile and the pancreas to secrete digestive enzymes. What's more, when a bolus of acidic chyme is released into the duodenum from the stomach, the acid causes duodenal epithelial cells to release **secretin**, a hormone that stimulates the pancreas to secrete bicarbonate-rich juice to neutralize the acid.

The Role of the Large Intestine

The large intestine (Fig. 11.1A) extends from the ileocecal valve of the small intestine to the anus. In descending order, it consists of the cecum, the colon, the rectum, and the anus. The appendix is a long, thin, blind pouch extending from the cecum. The function of the appendix is unclear. Some speculate that it serves to hold a specimen of normal intestinal flora with which to repopulate the bowel with normal flora after disease-related disruption of the usual mix of intestinal flora.

The colonic mucosa contains no villi and has no digestive function. Its function is to absorb water and a few vitamins, to compact feces, and to hold them for elimination.

Case Notes

11.4 Did Melanie's tumor originate in the large or small intestine?

Intestinal Bacteria Are Beneficial

Shortly after birth, an individual's intestinal tract becomes populated by billions of bacteria from the environment. Most of them inhabit the colon and live there in a natural and mutually beneficial, symbiotic relationship with the body. They are a mixture of bacteria that require oxygen (*aerobic*) and others for which oxygen is toxic (*anaerobic*). Intestinal bacteria produce significant amounts of vitamin K and folic acid. They are an important guard against bacterial infection—they are so numerous and have such a large claim on nutrients, that a large dose (inoculum) of infective bacteria is required to establish a foothold; ingestion of a few pathogenic bacteria is not likely to establish infection. Indeed, bacterial cells in the colon outnumber the entire body's own cells 10–1.

Altering the balance or concentration of normal flora can produce ill effects, usually due to overgrowth of a certain strain of bacteria. The most common cause is antibiotic therapy for a nonintestinal infection, which kills some populations of the flora and allows others to proliferate.

Pop Quiz

11.1 What is the outermost layer of the small intestine?

11.2 Which intestinal cells secrete hormones?

11.3 Name the three mesenteries.

11.4 Dietary carbohydrates are broken into what compounds for absorption?

11.5 How does fat absorption differ from protein and carbohydrate absorption?

11.6 Where in the intestinal epithelium are digestive enzymes located?

11.7 How are intestinal bacteria useful?

Signs and Symptoms of Gastrointestinal Disorder

Abdominal discomfort and pain are among the most common reasons people seek medical care. Mild, transient abdominal complaints are common and often of no consequence. Acute, severe abdominal pain, however, is usually a symptom of intra-abdominal disease. It may be the sole signal of a need for surgery and quick decisions are required.

Gastrointestinal Disorder Can Produce a Variety of Classic Symptoms

Anorexia is lack of appetite and is frequently a sign of intestinal disease. Nevertheless, it may be due to mental illness, stress, or other psychologic condition, or it may be a side effect of medication or a symptom of a nonintestinal condition—patients with widespread cancer, kidney failure, or other severe disease are often anorexic.

Nausea is an unpleasant sensation with an urge to vomit. It can be triggered by any of the physical or mental stimuli of vomiting (below).

Vomiting (emesis) is the forceful ejection of contents from the stomach or upper intestine. It is usually preceded by nausea and is a complex, coordinated protective reflex regulated by a vomiting center in the brainstem. It can be stimulated by unpleasant sights, smells, or tastes, gastric or intestinal irritation or obstruction, the effect of certain motions on the inner ear, some drugs and toxins, hormonal changes such as occur in pregnancy, and increased intracranial pressure. The reflex begins with a deep breath. The glottis (vocal chords) closes to protect the lower airways and the palate rises to seal the nasopharynx. The lower esophageal sphincter relaxes, the abdominal muscles and diaphragm contract, and the stomach and upper intestine begin reverse peristalsis.

The character of vomitus is important. Vomiting undigested food may indicate an obstruction near the pyloric sphincter. Yellow or green vomitus indicates the presence of duodenal bile. Dark brown vomitus suggests an origin point below the duodenum and may indicate intestinal obstruction. Bloody vomitus (*hematemesis*) will be addressed in further detail later.

Dysphagia is difficulty swallowing and is the most common sign of esophageal disease. It can also be caused by head injury, dementia, or another neurological disorder.

Belching is the passing of gas from the mouth. When gas is passed from the anus, it is termed **flatulence**. Most intestinal gas is swallowed air. The remainder is due to bacterial alteration of food. Excess intestinal gas also may be a sign of *lactose intolerance*, discussed later in this chapter.

Diarrhea is famously difficult to define with precision because bowel habits vary greatly. A convenient clinical definition is thinner and more frequent bowel movements than normal. **Dysentery** is low-volume, bloody, painful diarrhea. Diarrhea may be accompanied by **steatorrhea,** fatty stools. They are typically abundant, loose, and malodorous, and associated with *malabsorption syndromes*. Diarrheal diseases and malabsorption syndromes are discussed later in this chapter.

Constipation is difficulty passing stool. It is usually caused by compacted, dry, hard fecal matter. The causes are many: weak peristalsis in the elderly; inadequate fluid intake; lack of dietary fiber; neurologic disorders (e.g., paraplegia or multiple sclerosis may interfere with peristalsis); and purposeful disregard of the urge to defecate. Opiate pain relievers and some other drugs are notorious for slowing and weakening peristalsis and allowing too much water to be absorbed from feces. A fecal **impaction** is compacted feces that cannot be passed naturally and may require an enema or other intervention for removal.

Case Notes

11.5 Regarding Melanie's glottis and lower esophageal sphincter when she was vomiting immediately, what was the state of each: open or closed?

There Are Two Types of Intestinal Bleeding

Intestinal bleeding falls into two major categories (Fig. 11.3). **Upper gastrointestinal bleeding** is from the esophagus, stomach, or the first few centimeters of the duodenum, where peptic ulcers usually appear. It may present as bloody vomitus or as blood in the stool. The most common causes of upper GI bleeding are, in order, acute hemorrhagic gastritis, peptic ulcer of the duodenum or stomach, esophageal tears caused by vomiting, esophageal varices, and vascular malformations.

Lower gastrointestinal bleeding originates anywhere in the bowel below the first few centimeters of the duodenum. Blood may be bright red or dark brown to black from alteration by intestinal bacteria. Some bleeding is very slow, does not produce visible change in stool, and requires stool testing for detection. The most common causes (not including hemorrhoids and other anal disease) are: inflammatory bowel disease or gastroenteritis, colonic diverticulosis, neoplasms, and colonic angiodysplasia.

Case Notes

11.6 Would Melanie's bleeding be classified as lower or upper GI bleeding?

Rapid intestinal bleeding can be fatal and is characterized by weakness, fainting, and shock. Intestinal malignancy is often the cause of slow intestinal bleeding. Slow intestinal bleeding is often clinically silent and, if persistent, can cause iron deficiency anemia.

Remember This! Gastrointestinal bleeding is so important it warrants immediate attention in every instance and should be considered suspicious for intestinal malignancy until proven otherwise.

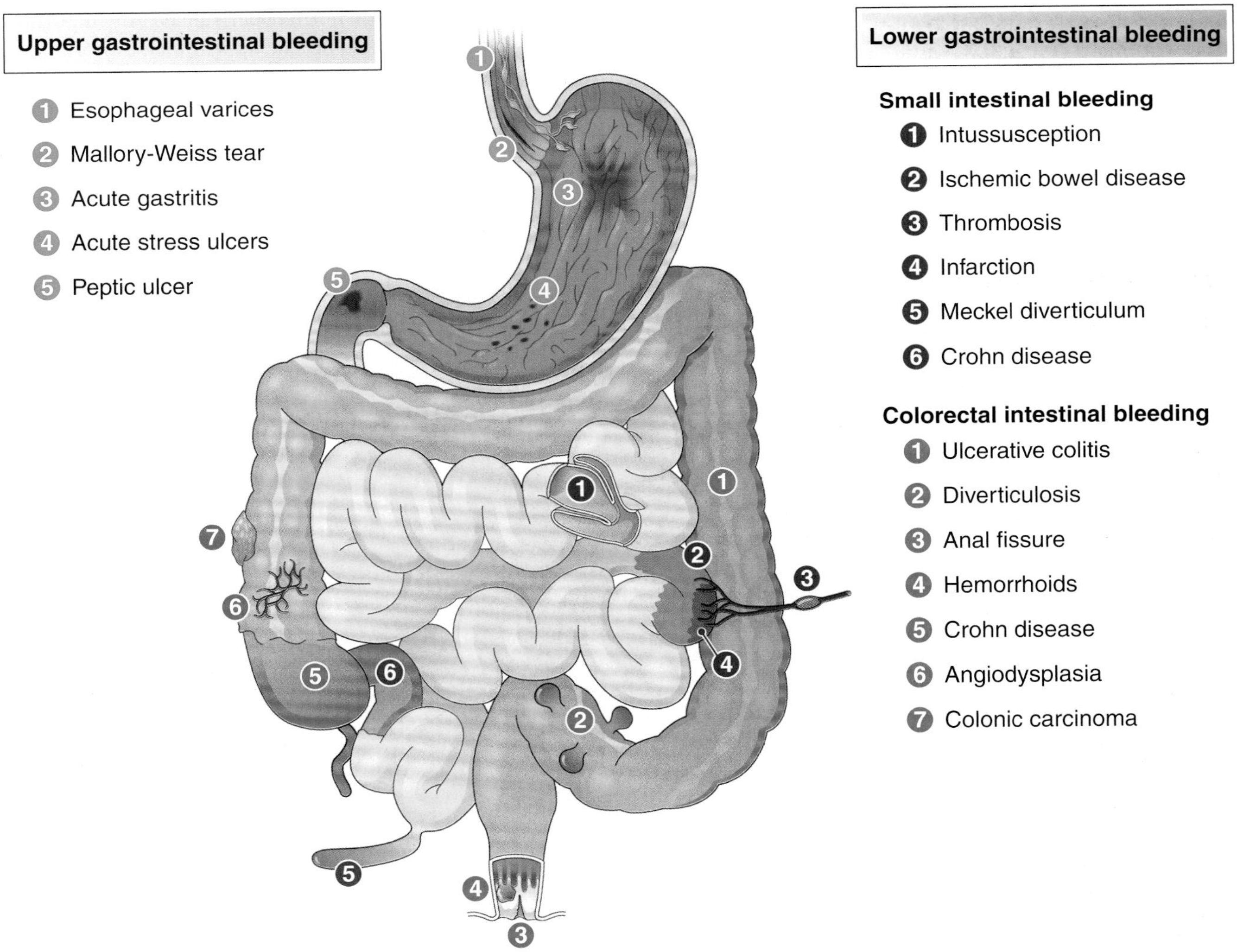

Upper gastrointestinal bleeding

1. Esophageal varices
2. Mallory-Weiss tear
3. Acute gastritis
4. Acute stress ulcers
5. Peptic ulcer

Lower gastrointestinal bleeding

Small intestinal bleeding

1. Intussusception
2. Ischemic bowel disease
3. Thrombosis
4. Infarction
5. Meckel diverticulum
6. Crohn disease

Colorectal intestinal bleeding

1. Ulcerative colitis
2. Diverticulosis
3. Anal fissure
4. Hemorrhoids
5. Crohn disease
6. Angiodysplasia
7. Colonic carcinoma

Figure 11.3 **Causes of gastrointestinal bleeding.** (Reproduced with permission from Mulholland MW, Maier RV, et al. *Greenfield's Surgery Scientific Principles and Practice*. 4th ed. Philadelphia (PA): Lippincott Williams & Wilkins; 2006.)

Intestinal bleeding may manifest in vomit or stool. **Hematemesis** is bloody vomiting and is a sign of upper GI bleeding, usually from the lower esophagus, stomach, or upper duodenum. Vomited blood may be bright red, indicating fresh bleeding, or black "coffee grounds" material, indicating that blood has been in the upper GI tract long enough to be altered by gastric acid. **Hematochezia** is the presence of red blood in stool. Unaltered *red* blood *mixed with stool* usually originates from lesions in the lower colon or rectum. Blood from bleeding hemorrhoids or anal fissures is usually bright red and appears *on*, not *in*, stool. (A note of caution: hemorrhoids and anal fissures are very common; therefore, clinicians should never assume that either is the cause of rectal bleeding until other, more serious lesions [colon cancer] have been excluded. Just because a patient has hemorrhoids doesn't mean they cannot have colon cancer at the same time.) **Melena** is dark, nearly black (tarry) stool discolored by altered blood. It may be caused by bleeding from any intestinal site, including the esophagus.

Occult bleeding is not visible to the naked eye and must be detected by a simple laboratory test, as discussed in *The Clinical Side*, "Stool Occult Blood Test." It occurs when blood slowly seeps into any part of the GI tract from any cause (see Fig. 11.3). Annual occult blood testing of stool is simple, cheap, and effective: if repeated regularly over a period of 10 or more years, it will detect precancerous lesions of the colon and prevent about one-third of colon cancers.

Case Notes

11.7 Was Melanie's rectal bleeding melena or hematochezia?

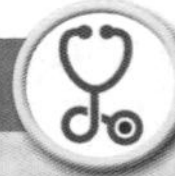

The Clinical Side

STOOL OCCULT BLOOD TEST

Blood in stool that is invisible to the naked eye can be detected by a simple chemical test. All adults over 50 should be tested regularly. At least three stools should be tested from separate days. Any positive test result warrants further studies to rule out sources of slow bleeding such as colon cancer or colon polyps, diverticula, esophageal varices, peptic ulcer, or other intestinal lesions.

The sensitivity of a single occult blood exam is low, but with repeated examinations using the latest chemical methods, the sensitivity of the test in detecting adenoma or carcinoma rises above 50%. False negatives are common because bleeding from polyps or cancers is often limited and irregular. A complete colon exam by direct colonoscopy or radiographic imaging—recommended once every 5–10 years for persons over age 50 (some say 40)—detects many of the lesions missed by occult blood testing.

Normal Intestinal Function Requires Constant Peristalsis

Peristalsis may be interrupted by paralysis or mechanical obstruction. In either instance, intestinal contents cannot proceed down the GI tract. Both causes are serious and may quickly become an emergency.

Ileus

Ileus is lack of peristalsis—intestinal paralysis, in other words. It is a fairly common condition of poorly understood etiology that is associated with the following:

- Postoperative state after abdominal surgery
- Appendicitis, gallbladder disease, peritonitis and other intra-abdominal inflammations
- Intestinal ischemia
- Post spinal cord injury
- Hypokalemia (low blood potassium)

Signs and symptoms of ileus include vomiting, abdominal pain, lack of bowel movements (*obstipation*), and lack of the usual tinkling, gurgling abdominal bowel sounds associated with normal peristalsis. An important radiologic finding in ileus is the appearance of horizontal air-fluid interfaces in loops of paralyzed bowel (Fig. 11.4). Treatment is alleviation of the causative condition. Insertion of a nasogastric tube may relieve dangerous build up

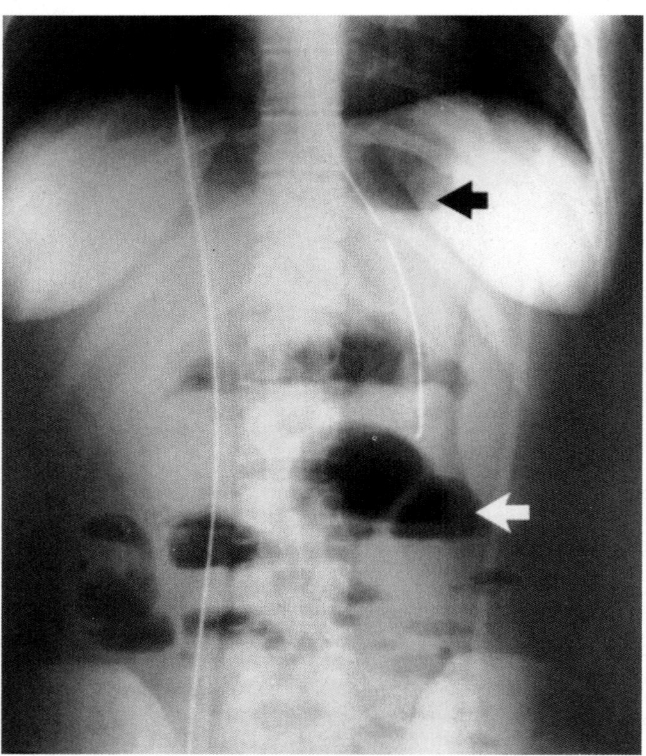

Figure 11.4 **Ileus.** Radiograph of female patient sitting upright. Lack of peristalsis allows intestinal gas and fluid to separate, creating a smooth interface between the two. Black arrow is a bubble of gas in the stomach. White arrow is bubbles of intestinal gas.

of intestinal gas that otherwise would escape through the mouth or anus.

Mechanical Obstruction

Mechanical obstruction is defined as physical obstruction of the passage of intestinal contents. The four most common causes of mechanical obstruction are shown in Figure 11.5:

- *Adhesions:* Abdominal surgery, infection, or other inflammation very commonly leave bands of fibrous scar tissue (adhesions) in which loops of bowel may become entangled, trapped, and obstructed.
- *Intussusception:* **Intussusception** is a telescoping of bowel, in which the distal (downstream) segment swallows the proximal one. This occurs briefly and regularly in normal people without consequence. Pathologic intussusception occurs when the swallowed segment becomes trapped. The swallowed bowel carries its blood supply, which may become obstructed at the mouth of the swallowing segment.
- *Volvulus:* The intestines are attached to and suspended from the aorta by the mesentery, through which blood vessels travel. Collectively the mesentery and vasculature are called the vascular pedicle (stalk) or mesenteric root. A **volvulus** is a twisting of a segment

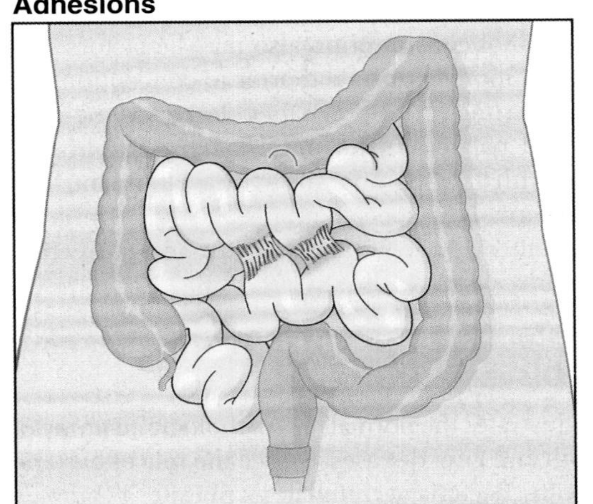

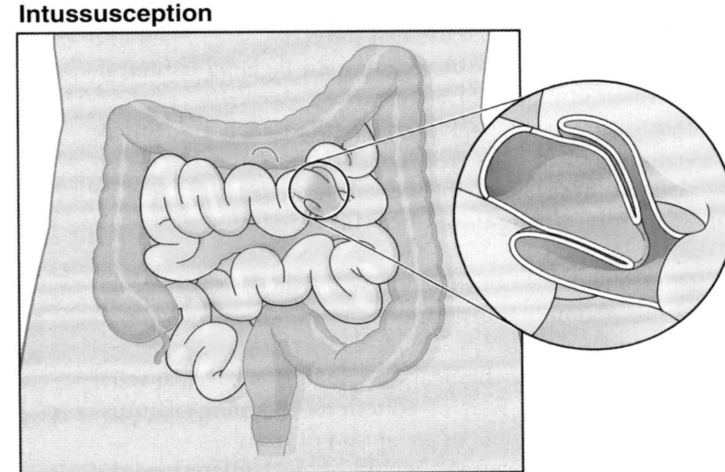

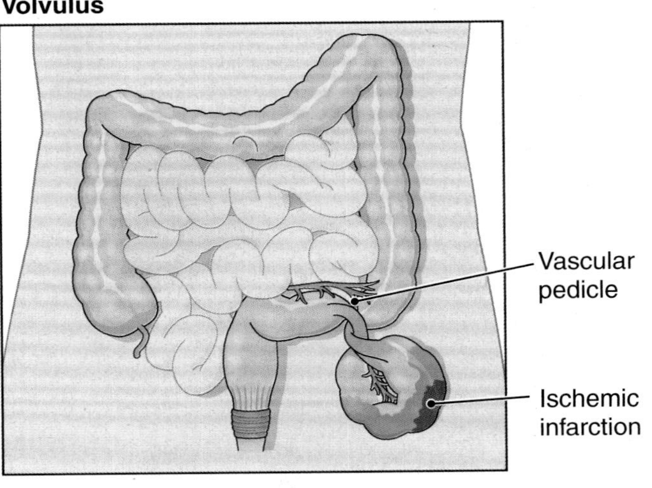

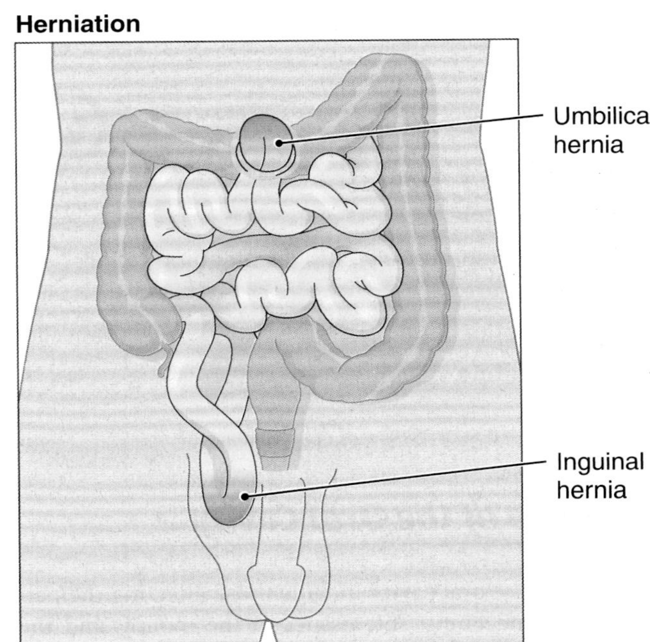

Figure 11.5 **Causes of mechanical intestinal obstruction.**

of bowel on its pedicle. The result can be mechanical obstruction or ischemia and infarction.

- *Hernias:* A **hernia** is a protrusion of a piece of anatomy, bowel in this instance, through a dilated anatomic space such as the esophageal hiatus in the diaphragm or a defect such as a weakened surgical scar. Hernias are a concern because they are common, because loops of bowel may become trapped in them, and because blood flow may become obstructed and cause bowel infarction.

  A weakness in the abdominal wall or the diaphragm may allow a pouch of peritoneum to push through the opening, which forms a sac into which loops of bowel or omentum can slide. Small hernias occur frequently in the umbilicus, a weak point where fetal umbilical blood vessels penetrated (*umbilical hernia*). As the fetus grows, the testes descend to the scrotum from the abdomen, creating a channel (the inguinal canal) through which the spermatic cord passes in adulthood. Intra-abdominal pressure can force the canal open and bowel can slide into it, creating an *inguinal hernia*, illustrated in Figure 11.5.

  Pressure at the neck of the hernia pouch may impair venous return, causing edema and entrapment (**incarcerated hernia**) of the bowel segment. Ischemia or infarction (**strangulated hernia**) may follow.

Clinically, bowel obstruction is characterized by pain, vomiting, abdominal distention, lack of stools, and hyperactive bowel sounds.

Treatment for mechanical obstruction is surgical relief of the obstruction: lysis of adhesions, undoing of intussusception or volvulus, or reduction of hernia.

Potential complications include bowel infarction: the anatomic deformity frequently stretches or twists bowel blood vessels in a way that can occlude blood flow.

Pop Quiz

11.8 Define dysentery.

11.9 Define steatorrhea.

11.10 Melena usually implies bleeding from where?

11.11 Define ileus.

11.12 Define volvulus.

Diseases of the Oral Cavity

Diseases of the oral cavity include those affecting the palate, teeth, and gums, soft tissues of the mouth, and the salivary glands.

Congenital Anomalies May Affect Soft Tissue and Bone

Cleft lip and **cleft palate** are related congenital malformations that arise from failure of embryologic structures to fuse during the first trimester of pregnancy (Fig. 11.6). The mildest form of defect is a split uvula. More significant clefts may involve the soft tissue of the lip or the soft palate, or the condition may manifest as a fissure along the midline of the roof of the mouth—that is, the bone of the hard palate. The defect may be bilateral, one cleft on each side of the midline extending from each nostril. Cleft palate interferes with feeding and speech development. About 1 in every 750 infants is affected.

A mix of genetic and environmental factors appears to contribute to cleft lip and palate. Having one affected child increases the chance of having a second affected child. Maternal smoking and alcohol use increase the risk, and fetal exposure to certain viruses and to maternal smoking or alcohol consumption also may be factors. Folic acid dietary supplements taken prior to conception and during the first trimester of pregnancy decreases the risk.

Cleft lip and palate are not only disfiguring but also can interfere with feeding and speech development. Initial treatment involves special nipples to keep milk or formula from entering the nasal cavity. Surgical correction is effective.

Poor Oral Hygiene Promotes Tooth and Gum Disease

Figure 11.7 illustrates the normal and pathologic anatomy of common tooth and gum diseases. Notice the role of bacteria in dental disease. Bacteria accumulate as **plaque**, a complex

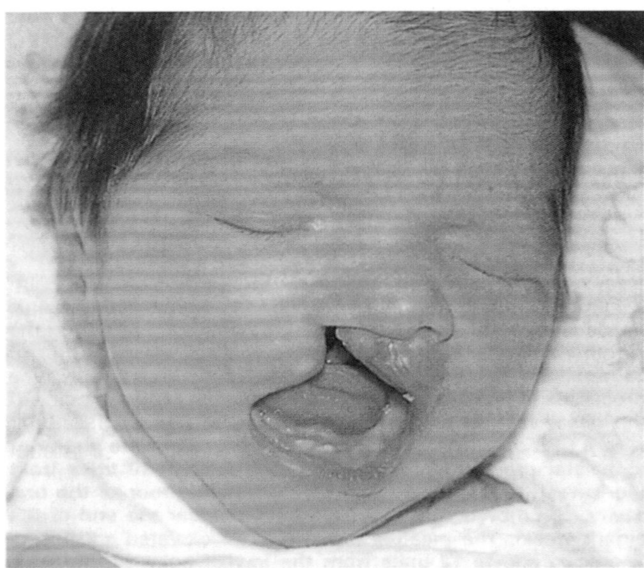

Figure 11.6 **Cleft lip.** (Reproduced with permission from Moore KL, & Dalley AF II. *Clinical Oriented Anatomy*. 4th ed. Baltimore (MD): Lippincott Williams & Wilkins; 1999.)

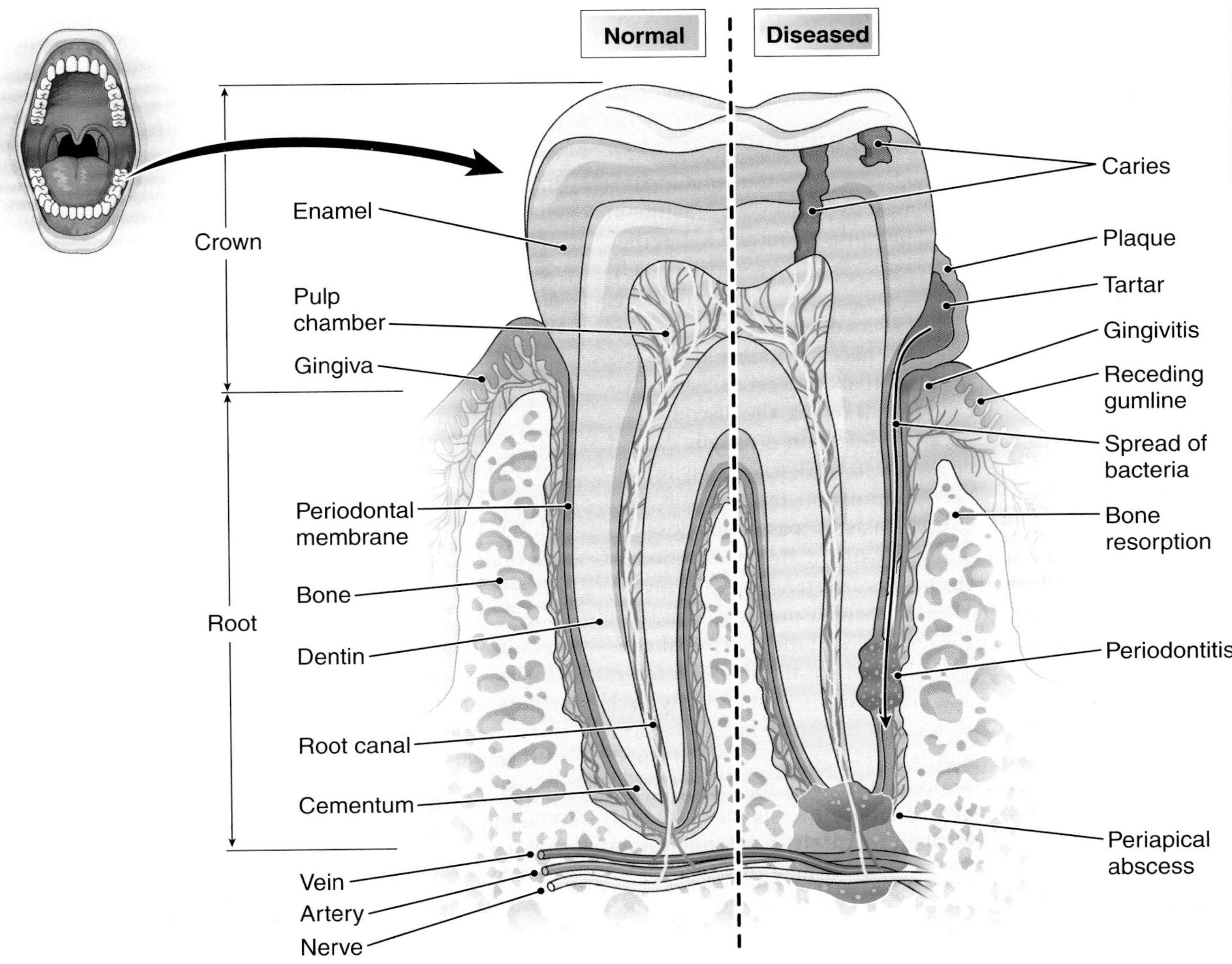

Figure 11.7 **Normal and pathologic anatomy of a tooth.** Caries is caused by bacteria that erode enamel and invade tooth structure. Periodontal disease results from bacterial invasion of gingival pockets around the root.

film of bacteria, dead cells, food debris, and mucus that builds at the gum-tooth margin. If not removed, plaque calcifies as **tartar**. Plaque and tartar are both irritants, and their accumulation promotes dental caries and gingivitis.

Caries are an erosion of tooth enamel caused by bacterial digestion of dietary carbohydrates, which produces tooth-destroying acid. Dental caries is second only to the common cold as a widespread disorder. Although the primary risk factor is poor oral hygiene, a high-sugar diet and genetic predisposition are also factors. Caries can be prevented by regular brushing and flossing, periodic dental cleanings to remove accumulations of tartar, and avoiding sugary drinks and snacks. An important public health measure is fluoridation of public drinking water, which improves the resistance of enamel to bacteria. Prevention is the best treatment, but fillings may be required to restore normal anatomy and avoid enlargement of the defect.

Gingivitis is inflammation of the superficial gums (gingiva). The gums may bleed, swell, and be tender. As gingivitis progresses, gums retract, exposing more of the tooth. Gum retraction progresses with age and is the source of the phrase "long in the tooth" to describe an elderly person. Treatment of gingivitis begins with a thorough dental cleaning to remove tartar deposits. Strict oral hygiene must be maintained, and a special mouth rinse may be recommended.

Untreated gingivitis may proceed to **periodontitis**, a deeper inflammation and infection of soft tissues around the tooth root. Deep-seated inflammation can loosen dental ligaments, allowing deeper bacterial invasion, which may infect the pulp (the soft central tissue of the tooth). Since pulp contains blood vessels and nerves, pulp infections are usually painful. Infection of the root produces a *periapical abscess*, which usually requires surgical drainage. Other signs and symptoms of periodontitis are bad breath, swollen gums that bleed easily, and loose teeth. Indeed, periodontal disease causes far more tooth loss than does dental caries.

Rigorous oral hygiene can stop or reverse periodontal disease. Nevertheless, root canal surgery may be required to save an infected tooth. The root is entered through the crown and the infected canal is drained and cleaned. Blood vessels and nerves are destroyed and the empty canal is filled with an inert substance.

Lesions of the Mouth Are Common

Aphthous ulcers (*canker sores*) are common, small, painful, shallow ulcers of the oral cavity. They occur mainly in children and young adults. The cause is unknown, but they are thought to be triggered by stress, fever, nutrient deficiencies, or certain foods. In some cases, aphthous ulcers are associated with other disorders of the GI tract, such as Crohn disease. No treatment is necessary, since the ulcers are self-limiting and disappear in about a week. Nevertheless, a simple salt-water gargle can relieve the discomfort.

Oral **herpesvirus** (Fig. 11.8) infection is usually caused by the *herpes simplex virus type 1 (HSV-1)*, which infects more than half of the U.S. population by the time they reach their 20s. The virus is usually passed by kissing, though it can be transmitted sexually. Initial infection is asymptomatic, but the virus finds a permanent home in the fifth cranial (trigeminal) nerve, which provides sensation to the face and lips. The virus settles in the trigeminal ganglion at the base of the skull and, when stimulated by fever, sunlight, cold, trauma, or infection, it can multiply and migrate out nerve axons to erupt in nerve endings in skin or mucosa as a *cold sore* or *fever blister*—a cluster of small vesicles. These vesicles soon rupture, leaving a small painful ulcer for a week or two, often on the lips or chin, and sometimes on the cheeks or in the nostrils. In children or immunodeficient hosts, the infection may disseminate to cause widespread visceral lesions or even fatal encephalitis. Although no treatment is available for the lesions, antiviral ointments can help shorten the outbreak and topical anesthetics can be used for pain relief. Note that genital herpes is usually caused by HSV-2, less commonly by HSV-1, and is passed by sexual contact; otherwise the pathologic processes of oral and genital herpes are the same.

Candida albicans is a species of fungus that, in small amounts, normally inhabits the mouth. It causes disease only when normal protective mechanisms are impaired by immune deficiency, diabetes mellitus, antibiotic or steroid therapy, or anemia. The impairment of normal protective mechanisms allows overgrowth, a condition called **candidiasis** of the mouth (also called *thrush*) (Fig. 11.9). It presents as a fuzzy white membrane or curd composed of matted fungi and acute inflammatory cells. Rarely, infection may extend into the esophagus or disseminate via the blood stream. Treatment of oral lesions is often unnecessary, though eating live-culture yogurt may help. In severe cases, an antifungal mouthwash may be advised.

Leukoplakia is a clinical term that refers to a small white patch of oral mucosa. It occurs most commonly in older adults. When chronically irritated, squamous cells lining the oral cavity undergo metaplasia and produce *keratin*, a dense, protective protein normally found in the epidermis (the outer layer of skin). The result is a superficial cap of keratin (*hyperkeratosis*), which is responsible for the white clinical appearance. Leukoplakia is associated with chronic irritation from tobacco use (especially pipe smoking, or the use of snuff or chewing tobacco), alcohol abuse, and rough teeth or ill-fitting dentures. In most cases of leukoplakia, the pathologic findings are benign, but a few lesions are precancerous or malignant. Treating the underlying condition is necessary. Biopsy or surgical removal should be considered in those at high risk for oral carcinoma.

Almost all oral cancers are **squamous cell carcinomas**. Most occur in middle-aged to older adults. The most common site is the border of the lower lip (Fig. 11.10), but the floor of the mouth and the lateral aspect of the tongue are

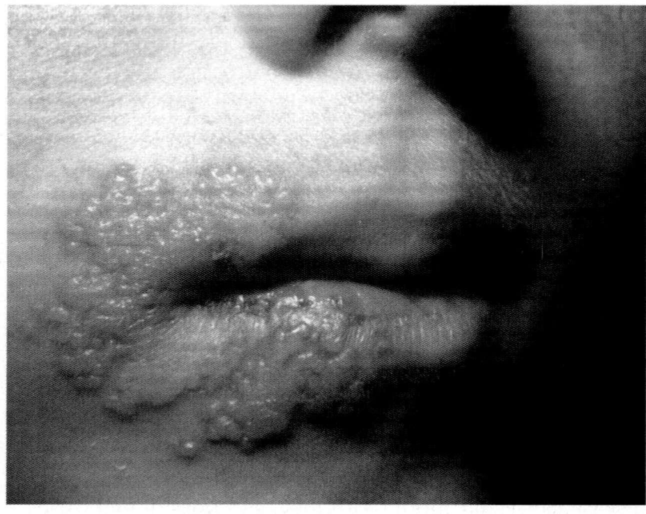

Figure 11.8 **Cold sores (oral herpesvirus).** An unusually large crop of confluent vesicles.

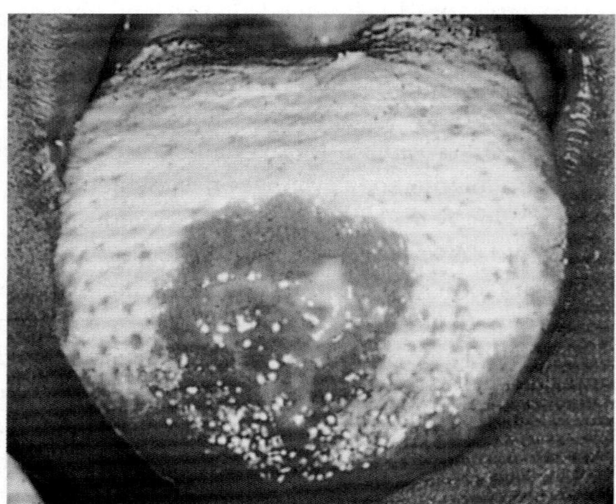

Figure 11.9 **Oral candidiasis (thrush).** The fungi have formed a white mat on this patient's tongue. (Reproduced with permission from Weber J, Kelley J. *Health Assessment in Nursing.* 2nd ed. Philadelphia (PA): Lippincott Williams & Wilkins; 2003.)

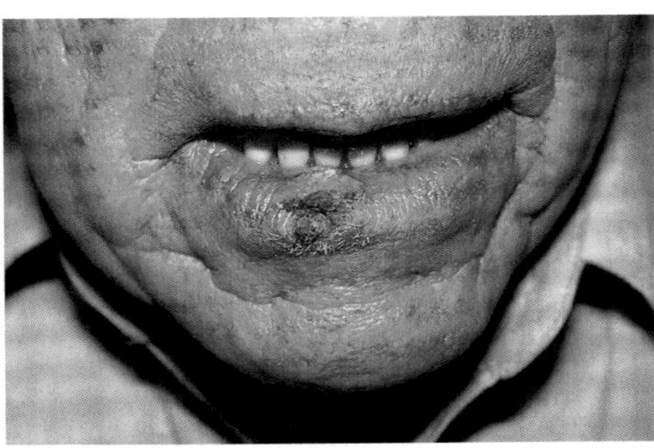

Figure 11.10 **Squamous carcinoma of the lower lip.** (Reproduced with permission from Goodheart HP, MD. *Goodheart's Photoguide of Common Skin Disorders*. 2nd ed. Philadelphia (PA): Lippincott Williams & Wilkins; 2003.)

also common sites. Oral cancers are typically associated with poor oral hygiene, alcohol abuse, and tobacco use. Despite the ease of visibility and access to the oral cavity, oral cancers are often missed by nondental professionals, who tend to abandon the mouth to dentists and oral hygienists. Treatment is surgical excision. Nearly all patients with lip cancer survive five years; by contrast, of those with carcinoma of the floor of the mouth, only about one-third survive five years.

Diseases of Salivary Glands Include Inflammation and Neoplasms

Saliva is produced by salivary glands (Fig.11.11). The *major salivary glands* are paired. Small *minor salivary glands* are scattered about the floor of the mouth. Disorders involving salivary glands include inflammation and neoplasms.

Sialadenitis is inflammation of the salivary glands. In acute cases, the etiology is usually infection with the streptococcus bacterium or the mumps virus. Acute sialadenitis usually resolves without treatment or sequelae. In contrast, chronic sialadenitis is usually caused by autoimmune disease or by stones in the gland duct. The parotid gland is most often affected. Autoimmune sialadenitis is usually seen as a part of **Sjögren syndrome**, an autoimmune inflammation of salivary and lacrimal glands in which inflammatory scarring replaces the normal acinar structure, drying up tears and saliva and producing dry eyes (*conjunctivitis sicca*) and dry mouth (*xerostomia*). Sialadenitis may also occur as a component of systemic collagen-vascular disease, such as systemic lupus erythematosus (SLE).

Salivary gland tumors are uncommon. Most are benign and occur in the major glands, especially the parotid gland of adults age 40–60. Those arising in minor salivary glands are more likely to be malignant. Of the various types of benign and malignant tumors of the salivary glands, the most common is **pleomorphic adenoma**. They are often called *mixed tumor* because of their varied microscopic appearance, and almost all are benign. However, they can grow very large and they must be removed. The surgery is challenging because a branch of the facial nerve passes through the parotid and can be damaged during removal by even the most attentive surgeon. Avoiding the facial nerve yet achieving complete excision is difficult—about 10% of pleomorphic adenomas are incompletely removed and recur. The prognosis is good for most salivary gland tumors—average five-year survival is about 90%.

Pop Quiz

11.13 True or false? Most tooth loss is caused by caries.

11.14 What is the clinical term for oral Candidiasis?

11.15 What is the most common site for oral squamous carcinoma?

11.16 Define Sjögren syndrome.

11.17 True or false? Pleomorphic adenoma is almost always malignant.

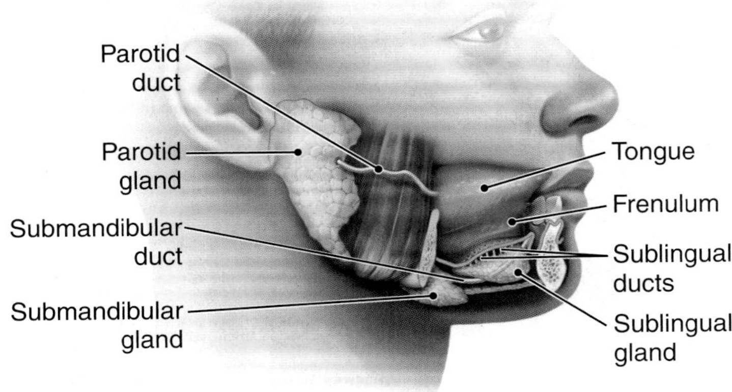

Figure 11.11 **Salivary glands.** Salivary glands secrete saliva into the oral cavity through small ducts. (Reproduced with permission from McConnell TH, Hull KL. *Human Form Human Function: Essentials of Anatomy & Physiology*. Baltimore (MD): Wolters Kluwer Health; 2011.)

Diseases of the Esophagus

Movement of food from mouth to stomach requires coordinated motor function of the esophagus. Symptoms of esophageal disease include **dysphagia** (difficulty swallowing), pain, and bleeding. Almost all esophageal disease is associated with dysphagia, which may be due to hernia of the upper stomach through the diaphragm, an obstructing scar, a tumor, or abnormal peristalsis secondary to neurologic disease such as stroke or Parkinsonism. Esophageal pain occurs substernally, and can be crampy or burning, features that make it difficult to distinguish from cardiac pain. Rapid bleeding may be manifest by alarming bloody vomitus. Slow bleeding may appear as "coffee grounds" vomiting of altered blood or by melena.

Disorders of Structure Affect Function

The most common congenital defect is **atresia**, failure of the esophagus to develop normally in the embryo. In some cases, the esophagus ends in a pouch rather than connecting to the stomach. Atresia may also be part of a more complex defect, *esophagotracheal fistula*, in which an opening exists between the two structures. It presents with the first attempted feeding after birth, when milk is regurgitated or initiates a fit of coughing. Surgical repair is necessary.

Achalasia is spasm of the lower esophageal sphincter. A motility disorder, it is due to disappearance of autonomic ganglion cells in the muscular wall, the absence of which prevents normal relaxation after each peristaltic wave. Achalasia is a rare disorder and the cause is poorly understood. It may be related to autoimmunity or abnormal immune reactions to viruses. It usually begins between ages 20 and 40 and presents as slowly progressive dysphagia and esophageal pain. It is typically chronic and intermittent, and causes partial obstruction in the lower esophagus near the esophageal hiatus. Treatments include dilation, chemical denervation of remaining autonomic connections, and surgery to release spastic muscle fibers.

Hiatal hernia is a protrusion of part of the stomach superiorly into the chest through the esophageal hiatus. Radiographic studies suggest that up to 10% of adults have some degree of hiatal hernia. The majority of these patients are asymptomatic, but about 10% experience dysphagia, pain, or reflux of gastric acid into the lower esophagus. Asymptomatic patients do not need treatment. Those with chronic symptoms require surgery.

Severe and frequent retching or vomiting, as in bulimia, for example, may cause esophageal (or gastric) *laceration* (also known as **Mallory-Weiss syndrome**). Lacerations usually occur near the gastroesophageal junction (Fig. 11.12) and can be associated with life-threatening hemorrhage. Bleeding may be halted briefly by an esophageal balloon, but emergency surgery is required.

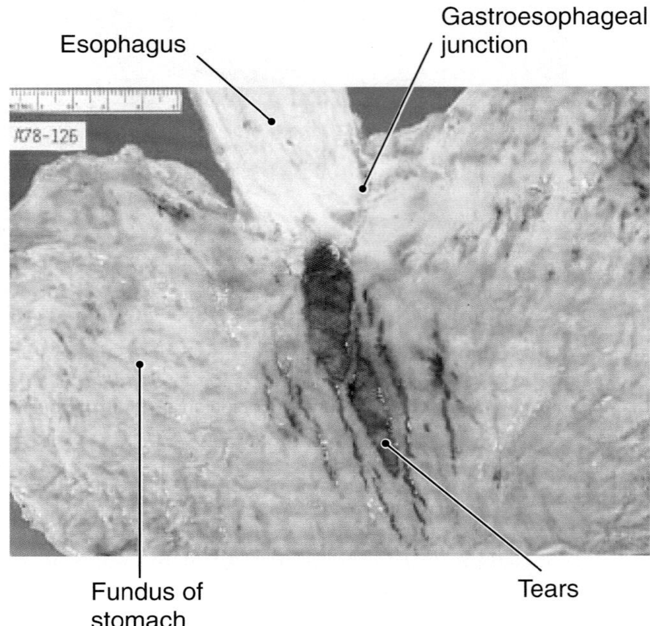

Figure 11.12 **Mallory-Weiss syndrome.** Gastroesophageal tears occur from vomiting or retching.

A dilated vein is a *varix*. **Esophageal varices** are like hemorrhoids—dilated veins full of blood (Fig. 11.13). The cause is almost always *cirrhosis of the liver*—a severe scarring of the entire liver that obstructs normal flow of portal blood on its way to the heart from the intestines. Esophageal veins are an important bypass route for blood to get back to the heart around the obstructed liver flow; however, this extra blood flow causes the veins to balloon outward, increasing the likelihood that they will rupture. Patients known to have cirrhosis can be presumed to

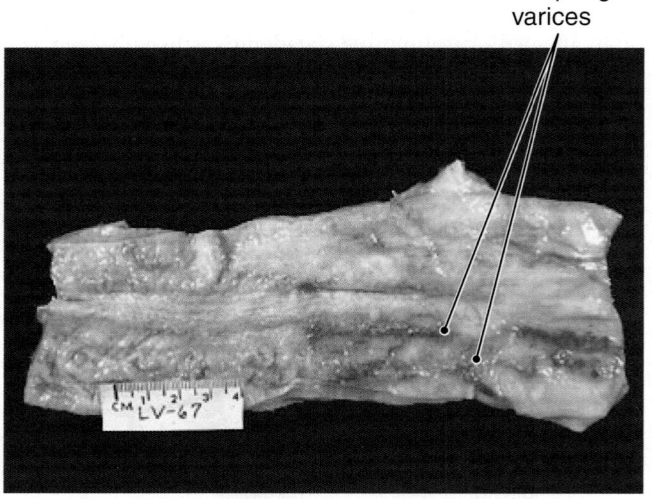

Figure 11.13 **Esophageal varices.** Veins in this postmortem specimen are much smaller than during life. The patient had portal hypertension caused by cirrhosis of the liver.

have esophageal varices. Typically the varices produce no symptoms until rupture, and when they do, the bleeding can be horrific and require emergency treatment such as balloon tamponade or surgery. Among patients with advanced cirrhosis, half will die of ruptured varices, many of them with the first bleeding episode.

Esophagitis is inflammation of the esophagus. It affects about 10% of Americans. Alcohol abuse and smoking are risk factors. It is most often caused by gastric acid refluxing upward from the stomach, a condition called *reflux esophagitis*, discussed in more detail below. Infectious esophagitis is usually due to an opportunistic viral or fungal infection in patients with impaired immunity from HIV/AIDS, lymphoma, leukemia, severe neutropenia, and steroid or other immunosuppressive drug therapy. An autoimmune disorder can also cause esophagitis. Chest pain and painful swallowing (odynophagia) are common. Treatment is correction of the underlying disorder and antimicrobial therapy if appropriate.

Carcinoma of the Esophagus Is More Common in Males

Carcinoma of the esophagus accounts for about 4% of malignant neoplasms in the United States, but the ratio of affected males to females is 4:1. Genetic factors are important: the incidence in Iran, parts of Asia, and Africa are many times higher, and in the United States the prevalence in African Americans is roughly triple that of Caucasians. Environmental factors are also important—tobacco use and alcoholism greatly increase risk.

About half of esophageal carcinomas arise from the lining epithelium in the upper esophagus as *squamous cell carcinomas*. The other half are *adenocarcinomas* that arise near the gastroesophageal junction and are strongly associated with chronic *gastroesophageal reflux disease* (discussed below). Other risk factors include achalasia, and dietary deficiencies of certain vitamins and minerals. Esophageal carcinomas tend to invade and metastasize early. Though less common than colon or stomach cancer, they are important because they are so deadly: fewer than 5% of patients survive two years after diagnosis. Early detection is best accomplished by careful monitoring of patients with achalasia and chronic esophagitis. Treatment may include surgery, endoscopic techniques, chemotherapy or radiation depending on the clinical stage.

Gastroesophageal Reflux Disease Is Common

Gastroesophageal reflux disease (GERD) is due to chronic reflux of gastric acid into the lower esophagus. About 30% of the U.S. adult population is affected. GERD is caused by incompetence of the lower esophageal sphincter (LES). Factors contributing to LES incompetence include anatomic abnormality of the esophageal hiatus, obesity, alcohol, smoking, caffeine, high-fat diet, and certain drugs known to relax the LES.

Substernal burning pain (heartburn) is the most common symptom of GERD and may be associated with regurgitation of gastric contents into the mouth. Painful swallowing is common. Bleeding is uncommon, but can be severe.

A detailed history points to the diagnosis, and a successful trial of treatment confirms the diagnosis. Treatment for GERD includes raising the head of the bed, avoiding intake of food within three hours of bedtime, cessation of smoking and caffeine intake, weight loss for patients who are overweight or obese, and therapy with drugs that inhibit gastric acid production. Repeated balloon dilation may be required for patients with strictures. Patients who do not improve may require surgery to tighten the LES.

Patients who do not improve require further investigation. Endoscopy with biopsy is the preferred initial test. Patients with unremarkable endoscopy and persistent symptoms require further investigation and treatment.

GERD may cause chronic esophagitis, esophageal ulcers, scarring with stricture, and change (metaplasia) of esophageal epithelium from squamous to columnar (*Barrett metaplasia* or *Barrett esophagus* [Fig. 11.14]).

Patients with biopsy-proven **Barrett metaplasia** deserve close follow-up. Barrett is a precursor condition that is associated with increased risk of esophageal adenocarcinoma, which can be reliably detected only by biopsy. Repeated endoscopy and biopsy may be required for follow-up of patients with dysplasia of the metaplastic epithelium. Laser ablation or surgery may be required.

Pop Quiz

11.18 Define achalasia.

11.19 What is the cause of almost all esophageal varices?

11.20 True or false? The majority of people with GERD develop adenocarcinoma of the esophagus.

11.21 What term is used to describe change from one kind of epithelium to another (i.e., squamous to columnar)?

Diseases of the Stomach

Diseases of the stomach owe largely to the fact that the stomach produces very strong acid and acts as a holding tank for acidic chyme. Most gastric disease causes pain or bleeding, though gastric cancer owes its reputation as a deadly disease to the fact that it is initially silent and far advanced by the time it becomes symptomatic.

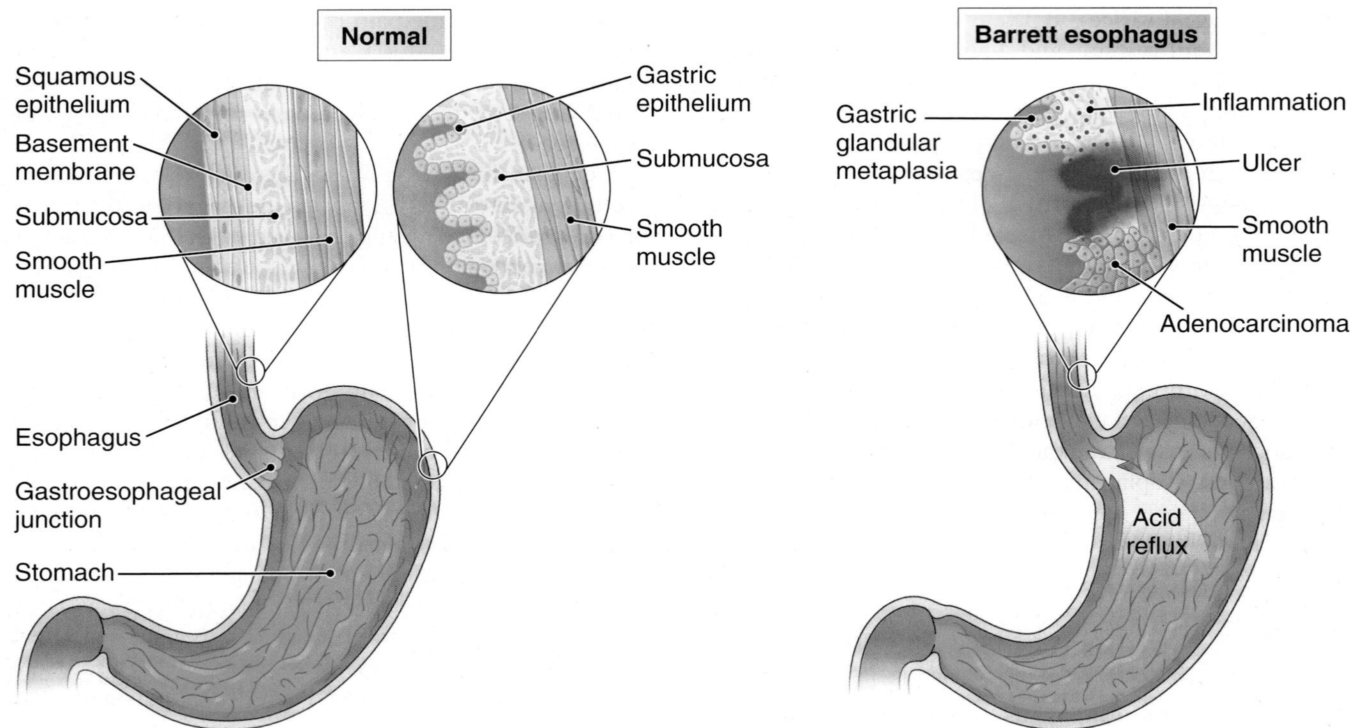

Figure 11.14 **Barrett esophagus.** Normal esophagus is lined by layers of flat, squamous epithelium. Normal stomach is lined by tall, columnar cells. Chronic reflux of gastric acid (GERD) evokes change (metaplasia) of normal esophageal squamous epithelium into gastric epithelium (Barrett metaplasia). Esophageal ulcers and adenocarcinoma may arise in areas of Barrett metaplasia.

Gastric discomfort or pain (**dyspepsia**, *indigestion*) usually occurs high in the abdomen, just below the end of the sternum (deep to the xiphoid process) and therefore may be mistaken for cardiac pain (angina). Vomiting is also a common gastric symptom, but is a reflex stimulated by many nongastric conditions. Gastric bleeding may result in *hematemesis* (discussed earlier). Most gastric hematemesis looks like "coffee grounds," because the color and consistency of the blood has been altered by gastric acid. If gastric blood passes through the entire lower GI tract, it manifests as black stool (*melena*).

Congenital Pyloric Stenosis Causes Newborn Intestinal Obstruction

The pyloric sphincter is a thick ring of gastric smooth muscle that surrounds the lumen of the gastroduodenal junction. **Pyloric stenosis** is obstruction of the stomach outlet due to hypertrophy of the sphincter muscle.

Pyloric stenosis affects 1 of 250 newborns and is more common among males (particularly firstborn males) than females by a 4:1 ratio. It usually presents at about three to five weeks of age. The etiology is uncertain, but a genetic component is clear because siblings and offspring of affected infants are at increased risk.

The cardinal symptom is bile-free-projectile vomiting shortly after eating. Until dehydration occurs, the child otherwise seems completely normal and has none of the other signs or symptoms (fever, fussiness, and so on) that accompany vomiting caused by other illnesses.

Diagnosis is by abdominal sonography. Surgery is curative: a longitudinal incision through the muscle relaxes the outlet and the infant resumes feeding within a day.

Acute Gastritis Is Inflammation of the Gastric Mucosa

Gastritis is inflammation of the gastric mucosa. It is caused by any of several conditions—bacterial infection by *Helicobacter pylori*, alcohol, stress, chronic use of nonsteroidal anti-inflammatory drugs (NSAIDs) such as aspirin, uremia, shock, and autoimmune disease. Acute gastritis is classified as erosive or nonerosive based on the severity of mucosal injury. Chronic gastritis involves mucosal atrophy as well. The pathogenesis of gastritis is poorly understood, a fact emphasized by the variety of conditions that may cause it.

Acute nonerosive gastritis is a transient inflammation of the gastric mucosa (Fig. 11.15) without ulceration. It can be due to chronic use of nonsteroidal anti-inflammatory drugs, binge drinking, uremia, steroid use, chemotherapy, or age-related loss of the normal layer of mucus that protects the mucosa.

With more severe inflammation, superficial mucosal defects may appear and the diagnosis becomes **acute**

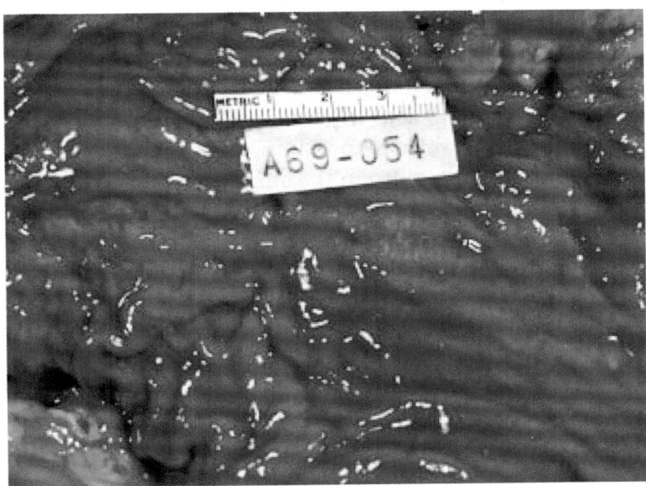

Figure 11.15 **Acute gastritis.** The inflamed gastric mucosa is markedly hyperemic (normal mucosa is pink–gray).

erosive gastritis (Fig. 11.16). Acute defects are also associated with stressful clinical conditions such as severe trauma, sepsis, major surgical procedures, grave illnesses, extensive burns, brain trauma or surgery, and chronic exposure to corticosteroids. If the defects are superficial, they are called *erosions*; deeper ones are called *peptic ulcers*. Defects due to stress such as burns or other trauma are called *Curling ulcers*. Defects owing to brain trauma or tumor are called *Cushing ulcers*.

Acute gastritis, with or without erosions or ulcers, is usually associated with upper abdominal pain, nausea, and vomiting. Bleeding is common and may be severe. For most cases, treatment consists of removing the offending stimulus and administration of drugs to suppress gastric acid secretion. Bleeding requires endoscopic hemostasis or surgery.

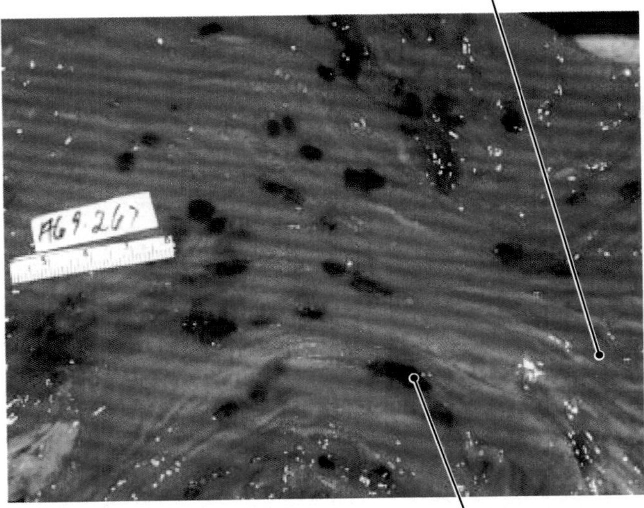

Figure 11.16 **Acute gastric stress ulcers.** Multiple superficial ulcers in a patient with brain injury. Altered blood on the ulcer's surface is black.

Chronic Gastritis Is Caused by Infection or Autoimmune Disease

Most gastritis is chronic and associated with varying degrees of gastric atrophy. **Chronic gastritis** (Fig. 11.17) is asymptomatic and often goes undiagnosed. It is usually discovered by endoscopic study for symptoms caused by complications. Chronic gastritis is usually caused by *Helicobacter pylori* infection (over 90% of cases). Cigarette smoking and alcohol abuse also play a role. It can also be caused by *autoimmune gastritis*, as part of a syndrome known as *pernicious anemia* (Chapter 7).

H. pylori is a gram-negative bacterium adapted to live in strong acid. In developing countries, most people are infected as children, but, in other nations, new infections occur mainly in adults. About half of American adults over age 50 are infected; only about 10% of infected adults, however, develop disease.

H. pylori attach themselves to the gastric mucosa (Fig. 11.18). In the gastric antrum, this stimulates increased secretion of gastrin, which in turn stimulates acid secretion. When the body of the stomach is infected, the result is mucosal atrophy and increased risk of gastric carcinoma or lymphoma.

About 85% of infected patients will have anti-*H. pylori* antibodies in their blood. In some instances, endoscopic biopsy is required to demonstrate presence of the organism attached to gastric mucosa.

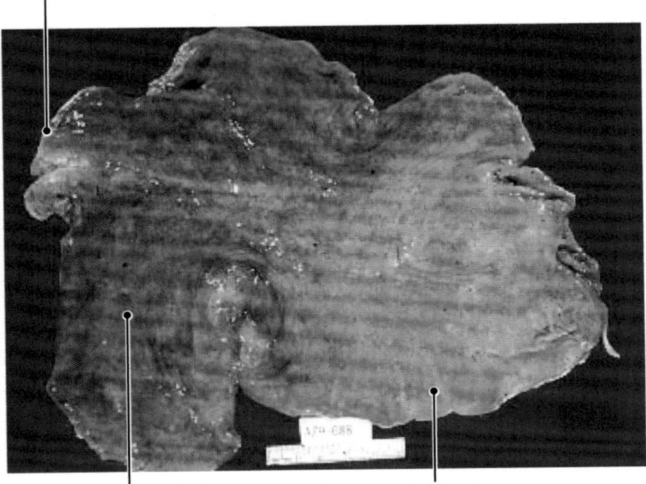

Figure 11.17 **Chronic atrophic gastritis.**

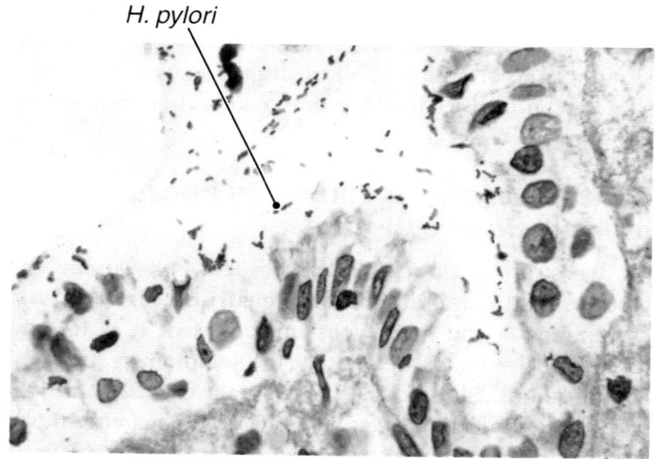

Figure 11.18 **Helicobacter pylori.** Organisms present in the mucous layer on the gastric mucosal surface. (Reproduced with permission from Mills SE. *Histology for Pathologists.* 3rd ed. Philadelphia (PA): Lippincott Williams & Wilkins; 2007.)

Patients with gastritis, ulcer, or cancer should be treated until the organism is eradicated. Eradication requires multidrug therapy, typically multiple antibiotics plus acid suppressants. The role of *H. pylori* in cancer is the rationale for treating asymptomatic patients. Vaccines are under development.

A radioactive urea test is used to confirm cure. *H. pylori* metabolizes radioactive urea into radioactive CO_2, which is detected by breath analysis. A negative test is considered proof of cure.

Autoimmune gastritis accounts for <10% of gastritis and occurs when autoantibodies attack the hydrochloric acid-producing parietal cells of the gastric epithelium. In addition to making acid, the parietal cells normally produce *intrinsic factor*, which is important for the eventual absorption of vitamin B_{12} in the small intestine. When the immune system destroys parietal cells, both acid production and the ability to absorb B_{12} are impaired. Since B_{12} is important for red blood cell production, anemia ensues. Over time, the patient may also develop neurological deficits, including confusion that can be misdiagnosed as dementia. The syndrome of autoimmune gastritis, B_{12} deficiency, and anemia is still sometimes called *pernicious anemia* because it was so serious or fatal before it was discovered to be due to B_{12} deficiency and therefore treatable. No treatment is necessary other than B_{12} injections.

Peptic Ulcers Are Deep Mucosal Defects

A **peptic ulcer** (Fig. 11.19) is a deep defect of gastric, duodenal, or esophageal mucosa, usually solitary. It is a somewhat common condition: each year about half a million Americans (about 1 in 600) develop a peptic ulcer. The incidence is higher in men.

Most peptic ulcers occur in the gastric antrum or first few centimeters of the duodenum; however, they may occur in the esophagus with GERD. Infection by *H. pylori* and chronic use of NSAIDs are the most common causes. Both increase acid secretion and weaken mucosal repair mechanisms. Cigarette smoking and alcohol abuse are risk factors. Psychological stress, family history, and personality traits also play a role.

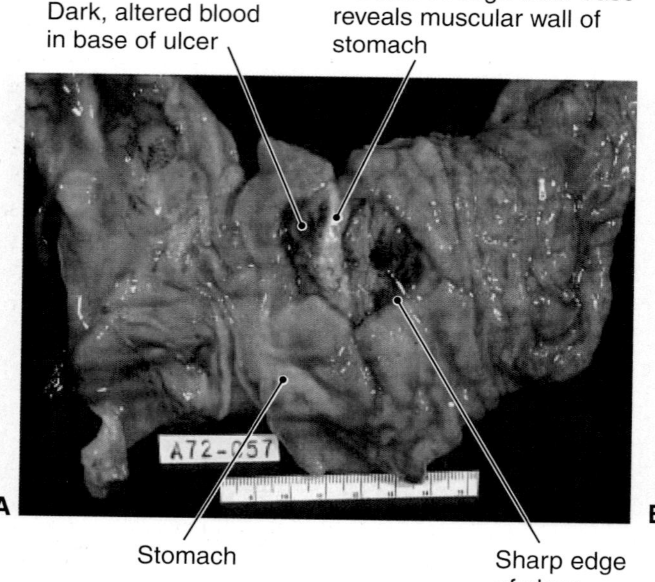

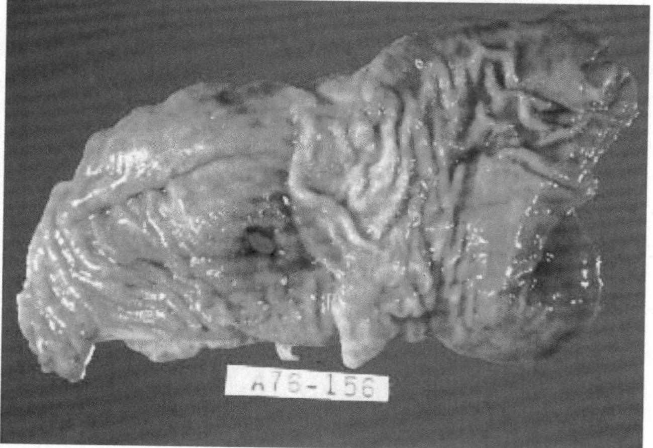

Figure 11.19 **Chronic peptic ulcer of stomach. A.** (preserved specimen). The ulcer has been incised to reveal the muscular wall. Note that the ulcer extends down to but not into muscular wall. Altered blood in the ulcer base is black. **B.** (fresh specimen). Perforated acute peptic ulcer.

Peptic ulcers typically cause a penetrating, burning pain high in the abdomen, but some remain asymptomatic until hemorrhage or bowel perforation occurs. The pain typically is relieved by food or antacids. Weight loss, nausea, and vomiting are common.

Peptic ulcers are by nature chronic and recurrent—some patients will heal completely, only to develop ulcers again. Especially noteworthy are recurrent ulcers due to the **Zollinger-Ellison syndrome**, in which pancreatic islet tumors secrete gastrin, which stimulates marked gastric acid production and recurrent ulcers that resist medical treatment. Surgical removal of the tumors is required.

Diagnosis of peptic ulcer requires imaging or endoscopy or both. Endoscopy offers a chance for biopsy to prove *H. pylori* infection and rule out malignancy.

Treatment of peptic ulcers with modern drugs is usually effective and relies mainly on drug control of gastric acid secretion and antibiotic therapy for *H. pylori* infection. If *H. pylori* infection is eradicated, only 10–20% of patients will develop another ulcer.

Complications include duodenal ulcers that penetrate into the pancreas, causing acute pancreatitis. A fairly common serious complication is bleeding from erosion of blood vessels in the bowel wall. Some patients may develop mechanical obstruction of the gastric outlet. Complete perforation of the gastric or duodenal wall causes release of strong acid and bacteria into the abdominal cavity. Shock, sepsis, and peritonitis may occur. Finally, peptic ulcers increase by three to six times the risk for gastric carcinoma later in life.

Remember This! Infection with *Helicobacter pylori* is the cause of most chronic atrophic gastritis and peptic ulcers.

The Etiology of Stomach Cancer Is Multifactorial

Almost all malignancies of the stomach are adenocarcinomas (Fig. 11.20), which arise from gastric epithelium. In the 1930s, gastric carcinoma was the number one cancer killer in the United States, but in 2010 it ranked far down the list, causing about 10,000 deaths per year. The cause for this decline is unknown. Worldwide, however, gastric carcinoma still causes about as many deaths as lung cancer. Genetic factors appear to be the reason stomach cancer is about 10 times more common in Japan, Chile, and Iceland than in the United States. Nevertheless, immigrants from those nations who move to nations with lower incidence have less risk, which suggests environmental factors are important, too.

Risk factors for gastric carcinoma are 1) *H. pylori* infection, 2) a diet high in smoked, pickled, or salt-preserved food, 3) use of nitrite food preservatives, and 4) a diet low in fresh fruits and vegetables.

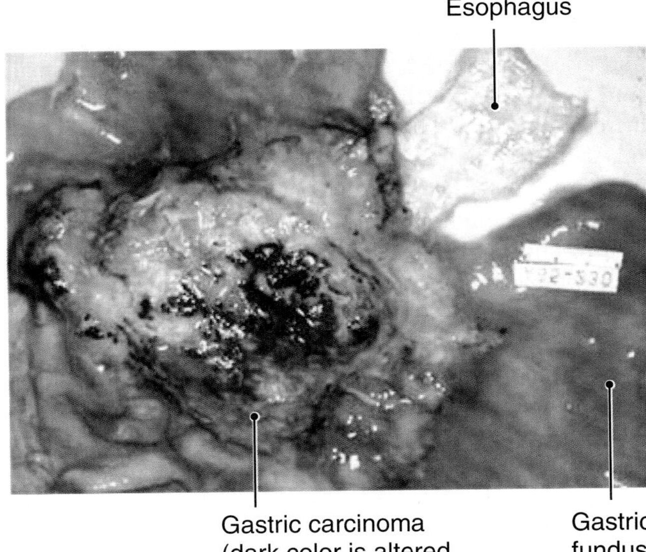

Figure 11.20 Carcinoma of the stomach. Altered blood on the tumor's surface is black.

In keeping with the fact that chronic gastritis is a predisposing factor and usually occurs in the gastric antrum, more than half of gastric carcinomas also occur in the antrum. Several growth patterns are recognized, but in general those that are exophytic (protrude into the lumen) are less lethal than those that burrow into the wall.

Gastric carcinomas are often asymptomatic. Patients with symptoms of peptic ulcer or its complications should be investigated for gastric carcinoma. Diagnosis requires endoscopic biopsy.

Gastric carcinoma commonly metastasizes first to regional lymph nodes and then to the liver. Also, by the time it produces gastric discomfort or weight loss, gastric carcinoma is usually too advanced for curative surgery. For these reasons, five-year survival is about 10%, although new therapies offer some hope for improved survival. For example, *epidermal growth factor* (EGF) is a protein that promotes epidermal growth in normal tissues. It is also capable, however, of promoting growth of epithelial malignancies such as gastric carcinoma if tumor cells have EGF-receptors. Some studies show improved survival in patients treated with drugs that block EGF-receptors.

Primary Gastrointestinal Lymphoma Often Arises in the Stomach

Lymphomas of the GI tract may be primary or secondary. Secondary GI lymphomas are those that begin in the bone marrow or lymph nodes and spread to the GI tract. This section focuses on lymphomas originating in the GI tract.

Primary gastrointestinal lymphomas are those that originate in the GI tract. The stomach is the most common site (60%), followed by the small intestine (25%), and colon (10%). The lymphomas may be B- or T-cell type and arise from MALT, such as Peyer patches of the small intestine. Paradoxically, however, most MALT lymphomas arise in the stomach, which normally contains no organized MALT patches. Over 90% of patients with gastric lymphoma have *H. pylori* infection and it is speculated that gastric lymphomas arise in MALT patches organized as a reaction to the infection. Some GI lymphomas arise in response to long-standing malabsorption syndromes (discussed below) or in immunodeficient states such as HIV/AIDS.

Signs and symptoms are those of almost any intestinal neoplasm: abdominal pain and bleeding.

Tumor behavior varies according to histologic type and location. Low-grade tumors have a relatively good prognosis and gastric lymphomas tend to have a significantly better outlook than those elsewhere in the GI tract.

Treatment varies according to histologic type, grade, and clinical stage. *H. pylori* should be treated with antibiotics, and may lead to regression of lymphoma. If not, radiation and chemotherapy may be employed.

Case Notes

11.8 **Was Melanie's tumor a lymphoma?**

Pop Quiz

11.22 True or false? *H. pylori* is the cause of most acute nonerosive gastritis.

11.23 True or false? *H. pylori* infection is the cause of most chronic atrophic gastritis.

11.24 True or false? *H. pylori* infection is the cause of most peptic ulcers.

11.25 True or false? *H. pylori* infection is a risk factor for gastric adenocarcinoma and lymphoma.

Congenital Anomalies of the Small and Large Bowel

About 2%–3% of people have a **Meckel diverticulum** (Fig. 11.21), an appendix-like blind pouch opening onto the distal ileum. It is an embryologic remnant that often contains islands of gastric tissue or pancreatic tissue.

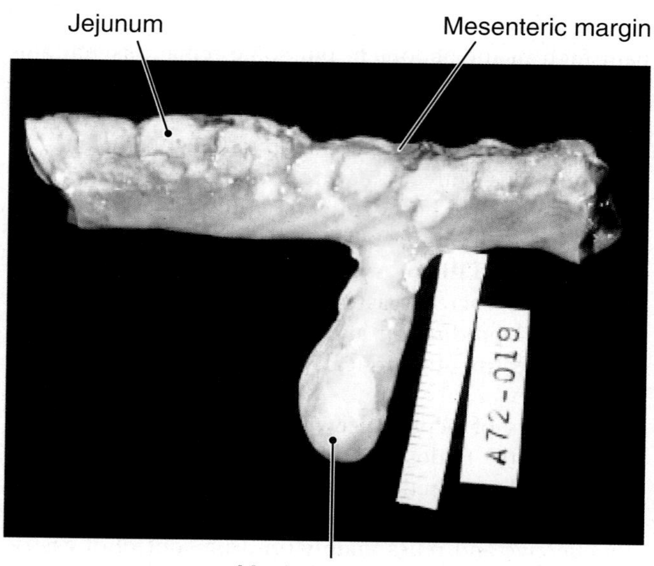

Figure 11.21 **Meckel diverticulum of the jejunum.** Incidental finding at autopsy.

Rarely, fecal matter becomes impacted into it and it becomes acutely inflamed like an appendix. Symptoms are uncommon but include bleeding, bowel obstruction, and inflammation. Diagnosis is usually made at surgery for severe, acute unexplained abdominal pain. Treatment is surgical resection.

Congenital **atresia** (complete obstruction) or **stenosis** (partial obstruction) are rare and can involve any part of the bowel including the anus. Treatment is excision of the affected segment and reanastomosis.

Like all other hollow structures, the abdominal cavity forms from a trough. The edges of the trough rise up, fold inward and fuse to form a tube. Failure of the edges to close during prenatal development leads to congenital defects. **Umbilical hernia** is a finger-size opening in the abdominal wall at the umbilicus. It can be palpated just deep to the skin. Intra-abdominal pressure causes an outward ballooning of peritoneum. A loop of bowel may protrude (herniate) into the defect. Most umbilical hernias are small and close spontaneously early in life, but larger ones may require surgical closure.

Larger defects occur in about 1 of every 2,000 newborns. **Omphalocele** (Fig. 11.22) is a midline defect in which herniated viscera are covered by a thin peritoneal membrane. It may be small (only a few loops of intestine) or may contain most of the abdominal viscera (intestine, stomach, liver). Immediate dangers are drying of the viscera and infection of the peritoneum. About three in four infants with omphalocele have other congenital anomalies, including bowel atresia, cytogenetic chromosomal abnormalities (e.g., Down syndrome), and developmental abnormalities of the heart and genitourinary system. Omphalocele can be detected by routine prenatal

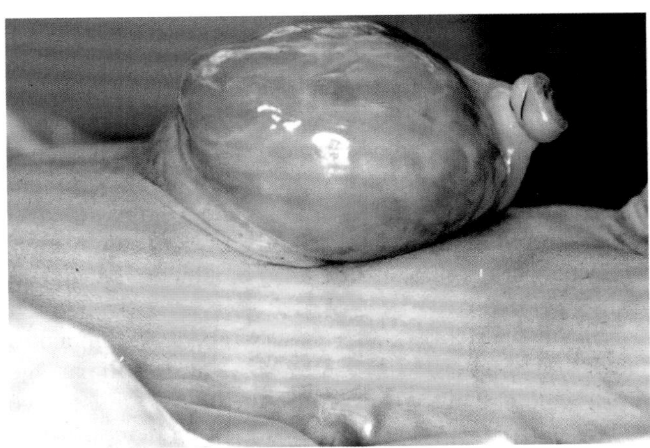

Figure 11.22 **Omphalocele Newborn infant**. Base of penis is at right margin of photo. Protruding from the abdominal wall defect is small bowel encased in parietal peritoneal sac. The base of the amputated umbilical cord visible at the right edge of the sac. (Image courtesy of Douglas Katz, MD.)

sonogram. Surgical correction is required. **Gastroschisis** is a related, larger defect in which the intestines and other viscera protrude herniate through the largely absent abdominal wall. No membrane covers the protruding viscera. Diagnosis and treatment are similar to that for omphalocele.

By far, the most important developmental abnormality of the bowel is **congenital megacolon** or **Hirschsprung disease** (Fig. 11.23). It is due to genetic absence of the autonomic ganglionic neural plexus in the smooth muscle of the colon wall. Deprived of ganglionic neural control, no peristalsis occurs in the affected segment, feces cannot pass, and the upstream colon distends with fecal material. The lower colon and rectum are usually involved as well. Hirschsprung disease predominantly affects males and occurs about once in 5,000 live births. The principal threat to life is an overgrowth in the distended segment of toxic bacteria, which produce severe intestinal inflammation. Surgical excision of the aganglionic segment is curative.

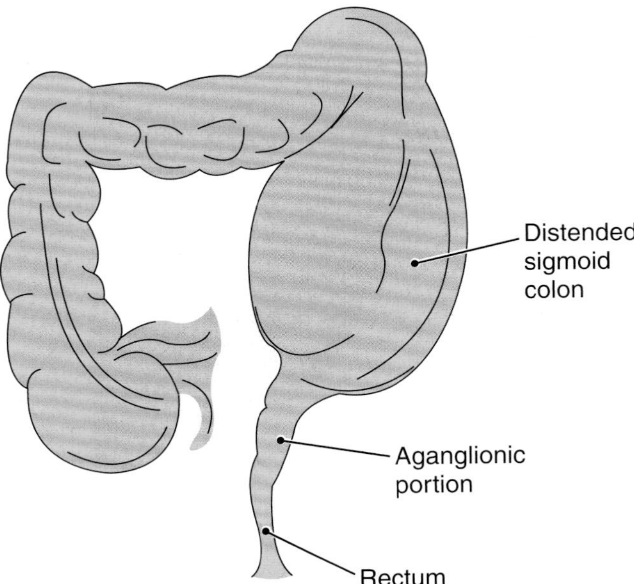

Figure 11.23 **Hirschsprung disease (aganglionic megacolon).** The distal portion of the bowel lacks nerve innervation. Because there is no peristalsis in this narrowed segment, the bowel proximal to it distends markedly. (Reproduced with permission from Pillitteri, A. *Maternal and Child Nursing*. 4th ed., Philadelphia (PA): Lippincott Williams & Wilkins; 2003.)

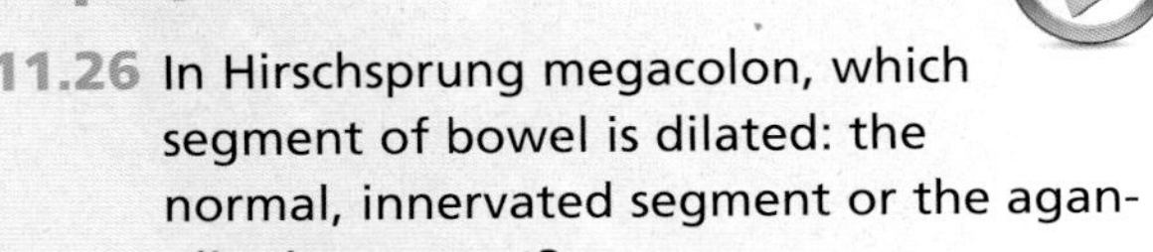

Pop Quiz

11.26 In Hirschsprung megacolon, which segment of bowel is dilated: the normal, innervated segment or the aganglionic segment?

11.27 True or false? An omphalocele is a midline defect where intestines and/or other organs are extruded through the abdominal wall and into a small sac.

Vascular Diseases of the Small and Large Bowel

The small and large bowel are richly vascular and supplied by the celiac and superior and inferior mesenteric arteries. **Ischemic vascular disease** of the bowel is most common in elderly patients with atherosclerosis that involves the celiac or superior mesenteric arteries. Chronic ischemia is common and produces few symptoms. Acute ischemia is less common and can be caused by thrombosis, embolism, or vasculitis, or by the twisting of bowel loops (**volvulus**) on the vascular pedicle (Fig. 11.24). Ischemia or infarction also can occur without complete vessel occlusion in patients with atherosclerosis of the intestinal vascular supply who develop low cardiac output due to shock, myocardial infarction, or congestive heart failure.

Early diagnosis may allow surgical reopening of obstructed vessels. With vascular occlusion, however, it is difficult to make the diagnosis in time to save the bowel. The mortality rate approaches 90% for those who have bowel infarction.

Angiodysplasia is a small, tortuous collection of small blood vessels (somewhat like a hemangioma) usually found in the mucosa or submucosa of the right (ascending) colon or cecum. These vessels are very prone to bleeding, and account for about 20% of lower intestinal bleeding, especially in older adults. Most are probably congenital defects.

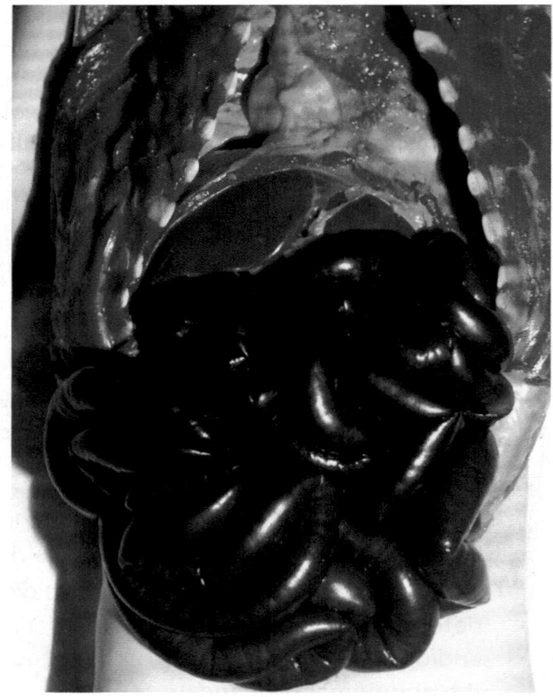

Figure 11.24 **Volvulus with infarction of small bowel.** The intestine in this child twisted on its vascular pedicle and occluded the superior mesenteric artery, which infarcted the entire small bowel. (Reprinted with permission from Rubin E. *Pathology*. 4th ed. Philadelphia (PA). Lippincott Williams & Wilkins; 2005.)

Hemorrhoids are dilated anal veins (*varices*). They affect about 5% of adults. *Internal hemorrhoids* lie within the anal canal. *External hemorrhoids* protrude from the anal orifice (Fig. 11.25). Hemorrhoids occur mainly in persons over age 50. Some people have a familial tendency to develop them. The principal cause is straining at stool in chronically constipated older adults. Hemorrhoids may also develop from the venous stasis of pregnancy. Rarely, hemorrhoids may be a sign of obstructed portal blood flow due to cirrhosis of the liver.

The anus is richly endowed with nerves, which makes hemorrhoids especially painful, particularly with passage of stool. The slang term "*a pain in the . . .*" must have been coined by someone suffering from hemorrhoids. Other signs and symptoms include anal itching, one or more tender lumps near the anus, and bleeding. Note, however, that blood from hemorrhoids is *bright red* and on the toilet tissue or the stool *surface*, whereas bleeding higher in the GI tract is mixed with stool and may be altered to brown–red or black.

Case Notes

11.9 **Why was the blood in Melanie's stool not likely to be from hemorrhoids?**

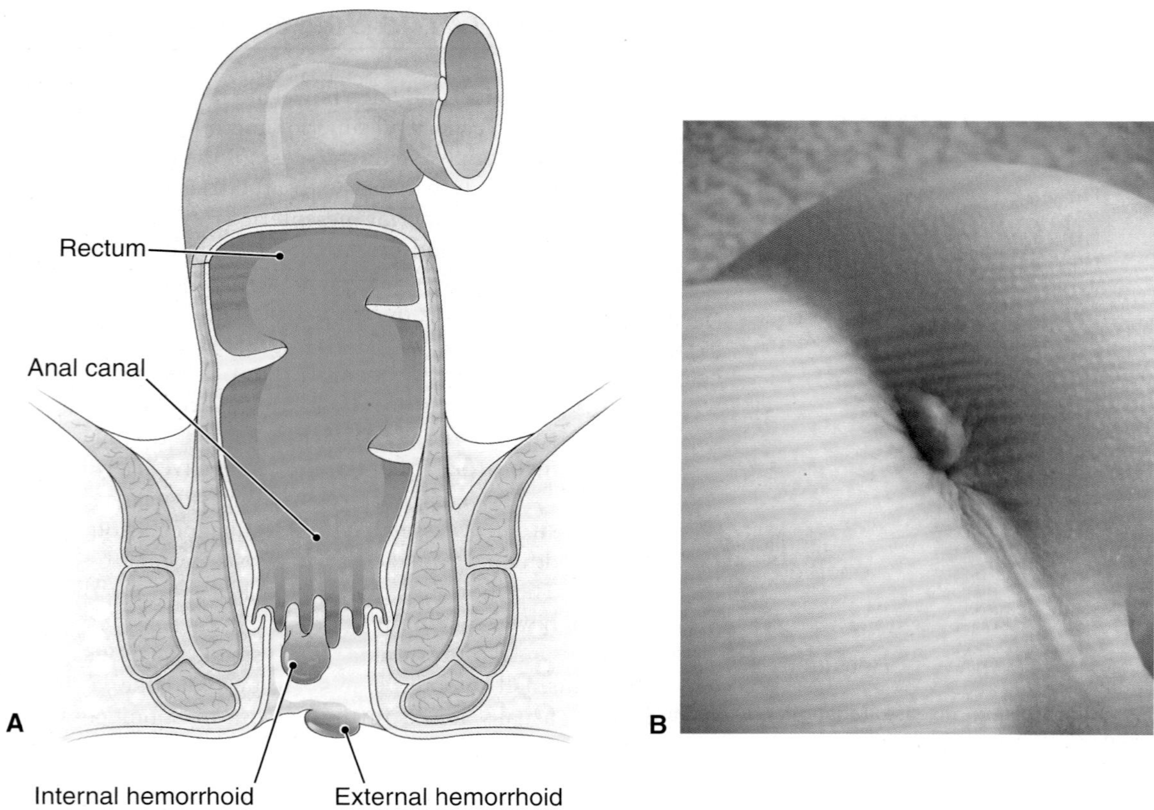

Figure 11.25 **Hemorrhoids. A.** Internal and external hemorrhoids. **B.** Clinical photo of protruding external hemorrhoid. (Image **B** courtesy of Michael J. Wilsey, Jr., MD.)

In mild cases, an over-the-counter ointment can help relieve the itching and pain of hemorrhoids. Warm baths may also help. Infrared heat coagulation may shrink hemorrhoids. Surgical excision of the dilated veins is curative.

Complications of hemorrhoids are thrombosis, strangulation, and infarction, all of which are very painful.

Pop Quiz

11.28 True or false? Angiodysplasia accounts for <5% of cases of lower GI bleeding.

Infectious Diseases Affecting the Small and Large Bowel

Acute **gastroenteritis** is clinically defined as inflammation of the lining of the stomach and small and large intestines. Nevertheless, with the exception of *H. pylori*, which preferentially infects the highly acidic environment of the stomach, most GI infections involve the friendlier confines of the small and large bowel. Because the stomach is less often involved, some prefer the term *enterocolitis*.

About half of the U.S. population will suffer a bout of gastroenteritis each year. Although gastroenteritis may follow ingestion of chemical toxins (e.g., illicit drugs, household chemicals, plant substances), most cases are infectious. Like most infectious disease, gastroenteritis may be episodic or epidemic; that is, it may occur in one person, or it may cause widespread waves of illness by transmission from one person to the next. Viruses and bacteria, which cause most cases in the developed world, tend to produce acute illness; parasites and protozoa, which cause most cases in developing nations, are often associated with chronic or recurrent disease.

Bacteria and Viruses Cause Most Infectious Diarrhea

In general, gastroenteritis due to viruses or bacteria usually produces only mild mucosal inflammation. Symptoms include anorexia, nausea, vomiting, diarrhea, and abdominal discomfort. For otherwise healthy adults, this is usually nothing more than an unpleasant inconvenience that resolves spontaneously. In vulnerable populations, however, gastroenteritis is a much different story. According to the World Health Organization (WHO), diarrhea causes death by dehydration of about 3,000 persons *per day*, mostly children in underdeveloped nations.

Diagnosis is by clinical presentation or by stool culture. Treatment is symptomatic, although in cases with severe diarrhea, fluid and electrolyte replacement may be required. Some infections require specific antimicrobial therapy.

Viral Gastroenteritis

Rotavirus and **norovirus** are the main causes of acute viral gastroenteritis in the United States. They infect intestinal villi and cause exudation of fluids and electrolytes.

Rotavirus is the leading cause of diarrhea in young children. Because the diarrhea can be severe, dehydration may develop quickly, and hospitalization with IV fluid support may be necessary. New vaccines against rotavirus are available for newborns.

Norovirus (also called *Norwalk virus*) affects older children and adults. It is the most common cause of acute gastroenteritis in the United States and has been associated with epidemics of diarrhea in nursing homes, on cruise ships, at summer camps, on college campuses, and in other places where food is prepared for groups. It can cause diarrhea or vomiting, and typically resolves spontaneously within about three days.

Bacterial Gastroenteritis

Bacterial gastroenteritis is less common than viral gastroenteritis, but is often more severe and protracted. Bacteria cause gastroenteritis by several mechanisms. Given the right environment and enough time, some bacteria (e.g., *Staphylococcus aureus*) produce an exotoxin that is ingested in contaminated food—for example, potato salad left unrefrigerated for several hours during a family barbecue on a hot afternoon (Fig. 11.26A). The exotoxin directly damages intestinal epithelium, rapidly producing gastroenteritis without bacterial infection. Exotoxins generally cause acute nausea, vomiting, and diarrhea within a few hours of ingestion. Symptoms disappear within a day or so.

In contrast, some bacteria produce toxins after ingestion. For instance, *Vibrio cholera*, the agent of *cholera*, adheres to the intestinal mucosa, where it produces enterotoxins that impair intestinal absorption and cause secretion of electrolytes and water (Fig. 11.26B). *Clostridium difficile*, the agent of *pseudomembranous colitis* (discussed shortly) produces a similar toxin.

Other bacteria (e.g., *Shigella*, *Salmonella*, *Campylobacter*, and some species of *E. coli*) invade the mucosa of the small intestine or colon, and cause ulceration, bleeding, and secretion of electrolytes and water (Fig. 11.26C).

Species of *Salmonella* and *Campylobacter* are the most common bacterial causes of diarrheal infection in the United States. Both are most frequently acquired through consumption of undercooked poultry or juices from raw poultry. Undercooked eggs, processed meats, peanut butter, alfalfa sprouts, and many other foods can also transmit salmonella. The diseases associated with these two agents are as follows:

- **Campylobacteriosis.** There are about 500 species of *Campylobacter*, but just one, *Campylobacter jejuni*, is responsible for most illness. Campylobacteriosis is

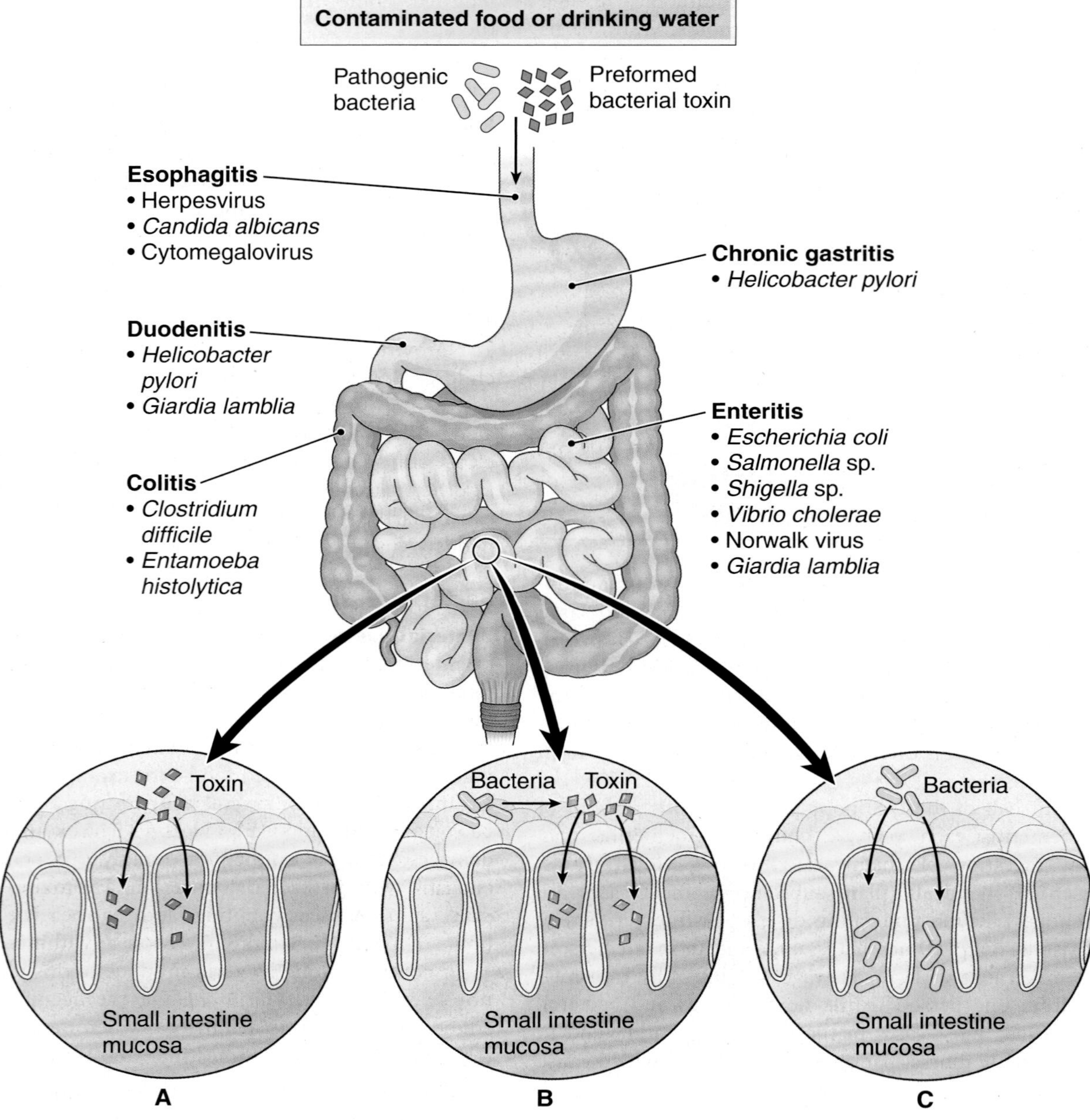

Figure 11.26 **Mechanisms of bacterial enterocolitis.** Diarrhea can be caused by **A.** bacterial toxin formed in food before ingestion, **B.** toxin formed in the intestinal tract after infection, or **C.** direct invasion of infective organisms in the bowel wall.

self-limiting, and typically resolves within about five days without medical treatment.

- **Salmonellosis.** *Salmonella enterica* has many subtypes that cause a variety of types of salmonellosis. By far, the most common symptoms are sudden fever, chills, nausea, vomiting, and diarrhea. Diagnosis is confirmed by stool culture of the organism.
- **Typhoid fever.** *Salmonella typhi* causes a syndrome of slow onset of GI and systemic symptoms including fever, headache, sore throat, splenomegaly, bloating, constipation or diarrhea, and skin rash. Diagnosis is confirmed by blood culture of the organism. In the United States, typhoid fever is far less common than salmonellosis.

Species of *Shigella* are the third most common bacterial cause of diarrheal infection in the United States. Infection is usually transmitted person to person by oral-fecal contamination from unwashed hands, plates, or utensils. *Shigella* species cause **shigellosis**, also called *bacillary dysentery*, another epidemic form of gastroenteritis.

Several different *subtypes* of *Escherichia coli* also commonly cause infectious diarrhea. The epidemiology and clinical manifestations vary depending on the type:

- **Enterohemorrhagic subtype.** The most common in the United States is *enterohemorrhagic E. coli*, particularly the O157:H7 subtype. It causes bloody diarrhea (hemorrhagic colitis), and is transmitted by undercooked ground beef, unpasteurized milk and juice, and contaminated water. Person-to-person transmission is common in day care settings. *Hemolytic-uremic syndrome* is a serious complication that develops in 2–7% of cases, most commonly among the very young and old. It consists of thrombocytopenia, hemolysis, and renal failure.
- **Other subtypes.** *Enterotoxigenic E. coli* produces toxins that cause watery diarrhea. It is the most common cause of **traveler's diarrhea**. *Enteropathogenic E. coli* also causes watery diarrhea, particularly in nurseries. *Enteroinvasive E. coli* causes diarrhea, primarily in the developing world, but is rare in the United States.

Pseudomembranous colitis is an uncommon, severe inflammation of the colonic mucosa usually seen in elderly patients. It is due to an enterotoxin produced by *Clostridium difficile*. *C. difficile* is normally present in about 5% of healthy adults and from 15% to 70% of newborns. The usual cause is *broad-spectrum antibiotic therapy*, which in some patients alters the intestinal flora such that *C. difficile* overgrows pathologically and secretes a potent toxin that damages colonic mucosa. The resulting inflammatory exudate forms a membrane of pus and dead tissue that clings to the mucosal surface, hence the name of the condition. Pseudomembranous colitis can affect young or old, and most patients have no history of previous GI problems. Diagnosis is confirmed by laboratory detection of *C. difficile* toxin in stool.

A somewhat similar condition, **necrotizing enterocolitis**, can affect immature or low birth weight infants in the first week of life. The cause is unknown and is characterized by acute, necrotizing inflammation involving the small bowel and colon.

Diagnosis of bacterial infection is confirmed by stool culture. Nevertheless, immunologic tests of stool for toxins and other antigens are becoming more common. Antibiotic therapy is usually effective, and fluid support is important. Without proper medical attention, especially in children, death may occur due to dehydration, sepsis, or intestinal perforation.

Intestinal Protozoa Also Cause Infectious Diarrhea

In developing nations, *protozoa* and *parasites* are the most common offenders in infectious diarrhea. Protozoa are single-cell nucleated life-forms, most of which are motile. They may infect almost any tissue. The most important intestinal pathogens are *Entamoeba histolytica*, *Giardia lamblia*, and *Cryptosporidium*.

- *E. histolytica* is the cause of **amebic dysentery**. The organism burrows deeply into the colonic wall, and in about half of cases spreads up the portal vein to the liver to produce hepatic amebic abscesses.
- *Giardia* is a noninvasive protozoan that mainly affects the duodenum and small bowel and may produce an acute diarrhea or a chronic malabsorption syndrome.
- *Cryptosporidium* can cause gastroenteritis in any population group, but both *Cryptosporidium* and *Giardia* are common causes of opportunistic infection in immunodeficient patients (e.g., those with HIV/AIDS infection).

Intestinal protozoa are spread by oral-fecal contamination and are therefore most common in developing nations with poor sanitation and water treatment. They also may occur in the United States in institutions and day care centers if sanitation standards are not observed. Some protozoa cause opportunistic infections in patients with AIDS (Chapter 3).

Clinical differentiation among viral, bacterial, and protozoal infection is difficult. Diagnosis requires stool testing for parasite antigens or microscopic examination of stool for organisms. Reliable fecal antigen tests are available for *E. histolytica*, *Giardia*, and *Cryptosporidium*.

Pop Quiz

11.29 True or false? Most acute gastroenteritis is caused by viruses and resolves without treatment.

11.30 What is the cause of most traveler's diarrhea?

11.31 What is the usual cause of pseudomembranous (*C. difficile*) colitis?

Malabsorption Syndromes

Digestion occurs in three phases:

- *Luminal phase*: intraluminal breakdown of fat, carbohydrate, and protein by enzymes with the help of bile salts to solubilize fat

- *Epithelial phase*: digestion by enzymes in intestinal epithelial cells with absorption of end-products into blood
- *Lymphatic phase*: lymphatic transport of absorbed fat

Malabsorption syndrome is poor digestion or absorption of dietary substances with excess fecal excretion of nutrients, including minerals and water. The result is nutritional deficiency and GI and other symptoms. Some conditions affect many nutrients; others have a narrow effect.

Luminal phase digestion is particularly affected by severe pancreatic disease. Lack of pancreatic lipase is most critical because other intestinal enzymes are available to digest carbohydrate and protein. Liver or biliary disease that decreases the availability of bile salts to emulsify fat also impairs luminal fat digestion. Because bacteria and pH are important in digestion, alteration of acid/base balance, or makeup of gut bacteria content can affect luminal phase digestion. A common cause of luminal phase malabsorption is cystic fibrosis (Chapter 22)—thickened pancreatic secretions block the flow of pancreatic enzymes, including lipase.

Epithelial phase digestion can be affected by lack of mucosal enzymes (e.g., lactose intolerance), mucosal inflammation (e.g., chronic inflammatory bowel disease), or immune reaction to dietary content (e.g., gluten sensitivity).

Lymphatic phase digestion can be affected from blockage of lymphatic ducts by scar, tumor, or infection, or by congenital defect of the lymphatic system.

Signs and symptoms common to malabsorption syndromes include diarrhea, fatty stools (steatorrhea), bloating, and excess gas. Patients may lose weight despite an adequate diet. Chronic diarrhea is the most common symptom. Steatorrhea is a trademark of malabsorption and can be particularly troubling due to bulky, frothy, yellowish, greasy and very malodorous stools. Mineral (e.g., iron) and vitamin (B_{12}) deficiency may occur in severe cases, each of which will have its own particular signs and symptoms.

Diagnosis begins with clinical suspicion—chronic diarrhea, steatorrhea, weight loss, or anemia in some combination. Other medical history will point more particularly at underlying causes. Laboratory measurement of fecal fat output is a standard test for steatorrhea. Administration of oral D-xylose (an inert sugar) and measurement of blood and urinary D-xylose is a good index of intestinal epithelial health: D-xylose is passively absorbed by intestinal epithelium and does not require action by pancreatic enzymes. Low blood and urine levels suggest impaired mucosal function. Endoscopy may be required to determine the character of intestina flora or to biopsy intestinal mucosa.

Patients with malabsorption syndrome often have broad nutritional deficiencies that can cause problems in multiple organ systems:

- *Hematopoietic disorders*: anemia due to failure to absorb iron, B_{12}, or folic acid, and bleeding tendency due to failure to absorb vitamin K
- *Musculoskeletal disorders*: weak, brittle bones and tetany (muscle spasms) from defective calcium and vitamin D absorption
- *Hormonal disorders*: amenorrhea, impotence, and infertility from malnutrition
- *Skin disorders*: purpura from vitamin K deficiency; osmotic edema from low albumin due to protein deficiency; various other skin disorders due to other nutrient deficiencies
- *Nerve disorders*: peripheral nerve disease (peripheral neuropathy) from vitamin A and B_{12} deficiency

Case Notes

11.10 Melanie's total blood protein was low. Presuming that this was due to failure to absorb dietary nutrients, which phase of digestion might have been responsible?

Carbohydrate Intolerance Is Due to Lack of Mucosal Enzymes

Carbohydrate intolerance is an inability to metabolize certain sugars because of a lack of enzymes in the intestinal mucosal epithelium. Symptoms are diarrhea, abdominal discomfort, and excess gas. Undigested sugars remain in the bowel. This increases luminal osmotic pressure, which causes water to remain in the lumen and watery diarrhea to result. In addition, bacteria metabolize the excess sugar, which releases hydrogen gas and results in flatulence.

The most common variety of carbohydrate intolerance is acquired *lactase deficiency*. Lactase levels are high in infants so they can digest milk. In most ethnic groups, lactase disappears as an individual matures, with the exception of people of northern European ancestry. The ethnic diversity in the United States, along with the prominence of dairy products in the U. S. diet, make **lactose intolerance** the most common carbohydrate deficiency in the United States.

Signs and symptoms usually begin in childhood with diarrhea and gas after milk consumption. Affected adults react similarly. The key to diagnosis is a careful history. A hydrogen breath test may be helpful. A standard dose of lactose is administered and, after a suitable delay, breath is analyzed for hydrogen gas. Treatment is to avoid milk and other dairy products, to consume products with predigested lactose, or to use lactase enzyme supplements immediately before meals containing dairy products.

Celiac Sprue Is Caused by Gluten Sensitivity

Celiac sprue is a malabsorption disease prompted in genetically susceptible people by an immunologically mediated mucosal inflammatory reaction to gluten, a protein found in wheat, rye, and barley. Gluten-sensitized T cells react with dietary gluten to produce inflammation and atrophy of mucosal villi. Persons of northern European ancestry are most often affected. About 10%–20% of patients have an affected relative. Females are more often affected than males. Celiac sprue is also more prevalent in people with Type I diabetes, autoimmune disease of the thyroid, and Down syndrome.

Celiac sprue can develop at any point in life, from infancy to adulthood. Onset is often noticed with an infant's or toddler's first exposure to wheat cereals. A cardinal sign at any age is weight loss. The stools are typically bulky, soft, tan, and malodorous. Although chronic diarrhea or steatorrhea is common, the patient may have constipation or no bowel disorder. Some patients may develop osteoporosis because of calcium and vitamin D loss in stool. Electrolyte imbalances may prompt seizures and a misdiagnosis of epilepsy. Other unusual signs and symptoms include an itchy skin rash called *dermatitis herpetiformis*, missed menstrual periods, hair loss, and joint pain.

Diagnosis begins with clinical suspicion based on a thorough medical history. An affected relative is an important clue. Celiac sprue should be suspected in any patient with iron deficiency who has no evidence of GI bleeding. A small-bowel biopsy with demonstration of atrophy of villi is confirmatory but may also be found in some other malabsorption syndromes. Antigluten antibodies can be demonstrated in the blood of almost all patients.

Treatment is adherence to a strictly gluten-free diet. Gluten is so widely present, especially in processed foods, that professional nutritional counseling is advised. Vitamin and mineral supplementation is usually required. Refractory disease may require steroid therapy.

About one in four children with celiac disease will die if gluten is not eliminated from the diet. Adult deaths are rare; however, intestinal lymphomas and adenocarcinomas develop in some patients after years with disease.

Tropical Sprue Is Probably Due to Intestinal Infection

Tropical sprue is an acquired malabsorption syndrome, probably caused by intestinal infection. It is characterized by diarrhea, steatorrhea, and macrocytic anemia.

Tropical sprue occurs mainly in the Caribbean, southern India, and Southeast Asia. Transient travelers are not affected, but long-term visitors may be. Although the cause is unclear, it is probably caused by chronic small bowel infection by toxic strains of *E. coli*.

Patients usually present initially with acute diarrhea, fever, and malaise. Chronic diarrhea and steatorrhea typically follow. Nutritional deficiencies, especially of folate and vitamin B_{12}, develop after months or years, and can cause macrocytic anemia.

If the clinical history is suspicious, demonstration of atrophic villi by endoscopic biopsy supports the diagnosis. Celiac disease and parasitic infection must be excluded. Negative blood tests for antigluten solidify diagnostic certainty.

Treatment is oral tetracycline antibiotic for up to six months depending on response. Relapse may occur in some patients. Failure to respond after a month or two of therapy suggests another diagnosis should be sought. Folate and B_{12} supplement may be required.

There Are Many Other Causes of Malabsorption

The process of digestion and absorption is complex and subject to disruption at many points. The following are a few other common causes of malabsorption.

Change in the type and number of small bowel bacteria can cause malabsorption. **Bacterial overgrowth syndrome** can be caused by local abnormalities of intestinal anatomy, altered motility, or change of pH due to lack of gastric acid. The most common cause is anatomic alterations that promote stasis of intestinal contents: surgical alterations of the stomach and duodenum, diverticula, partial obstruction, or intestinal motility problems due to neurologic disease. The excess bacteria consume nutrients and bile salts, which impairs fat absorption. Many patients are asymptomatic. Diagnosis is by endoscopic culture of small bowel contents. Positive *C-xylose breath test* is confirmatory—radioactive C-xylose is administered orally and breath is sampled for the presence of radioactive bacterial metabolites. Oral antibiotic treatment is effective.

Extensive surgical resection of small bowel is the cause of **short bowel syndrome**. Symptoms depend on the amount of bowel resected. Diarrhea and nutritional deficiencies are common. Treatment is by transplant or by frequent small meals and antidiarrheal drugs to slow intestinal motility.

Malabsorption can also be caused by any chronic disease of the intestine: inflammatory bowel disease (see below), chronic ischemia, deposits of amyloid protein (Chapter 3), radiation enteritis, and many others.

Pop Quiz

11.32 What is the cause of most luminal phase malabsorption?

11.33 True or false? Most newborns are lactase deficient.

11.34 True or false? Celiac sprue is probably an infectious disease.

Inflammatory Bowel Disease

Inflammatory bowel disease (IBD) is a chronic condition characterized by chronic inflammation at various sites in the GI tract. Inflammation is the result of a cell-mediated immune response in the bowel mucosa. The exact cause is unknown; however, evidence suggests that normal intestinal bacteria trigger an immune reaction in genetically susceptible patients. No particular environmental, dietary, or infectious basis has been identified.

Crohn Disease and Ulcerative Colitis Are Similar

Two varieties of IBD are recognized. Though they have many similarities, they can be distinguished in most cases (Tab. 11.2, Fig. 11.27): **Crohn disease** can affect any portion of the GI tract, but usually begins in and affects the small bowel, whereas **ulcerative colitis (UC)** is confined to the colon, and usually begins in the rectum. Some cases are indeterminate and neither diagnosis perfectly fits the signs and symptoms.

Remember This! Crohn disease and UC are closely related conditions caused by immune-mediated inflammation.

Table 11.2 Comparison of Crohn Disease and Ulcerative Colitis

Crohn Disease	Ulcerative Colitis
Anywhere in GI tract (small bowel is involved in 80% of cases).	Disease is confined to the colon.
Colonic involvement is usually right-sided.	Rectosigmoid is always involved.
Gross rectal bleeding is uncommon.	Gross rectal bleeding always occurs.
Fistulas are common.	Fistulas do not occur.
Perianal lesions are significant in 25%–35% of cases.	Significant perianal lesions never occur.
"Skip areas" present between diseased segments.	Bowel wall is affected uniformly. No "skip areas."
Inflammation involves full thickness of bowel wall.	Inflammation is usually confined to mucosa.
Granulomas relatively common.	Generally no granulomas.

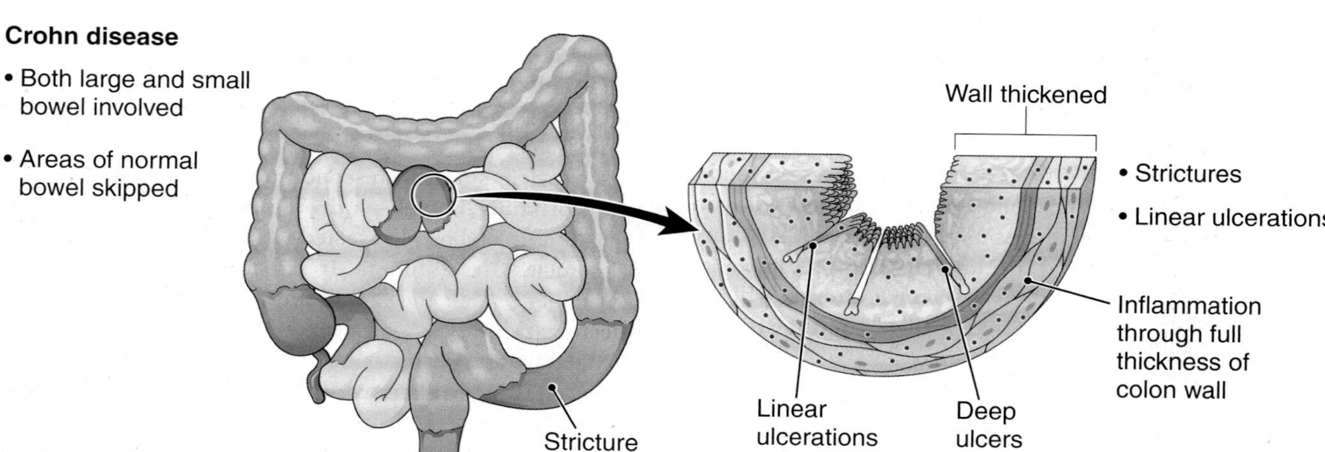

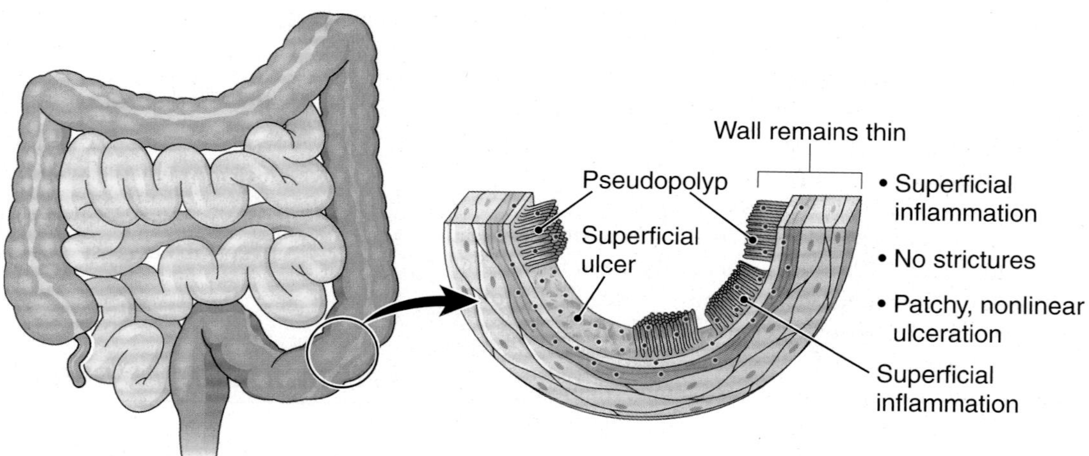

Figure 11.27 **Crohn disease and ulcerative colitis contrasted.** The two drawings illustrate differences in the anatomic location in the intestine and the differing character of bowel wall inflammation.

IBD may affect people of any age, but usually begins in teenagers or young adults. It is most common in whites of European ancestry. The sexes are equally affected. A distinct familial tendency is present, especially for Crohn disease. Oddly, cigarette smoking is a risk factor in Crohn disease, but decreases risk for UC. Aspirin and other NSAIDs may exacerbate IBD.

Pathology

The pathology of *Crohn disease* is characterized by a sharply segmented inflammation that is marked in one segment of bowel and skips the next length before occurring again. As shown in Figure 11.28, the full thickness of the bowel wall is involved from mucosa through to the peritoneal surface, a feature that produces bowel segments that are stiff like a rubber hose. Microscopically, intense chronic inflammation with formation of granulomas is seen. The inflammatory reaction has a burrowing quality that leads to bowel wall fissures and abscesses.

Case Notes

11.11 The lesions in Melanie's small bowel were separated from one another by segments of normal bowel. Is this typical of Crohn disease or UC?

11.12 Would the inflammatory reaction in Melanie's bowel wall be confined to the mucosa?

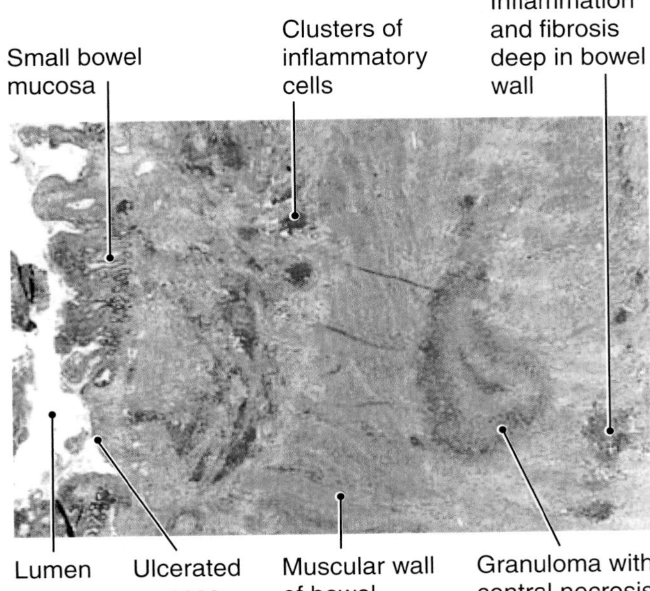

Figure 11.28 **The small bowel in Crohn disease.** The inflammatory reaction extends deep into the bowel wall, where a large granuloma is present.

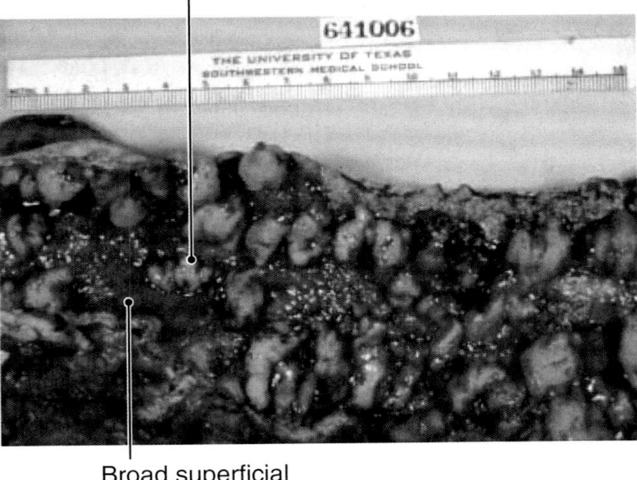

Figure 11.29 **The colon in chronic ulcerative colitis.** Polypoid islands of intact mucosa are surrounded by mucosal ulcers.

The pathology of *UC* is characterized by intense inflammation in the anus and rectosigmoid colon. Typically the process spreads as broad, superficial ulcers (Fig. 11.29) that merge to leave stranded small polypoid islands of inflamed mucosa. Microscopically, the mucosa is ulcerated and chronically inflamed but the inflammation does not extend deep into the bowel wall (Fig. 11.30). No granulomas are present.

Signs and Symptoms

The signs and symptoms most commonly found with IBD are chronic abdominal pain and diarrhea.

Extraintestinal involvement of other organs is common in both Crohn disease and UC. Some of these conditions appear and remit with the intensity of IBD activity. These include acute, transitory arthritis in the arms and legs; oral lesions; and skin disorders. Other conditions are closely associated with IBD but are independent of IBD flare-ups. Discussed elsewhere in this text, these include joints (ankylosing spondylitis), eye (uveitis), and liver (sclerosing cholangitis). Primary sclerosing cholangitis is strongly associated with IBD and may appear many years before or concurrently with onset of bowel disease.

Case Notes

11.13 Did Melanie have extraintestinal symptoms?

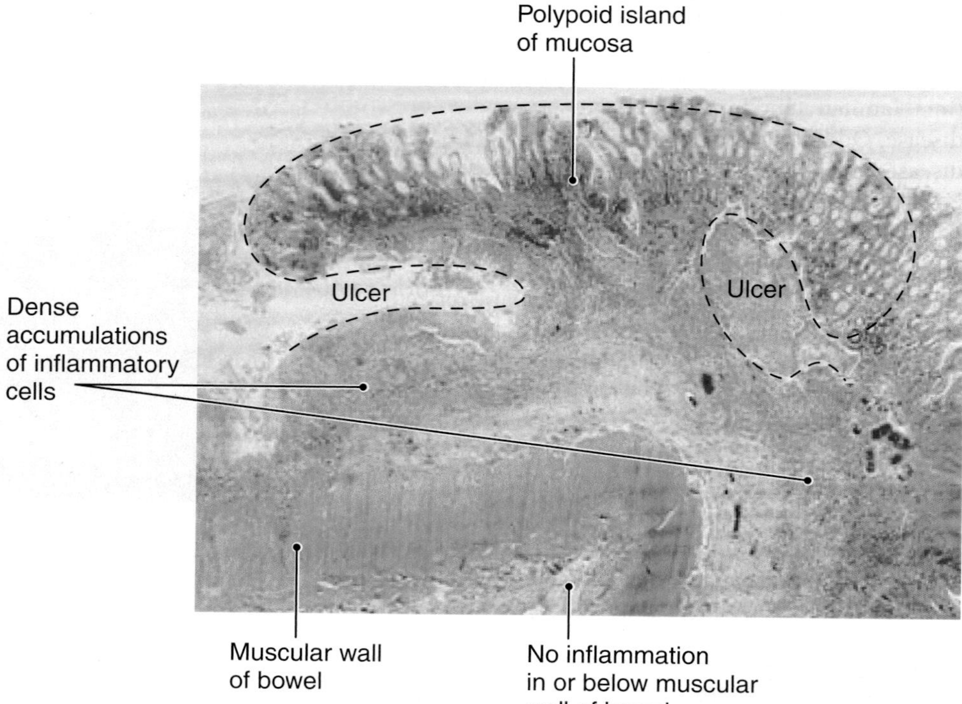

Figure 11.30 The colon in chronic ulcerative colitis. Ulcers undermine the mucosa, leaving polypoid islands of intact mucosa. Dotted line demonstrates polypoid island of remaining mucosa.

Diagnosis and Treatment

Diagnosis depends on clinical history, the anatomic site of bowel disease, and the character of extraintestinal involvement.

Treatment is mainly medical. Low-bulk, low-fat diet and nutritional supplements may be required. During severe exacerbations, total parenteral nutrition may be used. Mainstays of drug treatment are antibiotics, steroids, and other or anti-inflammatory agents, and immunosuppressive drugs. Surgical resection of severely diseased bowel may be required. Total colectomy with ileostomy may be required in some instances, particularly with severe UC. Colectomy removes the toxic site and prevents the development of colon cancer.

Complications and Prognosis

Complications are common. Some are consequences of disrupted bowel physiology, which mainly occur in severe Crohn disease of the small bowel. Malabsorption may be caused by extensive surgical removal of diseased bowel, or inflammation may create a malabsorption syndrome with associated vitamin and nutrient deficiencies. Anemia, hypocalcemia, clotting disorders, and osteoporosis may occur. Some patients with UC may develop *toxic colitis*, an especially severe episode in which perforation and peritonitis may occur. Figure 11.31 illustrates some of the complications of UC.

Patients with long-standing UC are at high risk for development of *carcinoma of the colon*. Colon carcinoma is much less likely with Crohn disease. A well-defined sequence of progressive mucosal dysplasia, carcinoma in situ, and invasive carcinoma occurs in some cases. Occasionally the risk is great enough to warrant prophylactic complete excision of the colon (total colectomy).

Irritable Bowel Syndrome Is Difficult to Define

Irritable bowel syndrome (IBS) is a combination of intestinal symptoms that, like diarrhea, is difficult to define. It was first recognized in 1892 and called "mucous colitis." The various names for it give a feel for the nature of the condition: spastic colon, irritable colon, and nervous colon. It is a common disorder, and part of its importance lies in the fact that it can mimic IBD. Nevertheless, IBS is a functional disorder and, like *fibromyalgia*, offers no objective pathologic findings or laboratory abnormalities.

IBS typically begins in teenagers or young adults and is characterized by abdominal pain, bloating, and altered frequency of bowel habits; some patients have diarrhea, others constipation. Symptoms do not waken a sleeping patient. Other symptoms include headache, fibromyalgia-like pain in other body parts, painful intercourse. Psychological problems are common. Weight loss, bleeding, and vomiting do not occur with IBS and suggest another diagnosis. Temporary relief of symptoms occurs with bowel movements. Diagnosis is by exclusion of other conditions.

Treatment is supportive and includes psychological support and dietary measures, including increased fiber intake. The effectiveness of fiber is controversial because 40–70% of patients improve with placebo. Diarrhea or constipation should be treated accordingly.

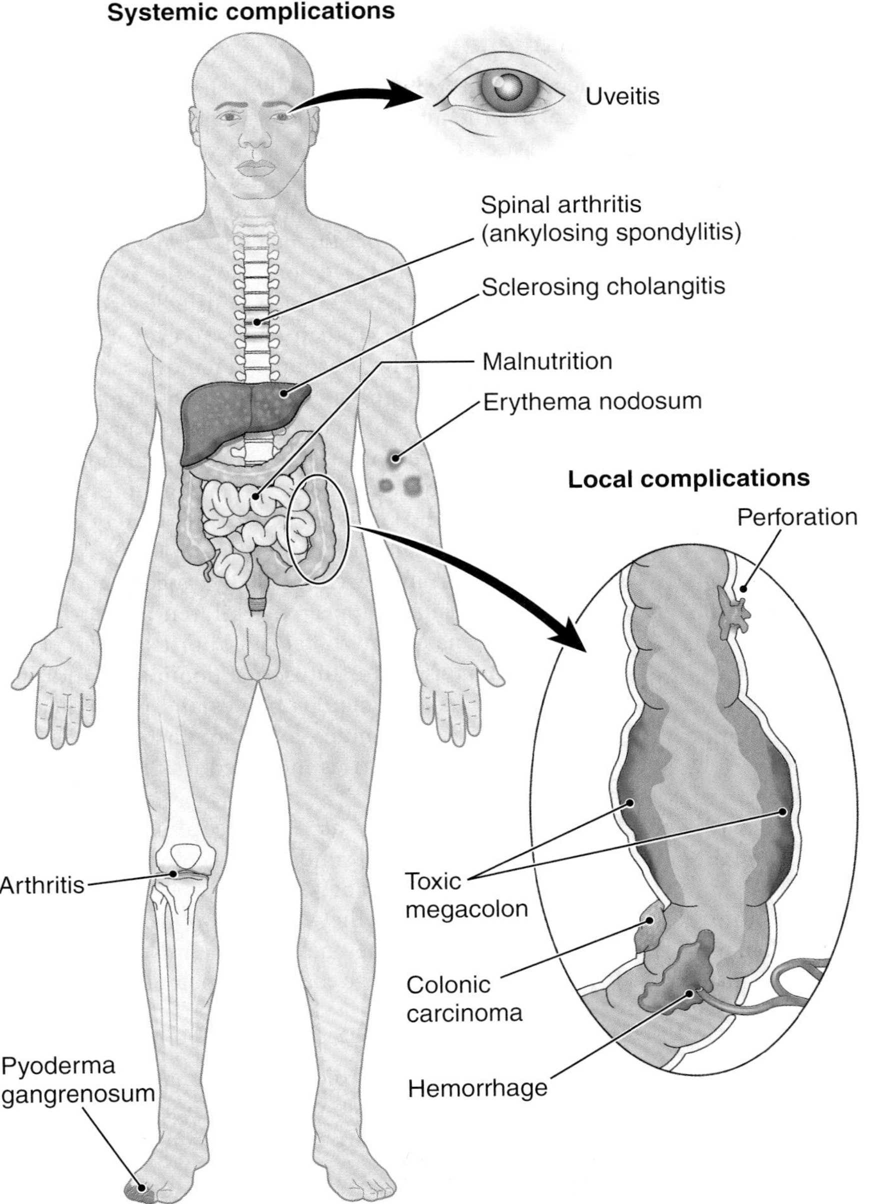

Figure 11.31 **Complications of ulcerative colitis.**

Pop Quiz

11.35 What distinguishes irritable bowel syndrome from other intestinal conditions?

11.36 What is the probable etiology of IBD?

11.37 Which is more often associated with risk for colon cancer: UC or Crohn disease?

11.38 List several extraintestinal manifestations of IBD.

Neoplasms of the Large and Small Bowel

Neoplasms of the small bowel account for <1% of intestinal neoplasms; however, malignant tumors of the colon comprise the second most common cause of cancer death among Americans, exceeded only by lung cancer. Common though they are, colon cancers are far outnumbered by benign growths, many of which are precancerous. This places a premium on early detection and removal of benign neoplasms. Most colonic neoplasms, benign or malignant, protrude into the bowel lumen and can be detected by X-ray imaging or colonoscopy. About 25% can be detected by digital rectal examination, and another sizeable fraction can be detected by simple screening tests for occult blood in stool.

Remember This!

- **Apart from skin, the colon is host to more *neoplasms* (benign and malignant) than any other organ in the body.**
- **Most carcinomas of the colon arise from colonic adenomatous polyps, most of which have been present for about 10–15 years before becoming malignant.**
- **Iron deficiency anemia in an adult male or post-menopausal female should be considered to be due to intestinal bleeding from an intestinal carcinoma until proven otherwise.**

About 20% of colon cancers have an element of genetic predisposition, which is most evident in *familial polyposis syndromes* and *hereditary nonpolyposis colonic carcinoma* (HNPCC), discussed below. Nevertheless, diet is the most important risk factor. Populations with a low-fiber, high-fat diet have a high incidence of colon cancer. Those with a high-fiber, low-fat diet have a low incidence. Experts speculate that fat may interact with intestinal bacteria to produce carcinogens. Certain diseases predispose patients to colon cancer, most notably long-standing UC.

Though much remains unknown, oncogenes, tumor suppressor genes, and apoptosis appear to play an important role. Activation of oncogenes, deletion or inactivation of tumor suppressor genes, and failed apoptosis seem to conspire to produce an overgrowth of epithelium that forms a benign neoplastic polyp. From this point, a "second hit" of abnormal genetic influence appears to transform the benign polyp into a colon cancer.

Non-Neoplastic Polyps Are Not Premalignant

Remember that a **polyp** is merely a shape, a projection of tissue above the mucosa. Polyps occur frequently in the GI tract and are classified according to whether or not they have a stalk (pedunculated or sessile), their microscopic appearance (hyperplastic or adenomatous), and their nature (neoplastic or non-neoplastic; benign, or malignant). They are most common in the colon. Most are asymptomatic except for minor bleeding, which is usually occult. Their clinical importance lies in their ability to evolve into colon cancer. Therefore, early detection and removal is important.

Hamartomatous polyps are rare, non-neoplastic polypoid accumulations of mature but disorganized normal tissue normally present at the site (e.g., glands, blood vessels, smooth muscle). They are one manifestation of several familial syndromes that include a variety of other defects: skin, epithelial, neural and bone lesions; tumors in other organs; increased risk of cancer; and other features. They usually appear in children and are a few centimeters in maximum dimension. For example, *Peutz-Jeghers syndrome* is a rare autosomal dominant syndrome of multiple GI hamartomatous polyps and pigmented lesions of skin and oral mucosa. Although not associated with bowel cancer, it carries increased risk for cancers of many other organs.

Hyperplastic polyps are non-neoplastic accumulations of epithelial cells found in the colonic mucosa of elderly adults. Their etiology is unknown. They are common, about 5 mm, and they are not premalignant. They are significant in that they must not be mistaken for sessile adenomas, which have malignant potential.

Adenomatous Polyps Are Premalignant

Adenomatous polyps (colonic adenomas) are premalignant neoplasms of colonic epithelium (Fig. 11.32). Like colon cancer, they are most prevalent in developed

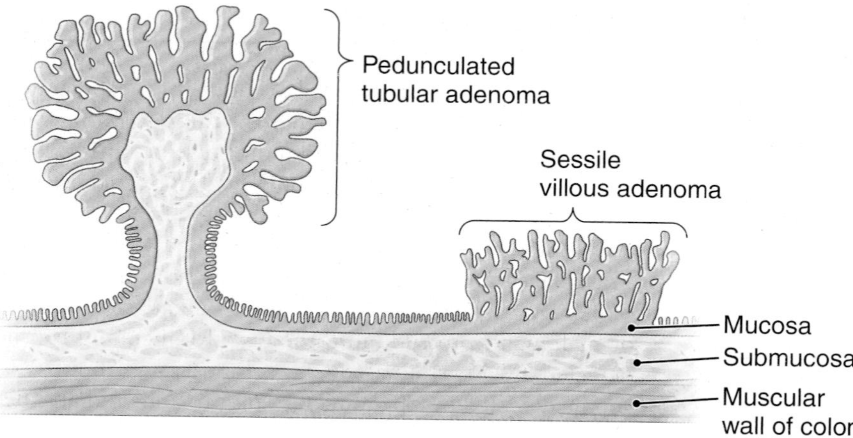

Figure 11.32 **Adenomatous polyps.** Tubular adenomas are usually pedunculated. Villous adenomas are sessile.

nations with low-fiber, high-fat diets. About half of American adults harbor at least one adenomatous polyp. For those over 65, half have two or more. Males are affected slightly more often. The presence of adenomatous polyps in a family member increases risk.

Half of all adenomatous polyps occur in the rectosigmoid colon and can be detected by simple office endoscopy or digital rectal examination. The remaining half are scattered through the remaining colon, a pattern that matches the distribution of colon cancers. They vary from tiny to thumb-size and their epithelium is often dysplastic (Fig. 11.33). It takes 10–15 years, however, for them to become fully malignant and capable of metastasis.

Most adenomas are asymptomatic when small. As they enlarge, they tend to bleed, often subclinically so that bleeding can be detected only by stool analysis for occult blood.

Tubular adenomas (Fig. 11.34) are by far the most common (75%) variety of adenomatous polyp. They typically have a smooth surface, are <2 cm, and have a narrow stalk. Small ones may be sessile or nearly flat, which makes them difficult to see during endoscopy. Microscopically, they are composed of crowded glands. About one-fourth have foci of premalignant dysplasia. Resection is curative. Nevertheless, larger ones may contain invasive adenocarcinoma.

Villous adenomas (Fig. 11.35) are less common (10% of adenomatous polpys) and found mainly in the rectosigmoid. Typically, they are larger than tubular adenomas, have a broad base and a shaggy, fernlike surface composed of finger-like projections of epithelium. Risk of dysplasia and carcinoma rises dramatically with increasing size. One-third contain foci of invasive carcinoma.

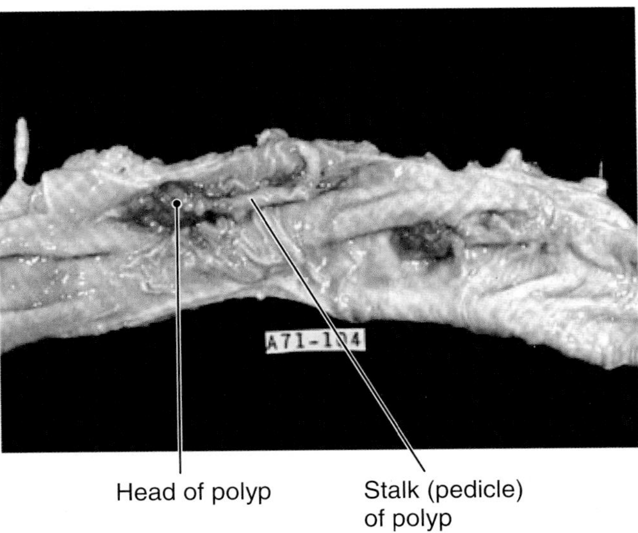

Figure 11.34 Pedunculated tubular adenomas of the colon. These tubular adenomas (adenomatous polyps) have unusually long pedicles.

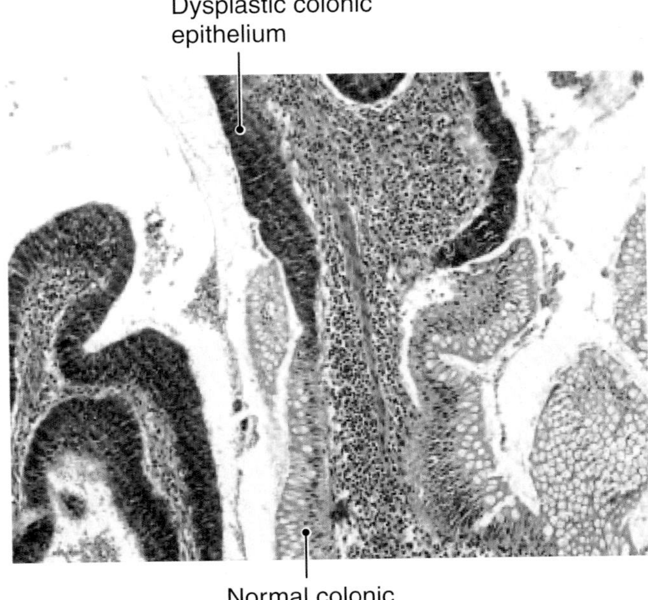

Figure 11.33 Dysplastic (premalignant) change in the epithelium of a colonic adenoma. Dysplastic cells have large, dark nuclei and have lost their ability to make mucin.

Tubulovillous adenomas (15%) have tubular and villous components and have intermediate risk of dysplasia and invasive carcinoma.

Familial Adenomatous Polyposis Always Leads to Colon Cancer

Familial adenomatous polyposis (FAP) syndrome (FAP, Fig. 11.36) is an uncommon autosomal dominant disorder that develops in teenagers with a defect in the APC gene (long arm, chromosome 5). A minimum of 100 polyps is necessary to diagnose FAP; however, thousands may

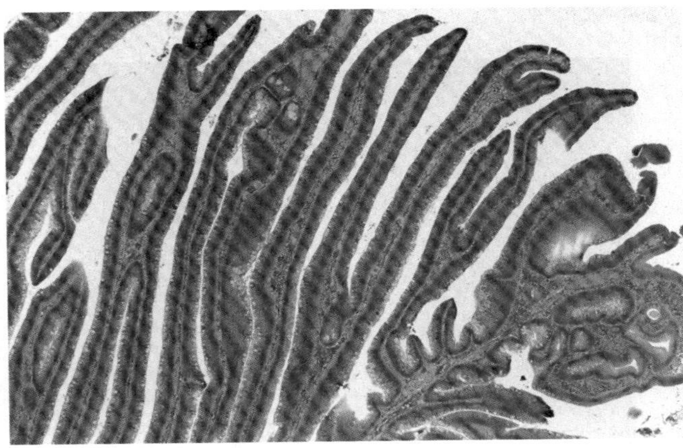

Figure 11.35 Villous adenoma. These are sessile adenomas with long, fern-like fronds. (Reproduced with permission from Mulholland MW, Maier RV, et al. *Greenfield's Surgery Scientific Principles and Practice*. 4th ed. Philadelphia (PA): Lippincott Williams & Wilkins; 2006.)

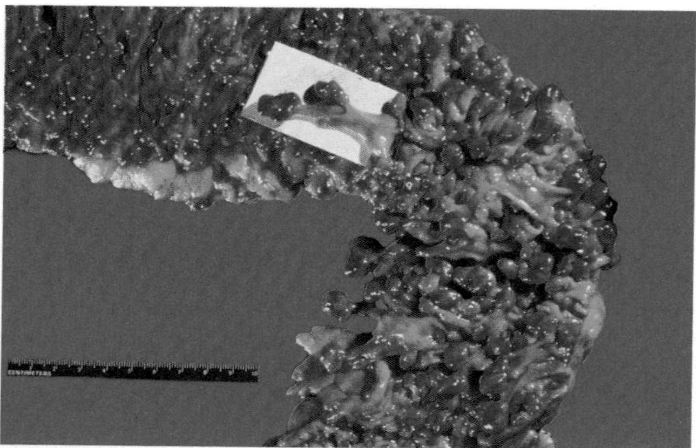

Figure 11.36 **Familial adenomatous polyposis syndrome.** A minimum of 100 polyps must be present. (Reproduced with permission from Mulholland MW, Maier RV, et al. *Greenfield's Surgery Scientific Principles and Practice*. 4th ed. Philadelphia (PA): Lippincott Williams & Wilkins; 2006.)

be present. Microscopically, they are identical to sporadic adenomatous polyps. Left untreated, 100% of those with FAP will develop colon cancer, often before age 30. Treatment is total colectomy. Extraintestinal manifestations are common and provide clues to early diagnosis: darkly pigmented retina, osteomas of the mandible and long bones, extra teeth and other dental abnormalities, and benign skin tumors and cysts.

Colon Cancer Is the Second Most Common Cause of Cancer Death

Almost all **colon carcinomas** are adenocarcinomas: gland-forming malignant neoplasms of colon epithelial cells.

The American Cancer Society estimated that in 2013 153,000 Americans would develop colon cancer and 51,000 would die of it, making it second only to lung cancer as the most common cause of cancer death. The tragedy behind this statistic is that most of these deaths could have been avoided with timely screening and excision of precancerous lesions.

Pathology and Pathogenesis

Colon cancer does not leap into being in an instant. Years before development of an invasive malignancy, the colonic epithelium becomes progressively abnormal, usually in the form of an adenomatous polyp, which then becomes dysplastic and passes through a stage of carcinoma in situ before becoming invasive.

The distribution of colon cancers is similar to the distribution of adenomatous polyps—nearly half are in the rectosigmoid colon within easy reach during an office visit. Nevertheless, growth patterns vary. Tumors in the right (ascending) colon tend to be exophytic, bulky masses that protrude into the lumen (Fig. 11.37A). Those in the left (descending) colon and rectosigmoid colon are more likely to be dense and constrict the lumen like a napkin-ring (Fig. 11.37B). Their microscopic appearance is similar.

Colon carcinomas grow by direct extension through the bowel wall and spread beyond the colon by invasion of lymphatics and blood vessels. The most common sites of metastasis are lymph nodes, liver (via the portal circulation), lungs, and bones. About one-third of cases are beyond cure at the time of initial diagnosis.

Hereditary nonpolyposis colorectal carcinoma syndrome (*HNPCC* or *Lynch syndrome*) accounts for about 3%–5% of colon cancers. It is an autosomal dominant genetic disorder characterized by colon cancer and cancer in multiple other organs. Colon cancers in HNPCC are not preceded by formation of adenomatous polyps. HNPCC colon cancers arise at an earlier age than sporadic colon cancers. Most occur in the right (ascending) colon.

Signs and Symptoms

Early colon cancer is asymptomatic. Many, if not most, cases have a poor prognosis by the time they bleed visibly, cause abdominal pain from obstruction or perforation, or

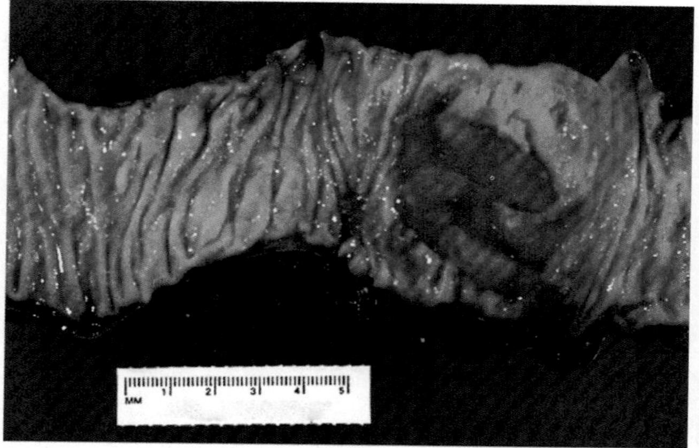

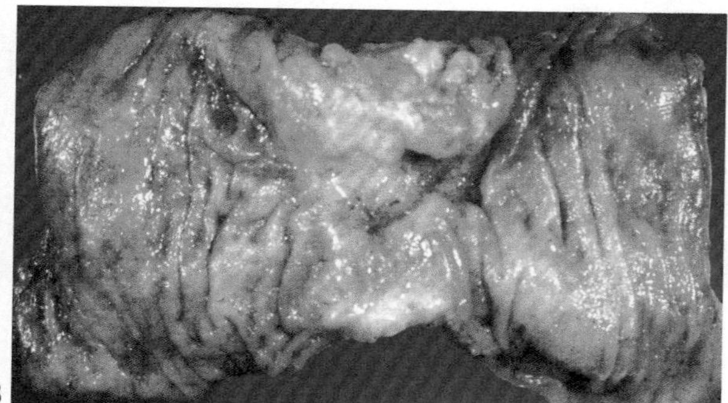

Figure 11.37 **Carcinoma of the colon. A.** Carcinomas of the right (ascending) colon tend to be bulky masses that protrude into the lumen. **B.** Carcinomas of the left (descending colon) tend to be constricting, "napkin ring" growths.

cause other symptoms. Despite readily available methods for early detection (digital rectal exam, stool occult blood test, office endoscopy) most colon cancers go undetected for a long time. Cancers in the ascending colon tend to bleed slowly and may be discovered only because of fatigue and listlessness due to iron deficiency anemia. For this reason, careful practitioners rely on this rule: *iron deficiency anemia in an adult male or postmenopausal female is intestinal carcinoma until proven otherwise*. Cancers in the descending or sigmoid colon may also remain asymptomatic and bleed slowly, but are more likely to produce visible bleeding, altered bowel habits, including small stools and a feeling of incomplete bowel movements, and left lower quadrant discomfort and cramping.

Diagnosis and Treatment

The ideal screening test for any disease is inexpensive, sensitive (few false negatives), and capable of detecting a serious but potentially curable disease. The fecal occult blood test (FOBT) fits two of these criteria: it costs a few dollars and screens for a deadly but completely curable disease. Although a single FOBT is not very sensitive, when performed annually over a 10-year period, the test will detect about half of colon cancers and reduce colon cancer deaths by about 30%. Nevertheless, this leaves many curable tumors undiagnosed. The U.S. Preventive Services Task Force recommends that adults aged 50–74 years be screened in one of the following ways:

- Every year with FOBT and once every 10 years with colonoscopy
- Every 5 years with FOBT plus sigmoidoscopy

These exams will detect the majority of polyps and cancers. For some people with risk factors, screening begins at age 40.

Surgery with hope of cure is possible in about 70% of patients. Chemotherapy increases survival in patients with lymph node metastases.

Complications and Prognosis

The most important prognostic factor in colorectal carcinoma is the clinical stage of the neoplasm at the time of diagnosis. The current accepted scheme is that of the American Joint Committee on Cancer (AJCC). It follows the tumor, nodes, metastasis (TNM) method widely in use to stage other cancers and is detailed in Table 11.3 and Figure 11.38.

Other Tumors of the Gastrointestinal Tract Are Uncommon

Carcinoid tumor is a rare neoplasm of mature adults that arises from neuroendocrine cells. About half arise in the small bowel and another quarter in the appendix. A few arise in the tracheobronchial tree. Most are benign, many discovered incidentally; however, some are locally invasive and a few metastasize.

Although made up of neuroendocrine cells, most carcinoids are endocrinologically inert. Only a few produce hormones. The type of hormone depends on the site of origin. For example, gastric carcinoids can secrete gastrin and give rise to Zollinger-Ellison syndrome, mentioned earlier in this chapter. *Carcinoid syndrome* develops in about 10% of cases, usually in patients with metastatic tumor. It is due to release of vasoactive substances and features skin flushing, abdominal pain, and diarrhea. Diagnosis is by clinical picture, detection of a mass, and by detection of hormone products in urine. Treatment is surgical excision. For malignant tumors, the average survival interval is 10–15 years.

Table 11.3 *Staging Colorectal Cancer*

Stage	Tumor Maximum Penetration	Regional Lymph Node Metastasis	Distant Metastasis	Five Year Survival
0	Carcinoma in situ	No nodal metastasis	None	100%
I	Tumor confined to mucosa	No nodal metastasis	None	93%
II	Tumor penetrates all layers of colonic wall	No nodal metastasis	None	72–85%
III	Any tumor *not* invading beyond colon **or** Any tumor invading beyond colon	Any nodal metastasis **or** No nodal metastasis	None None	44–83%
IV	Any tumor	With or without nodal metastasis	Any site	8%

Source: Slightly modified and substantially abbreviated from American Joint Committee on Cancer, AJCC, 7th edition, 2010.

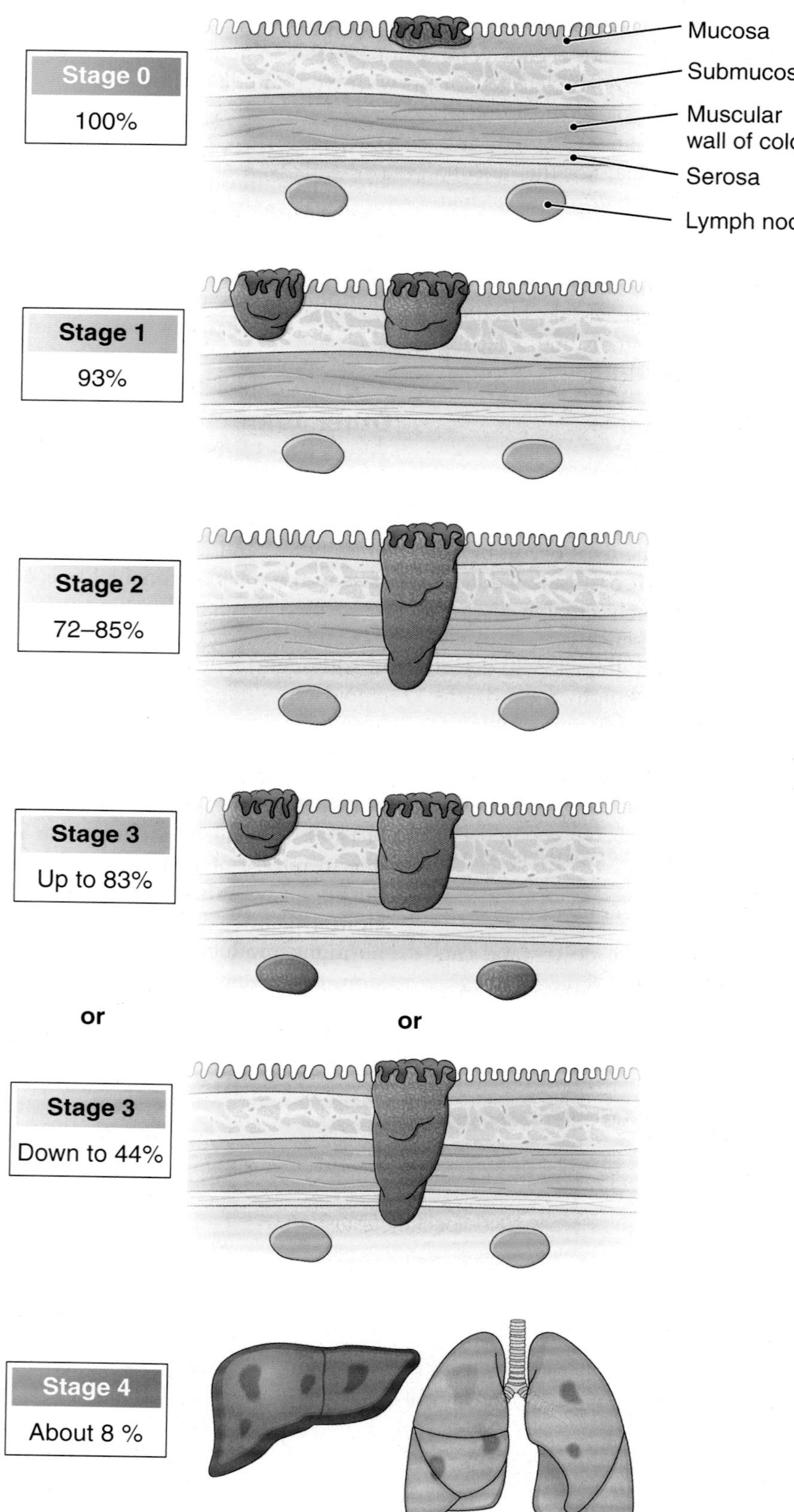

Figure 11.38 **AJCC staging system for colonic carcinoma.** Approximate five-year survival figures for each stage. Table 11.3 describes the degree of tumor invasion and spread that characterize each of the stages.

Gastrointestinal stromal tumors (GIST) are tumors of the GI tract derived from mesenchymal precursor cells in the intestinal wall. About half arise in the stomach. The average patient is about 50–60 years old. GIST are caused by mutations of a growth factor receptor gene, although some owe to previous radiation therapy to the abdomen for another tumor. They grow slowly and may be locally aggressive or frankly malignant. Most are discovered because of the effect of a tumor mass. Symptoms vary with location but include bleeding, pain, and obstruction. Diagnosis is usually by endoscopic biopsy of the mass. Treatment is surgical removal. The effectiveness of radiation and chemotherapy is not established, but biological drugs appear promising (see *Molecular Medicine*, "Hired Guns to Fight Inflammation: The New Biologicals").

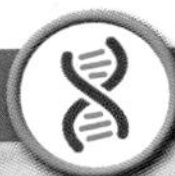

Molecular Medicine

HIRED GUNS TO FIGHT INFLAMMATION: THE NEW BIOLOGICALS

Corticosteroids have long been used to treat inflammatory conditions, but new, more targeted therapies are being developed to treat these diseases. A new class of drugs called *biologicals* are actually antibodies that can bind to very specific targets. They derive their name from the fact that they are produced not by chemistry but by biological processes. For example, tumor necrosis factor (TNF) is a soluble protein that promotes inflammation. Anti-TNF drugs are antibodies that bind to and inactivate TNF and are being used to treat IBD. Other targeted biological drugs are being developed to treat other inflammatory diseases and certain cancers.

Pop Quiz

11.39 True or false? All colonic polyps are neoplastic.

11.40 Which is more likely to proceed to malignancy: tubular adenoma or villous adenoma?

11.41 True or false? All adenomatous polyps are premalignant.

11.42 True or false? Hyperplastic polyps are not premalignant.

11.43 What lesion precedes most colon cancers?

11.44 True or false? Colon cancer is the number one cancer killer in the United States.

11.45 True or false? A single FOBT will detect most colon cancers.

11.46 What percentage of adenomatous polyps and colon cancers occur in the rectosigmoid colon?

11.47 About how long does it take for an adenomatous polyp to evolve into colonic carcinoma?

11.48 What type of cells give rise to GIST tumors?

11.49 What is the triad of symptoms seen in patients with carcinoid syndrome?

Case Notes

11.14 **How was Melanie's case typical of Crohn disease?**

11.15 **How was Melanie's case not typical of Crohn?**

11.16 **What was the clinical stage of Melanie's colonic carcinoma? Stage III.**

Colonic Diverticulosis and Anorectal Conditions

A *diverticulum* is a blind pouch with a mouth opening onto the lumen of a space, in this instance the colon. *Congenital* colonic diverticula are rare and represent a blind pouch of normal colon protruding to one side. In contrast, *acquired* diverticula are very common.

Diverticulosis Can Lead to Diverticulitis

Colonic diverticulosis (Fig. 11.39) is characterized by multiple, small, outward protrusions of colonic mucosa through the muscular wall that arise at the weak points where small blood vessels penetrate from the external surface. They are usually found incidentally during colonoscopy or barium enema imaging study. They occur mainly in populations with a low-fiber diet (developed nations), and are rare in people who eat a high-fiber diet. They are uncommon before age 30, but by age 60 are present in at least half of the population in developed nations. They are found almost exclusively in the sigmoid colon, presumably from straining

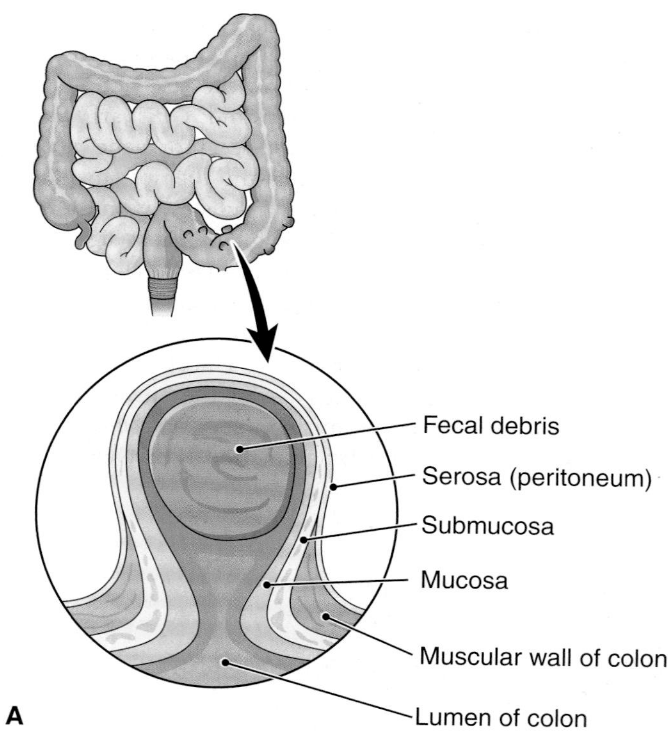

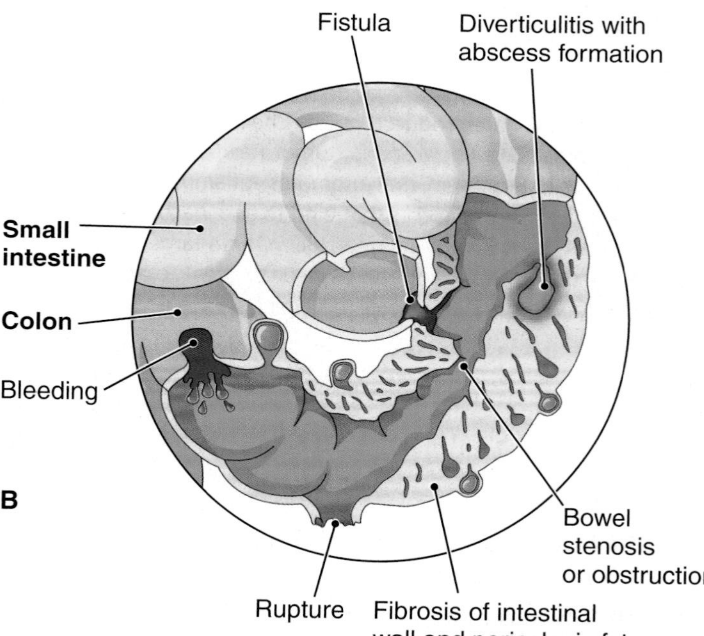

Figure 11.39 **Colonic diverticulosis and diverticulitis. A.** Detail of the anatomy of an acquired diverticulum. **B.** Complications of diverticular inflammation (diverticulitis).

to pass compacted stool, as is common with a low-fiber diet. Most are asymptomatic and are discovered incidentally at autopsy, during colorectal endoscopy, or by colon X-ray studies. Treatment is not necessary unless diverticulitis occurs.

Diverticulitis is an inflamed diverticulum. Colonic diverticula typically trap feces and seeds or other indigestible matter, which over time irritate the diverticulum, promote inflammation, and allow intestinal bacteria to invade through the thin wall of the pouch (Fig. 11.40). Diverticulitis is characterized by fever and low, left-side abdominal pain. Perforation into the abdominal space can produce peritonitis. Other complications include hemorrhage, abscess, fistulous connections to small bowel loops or bladder, colonic stenosis, and the formation of inflammatory masses that clinically mimic colonic carcinoma.

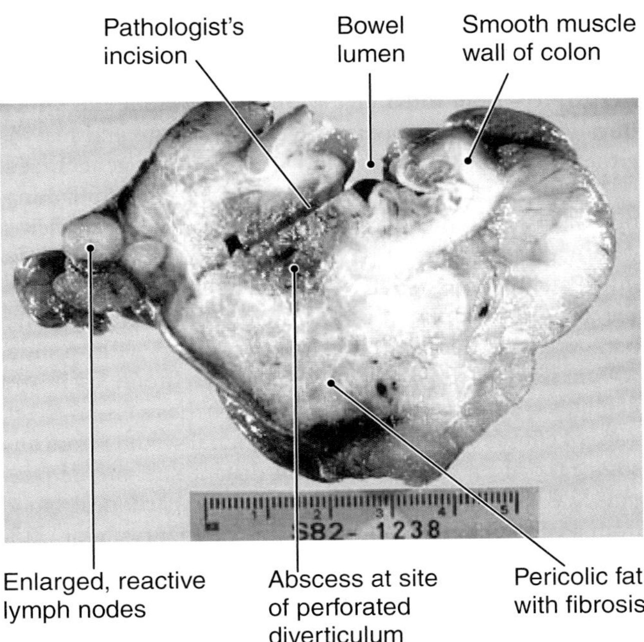

Figure 11.40 **Acute and chronic diverticulitis.** In this cross-section of the colon, the opened bowel lumen appears at top center. The pathologist's incision extends from the lumen into an abscess that has obliterated the diverticulum. Fibrosis in pericolic fat is evidence of long-standing inflammation.

Clinical suspicion should be high in patients with known diverticula. Abdominal imaging studies are usually conclusive, though exploratory surgery may be necessary when the cause of abdominal pain and fever is unclear. Treatment includes a high-fiber diet. Most bleeding stops spontaneously, but persistent bleeding may require surgical or angiographic hemostasis. Severe cases may require surgical drainage or excision of the affected segment. For acute cases, liquid diet and broad spectrum antibiotic therapy is usually sufficient. Patients also should be encouraged to increase dietary fiber.

Anorectal Conditions Are Common

Hemorrhoids are common and were discussed earlier. An **anal fissure** is a longitudinal tear in the anal mucosa. Almost all arise from straining to pass large, hard stools. They can be quite painful, but usually heal quickly and without therapy. Nevertheless, they may bleed. Blood from an anal fissure is bright red and appears on toilet tissue or the surface of stool.

An **anorectal abscess** usually forms in an *anal crypt*. Crypts are tiny mucosal pouches containing glands that secrete mucus to lubricate fecal passage. They sit at the squamocolumnar junction where the squamous epithelium of the anal canal meets the glandular epithelium of the rectum. Anorectal abscess arise from bacterial invasion of the wall of the crypt pouch. Signs and symptoms include a painful mass that may be deep or superficial. Surgical drainage is required.

An **anal fistula** is a tubular tract from the anus to some other surface, usually perianal skin. They may form from an abscess or de novo. Signs and symptoms include a painful swelling and an opening to skin (or interior surface, such as bladder mucosa). Surgery is usually required.

Pilonidal cyst (*pilonidal sinus*) is a cyst, pit, or blind pouch in the midline skin posterior to the anus near the coccyx, which occurs almost exclusively in young, hirsute, white males. The cause is not known. They are prone to become irritated or infected and form an acute abscess or chronically infected, draining sinus tract. A pilonidal cyst is typically palpable and quite painful, especially when the patient is seated. Antibiotic therapy and local heat may offer relief but surgical drainage and excision is often required. These cysts have a tendency to recur.

Proctitis is inflammation of the anal mucosa. IBD, infection, and radiation are common causes. Infectious proctitis is often sexually transmitted. The condition is more common in immunocompromised patients. Radiation proctitis may follow radiotherapy for prostate cancer in men or pelvic cancer in women. Pain and bleeding are common symptoms. Diagnosis may require endoscopic biopsy and culture. Treatment depends on etiology.

Pop Quiz

11.50 True or false? Most colonic diverticula occur in the transverse colon.

11.51 Are colonic diverticula more likely to be single or multiple?

Diseases of the Appendix and Peritoneum

The appendix is a finger-size blind pouch arising from the cecum. It has no apparent function, but nevertheless looms large in medical practice because the differential diagnosis of acute appendicitis is difficult, requiring consideration of a very broad range of acute medical and surgical conditions.

Appendicitis Is Inflammation of the Appendix

Acute appendicitis is acute inflammation of the appendix (Fig. 11.41). It is the most common cause of acute abdominal pain requiring surgery—at some point 5% or more of the population will have appendicitis. Teenagers

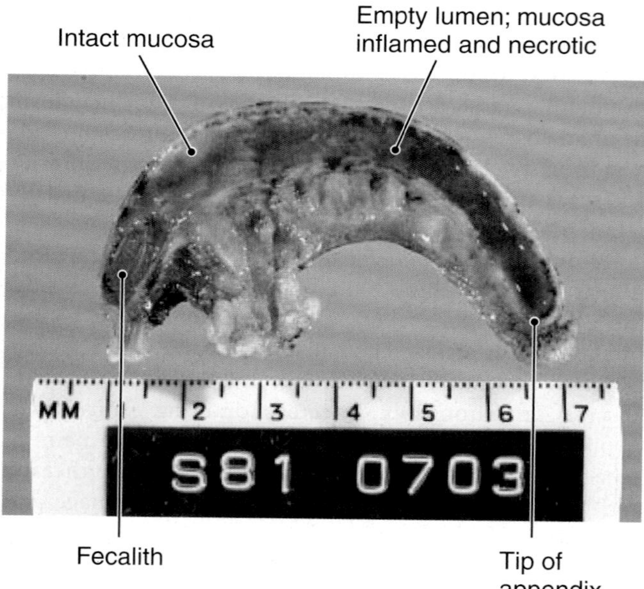

Figure 11.41 **Acute appendicitis.** A fecalith is wedged into the mouth of the appendix (left).

and young adults are most often affected. The appendix may also be affected by IBD and tumors.

Most cases are presumed to be due to obstruction of the lumen by hyperplasia of lymphoid (MALT) patches in the mucosa. Impacted feces (*fecalith*, Fig. 11.41), a foreign body, or intestinal parasitic worms also may be responsible, but often no anatomic cause can be identified. As pressure increases behind the obstruction, blood flow into the appendix is hindered and edema, ischemia, necrosis, and bacterial overgrowth follow. Necrosis, gangrene, and perforation may occur.

Classic appendicitis begins as epigastric or periumbilical pain followed by nausea, vomiting, and anorexia. In a few hours, pain shifts to the right lower quadrant. Pain intensifies with cough and motion. Low-grade fever is common.

Unfortunately, this classic presentation occurs in <50% of patients. Some cases may be silent, especially in the elderly or debilitated. The differential diagnosis includes other causes of abdominal pain such as fallopian tube infection, ectopic pregnancy, and the low abdominal pain normally associated with ovulation. Because signs and symptoms vary widely, and because delay of surgical intervention risks the very serious hazard of rupture and peritonitis, it is accepted that 10%–20% of abdominal surgery for presumptive appendicitis will find some other disease process or nothing. Appendicitis is a surgical emergency; however, for patients without access to surgery, antibiotic therapy is usually lifesaving. Without surgery or antibiotics, mortality is >50%.

Peritonitis Is Inflammation of the Peritoneum

Peritonitis is an inflammation of the peritoneum, which lines the abdominal cavity. It is usually acute and may be either infectious or sterile, and either local or generalized.

Peritonitis can develop as an extension from inflammation of any abdominal or pelvic organ, such as appendicitis, diverticulitis, pancreatitis, or salpingitis. *Infectious* peritonitis usually arises as a result of bacteria escaping through the wall of some part of the GI tract, as for example with a perforated gastric ulcer or acute appendicitis with rupture. Ascitic fluid in the abdomen, especially chronic ascites in debilitated patients (as with alcoholic cirrhosis) is, in effect, a sac of culture media that awaits bacterial seeding from any source, local or via blood from a distant site. *Sterile* peritonitis is due to chemical irritation. Intraperitoneal blood from any source (e.g., trauma, ruptured aneurysm, or ectopic pregnancy) is irritating and causes peritonitis. In acute pancreatitis, digestive enzymes may be spilled into the peritoneum where they incite a severe inflammatory reaction.

In most cases of peritonitis, the inflammation is acute—a purulent inflammatory exudate spreads throughout the abdomen. Healed peritonitis leaves bands of fibrous scar tissue (*adhesions*) that may later cause intestinal obstruction by trapping loops of bowel.

Peritonitis features abdominal pain, tenderness, and spasm of abdominal muscles to form a rigid abdominal wall. The differential diagnosis of peritonitis is difficult because abdominal pain is among the most difficult challenges in medical diagnosis and beyond the scope of this textbook. Treatment depends upon the cause and is as varied as the causes.

Peritoneal Carcinomatosis Usually Arises from Abdominal Malignancies

Carcinomas of abdominal or pelvic viscera may spread widely on the surface of the peritoneum to cause a secondary form of cancer called **peritoneal carcinomatosis**. It is a common complication of abdominal malignancy. In some cases, however, no primary site can be identified and the tumor is presumed to arise de novo from peritoneum. The condition is common in patients with ovarian or pancreatic cancer. Abdominal aching, cramping, and bloating due to fluid accumulation are all common indicators.

Pop Quiz

11.52 What are the three features of peritonitis?

11.53 True or false? Most appendicitis begins with obstruction of the lumen.

Case Study Revisited

"Her intestines are acting much worse this time." The case of Melanie K.

Melanie first became ill at age 21 with a chronic ailment characterized by intestinal symptoms: fever, diarrhea, abdominal pain, and bloody stools. Lack of international travel and negative stool cultures excluded infection. Fever and bloody stools exclude the possibility of IBS because IBS is purely a functional disease without objective laboratory or physical abnormalities.

Age, a relative with a chronic intestinal ailment, the presence of arthritis with flare-ups, and the chronic nature of the illness suggested IBD. X-ray studies showed disease mainly in her small bowel. A diagnosis of Crohn IBD was made but biopsy proof was lacking until her surgery five years later.

At the time of her hospitalization five years later, she was anemic (low hemoglobin and hematocrit) and suffering from nutritional deficiency (low blood protein). The anemia can be explained by chronic blood loss from intestinal bleeding that depleted iron stores more rapidly than they could be replenished by diet. Also, bowel disease could have interfered with iron absorption. Low serum iron confirmed the diagnosis of iron deficiency anemia. Low blood protein could be due to inadequate diet or epithelial phase malabsorption of nutrients due to mucosal inflammation. Both are probably responsible. Low body mass index confirms the suspicion of malnutrition.

Surgery produced proof of Crohn disease in the pathology specimen. The full thickness of the bowel wall was inflamed. By contrast, UC involves only the mucosa. That a fistula was present and inflammation spread to pelvic organs and peritoneum was also consistent with Crohn disease.

The big surprise in this case was an adenocarcinoma of the colon (cecum). Though not unheard of in Crohn, it would not have been a surprise if she had UC. In retrospect, the degree of rectal bleeding was a clue that something else was going on. Rectal bleeding is much more common in UC, but in this case was easily explained by bleeding from the colon cancer.

Chapter Challenge

CHAPTER RECALL

1. The myenteric plexus is contained within which of the following?
   A. Mucosa
   B. Submucosa
   C. Serosa
   D. Muscularis propria
2. Which of the following statements regarding the bacteria in the GI system are true?
   A. They produce vitamin K, but not folic acid.
   B. They serve no purpose in GI immunity.
   C. They outnumber the body's own cells 5–1.
   D. When the flora is altered by antibiotics, it can lead to diarrhea.
3. Concerning aphthous oral ulcers, which is true?
   A. They are associated with periodontitis.
   B. The cause is unknown.
   C. They are caused by herpesvirus.
   D. They are caused by *Candida.*
4. Which of the following is a condition that involves the stomach?
   A. Peptic ulcer
   B. Malabsorption syndrome causing steatorrhea
   C. *Clostridium difficile* ulceration
   D. Crohn disease
5. Which of the following is associated with an increased risk of esophageal carcinoma?
   A. *Candida* infection
   B. Herpesvirus infection
   C. Achalasia
   D. Hiatal hernia
6. Which of the following is a cause of luminal phase malabsorption syndrome?
   A. Chronic pancreatitis
   B. Gluten-sensitive enteropathy (celiac sprue)
   C. Whipple disease
   D. Tropical sprue

7. Which of the following is a cause of ileus?
   A. Postoperative state after abdominal surgery
   B. Hypokalemia
   C. Intestinal ischemia
   D. All of the above

8. A telescoping of bowel, in which the distal segment swallows the proximal one, is best known as which of the following?
   A. Intussusception
   B. Hernia
   C. Volvulus
   D. Ileus

9. True or false? There are objective findings in IBS.

10. True or false? Diverticula are thin outpouchings of the mucosa, submucosa, and muscle.

11. True or false? *Helicobacter pylori* infection is the most common cause of chronic gastritis and peptic ulcer disease.

12. True or false? Carcinoma of the colon kills more people annually than breast cancer.

13. True or false? The facial nerve passes through the parotid and can be damaged during removal of even benign adenomas.

14. True or false? Most peptic ulcers occur in the stomach or duodenum.

15. Match the following diseases with their causative agents:
   i. Shigella
   ii. Rotavirus
   iii. *Enterotoxigenic* Escherichia coli (ETEC)
   iv. Enterohemorrhagic Escherichia coli (EHEC)
   v. Entamoeba histolytica
   A. The leading cause of diarrhea in children
   B. Bloody *bacillary dysentery*
   C. May spread to liver via portal vein to produce hepatic amebic abscesses
   D. Traveler's diarrhea
   E. Hemorrhagic colitis transmitted by undercooked ground beef

16. Match the following hormones with their actions:
   i. Gastrin
   ii. Gastric Inhibitory peptide
   iii. Cholecystokinin
   iv. Pepsinogen
   v. Secretin
   A. Zymogen converted to active form to digest protein
   B. Stimulates secretion of hydrochloric acid
   C. Stimulates release of insulin by pancreatic islands of Langerhans
   D. Stimulates release of bicarbonate from pancreas to neutralize acidic chyme
   E. Stimulates secretion of pancreatic enzymes and release of bile from gallbladder

17. What type of bleeding would you expect in the case of hemorrhoids?
   A. Melena
   B. Hematemesis
   C. Hematochezia
   D. None of the above

18. Which of the following is the first-line treatment of primary GI (MALT) lymphomas?
   A. Surgery
   B. Chemotherapy
   C. Radiation
   D. Antibiotics

CONCEPTUAL UNDERSTANDING

19. After receiving antibiotics to treat his bladder infection, your patient begins complaining of diarrhea. What test do you order to confirm your suspicions, and what happened to cause his diarrhea?

20. Your brother calls you to ask about his stomach pain. He tells you it began a few hours ago around his umbilicus, but now the pain is in his right lower quadrant. He also complains of nausea, vomiting, and a fever. Why is surgery the right choice in treating him?

APPLICATION

21. Discuss the following precursor lesions and their role in malignancy.
   A. Leukoplakia
   B. Barrett esophagus
   C. *H. pylori* and chronic gastritis
   D. Polyps

22. Describe the pathogenesis of Hirschsprung disease, and how it is treated.

23. Compare and contrast Crohn disease and UC and name some of their extraintestinal manifestations.

CHAPTER

12

Disorders of the Liver and Biliary Tract

Contents

Chapter Objectives

After studying this chapter, you should be able to complete the following tasks:

THE NORMAL LIVER

1. Explain the function and structure of the liver circulatory systems.

THE LIVER RESPONSE TO INJURY

2. Discuss the complications associated with liver injury.

VIRAL HEPATITIS

3. Compare and contrast the transmission route, incubation time, clinicopathologic syndromes associated with, and diagnostic findings of HAV, HBV, and HCV, and briefly comment on the clinical significance of infection with HDV and HEV.

NON-VIRAL INFLAMMATORY LIVER DISEASE

4. Name the nonviral causes of inflammatory liver disease.

TOXIC LIVER INJURY

5. Using examples from the text, compare and contrast dose- and nondose-related liver reaction; briefly discuss Reye syndrome.
6. Describe the acute and chronic changes induced in the liver by alcohol abuse.

METABOLIC LIVER DISEASE

7. Discuss the etiology of metabolic liver disease, distinguishing nonalcoholic fatty liver disease, hemochromatosis, Wilson disease, and Alpha-1 antitrypsin deficiency from one another, and identify the signs/symptoms, diagnosis, treatment, and complications of each as applicable.

DISEASE OF INTRAHEPATIC BILE DUCTS

8. Compare and contrast secondary biliary cirrhosis with primary biliary cirrhosis and sclerosing cholangitis.

CIRCULATORY DISORDERS

9. Name the causes of prehepatic, intrahepatic, and posthepatic obstruction of blood flow.

TUMORS OF THE LIVER

10. List the tumors that can arise in the liver.

DISORDERS OF THE GALLBLADDER AND EXTRAHEPATIC BILE DUCTS

11. Describe the etiologies, risk factors, symptoms, and complications of extrahepatic bile duct obstruction.

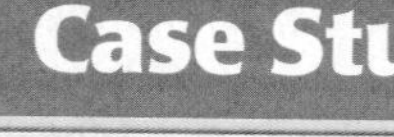

"I didn't give it a second thought." The case of Ling C.

Chief Complaint: Increased liver enzymes in blood

Clinical History: Ling C. was a 58-year-old banker referred to the office of a liver disease specialist. The entry on her appointment sheet says "Hepatitis C?"

The patient was asymptomatic, but when she was 28 years old, she gave birth via Caesarian section and required transfusion of two units of packed RBCs. About two months later, she experienced an episode of yellow skin, dark urine, pale stools, anorexia, nausea, and vomiting, with vague right upper abdominal discomfort. An infectious disease specialist told her that she had "non-A, non-B" hepatitis. She was ill for several weeks, but after three months was told she was completely recovered and discharged from care.

"I didn't give it a second thought," she added. "After it was all over, I felt completely normal." Her current medical episode began during a change of employment when she took an insurance physical examination that revealed mildly increased levels of liver enzymes in her blood. Complete blood count (CBC), urinalysis, and other blood chemistries were unremarkable.

Further questioning revealed that she was employed full time and led an active life, but admitted to periods of fatigue and "the blues." She had not needed to see a physician in many years except for her annual gynecologic exam. She denied using intravenous drugs or having sex with anyone but her husband. She said her alcohol intake was an occasional cocktail at a social event and a glass of wine now and then with dinner. She proudly said, "I've never smoked a cigarette." In college she "experimented" with marijuana but never injected drugs. She was not taking any medication except a daily multivitamin.

Physical Examination and Other Data: Ling appeared her stated age and was articulate and cooperative. She was very anxious about what might be wrong. Vital signs and physical examination were unremarkable. Neither liver nor spleen could be palpated. No jaundice was noted. Her skin showed no evidence of spider angiomata, palmar erythema, or bruises. She did not have hemorrhoids. A vaginal examination was not performed. The blood studies showed mild increases of liver enzymes and the presence of HCV-RNA and anti-Hbc antibody. No autoantibodies were present. Hemoglobin, hematocrit, bilirubin, alkaline phosphatase (AP), lipids, iron, and proteins were normal.

Clinical Course: She was informed that she had chronic hepatitis C infection that she very likely contracted from her postpartum blood transfusion 30 years earlier. She refused the offer of a liver biopsy but agreed to interferon therapy, which was administered intravenously three times a week for a year. She tolerated treatment well and had no side effects. At the conclusion of therapy, liver enzymes were normal, and HCV-RNA was no longer detectable. Follow-up laboratory studies remained normal for two years after therapy, and she was discharged back to the care of her usual physician.

Two of every three deaths are premature; they are related to the loafer's heart, smoker's lung and drinker's liver.

DR. THOMAS J. BASSLER, PATHOLOGIST; QUOTED BY JAMES FIXX IN THE COMPLETE BOOK OF RUNNING (RANDOM HOUSE, 1977)

The liver is a metabolic powerhouse because of the variety of its tasks and the volume of product it processes. To perform these tasks the liver must be large, and it is: by weight it is the largest of the viscera. It must also be richly supplied with blood, and it is: through the portal vein it receives all blood leaving the intestine, which filters through the liver for processing before flowing into the vena cava. It also receives an abundance of arterial blood from the aorta.

The Normal Liver

Figure 12.1 illustrates the anatomy of the liver, bile ducts, and portal venous system. The **portal venous system** gains its name from the liver acting as a gate (a portal) through which blood must pass before entering the general circulation: venous blood goes from one capillary system (the intestine) and passes upward through the **portal vein** through a second capillary system (the liver) and then flows into the hepatic vein and the inferior vena cava. The liver also receives arterial blood from the hepatic artery. This oxygenated blood bathes hepatocytes then merges with portal venous blood for return to the general circulation.

Because of the portal venous system, nutrients absorbed by the intestine do not enter the general circulation directly. Carbohydrates and proteins first flow to the liver via the portal vein. Fat-bearing chylomicrons are absorbed not into blood but into intestinal lymphatics, which flow up the thoracic duct and empty into the left subclavian vein.

Case Notes

12.1 We presume Ling C's hepatic and intestinal anatomy was normal. What blood vessel connects her intestines to her liver?

The Liver Is a Ducted Gland Organized into Lobules

Upon entering the portal circulation, blood and freshly absorbed nutrients are brought into close contact with the main functional cells of the liver (**hepatocytes**). Liver cells are formed into plates one or two cells thick that are sandwiched between large venous capillaries (**hepatic sinusoids**). Hepatic sinusoids have no basement membrane and are therefore much more permeable than other capillaries, so that even large protein and lipid molecules cross freely. Venous sinusoid walls contain fixed macrophages known as **Kupffer cells**, which, unlike other macrophages, do not move about but remain in place to filter portal blood.

The plates of hepatic cells are arranged into **hepatic lobules** (Fig. 12.1B). In the middle of each lobule is a **central vein** surrounded by hepatocytes. Woven into the lobules are tiny **bile canaliculi**, which coalesce into small **bile ducts** at the periphery of the lobule. The corners of each lobule are defined by several **portal triads** consisting of 1) a branch of the hepatic artery bringing blood from the aorta, 2) a portal vein carrying blood from the GI tract, and 3) a small bile duct that carries bile out of the liver. Blood entering the lobule from the hepatic artery and portal vein flows into venous sinusoids, percolates through hepatic plates, and is collected in the central vein for delivery to the general circulation.

Remember This! The circulation of blood through the intestines and liver is unusual: blood from one capillary system, the intestinal, flows into another capillary system, the hepatic, before returning to the heart.

The liver acts as a large gland that secretes bile into the intestines. **Bile** is a mixture of metabolic waste and *bile acids*, compounds derived from cholesterol that emulsify dietary fat into microscopic droplets that blend easily with water so the fat can be absorbed by the intestinal mucosa. Bile is excreted by hepatocytes into a network of small intrahepatic bile ducts that carry it out of the liver and into the **common bile duct** (hepatic duct), which connects to the intestine at the **ampulla of Vater** in the duodenum. A reserve of bile is held in the **gallbladder** and discharged after meals. Figure 12.2 illustrates that much of the bile acid excreted into the intestine is reabsorbed by the small intestine and sent back to the liver for reuse, a process known as the *enterohepatic circulation*. Only a small amount of bile acid finds its way into feces.

Case Notes

12.2 Nervous about her appointment, Ling ate a big bowl of ice cream the night before. What liver secretion helped break down the fat in the ice cream?

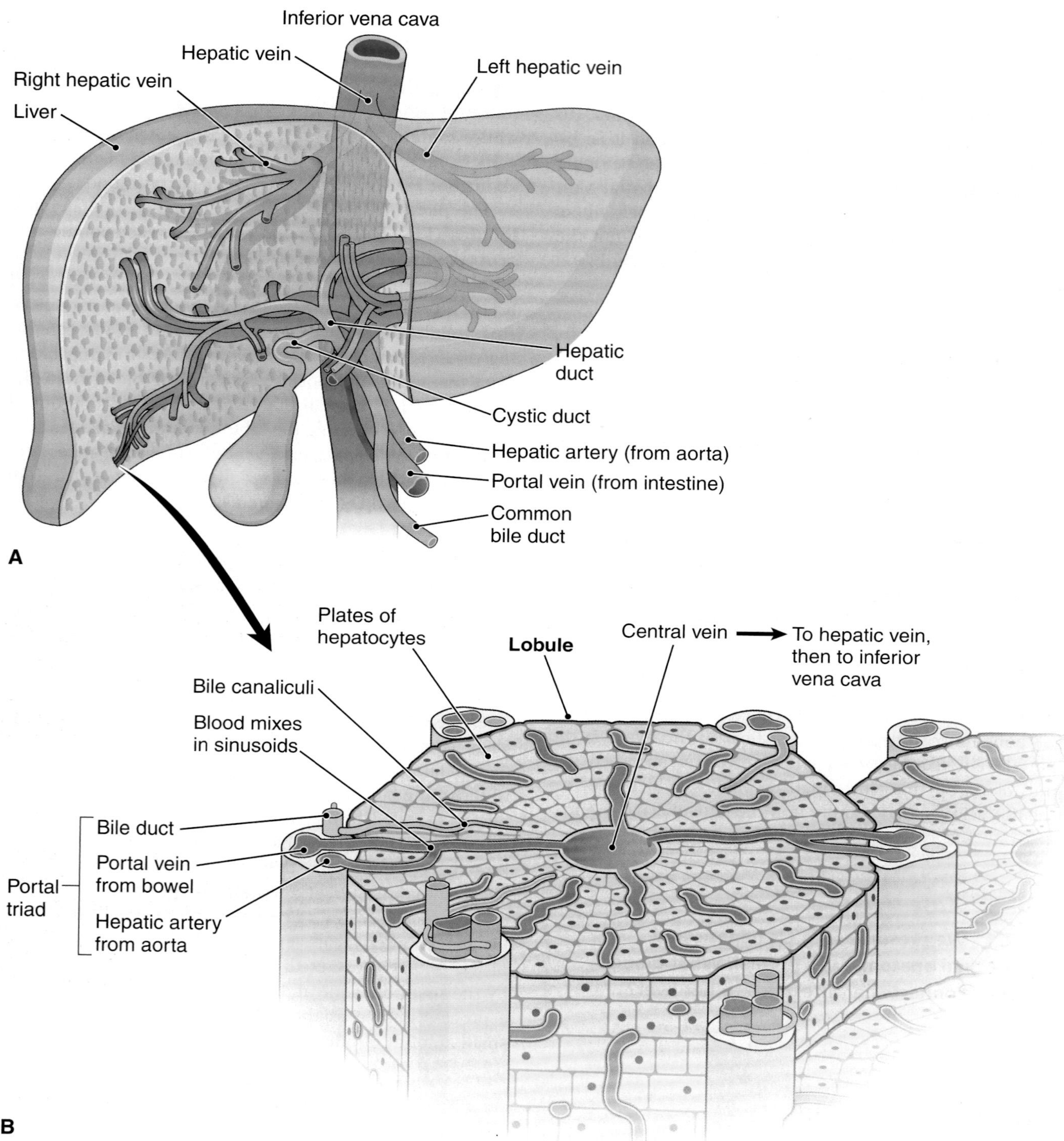

Figure 12.1 **The liver, portal venous system, and bile ducts. A.** The liver and biliary system. **B.** The hepatic lobule. Blood flows into the central vein from branches of the portal vein and hepatic artery clustered in portal triads at the edge of the lobule. Bile flows in the opposite direction—from the interior of the lobule to bile ducts in the portal triads.

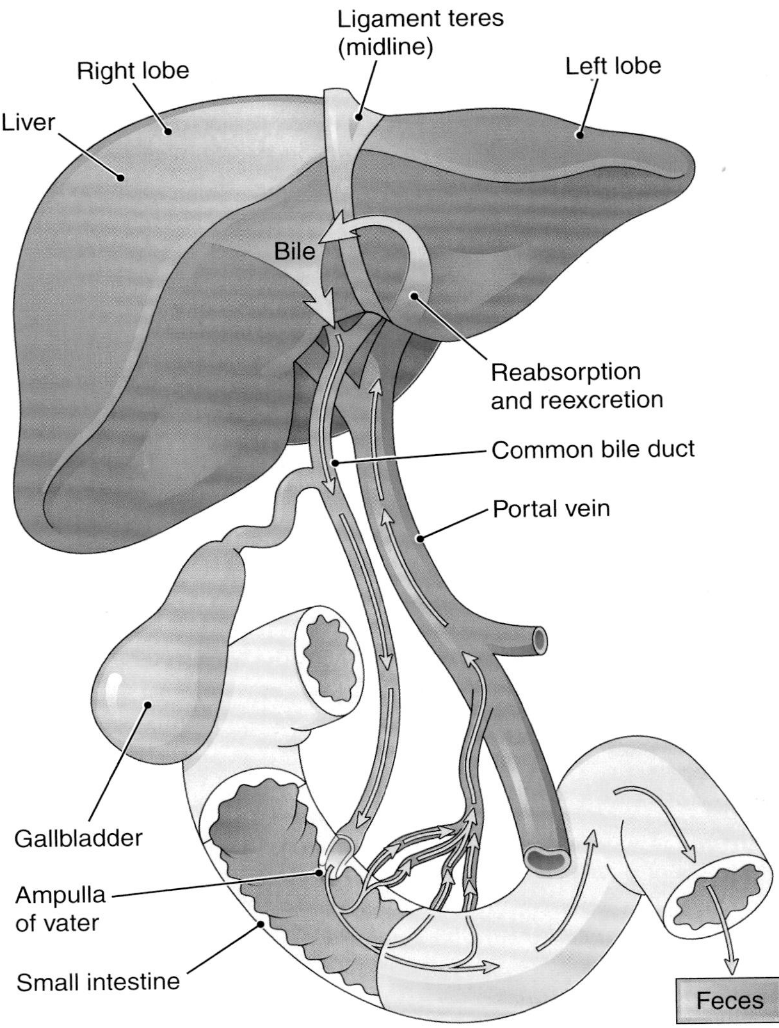

Figure 12.2 **The enterohepatic circulation.** Bile acids are secreted into bile, absorbed back into blood by the intestine, and recirculated via the portal vein for remetabolism by the liver.

The Liver Has Diverse Functions

As outlined in Table 12.1, the liver has five main functions: 1) carbohydrate metabolism; 2) lipid metabolism; 3) protein metabolism; 4) waste management, detoxification, and drug metabolism; and 5) storage of vitamins, iron, carbohydrate, and fat.

Carbohydrate Metabolism

Dietary carbohydrates are broken down by the intestine into monosaccharides (glucose, fructose, and galactose), which are absorbed by the intestinal mucosa and delivered to the liver in portal blood. The liver modulates blood glucose concentration by removing or adding glucose to blood. It (and other tissues) utilizes blood glucose as an energy source to power its metabolic activity. The liver removes excess glucose from blood, polymerizes it into glycogen, and stores it. Glycogen is available for reconversion into glucose if blood glucose falls and is unable to meet metabolic demand.

Lipid Metabolism

Dietary fat (mainly triglyceride with some cholesterol) is converted in the intestine into free fatty acids (FFA) and monoglycerides. These are absorbed by intestinal mucosa, which reassembles the triglycerides. The triglycerides are bundled with cholesterol as chylomicrons. Chylomicrons are absorbed into intestinal lymphatics (not portal blood) and delivered to the liver, where the triglyceride and cholesterol are repackaged into lipoproteins (Chapter 8) and secreted into blood. Some cholesterol is synthesized into bile salts and excreted into bile. Some triglyceride is broken down into FFA and then into ketones to be burned for energy by the liver or other tissues (as in diabetic ketoacidosis, Chapter 13). By various metabolic steps, some triglyceride is converted into glucose or cholesterol.

Protein Metabolism

Dietary protein is broken down into amino acids and short polypeptides, absorbed by the intestinal mucosa and

Table 12.1

Metabolic Task	Liver Action
Carbohydrate metabolism	• Conversion of excess blood glucose to stored glycogen • Breakdown of stored glycogen into glucose for secretion into blood

Lipid metabolism	• Synthesis and excretion of lipoproteins (Chapter 8) into blood
	• Breakdown of triglycerides into fatty acids, which can be further metabolized:
	  • Into ketones for fuel
	  • Into glucose and cholesterol
	• Synthesis of bile acids
	• Excretion of cholesterol as bile acids

Protein metabolism	• Synthesis and secretion into blood of albumin, transport proteins, and blood coagulation (clotting) factors
Waste management, detoxification and drug metabolism	• Clearance and excretion of drugs, metabolic byproducts (e.g., bilirubin, ammonia), and hormones (e.g., estrogen)
Storage	• Stores vitamins, iron, carbohydrate, and fat

delivered to the liver in portal blood. With the exception of immunoglobulins, the liver synthesizes most plasma proteins—albumin, coagulation factors, transport proteins, and many others.

Waste Disposal

Bilirubin is an intensely yellow pigment, most of which is produced in the spleen from the hemoglobin of old RBCs the spleen has removed from the circulation. This fresh bilirubin (*unconjugated bilirubin*) is not water soluble and is tightly bound to albumin for transport to the liver. In the liver, bilirubin is joined (conjugated) to glucuronide to make water-soluble *conjugated bilirubin*, which is excreted in bile. Increased blood bilirubin (hyperbilirubinemia) of either type causes yellow discoloration of skin (**jaundice**) and sclera (**icterus**, Fig. 12.3). Because it is tightly bound to albumin, unconjugated bilirubin does not spill into urine, even when blood levels are high. Nevertheless, conjugated bilirubin is readily excreted into urine (*bilirubinuria*), which gives normal urine its faint amber color and accounts for the dark amber urine of patients with jaundice.

The liver also clears (cleans) blood of *ammonia*, a product of protein metabolism, by converting it into urea, which is excreted by the kidneys. It captures and excretes *chemicals*, *toxins* (especially drugs), and *hormones* (especially estrogen) into bile.

Finally, the liver synthesizes cholesterol into *bile acids*—the main way by which the body rids itself of cholesterol. **Bile acids**, the main constituent of bile, emulsify fat like soap does grease, blending it with water for absorption. Nevertheless, most bile acids and the cholesterol they contain are reabsorbed by the intestinal mucosa and returned to the blood (a loop called the *enterohepatic circulation, Fig. 12.2*). The enterohepatic circulation is very important in cholesterol metabolism—most cholesterol absorbed from the intestine is not from diet but from reabsorption of bile acids. A class of drugs can lower blood cholesterol by blocking intestinal cholesterol absorption. Obstruction of bile excretion is referred to as "cholestasis."

Remember This! Conjugated bilirubin is water soluble. Unconjugated is not.

Storage

The liver stores an abundance of glycogen, fat, vitamins, and iron.

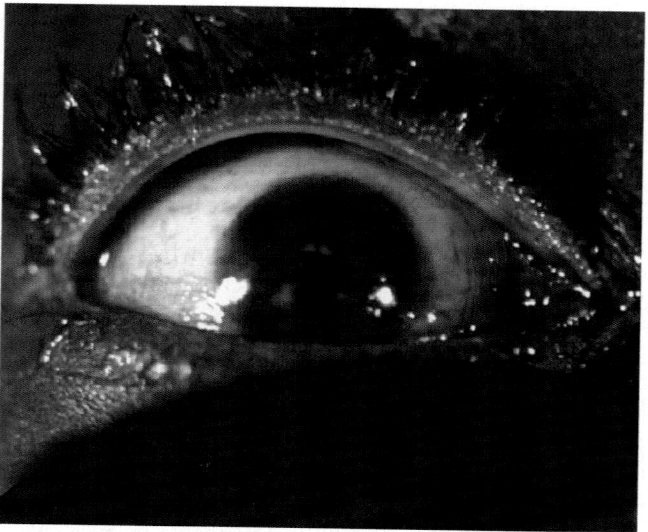

Figure 12.3 **Scleral icterus of hyperbilirubinemia.**

Case Notes

12.3 One of Ling's symptoms from the episode of hepatitis 30 years earlier was yellow skin. 1) What is the name of that condition? 2) What is the name of the increased blood compound? 3) Where does it originate?

Pop Quiz

12.1 True or false? The liver produces all plasma proteins.

12.2 Name the two blood supplies of the liver.

12.3 What cells are responsible for portal blood filtration?

The Liver Response to Injury

Most liver disease is chronic and progresses insidiously. Because the liver has a very large functional reserve, by the time symptoms appear, disease is often far advanced. The most important liver diseases are viral hepatitis, alcoholic liver injury, nonalcoholic fatty liver disease (NAFLD), and malignancy.

The great variety of diseases that may affect the liver usually emerge clinically as one of just four *clinical syndromes of liver disease*: 1) jaundice and cholestasis; 2) cirrhosis; 3) portal hypertension; or 4) hepatic failure.

Laboratory evaluation of blood is critical in the diagnosis and management of liver disease. *The Clinical Side*, "Liver Function Tests," provides the most common lab tests.

The Clinical Side

LIVER FUNCTION TESTS

The most useful laboratory tests for liver function are the following:

- **Enzymes:** In keeping with its metabolic role, the liver is packed with enzymes. In liver disease, these enzymes are washed into blood from damaged or dead cells. Even mild liver-cell injury can cause minor increases in levels of liver enzymes. Elevation of lactic dehydrogenase (LDH), aspartate aminotransferase (AST), and alanine aminotransferase (ALT) suggests hepatic cellular damage. Alkaline phosphatase (AP) and gamma glutamyl transpeptidase (GGT) also may be increased in liver disease, but they tend to be highest in conditions mainly affecting the bile ducts.
- **Bilirubin:** The liver metabolizes and excretes bilirubin into the bile ducts. If hemolytic disease has been excluded, increased levels of blood bilirubin usually indicate at least moderate liver or bile duct disease.
- **Albumin:** The liver makes all plasma albumin. Low levels are characteristic of moderate to serious liver disease.
- **Coagulation tests:** The liver makes most of the coagulation proteins (Chapter 6). Liver disease can cause abnormal (prolonged) prothrombin time and partial thromboplastin time.
- **Hepatitis virus antigens and antibodies:** Each type of hepatitis virus (discussed below) is distinguished by characteristic patterns of virus antigens and antibodies in blood.
- **Autoimmune antibodies:** Antimitochondrial antibodies in blood are characteristic of primary biliary cirrhosis. The two most common are antismooth muscle antibodies and anti-liver-kidney-microsomal (anti-LKM) antibody, which is characteristic of chronic autoimmune hepatitis. Both are discussed below.

Case Notes

12.4 Which of the syndromes of liver disease did Ling present with when she was ill 30 years earlier?

Jaundice and Cholestasis Typically Occur Together

As discussed earlier, **jaundice** is a yellow discoloration of skin due to increased blood bilirubin. It usually becomes visible when blood bilirubin level is > 2 mg/dL (normal < 1.2 mg/dL). Jaundice is usually accompanied by **cholestasis** (obstruction in the excretion of bile).

Etiology of Jaundice

Jaundice develops as a consequence of an imbalance between the production and excretion of bilirubin. The mechanisms responsible can be the following:

- Excess production of unconjugated bilirubin
- Decreased hepatic uptake of unconjugated bilirubin
- Defective hepatocellular conjugation of bilirubin
- Defective hepatocellular excretion of conjugated bilirubin
- Obstructed bile flow of conjugated bilirubin

As Figure 12.4 illustrates, jaundice can be etiologically traced to one of three conditions:

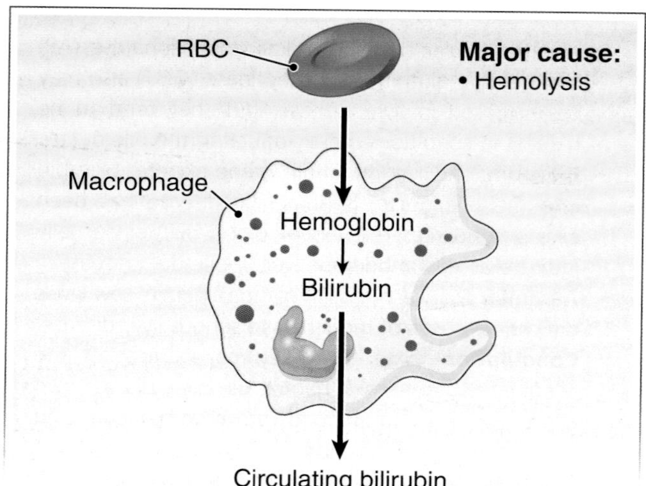

A Prehepatic jaundice (unconjugated hyperbilirubinemia)

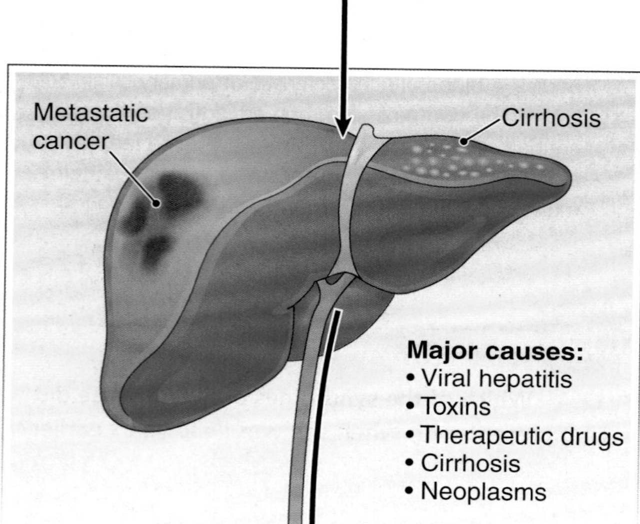

B Hepatic jaundice (unconjugated or conjugated hyperbilirubinemia)

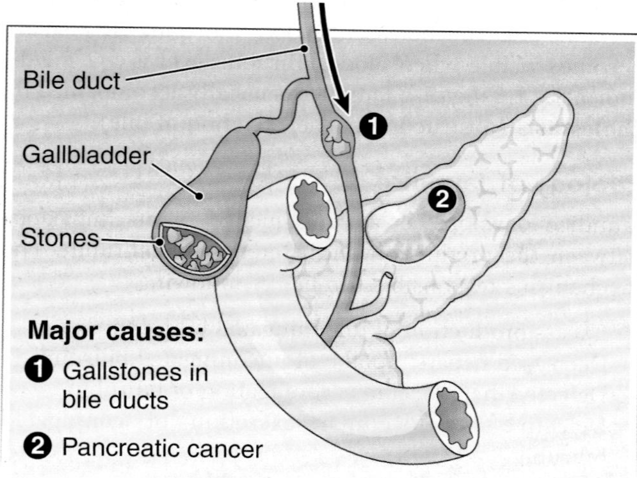

C Posthepatic jaundice (conjugated hyperbilirubinemia)

Figure 12.4 **Three types of jaundice. A.** Prehepatic jaundice causes increased levels of unconjugated bilirubin in blood. **B.** Hepatic jaundice may be caused by interference with the liver's ability to conjugate bilirubin or to secrete it after conjugation; increased levels of blood bilirubin may be of either conjugated or unconjugated type. **C.** Posthepatic jaundice is caused by obstruction of bile flow inside or outside of the liver; increased levels of blood bilirubin are of conjugated type.

- Overproduction of bilirubin (*prehepatic jaundice*), as occurs with hemolytic anemia. Blood *unconjugated* bilirubin is increased.
- Defective liver functioning (*hepatic jaundice*), as occurs with viral hepatitis, drug interference with liver function, genetic defects of bilirubin metabolism, or cirrhosis. Blood *unconjugated* or *conjugated* bilirubin is increased depending on the nature of the defect.
- Biliary obstruction (*posthepatic jaundice*), as occurs when pancreatic cancer or gallstones occlude the common bile duct. Blood *conjugated* bilirubin is increased.

Pathophysiology of Jaundice

The most important distinction between unconjugated and conjugated hyperbilirubinemia, besides the differences in cause, is their water solubility. Because it is water insoluble and tightly bound to albumin, little or no unconjugated bilirubin spills into urine. Nevertheless, a tiny fraction remains unbound and can diffuse into tissues. As a consequence, in *hemolytic disease of the newborn* (Chapter 22), some unconjugated bilirubin deposits in the newborn brain and may cause devastating neurologic damage (*kernicterus*). Nevertheless, even in normal newborns, the hepatic apparatus for bilirubin conjugation is immature and virtually every newborn experiences transient unconjugated hyperbilirubinemia for a few days (*physiologic jaundice of the newborn*, Chapter 22). Ordinarily, it has no lasting effect and requires no treatment.

Hyperbilirubinemia can be caused by *genetic defect*. The most common cause of increased *unconjugated* bilirubin in blood is **Gilbert syndrome** (pronounced "jeel-bear" in the French manner), a very common and harmless autosomal recessive condition that is the result of mild deficiency of the enzyme glucuronyl transferase (UGT1A1), which normally conjugates bilirubin, making it more water soluble. It is usually not detected until adolescence or adulthood, when the problem is amplified by an intercurrent illness, exposure to certain drugs, vigorous exercise, or prolonged fasting. The liver is morphologically normal. No treatment is necessary. A second genetic cause of unconjugated hyperbilirubinemia is **Crigler-Najjar syndrome**, which also owes to genetic defect of UGT1A1. Two varieties exist, one of which causes death in infancy; the other is innocuous and needs no treatment. The liver is morphologically normal in both.

Conjugated hyperbilirubinemia may also owe to genetic defect. **Dubin-Johnson syndrome** is an innocuous autosomal recessive condition in which the liver is deeply pigmented. **Rotor syndrome** is an autosomal recessive condition in which the hepatocellular secretory apparatus appears to be defective. The liver is morphologically normal. Neither needs treatment.

Pathophysiology of Cholestasis

Cholestasis is the general term for a pathologic condition of impaired bile formation and bile flow that leads to accumulation of bile pigments in the liver. It can be caused by intrahepatic or extrahepatic bile flow obstruction or by defective hepatocyte bile secretion. It may result from liver disease, biliary obstruction, drug interference with bile secretion, pregnancy, and a variety of other conditions. It is usually accompanied by jaundice and sometimes by severe pruritus (itching) because of the deposition of bile acids in the skin. Because bile is the means by which the body rids itself of excess cholesterol, blood cholesterol levels may become markedly elevated and associated with yellow deposits of cholesterol in skin (*xanthomas*). Lack of bile acids in the bowel may also cause fat malabsorption syndromes (Chapter 11). Because bile duct epithelium is rich in AP and gamma glutamyl transpeptidase (GGT), a characteristic laboratory finding is marked increase of blood levels of these enzymes. Typically, levels of other liver enzymes are usually normal or only mildly increased.

Cirrhosis Is Patterned Scarring of the Liver

Cirrhosis (Figs. 12.5 and 12.6) is a widespread scarring of the liver that is progressive, irreversible, and incurable. The common end-stage of many chronic liver diseases, cirrhosis is among the top 10 causes of death in the western hemisphere.

About 65% of cases result from alcoholism and chronic viral hepatitis. In about 25% of cases, the cause is unknown (*cryptogenic cirrhosis*). An important growing cause of cirrhosis is fatty liver disease, which is associated with obesity and other forms of metabolic injury. Less common causes of cirrhosis are genetic hemochromatosis and diseases of bile ducts.

Pathology and Pathophysiology

Cirrhosis is characterized anatomically by a three-dimensional web of interconnecting bands of scar tissue that divide the liver into small nodules of viable liver lobules. The liver possesses remarkable regenerative power and, as the trapped lobules attempt to regenerate, they swell to form nodules. At the same time, the scar tissue is maturing and contracting. As a result, intrahepatic pressure rises, further damaging liver cells; the liver becomes tense and stiff; portal blood flow is obstructed; and portal blood pressure rises (*portal hypertension*, discussed below). As a consequence, portal blood flow diverts (shunts) around the

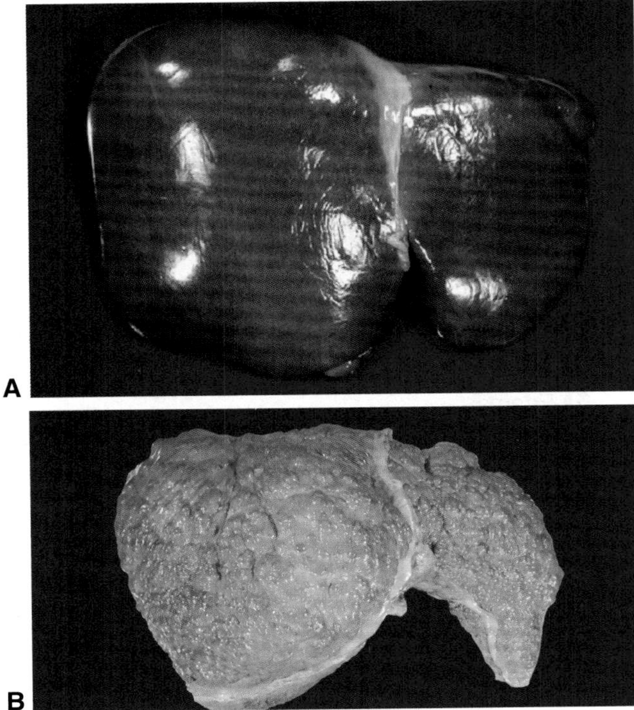

Figure 12.5 **Cirrhosis. A.** Normal liver. **B.** Cirrhosis. Note the small size of the cirrhotic liver.

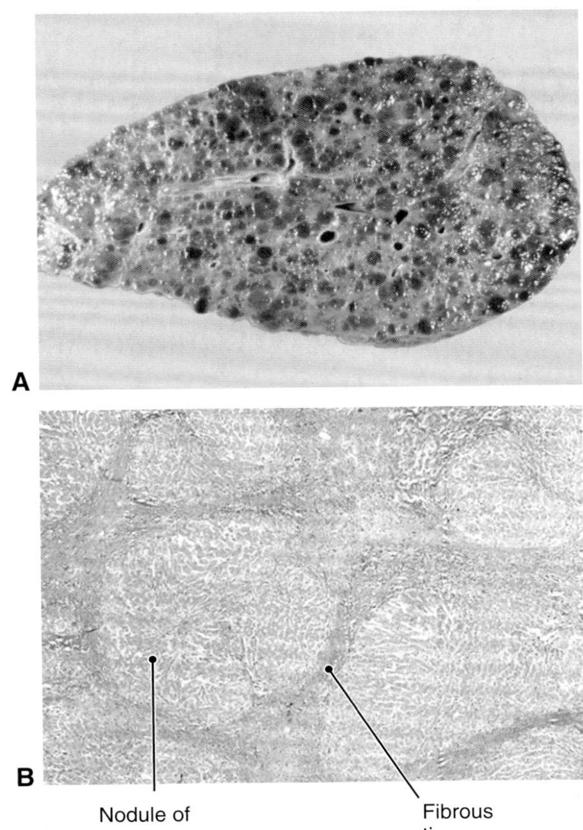

Figure 12.6 **Cirrhosis. A.** Gross section. **B.** Microscopic study. Note the nodular pattern in both specimens. The liver is divided into nodules by a web of fibrous (scar) tissue. Dark discoloration of some nodules is caused by the accumulation of bile pigment in lobules. The cause of cirrhosis in this patient is unknown.

liver through alternative (collateral) vessels in the GI tract, spleen, and skin. Poor hepatic perfusion further damages hepatocytes.

Regardless of cause, there are only two anatomic types of cirrhosis:

- **Portal cirrhosis** is by far the most common and is caused by chronic diffuse liver cell injury, such as alcoholism or viral hepatitis. Scar tissue disrupts the lobular anatomy and does not follow the anatomic outlines of the lobules.
- **Biliary cirrhosis** is uncommon and is caused by chronic disease of the biliary tree, such as primary biliary cirrhosis or chronic biliary obstruction and inflammation. The pattern of scars follows the outline of hepatic lobules.

Signs and Symptoms

About half of patients with cirrhosis remain asymptomatic for many years. When symptoms first occur, they are often nonspecific: weakness, weight loss, and fatigue. Later, however, signs and symptoms of hepatic failure begin to appear—jaundice, ascites, coagulation defects, and so on. Progression is inevitable. Death occurs from hepatic coma, hemorrhage attributable to portal hypertension (below) and coagulation defects, or development of hepatocellular carcinoma (HCC). Figure 12.7 summarizes the clinical features of cirrhosis.

In early cases, portal and biliary cirrhosis are easy to distinguish by microscopic examination of liver biopsy tissue, but as disease progresses, the distinctions often disappear. In early cirrhosis, the liver may be large, but,

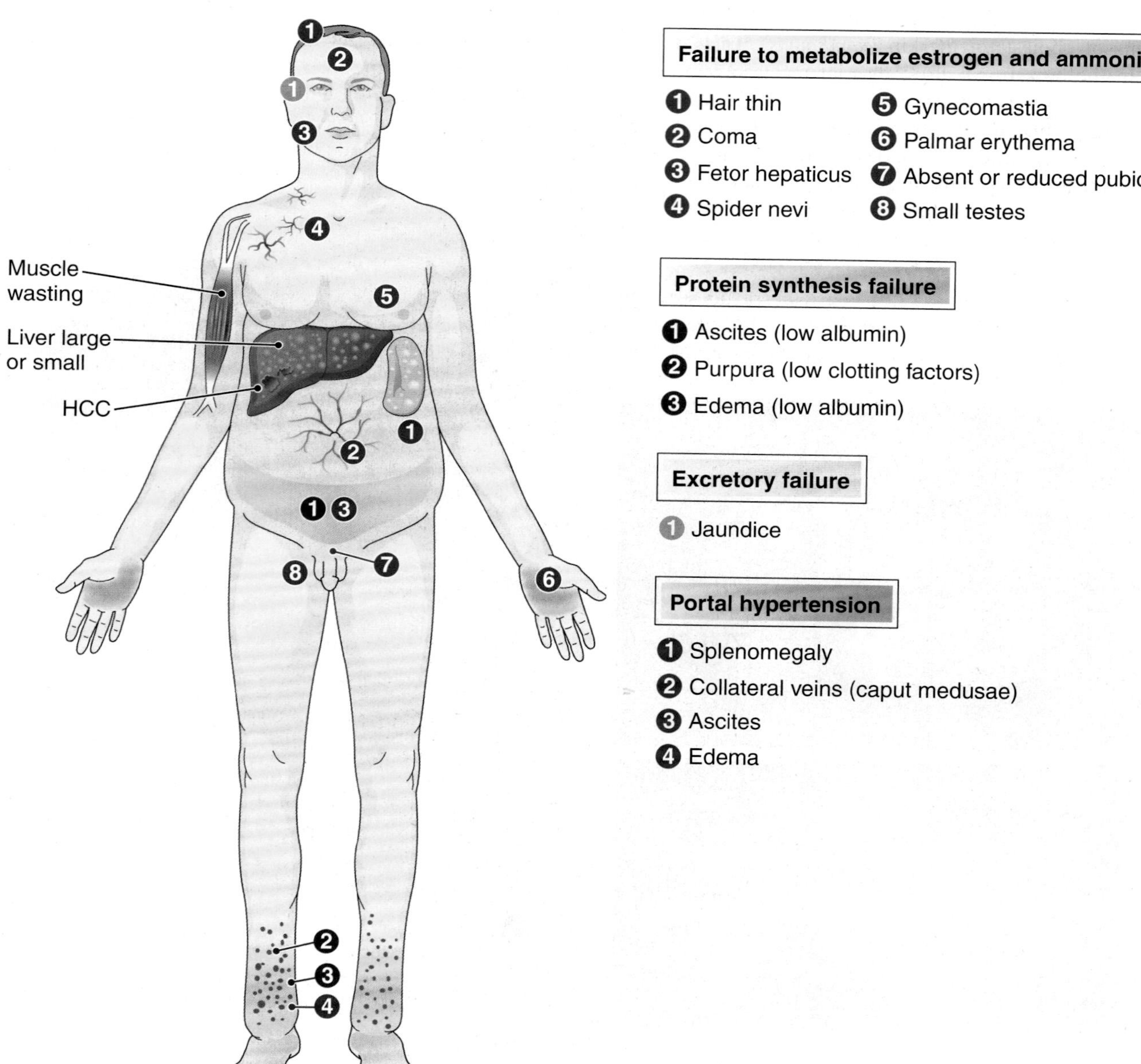

Figure 12.7 **Clinical features of cirrhosis.**

as scarring progresses, it shrinks to less than normal size. In the end, the cause of most cases of cirrhosis cannot be determined by study of the liver: clinical findings and history are of paramount importance.

Diagnosis and Treatment

Cirrhosis is typically diagnosed when patients present with signs and symptoms of liver disease and a liver biopsy is performed. Treatment is supportive. Liver transplant is the only effective therapy for fully developed cases and is reserved for those in hepatic failure. Because of America's dramatically rising rates of obesity, in the near future fatty liver disease will likely overtake viral hepatitis as the most common indication for liver transplant. Indeed, the liver transplant system in the United States may not be capable of meeting the demand.

Portal Hypertension Is Caused by Obstruction to Portal Blood Flow

Portal hypertension is increased blood pressure in the portal venous system. It is caused by increased resistance to portal blood flow, which can occur at one of three points (Fig. 12.8): before blood reaches the liver (*prehepatic*), as it flows through the liver (*hepatic*), or after blood exits the liver (*posthepatic*).

Pathology and Pathophysiology

Prehepatic obstruction can be caused by thrombosis, narrowing (e.g., by scar tissue), or external pressure on the portal vein (e.g., by a tumor). Hepatic obstruction, usually owing to cirrhosis, is by far the most common. The most common causes of posthepatic flow restriction are severe right heart failure, restrictive pericarditis, and obstruction

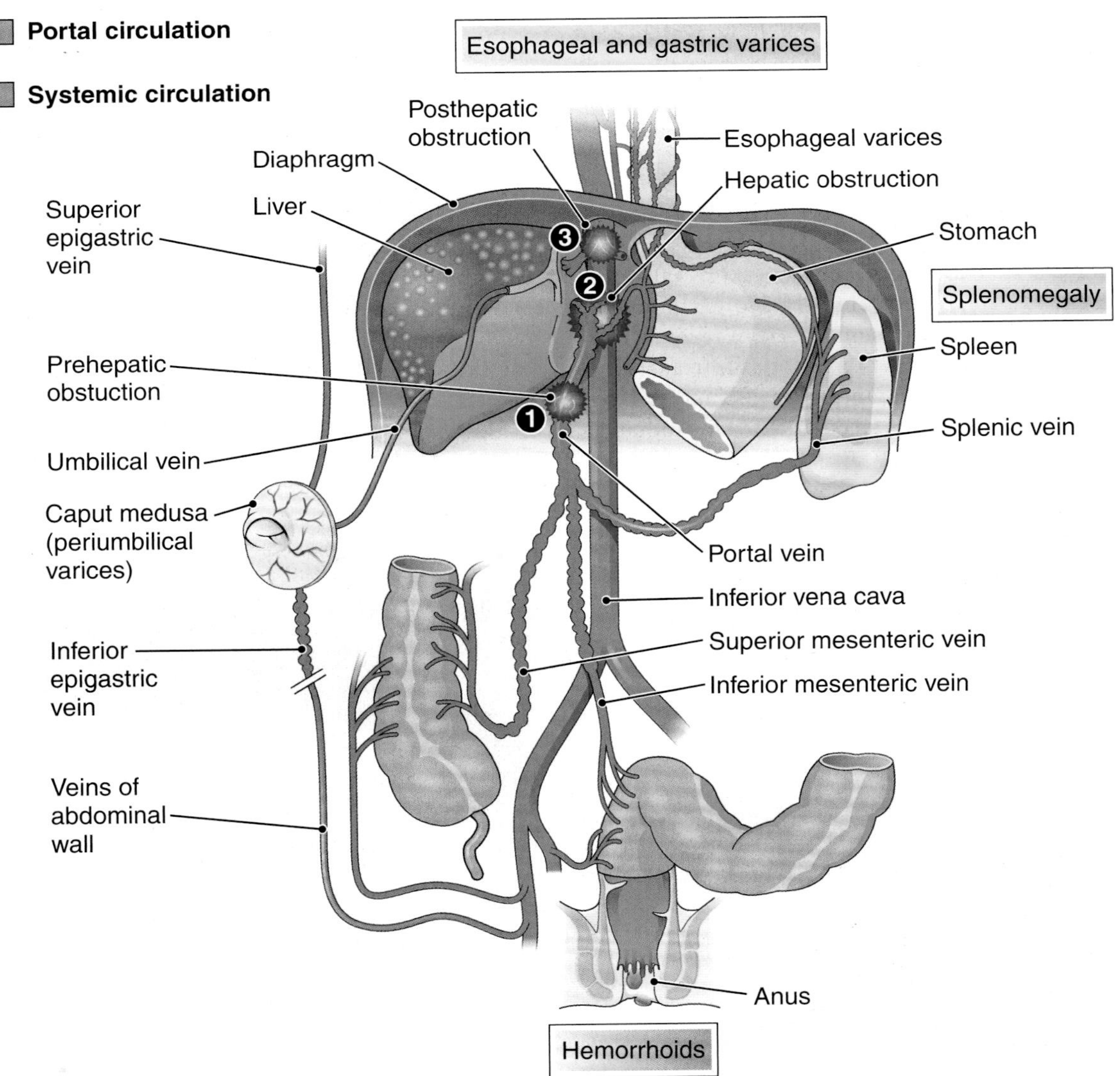

Figure 12.8 **Portal hypertension.** The hemodynamic consequences of obstructed portal blood flow.

of the hepatic vein by thrombosis or other cause. An important and poorly understood contributing cause is visceral arterial vasodilation and increased arterial blood flow into the viscera. In any case, portal pressure and flow are high, blood flow is diverted from the liver through alternate channels, and liver function declines.

Remember This! Cirrhosis is irreversible and always associated with portal hypertension.

Signs and Symptoms

The hemodynamic consequences of portal hypertension are ascites, portosystemic shunts, and splenomegaly.

Ascites (from Greek, *askos*, for bag) is an intraperitoneal accumulation of watery (serous) fluid (Chapter 6). It seeps into the peritoneal space mainly because of increased portal hemodynamic pressure, which is encouraged by low plasma osmotic pressure due, in turn, to low plasma albumin in patients with cirrhosis. Cirrhosis also causes marked increase of abdominal lymph flow, which may exceed thoracic duct capacity and cause seepage of lymph fluid into the peritoneal space. Ascites becomes clinically evident when about 500 ml of intraperitoneal fluid have accumulated; however, as Figure 12.9 illustrates, fluid accumulation may be massive.

Portosystemic shunts are diversions of blood around the liver through alternate channels into the systemic venous circulation. The main routes are via rectal veins, which present as *hemorrhoids* (Fig. 11.25, Chapter 11); esophageal veins, which present as *esophageal varices* (see Fig. 11.13, Chapter 11); retroperitoneal veins, which are not clinically apparent; and veins in the falciform ligament, which present as enlarged veins radiating around the skin of the umbilicus. The latter are known as *caput medusa*—literally snake-head—named after the female serpent-haired monster, Medusa, from Greek mythology.

Splenomegaly is enlargement of the spleen. The splenic vein empties into the portal system and increased portal pressure causes chronic passive congestion of the spleen (Fig. 12.10). Enlargement is often great enough for the spleen to become palpable below the rib cage. Massive splenomegaly may occur and be associated with hypersplenism (Chapter 7) and thrombocytopenia or pancytopenia.

Diagnosis and Treatment

Diagnosis is clinical. Treatment includes elimination of the cause, if possible (e.g., tumor obstruction of portal flow), beta-blockers to reduce hepatic resistance, or surgical shunting of blood from the portal system into the systemic circulation. Esophageal varices can be banded to prevent hemorrhage. For cirrhosis, liver transplant is the only life-saving option.

Hepatic Failure Is Usually Fatal

Hepatic failure is defined as a loss of hepatic metabolic function severe enough to cause hepatic encephalopathy (discussed below). Destruction of 80–90% of functional capacity is required. It may occur suddenly from acute injury such as a toxin, or it may appear slowly as a result of chronic liver disease. Without transplant, over 80% of cases are fatal.

Acute hepatic failure is uncommon. Accidental or deliberate ingestion of a large amount of acetaminophen is the cause of half of the acute cases in the United States. In descending order, the remaining incidents are due to other drugs, industrial chemicals and other toxins, autoimmune hepatitis, and viral hepatitis.

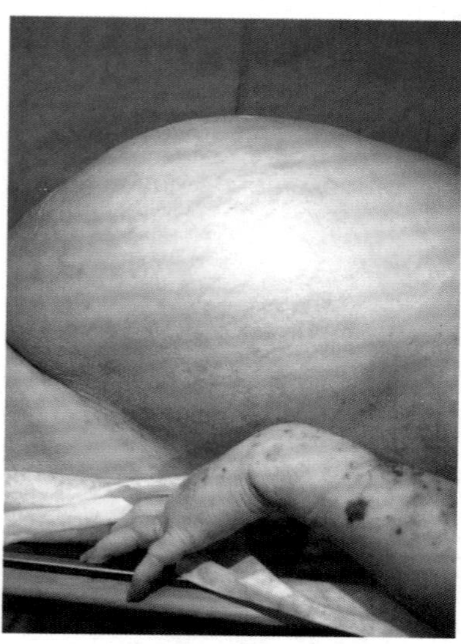

Figure 12.9 **Ascites.**

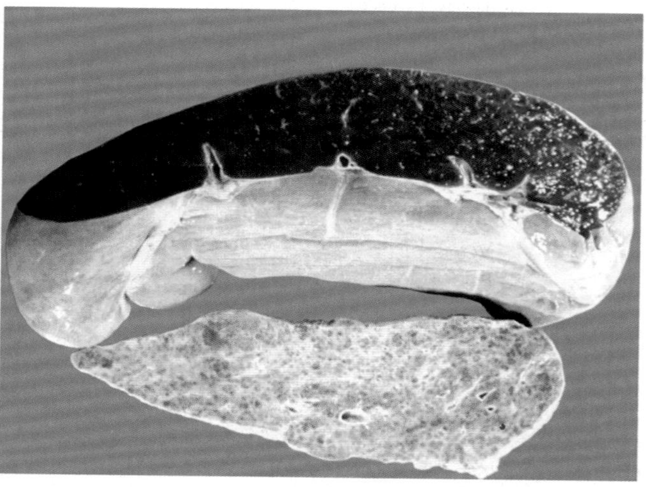

Figure 12.10 **Congestive splenomegaly in cirrhosis.** Both specimens are from the same patient. Note that the spleen (top) is much larger than the liver; normally the opposite is true.

Chronic liver disease, usually *cirrhosis*, is by far the most common route to chronic hepatic failure.

Signs and Symptoms

The signs and symptoms of chronic hepatic failure are similar, regardless of cause. Bilirubin excretion fails and jaundice appears. Low blood albumin encourages peripheral edema and ascites, which can become infected (*spontaneous bacterial peritonitis*). Loss of glycogen reserves makes patients vulnerable to hypoglycemia. A musty body and breath odor called *fetor hepaticus* develops. Accumulation of estrogen causes palmar erythema, development of spider angiomas (Chapter 8) of the skin of the upper chest and face, and gynecomastia (enlarged breasts) and hypogonadism in males (Chapter 16). Coagulation defects may lead to intestinal bleeding or hemorrhage from other sites.

As blood levels of ammonia and other toxic products rise, patients with hepatic failure develop a form of brain dysfunction called **hepatic encephalopathy**. This syndrome of reduced and disordered consciousness is associated with a variety of motor defects. Neurologic signs include rigidity, hyperreflexia, and, rarely, seizures. Coma usually follows. A characteristic neurologic sign is *asterixis*, a rapid extension-flexion motion of the head and extremities that can be demonstrated with a simple test in which the arms are held extended and the hands dorsiflexed. A pulsating, flapping, or hand waving motion (called the "hepatic flap") constitutes a positive test.

Patients with hepatic failure are also subject to renal and respiratory failure. **Hepatorenal syndrome** is the development of renal failure in a patient with severe chronic liver disease in whom no other cause for renal failure can be found. The mechanism linking the two disorders is obscure. **Hepatopulmonary syndrome** is a syndrome of respiratory failure in patients with liver failure. Again, the cause is obscure.

Diagnosis and Treatment

Diagnosis is clinical and supported by laboratory findings and, if needed, liver biopsy. Treatment of the underlying cause usually reverses mild cases. Nonsurgical treatment is exceptionally complex and beyond the scope of this discussion. Liver transplant may be life saving, but many patients are in no shape to tolerate surgery.

Case Notes

12.5 Ling was examined to see if she had hemorrhoids. Why was this important?

12.6 With her episode of hepatitis and jaundice, which type of bilirubin was most likely elevated: unconjugated, conjugated, or both?

Pop Quiz

12.4 True or false? Hepatic failure occurs after 80–90% of the liver's functional capacity is lost.

12.5 True or false? Cirrhosis is reversible.

12.6 True or false? Water-soluble bilirubin becomes elevated with obstruction of bile flow.

12.7 Name the consequences of portal hypertension.

12.8 What is the cause of pruritus in patients with cholestasis?

Viral Hepatitis

Viral hepatitis is infection by one of the several viruses that preferentially infect the liver (hepatotropic): hepatitis viruses A, B, C, D, and E, which are designated HAV (for hepatitis A virus), HBV, and so on. Other viruses can incidentally infect the liver and cause hepatitis, most notably the cytomegalovirus, Epstein-Barr virus (EBV) (the cause of infectious mononucleosis), or sometimes herpes simplex virus (HSV).

Hepatitis viruses are distinguished from one another according to the following clinical characteristics (summarized in Table 12.2):

- *Mode of transmission*: Is the virus transmitted by oral-fecal contamination, close personal contact (e.g., sexual intercourse), contaminated water, or blood contamination (needlestick or transfusion)?
- *Length of incubation period*: What is the length of time from infection to symptomatic disease?
- *Carrier state*: After recovery from acute infection, does the virus linger, so that an apparently healthy person continues to infect others?
- *Chronic hepatitis*: Can the virus cause chronic hepatitis?
- *Fulminant hepatitis*: Can the virus cause a sudden, catastrophic hepatitis?
- *Hepatocellular carcinoma*: Is infection associated with increased risk of HCC?

Case Notes

12.7 Which mode of transmission was most likely for Ling's hepatitis?

Hepatitis Presents as One or More Clinicopathologic Syndromes

Viral hepatitis can cause several clinicopathologic syndromes. Nevertheless, not every hepatitis virus can produce

Table 12.2 Characteristics of the three most common hepatitis virus infections in the United States (Figures vary geographically)

Characteristic	Hepatitis A	Hepatitis B	Hepatitis C
Estimated new cases per annum in the US (2009)*	21,000	38,000	21,000
Estimated number of chronic infections in the US (2009)*	0	1,000,000	3,000,000
Transmission			
Route	Fecal-oral	Parenteral or close contact	Parenteral or close contact
Vertical transmission (from mother to child during childbirth)	No	Yes	?
Incubation period	3–6 weeks	2 weeks–6 months	2 weeks–6 months
Viremia	Very brief	Months	Months
Fulminant hepatitis	Rare	Yes	Rare
Carrier state**	No	Yes, <1%	Yes, 10–40%
Chronic hepatitis	No	5–10%	>50%
Vaccine available	Yes	Yes	No

*Includes asymptomatic and unreported cases. Most cases are asymptomatic and only a small percentage (~10%) of cases are reported to public health officials.
**In endemic areas in developing nations, the carrier state develops in about 90% of HBV and HVC infections.

each syndrome, and some of these clinical syndromes can be caused by diseases other than viral hepatitis.

Acute Viral Hepatitis

Acute asymptomatic hepatitis with recovery is common, undiagnosed as it occurs, and is found by incidental detection of abnormal blood evidence such as increased liver enzymes. Worldwide, most HAV and HBV childhood infections escape detection and are verified later by presence of anti-HAV or anti-HBV antibodies.

Acute symptomatic hepatitis with recovery can be caused by HAV, HBV, HBC, or HEV. The illness typically evolves through four clinical stages:

- *Incubation* usually lasts a few weeks. Peak infectivity occurs about the time symptoms appear.
- The *prodromal phase* is without jaundice and features constitutional symptoms, including malaise, fatigability, nausea, and anorexia. Nevertheless, right upper-quadrant pain, low-grade fever, headache, skin rash, vomiting, diarrhea, or muscle and joint aches may also occur.
- The *symptomatic, jaundiced phase* begins as jaundice appears and other symptoms fade. The jaundice reflects a rise in conjugated bilirubin. Because conjugated bilirubin is water soluble, it is excreted in urine, causing a brown discoloration. Nevertheless, as less bilirubin is getting into the gut, stools may be pale. With HAV infection, most adults become jaundiced, but most children do not. About half of patients with HBV infection become jaundiced, while patients with HCV infection are rarely jaundiced.
- *Convalescence* begins as jaundice fades, infectivity disappears, and antibodies appear in blood to confer immunity.

Acute viral hepatitis with fulminant liver failure denotes explosively acute liver disease that progresses to encephalopathy in a very short time, usually a few weeks. Fulminant hepatitis (Fig. 12.11) accounts for more than half of fulminant liver failure, most of which are associated with HAV or HBV infections, and occasionally HEV infections in pregnant women.

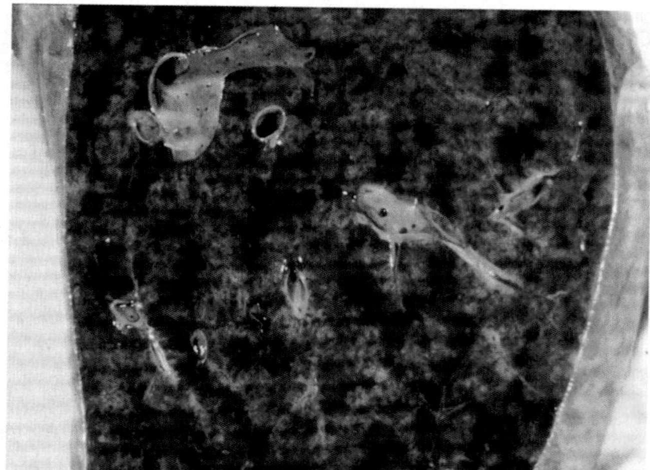

Figure 12.11 **Hepatitis with massive hepatic necrosis and fulminant liver failure.** Dark spots are hemorrhagic necrosis around central veins; red areas are nonhemorrhagic necrosis.

Case Notes

12.8 What phase of illness followed Ling's symptomatic, jaundiced phase?

The Carrier State

The **carrier state** is defined as *asymptomatic* infection in a patient who harbors the virus and is therefore *capable of infecting others*. The percentage of infected people who become carriers varies greatly from one type of viral hepatitis to another. For example, few patients infected with hepatitis B virus (HBV) become carriers; conversely, many of those with hepatitis C virus (HCV) develop chronic infection, which may be symptomatic or asymptomatic. If they are asymptomatic, they fit the definition of the carrier state. If symptomatic, they are said to have *chronic viral hepatitis*. Both conditions are contagious.

Chronic Viral Hepatitis

Chronic viral hepatitis is defined as viral hepatitis proven by liver biopsy, with six months or more of laboratory or clinical evidence of disease activity. Not all patients with chronic hepatitis have chronic viral hepatitis—autoimmune hepatitis and alcoholic hepatitis, discussed below, are also examples.

About 10% of patients with hepatitis B infections develop chronic hepatitis, whereas >50% of patients with *untreated* hepatitis C do so. Most patients with chronic hepatitis show few specific clinical signs and symptoms, and the extent of disease is revealed only by laboratory tests. The most common complaint is fatigue. Physical findings are minimal and only uncommonly include spider angiomas, palmar erythema, mild liver enlargement and tenderness, and mild splenomegaly due to portal hypertension or reactive hyperplasia developed secondary to the immune response to infection. Blood studies often show increased levels of hepatic enzymes but few other changes. Some patients with chronic HBV or HCV hepatitis may develop circulating immune complexes resulting in vasculitis or glomerulonephritis (Chapter 15). Other complications from long-standing infection include cirrhosis and HCC.

HBV chronic hepatitis is an important problem because younger patients are more likely to develop chronic hepatitis. Without drug therapy, disease progression is certain. Though cure is rare, progression can be arrested in many instances.

HCV infection is the most common cause of chronic viral hepatitis. The infection is often subclinical, but patients are nevertheless at risk of developing cirrhosis and deserve treatment with available drugs. Cure is possible.

HIV/AIDS coinfection often occurs with chronic hepatitis because the epidemiology and modes of transmission are similar. Among patients with HIV infection, about 10% are also infected with HBV and 30% with HCV. HIV infection increases the severity of liver chronic hepatitis and can make the achievement of a cure more difficult.

Case Notes

12.9 Which hepatitis syndrome did Ling manifest after her Caesarian section?

12.10 Does Ling fit the criteria to be called a carrier?

12.11 Did Ling show any of the criteria of cirrhosis or portal hypertension?

Hepatitis A Virus (HAV) Causes Epidemic Hepatitis

HAV is the cause of epidemic hepatitis and is the most common form of *clinically recognized* hepatitis. Worldwide, it is the most common type of hepatitis. About 21,000 new infections were estimated in the United States in 2009, but only a minority were diagnosed and even fewer were reported to public health authorities. HAV is a benign, self-limited disease that requires only supportive treatment and public health measures to limit spread, which is primarily by oral-fecal contamination of water or food. Shared food utensils, kissing, handshaking, and sexual activity are less common modes of transmission. Because the virus is present in blood (viremia) only for a very short time, spread by transfusion or needlestick is exceptionally rare, so rare that blood for transfusion is not screened. HAV does not cause chronic hepatitis or a carrier state and only rarely is the cause of fulminant hepatitis. Accordingly, the fatality rate is on the order of 0.1%. Most infections are asymptomatic or feature mild constitutional symptoms. Jaundice is common and mild. Most victims are children or young adults. Evidence of infection increases with advancing age until, in the United States, about half of the population shows evidence of previous infection.

As Figure 12.12 illustrates, the virus infects the liver and quickly begins to be shed in feces. Viremia is so short that risk of blood-borne transmission is very low. Jaundice, increased liver enzymes in blood, and the appearance of **IgM anti-HAV** antibodies are clinical markers of disease progress. Recall from Chapter 3 that IgM antibodies are acute phase antibodies, whereas IgG antibodies appear later and confer immunity.

Diagnosis of acute infection is clinical and by detection of anti-HAV (IgM) antibodies in blood. Presence of **IgG anti-HAV** is evidence of immunity due to vaccination or prior infection. Treatment is supportive.

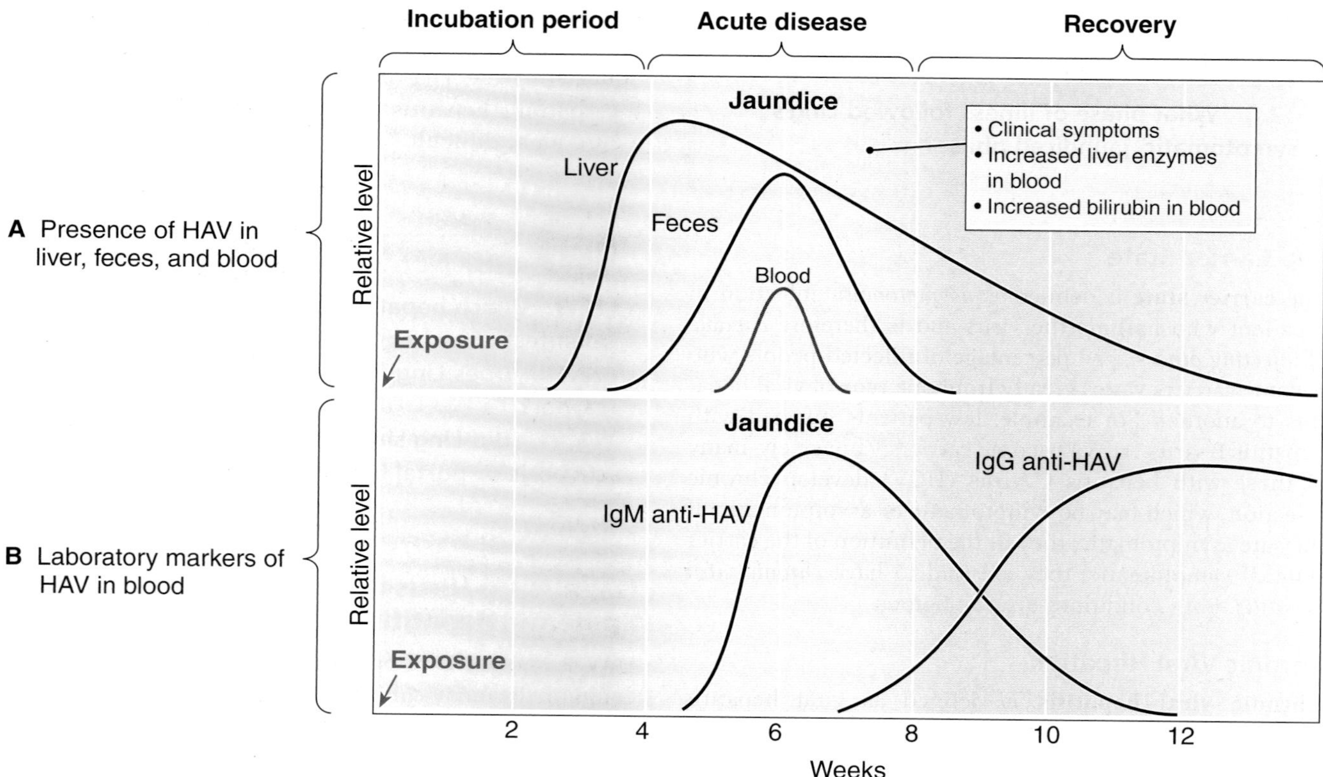

Figure 12.12 **Hepatitis A: clinical phases and blood markers of infection. A.** Infection of the liver is followed quickly by the appearance of virus in blood and feces. **B.** Jaundice or other symptoms of acute infection are accompanied by the appearance of IgM-type acute phase antibodies in blood. The appearance of IgG-type antibodies signals recovery and immunity against reinfection.

Hepatitis B Virus (HBV) Has Infected One-Third of the World Population

HBV is a much more serious disease than hepatitis A because it is more prevalent and causes more extensive and chronic liver disease. According to the CDC about 38,000 new infections were estimated in the United States in 2009, but most cases are asymptomatic and go undiagnosed and unreported. It is the second most common cause of *clinically recognized* hepatitis. One-third of the world's population shows evidence of current or prior infection. Prevalence is highest in Asia and Southeast Asia, where most cases are spread perinatally from mother to child. In areas with intermediate prevalence, spread is horizontal among children living in close quarters, and typically occurs through minor breaks in skin and mucus membranes. Prevalence in Europe, North America, and Australia is <2%, and transmission is usually among adults by sexual contact or needlestick. In the United States, new cases have fallen dramatically because of improved public awareness and vaccination. Transfusion spread is now very low due to prohibition of paid blood donations (offering a tangible reward for blood donation is an incentive to lie about medical history) and rigorous screening for blood evidence of infection.

Remember This! One-third of the world's population has evidence of hepatitis B infection.

The incubation period for HBV varies greatly from a few weeks to six months. Figure 12.13 illustrates outcomes of infection. Most infections do not come to medical attention because they are asymptomatic or cause minor constitutional symptoms without jaundice. Symptomatic infections appear as a syndrome of acute hepatitis that resolves quickly with supportive care. Fulminant hepatitis with liver failure is rare. A carrier state evolves in <10% of infections, usually in neonates and people with impaired immunity.

Laboratory tests for hepatitis markers (antigens and antibodies) are critical in the diagnosis and management of hepatitis B. As depicted in Figure 12.14, the viremia of acute infection is indicated by detection in blood of a particular hepatitis B antigen, **hepatitis B surface antigen**, designated **HBsAg**. HBsAg is the first marker to appear and is an indicator of viremia and, therefore, of infectivity. Hepatitis B viremia may last for many weeks in acute infection and for years in chronic infection (Fig. 12.14B). It is transmitted in blood, saliva, and semen and can be spread by heterosexual or homosexual contact, blood transfusion, renal dialysis, needlestick accidents among healthcare workers, and intravenous drug use. Pregnant women with HBV may infect the fetus in utero or during vaginal delivery (vertical transmission). In some cases the method of infection is not known.

Diagnosis of acute infection is clinical, with confirmation by liver biopsy and by detection of HBsAg in blood.

Hepatitis B infection
Symptomatic acute hepatitis
90%
Recovery
10% Chronic
hepatitis
1%
ACUTE LIVER
FAILURE AND DEATH
HCC
Chronic hepatitis
1%
CHRONIC HEPATITIS
AND CIRRHOSIS
10–30%
65%
Subclinical
infection
35%
Symptomatic
acute hepatitis
70–90%
Asymptomatic
carrier state
100%
90%
RECOVERY
2–6% annually

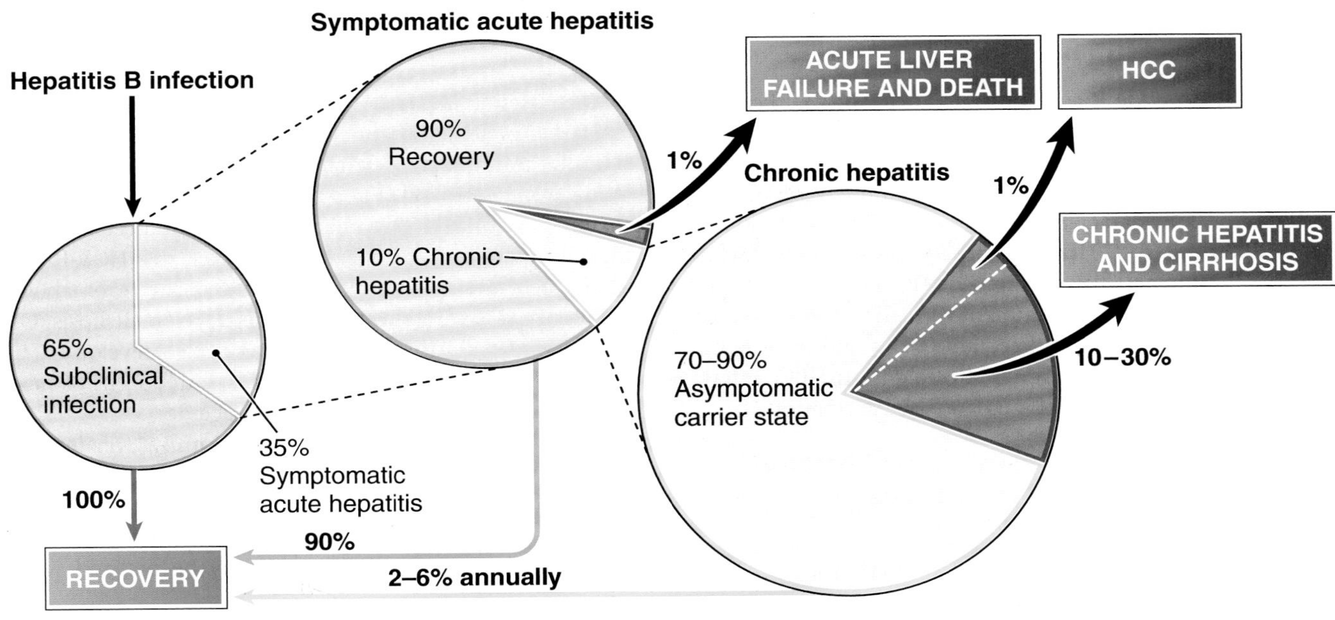

Figure 12.13 **Outcomes of hepatitis B infection.**

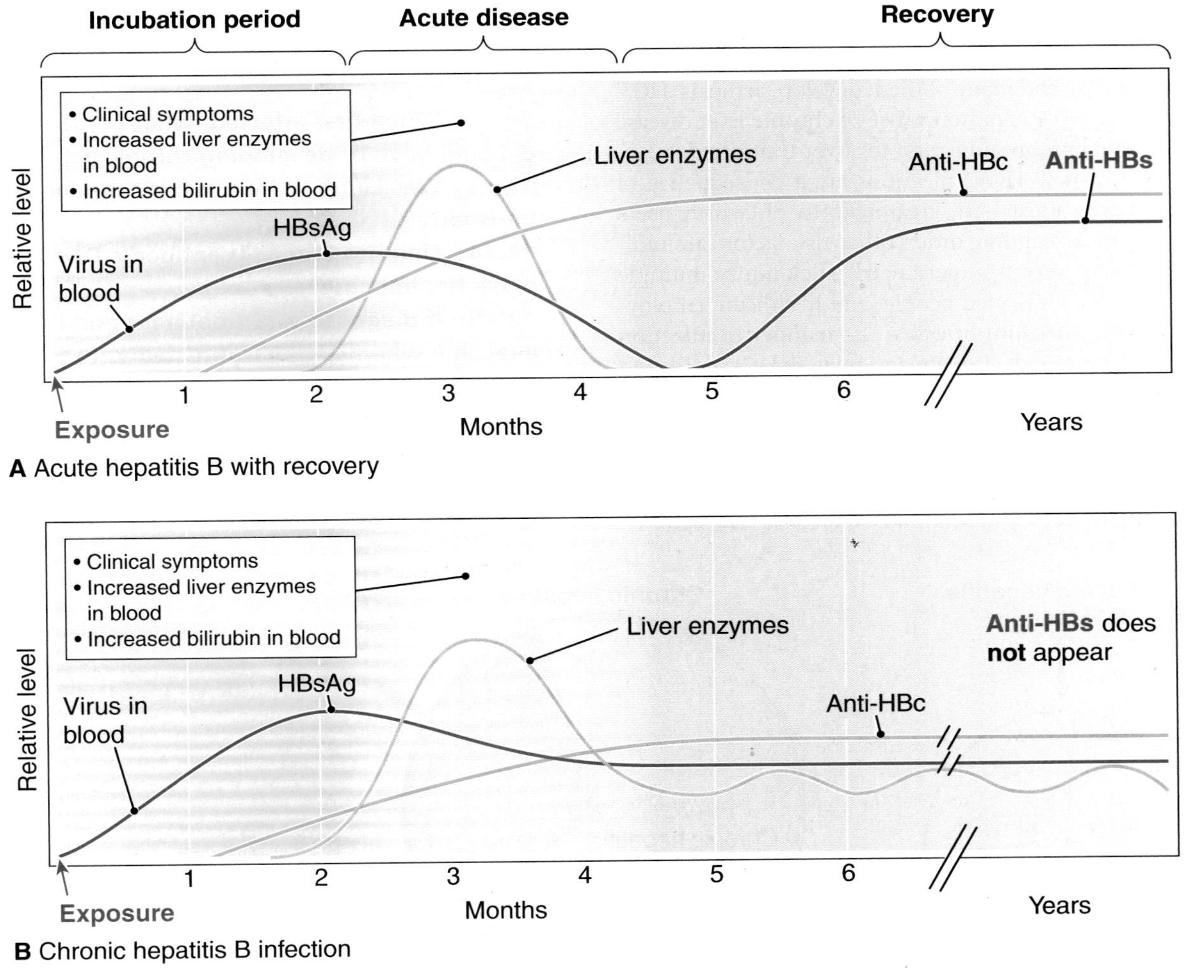

Incubation period
Acute disease
Recovery
• Clinical symptoms
• Increased liver enzymes in blood
• Increased bilirubin in blood
Liver enzymes
Anti-HBc
Anti-HBs
HBsAg
Virus in blood
Relative level
1
2
3
4
5
6
Exposure
Months
Years
A Acute hepatitis B with recovery
• Clinical symptoms
• Increased liver enzymes in blood
• Increased bilirubin in blood
Liver enzymes
Anti-HBs does not appear
HBsAg
Virus in blood
Anti-HBc
Relative level
1
2
3
4
5
6
Exposure
Months
Years
B Chronic hepatitis B infection

Figure 12.14 **Hepatitis B: clinical phases and blood markers of infection. A.** Acute infection is characterized by rapid appearance of the virus in blood before symptoms appear, disappearance of the virus from blood, and the appearance in blood of antibodies to hepatitis B surface antigen (HBsAg). **B.** Chronic hepatitis is signaled by continuing jaundice or clinical symptoms, or the continued presence of virus in blood (as is indicated by the detection in blood of HBsAg).

Antibody to hepatitis B core antigen (**anti-HBc**) is the first antibody to appear and is useful as an early indicator of HBV infection. The appearance of *antibody to hepatitis B surface antigen* (**anti-HBs**) marks the beginning of recovery and is not usually detectable until viremia (HBsAg in blood) has disappeared. Anti-HBs does not appear in patients who develop chronic hepatitis B (Fig. 12.14B) or hepatitis B carrier state. Antiviral drug treatment of certain patients may be effective in eliminating detectable virus and improving clinical outcomes. Vaccination is effective. Anti-HBs confers immunity and is the antibody created by vaccination.

Hepatitis C Virus (HCV) Infection Usually Progresses to Chronic Liver Disease

HCV is a major cause of chronic liver disease (chronic hepatitis, cirrhosis, and hepatocellular carcinoma). About 20,000 new cases are estimated to occur each year, but like hepatitis A and B, most go undiagnosed and unreported. Nearly 2% of the U.S. population has blood antibodies and about 1% are chronically infected, which makes HCV the most common blood-borne infection in the United States. In more than half of those infected, virus is detectable in the blood, indicating a chronic carrier state. In sharp contrast to HAV and HBV infection, most *untreated* HCV infections progress to chronic disease and many of them develop cirrhosis. HCV infection is the most common cause of chronic liver disease and the most common indication for liver transplant.

Over half of new HCV infections are a consequence of intravenous drug abuse—the great majority of IV drug users are infected. In descending order, other risk factors are multiple sex partners, recent surgery, needlestick injury, multiple contacts with HCV-infected people, and healthcare employment. In about one-third of cases, the manner of infection cannot be determined. Transfusion-related HCV infection has nearly disappeared due to rigorous blood bank practices. Figure 12.15 depicts outcomes of HCV infection.

The incubation period is variable but is usually 6–12 weeks. Diagnosis of acute infection is clinical and confirmed by detection in blood of viral RNA (**HCV-RNA**). In acute infection (Fig. 12.16A), **anti-HCV** appears promptly as a marker of acute immune response and persists but does not confer immunity. Over half of patients with HCV progress to chronic infection (Fig. 12.16B). Many of these patients remain asymptomatic, but others have nonjaundiced relapses with mild symptoms, reappearance of detectable HCV-RNA, and elevated levels of liver enzymes. After 20 years, about 25–35% of those with chronic hepatitis develop cirrhosis. Of those developing cirrhosis, a small percentage develop HCC each year. HCV is a mutating RNA virus with dozens of subtypes, which has frustrated hope for a vaccine.

Diagnosis is clinical, with confirmation by liver biopsy and detection of blood markers. Treatment is with a combination of antiviral drugs. Results vary according to the genotype of the virus and if the infection is new or chronic. Cure rates of 70–80% may be realized with prompt treatment of new infections.

Remember This! Most patients infected by HCV who are *not treated* develop chronic hepatitis.

Case Notes

12.12 When first infected, what percent chance did Ling have of developing chronic hepatitis?

12.13 Was Ling's two-month incubation period unusual?

12.14 Ling has anti-HCV antibody. Does this make her immune?

12.15 If diagnosis and treatment had been available when Ling was infected with HCV, was it more likely than not that she would develop chronic hepatitis?

12.16 Why was Ling not given a vaccine for hepatitis C after her initial episode of jaundice?

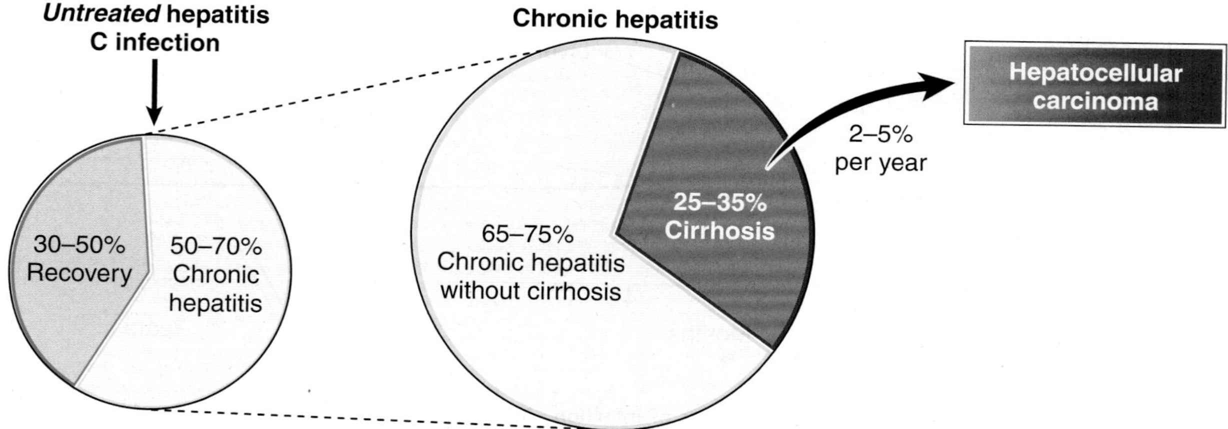

Figure 12.15 Outcomes of *untreated* hepatitis C infection.

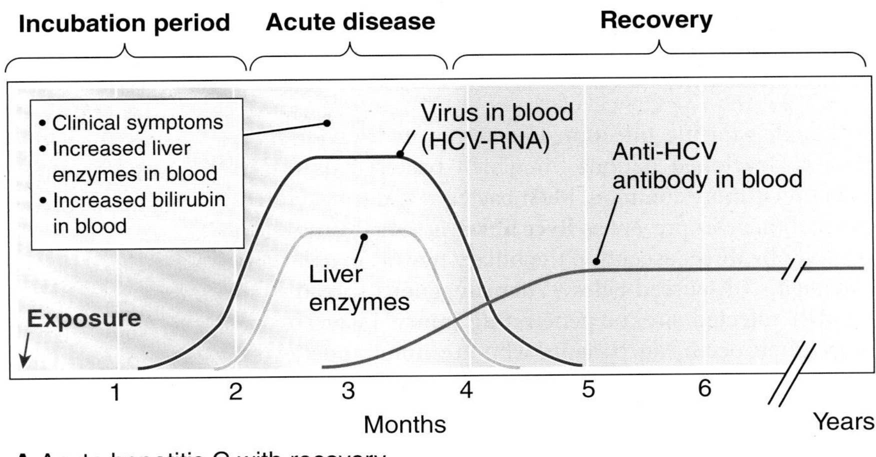

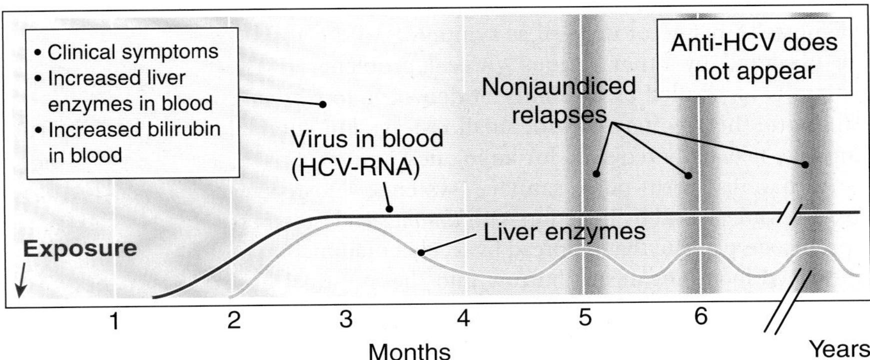

Figure 12.16 **Hepatitis C: clinical phases and blood markers of infection. A.** Acute infection with recovery is characterized by permanent disappearance of clinical symptoms and disappearance of the virus from blood (as is indicated by inability to detect HCV RNA—HCV-RNA—in blood). **B.** Chronic hepatitis is characterized by reappearance of jaundice or clinical symptoms and persistent evidence of the virus in blood, as is indicated by detection in blood of HCV RNA (HCV-RNA). The carrier state is indicated by asymptomatic persistent evidence of the virus in blood.

Other Hepatitis Virus Infections are Uncommon

Hepatitis D Virus (HDV) is peculiar in that it cannot infect without HBV. It can coinfect at the same time HBV is acquired or it can superinfect someone previously infected with HBV. With coinfection, the clinical syndrome is that of the usual HBV infection, the immune system successfully overcomes both of the viruses, and the patient recovers. On the other hand, HDV can superinfect someone who is already a chronic carrier of HBV, in which case the asymptomatic HBV carrier develops acute hepatitis. Most of such cases progress to chronic B + D hepatitis. Most of these infections occur among patients who inject illegal drugs. Patients in both of these groups have multiple opportunities for infection—first by HBV infection, then by HDV infection on a subsequent injection or transfusion. Formerly, hemophiliacs were frequently infected because of their need for intravenous coagulation therapy, but rigorous protective measures by blood banks have eliminated the problem.

Hepatitis E virus (HEV) infection is rare in the United States, but it is the most common form of epidemic hepatitis in India, where it is more common than hepatitis A. Like hepatitis A, it is transmitted by food and water and causes epidemics from time to time in Asia and Africa. The disease usually is mild and self-limiting, but it is exceptionally dangerous in pregnant women, in whom 20% of cases are fatal. It does not appear to have a carrier state and does not cause chronic hepatitis.

Pop Quiz

12.9 True or false? The hepatitis viruses (A-E) are the only viruses capable of infecting the liver.

12.10 True or false? HCV causes epidemic hepatitis, and is responsible for the majority of chronic hepatitis.

12.11 Which hepatitis is of special concern in pregnant women?

Non-Viral Inflammatory Liver Disease

Although parasitic infection is common worldwide, it is rare in developed nations, in which bacterial or fungal infection is more common. Most bacterial and fungal infections of the liver present as **liver abscess**. Organisms reach the liver by direct ascent up the biliary tree, as in *ascending cholangitis* (discussed below), hematogenous spread from another infected site, or penetrating injury. Liver abscess most often occurs in patients who are immunodeficient, who are on cancer chemotherapy, or who are very old or severely debilitated from chronic disease. Fever and hepatomegaly are usually present but are not specific enough to add much value to the differential diagnosis. The mortality rate is high. Often this is because the patient's underlying condition is serious; however, it is sometimes because the diagnosis is missed or delayed as symptoms of the abscess are obscured by other serious clinical problems or the patient is too dulled by disability or dementia to respond. Antibiotic therapy may control small lesions, but surgical drainage is usually required for large ones.

In nations with poor sanitary systems, most liver abscesses are caused by infection with *Entamoeba histolytica*, a protozoan parasite that is spread by fecal contamination of unwashed food. Organisms burrow into the intestinal wall and spread up the portal vein to infect the liver.

Schistosomiasis (Chapter 4) is a parasitic disease caused by *Schistosoma* species, tiny freshwater parasites with an unusually complex life cycle and an ability to infect many organs. It is widespread in South America, the Middle East, and Africa. One variety infiltrates the portal venous system, inciting a chronic immune reaction that leads to portal hypertension and cirrhosis.

Autoimmune hepatitis is a syndrome of chronic, progressive hepatitis not associated with a viral infection, although its microscopic features are indistinguishable from those of chronic viral hepatitis. It may be indolent or may progress to fulminant hepatitis with liver failure. It accounts for about 20% of cases of chronic hepatitis. The immune mechanism is a delayed T-cell–mediated (Chapter 3) reaction. The environmental trigger is often unknown but may owe to viral infection or certain drugs.

In autoimmune hepatitis, nearly 80% of patients are women, mostly middle-aged adults. The clinical picture varies from mild to severe. As a rule, no blood markers of viral hepatitis are present, but a few patients may have false-positive anti-HCV antibody test results. Most patients have high titers of autoantibodies, such as antinuclear, antismooth muscle, or antimitochondrial antibodies. In more than half of patients, some other autoimmune disease is present, such as ulcerative colitis (UC), Sjögren syndrome, thyroiditis, systemic lupus erythematosus (SLE), or rheumatoid arthritis (RA). As with many autoimmune diseases, there is an increased frequency of association with certain HLA genotypes. Most patients respond well to immunosuppressive therapy, but a few patients progress to cirrhosis.

Diagnosis is clinicopathologic, taking into consideration the clinical picture, laboratory findings including autoantibodies, and the liver biopsy. Steroids and immunosuppressive drugs are mainstays of treatment.

Case Notes

12.17 Ling had anti-HCV in her blood, a condition that may occur in autoimmune hepatitis. Is there other evidence for or against the possibility of autoimmune hepatitis?

Pop Quiz

12.12 True or false? Autoimmune hepatitis is indistinguishable from viral hepatitis on microscopy.

12.13 What infectious etiology is responsible for liver abscesses in nations with poor sanitary systems?

Toxic Liver Injury

Injury from toxins or drugs should always be suspected in the differential diagnosis of liver disease, as the liver metabolizes and excretes most drugs and other exogenous compounds, almost any of which in sufficiently large amounts can cause liver damage. Toxic liver injury accounts for about 10% of adverse drug reactions and is the most common cause of acute fulminant liver failure.

A Wide Variety of Toxins Cause Liver Damage

There are two types of toxic liver reactions. First are those that are predictable and **dose-related**; that is, liver damage is certain if enough toxin is present. Historically, most cases of liver toxicity arose in industrial settings, but improved occupational safety regulations have nearly eliminated the problem. With the exception of alcohol abuse, acute, dose-related liver injury is uncommon today. When it happens, it is usually the result of large doses of chemotherapy agents or of accidental or suicidal doses of drugs. Acetaminophen (Tylenol®) accounts for half of cases of acute fulminant liver failure. Activated charcoal avidly absorbs acetaminophen and should be administered orally if the patient arrives for care within one hour of ingestion. Oral

N-acetylcysteine may be helpful in blunting the toxic effect of acetaminophen.

Second, and much more common, is unpredictable and **nondose-related** toxic injury, where the damage is out of proportion to the dose. These reactions, also called *idiosyncratic reactions*, occur when the individual cannot metabolize a chemical as well as other persons can. The chemical may initiate autoimmune hepatitis. Although microscopically idiosyncratic reactions are indistinguishable from chronic viral hepatitis, laboratory markers of virus infection are present in patients with viral hepatitis. Idiosyncratic reactions have been attributed to a long list of drugs, among them sulfonamide antibiotics, isoniazid (an antituberculosis drug), halothane (a gas anesthetic), and chlorpromazine (a tranquilizer).

Remember This! Half of all cases of acute liver failure are caused by acetaminophen.

Symptoms of acute toxic injury span the continuum of liver injury from almost imperceptible to fulminant liver failure, and onset ranges from instantaneous to weeks after exposure. Drug-induced hepatitis is clinically and pathologically indistinguishable from chronic viral hepatitis. Diagnosis is confirmed by absence of hepatitis markers in blood. Patients with drug- or toxin-induced liver disease usually recover upon withdrawal of the agent.

Reye syndrome is a special category of liver injury related to aspirin, although a direct, causal relationship with aspirin has not been established. It is a combination of fatty liver and acute brain dysfunction (encephalopathy) in children that usually develops a few days after an acute viral illness treated with aspirin. Onset is heralded by severe vomiting, lethargy, irritability, and hepatomegaly. Jaundice is usually absent initially. About 25% of these youngsters progress to coma. Death may be attributable to liver or to neurologic disease. The disease is more complex than simple aspirin toxicity because the doses consumed are far too small to be toxic. Public information campaigns advising parents to use acetaminophen instead of aspirin have led to a sharp decline in Reye syndrome in the United States.

Alcohol Abuse Is the Leading Cause of Liver Disease

Alcohol abuse is a fact of antiquity and is still the leading cause of liver disease in industrialized countries today. About 20 million Americans abuse alcohol (about 10% of adults) and about 25% of hospitalized patients have some alcohol-related problem. Short-term ingestion of 80 gm of alcohol (more or less about six beers, six standard cocktails, or six glasses of wine) produces mild, reversible fatty liver. Consistent ingestion of twice this amount over many years is likely to produce severe injury.

The History of Medicine, "Famous People with Alcoholism," provides a glimpse at the lives of several well-known individuals who have abused alcohol.

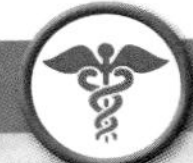

The History of Medicine

FAMOUS PEOPLE WITH ALCOHOLISM

Many famous American writers have struggled with alcohol abuse and dependency. Poet and short story writer Edgar Allan Poe (1809–1849), perhaps most famous for his haunting poem *The Raven*, fell dead on the streets of Baltimore at age 40, apparently from complications of alcohol abuse. F. Scott Fitzgerald (1896–1940), author of the classic American novel *The Great Gatsby*, was notorious for his heavy drinking and died of a massive heart attack at age 44. Novelist, poet, and film critic James Agee (1909–1955) suffered a similar fate. Of course, literary figures aren't alone in battling alcohol abuse. Entertainers, politicians, and many others in the public spotlight have fought the same demons, including one particularly inspiring star athlete.

At the 2000 Olympics in Sydney, Australia, Native American Jim Thorpe (1888–1953) was voted the greatest athlete of the 20th century, a fact that astonished legions of sports-crazed Americans who had never heard of him.

Here's why. In the 1912 Olympics, Thorpe won gold medals in the decathlon and pentathlon (which together encompass 15 sports); he played professional baseball, hitting for a lifetime average of 0.252 in six seasons with the Giants, Braves, and Reds; he played professional football, playing on both offense and defense and scoring 25 touchdowns in one season for the Canton Bulldogs, after which he became president of what would later become the National Football League; in 1950, he was named by the Associated Press as the greatest football professional ever.

He was formidable at every sport he tried: basketball, lacrosse, hockey, archery, handball, tennis, boxing, wrestling, bowling, billiards, darts, shooting, golf, gymnastics, and swimming. He even won first place in a school dance contest while a student at Carlisle (Pennsylvania) Indian School. In 1941, on a return trip to Carlisle, Thorpe stood at midfield and drop-kicked a football over the goal. He then turned and placekicked a second ball for a successful field goal at the other end of the field—at the age of 52.

In a triumph of legalism over justice, Thorpe's Olympic Medals were stripped from him in 1913 because it was found he had played semiprofessional baseball, something he did not hide like others, who played under false names. Thorpe's Olympic medals were restored by the International Olympic Committee in 1983. That was too late for Thorpe. He had battled alcohol for decades and died penniless in 1953. Thorpe's alcohol dependence takes nothing from his accomplishments. If anything, it makes them all the more remarkable because he triumphed despite the burden.

Women are more prone to develop alcoholic liver injury than men. For an equivalent amount of ingested alcohol, they develop higher blood alcohol because they have less body mass and relatively less body water than men (Chapter 6). Perhaps due to the influence of estrogen, which is metabolised by the liver, the female liver is more susceptible to alcohol injury.

Genetics also plays a role in liver injury. Persons of African descent are more vulnerable than Caucasians despite the fact that alcohol consumption is similar in the two groups.

The best evidence linking alcohol to liver disease is epidemiologic: 1) evidence shows a direct relationship between the amount of alcohol consumed and the development of cirrhosis; and 2) during prolonged shortages of alcohol there is less cirrhosis—in the United States during Prohibition (1919–1933) and in France during World War II (1939–1945), deaths from cirrhosis declined. As a rule, the amount of alcohol necessary to produce cirrhosis is about 200 grams of ethanol per day—the approximate amount in one pint (near 500 ml) of whiskey, gin, or vodka or two bottles of wine—and consumed regularly for 10–16 years.

Alcohol directly damages hepatocytes. Alcohol *abuse* produces three distinct lesions: fatty liver (>95%), alcoholic hepatitis (about 20%), and cirrhosis (about 15%), which usually occur in sequence. Not to be forgotten in this discussion is the other damage done by alcohol abuse—social disruption, cancers of the oral cavity and esophagus, pancreatitis, cardiomyopathy, fetal alcohol syndrome, brain damage, and accidents of every kind.

Treatment is abstention.

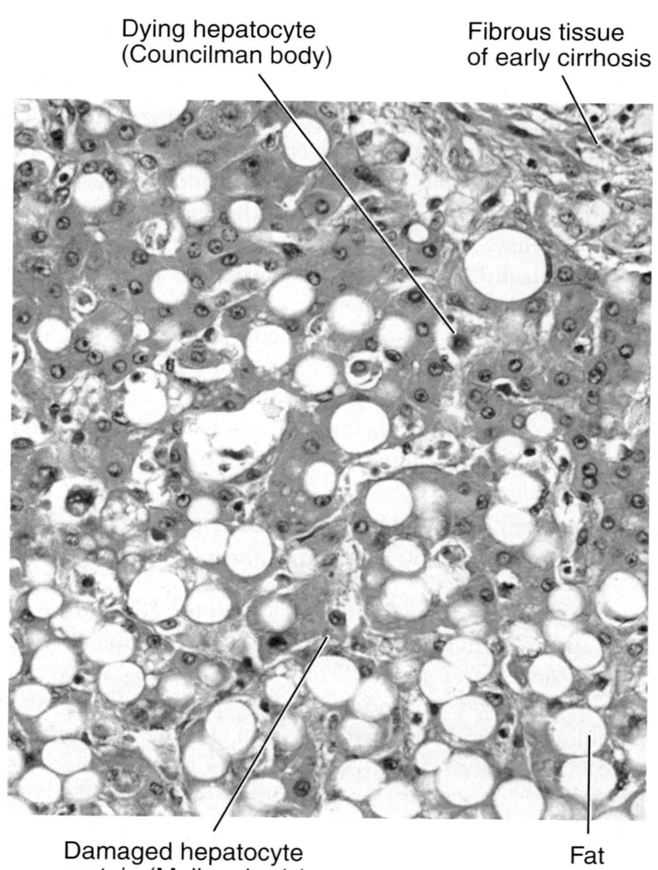

Figure 12.17 **Alcoholic liver.** Fatty liver (steatosis) and alcoholic hepatitis. Large clear areas are hepatocytes filled with fat. Hepatitis is indicated by necrotic liver cells (Councilman bodies), intracellular degenerative inclusions (Mallory alcoholic hyaline), and fibrosis. Nonalcoholic steatohepatitis (NASH) can be indistinguishable from this pathologic picture.

Fatty Liver

Virtually all alcoholics develop fatty livers. The first sign of alcohol injury is fatty degeneration of hepatocytes, also known as **steatosis**, as is depicted in Figure 23.10 (Chapter 23) and Figure 12.17. In severe cases, the liver is enlarged (sometimes two or three times normal size), yellow, and greasy. Exactly how alcohol causes fatty liver is not completely clear but appears related to intracellular lipid transport. Why some patients get simple fatty liver and others steatohepatitis is a mystery. Withdrawal will reverse the steatosis, but not the scarring and cirrhosis, if it is present.

Patients with fatty liver are usually asymptomatic, though they may have mild elevations of liver enzyme levels in blood. Elevations of liver enzyme levels indicate that even though fatty liver is fully reversible, hepatocytes are being damaged. Continued damage may lead to increasingly severe liver disease. Figure 12.17 presents evidence of damaged hepatocytes: dying hepatocytes appear as small, round, dark cells (*Councilman bodies*), and clumps of damaged protein appear as irregular reddish deposits (*Mallory bodies*).

Alcoholic Hepatitis

Alcoholic hepatitis is a more severe form of liver injury than fatty liver. The pathologic findings are called **steatohepatitis**, and are characterized by steatosis, inflammation, hepatocyte necrosis, and early fibrosis, which can progress to cirrhosis if alcohol abuse continues. Why some patients progress from fatty liver to alcoholic hepatitis is not known.

Clinical features depend on the degree of liver injury. Occasionally, alcoholic hepatitis may appear so suddenly that bile duct obstruction or viral hepatitis is suspected. Malaise, anorexia, right upper quadrant pain, and jaundice are common. Leukocytosis and fever may be present, depending upon the extent of liver cell necrosis. Blood enzyme levels are moderately elevated. Each bout of alcoholic hepatitis carries a 10–20% chance of death, not merely from liver disease, but also from intestinal hemorrhage, pancreatitis, and other alcohol-related problems. Abnormal clotting tests, low blood albumin, or clinical signs of hepatic failure are a bad prognostic sign because they do not become evident until the liver is severely damaged.

Pathologically, *alcoholic steatohepatitis* can be indistinguishable from *nonalcoholic steatohepatitis* (NASH) except for a clinical history of alcohol abuse.

Established alcoholic hepatitis may not be reversible even with complete abstention from alcohol. Among those who quit drinking completely, one in five will nevertheless progress to cirrhosis. Patients who continue to drink usually develop cirrhosis within a few years.

Alcoholic Cirrhosis

Alcoholic cirrhosis is the final and irreversible stage of alcoholic liver disease and is similar clinically and anatomically to other forms of cirrhosis discussed earlier. Although most alcoholics do not develop cirrhosis (only about 15% do), alcoholic cirrhosis is second only to chronic viral hepatitis as a cause of adult liver transplantation in the United States. Moreover, few alcoholics escape portal hypertension and other forms of liver damage, upon which are piled the train wreck of pancreatitis, encephalopathy, and gastric ulcers; cancers of the mouth, throat, and esophagus; increased risk for motor vehicle and other accidents, and social and financial ruin.

Case Notes

12.18 Was there anything in Ling's background to suggest the possibility of alcohol-related liver disease?

Pop Quiz

12.14 True or false? Among alcoholics who quit drinking completely, one in five will nevertheless progress to cirrhosis.

12.15 True or false? The majority of alcoholics develop cirrhosis.

12.16 How does an idiosyncratic reaction differ from a predictable reaction?

Metabolic Liver Disease

A small number of liver diseases are caused by inherited or acquired metabolic disorders.

Non-Alcoholic Fatty Liver Disease Is Very Common

Nonalcoholic fatty liver disease (NAFLD) is a group of related conditions featuring fatty liver in patients who consume very little or no alcohol. It is arguably the most common liver disease in the United States. It is closely associated with some features of the *metabolic syndrome* (Chapter 23)—obesity, hyperlipemia, and prediabetic insulin resistance (Chapter 13). An estimated two-thirds of all obese persons have some degree of NAFLD. Pathologic changes in the liver vary from minimal steatosis without inflammation, to steatosis with minor inflammation, to severe *steatohepatitis*. **Nonalcoholic steatohepatitis (NASH)** affects men and women equally. It may progress to cirrhosis and is probably the cause of most cirrhosis of "unknown" origin.

Patients with simple steatosis are usually asymptomatic but may have elevated liver enzymes. Patients with more significant liver involvement may have hepatomegaly and fatigue. Many patients are obese or have metabolic syndrome. Diagnosis is by liver biopsy and imaging studies to demonstrate liver fat. Treatment addresses underlying risk factors such as obesity, insulin resistance, and hyperlipemia.

Case Notes

12.19 Was there any reason to suspect that Ling might have had NAFLD?

Hemochromatosis Is Surprisingly Common

Hemochromatosis is a hereditary iron storage disease, which features accumulation of excessive iron in the liver, heart, and pancreas. It is frequently referred to as primary or hereditary hemochromatosis to distinguish it from **hemosiderosis**, an acquired excess of stored iron that may be referred to as secondary hemochromatosis. Hemosiderosis is usually the result of repeated blood transfusions given as treatment for sickle cell anemia, thalassemia, or aplastic anemia.

Although the small intestine avidly absorbs iron, there is no specialized excretory pathway for iron. Women regularly shed iron with the blood they lose with each menstrual period, but in men there is little physiologic opportunity for iron loss. Most body iron reserves are stored in the liver, which therefore is directly affected by iron overload.

Hemochromatosis is an autosomal recessive disorder caused by abnormally high iron absorption from the intestine. It is surprisingly common: among people of northern European ancestry—about 1 in 10 persons are heterozygous carriers of the faulty gene, and about 1 in 200 persons is diseased (homozygous), making hemochromatosis one of the most common inborn errors of metabolism in the United States.

Hemochromatosis usually does not become symptomatic until adulthood because it takes many years to accumulate enough iron to cause damage. Men are affected 10 times more often than women. Cirrhosis is universal in untreated cases. As Figure 12.18 illustrates, full blown

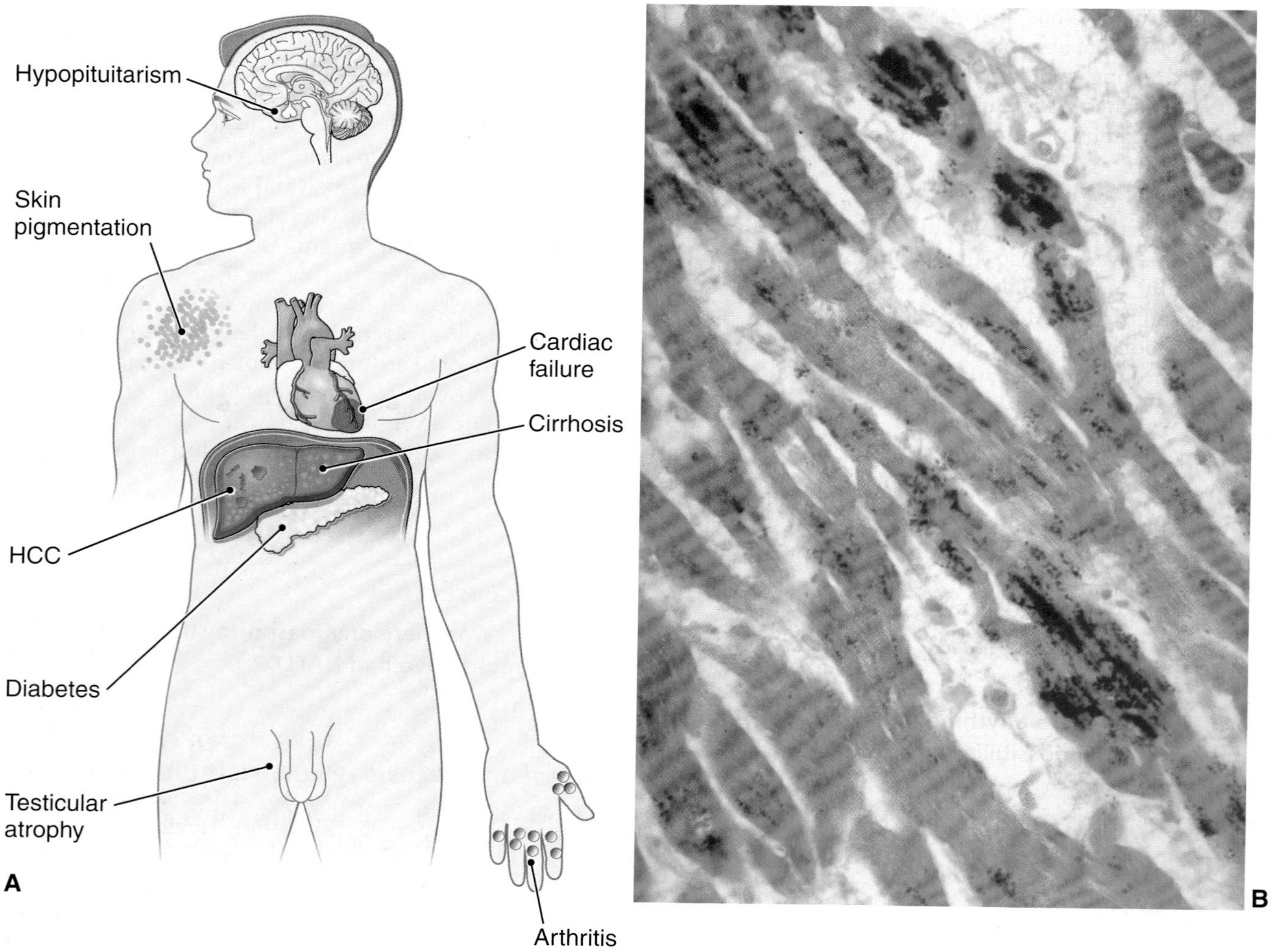

Figure 12.18 **Hemochromatosis A.** Complications of hemochromatosis. **B.** Iron stain of myocardium.

cases result in iron deposits in the liver causing cirrhosis; in the pancreas, diabetes; in cardiac muscle, heart failure; in skin, brown pigmentation; in joints, arthritis; and in the pituitary, pituitary failure. In some patients, the first complaint is hypogonadism, the origin of which is not well understood.

Diagnosis depends on finding clinical features or markedly increased levels of blood iron, ferritin, and transferrin in the absence of another known cause. It is confirmed by liver biopsy showing marked iron overload. Screening family members of the patient is very important. If the diagnosis of primary hemochromatosis is made early, most patients can expect to live normal lives if the excessive accumulation of iron is removed by periodic bleeding (phlebotomy). Patients with transfusion hemosiderosis who continue to need blood because of their underlying anemia can be treated effectively with injectable chemicals that bind (chelate) iron in a form that allows iron excretion in urine.

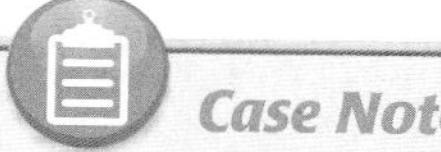

12.20 Was there any evidence to favor or disfavor hemochromatosis in Ling's case?

Wilson Disease Is a Disorder of Copper Metabolism

Copper is absorbed in the gut and excreted in bile. Absorbed copper is carried by albumin to the liver, where it is bound to *ceruloplasmin*, the copper transport protein, and secreted back into blood for metabolic distribution. Excess copper is secreted into bile. **Wilson disease** is a rare autosomal recessive inherited disorder that results in impaired excretion of copper into bile, failure of copper to attach to ceruloplasmin, and failure of ceruloplasmin secretion into blood. The result is a toxic accumulation of copper, mainly in the brain and liver.

First symptoms may occur at any age but are usually manifest by the young adult years. The earliest manifestation is usually acute or chronic liver disease. Other signs include behavioral oddities, psychosis, or tremors and abnormal gait. The liver may show fatty change and chronic hepatitis or cirrhosis, changes that combined with the neurologic symptoms may result in misdiagnosis of alcoholic liver disease. Copper deposits in the eye occur as a brown-green arc (*Kayser-Fleischer ring*) where the sclera meets the cornea. The diagnosis of Wilson disease rests on finding decreased serum ceruloplasmin, increased liver copper deposits, and increased urine excretion of copper. Blood levels of copper are variable. Treatment is by chelation with penicillamine, which binds (chelates) copper for urinary excretion. Although many patients given long-term copper chelation therapy do well, in some patients liver disease is relentless, and liver transplantation offers the only hope.

Hereditary Alpha-1 Antitrypsin Deficiency Causes Liver Disease and Emphysema

Alpha-1 antitrypsin (AAT) is an enzyme that was discussed in Chapter 10 because of its importance in the pathogenesis of emphysema caused by smoking. AAT is a protein made by the liver that inhibits the action of trypsin and other protein-digesting enzymes that are released by neutrophils in acute inflammatory reactions. AAT deficiency is an inherited disorder that results in low levels of AAT activity in the lungs and accumulation of excessive amounts of defective AAT in the liver, which appear in liver cells as distinctive protein globules and damage liver cells by an unknown mechanism.

About 10–20% of infants with AAT deficiency develop *neonatal hepatitis and cholestasis* (Chapter 22). Nevertheless, in most patients liver disease does not appear until hepatitis or cirrhosis appear in adolescence or adult life. Patients who have never smoked or who do not have occupational exposure have normal life expectancy but many will develop mild emphysema. The most common causes of death are emphysema and cirrhosis.

The diagnosis is made by finding low levels of blood AAT activity and characteristic microscopic evidence of AAT accumulation in hepatocytes. Some patients may warrant treatment of their pulmonary disease with replacement AAT. Smokers should stop smoking. Those with impaired lung function need standard emphysema treatment. Treatment of liver disease is supportive.

Pop Quiz

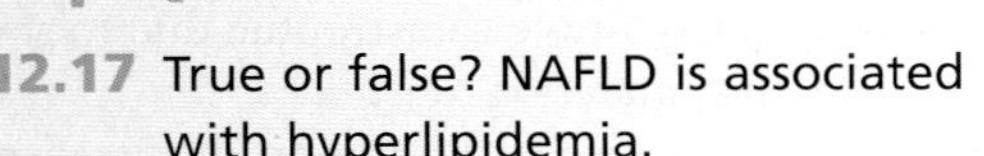

12.17 True or false? NAFLD is associated with hyperlipidemia.

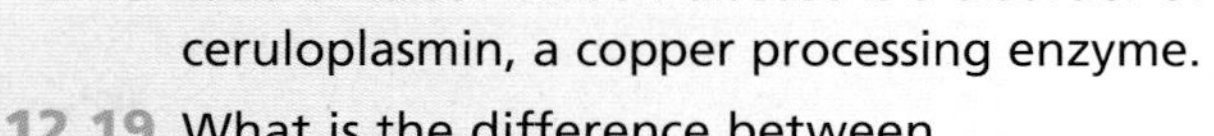

12.18 True or false? Wilson disease is a disorder of ceruloplasmin, a copper processing enzyme.

12.19 What is the difference between hemochromatosis and hemosiderosis?

12.20 What organ, aside from the liver, is commonly affected in AAT deficiency?

Disease of Intrahepatic Bile Ducts

The biliary tree can be the primary site of liver disease. Nevertheless, intrahepatic biliary ducts are frequently involved secondarily in the diseases discussed heretofore.

Prolonged Biliary Obstruction Causes Secondary Biliary Cirrhosis

Prolonged obstruction in the extrahepatic biliary tree results in severe damage to the intrahepatic biliary system and to the liver in general. The most common cause is obstruction of the common bile duct by gallstones (discussed below), followed by cancer of the head of the pancreas, and by scars from prior surgical procedures. Pathologically, the initial change is cholestasis, which evolves into inflammation, then into scarring that extends outward until it results in **secondary biliary cirrhosis**. Obstruction may also allow bacteria to ascend the common duct to infect the biliary tree and liver (**ascending cholangitis**). Diagnosis of infection is clinical and by biopsy and imaging studies of the biliary system. Treatment is by antibiotics for infection and surgical relief of the obstruction.

Primary Biliary Cirrhosis Is an Autoimmune Disease

Primary biliary cirrhosis (Fig. 12.19) is an autoimmune disease that evolves from inflammatory destruction of intrahepatic bile ducts. Nearly 90% of patients also have another autoimmune disease such as SLE or Sjögren syndrome, and virtually all have high titers of antimitochondrial antibody in their blood. About 80% of patients are middle-aged women. Initial symptoms are fatigue and pruritus (due to cholestasis). Hepatomegaly is usually present. Skin hyperpigmentation and arthritis occur in about one-third of patients. Jaundice and spider angiomas appear late and suggest that cirrhosis is present and liver failure may be imminent. AP level is markedly elevated because of damage to the bile duct epithelium, and blood cholesterol is usually increased because of retained bile acids. Cholestasis often causes yellow cholesterol deposits in the eyelids (*xanthelasma*).

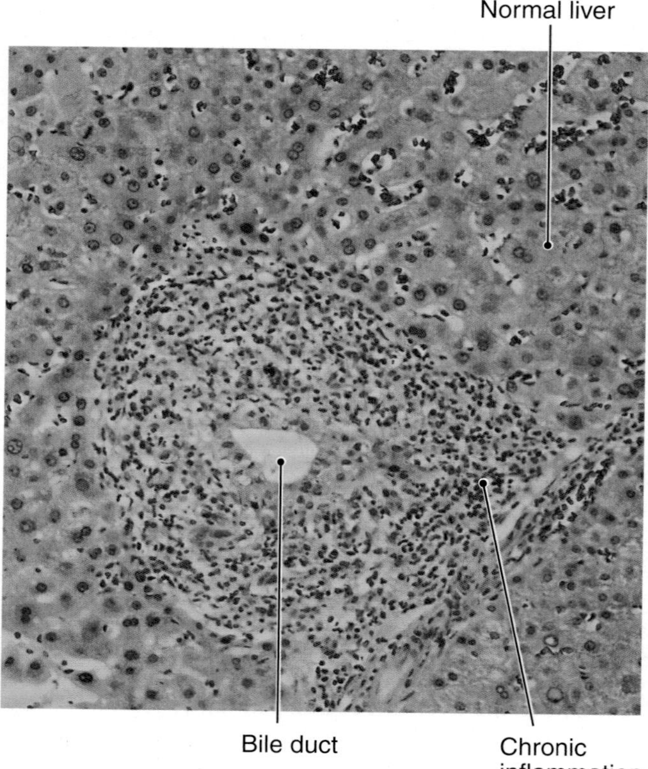

Figure 12.19 **Primary biliary cirrhosis.** Microscopic study of early stage showing a collar of chronic inflammatory cells (lymphocytes) around small bile duct.

Impaired bile excretion may also cause fat malabsorption syndrome (Chapter 11).

Diagnosis is by biopsy. Biopsy in early disease reveals accumulations of lymphocytes surrounding bile ducts. Later, bile duct scarring occurs and progresses to cirrhosis. Death results from cirrhosis, portal hypertension, and hepatic failure. The only effective treatment is liver transplantation.

Primary Sclerosing Cholangitis Affects Intrahepatic and Extrahepatic Bile Ducts

Primary sclerosing cholangitis is a chronic cholestatic liver disease caused by inflammation and fibrosis of intra- and extrahepatic bile ducts. Two-thirds of patients have ulcerative colitis (UC) (Chapter 11). Less often, other inflammatory bowel disease is present; however, in most cases of the other third, no underlying disease can be found. The pathology of sclerosing cholangitis is characterized by scarring of bile ducts inside and outside of the liver. Microscopically, findings in the liver are distinctive—onionskin fibrosis that encircles and eventually destroys the ducts.

Although most patients with UC are women, most patients with primary sclerosing cholangitis are men under age 40. The typical patient is an adult male with long-standing UC who slowly develops signs and symptoms of liver disease. Blood autoantibodies are varied and common and include antinuclear, antimitochondrial, antismooth muscle, and rheumatoid factor. Biliary cirrhosis is the end point. About 5% of patients develop primary biliary adenocarcinoma. Diagnosis is by liver biopsy supported by typical clinical and laboratory findings. Liver transplantation is the definitive treatment.

Case Notes

12.21 Did anything in Ling's case suggest the possibility of biliary tract disease?

Pop Quiz

12.21 True or false? Primary biliary cirrhosis is characterized by the presence of antismooth muscle antibodies.

12.22 What is the most common cause of secondary biliary cirrhosis?

Circulatory Disorders

Blood flow may be obstructed in the portal vein as it flows into the liver, as it flows through the liver, or in the hepatic vein as it flows out of the liver.

Limitation of blood flow *into* the liver may be arterial or portal. Obstruction of arterial flow through the hepatic artery is uncommon and usually due to atherosclerosis or thromboembolism. Liver infarction (Fig. 2.12A, Chapter 2) may occur, but because of the liver's dual blood supply, infarction may be avoided.

Limitation of portal blood flow may be due to obstruction of the extrahepatic portal vein. Portal hypertension occurs. Obstruction is usually caused by thrombosis associated with intra-abdominal disease, such as pancreatitis, trauma, cancer, abdominal surgery, or peritonitis. Slowly developing compromise of portal flow may be well tolerated until complications of portal hypertension arise. Widespread thrombosis of intrahepatic portal venules may also impair portal blood flow. Thrombi usually develop slowly; because of the liver's dual blood supply, the result is usually liver atrophy, not infarction. Acute portal vein occlusion, however, may prove catastrophic due to severe bowel congestion and infarction.

The most common cause of limitation of *intrahepatic* blood flow is cirrhosis. Another common cause is right heart failure with chronic passive congestion of the liver

(Fig. 6.9, Chapter 6). Severe congestion and sluggish flow in the central veins of the hepatic lobules causes centrilobular atrophy and hemorrhagic necrosis. Liver function is usually not much affected, but long-standing congestion may produce some fibrosis and impaired liver function. This is traditionally called *cardiac cirrhosis* though the degree of scarring and functional impairment is relatively minor compared to "real" cirrhosis.

Obstruction of blood flow *out* of the liver is caused by obstruction of one or more hepatic vein tributaries or the main hepatic vein near its juncture with the inferior vena cava. Obstruction of one large branch is usually asymptomatic, but occlusion of the main hepatic vein, called *Budd-Chiari syndrome*, causes severe congestion, intrahepatic hemorrhage, and hepatocellular necrosis. It is usually attributable to diseases associated with an increased tendency for intravascular coagulation and thrombosis, such as polycythemia vera (PV). It can also be prompted by pregnancy or oral contraceptive use, and coagulation disorders associated with a tendency to venous thrombosis (Chapter 6). Treatment is surgical. The mortality rate is high.

Pop Quiz

12.23 True or false? Liver infarction always occurs with obstruction of the hepatic artery.

12.24 True or false? The most common cause of limitation of intrahepatic blood flow is cirrhosis.

Tumors of the Liver

The most common neoplasm *in* (not "of") the liver is metastatic carcinoma (Fig. 12.20), usually from a primary malignancy in the colon, lung, breast, or pancreas. Primary liver cell carcinoma is uncommon in North America, but very common in some other regions.

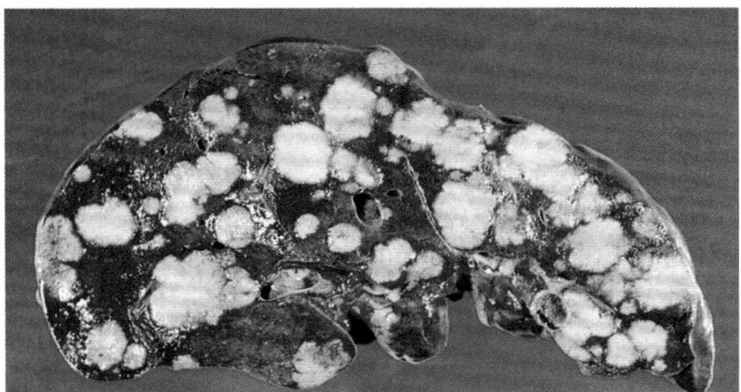

Figure 12.20 **Metastatic carcinoma in liver.** This patient had colon cancer, which metastasized up the portal vein to the liver.

The most common benign tumor *of* the liver is *cavernous hemangioma*, a vascular mass that is not neoplastic and is composed of dilated blood vessels. Cavernous hemangiomas are usually small and located immediately beneath the fibrous capsule of the liver.

Hepatic adenoma is a benign neoplasm of hepatocytes and is encountered most often in young women taking oral contraceptives. It may become quite large and may rupture, especially during pregnancy, causing life-threatening intra-abdominal hemorrhage. Regression occurs when contraceptive use stops.

Hepatoblastoma is a malignant tumor of hepatocytes that occurs in children. Treatment is surgery and chemotherapy. Five-year survival is 80%.

Hepatocellular carcinoma (HCC) is a malignant neoplasm of hepatocytes that is usually related to chronic HBV and HCV infections. Although rare in the United States, its incidence is very high in Africa and Asia, where hepatitis B is exceedingly common. Half of cases worldwide occur in China. Chronic hepatitis C with cirrhosis is the major cause in industrialized nations. HCC usually grows as a single massive neoplasm (Fig. 12.21). It has a marked tendency to invade hepatic veins and may snake its way up the hepatic vein and far into the vena cava. Hematogenous (blood borne) metastases are common.

The usual patient has pre-existing liver disease. HCC may be heralded by a sudden increase of liver size, sudden worsening of ascites, appearance of bloody ascites, or intense abdominal pain. About half of patients have increased levels of *alpha-fetoprotein* in the blood, although this is not a specific marker because increases are seen in cirrhosis, other liver diseases, pregnancy, and other conditions. Marked elevations, however, are rarely seen in any

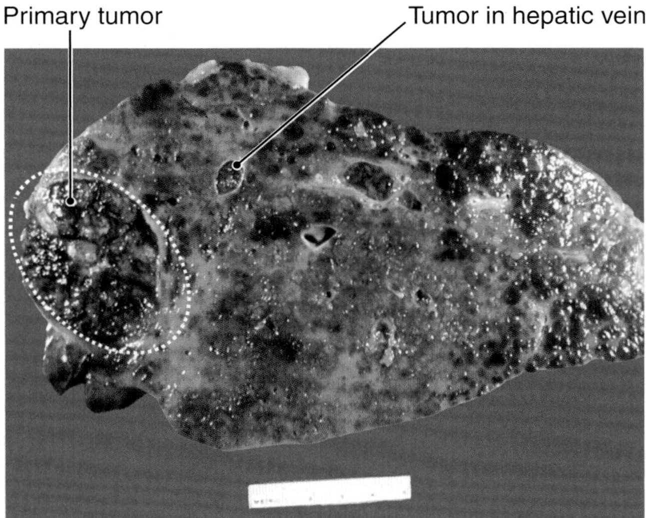

Figure 12.21 **Hepatocellular carcinoma.** The primary tumor is a single, large mass, which can be seen invading an intrahepatic branch of the hepatic vein. The liver is cirrhotic; cirrhosis is a major cause of HCC.

disease other than HCC. The prognosis for patients with HCC is grim; most patients die within a short period of time. Death usually follows profound wasting (cachexia), hepatic coma, or GI bleeding. HBV vaccinations have proven effective in lowering the incidence of HCC in areas where hepatitis B is acquired early in life.

Cholangiocarcinoma is a malignancy of bile duct epithelium. It may occur in the intrahepatic or extrahepatic bile ducts or in the gallbladder. Incidence is high in Asia and Southeast Asia. Risk factors include sclerosing cholangitis, HCV infection, and chronic liver schistosomiasis (parasites seen in Africa, Asia, and South America; Chapter 4). In the United States, however, most cases arise without known risk factors. Cholangiocarcinoma of the liver tends to be more aggressive than HCC—patients quickly develop severe cachexia, hepatic coma, and esophageal varices with fatal hemorrhage, and only 15% survive two years.

Case Notes

12.22 Does Ling's type of hepatitis put her at increased risk for HCC?

Pop Quiz

12.25 True or false? Most cases of cholangiocarcinoma in the United States arise without known risk factors.

12.26 Oral contraceptives are responsible for which hepatic tumor?

Disorders of the Gallbladder and Extrahepatic Bile Ducts

Recall that the biliary tree begins as tiny ducts that gradually grow larger as they merge, like rivers leading to the sea, until they form the common bile duct that exits the liver to connect with the duodenum at the ampulla of Vater. The gallbladder, attached to one side of the common bile duct, holds a reserve of bile that is discharged into the common bile duct after meals.

Gallstones Are the Most Important Problem of the Gallbladder

Disorders of the gallbladder are not complicated and are very common. Almost all gallbladder and biliary tract disease occurs as a result of inflammation closely related to the presence of gallstones.

Cholelithiasis (Gallstones)

Stones in the gallbladder or biliary tree are referred to collectively as **cholelithiasis**. Stones in the bile ducts are referred to as **choledocholithiasis**. The great majority of gallstones form in the gallbladder. Most patients have multiple stones, sometimes several dozen. In the United States, about one million new cases are diagnosed each year, half requiring surgery. The surgical mortality rate is <1%.

Most gallstones (80%) are *cholesterol gallstones*, which form when bile becomes oversaturated with cholesterol. Why some people develop gallstones and others do not is a mystery; however, there are certain well-known conditions associated with the development of cholesterol stones:

- *Age and sex*: Older people have more gallstones than younger ones do. In their reproductive years, women are three times more likely than men to have gallstones.
- *Weight*: Obese people are much more likely to develop gallstones; most are cholesterol stones.
- *Ethnic, hereditary, and geographic factors*: Cholesterol gallstones occur in about 75% of those of Pima, Hopi, and Navajo ancestry. A family history of gallstones imparts increased risk. Gallstones are more common in industrialized countries than in developing ones.
- *Drugs*: Oral contraceptives and estrogen therapy increase hepatic uptake and secretion of cholesterol.
- *Acquired conditions*: Any condition that causes decreased gallbladder motility (e.g., pregnancy, rapid weight loss, spinal cord injury) predisposes to gallstones.

Figure 12.22 illustrates pure **cholesterol gallstones**, which are semitranslucent, yellowish, and egg shaped. Cholesterol stones arise only in the gallbladder, but pigment stones may arise in the biliary tree as well.

Remember This! Most biliary tract disease is associated with gallstones.

Pigment gallstones (Fig. 12.23) account for the remaining 20% of gallstones. They are dark brown or black, have multiple flat surfaces, and are composed of bilirubin and bile substances other than cholesterol. The greatest risk factor for pigment gallstones is hemolysis of RBCs, as occurs with sickle cell anemia, which increases the amount of bilirubin delivered to the liver to be excreted in bile. Other risk factors for pigment gallstones are not so well understood.

A majority of patients with gallstones live a lifetime without symptoms. Gallstones usually do not cause symptoms until they begin to move through bile ducts. Large stones usually remain silently in the gallbladder. Small and midsized stones create most problems because they are small enough to pass from the gallbladder or intrahepatic duct, but are too big to pass out smoothly. Passage of a stone may cause extraordinarily painful cramps—*biliary colic*—in the right upper quadrant or upper abdomen,

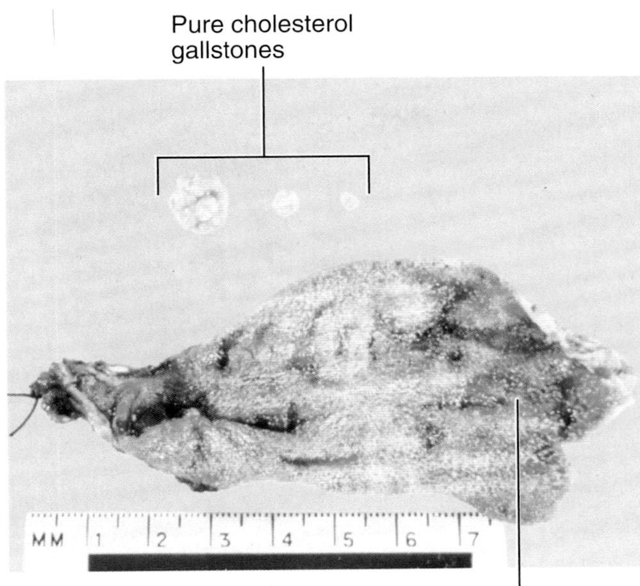

Figure 12.22 **Cholelithiasis (cholesterol gallstones) and chronic cholecystitis.** Normally gallbladder mucosa is green because of staining by normal bile. In this patient, cholesterol deposits caused a bright yellow coloration. Microscopic study of the gallbladder wall revealed chronic inflammation.

which is usually accompanied by nausea and vomiting. Fever, which does not occur in uncomplicated cholelithiasis, should arouse suspicion of ascending bacterial infection (*ascending cholangitis*), which is a threat when stones are passed or become lodged in bile ducts. Other complications include cholecystitis, pancreatitis, perforation, and empyema of the gallbladder.

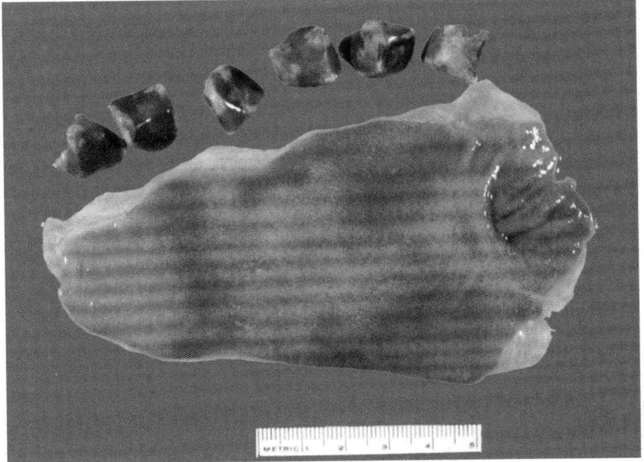

Figure 12.23 **Cholelithiasis (pigment stones) and chronic cholecystitis.** Normally gallbladder mucosa is green because of staining by normal bile. The lumen of this specimen contained mucus only; no bile was present, indicating that stones had blocked the cystic duct. Microscopic study of the gallbladder wall revealed chronic inflammation.

Because gallstones are often discovered during evaluation of other medical problems, finding asymptomatic stones forces a decision to leave them alone or to do surgery. Individual situations differ and stone behavior is unpredictable. Only about 2% of patients become symptomatic each year. Therefore, most patients elect to avoid surgery until symptoms occur.

Cholecystitis

Cholecystitis is inflammation of the gallbladder. *Acute cholecystitis* is the most common major complication of gallstones: >90% of cases are associated with stone obstruction of the neck of the gallbladder. Most patients have multiple stones. Bacterial infection usually is not present but may occur later and cause the lumen of the gallbladder to fill with pus (empyema), as depicted in Figure 12.24. On the other hand, acute cholecystitis can occur without stones: about 5–10% of gallbladders removed for acute cholecystitis contain no stones. Most of these patients have other significant conditions, such as pregnancy, burns, sepsis, or recent major surgery.

In acute cholecystitis, the gallbladder is enlarged, tense, and inflamed and in some instances may be necrotic or filled with pus. Clinically the presentation of acute cholecystitis can vary from persistent, rather mild right upper abdominal pain to severe, crampy pain (colic) associated with fever, nausea, vomiting, prostration, and leukocytosis. Jaundice suggests obstruction by a stone in the common bile duct. Mild attacks usually resolve in a few days or a week, but about 25% require immediate surgery.

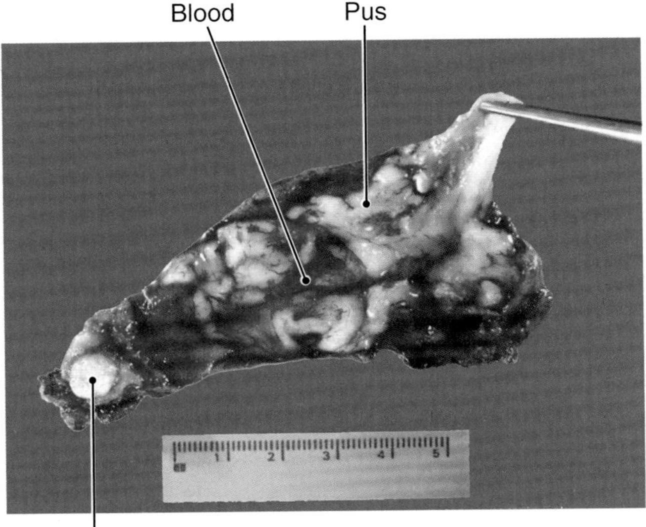

Figure 12.24 **Acute cholecystitis with empyema.** Gallbladder is filled with blood and pus. Note a pure cholesterol stone lodged in the gallbladder neck where the cystic duct arises.

As depicted in Figure 12.25, *chronic cholecystitis* may develop after numerous episodes of acute cholecystitis, but most often it occurs without a history of acute attacks. Most cases are nonbacterial: in only a third of cases can bacteria be cultured from the bile. Chronic cholecystitis is almost always associated with gallstones, but the exact role stones play is unclear. Obstruction is not necessary. Stones may be the result, not the cause, of the inflammation. At the very least, it appears that stones and inflammation coexist in gallbladders for many years.

Clinically, chronic cholecystitis is not as dramatic as an acute attack and is usually characterized by episodes of mild-to-moderate right upper quadrant pain with nausea, vomiting, and intolerance for fatty foods (because fatty foods stimulate the gallbladder to contract and send bile into the intestine to emulsify the fat). Most cases warrant surgery because complications can be severe—ascending cholangitis, gallbladder perforation with peritonitis, or septicemia (bacterial infection of blood).

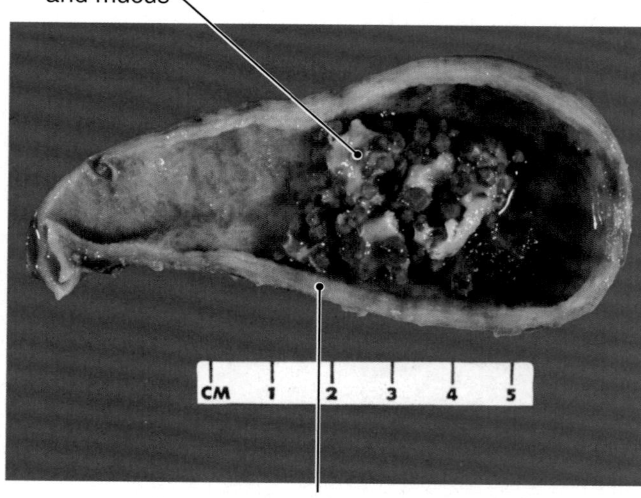

Figure 12.25 **Chronic cholecystitis and cholelithiasis.** Gallbladder contains mucus and numerous pigment stones. No normal bile is present. Note thick gallbladder wall, caused by chronic inflammation and fibrosis.

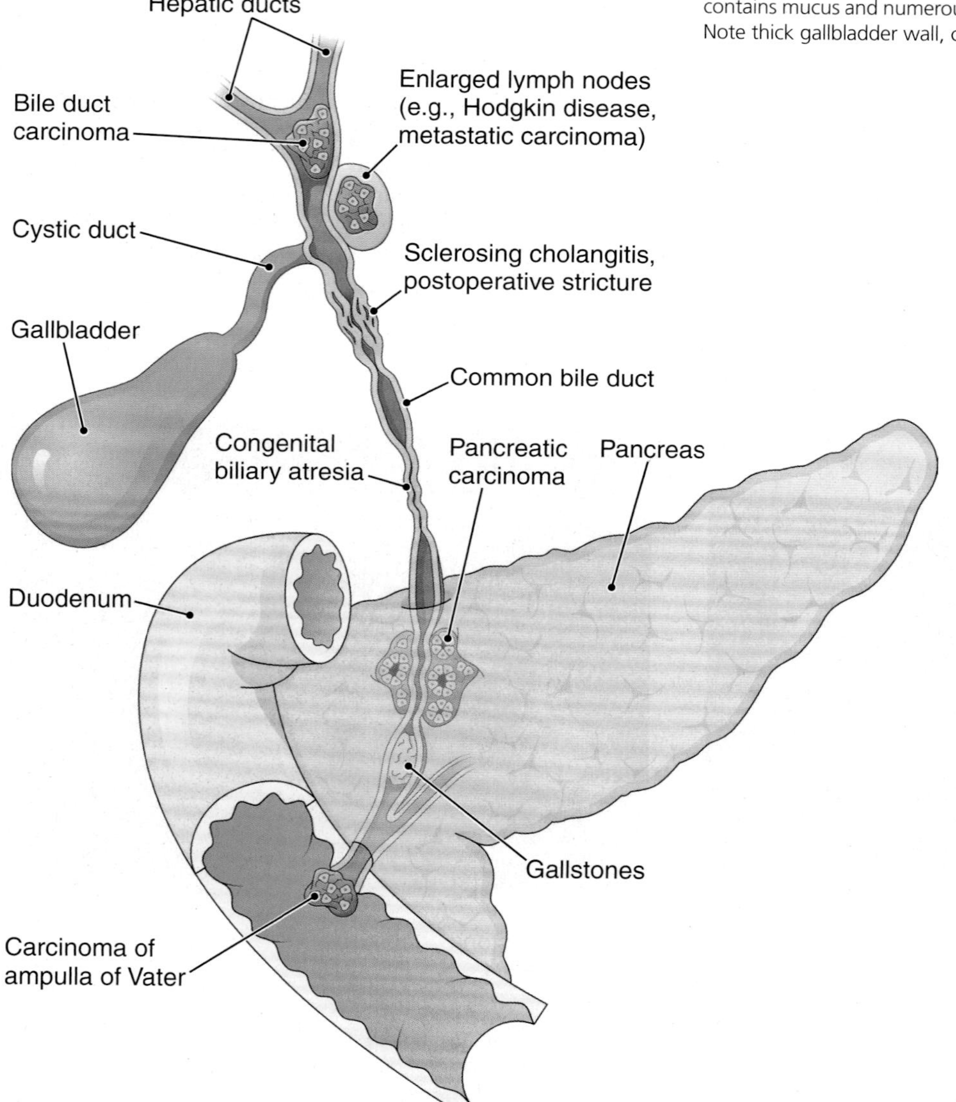

Figure 12.26 **Extrahepatic biliary obstruction.** The illustration shows the sites and causes of obstruction.

Tumors of the Gallbladder

Tumors of the gallbladder are uncommon. Most common are small, benign, mucosal papillary growths that occur with gallstones. Carcinomas of the gallbladder are adenocarcinomas of bile duct epithelium (*cholangiocarcinoma*) and are also associated with gallstones. At the time of discovery, most are beyond hope of cure, and five-year survival is <5%.

Obstruction Is the Most Important Problem of Extrahepatic Bile Ducts

Obstruction is the most important problem of the extrahepatic bile ducts. Figure 12.26 depicts the major causes. Gallstones are by far the most common cause of obstruction. Other causes include cancer of the head of the pancreas, pancreatitis, inflammatory disease of the ducts, and postoperative scarring. In industrialized nations, most gallstones form in the gallbladder, but in Asia there is a much higher prevalence of primary stone formation in ducts. Stones formed in the bile ducts are the main cause of *ascending cholangitis*, caused by intestinal bacteria that ascend the common bile duct into the liver. Not every patient with ductal stones develops ascending cholangitis, but ascending cholangitis almost never occurs without obstruction. Sepsis (bloodstream infection) is the most important clinical complication, far outweighing cholestasis. In its most severe form, obstruction may cause general sepsis and intrahepatic abscesses. Other acute complications of ductal stones and obstruction include acute pancreatitis and acute cholecystitis. Chronic obstruction may cause chronic liver disease with secondary biliary cirrhosis. Treatment is surgical.

Extrahepatic biliary atresia is an obstruction of extrahepatic bile ducts. A congenital condition (Chapter 22), it is not, strictly speaking, atresia (failure to develop) because most affected infants are born with patent bile ducts that become obstructed and scarred. The cause is unknown. It accounts for over half of children referred for liver transplantation.

Cholangiocarcinomas of the extrahepatic bile ducts are rare and usually fatal, but they are associated with a somewhat longer survival time than hepatic or gallbladder cholangiocarcinomas because they cause obstructive signs and symptoms earlier and are therefore detected earlier.

Pop Quiz

12.27 True or false? Most gallstones are pigment stones.

12.28 True or false? Acute cholecystitis only occurs in the presence of gallstones.

12.29 What is the difference between cholelithiasis and choledocholithiasis?

12.30 What disease is responsible for over half of children referred for liver transplant?

Case Study Revisited

"I didn't give it a second thought." The case of Ling C.

Ling C's case is straightforward and demonstrates recent progress in medicine. In retrospect, it is abundantly clear than Ling got transfusion-related hepatitis C with the birth of her first child 30 years earlier. In those days, the HCV had not been discovered, but hepatitis viruses A and B had been identified and laboratory tests had been developed to detect them. That she was told she had "non-A, non-B hepatitis" indicates she had been tested and found negative for HAV and HBV infection.

Transfusion-related hepatitis was common prior to the discovery of HCV in 1989 and the development of tests to screen donors and donated blood for evidence of HCV infection. Screening and the elimination of payment of donors for blood donations have reduced transfusion-related hepatitis virtually to zero (paid donors have an incentive to be untruthful about their medical history in order to receive payment). The only reward for blood donation in the modern era is coffee, a cookie, and the satisfaction of doing good.

After the discovery of HCV, there was no treatment available, which left most patients with a serious chronic disease for which little could be done. Further research has proven that interferon and, to a greater degree, the newly developed protease-inhibitor therapies, are successful in curing 70–80% of new infections and improving clinical outcomes in those with established chronic infection. Ling was one of the fortunate few with chronic infection who may have been cured.

Chapter Challenge

1. A 16-year-old Caucasian female presents to the ER via ambulance for suspected drug overdose. The patient's mother reports that her daughter locked herself in her room earlier that evening threatening suicide. On physical exam, the patient is pale and sweating; a basin in her lap holds partially digested white pills. The ER physician explains to the patient's mother that without immediate administration of charcoal and N-acetylcysteine, the patient could go into liver failure. What compound has the patient overdosed on?
   A. Acetaminophen
   B. Aspirin
   C. Alcohol
   D. Iron

2. Hepatitis B infection ________________.
   A. is the most common viral hepatitis in the United States.
   B. causes epidemics of infection.
   C. is the most likely hepatitis virus infection to cause chronic hepatitis and cirrhosis.
   D. is transmitted parenterally or by sexual contact.

3. A 53-year-old African American female with a past medical history significant for RA presents to the clinic. She complains of fatigue, nausea, dark urine, and loss of appetite. Pertinent positives on physical exam include an enlarged liver and jaundice. Her AST and ALT are elevated, while GGT and Alk Phos are normal. Her hepatitis panel is positive for anti-HCV, but her PCR is negative for virus. She is also positive for high titers of antismooth muscle antibodies. What is the patient's diagnosis?
   A. Acute viral hepatitis (HCV)
   B. Autoimmune hepatitis
   C. Alcoholic hepatitis
   D. Nonalcoholic fatty liver disease

4. You observe a 22-year-old Caucasian male on the psychiatric ward. His chart lists a diagnosis of schizophrenia. Over several days, you note that he also has several behavioral oddities, tremors, and an abnormal gait. On a hunch, you order a slit lamp exam, which reveals the presence of *Kayser-Fleischer rings.* These findings point to a diagnosis of which of the following diseases?
   A. Alpha-1 antitrypsin deficiency
   B. Nonalcoholic fatty liver disease
   C. Hemochromatosis
   D. Wilson disease

5. The pulsating, flapping motion of dorsiflexed wrists (asterixis) characterizes which hepatic syndrome?
   A. Hepatorenal syndrome
   B. Hepatopulmonary syndrome
   C. Hepatic encephalopathy
   D. Hepatic coma

6. A 20-year-old Hispanic male presents to his college clinic following a recent spring break trip to Cancun. He complains of nausea, vomiting, and diarrhea. His physical exam demonstrates marked jaundice. Pertinent labs include increased AST, ALT, (+) IgM HAV, (+) anti-HbS, (–) anti-HBc, and (–) anti-HCV. Which of the following explains his symptoms and laboratory findings?
   A. Acute HAV infection
   B. Acute HBV infection
   C. Acute HCV infection
   D. Chronic HBV infection

7. A 55-year-old morbidly obese male with a past medical history significant for hyperlipidemia and prediabetic insulin resistance returns to the clinic following a yearly checkup. His primary care doctor is concerned by his elevated AST and ALT. He denies alcohol consumption, previous history of hepatitis, and a history of autoimmune disease. His hepatitis panel is negative. A liver biopsy demonstrates marked fat deposition. What is his diagnosis?
   A. Alcoholic cirrhosis
   B. Chronic viral hepatitis
   C. Nonalcoholic fatty liver disease
   D. Autoimmune hepatitis

8. A 45-year-old obese Native American female presents to the ER complaining of severe cramping right upper abdominal pain, nausea, vomiting, and a mild fever. Her AST and ALT are normal, while GGT, alk phos, and conjugated bilirubin are all markedly elevated. Her CBC also reveals leukocytosis. On physical exam, an enlarged tense gallbladder is palpable. What is the most likely etiology?
   A. Cholelithiasis
   B. Cholangiocarcinoma
   C. Choledocholithiasis
   D. Cholecystitis

9. An autopsy performed on a 75-year-old Japanese male with a past medical history of PV demonstrates occlusion of the main hepatic vein with severe hepatic congestion, intrahepatic hemorrhage, and

hepatocellular necrosis. What is the proximal cause of these findings?
A. Thrombosis secondary to pancreatitis
B. Cirrhosis
C. Atherosclerotic thromboembolism
D. Budd-Chiari Syndrome

10. A 22-year-old nursing student rushes into the on-call room. She has been sick over the last week with a viral illness, and today her skin has a mild yellow tinge. You tell her it is time for a checkup with student health. She returns to work the next day with her blood work, which demonstrates normal AST, ALT, Alk Phos, and GGT, but an elevation of unconjugated bilirubin. What was her diagnosis?
A. Gilbert syndrome
B. Crigler-Najjar syndrome
C. Dubin-Johnson syndrome
D. Rotor syndrome

11. The enterohepatic circulation refers to which of the following?
A. Blood flow through hepatic sinusoids
B. Circulation of bile within the liver
C. Bile acid absorption from the intestine
D. Distribution of blood between liver arteries and veins

12. True or false? Unconjugated bilirubin is not water soluble and is attached to albumin for transport to the liver, where it is conjugated to glucuronide, becomes water soluble, and can be excreted in bile.

13. True or false? Wilson disease can be treated effectively by phlebotomy.

14. True or false? Esophageal varices are a direct consequence of portal hypertension.

15. True or false? The first stage of alcoholic liver disease is steatohepatitis.

16. Match the following neoplasms to their clinical and/or diagnostic findings:
i. Metastatic carcinoma
ii. Cavernous hemangioma
iii. Hepatic adenoma
iv. Hepatoblastoma
v. Hepatocellular carcinoma
vi. Cholangiocarcinoma
A. Malignant tumor of hepatocytes that occurs in children
B. The most common neoplasm *in* the liver
C. Benign neoplasm of hepatocytes encountered in young women taking oral contraceptives
D. Malignant bile duct epithelium
E. The most common benign tumor *of* the liver composed of dilated blood vessels
F. Malignant hepatic neoplasm with a marked tendency to invade hepatic veins; may also have increased levels of alpha-fetoprotein

CONCEPTUAL UNDERSTANDING

17. Name the major functions of the liver.

18. What are the risk factors that favor the formation of gallstones?

19. What are the components of a portal triad?

20. Explain the difference between primary biliary cirrhosis and sclerosing cholangitis.

APPLICATION

21. Explain why cirrhosis causes portal hypertension.

22. Hemochromatosis is commonly referred to as "bronze diabetes." Why?

23. A 65-year-old chronic alcoholic presents to the clinic. He is concerned by several physical changes that have occurred over the last year. He has enlarged breasts, red palms, and unusual blood-filled vessels on his upper chest and face. He prefers not to discuss his other related problem. Explain the cause of his findings and what his other problem might be.

24. A mother brings her six-year-old son into the clinic for evaluation of a sore throat and fever. You tell her that his symptoms are likely viral in nature, and caution her to avoid the use of aspirin. Why?

25. Are councilman bodies or Mallory bodies pathognomonic for any particular hepatic disease?

CHAPTER 13

Disorders of the Pancreas

Contents

Chapter Objectives

After studying this chapter, you should be able to complete the following tasks:

NORMAL PANCREATIC PHYSIOLOGY

1. Discuss the anatomy of the pancreas, and make a clear distinction between the digestive and the hormonal pancreas.
2. Explain the relationship of insulin, glucagon, somatostatin, and glucose to one another and to stored glycogen.

PANCREATITIS

3. Compare and contrast the etiology, clinical presentation, and complications of acute and chronic pancreatitis.

DIABETES

4. Compare and contrast the underlying etiology of Type I and Type II diabetes, paying special attention to its most important contributing factors where applicable.
5. List the accompanying signs and symptoms of diabetes, in addition to its diagnostic criteria.
6. Describe the complications of diabetes, noting the leading cause of mortality.
7. Discuss potential lifestyle modifications and available therapeutics in the treatment of diabetes.

PANCREATIC NEOPLASMS

8. Explain the clinical presentation and complications of adenocarcinoma of the pancreas, and give a reasonable estimate of the five-year survival rate.
9. Aside from adenocarcinoma of the pancreas, name the other pancreatic tumors and describe their diagnostic findings.

Case Study

"He's acting crazy." The case of Stanley B.

Chief Complaint: Weakness and confusion

Clinical History: Stanley B. was a 53-year-old Caucasian man brought to the emergency room because of weakness and confusion. "I don't know what's come over him; he's acting crazy," his wife said.

She said Stanley had been depressed and drinking to excess because he lost his job. She was especially worried that he might have cancer because he had recently lost 25 lb after being overweight for many years. The day before he had developed fever, chills, and back pain. During the night, he'd become short of breath and slept fitfully, getting up many times to urinate, a habit he developed about the time he lost his job several months ago. That morning, he vomited several times but had no diarrhea. When he became weak, confused, and combative, his wife brought him to the emergency room.

Mrs. B. went on to say that Stanley has been a heavy smoker all of his life. His mother had diabetes and died when she was about 60. He had no siblings. His father died of lung cancer a few years ago. She and her husband have two healthy adult children. Stanley's main employment has been as a long-haul truck driver, and he had no history of occupational exposures.

Physical Examination and Other Data: Stanley was a short, moderately obese man who was restless and had been restrained on a gurney. He seemed to understand he was in the hospital but not much of anything else. Vital signs were: BP 100/65, pulse 108, respirations 24 with a "driven" or "machine-like" quality, temperature 102°F. Physical exam was unremarkable except for his obtunded mental state and bilateral flank tenderness. Laboratory test results are summarized in the table.

Clinical Course: On arrival diabetes was the immediate suspicion, which was confirmed by laboratory tests that showed diabetic ketoacidosis, hyperglycemia, hyperkalemia, borderline low sodium, dehydration,

Laboratory results for Stanley B.

Blood tests

Test	Result	Normal Range	Interpretation
Hematocrit	50%	Male: 39–49	Dehydration?
WBC count	16.6 x 10^3 cells/μL	4.5–10.5	Infection
Neutrophils	82% with "7% bands"	60–70	Bacterial infection
Sodium	136 mEq/L	135–145	Sodium depletion
Potassium	5.1 mEq/L	3.5–5.0	High
Glucose	626 mg/dL	70–110	Hyperglycemia
Creatinine	3.2 mg/dL	0.6–1.2	Poor renal function
Blood pH	7.14	7.35–7.45	Acidosis
Blood osmolarity	305 mOsm/L	285–293	Dehydration
Glycohemoglobin (Hgba1c)	9.8%	<5.7%	Diabetes

Urinalysis

Test	Result	Normal Range	Interpretation
Bacteria	Many rods	None	Urinary tract infection
WBCs	Too numerous to count	Very few to none	Urinary tract infection
pH	3.3	4.8–5.2	Acidosis
Ketones	Strongly positive	Absent	Ketosis
Glucose	Strongly positive	Absent	Hyperglycemia
Albumin	Moderately positive	Absent	Diabetic nephropathy?

(*continued*)

"He's acting crazy." The case of Stanley B. (continued)

and urinary tract infection. He was treated with intravenous and subcutaneous insulin, antibiotics for urinary tract infection, and intravenous fluid and electrolytes. Five liters of normal saline with supplemental potassium were required in the first few hours to correct blood osmolarity and electrolyte abnormalities.

After 24 hours, Stanley's blood glucose was under control, his blood pH was nearly back to normal, and his temperature was 100.4°F. Blood pressure had recovered and was slightly hypertensive. Heart rate was 82, respirations 16, and creatinine had fallen to 2.1 mg/dL. On the third hospital day, a urine specimen cultured on admission grew abundant *E. coli*.

He continued to improve and was discharged on the sixth day with a supply of insulin and antibiotics, with provisions for ongoing care and education.

Those labouring with this Disease, [urinate] a great deal more than they drink, or take of any liquid ailment; and moreover they have always joyned with it continual thirst. . . . The Urine in all . . . was wonderfully sweet as it were imbued with Honey or Sugar. . . .

THOMAS WILLIS (1621–1675), ENGLISH PHYSICIAN, THE FIRST TO TASTE DIABETIC URINE AND FIND IT SWEET.

The **pancreas** is a tadpole-shaped organ about 5–6 inches (12–15 cm) long that is embedded in retroperitoneal fat of the midabdomen and lies across the front of the aorta just inferior to the stomach (Figs. 13.1 and 13.2). The head of the pancreas is nestled in the duodenal loop, and the tail rests near the spleen. Ducts lead from individual pancreatic glands (acini) and merge to form the pancreatic duct. The anatomy of the ductal system is variable, but in most people the main pancreatic duct merges with the common bile duct, and together they pass through the

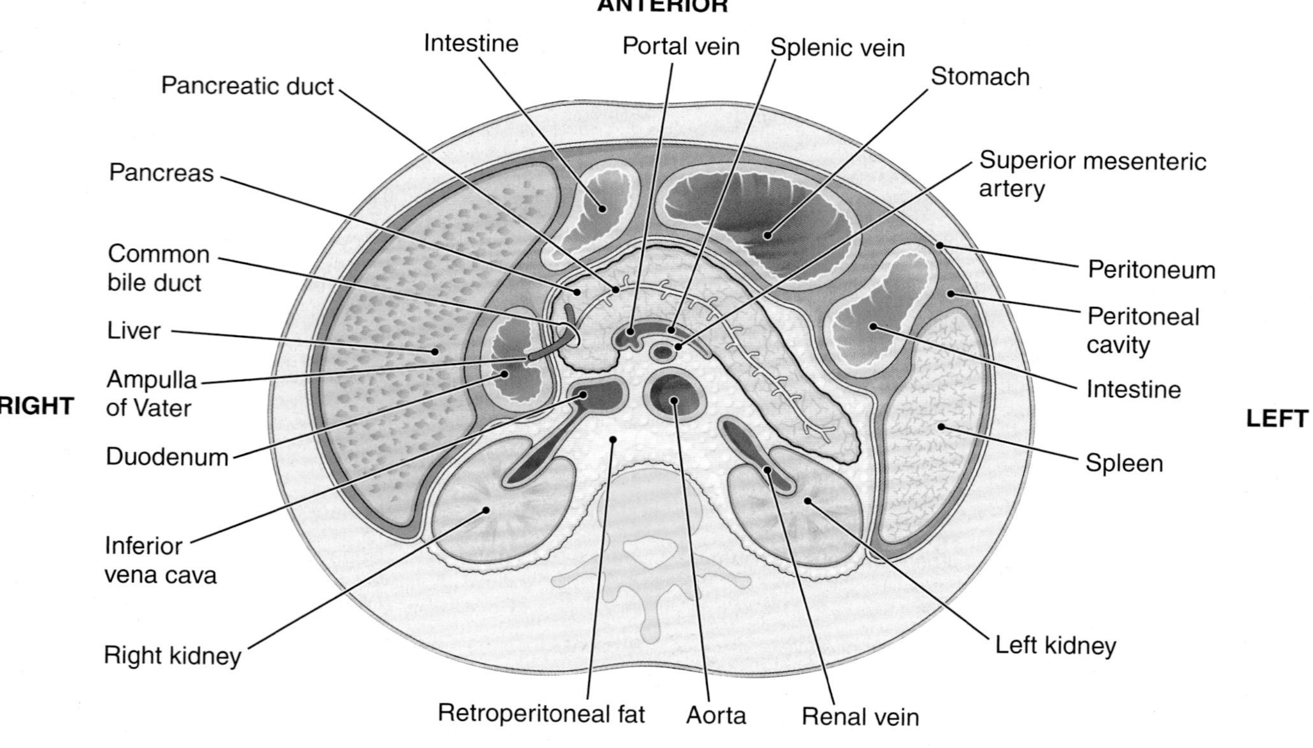

Figure 13.1 **The pancreas and its anatomic relationships.** Cross-section of the upper abdomen. View from inferior to pancreas, looking superiorly.

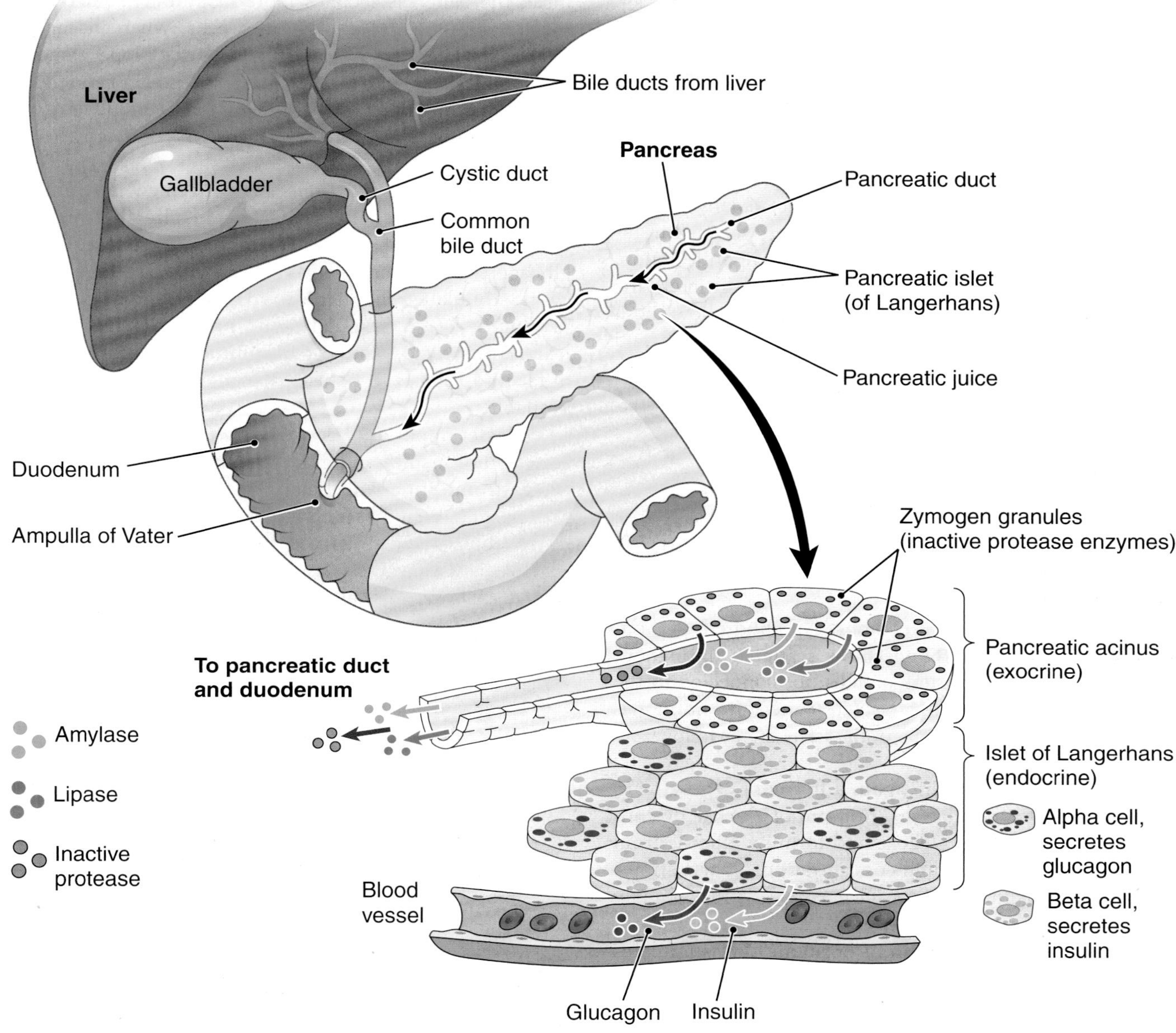

Figure 13.2 **Anatomic detail of the pancreas.**

head of the pancreas before emptying into the duodenum at the ampulla of Vater.

The pancreas is exceptional in three respects.

1. It is relatively inaccessible, hidden among soft organs and structures that give way to expanding pancreatic mass, making pancreatic tumors very difficult to diagnose early.
2. It has large functional reserves, so it is also difficult to make an early diagnosis of lost pancreatic function.
3. It is composed of two glandular systems: one exocrine, the other endocrine.

Normal Pancreatic Physiology

Anatomically, the pancreas is a single organ; functionally, however, it is two:

- Between 80% and 85% of pancreatic tissue functions as an *exocrine* organ that secretes pancreatic juice into ducts, which carry it to the intestine.
- Between 15% and 20% of pancreatic tissue functions as a ductless *endocrine* organ, which is composed of widely distributed small islands of tissue that secrete pancreatic hormones directly into blood.

The Exocrine Pancreas Excretes Digestive Juice into the Intestine

The **exocrine pancreas** is composed of glandular cells arranged into tiny pouches (acini) that empty their contents into ducts. The cells excrete about 2–3 liters of high pH (alkaline) **pancreatic juice** each day. This juice is a cocktail of about 20 digestive agents, water, bicarbonate, and mucus that is carried to the duodenum by the ducts. Many varieties of protein-digesting enzymes (*proteases*) are secreted in inactive form as **zymogens**. If they were active upon secretion, these enzymes would digest the organ before getting to the duodenum, a point to remember when reading below about pancreatitis. Nevertheless, **lipase**, which digests fat, and **amylase**, which digests carbohydrate, are secreted in active form because the walls of the pancreatic ducts are composed of protein and thus are impervious to the action of these two enzymes. As additional insurance against self-digestion, while still in the pancreas, pancreatic juice contains protease inhibitors, which become inactive in the intestine.

The Endocrine Pancreas Excretes Hormones into Blood

The **endocrine pancreas** is composed of hundreds of thousands of tiny **islets of Langerhans** scattered throughout the gland. Islets are clusters of cells not connected to the ductal system. Instead, they secrete pancreatic hormones directly into blood. The cells in the islets are as follows:

- **Alpha cells** secrete **glucagon**, a hormone whose main function is to stimulate liver output of glucose by converting glycogen to glucose and forming glucose from amino acids; at very high concentrations, it also stimulates the breakdown of fat for energy. It is functionally the opposite of insulin.
- **Beta cells** secrete **insulin**, a hormone that stimulates cell uptake of glucose from blood, thereby lowering blood glucose levels.
- **Delta cells** secrete **somatostatin**, a hormone that inhibits glucagon and insulin secretion and slows peristalsis in the gastrointestinal and biliary systems.
- **PP cells** secrete **pancreatic polypeptide**, which acts on the stomach to stimulate the secretion of gastric enzymes and on the small intestine to inhibit motility.

As Figure 13.3 illustrates, the level of blood glucose is controlled by the opposing effects of insulin and glucagon. Effective regulation of the levels of these two islet hormones is absolutely critical to health and metabolic functions throughout the body.

Insulin is a gatekeeper hormone that acts on cell membranes to allow glucose to enter cells, where it can be burned for energy. A negative-feedback loop regulates insulin and glucose—high blood glucose causes increased pancreatic insulin secretion; low blood glucose causes decreased insulin secretion. As blood glucose rises after a meal, the pancreas secretes more insulin. This facilitates the uptake of blood glucose into cells, where it can be burned for energy. Physical exercise burns blood glucose. As blood levels of glucose decline, so does beta-cell release of insulin. An injection of insulin forces blood glucose levels down because it allows glucose to enter cells.

A similar homeostatic relationship exists between blood glucose and *glucagon*. It is convenient to think of glucagon as a "backup" system for insulin that releases energy from body stores. When blood glucose drops, glucagon makes energy available to cells in three ways: 1) it stimulates the liver to convert stored glycogen to glucose, 2) it stimulates the production of glucose from amino acids, and 3) it stimulates the breakdown of fat into *ketones* to be used for energy if glucose is not available.

Of lesser importance is *somatostatin*, which inhibits the secretion of insulin and glucagon and slows peristalsis in the gastrointestinal and biliary systems. These inhibitory actions guarantee that food is absorbed slower rather than faster; thus, glucose derived from food is not used too quickly by tissues and is available over a longer period of time. Somatostatin is also secreted by the pituitary gland (Chapter 14) and inhibits the activity of growth hormone (the activity from which its name is derived).

Case Notes

13.1 Which pancreatic cells in Stanley were defective?

13.2 Why was Stanley administered intravenous and subcutaneous insulin?

Pop Quiz

13.1 True or false? The endocrine pancreas secretes digestive juices into the small intestine.

13.2 The common bile duct and main pancreatic duct empty into the small intestine through the ______________.

13.3 What cells make up the pancreatic islets, and what do they secrete?

Pancreatitis

Pancreatitis is a very serious disease. The five-year mortality rate for acute pancreatitis is 5%, and for chronic pancreatitis 50%.

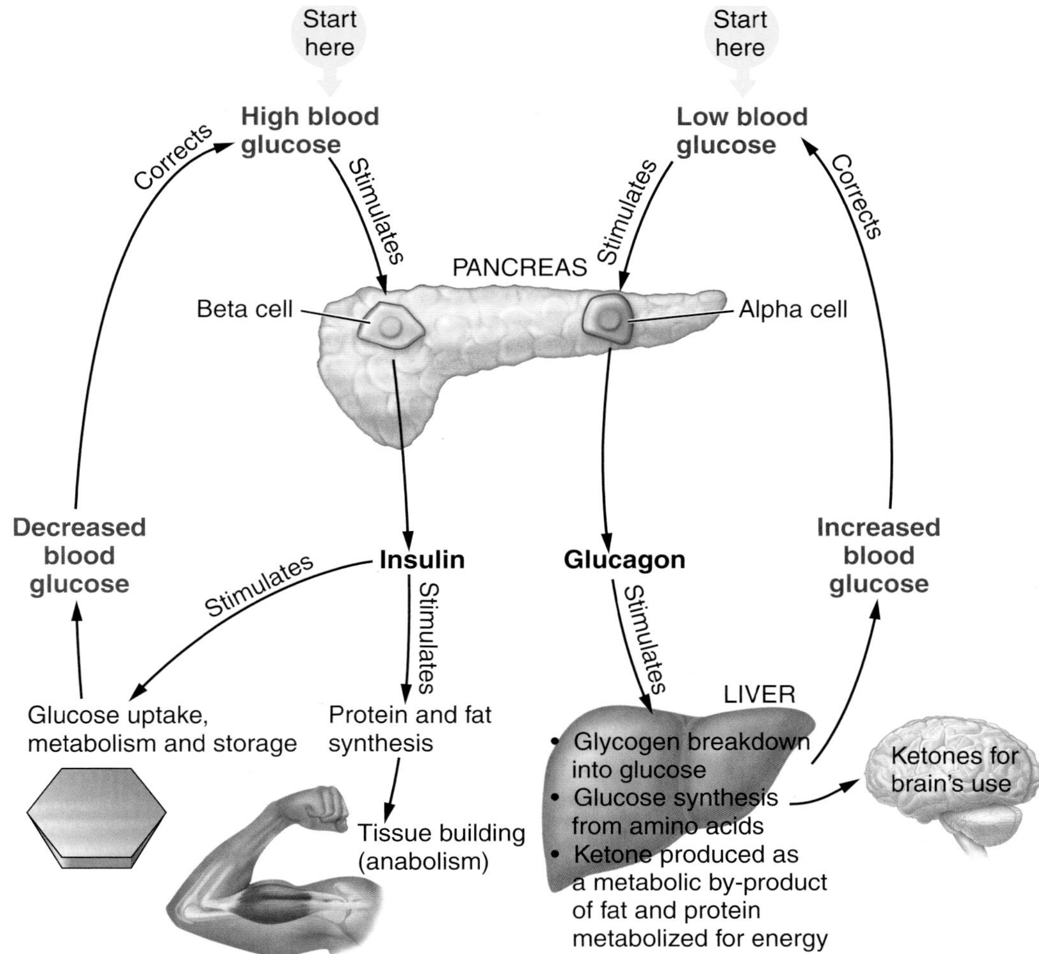

Figure 13.3 **Glucose, glycogen, insulin and glucagon metabolism.** Insulin promotes lower blood glucose by increasing peripheral cell glucose uptake. Glucagon promotes higher blood glucose by stimulating glycogen breakdown into glucose and glucose synthesis from amino acids. (Adapted with permission from McConnell TH, Hull KL. *Human Form Human Function: Essentials of Anatomy & Physiology.* Baltimore (MD): Wolters Kluwer Health; 2011.)

Acute Pancreatitis Causes Reversible Injury

(acute pancreatitis is). . . the most terrible of all calamities that occur in connection with the abdominal viscera. The suddenness of its onset, the illimitable agony which accompanies it, and the mortality attendant upon it render it the most formidable of catastrophes.

DR. B. MOYNIHAN, ANNALS OF SURGERY, 1925

Acute pancreatitis is acute, *reversible* inflammation of the pancreas. Figure 13.4 depicts the causes and mechanisms of injury in acute pancreatitis.

Normally pancreatic juice flows smoothly out of the ductal system and into the duodenum. A very small amount of juice escapes from the acini and finds its way into blood, where some of its enzymes can be measured to establish the expected or normal range. If more than a small amount of pancreatic juice seeps from the ducts into the substance of the gland, self-digestion of gland tissue, nerves, and blood vessels can occur, causing pain, bleeding, and the release of additional enzymes that digest additional tissue in a vicious circle.

Etiology and Pathogenesis

Conditions known to be associated with acute pancreatitis are listed below in order of frequency:

- *Alcohol abuse.* About two-thirds of cases are associated with chronic alcohol abuse. It appears that alcoholics have long-standing, smoldering subclinical pancreatitis that may suddenly flare into acute pancreatitis for uncertain reasons. Some of these also have gallstones.
- *Gallstones.* About half of patients with acute pancreatitis have gallstones (Fig. 13.5), and half of these patients suffer a second attack of pancreatitis if the stones are not removed.

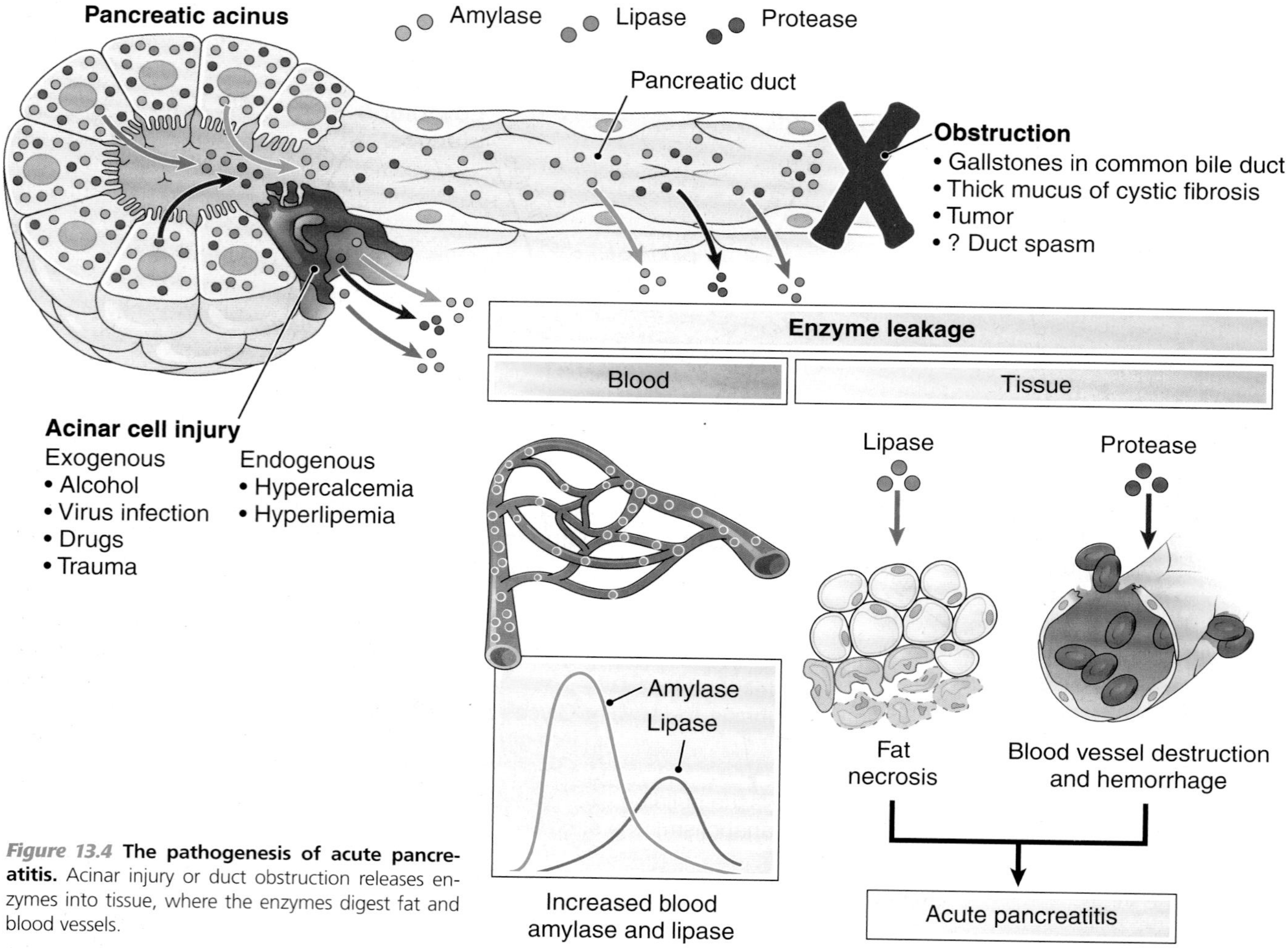

Pancreatic acinus
Amylase
Lipase
Protease
Pancreatic duct
Obstruction
• Gallstones in common bile duct
• Thick mucus of cystic fibrosis
• Tumor
• ? Duct spasm
Enzyme leakage
Blood
Tissue
Acinar cell injury
Exogenous
• Alcohol
• Virus infection
• Drugs
• Trauma
Endogenous
• Hypercalcemia
• Hyperlipemia
Amylase
Lipase
Increased blood amylase and lipase
Lipase
Protease
Fat necrosis
Blood vessel destruction and hemorrhage
Acute pancreatitis

Figure 13.4 **The pathogenesis of acute pancreatitis.** Acinar injury or duct obstruction releases enzymes into tissue, where the enzymes digest fat and blood vessels.

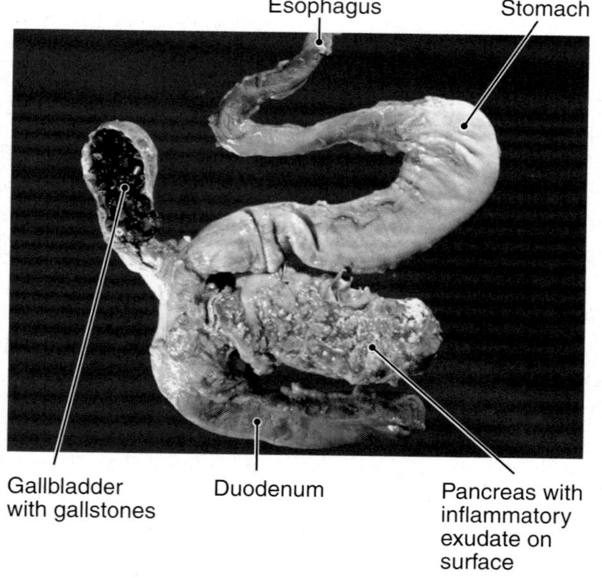

Figure 13.5 **Acute pancreatitis.** Dissection of esophagus, stomach, duodenum, gallbladder, and pancreas. The gallbladder is full of gallstones, and the surface of the pancreas is covered with an acute inflammatory exudate. Gallstones are an important cause of pancreatitis.

- *Unknown (idiopathic).* About 10% of cases have no known underlying cause.
- *Other causes.* The list is long and includes viral infections of the pancreas (e.g., mumps), blunt trauma to the upper abdomen, thiazide diuretics and other therapeutic drugs, high blood levels of lipids (especially high levels of triglycerides), scorpion stings, genetic defects of trypsin, and high levels of blood calcium (hypercalcemia).

The History of Medicine, "Did Alexander the Great Die of Pancreatitis?", examines a historic figure's death through the lens of these symptoms.

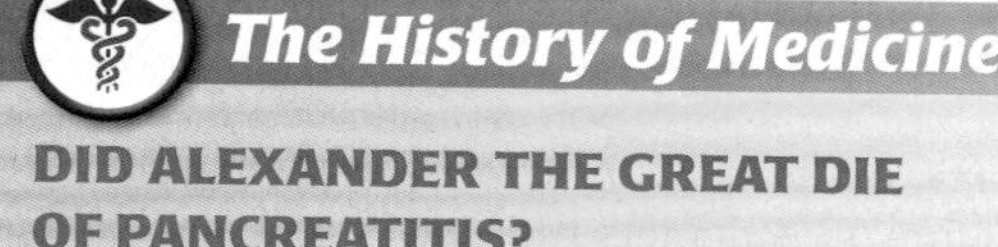

DID ALEXANDER THE GREAT DIE OF PANCREATITIS?

Alexander the Great (356–323 BCE)—the celebrated Greek who was arguably the greatest military leader in recorded history—conquered most of the known

Western world before he was 30 years old. His empire included what are now Greece, Turkey, Syria, Lebanon, Israel, Egypt, Iraq, Iran, Pakistan, Afghanistan, and northwest India. At age 32, he died in Babylon—now in southern Iraq—of an acute abdominal crisis that was keenly observed and recorded.

His illness featured sudden fever and acute upper abdominal pain and tenderness that erupted after a rich meal and a night of heavy drinking (the modern equivalent of multiple bottles of wine). The initial pain faded, but his abdomen remained tender. Pain and fever returned and fluctuated for several days, during which he bathed in cool water and continued to eat and drink. No skin rash or jaundice was reported. By the eighth day, he was semicomatose and seemed to be paralyzed. His abdomen was soft and nontender. He died on the 11th day.

Scholars have debated his death for more than two millennia. Pancreatitis is among the favorite diagnoses, but good cases have been made for poisoning (either purposeful or some contaminant—lead, perhaps—in the wine), biliary tract infection, malaria, perforated peptic ulcer, and a variety of intestinal infections including typhoid fever.

The initial lesion of acute pancreatitis is composed of multiple areas of edema, congestion, and acute inflammation. As autodigestion progresses, these foci become progressively inflamed, begin to bleed, and become necrotic and painful (Fig. 13.6). In its most severe form—acute hemorrhagic pancreatitis—bleeding is extensive, and the entire pancreas can be destroyed. A common outcome in survivors is the formation of a cyst by the fibrous "walling off" of inflammatory fluid and edema. Such cysts can be quite large and are termed **pancreatic pseudocysts** ("pseudo" because the cyst has no lining epithelium). Damage to islets of Langerhans may cause temporary diabetes.

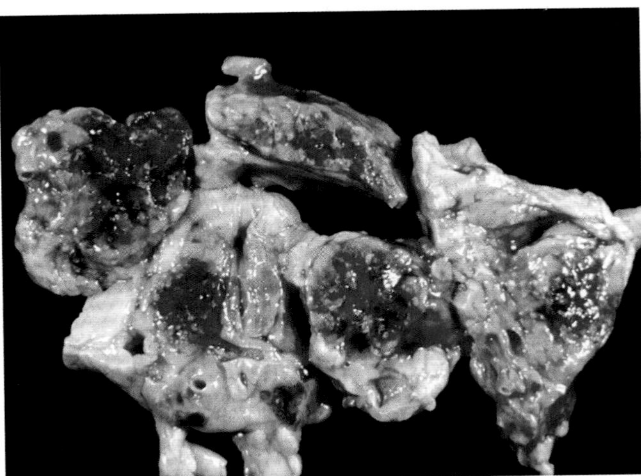

Figure 13.6 **Acute hemorrhagic pancreatitis.** Multiple cross-sections of the pancreas. Pancreatic injury or duct obstruction releases enzymes that digest fat and blood vessels, causing local hemorrhage.

Remember This! Of patients with acute pancreatitis, most are alcoholic, have gallstones, or both.

Signs and Symptoms

The typical patient with acute pancreatitis presents with severe upper abdominal pain radiating through to the back. Anorexia, nausea, and vomiting are usually present. The disease may progress rapidly to catastrophic vascular collapse and shock caused by pooling of blood and edema in the abdomen, or disseminated intravascular coagulation (Chapter 6). Renal failure and acute respiratory distress syndrome (Chapter 10) often develop. In many patients, the bloody mass of necrotic tissue becomes infected by intestinal bacteria, increasing mortality.

Diagnosis and Treatment

Diagnosis rests on the clinical picture plus laboratory tests. As detailed in *The Clinical Side*, "Laboratory Tests for Blood Amylase and Lipase in Pancreatitis," in the typical case, blood levels of amylase rise and fall quickly. Blood levels of lipase, however, are slow to rise, and they stay high days or weeks after blood amylase levels have returned to normal. Other laboratory tests are useful to round out the clinical picture. Blood calcium levels may fall as calcium is absorbed from blood by incorporation into the soap that forms as alkaline pancreatic juice mixes with necrotic peripancreatic fat, a process known as *saponification*. Blood bilirubin levels may rise because of obstructive jaundice, caused as pancreatic edema presses on the common bile duct.

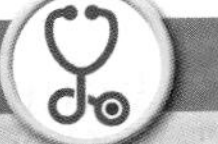

The Clinical Side

LABORATORY TESTS FOR BLOOD AMYLASE AND LIPASE IN PANCREATITIS

Analysis of blood amylase and lipase levels is very useful in the diagnosis of pancreatitis. As illustrated in the graph, after injury, amylase levels rise and fall quickly, whereas levels of lipase rise more slowly and remain elevated longer.

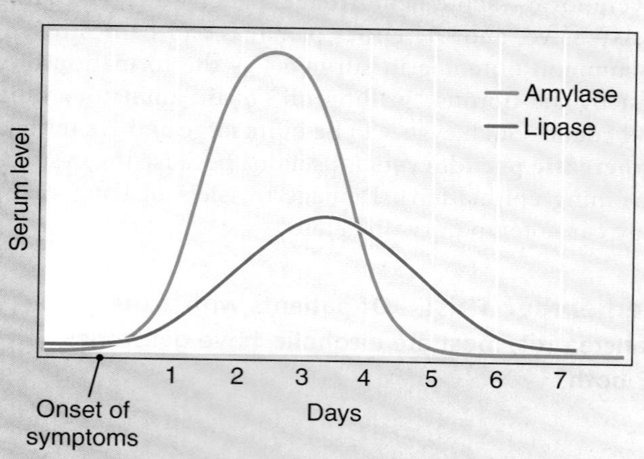

Amylase is found in high concentration in the pancreas and in salivary glands, and even minor inflammation or injury to either one causes release of significant amounts of amylase into the bloodstream. Blood amylase level is, therefore, a very sensitive test for pancreatic injury; that is, it is very likely to be above normal in pancreatitis or another pancreatic problem. It is not a very specific test, however, because it can also be increased by salivary gland inflammation or injury.

The opposite is true of lipase, which in pancreatitis or pancreatic injury is not released as quickly or in as great a quantity as amylase. Nevertheless, damage to no organ other than the pancreas releases enough lipase to cause elevated blood lipase levels. Thus, lipase level is a less sensitive and far more specific indicator of pancreatic injury or pancreatitis.

For these reasons, measurement of amylase and lipase levels are usually ordered together; that is, the combination provides high sensitivity and specificity.

Most patients with acute pancreatitis have increased levels of amylase and lipase, but timing is a factor. Amylase level rises within a few hours of pain onset and returns to normal in a few days. Lipase level usually increases slightly on the first day, but to a lesser extent than amylase, and it may remain elevated for a week or so. Patients with chronic pancreatitis may have normal blood amylase and lipase levels if prior injury has destroyed most of the pancreas.

The key to treatment of acute pancreatitis is to rest the gland by complete restriction of oral caloric intake. Supportive therapy includes total parenteral nutrition, intravenous fluids, and analgesics.

Acute hemorrhagic pancreatitis is a medical emergency, and prompt diagnosis is necessary to differentiate acute pancreatitis from perforated duodenal ulcer, acute cholecystitis, or other intraabdominal emergency. The mortality rate is about 5%.

Chronic Pancreatitis Is Associated with Irreversible Pancreatic Injury

Chronic pancreatitis is repeated episodes of symptomatic or subclinical acute pancreatitis that cause irreversible destruction and scarring. In many cases the acute episodes are well documented, but other cases may present with chronic pancreatitis and no history of prior acute attacks. Despite the close relationship between acute and chronic pancreatitis, they are distinctly different clinical syndromes and have different consequences, as is illustrated in Figure 13.7. As seen in Figure 13.8, in chronic pancreatitis the pancreas is obliterated by dense scar tissue, ducts are dilated, and gritty calcification (from calcium soap formation) may be abundant. Stones can form in pancreatic ducts, but they are not related to gallstones.

Etiology and Pathogenesis

Chronic alcohol abuse is the major or a contributing factor in two-thirds of the incidents of chronic pancreatitis. Alcohol is known to stimulate pancreatic enzyme production. Flare-ups of pancreatitis may be precipitated by binge drinking or by the use of opiates, which cause spasm of the sphincter muscle in the ampulla of Vater and obstruction of the flow of pancreatic juice. Gallstones also play a role in chronic pancreatitis. They are present in nearly half of cases, and about 5% of patients with gallstones develop pancreatitis. Chronic pancreatitis is also often a manifestation of *cystic fibrosis* (Chapter 22), a congenital disease that secondarily affects the pancreas beginning in childhood.

Recently, chronic autoimmune pancreatitis has been found to account for a small fraction of cases. It is typically

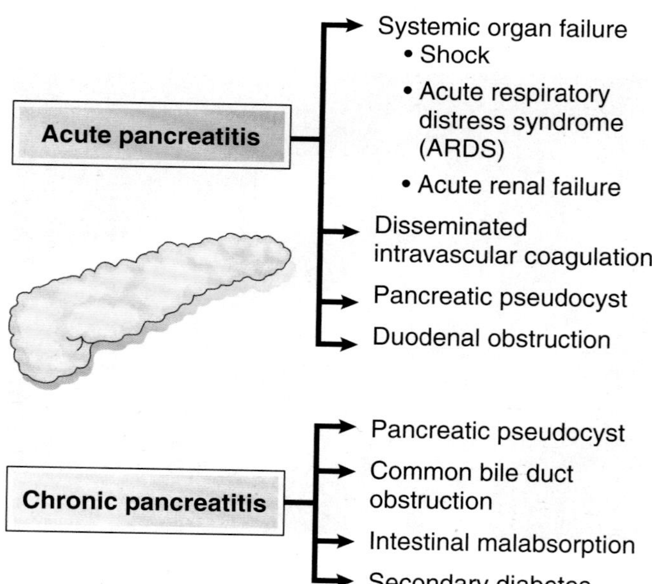

Figure 13.7 **The consequences of pancreatitis.** The consequences of acute and chronic pancreatitis are compared.

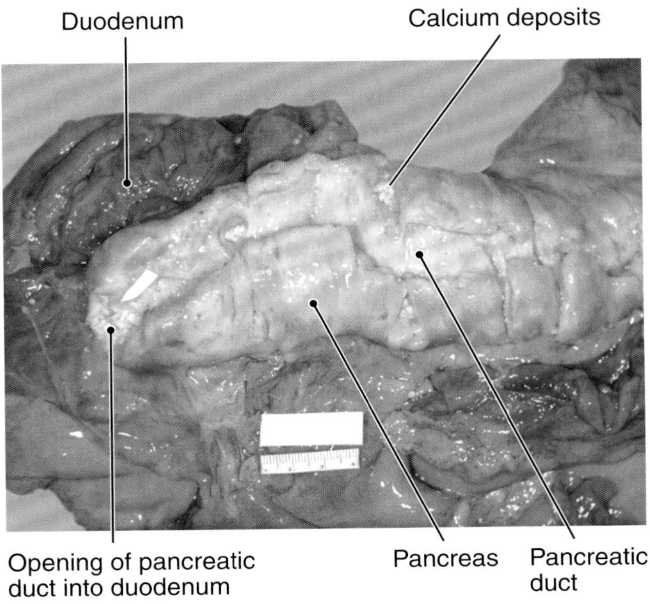

Figure 13.8 **Gross anatomy of chronic pancreatitis.** The pancreas is abnormally pale, dense, and fibrotic, and the pancreatic duct is dilated from chronic obstruction. The white marker indicates the opening of the pancreatic duct into the duodenum where a pancreatic stone (removed) obstructed the lumen.

diagnosed when radiologic imaging in a patient with mild symptoms of pancreatitis reveals what appears to be a pancreatic mass. On further investigation, the mass does not turn out to be cancer, but dense fibrosis (or sclerosis) of the pancreas. Another finding is an increase in a specific antibody called *immunoglobulin gamma type 4 (IgG4)* present in the tissue and subsequently the blood. The reasons for the increase in IgG4 are not entirely clear. Patients are treated with steroids and other immunosuppressants.

Signs and Symptoms

Some patients may have little more than obscure, nagging upper abdominal pain radiating through to the back, which does not initially suggest pancreatitis. Mild fever and modest elevation of blood amylase may occur. Some patients may develop mild jaundice from inflammatory edema pressing on the common bile duct. Other cases may not come to attention until the patient becomes diabetic from destruction of islets of Langerhans. Weight loss, sometimes dramatic, is common. Figure 13.9 illustrates the complications of chronic pancreatitis. In a few patients, the first manifestation is diabetes or fat malabsorption syndrome (Chapter 11) because of a lack of pancreatic digestive enzymes. Late in the course of the disease, severe chronic pancreatitis may destroy enough islets of Langerhans to render the patient diabetic.

Diagnosis and Treatment

Diagnosis requires a high degree of suspicion because symptoms are often nonspecific and mild. It is wise to remember that, in children, chronic pancreatitis is often a manifestation of *cystic fibrosis* (Chapter 22). The presence of elevated amylase and lipase are helpful in making a diagnosis, but normal levels do not rule out chronic

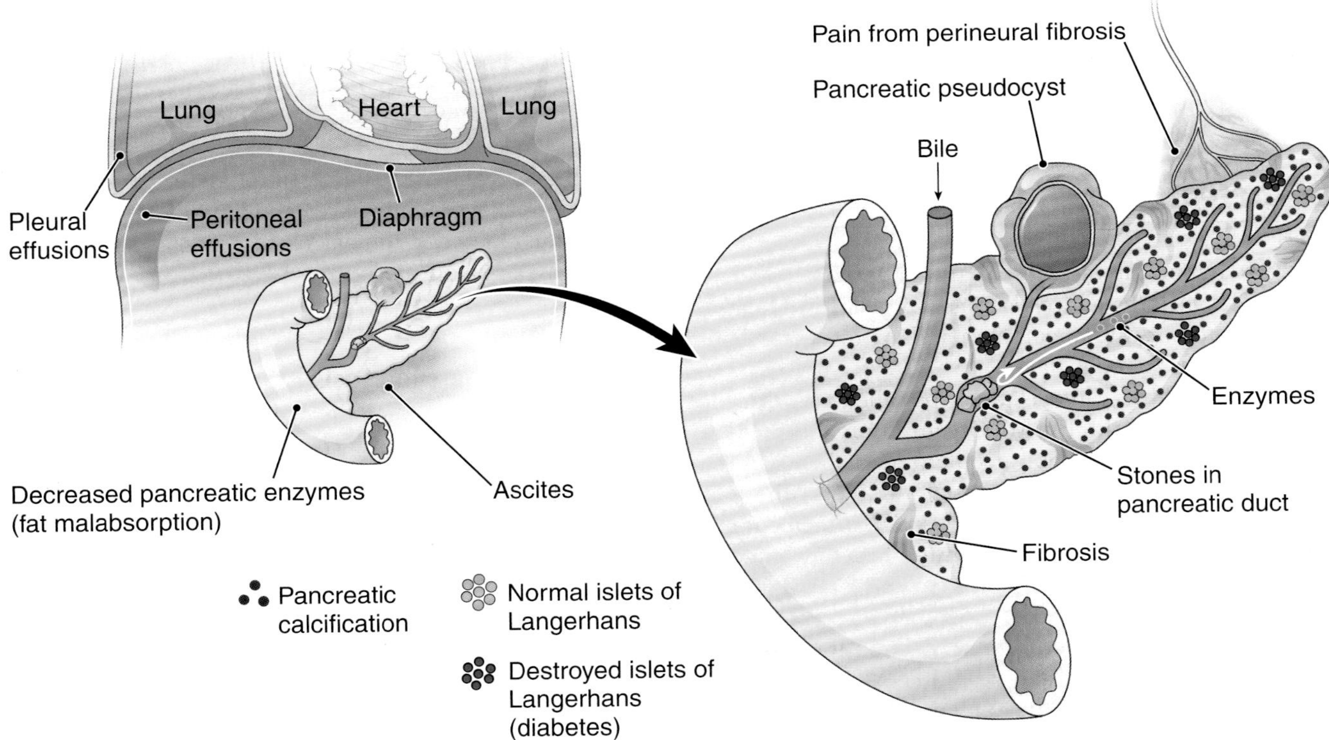

Figure 13.9 **Complications of chronic pancreatitis.**

pancreatitis as in some cases the gland is destroyed to such an extent that little normal, enzyme-bearing tissue remains and blood amylase and lipase levels are not elevated, despite continuing pancreatic damage and inflammation. Ultrasound scans and other abdominal imaging techniques may demonstrate ductal dilation or obstruction, pancreatic cancer, and destruction/scarring. Stippled calcification is a highly specific radiographic finding but occurs late and then only in about one-third of patients.

Treatment includes fasting, alcohol abstinence, IV fluid and nutrition, analgesia, oral pancreatic enzyme supplementation, and surgical drainage or relief of obstruction. Chronic pancreatitis is dangerous: within five years about 50% of patients die of their disease.

Case Notes

13.3 Is there any evidence that Stanley's diabetes might be due to chronic pancreatitis?

Pop Quiz

13.4 True or false? Acute and chronic pancreatitis are often treated with a pancreatectomy.

13.5 The specific test for pancreatitis is ________________ while the sensitive test is ________________.

13.6 What are the two main causes of both acute and chronic pancreatitis?

Diabetes

The two important diseases of the endocrine pancreas are *diabetes mellitus* and *endocrine neoplasms*. Endocrine pancreatic tumors are uncommon and are discussed later in this chapter.

Diabetes mellitus can reasonably be called a worldwide epidemic. The World Health Organization reported in 2011 that nearly 350 million people were diabetic. In the United States, over 25 million people—8.3% of the U.S. population—had diabetes in 2011, and the incidence is rising. One-third of these are not aware that they are diabetic. Among those over 65 years old, 27% are diabetic. The social and financial cost is stupefying: diabetes is the leading cause of chronic renal failure, nontraumatic lower limb amputations, and adult-onset blindness; and is a major contributor to the epidemic of atherosclerosis that accounts for virtually all adult cardiovascular disease and strokes.

Diabetes Mellitus Is Not a Single Disease Entity

Diabetes mellitus (usually shortened to "diabetes") is a disorder of insulin action or secretion (usually both) that results in high blood glucose (**hyperglycemia**). In addition to the 8.3% of the U.S. population who meet the criteria for diagnosis, another 35% of American adults have "prediabetes"—high blood glucose but not high enough to allow a diagnosis of diabetes.

The History of Medicine, "The Origin of the Word 'Diabetes'," recounts how the characteristics of this disease led to the names of its two primary subtypes.

The History of Medicine

THE ORIGIN OF THE WORD "DIABETES"

Diabetes is named for one of its distressing symptoms—the passage of large amounts of urine. The word was derived from a similarly pronounced Greek word, *diabetes*, which meant "excessive discharge of urine." The Greek *diabetes* was constructed from two roots, dia- meaning "through" + bainein, "to go," which referred to the large amount of fluid going through the body. Diabetes is first recorded in English in a medical text written around 1425.

In daily usage, "diabetes" means diabetes mellitus. *Mellitus* is Latin for "honeyed," which refers to the high glucose content of urine in uncontrolled diabetes mellitus and serves to distinguish diabetes mellitus from diabetes insipidus. *Insipidus* is Latin for tasteless or bland and has the same meaning in English. (Yes, physicians used to taste urine for diagnostic purposes.) *Diabetes insipidus* is a very rare condition (Chapter 14) caused by disease of the pituitary gland that, as in diabetes mellitus, causes production of profuse amounts of urine; however, the urine in diabetes insipidus does not contain glucose and therefore is tasteless or bland.

Definitions and Diagnosis

In nondiabetic healthy, people two-hour *fasting* blood glucose is tightly controlled in the range of 70–110 mg/dL. This is called the *normal range* or *reference range* (Chapter 1), which varies slightly from one laboratory to another according to technical factors.

According to the American Diabetes Association (ADA), *a diagnosis of diabetes is warranted if one of the three following criteria is met:*

1. Classic symptoms—increased urination (*polyuria*), increased thirst (*polydipsia*), and unexplained weight loss—*plus* random (any) blood glucose ≥200 mg/dL OR

2. Fasting (≥8 hr) blood glucose ≥126 mg/dL
   OR
3. Blood glucose ≥200 mg/dL two hours after a standard carbohydrate load (an oral dose of 75 gm of glucose). This challenge is called an **oral glucose tolerance test (OGTT)**. In clinical practice this standard is interpreted as: any glucose ≥200 mg/dL is diagnostic of diabetes. The exception, of course, would be someone receiving an intravenous infusion of glucose.

Patients are said to be **euglycemic** (having no evidence of diabetes or prediabetes) if they meet the following criteria:

1. *Fasting* blood glucose <100 mg/dL
   OR
2. *Peak* blood glucose <140 mg/dL during OGTT

Patients are said to be **glucose intolerant** or *prediabetic* if they meet the following criteria:

1. *Fasting* blood glucose 101–125 mg/dL
   OR
2. *Peak* blood glucose 140–199 mg/dL during OGTT

About 5–10% of glucose-intolerant patients progress to frank diabetes each year. They are at increased risk for cardiovascular complications, though the risk is not as high as it is for diabetics.

A word of caution is in order regarding the administration and interpretation of an OGTT. The test must be administered with strict attention to detail and should not be administered if prescribed conditions are not met. Even when conditions are ideal, results are often not reproducible. What's more, the standard test is not suitable for pregnancy, which requires a variant OGTT. The OGTT is losing support in favor of careful documentation of fasting blood glucose.

Case Notes

13.4 Which criteria do Stanley satisfy for the diagnosis of diabetes?

Classification of Diabetes

Though all diabetic patients share hyperglycemia as a defining feature, the basic abnormalities vary. There are two types of diabetes.

Type I diabetes is an autoimmune disorder featuring destruction of islets of Langerhans and an *absolute* lack of insulin. About 10% of cases are Type I. Most are diagnosed in patients younger than age 20; thus, in the past, Type I was often referred to as *juvenile diabetes*.

Type II diabetes is a multifactorial disease that features peripheral cell resistance to the effect of insulin and an inadequate secretory response (a *relative* lack of enough insulin). The great majority (90%) of cases are Type II. Although almost all of them occur in overweight adults, the current epidemic of childhood obesity is causing an increase of Type II diabetes in children. Thus, the previous designation of Type II as *adult-onset diabetes* has been discarded.

Diabetes can also be secondary to an underlying disease. Nevertheless, regardless of cause, *all diabetics face the same risks: cardiovascular, renal, neural, and ophthalmic disease.*

Figure 13.10 illustrates the age distribution (incidence) of new cases of Type I and Type II. Table 13.1 summarizes the differences in Type I and Type II diabetes.

Case Notes

13.5 What type of diabetes does Stanley have?

Type I Diabetes Is an Autoimmune Disease

Type I diabetes occurs when autoimmune destruction of beta cells causes a decrease in or absence of insulin production by the pancreatic islets of Langerhans. The evidence for autoimmune pathogenesis is clear: early in Type I diabetes the islets are infiltrated by T lymphocytes; in some patients, anti-insulin antibodies are present in blood; about 10% of patients have other autoimmune disease such as thyroiditis or pernicious anemia; and immunosuppressive therapy sometimes can ameliorate the disease.

Type I diabetes also has a genetic component. The *concordance rate* (both subjects have the same disease) is key evidence for genetic influence and is best reflected in

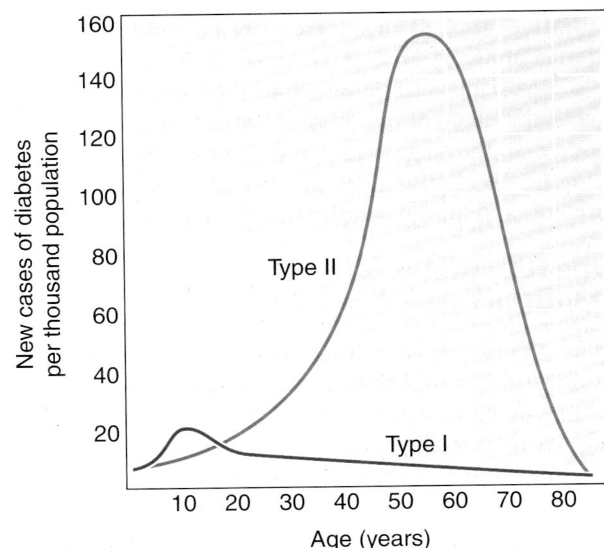

Figure 13.10 **Comparison of age distribution in Type I and Type II diabetes.** The figure shows the age at onset and relative numbers of new cases of both types of diabetes. Type II diabetes appears much later and is much more common than Type I.

Table 13.1 Comparison of Type I and Type II Diabetes

Criterion	Type I	Type II
Age at onset	Usually teenage years	Usually adult
Rapidity and intensity of onset	Sudden, severe	Slow, subtle
Body weight	Normal to underweight	Overweight or obese
Parents or siblings with disease	~20%	~60%
Autoimmune etiology	Yes	No
Islet pathology	Minimal inflammation or fibrosis	Amyloid deposits
Beta cells	Marked decrease	Near normal
Blood insulin level	Marked decrease	Normal or increased
Ketoacidosis episodes	Periodic	Rare
Clinical approach	Insulin and diet	Mainly diet and oral drugs; insulin in some patients

studies comparing monozygotic (identical) and dizygotic (nonidentical) twins. For Type I diabetes, the concordance rate in monozygotic twins is substantially higher than in dizygotic twins. Furthermore, Type I diabetes occurs most often in people of northern European ancestry and is less common in other ethnic groups, and a positive family history of diabetes is present in about 20% of Type I diabetics. About a dozen genes show association with Type I diabetes. The most notable is the locus of HLA genes on the short arm of chromosome 21, which accounts for about half of Type I genetic susceptibility. It is present in 95% of whites with Type I diabetes.

Environmental factors also play a role, especially viral infections. Epidemiologic links have been demonstrated with prior mumps, Coxsackie, rubella, and cytomegalovirus infections.

In Type I diabetes, biopsies of the pancreas show relatively little change, usually a slight accumulation of lymphocytes in the islets owing to the autoimmune reaction.

Figure 13.11 illustrates the interplay of genetics, environment, and autoimmunity in Type I diabetes.

Type II Diabetes is a Multifactorial Disease

Type II diabetes is caused by a complex mixture of genetic and environmental factors.

That genetic factors are more important in Type II diabetes than in Type I is indicated by the fact that the concordance rate for Type II disease among monozygotic twins is much higher than similar concordance rates among monozygotic twins with Type I diabetes. Also, about 60% of patients with Type II diabetes have a parent or sibling with the disease. The strong genetic influence is especially evident in some ethnic groups that have very high rates of Type II diabetes; for example, one-third to one-half of the population of the Pima tribe in Arizona has diabetes. Furthermore, about a dozen gene loci have been identified that show significant susceptibility association with Type II diabetes.

Environmental factors are also much more important in Type II diabetes than in Type I. Obesity is the single

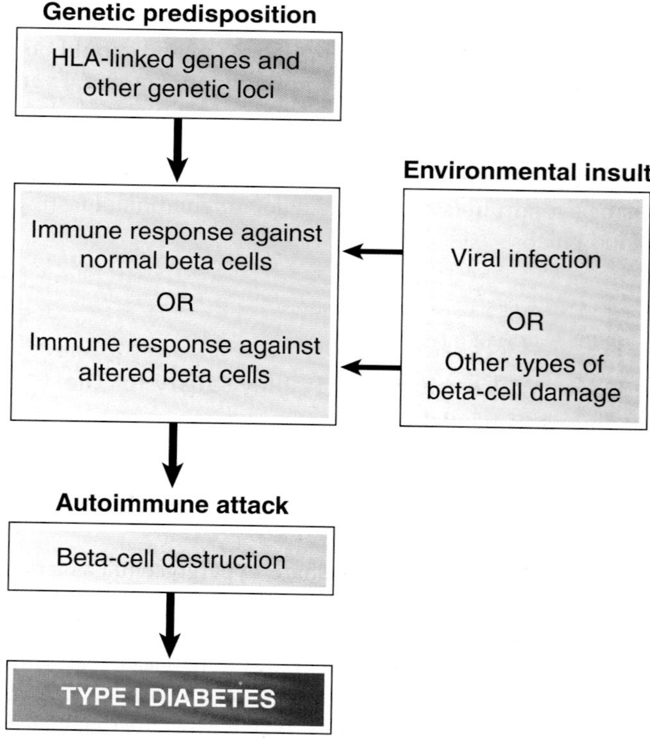

Figure 13.11 **The pathogenesis of Type I diabetes.** Type I diabetes is caused by autoimmune destruction of beta cells, which is induced by some type of environmental insult in genetically susceptible people.

most important environmental factor in Type II diabetes: 80% of Type II diabetics are obese. Precisely how obesity causes insulin resistance and beta-cell dysfunction is not yet clear, but research is focusing on adipose cell metabolism. In any case, the association is clear and strong.

In addition to obesity, a sedentary life style with little exercise and consumption of a diet high in processed carbohydrates are both implicated in Type II diabetes. Notice that this combination of factors is very uncommon in Type I diabetes.

Remember This! Obesity is an underlying cause of most Type II diabetes.

The aggregation of these genetic and environmental factors produces the two metabolic defects that characterize Type II diabetes:

1. *Decreased sensitivity of peripheral cells to the effect of insulin* (insulin resistance)
2. *Beta-cell dysfunction that prevents adequate insulin response* to decreased peripheral cell sensitivity and high blood glucose

In Type II diabetes, the islets are gradually replaced by amyloid (Chapter 3), an abnormal protein. The most important pathologic abnormalities caused by diabetes occur outside the pancreas.

Figure 13.12 illustrates the interplay of genetics, environment, and autoimmunity in Type II diabetes.

Case Notes

13.6 Is there evidence of genetic influence in Stanley's case?

13.7 Which environmental factor was most important?

13.8 Which is most likely: that Stanley has peripheral cell resistance to insulin or autoimmune destruction of his islets of Langerhans?

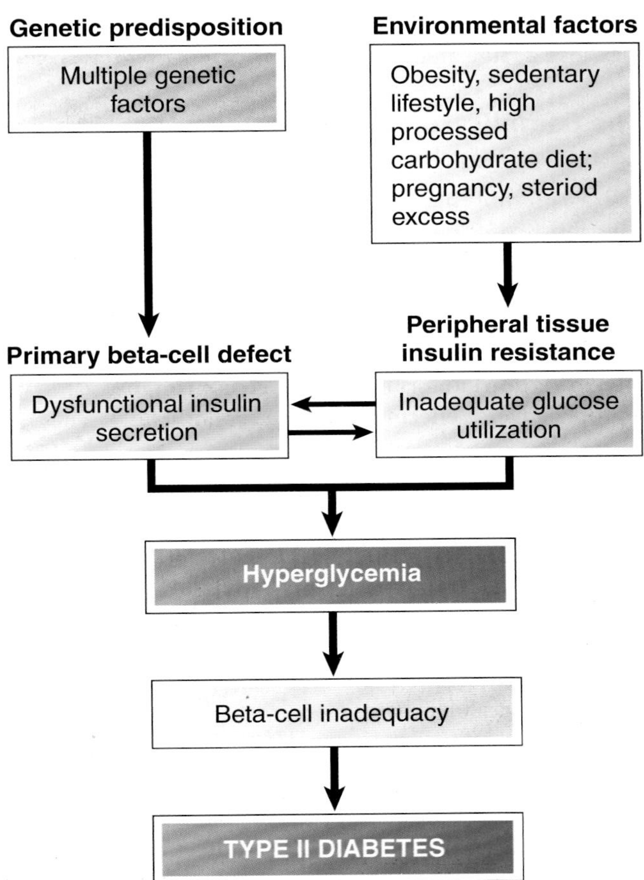

Figure 13.12 **The pathogenesis of Type II diabetes.** The primary mechanisms are peripheral tissue resistance to the effect of insulin, beta-cell inadequacy, and strong genetic susceptibility.

Prediabetes

In patients who develop Type II diabetes, peripheral tissues begin to resist the effect of insulin as much as 10 years before the diagnosis becomes apparent. As peripheral resistance increases, the pancreas secretes increased amounts of insulin to compensate, and blood glucose levels continue to remain normal or near normal. These patients are prediabetic (glucose intolerant), a state characterized by *high blood levels of insulin* and fasting blood glucose levels that are high-normal or slightly increased but not high enough to warrant a diagnosis of diabetes.

Secondary Type II Diabetes

Type II diabetes can be a product of conditions other than obesity. Normal pregnancy is associated with limited peripheral insulin resistance, and about 2–3% of women with otherwise normal pregnancies may develop gestational diabetes, which usually disappears after they give birth. About one-third of affected women will become frankly diabetic within 10 years. Infants born to women with diabetes tend to be large because maternal glucose crosses the placenta and stimulates fetal insulin output, which causes fat deposits and tissue growth. These large infants may suffer birth trauma or cause maternal injury as they pass through the birth canal. Those at greatest risk of gestational diabetes include obese patients, those with a family history of diabetes, and certain ethnic groups, especially Native Americans, African Americans, and Hispanics.

Diabetes may also be produced by drug therapy (especially steroids) and by some endocrine diseases (usually Cushing disease, Chapter 14). When diabetes is secondary to a specific condition, in most instances the diabetes disappears with correction of the underlying condition. For example, steroid therapy can cause temporary diabetes that disappears upon steroid withdrawal. Some obese patients with diabetes may revert to nondiabetic status if they lose a large amount of weight.

The Complications of Diabetes are Mainly Caused by Hyperglycemia

Just as multiple factors cause diabetes, multiple factors contribute to its complications. The most important contributor is abnormally high blood glucose, but comorbid conditions such as obesity, dyslipidemia, and hypertension also contribute.

Excess glucose binds to *extracellular* proteins (**glycosylation**) to form abnormal **glycoproteins** that have multiple adverse effects on vascular endothelium. They

- incite inflammation;
- promote thrombosis;
- loosen endothelial cells, allowing leakage of intravascular substances, including proteins and lipoproteins, into the vascular wall; or, in capillaries, through the wall and into surrounding tissue;
- stimulate proliferation of vascular smooth muscle cells, an important feature of atherosclerosis;
- promote vascular disease.

Abnormally high *intracellular* glucose also has an adverse effect on blood vessels. Glucose is metabolized intracellularly into sorbitol and other sugars in a manner that causes increased oxidative stress, an effect that is important in diabetic neuropathy (discussed below). High levels of glucose also stimulate the production of mediators that

- stimulate growth of new blood vessels (angiogenesis), an important aspect of diabetic retinal disease;
- promote thrombosis;
- promote vascular inflammation;
- promote vasoconstriction.

A distinctive pathologic lesion caused by hyperglycemia is **diabetic microangiopathy**. It is characterized by thickening of the basement membrane of small blood vessels. Blood flow and diffusion of essential substances is slowed. Diabetic microangiopathy is most visible in capillaries in skin, skeletal muscle, retina, and renal glomeruli. In the kidney, glomerular basement membranes and glomerular arterioles are most affected, and the changes are referred to as *diabetic nephropathy*. Retinal blood vessels are similarly damaged, and the changes are referred to as *diabetic retinopathy*. Though less visible in nerves, diabetic microangiopathy accounts for most *diabetic neuropathy*. These three complications are discussed later in this chapter.

Short-Term Effects of Diabetes

Despite the fact that the underlying pathologic processes in both types of diabetes take many years to do their damage, the first appearance of diabetes is often abrupt.

Type I onset is marked by increased urine ouput (*polyuria*), increased fluid intake (*polydipsia*), increased food intake (*polyphagia*), and in some cases by *ketoacidosis* (to be discussed shortly). Blood glucose levels rise above the renal threshold (about 180 mg/dL), and glucose spills into urine (*glycosuria*). Ill effects of glycosuria include wastage of ingested calories, water, and electrolytes. Urine containing a large amount of glucose has high osmotic pressure, which attracts water, so that urine output rises (*osmotic diuresis*). Frequent urination occurs, and increased water intake becomes necessary. Severe dehydration and electrolyte imbalances can occur.

Along with urinary water loss, the urine is also wasting electrolytes. Sodium and potassium balance are particularly disturbed. As blood H^+ concentration rises (acidosis, discussed below), cells absorb H^+ in exchange for K^+ to maintain electrical neutrality. The result is a flood of K^+ from intracellular to extracellular fluid, which causes plasma K^+ to rise. The excess plasma K^+ is excreted in urine. The result is a *total body deficit of* K^+. The continual flood of K^+ from cells keeps plasma K^+ normal or high despite the overall deficit.

Sodium balance is affected by the osmotic diuresis of glycosuria: Na^+ follows water into urine. The result is total body deficit of Na^+.

As calories are lost in urine, increased appetite offsets some of the loss, but so many calories are wasted that weight loss and muscle weakness are inevitable. The paradox of a ravenous appetite and weight loss is very suggestive of diabetes, especially after an overactive thyroid (*hyperthyroidism*, Chapter 14) has been ruled out.

As depicted in Figure 13.13, acidosis may occur and progress to coma if insulin is absent, because of either undiagnosed diabetes or insufficient insulin therapy, or if infection or physical activity increases the demand for insulin. Acidosis arises because, in the absence of glucose, the body must burn fat for fuel. The fat is broken down into fatty acids, which are transported to the liver and converted into ketones—small, acidic, glucose-size molecules, which are burned for fuel instead of glucose. The accumulation of ketones lowers blood pH (acidosis). Unburned ketones are excreted in urine and blown off by the lungs. This combination of metabolic disturbances produces **diabetic ketoacidosis**, which is characterized by the following:

- *Rapid, deep breathing* (Kussmaul respiration): the lungs labor to expel acid in the form of ketones and CO_2.
- *Glycosuria*: blood glucose levels exceed the renal threshold, and glucose spills into urine.
- *Acidosis*: low blood pH owing to ketone buildup.
- *Ketonuria*: excretion of ketones in urine.
- *Osmotic diuresis*: high urine output as glucose in the urine carries water with it.
- *Volume depletion*: the body loses water in urine.
- *Total body sodium and potassium depletion*.

Ketoacidosis is a serious and life-threatening event, which is most often seen in Type I diabetes. It can occur in Type II, but occurs less often and is usually less severe.

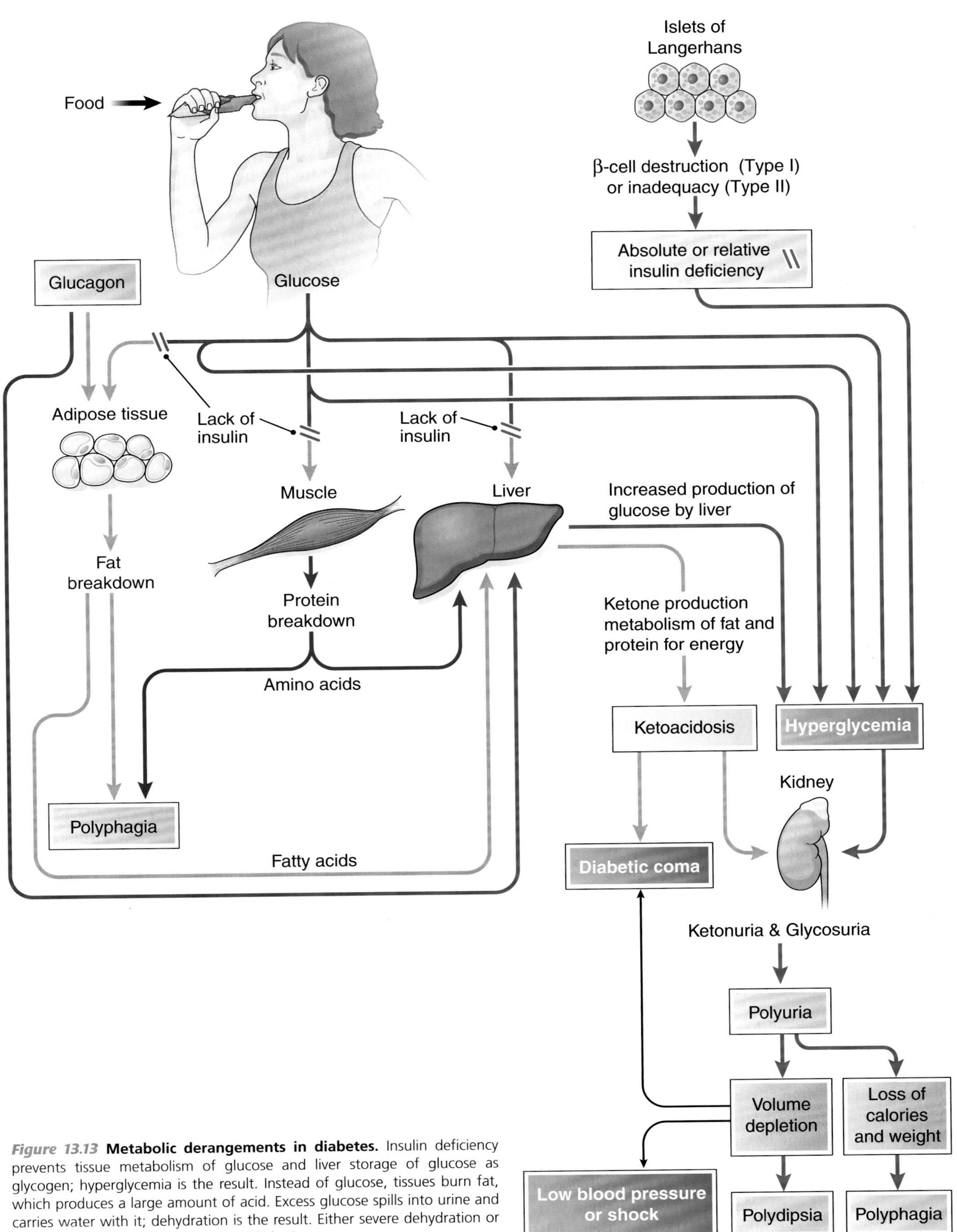

Figure 13.13 **Metabolic derangements in diabetes.** Insulin deficiency prevents tissue metabolism of glucose and liver storage of glucose as glycogen; hyperglycemia is the result. Instead of glucose, tissues burn fat, which produces a large amount of acid. Excess glucose spills into urine and carries water with it; dehydration is the result. Either severe dehydration or excessive amounts of acid can cause diabetic coma.

Ketoacidosis is typically accompanied by nausea and vomiting, which causes further electrolyte and water loss and distorted acid-base imbalance. Severe acidosis may produce coma. Even mild upsets of physiology, such as diarrhea, vomiting, injury, or infection, can rapidly push a patient with Type I diabetes into ketoacidosis.

A second type of diabetic coma can occur if water loss is especially severe and blood glucose levels rise extremely high. The combination of lost solvent (water) and increased solute (glucose) produces very high blood osmolarity and **hyperosmolar coma**. It is usually seen in elderly or debilitated patients with Type II diabetes who may suffer from dementia, stroke, or other afflictions of age and are unable to medicate themselves properly or to drink enough water to make up for fluid loss from prolonged osmotic diuresis. Hyperosmolar coma is not associated with the nausea, vomiting, and rapid respirations that are associated with ketoacidotic coma.

Case Notes

13.9 Which of the features of diabetic ketoacidosis did Stanley display?

Long-Term Complications of Diabetes

The long-term effects of diabetes owe almost entirely to vascular disease (Fig. 13.14). The two varieties of diabetic vascular disease are accelerated atherosclerosis and *diabetic microangiopathy*. Atherosclerosis accounts for the high risk in diabetes for myocardial infarction, stroke, and lower extremity gangrene. Microangiopathy is responsible for the adverse effect diabetes has on the eye (diabetic retinopathy), kidney (diabetic nephropathy), and peripheral nerves (diabetic neuropathy). It is these effects that account for the great majority of diabetic morbidity and mortality. They usually begin to appear 15–20 years after the onset of hyperglycemia.

Remember This! Hyperglycemia is the cause of most long-term complications of diabetes.

Complications are proportional to the severity and duration of hyperglycemia. Strict control of blood glucose levels is associated with fewer complications: patients have fewer strokes and heart attacks, and less kidney, peripheral nerve, and eye disease. A useful indicator of how effectively treatment is controlling blood glucose is one of the products of glycosylation. **Glycohemoglobin (Hgb A1C)** is formed by the attachment of glucose to globin, the protein part of hemoglobin. Glycohemoglobin is slowly metabolized and is an index of average blood glucose over the prior 120 days, the average life span of red blood cells. It is expressed as a percentage of total hemoglobin. To limit risk of long-term complications, the American Diabetes Association recommends that diabetics maintain blood glycohemoglobin below 7%.

Case Notes

13.10 Does Stanley's glycohemoglobin support the idea that he has been hyperglycemic for several months?

Atherosclerotic Vascular Disease

Atherosclerosis is directly promoted by diabetes. It is also promoted by comorbid conditions frequently found in diabetics: hypertension, obesity, and dyslipidemia. Compared to nondiabetics, diabetics have two to four times the risk for myocardial infarction, and four times the risk of stroke. Lower limb amputations for gangrene are about 200 times more common in patients with diabetes than in patients without diabetes.

Case Notes

13.11 Is Stanley at increased risk for stroke and myocardial infarction?

Kidney Disease

Diabetic nephropathy presents anatomically as *diabetic nephrosclerosis*. It is the most common cause of renal failure in the United States, affecting up to 20% of patients with diabetes. Nondiabetic nephrosclerosis (Chapter 15) is a "wear and tear" change that affects everyone but is accelerated by hypertension (Chapter 8). In patients with diabetes, nephrosclerosis is accelerated to an even greater degree. As Figure 13.15 illustrates, the diabetic kidney is shrunken and granular, and in some cases the glomeruli are also severely affected by nodular deposits of hyaline material (diabetic nodular glomerulosclerosis), which further affects kidney function. Genetics determines much of the frequency among ethnic groups. African Americans, Native Americans, and Hispanics are more likely to be affected than whites.

The earliest manifestation of diabetic nephrosclerosis is small amounts of albumin in urine (*microalbuminuria*). Microalbuminuria not only heralds diabetic nephropathy, it is also a marker for increased risk of atherosclerotic vascular disease and hypertension.

Case Notes

13.12 What evidence is there to suggest that Stanley may have diabetic nephropathy?

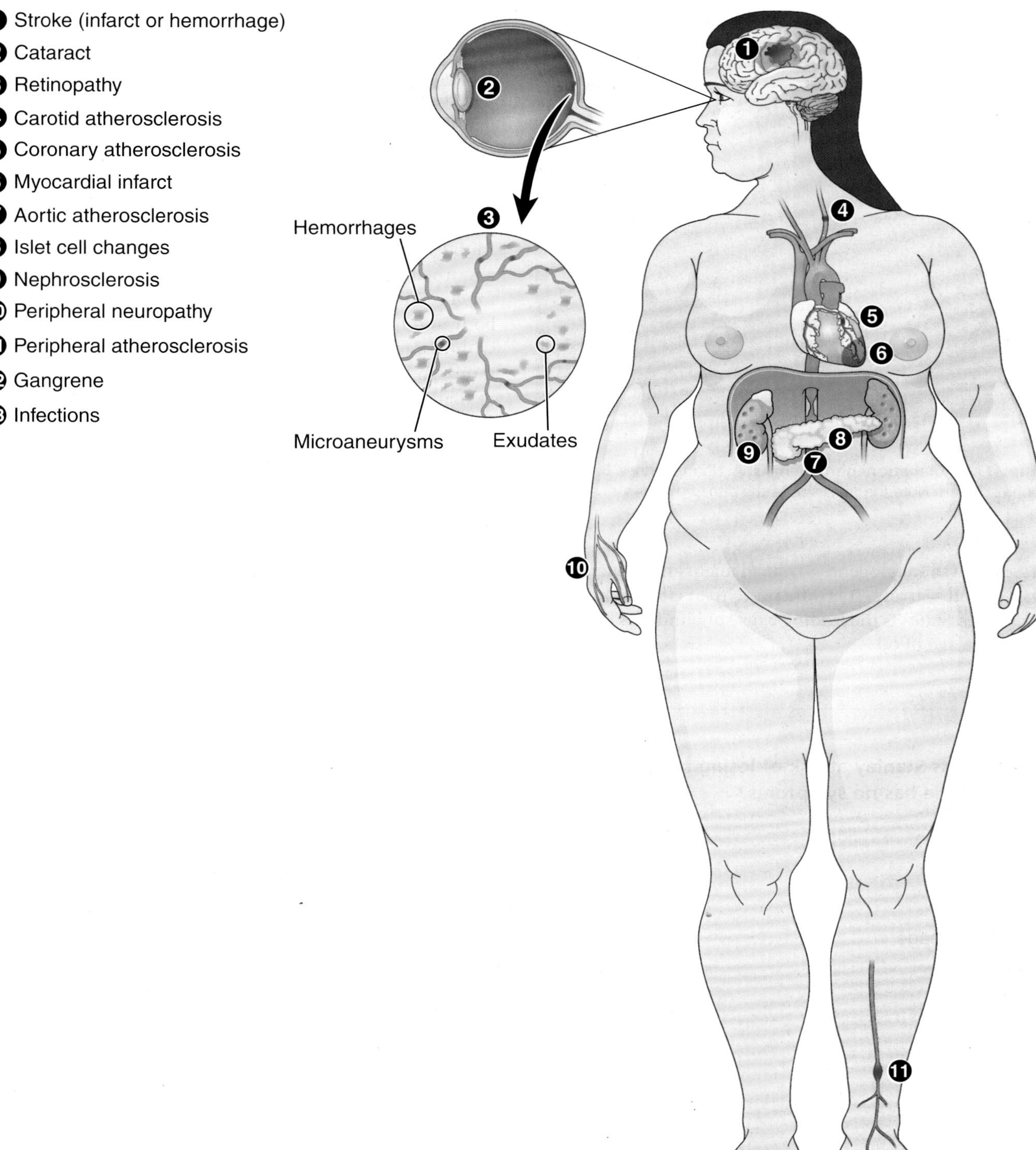

Figure 13.14 **Long-term complications of diabetes.**

Eye Disease

About three-fourths of patients with diabetes will have impaired vision. Diabetes is an important cause of impaired vision and blindness (Chapter 20). *Cataracts* are an opacification of the lens owing to the accumulation of glucose and its metabolic products, which act as solutes and attract water. Diabetes is also associated with *glaucoma*, a condition of increased intraocular pressure and optic nerve damage. Cataracts and glaucoma usually respond well to surgery or drug therapy; however, it is *diabetic retinopathy* (Fig. 13.16) that is most devastating. **Diabetic retinopathy** is a mixture of exudates, hemorrhages, edema, new blood

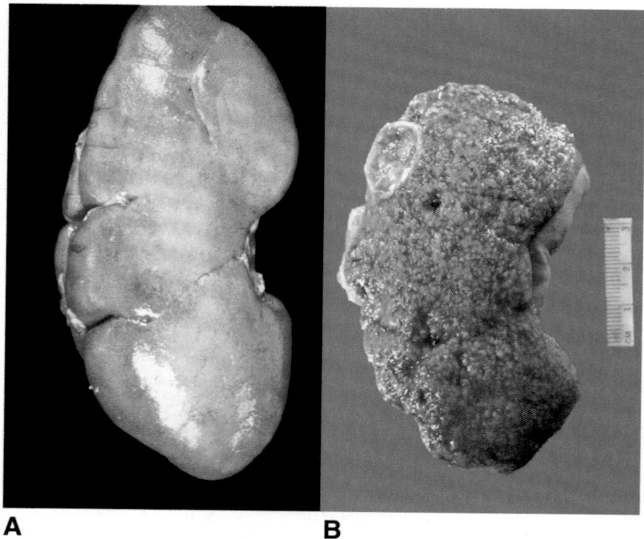

Figure 13.15 **Diabetic nephrosclerosis. A.** Normal kidney. **B.** Diabetic nephrosclerosis. Note the small size of the diseased kidney.

vessel growth (angiogenesis), small aneurysms (*microaneurysms*), and scarring. It is difficult to treat effectively and in the United States is the leading cause of blindness in people under the age of 60.

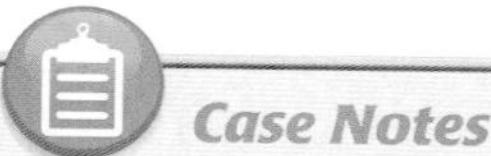

Case Notes

13.13 Is Stanley at risk of losing his sight even though he has no symptoms?

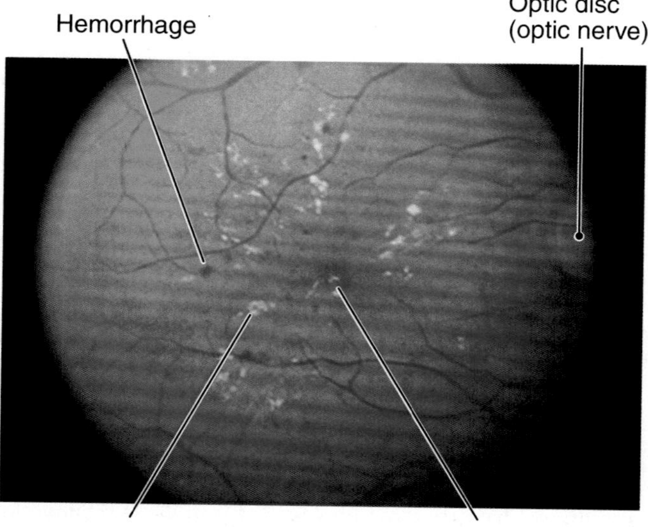

Figure 13.16 **Diabetic retinopathy.** Funduscopy of the right eye.

Peripheral Nerve Disease

The entire peripheral nervous system—motor, sensory, and autonomic nerves—is affected by **diabetic neuropathy**. It usually presents as *distal symmetric polyneuropathy*, mainly in the lower extremities, which are enveloped by a "stocking" neuropathy that is not confined to the distribution of any particular set of spinal nerves. The upper extremity may be involved by a similar "glove" neuropathy. Sensory functions are affected more than motor functions. Initially, patients suffer from nerve irritation, pain, and abnormal sensations, but later they lose the sense of fine touch, pain, and proprioception (the sense that indicates body and limb position, Chapter 20). As a result, patients with diabetes often ignore or are unaware of irritation or injury to the feet, an important factor in the development of diabetic foot ulcers and infections. Impaired sensation from lower limb joints can lead to severe wear-and-tear arthritis (*neuropathic arthritis* or *Charcot joint*) as patients clumsily damage joints without realizing they are doing so. Wristdrop or footdrop can indicate selective paralysis (palsy) of single nerves, but any peripheral or cranial nerve can be affected. Autonomic nerves may also be affected and include disturbances of bladder or bowel function and erectile dysfunction. A common autonomic dysfunction is postural hypotension—light-headedness or fainting—caused by lack of autonomically controlled vascular tone in the legs, which causes pooling of blood in the feet upon rising from a flat or sitting position.

Case Notes

13.14 Is Stanley at risk for diabetic neuropathy even though he has no symptoms?

Infections

Infections are a common problem in diabetes. The cause is multifactorial and owes to two main problems: impaired neutrophil and macrophage function and vascular disease that limit delivery of the circulating cells and molecules necessary for host defense. Patients are plagued by skin infections, pneumonia, urinary tract infections, and tuberculosis. What's more, infections in diabetics are likely to be more severe than in people who do not have diabetes. For example, an initially insignificant toenail infection in a patient with diabetes may be the first event in a downward spiral of deeper infection, gangrene, septicemia, and death.

Case Notes

13.15 Is Stanley's urinary tract infection related to his diabetes?

The Diagnosis of Diabetes Should Be Made According to Established Criteria

The initial diagnosis of Type I diabetes is often made because the patient unexpectedly presents with diabetic acidosis. On the other hand, patients with Type II diabetes often come to attention for polyuria, polydipsia, polyphagia, and weight loss. Some Type II patients are discovered accidentally when hyperglycemia or glycosuria are discovered in the course of laboratory testing for an unrelated complaint.

Whether patients are normal, prediabetic, or diabetic should be determined in accordance to established criteria, usually that of the ADA (discussed above). The most widely used diagnostic tool is the fasting blood glucose test, which should be confirmed by a repeat test if the result suggests prediabetes or diabetes. Glycohemoglobin is useful for confirmation: 5.7–6.4% confirms prediabetes; a value ≥6.5% is confirmatory of diabetes.

The diagnosis of *gestational diabetes* is a special case. There is no universally accepted standard for screening or diagnosis of gestational diabetes. Many caregivers prefer to administer an OGTT that is modified for use in pregnancy. Standards vary for interpretation of test results.

Treatment of Diabetes Depends on Calorie and Insulin Management

The main thrust of treatment is control of blood glucose, the level of which is a product of calorie intake, calorie burn, and the amount of insulin available.

There are three levels of control:

1. Diet and exercise
2. For Type I diabetics, insulin replacement
3. For Type II diabetics, oral hypoglycemic drug to increase insulin secretion, insulin, or both

During the day, the goal is blood glucose 80–120 mg/dL. At bedtime, the goal is 100–140 mg/dL. For glycohemoglobin, the goal is <7%.

Detailed discussion of diabetes treatment is beyond the scope of this chapter. In accomplishing these goals *it is not possible to overstate the importance of patient education* about the pathophysiology of diabetes, the interrelationship between diet, exercise, the effect of drugs, the importance of self-monitoring of blood glucose, and the signs of hyper- and hypoglycemia. *Hypoglycemia* (discussed further below) from an imbalance of insulin dose and caloric intake is one of the most common complications of insulin therapy, and is the most common cause of *documented* hypoglycemia. As a cautionary measure, most diabetics are urged to eat after taking their insulin and to carry a piece of candy in their pocket.

For overweight patients with Type II diabetes, weight reduction is exceptionally important and calls for diet and lifestyle counseling. The good news is that losing 10–30 pounds can lower average blood glucose, decrease the need for insulin or oral hypoglycemic drugs, and in some patients can return glucose metabolism to the previous nondiabetic state.

Diet and exercise must be matched. General guidelines for diabetic diet include a diet low in saturated fats and cholesterol that contains a moderate amount of carbohydrate. Though fat and protein contribute to caloric load, dietary carbohydrates are most important because they are most easily converted into glucose. Helpful in this regard is the **glycemic index**, a ranking of foods according to their ability to be converted quickly into glucose. By definition, pure glucose is ranked 100. Foods with high glycemic index (e.g., table sugar, white bread, raisins, and potatoes) are quickly converted into glucose, push blood glucose high, and should be consumed sparingly. Foods with a low glycemic index (e.g., whole grains, nuts, and vegetables) are favored. Exercise should be calibrated according to caloric intake, and vice versa.

Oral hypoglycemic drugs increase the output of insulin by the pancreas, increase peripheral cell sensitivity to insulin, or impair gastrointestinal absorption of glucose. Drugs with differing mechanisms may be synergistic.

Treatment of diabetic ketoacidosis requires expert clinical management. It relies mainly on insulin and intravenous fluids to correct volume and electrolyte imbalances. Because of their total body K^+ deficit, most need K^+ supplementation despite normal plasma K^+.

Case Notes

13.16 Apart from taking insulin and otherwise managing his diabetes, what are the most important things Stanley can do to improve his health?

Pop Quiz

13.7 True or false? Type I diabetes can be cured by weight loss.

13.8 Diabetic coma is caused by what two mechanisms?

13.9 With classic symptoms, what glucose level is required for a diagnosis of diabetes?

Pancreatic Neoplasms

Neoplasms of the pancreas are cystic or solid, benign or malignant, and arise from either the exocrine or the endocrine pancreas. About 95% of pancreatic neoplasms are solid, malignant tumors arising from the ductal network of the exocrine pancreas.

Cystic Neoplasms Are Uncommon and Usually Benign

Most cysts of the pancreas are benign inflammatory pseudocysts formed as a result of pancreatitis. About 10% of cysts are cystic neoplasms, which account for <5% of pancreatic tumors.

Serous cystadenomas account for 25% of cystic neoplasms. They are benign, filled with thin, clear, watery fluid, and lined by epithelium derived from pancreatic duct epithelium. Two-thirds of patients are women, most of them >60 years old. Patients usually present with mild pain and an abdominal mass. Surgical excision is curative.

Mucinous cystic neoplasms account for the remaining 75% of cystic neoplasms. They are filled with stringy, thick mucus and lined by columnar, mucus-producing cells derived from ductal epithelium. The cysts are surrounded by characteristic ovarian-like supporting stromal cells. Almost all patients are women. In contrast to their serous counterpart, mucinous cystic neoplasms tend to be larger and pancreatic cancer is found in one-third of them.

Intraductal papillary mucinous neoplasms are rare tumors that may be benign or malignant. They may be multiple. They are more common in men than in women. Symptoms arise from duct obstruction.

Differentiating serous versus mucinous and benign versus malignant usually requires surgical excision of the mass.

Pancreatic Carcinoma Is Common and Lethal

In the discussion that follows, pancreatic carcinoma refers only to adenocarcinomas that arise in ducts of the digestive (exocrine) pancreas—tumors of the islets of Langerhans of the hormonal (endocrine) pancreas are discussed separately. Although some of these endocrine tumors may be malignant, among professionals they are usually not included when the term "pancreatic cancer" is used.

Pancreatic carcinomas are dense, scar-filled tumors, most of which arise in the head of the pancreas and cause jaundice by obstructing the common bile duct. Tumors of the body and tail of the pancreas (Fig. 13.17) have fewer opportunities to invade sensitive structures and may be quite large or have distant metastases at time of discovery. Local lymph nodes and the liver are the foremost sites of metastasis.

In 2011, cancer of the pancreas was tied with carcinoma of the prostate as the fourth most common cause of death in the United States behind lung, colon, and breast. Almost all are invasive carcinomas derived from the lining epithelium of pancreatic ducts. It is one of the most lethal of all cancers: about half of patients die within three months of diagnosis and only about 5% survive five years.

Cancer of the pancreas usually affects men and women in equal numbers, mostly between ages 60 and 80. We know little about what causes it except for one thing—smokers have about twice the risk of nonsmokers. It is sometimes associated with chronic pancreatitis, but it is difficult to know which causes which: some small pancreatic cancers are known to block ducts and incite pancreatitis. Too, it is sometimes associated with diabetes, which raises a similar chicken-egg question. Elderly patients with new-onset diabetes should be examined with pancreatic cancer in mind.

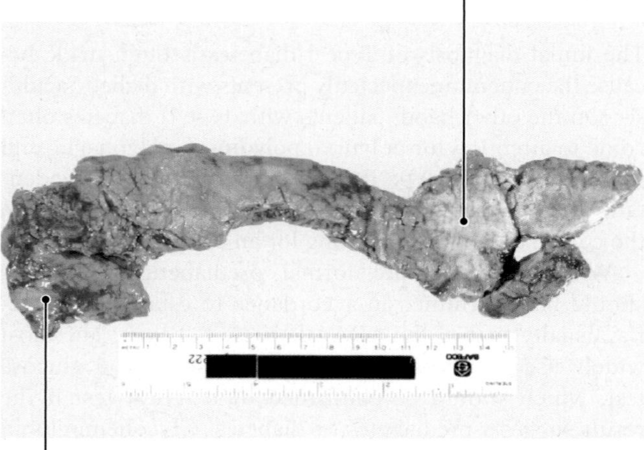

Figure 13.17 **Pancreatic carcinoma.** This example is in the tail of the gland; most occur in the head.

Signs and Symptoms

Pancreatic cancer is insidious, usually causing few symptoms until it has progressed beyond much hope for resection for cure. As with carcinoma of the cervix (and other epithelia), pancreatic cancer begins with dysplasia of the ductal epithelium and progresses through carcinoma in situ to invasive cancer. Unfortunately, no technique that would be the pancreatic equivalent of a Pap smear yet exists to screen patients. Certain blood markers are elevated, but they are far too insensitive to serve screening purposes.

Remember This! Pancreatic cancer is among the most lethal of malignancies.

Figure 13.18 depicts the clinical picture of pancreatic carcinoma. Upper abdominal pain or back pain is the first symptom; however, by the time pain occurs, it is too late—almost all pancreatis carcinomas will have metastasized. The clinical course is typically progressive and rapidly fatal. Painless obstructive jaundice may be the initial sign if the tumor obstructs the common bile duct. Unexplained weight loss should always suggest a hidden malignancy, especially visceral cancer, and most especially pancreatic cancer. *Migratory thrombophlebitis* (Chapter 6) is the formation of intravenous thrombi at various points without apparent cause. It is sometimes referred to as Trousseau sign, and is often a signal of hidden (occult)

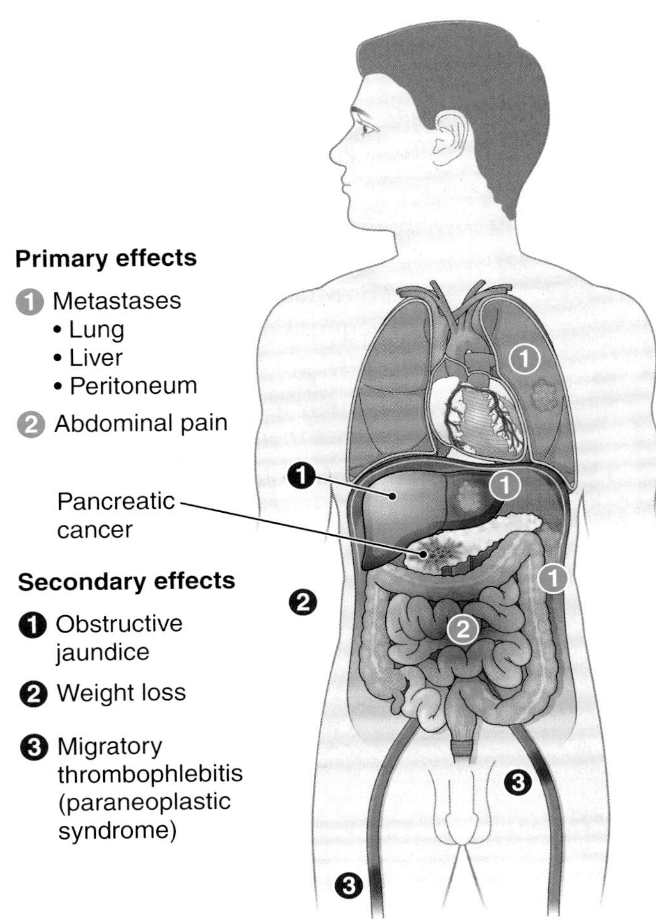

Figure 13.18 **Complications of carcinoma of the pancreas.**

cancer. It may prove an early diagnostic clue that a pancreatic (or other visceral) cancer is present.

Diagnosis and Treatment

Diagnosis requires imaging techniques and biopsy. At time of diagnosis, fewer than 20% of tumors are resectable with any hope of cure. Unfortunately, most patients succumb within 3–9 months. The remainder are biopsied for diagnosis and may have palliative surgery.

Islet Cell Tumors are Usually Benign and Functional

Other than diabetes, the only significant diseases of the endocrine pancreas are tumors of islet cells and related cells that occur in the pancreas and nearby fat. They are usually benign but can be malignant. They usually produce hormones, may be single or multiple, and account for about 2% of pancreatic neoplasms.

Beta-cell tumors (**insulinomas**) are the most common; 90% are benign. They usually occur as a single, small, tumor mass in the pancreas, and can secrete enough insulin to produce **hypoglycemia**.

Hypoglycemia causes autonomic nervous system symptoms such as nervousness, sweating, irregular heartbeats, tremor, and hunger. Blood insulin is high, but in most cases the hypoglycemia is mild. A diagnosis of hypoglycemia requires blood glucose <50 mg/dL in adults or 40 mg/dL in children. Symptoms should be relieved by parenteral glucose or a carbohydrate meal. Hypoglycemia can be very dangerous or fatal because it can cause irreversible damage to the cerebral cortex—with the exception of ketones in diabetic ketoacidosis, the brain cannot burn anything other than glucose.

Other than inadvertent hypoglycemia in diabetics, there are few other causes of *documented* hypoglycemia. *Alcoholic hypoglycemia* occurs in alcoholics who have not eaten in a long time and then ingest alcohol. Alcoholics are vulnerable under these circumstances. Because of the long period without food, the alcoholic's blood glucose is being derived from conversion of liver glycogen into glucose, a process that is interrupted by the toxic effect of alcohol on the liver. Liver output of glucose stops, and the result is hypoglycemia.

To deliberately create hypoglycemia, some patients may inject themselves with illicitly obtained insulin or diabetics may inject extra insulin. This behavior is a well-recognized variant of the psychiatric disorder *Munchausen syndrome*—the deliberate creation or simulation of illness to gain attention and sympathy.

Reactive hypoglycemia is hypoglycemia that follows a meal. Documented cases are very rare. Most of these occur in children with hereditary enzyme deficiencies. Hypoglycemia is said to occur because insulin production by the pancreas "overshoots" and pushes glucose levels too low. Most experts doubt that it occurs in people who have no underlying medical condition. The topic is somewhat controversial, however, as *The Clinical Side*, "Hypoglycemia," shows.

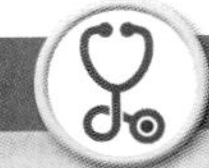

The Clinical Side

HYPOGLYCEMIA

A cautionary note about hypoglycemia is in order. From the text discussion, it should be clear that hypoglycemia is a complex physiologic matter. Apart from the very real risk of hypoglycemia in diabetics taking insulin, there are few instances of genuine hypoglycemia: where blood glucose level is *documented* to be <50 mg/dL in an adult or 40 mg/dL in a child. In such cases, the underlying cause is usually clear. Documented hypoglycemia is exceptionally rare in the absence of insulin therapy of diabetes.

Nevertheless, some ill-informed people believe hypoglycemia is a very common problem. In these circles, strict diagnostic criteria are not required, and *undocumented*, presumed hypoglycemia is offered as the cause of dizziness, weakness, headaches, cold sweats, trembling, nervousness, irritability, sleeplessness, confusion, impotence, depression, irregular bowel habits, difficulty concentrating or handling stress or fears, apprehensions, and dozens of other ailments.

A second type of hormone overproduction by the pancreas is **Zollinger-Ellison syndrome**, a constellation of clinical findings resulting from **gastrinomas**, which arise with equal frequency in the pancreas or nearby in the stomach or duodenum. The cell of origin is a mystery. Most are microscopically benign, but occasionally they metastasize. They produce large amounts of gastrin, causing marked increases of gastric acid production and recurrent peptic ulcers and duodenal ulcers. These ulcers are identical to peptic ulcers associated with *Helicobacter pylori* infection, except that they may be multiple and are resistant to medical therapy. Surgical excision of the tumor is curative.

Tumors of alpha cells (*glucagonoma*) and delta cells (*somatostatinoma*) are exceptionally rare. Treatment of endocrine neoplasms of the pancreas is surgical excision.

Pop Quiz

13.10 True or false? Most pancreatic neoplasms are malignant.

13.11 The neoplasm of the pancreas which has ovarian-like stromal cells is called ______________________________.

13.12 On average, how long do most patients live after a diagnosis of pancreatic adenocarcinoma?

13.13 True or false? Ninety percent of insulinomas are benign and are therefore not dangerous.

13.14 What tumor might you suspect in a patient with ulcers that are resistant to medical therapy?

Case Study Revisited

"He's acting crazy." The case of Stanley B.

That Stanley had diabetes was abundantly clear from the clinical and laboratory evidence on admission. His history was consistent with the diagnosis of diabetes: he had lost a significant amount of weight without trying, and he was getting up many times at night to urinate. Both of these are associated with glycosuria—glucose was going into the toilet and carrying calories and large amounts of water with it. Confirming laboratory evidence was clear: his glucose was >200 mg/dL, he had glucose in his urine, and his glycohemoglobin was elevated.

That he was in diabetic ketoacidosis was also clear. First, he was confused and combative, a sign he was nearing diabetic coma. Second, he had Kussmaul respirations, which have a forced quality somewhat like breathing after hard exercise. Third, his urine and blood pH were abnormally acidotic, and his urine was strongly positive for ketones.

The high WBC, neutrophilia, and left shift (Chapter 7) were explained by the urinary tract infection. That he had bilateral flank tenderness suggests that the infection was in his kidneys (pyelonephritis, Chapter 15). The elevated hematocrit suggested he was dehydrated and hemoconcentrated, a point confirmed by high blood osmolarity due to the osmolar effect of high blood glucose.

Stanley's plasma sodium and potassium require special comment. The marginally low blood sodium level resulted from the flushing of salt out in urine because of osmotic diuresis associated with severe glycosuria, which tended to drive sodium down. On the other hand, he was dehydrated and hemoconcentrated, which would tend to drive sodium upward. From experience, his physicians knew that, despite his marginally low plasma sodium, total body sodium was depleted. Therefore, his rehydration included sodium to correct the imbalance.

His plasma potassium level also required careful attention. Though it was high, his physicians knew that he was potassium depleted. This paradox of potassium depletion and high plasma potassium is explained by the fact that, in diabetic acidosis, K^+ cannot enter cells without insulin and excess H^+ (acidosis) enter cells in exchange for K^+. Blood K^+ rises from both of these forces and spills into urine, which causes total body K^+ deficit. When acidosis is corrected by insulin, K^+ reenters cells and plasma K^+ falls; hence the need for potassium supplementation in his intravenous fluids.

The high creatinine could be attributed to two things: low renal blood flow due to dehydration and/or diabetic nephropathy. Notice that his creatinine

"He's acting crazy." The case of Stanley B. (continued)

fell significantly after he was rehydrated, which improved renal blood flow. But it did not fall back into the normal range, suggesting that something else, almost certainly diabetic nephropathy, was also contributing.

The odd thing about this case was that Stanley presented with diabetic ketoacidosis, a presentation that usually occurs in Type I diabetes. This could be either a rare case of Type I diabetes first diagnosed in an older adult, or a rare case of Type II first presenting with ketoacidosis. Blood insulin assay would answer the question, but it was not performed. Near normal insulin would have proved Type II, low insulin Type I. His obesity, however, strongly argues in favor of Type II diabetes. The question is somewhat academic: he needed insulin immediately, and he may need it regularly.

Finally, this patient was a cardiovascular time bomb waiting to explode. Despite losing 25 pounds, he was still obese. What's more, he was a smoker and hypertensive. Although we do not know his blood lipid profile, we can predict that he probably suffered from *metabolic syndrome* (Chapter 23), which is commonly associated with Type II diabetes.

Chapter Challenge

CHAPTER RECALL

1. A 65-year-old Hispanic female presents to the clinic complaining of mild abdominal pain, nausea, and vomiting. Physical exam is notable for absence of jaundice and the presence of an abdominal mass. She is sent for CT imaging which reveals a cyst. Subsequent fine needle aspiration of the cyst, guided by ultrasound, reveals thin, clear, watery fluid and pieces of pancreatic duct epithelium. What is your diagnosis?
   A. Pseudocyst
   B. Serous cystadenoma
   C. Mucinous cystic neoplasm
   D. Intraductal papillary mucinous neoplasms

2. While volunteering at a summer camp for diabetics, you observe one of your students who appears ill. He is pale, sweating profusely, and trembling. When you take his wrist, his skin is cool and clammy to the touch, and his heartbeat is erratic. What is the likely cause of his symptoms?
   A. Presence of an insulinoma
   B. Complications of new onset diabetes
   C. Injection of too much insulin
   D. Hyperglycemia

3. Which of the following statements concerning Type II diabetes is true?
   A. Pancreatic islets are infiltrated by T lymphocytes.
   B. It features an absolute lack of insulin.
   C. It is characterized by periodic episodes of ketoacidosis.
   D. The islets are gradually replaced by amyloid.

4. A 54-year-old African American male presents to the ER with nausea, vomiting, weight loss, and upper abdominal pain radiating to the back. Physical exam demonstrates a well-developed, nonobese male with moderate abdominal tenderness; you note a mild scleral icterus (yellowing of the eyes). A CT demonstrates a large pancreatic mass, and blood studies are remarkable for elevation of nonalbumin protein, which is determined to be IgG4 on additional testing. What is the most likely etiology of his pancreatitis?
   A. Autoimmune
   B. Gallstones
   C. Malignancy
   D. Alcohol abuse

5. Which of the following structures is a cyst lacking lining epithelium?
   A. Serous cystadenoma
   B. Mucinous cystic neoplasm
   C. Pseudocyst
   D. Intraductal papillary mucinous neoplasms

6. A 45-year-old Caucasian female presents for evaluation of a right leg pain. Physical exam reveals a jaundiced, gaunt woman with a right leg that is twice the size of the left. Her physical exam is also positive for abdominal tenderness. On further

questioning, the patient confirms recent unintentional weight loss. In the context of these textbook symptoms, you recognize the blood clot in her leg as Trousseau sign. Which of the following tumors is responsible for her symptoms?
A. Pancreatic adenocarcinoma
B. Zollinger Ellison Gastrinoma
C. Insulinoma
D. Intraductal papillary mucinous neoplasms

7. All of the complications of diabetes are caused by which one of the following?
A. Circulating ketones
B. Autoimmunity
C. Hyperglycemia
D. Atherosclerosis

8. True or false? A fasting blood glucose of ≥126 mg/dL is diagnostic of diabetes.

9. True or false? Women with gestational diabetes are not at increased risk of developing diabetes.

10. True or false? Chronic pancreatitis is one possible cause of diabetes.

11. Match the following hormones with their mechanism of action.
i. Insulin
ii. Glucagon
iii. Pancreas polypeptide
iv. Somatostatin

A. Inhibits glucagon and insulin secretion; slows GI and biliary peristalsis
B. Stimulates cell uptake of glucose from blood
C. Stimulates gastric enzymes secretion and inhibits small bowel motility
D. Stimulates liver output of glucose (via glycogen breakdown or amino acid conversion) and breakdown of fat for energy

CONCEPTUAL UNDERSTANDING

12. What methods are available for diagnosing a patient with chronic pancreatitis in the absence of elevated amylase and/or lipase?

13. Name the two types of diabetic coma and the pathogenesis of each.

14. Most of the enzymes secreted by the exocrine pancreas are inactive when secreted. How is this accomplished and what are the exceptions?

APPLICATION

15. Why is it important for diabetics to perform foot checks?

16. At his three-month follow-up, your patient reports that his diabetes has been well controlled. Although his lab results reveal normal blood glucose today, his HgbA1C is 10.3%. What advice should you offer your patient?

CHAPTER 14

Disorders of the Endocrine Glands

Contents

Chapter Objectives

After studying this chapter, you should be able to complete the following tasks:

THE NORMAL ENDOCRINE SYSTEM

1. Using examples from the text, explain homeostatic negative feedback loops.

DISORDERS OF THE PITUITARY GLAND

2. Classify the types of functioning pituitary adenomas according to cell of origin, hormone produced, and clinical findings; include a description of mass and stalk effect.
3. Describe the presentation of hypopituitarism and catalog the potential underlying etiologies.
4. Compare and contrast diabetes insipidus and syndrome of inappropriate ADH secretion.

DISORDERS OF THE THYROID GLAND

5. Categorize the diseases of the thyroid—goiter, euthyroid sick syndrome, thyrotoxicosis, Grave disease, cretinism, myxedema, Hashimoto thyroiditis, and subacute granulomatous

thyroiditis—as hyperthyroid, euthyroid, or hypothyroid, and give their characteristic features and diagnostic findings.

DISORDERS OF THE ADRENAL CORTEX

6. Discuss the etiology, clinical presentation, and diagnostic findings of Cushing syndrome, primary hyperaldosteronism, congenital adrenal hyperplasia, and causes of adrenocortical failure including Addison disease.

DISORDERS OF THE ADRENAL MEDULLA

7. Explain why patients with pheochromocytoma have high blood pressure.

DISORDERS OF THE PARATHYROID GLANDS

8. Distinguish hypo- from hyperparathyroidism using signs and symptoms, and offer a brief profile of the possible laboratory abnormalities.

MULTIPLE ENDOCRINE NEOPLASIA SYNDROMES

9. Compare and contrast the MEN syndromes.

Case Study

"I'm running out of gas." The case of Azadeh N.

Chief Complaint: Tiredness, swollen feet

Clinical History: Azadeh N. was a pleasant, upbeat 53-year-old woman who worked as a receptionist in a medical office. She frequently asked questions of physicians about her type I diabetes and minor ailments. One day she complained about feeling tired and down in the dumps, and the physician recalled she had seemed less outgoing lately and had missed several days of work, both unusual for her. He suggested she make herself an appointment for the next week and he would see her as a regular patient.

Before seeing her the next week, he reviewed her chart. She had a rather full chart, mainly entries regarding recent downward adjustments of her insulin and high blood pressure medicines, but nothing else recently other than a minor vaginal infection and upper respiratory complaints. In the exam room, he asked her to tell him what was bothering her most.

"I'm running out of gas," she said with a sigh, pausing to gather strength for the next sentence. "I guess I'm just too old for this job. It's my legs; they are so swollen and heavy even though I'm very regular about my water pills," she said, referring to the diuretics she took for blood pressure control and edema in her feet. "I'm just so tired I can't find the energy sometimes to comb my hair. Not that it'll do much good," she said, running fingers through thinning hair to collect some strands, which she held out for him to see. "My hair is falling out, too. I'm just falling apart, I guess," she said.

The remainder of the history and review of systems revealed only that she had increased her daily laxative dose lately to avoid constipation.

Physical Examination and Other Data: Vital signs were: BP 110/78, HR 64, respirations 12, and thermographic middle ear temperature was 97.4°F.

During the examination, the physician asked if she noticed any change in her appearance. "Oh, yes, my face seems to be getting fat. I'm sensitive about my appearance and it's something that has bothered me for quite some time. These bags under my eyes are just terrible, too," she said, managing a rare laugh. "I seem to be getting old before my time."

Her thyroid was slightly and uniformly enlarged and nontender. She had no palpable cervical lymph nodes. Heart sounds were barely audible. A few crackling rales were heard with each inspiration, but her chest was otherwise quiet. Her abdomen was soft, and no masses were palpable. Her skin was dry and scaly, especially on her lower legs, where she had some poorly outlined nodules in the pretibial skin and moderate pitting edema of the ankles and feet.

"Well," the physician said, "nothing alarming. Let's do an ECG and some lab tests and we'll talk again."

Later in the day, the results were available. A complete blood count revealed normal values. Standard blood chemistry tests revealed that the only abnormal value was blood glucose 318 mg/dL, consistent with her diabetes. Blood creatinine was slightly elevated. The thyroid test results were:

T4	1.1 mcg/dL	normal: 5.0–11.0
T3	22 ng/dL	normal: 95–190
TSH	17 mIU/L	normal: 0.4–6.0

Urinalysis showed a moderate amount of glucose and a small amount of albumin in her urine. The ECG was unremarkable except for low voltage across all leads.

"I'm running out of gas." The case of Azadeh N. (continued)

Clinical course: The physician quickly concluded she had hypothyroidism. Before beginning therapy, blood was collected for antithyroid and other autoantibody tests. Antithyroid antibodies were detected; no other autoantibodies were present. When questioned about her family medical history, she recalled that an aunt had rheumatoid arthritis (RA). Further questioning revealed that her daily insulin requirement had lessened and her usual dose tended to make her hypoglycemic, and that another clinic physician had lowered her blood pressure medicine dosage because she developed orthostatic hypotension and felt faint sometime when rising from a seated position.

She was prescribed oral thyroid hormone (L-thyroxine, T4) replacement therapy. She responded nicely and soon seemed her old self, full of energy and laughter. She lost about five pounds, her pedal edema and pretibial nodules disappeared, and her hair stopped shedding. Her thyroid gland remained slightly enlarged but did not present a cosmetic problem. Her insulin requirement increased and she returned to her former dosage. She no longer felt faint when standing up suddenly, and her blood pressure returned to hypertensive levels necessitating upward adjustment of antihypertensive drugs to previous levels.

War will never cease until babies begin to come into the world with larger cerebrums and smaller adrenal glands.

H. L. MENCKEN (1881–1956), FAMOUSLY CRABBY AMERICAN JOURNALIST AND LINGUIST

Recall from Chapter 2 that *endocrine* molecules are signaling agents that are secreted and then absorbed directly into blood for distribution throughout the body to exert an effect on distant cells. **Hormones** are endocrine molecules. The **endocrine system** comprises the pituitary and its target organs—thyroid gland, adrenal glands, testes, and ovaries—and the parathyroid glands (which are not under the control of pituitary hormones). The pituitary gland also influences the functions of organs that are not part of the endocrine system: milk formation in the breast, uterus contractions in pregnancy, bone and muscle growth in children, and water retention by the kidney. Figure 14.1 illustrates the relationships of the major endocrine glands and their target organs. Note that other organs and tissues can secrete hormones. For example, the pancreas secretes insulin, the kidney secretes renin and erythropoietin, and the stomach secretes gastrin.

Endocrine disorders are generally of two types:

1. *Over- or underproduction* of hormone with associated effect on target organs
2. *Mass lesions,* often tumors, which may be
   - nonfunctional and exert local pressure (called **mass effect**) on the gland or surrounding tissue, which can interrupt or alter function or slowly crush the tissue out of existence;
   - functional and secrete hormones.

Diabetes, discussed in Chapter 13, is the most important endocrine disease; those discussed in this chapter are far less common.

The Normal Endocrine System

The endocrine system maintains metabolic equilibrium by continuously adjusting mutually opposing forces, a process known as *homeostasis.* It does this by secreting hormones that stimulate a target organ, which in turn secretes its own hormone(s) to achieve the desired end effect. The target organ hormone in turn inhibits the organ that produced the original hormone, an action called *negative feedback* (Chapter 2).

Remember This! Homeostatic negative feedback loops are extremely important in endocrine disease.

The Pituitary Secretes Multiple Hormones

The pituitary gland sits at the base of the skull in a bony cradle, the sella turcica, arguably the most important intersection in the body—directly between the ears, encircled by the arteries of the circle of Willis, between the optic nerves, anterior to the brainstem, and between the internal carotid arteries. It consists of two parts—the anterior pituitary (the adenohypophysis), which comprises 80%, and the posterior pituitary (the neurohypophysis), which makes up 20%. Figure 14.2 illustrates the pituitary gland and the hormones it secretes, which are also tabulated in Table 14.1.

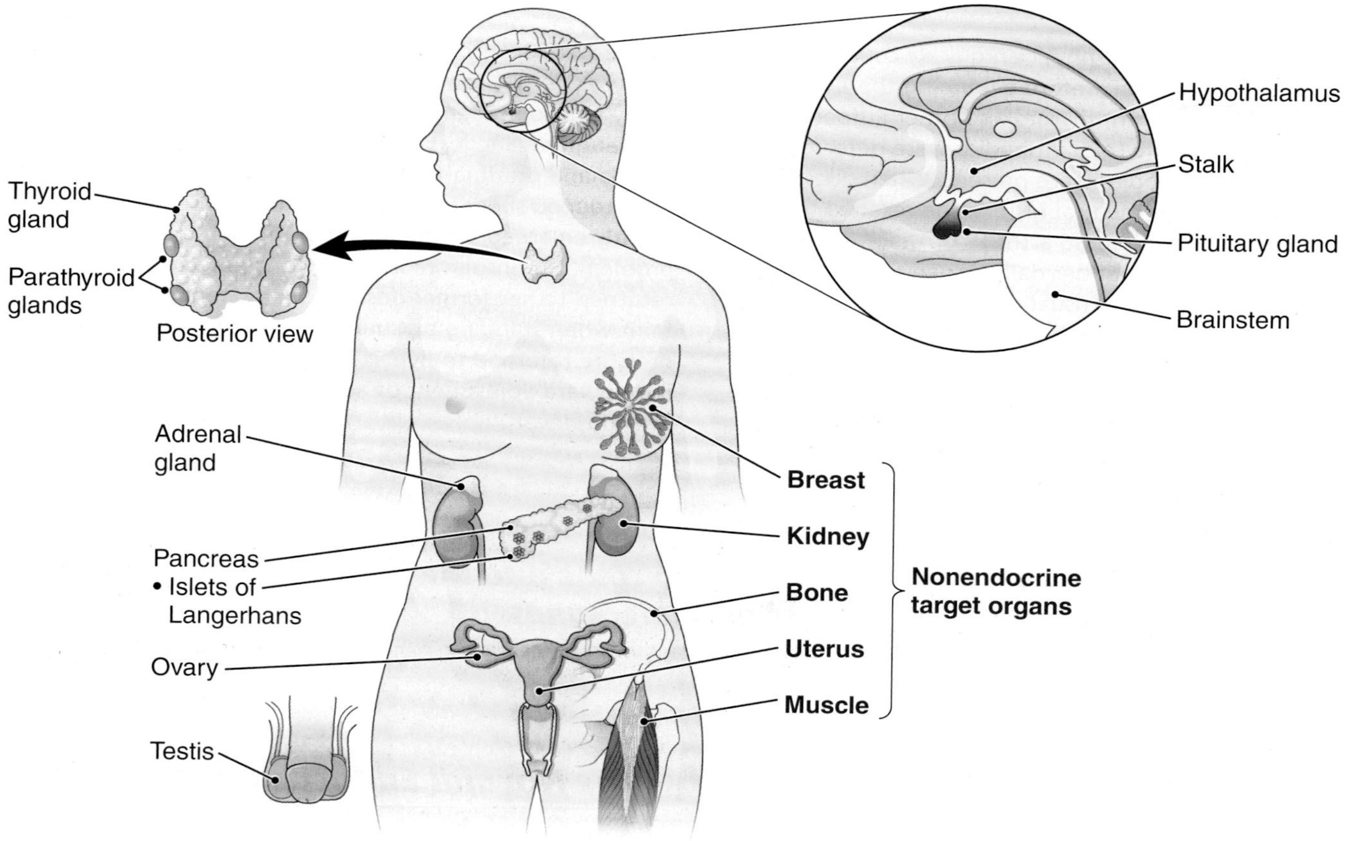

Figure 14.1 **Major endocrine glands and target organs.**

Case Notes

14.1 Is Azadeh's thyroid controlled by the anterior or the posterior pituitary?

Case Notes

14.2 Which hypothalamic hormone initiates stimulation of Azadeh's thyroid gland?

The hypothalamus is an area of the brain immediately above the pituitary gland. It controls the pituitary via the pituitary stalk, which extends directly from the hypothalamus to the pituitary. The hypothalamus secretes *releasing hormones* that are carried to the *anterior* pituitary by a network of small veins. **Releasing hormones** act on the anterior pituitary to control the secretion of its hormones, which in turn act on the target organ. For example, the hypothalamus secretes *thyrotropin-releasing hormone (TRH)*, which stimulates pituitary release of *thyroid-stimulating hormone (TSH)* from the anterior pituitary. TSH then enters the bloodstream and acts on the thyroid gland, causing it to release its hormones. With one exception, the hypothalamus *stimulates* the pituitary to release its hormones. Hypothalamic influence on prolactin is the exception: the influence of the hypothalamus *inhibits* the release of prolactin from the pituitary.

The Anterior Pituitary

The *anterior* pituitary is composed of glandular epithelial cells. There are five types of cells:

- **Somatotrophs**, which produce *growth hormone (GH)*
- **Lactotrophs**, which produce *prolactin*
- **Corticotrophs**, which produce **pro-opiomelanocortin (POMC)**, the precursor molecule from which both *adrenocorticotrophic hormone (ACTH)* and *melanocyte-stimulating hormone (MSH)* are derived
- **Thyrotrophs**, which produce *thyroid-stimulating hormone (TSH)*
- **Gonadotrophs**, which produce *follicle-stimulating hormone (FSH)* and *luteinizing hormone (LH)*

Anterior pituitary hormones affect two types of targets:

- *Organs that have endocrine activity*—adrenal glands, thyroid gland, ovary, and testis—which release their

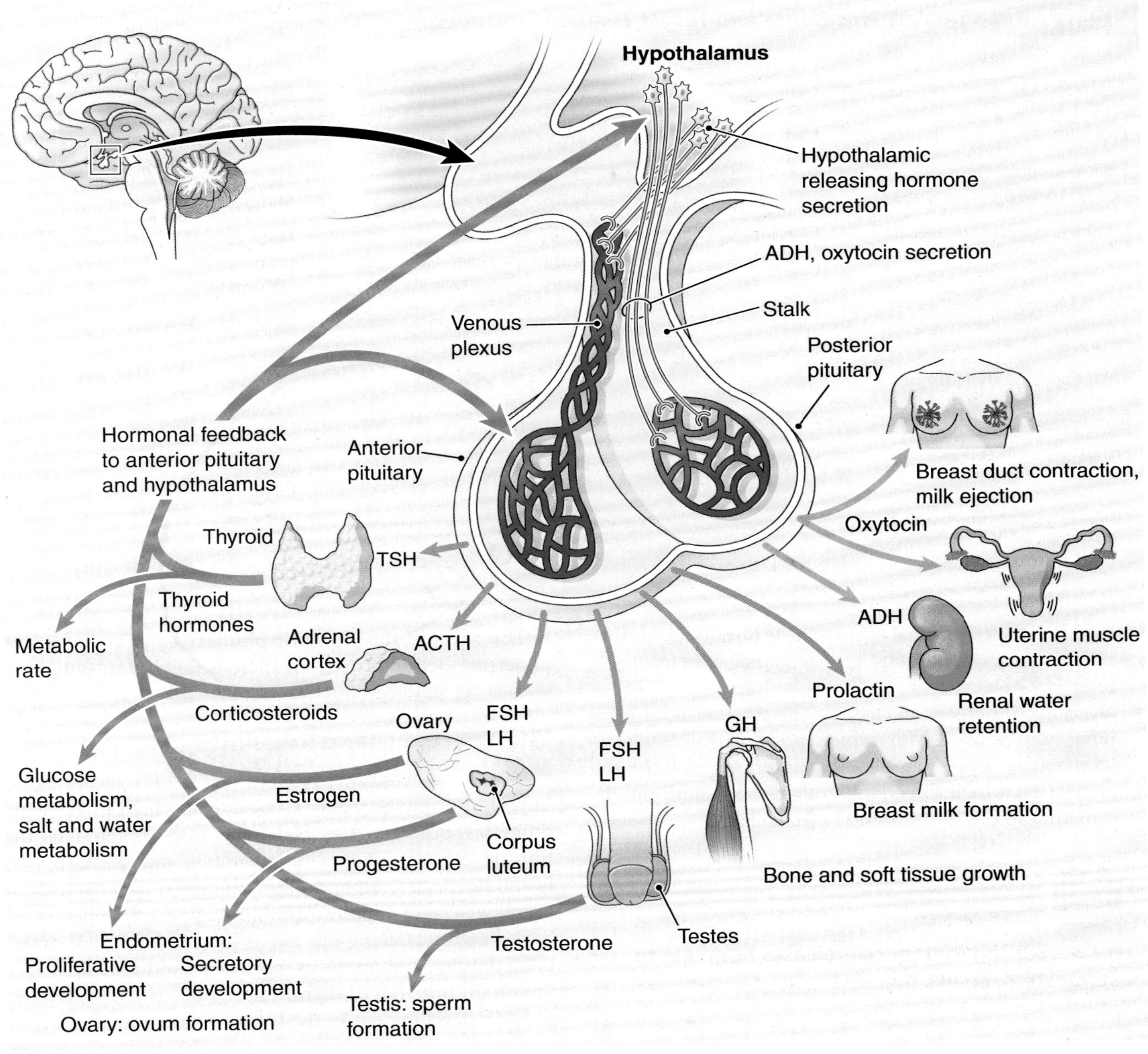

Figure 14.2 **Hypothalamus, pituitary gland, and target organs and tissues.**

Table 14.1 *Pituitary Hormones and Target Tissues*

Anterior Pituitary Hormones

Hormone	Cell	Target Tissue	Effect on Target
*Adrenocorticotrophic hormone (ACTH)	Corticotroph	Adrenal cortex	Secrete steroid hormones
Thyroid-stimulating hormone (TSH)	Thyrotroph	Thyroid gland	Secrete thyroxine (T4) and triiodothyronine (T3)
Growth hormone (GH, somatotropin)	Somatotroph	All tissues	Tissue growth

(continued)

Table 14.1 Pituitary Hormones and Target Tissues (Continued)

Hormone	Cell	Target Tissue	Effect on Target
Anterior Pituitary Hormones			
Prolactin	Lactotroph	Breast glands	Milk formation
Follicle-stimulating hormone (FSH)	Gonadotroph	Ovary: germ cells Testis: Sertoli cells	Stimulate ovulation Stimulate sperm formation
Luteinizing hormone (LH)	Gonadotroph	Ovary: granulosa and theca cells Testis: Leydig cells	Form corpus luteum and secrete progesterone and estrogen Secrete testosterone
*Melanocyte-stimulating hormone (MSH)	Corticotroph	Melanocytes in skin, retina, meninges and other sites	Increases melanin production
Posterior Pituitary Hormones			
Antidiuretic hormone (ADH)	Modified brain cells	Kidney tubules	Conserve water
Oxytocin	Modified brain cells	Breast ducts Uterus	Eject milk Contraction

*ACTH and MSH are derived from a single precursor molecule, *pro-opiomelanocortin (POMC)*, which is metabolized into several pieces, one of which is ACTH and another is MSH.

own hormones for final effect. These hormones in turn interact with the pituitary gland in a negative feedback loop.

- *Nonendocrine organs and tissues*—breast, uterus, kidney, bone, and muscle—for which no negative feedback loop exists. For example, the anterior pituitary secretes GH, which directly stimulates bone and muscle growth; there is no "shut off" mechanism.

Case Notes

14.3 Which pituitary cell releases hormone to stimulate Azadeh's thyroid?

The Posterior Pituitary

The *posterior* pituitary (or neurohypophysis) is composed of modified brain cells. The two hormones of the posterior pituitary (*antidiuretic hormone [ADH]* and *oxytocin*) are actually synthesized in the hypothalamus then travel down nerve axons within the pituitary stalk to the posterior pituitary, where they are stored in the tips of the axons. Upon receiving a hypothalamic nerve impulse, the hormones are released directly into the systemic circulation.

Antidiuretic hormone (ADH) acts on renal tubules to reabsorb water, which concentrates urine and conserves water. **Oxytocin** acts on smooth muscle in breast ducts to eject milk in lactating women and in the uterus to cause contractions during childbirth.

Disorders of the posterior pituitary consist of over- or underproduction of ADH as there is no clinical syndrome of over- or underproduction of oxytocin.

The Thyroid Gland Regulates Metabolic Rate

Thyroid hormones regulate the rate at which physiologic processes proceed—the metabolic rate—much like the throttle for an engine. For example, increased thyroid hormone causes, among other things, the heart to beat faster. Just as a rapidly running engine consumes more fuel, a high metabolic rate burns more calories, consumes more oxygen, and produces more heat. Additionally, a very important function of thyroid hormones is the promotion of brain development in the fetus.

The **thyroid gland** sits just under the skin in the anterior neck, above the breastbone (sternum), below the larynx, and in front of the trachea. It has two lobes, one on either side of the trachea, which are joined inferiorly by a narrow strip of thyroid, the isthmus. The thyroid is composed of thousands of tiny spaces (**follicles**) formed of thyroid epithelial cells, which synthesize thyroid hormones. The follicles are filled with **colloid**, a gelatinous fluid. The colloid contains a specialized protein, **thyroglobulin**, which binds thyroid hormones until they are released from these stores into the blood. In this regard, the thyroid is unique among endocrine glands, as it stores a big reserve of hormone.

The thyroid gland secretes two major thyroid hormones, one with four iodine molecules, the other with three. The most abundant thyroid hormone is **thyroxine** (**tetraiodothyronine**, or **T4**). (*Note*: The molecularly correct name for T4 is **L-thyroxine**, the levo [left] isomer; the mirror-image dextro [right] isomer is metabolically inactive.) Less abundant, but more potent, is **triiodothyronine** (**liothyronine**, or **T3**). Patients with normal thyroid function (normal metabolic rate, normal blood levels of T4 and T3) are said to be **euthyroid**; those with high blood levels of thyroid hormone are hypermetabolic and are **hyperthyroid**; those with low blood levels of thyroid hormone are hypometabolic and are **hypothyroid**. T4 and T3 are transported to peripheral tissues bound to a specialized blood protein, **thyroxine-binding globulin (TBG)**. To be metabolically active, however, T3 and T4 must detach from TBG. Thus, *free* T4 and T3 determine metabolic rate.

A classic negative feedback loop regulates thyroid function (Fig.14.3). The hypothalamus secretes TRH, which causes the pituitary gland to secrete TSH, which in turn stimulates the thyroid gland to secrete T4 and T3, which act to upregulate the metabolic rate. T4 and T3 then stimulate the hypothalamus and pituitary gland to decrease output of TRH and TSH.

Most of the hormone secreted by the thyroid gland into the blood is T4. T4 lacks the metabolic wallop of T3, however, which is secreted in lesser quantity and circulates in blood at lower concentration than T4.

Thyroid follicles also contain a population of **parafollicular cells (C cells)** that synthesize and secrete **calcitonin**, a hormone that promotes absorption of calcium by bones and prohibits bone resorption by osteoclasts (Chapter 18).

Case Notes

14.4 **In a normal individual, are the thyroid hormones released by Azadeh's gland freshly synthesized or released from stores?**

14.5 **Name the cells that synthesize Azadeh's thyroid hormones.**

14.6 **Is Azadeh's thyroglobulin located in her thyroid or her blood?**

14.7 **Why is Azadeh's TSH high?**

The Adrenal Cortex Secretes Corticosteroids

As the name suggests, the **adrenal glands** sit atop the kidneys. As is illustrated in Figure 14.4, the adrenals are two organs in one: an outer *cortex*, under control of the pituitary gland, and an inner *medulla*, linked directly to and controlled separately by the autonomic nervous system. Extensive damage to the adrenals causes clinically

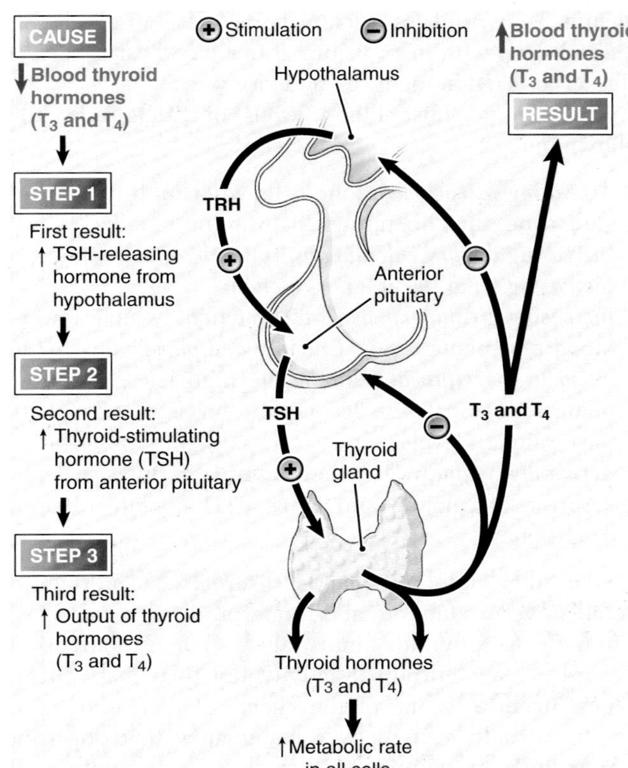

Figure 14.3 **Control of thyroid hormone output.**

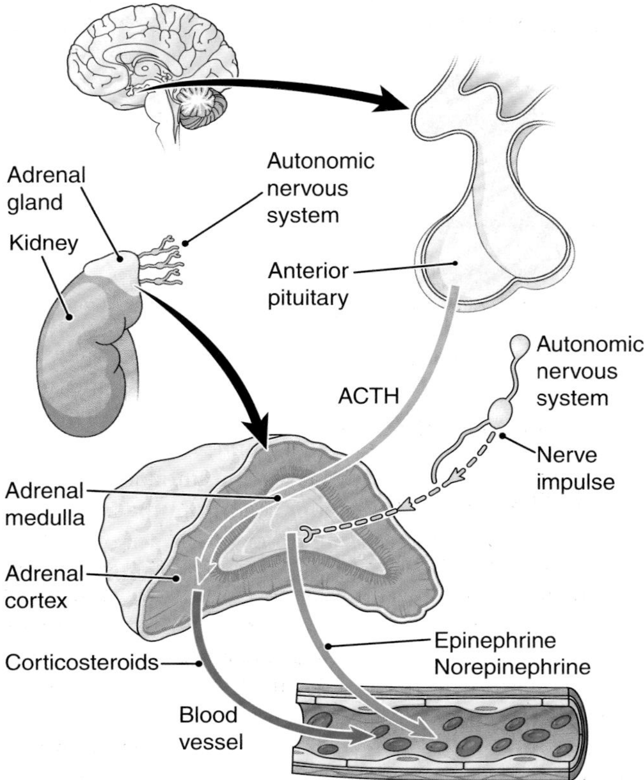

Figure 14.4 **Normal adrenal gland.** The cortex and the medulla secrete hormones directly into blood—the cortex under command of pituitary ACTH, the medulla under command of autonomic nerve impulses.

significant loss of cortical hormones; the loss of medullary function is insignificant because other systems compensate efficiently for the loss.

The **adrenal cortex** comprises 90% of the gland. It has three distinct layers: a thin outer *zona glomerulosa*; a broad middle layer, the *zona fasciculata*; and a thin inner layer, the *zona reticularis*. Each layer is composed of epithelial cells that respond to pituitary output of ACTH, which stimulates release of three **corticosteroids**:

1. **Mineralocorticoids** (principally **aldosterone**) are secreted by the zona glomerulosa. They act on the kidney to retain sodium (Na^+) and water and excrete potassium (K^+), actions that increase blood volume and blood pressure (Chapter 8) and decrease potassium (hypokalemia).
2. **Glucocorticoids** (mainly **cortisol**) are secreted by the zona fasciculata. They do the following:
   - *Increase glucose production* by stimulating breakdown of liver and muscle glycogen into glucose.
   - *Stimulate the degradation of protein into amino acids and fat into fatty acids.* The amino acids and fatty acids are then available for energy production.
   - *Inhibit peripheral glucose utilization* to ensure that adequate glucose is available for the brain.
   - *Suppress immune reaction and limit inflammation* to lessen the stress of injury (disease).
3. **Sex steroids** (*estrogens* and *androgens* less potent than those secreted by the ovaries and testes), which have a variety of effects on bone, muscle, brain, and genitalia, are secreted by the zona reticularis.

Disorders of the cortex are over-and underproduction of hormones, each of which can be serious or fatal. Cortical neoplasms may come to attention by overproduction of hormones, or by mass effect.

The Adrenal Medulla Is Anatomically and Functionally Distinct from the Cortex

The **adrenal medulla** is embryologically, anatomically, and functionally separate from the cortex. It forms the small central part of each adrenal gland, comprising about 10% of gland weight. It is completely surrounded by cortex, and is directly connected by nerve fibers to the autonomic nervous system (Chapter 19). Upon command from the autonomic nervous system, it secretes hormones that act on cardiac muscle, smooth muscle, and glands to control involuntary functions such as heart rate, blood pressure, sweating, and bowel peristalsis.

The medulla is formed of **chromaffin cells**, neuroendocrine cells derived from the embryologic neural crest that develops into brain and peripheral nerves. Clusters of chromaffin cells (called the *paraganglionic system*) are also found in the wall of the aorta and major blood vessels (e.g., the carotid body), the urinary system, and ganglia of the autonomic nervous system. Those in the walls of arteries serve as chemoreceptors sensitive to pH and oxygen tension in the regulation of respiration. The function of the others is unknown.

The chromaffin cells secrete **catecholamines**, chemicals that act in various ways to help the body adapt to sudden stress. **Epinephrine**, the most important of these compounds, is released from the medulla upon stimulation by nerve signals from the autonomic nervous system. Epinephrine stimulates heart rate, dilates bronchioles and coronary arteries, constricts peripheral blood vessels, increases mental alertness and respiratory rate, and increases the metabolic rate. **Norepinephrine** is a second catecholamine secreted by the medulla. Its very powerful effect causes constriction of small blood vessels, increasing peripheral resistance and raising blood pressure.

The most important disorders of the adrenal medulla are tumors, many of which come to attention because of overproduction of these catecholamines.

The Parathyroid Glands Regulate Calcium Metabolism

Normally, there are four **parathyroid glands**, one each behind the upper and lower poles of the right and left thyroid lobes; however, they may be embedded in the thyroid gland, and several extra parathyroids can be present in the nearby neck or upper chest. The parathyroids are tiny, about the size of a grain of rice, and are composed of glandular epithelial cells. They do not operate under the control of the pituitary gland. Rather, their output of **parathormone (PTH)** is controlled by the level of free (ionized) blood calcium. PTH regulates calcium homeostasis in a negative feedback loop with free calcium: if free blood calcium level falls, PTH secretion increases, and vice versa.

PTH acts to raise blood levels of calcium by the following:

- *Activating osteoclasts*, bone cells whose job it is to resorb bone, thus liberating calcium into blood;
- *Increasing dietary calcium absorption by the intestine;*
- *Increasing renal retention of calcium;*
- *Increasing urinary phosphate excretion*, which lowers blood phosphate levels. *Calcium and phosphate exist in blood in a reciprocal relationship*: high levels of phosphate reduce calcium levels; low levels of phosphate raise calcium levels;
- *Activating vitamin D*, which stimulates intestinal absorption of calcium and helps PTH liberate calcium from bones.

Like other endocrine glands, disorders of parathyroid include overproduction and underproduction of PTH. Tumors of parathyroids almost always come to attention because of their hormonal activity, not their mass effect. **Hypercalcemia** is one of the effects of increased PTH, but it is usually caused by a malignancy that does not involve the parathyroids. Nevertheless, nonparathyroid malignancy is the most common cause of hypercalcemia. Instead, tumors may cause hypercalcemia by secreting

PTH-related peptides (PTH-rp) or by destruction of bone by local invasion or metastasis.

Remember This! The parathyroids are not regulated by the pituitary.

Pop Quiz

14.1 True or false? The hypothalamus stimulates the release of all pituitary hormones.

14.2 True or false? Colloid found in the follicles contains TBG which binds thyroid hormones until they are released from stores into blood.

14.3 True or false? Nonparathyroid malignancy is the most common cause of hypercalcemia.

14.4 Which hormone is responsible for stimulating ovulation, and where is it made?

14.5 Name the hormones made in the adrenal gland.

Disorders of the Pituitary Gland

Of the two lobes of the pituitary gland, the anterior is far more often involved by disease. The posterior pituitary is much less affected. Pituitary disease manifests in three ways.

Hyperpituitarism is excretion of excess trophic hormones and can be caused by hyperplasia, adenoma, or carcinoma of any of the cell types of the anterior pituitary. Adenomas are the most common cause. *Hyperpituitarism is much more common than hypopituitarism.* Disease usually presents with symptoms traceable to excess hormones being excreted by the target organ. For example, a common manifestation of hyperpituitarism is oversecretion of prolactin.

Hypopituitarism is deficiency of trophic hormone excretion and is usually due to a local destructive process, which includes infarction, surgery, radiation, inflammation, and nonfunctional pituitary adenomas (which crush the gland). Disease usually presents as a deficiency of hormones excreted by the target organ.

Some pituitary disease presents first as manifestations of local mass effect, which is usually evident as radiographic abnormalities of the sella turcica. The expanding pituitary mass erodes bone and may press on the optic nerves to produce diplopia and other ocular problems and visual field defects, especially loss of lateral vision, a condition known as *bitemporal hemianopsia* (Chapter 20). Finally, increased intracranial pressure is common and may present as headache, nausea, and vomiting. Sometimes mass effect produces **stalk effect**, a term applied to the effect when tumor mass blocks the *inhibitory* effect of the hypothalamus on prolactin secretion. The result is excess prolactin secretion.

Pituitary Adenomas Usually Cause Hyperpituitarism

Most hyperpituitarism results from pituitary adenomas, benign neoplasms that occur only in the anterior pituitary (Fig. 14.5). Surprisingly, pituitary adenomas are very common: about 15% of people have one. Almost all are small (*microadenomas*), nonfunctional, and persist a lifetime without ill effect. Because these and tumors in other glands are usually discovered by high-resolution imaging incidental to some other investigation, they are often irreverently referred to as "*incidentalomas*."

As detailed in Table 14.2, most adenomas that come to medical attention are functioning adenomas composed of a single cell type secreting a single hormone. Adenomas occur most frequently in men between ages 20 and 50 years. They occur as solitary lesions that come to medical attention because of excessive hormone production or mass effect. Most occur as discrete nodules, but a few are locally aggressive and invade bone, sinuses, or brain. Carcinomas are very rare.

Prolactinoma

Prolactinoma is the most common functioning pituitary tumor, accounting for about 30% of adenomas. Even small prolactinomas can secrete enough prolactin to become

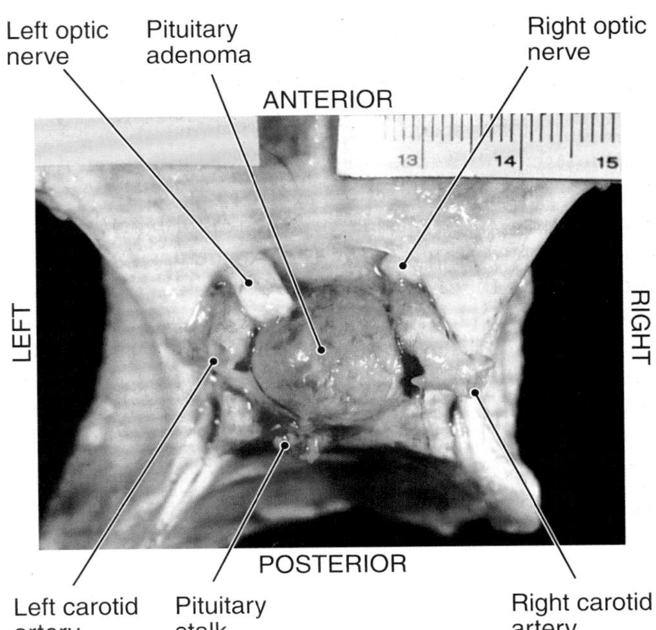

Figure 14.5 **Pituitary adenoma.** View from above, looking down from inside the cranium.

Table 14.2 Classification of Pituitary Adenomas

Pituitary Cell Type*	Hormone	Approximate Percent of all Adenomas	Tumor Type	Effects
Lactotroph	Prolactin	~30%	Prolactinoma	Females: unexpected milk secretion or amenorrhea Males or females: sexual dysfunction, infertility
Various cells	None	~25–30%	Null cell adenoma	Mass effect or stalk effect
Corticotroph	ACTH MSH	~15%	ACTH adenoma	Cushing disease; Nelson syndrome
Somatotroph	GH	~15%	GH cell adenoma	Gigantism in children; acromegaly in adults
Gonadotroph	LH, FSH	~10%	Gonadotroph adenoma	Hypogonadism, mass effect, hypopituitarism
Thyrotroph	TSH	~1%	TSH adenoma	Hyperthyroidism

*Each cell type may produce nonfunctioning adenomas that present with mass effect and hypopituitarism due to destruction of the gland. Some adenomas may produce more than one hormone (most commonly a combination of GH and prolactin).

symptomatic, and as a general rule the larger the tumor the more hormones it produces. It causes **galactorrhea**, milk secretions from the breast of a male or nonpregnant female. Other symptoms in women include cessation of menstruation (amenorrhea), infertility, and loss of sexual drive. The main symptoms in men are decreased sexual drive and impotence. The diagnosis is much easier to make in menstruating women because of menstrual symptoms, usually amenorrhea. In nonmenstrual women and in men, the tumor may not become evident until mass effects bring it to attention.

Diagnosis is confirmed by finding high levels of prolactin in blood and radiographic abnormalities of the gland or sella turcica. Any mass in the pituitary or in the suprasellar space immediately above it, however, may interfere with the normal *inhibitory* influence of the hypothalamus on prolactin secretion and thereby cause excess prolactin secretion. Also, increased blood prolactin secondary to high-dose estrogen therapy, pregnancy, renal failure, thyroid gland failure, lesions of the hypothalamus, and some drugs, can present with symptoms similar to those caused by a prolactinoma. These conditions must be ruled out before presuming that a pituitary mass is a prolactinoma.

Treatment of small prolactinomas is controversial. Asymptomatic patients with mildly elevated prolactin may be merely observed. Symptomatic prolactinomas can be treated with drugs or surgery.

Null Cell Adenoma

Null cell adenomas do not secrete hormones and come to attention because of mass effect. They are second in number only to prolactinomas and comprise about 25–30% of pituitary adenomas. They can originate from any of the cell types in the anterior pituitary. Destruction of the normal gland by the expanding mass may lead to hypopituitarism, discussed below. Although they do not secrete hormones, they often come to attention because of excess prolactin secretion and associated galactorrhea due to their interference with the normal *inhibitory* influence of the hypothalamus on prolactin secretion. Diagnosis is based on radiographic demonstration of a pituitary mass, and a clinical picture and blood hormone levels consistent with hypopituitarism. Treatment may include surgical or radiotherapeutic ablation of the mass and hormone replacement therapy.

ACTH Adenoma

ACTH adenomas account for about 15% of pituitary adenomas. They are associated with excessive secretion of cortisol and related hormones from the adrenal cortex. The effects are dramatic and produce a combination of clinical findings known as *Cushing syndrome,* which is discussed in detail later in this chapter.

If the ACTH adenoma is microscopic, it may go undetected. In such cases, the patient's adrenals may be removed in an attempt to treat the Cushing syndrome. Removal of the adrenals results in a loss of the inhibitory effect of adrenal corticosteroids on pituitary ACTH production. This may cause *Nelson syndrome*—the rapid growth of the missed tiny adenoma as it secretes ever-increasing amounts of ACTH in an effort to increase cortisol secretion from adrenal glands that no longer exist. The mass effect may be locally destructive, and functionally, the adenoma makes large amounts of POMC, the precursor of both ACTH and MSH. The ACTH production is of no consequence because the adrenals are absent, but the increased output of MSH causes marked darkening of the skin.

Diagnosis of ACTH adenoma requires demonstration of a pituitary lesion and high levels of blood ACTH. Treatment may include surgical or radiographic ablation of the adenoma and drug therapy to block the effect of excess steroids.

Growth Hormone Adenoma

Growth hormone (GH) adenomas secrete GH and are second only to prolactinomas among *functioning* adenomas of the anterior pituitary. Many GH adenomas also secrete prolactin. Often the early clinical manifestations are subtle (e.g., a change of shoe or hat size in an adult). They are often diagnosed because of mass effect and may become quite large. GH produces many of its effects by stimulating liver production of *insulin-like growth factor-1* (IGF-1, also called *somatomedin C*).

Excessive production of GH causes two syndromes. **Acromegaly** is a syndrome that occurs when abnormal secretion of GH occurs in adults after bone growth plates disappear. It is characterized by conspicuous growth of bones in the hands, feet, face, skull, and jaw; growth of liver, heart, thyroid, adrenals, and other viscera; and expansion of the skin and soft tissue. Patients (Fig. 14.6) have prominent brows and chin, gapped teeth (teeth become separated as the jaw lengthens), and huge feet and hands with thick fingers. Nevertheless, they are not exceptionally large or tall. Skin and soft tissue growth adds to the coarse facial appearance. Other problems (Fig. 14.7) associated with acromegaly are secondary Type II diabetes (caused by insulin resistance by peripheral tissues), hypertension, muscle weakness, heart failure, arthritis, and osteoporosis (Chapter 18). **Gigantism**, a general increase in body size, with especially long arms and legs, occurs when a child or teenager develops an adenoma that secretes GH before growth plates close at the ends of long bones. Patients with gigantism usually have some features of acromegaly.

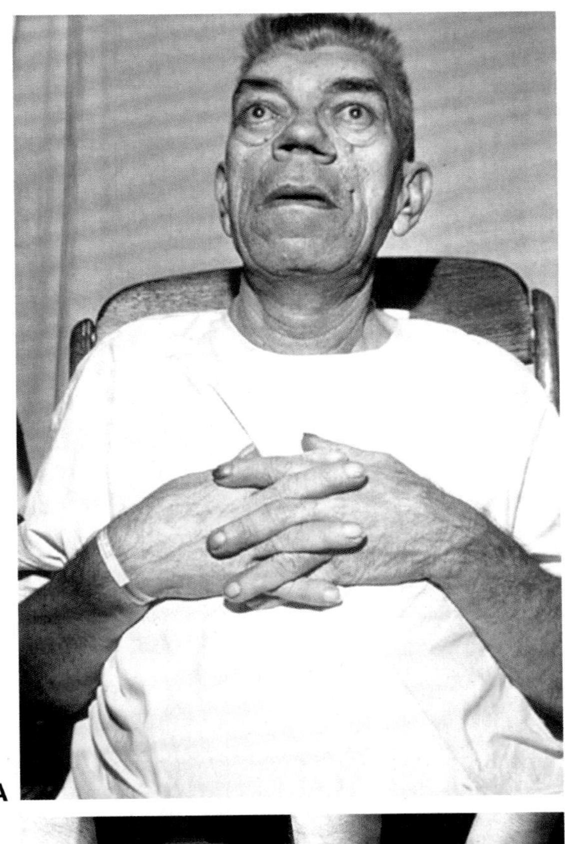

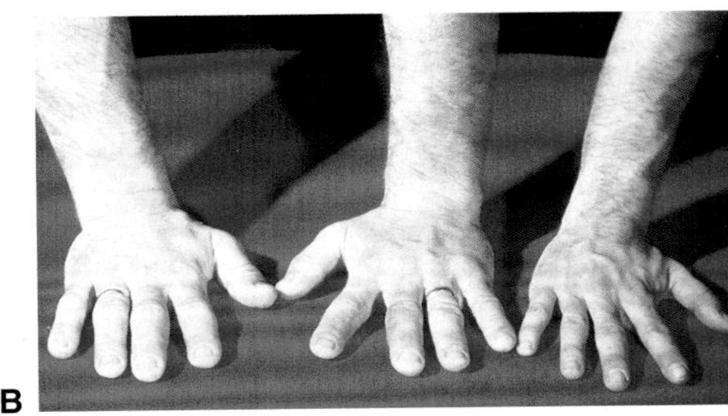

Figure 14.6 **Acromegaly.** Acromegaly is caused by oversecretion of GH in adults, after normal bone growth has stopped. **A.** Note coarse facial features. **B.** Patient's large hands at left; single normal hand at right.

Diagnosis depends on clinical circumstances, radiographic studies of skull and hands for evidence of abnormal bone growth, and the presence of increased blood GH and IGF-1. A sensitive test for GH adenoma is the failure of a glucose meal to suppress GH production.

Treatment may include surgical or radiologic ablation of the adenoma. If surgery is contraindicated because of heart failure or other complications, drug therapy can be effective to block the effect of GH or prevent its secretion.

Gonadotroph Adenoma

Gonadotroph adenomas secrete LH and FSH and comprise about 10% of anterior pituitary adenomas. They occur most commonly in middle-aged men and women. Hormone secretion varies greatly and is often minimal. They usually do not produce a recognizable syndrome related to hormone excess. For this reason, they may go undiagnosed for many years and come to attention only because of mass effect. Paradoxically, the mass effect can be destruction of the remaining gland and a *decrease* of LH and FSH secretion, the result of which is gonadal hypofunction: apathy and decreased libido in men and amenorrhea in menstruating women.

Diagnosis depends on the clinical picture, laboratory assessment of blood LH and FSH levels, and radiographic imaging of the sella turcica. Treatment may include surgical or radiotherapeutic ablation of the adenoma and hormone replacement.

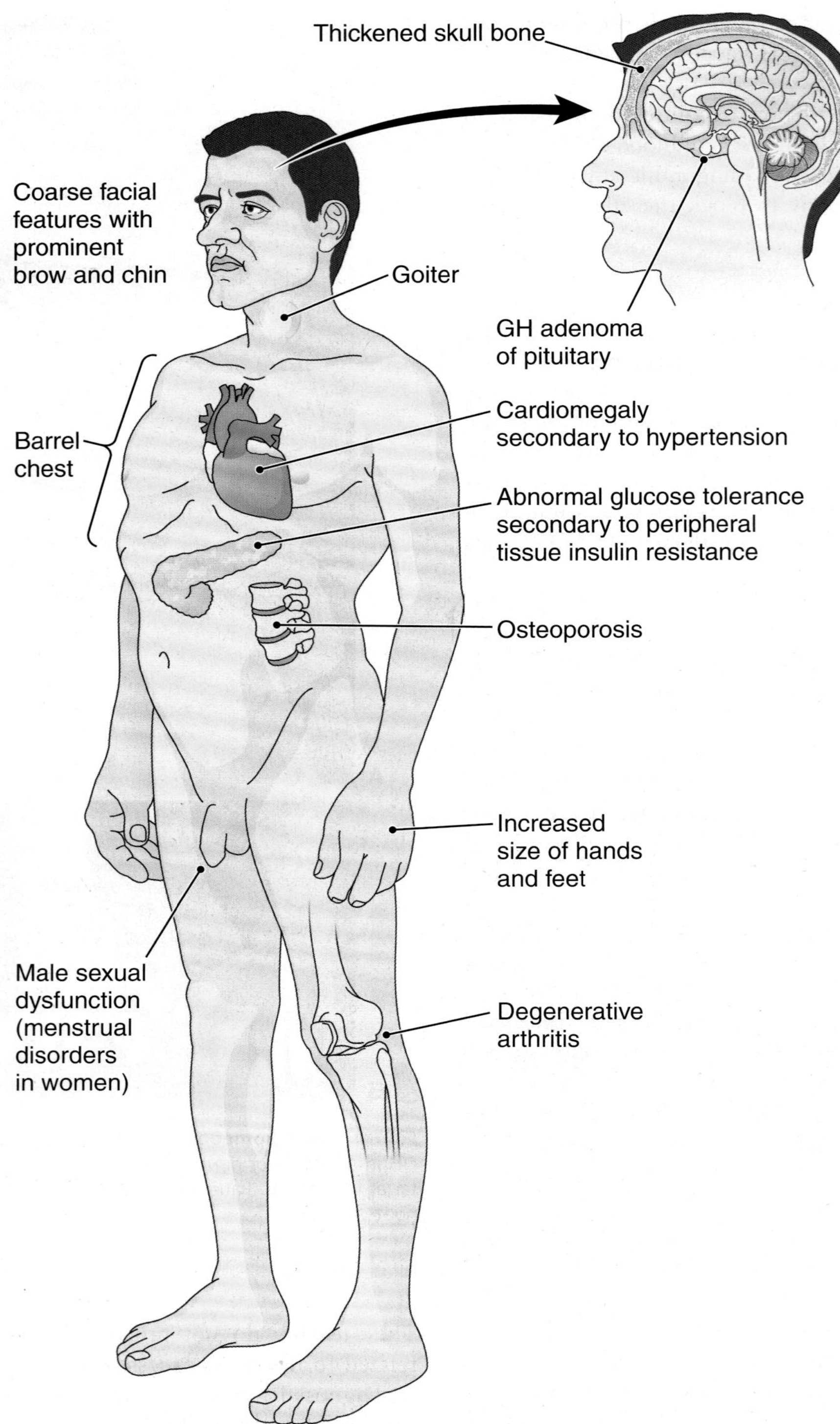

Figure 14.7 **Clinical manifestations of acromegaly.**

TSH Adenoma

TSH adenomas secrete TSH and are rare, comprising 1% or less of pituitary adenomas. TSH production stimulates thyroid release of T3 and T4, which causes *hyperthyroidism* (discussed below). Diagnosis is based on the clinical presence of hyperthyroidism associated with increased blood TSH and radiographic imaging of the sella turcica. Treatment may include surgical or radiotherapeutic ablation of the lesion and drug treatment to counteract the effects of increased T3 and T4.

Hypopituitarism Is Usually Due to Destruction of the Anterior Pituitary

Hypopituitarism is decreased secretion of pituitary hormones. Most are failure of the anterior pituitary and do not involve the posterior pituitary. Nevertheless, if there is evidence of failure of the posterior pituitary in the form of *diabetes insipidus (DI)* (discussed below), the pathologic lesion is almost always in the hypothalamus, not in the pituitary.

About 75% of the anterior pituitary must be destroyed for hormonal deficit to become symptomatic. The most common causes of pituitary failure are the following:

- *Tumors* and other masses, usually pituitary adenomas.
- *Brain trauma* and subarachnoid hemorrhage (Chapter 19).
- *Surgery or radiation*: surgical or radiologic ablation of an adenoma may damage the remaining normal gland.
- Sudden pituitary hemorrhage (*pituitary apoplexy*), usually as a consequence of some other pathologic process in the pituitary.
- *Ischemic infarction of pregnancy (Sheehan syndrome)*. The physiologic demands of pregnancy cause pituitary hyperplasia and increase the need for blood flow through the portal venous plexus that extends through the stalk to carry releasing hormones from the hypothalamus to the anterior pituitary (Fig. 14.8). Obstetrical hemorrhage and shock may cause infarction of the anterior pituitary. The posterior pituitary is usually spared because it receives direct arterial flow from other sources. The diagnosis should be suspected in a woman who is unable to breastfeed and does not resume normal menstrual periods after pregnancy (provided, of course, she is not pregnant again). Some women may become hypothyroid from lack of TSH.
- *Suprasellar or hypothalamic cysts and tumors.*
- *Empty sella syndrome.* Sometimes the sella is empty of anterior pituitary tissue. There are two varieties. *Primary* empty sella is caused by a defect in the meningeal membrane that covers the superior surface of the sella. This herniation allows cerebrospinal fluid to enter the sella and destroy the gland by slow pressure. Typically, this occurs in obese women with multiple pregnancies. *Secondary* empty sella syndrome owes to surgical removal or spontaneous necrosis of an adenoma.
- *Hypothalamic lesions:* Locally developing tumors and cysts, or metastatic malignancy.
- *Inflammatory conditions*, usually chronic disease such as tuberculous meningitis or sarcoidosis.

The clinical presentation of anterior pituitary hypofunction is usually insidious and depends upon which hormones are most deficient. Usually only one or two hormones are deficient, and sometimes only mildly so. Patients typically become easily fatigued, lose weight, and are mildly anemic. Target organs—adrenal cortex, thyroid gland, testes, and ovary—atrophy, and patients suffer from lack of cortisol, thyroxine, and testosterone or estrogen. Often the effect on organs of sexual function calls attention—patients may develop amenorrhea, loss of libido, atrophic gonads, and erectile dysfunction. In postpartum women, failure to lactate may be the first sign. The diagnosis is often difficult to make because the symptoms are nonspecific.

Diagnosis is clinical and supported by radiographic imaging of the sella and blood hormone assays. Treatment is hormone supplementation and elimination of the cause.

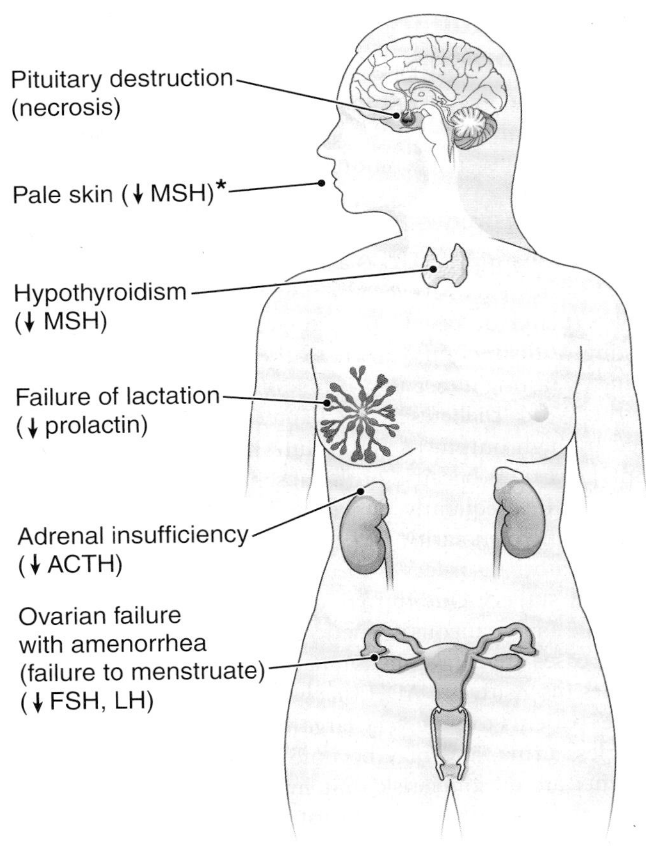

Figure 14.8 **Clinical manifestations of Sheehan syndrome.** Sheehan syndrome is caused by hemorrhagic destruction of the pituitary in pregnancy.

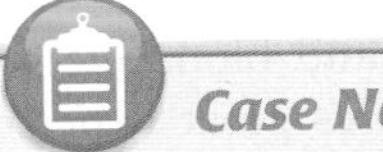

Case Notes

14.8 How do we know that Azadeh's hypothyroidism is not due to pituitary failure?

Posterior Pituitary Syndromes are Uncommon

There are but two syndromes of posterior pituitary function: secretion of too little or too much ADH. Syndromes related to oxytocin secretion are not known.

Diabetes Insipidus

Diabetes insipidus (DI) is a syndrome of ADH deficiency and features excessive production of dilute urine. *Insipid* means bland or tasteless, as opposed to *mellitus*, sweet tasting, a distinction known to the ancients, who tested urine by tasting it (see the *History of Medicine*, "The Origin of the Word 'Diabetes'," in Chapter 13). DI is characterized by high output of very dilute urine (specific gravity [SpG] ~ 1.002) because of the absence of ADH secretion. Patients are frequently dehydrated and have high blood sodium and osmolarity. DI can be caused by head trauma, inflammatory disorders of the brain or pituitary, tumors, or pituitary surgery. One-third of cases appear to be caused by sporadic (spontaneous) genetic defects of ADH synthesis. A few cases are caused by a renal defect that renders renal tubules insensitive to ADH (*nephrogenic DI*). Whatever the cause, patients excrete very large volumes of dilute, nearly colorless urine, and may become dehydrated. Debilitated patients are at some risk, but most patients can remain hydrated by drinking a lot of water.

Diagnosis is clinical and supported by low urine specific gravity and high blood sodium and osmolarity. A water-deprivation test is confirmatory. Under strict observation (serious dehydration may occur), the patient is deprived of water. Body weight, blood sodium and osmolarity, and urine specific gravity are tracked until orthostatic hypotension and tachycardia appear, 5% of body weight is lost, or urine specific gravity does not rise >0.001 in sequential specimens.

Treatment is ADH replacement by a synthetic analog.

Inappropriate ADH Secretion

The **syndrome of inappropriate ADH secretion (SIADH)** is associated with excessive ADH production, usually from a nonpituitary neoplasm (e.g., small cell carcinoma of the lung). Nevertheless, it may occur in a very wide variety of other conditions, including brain, pulmonary, and endocrine disorders. Symptoms are essentially due to water intoxication (Chapter 6): hyponatremia and cerebral edema with associated neurologic problems. Laboratory findings include having low serum sodium (below 135 mEq/L, hyponatremia) while having concentrated urine with high urine sodium (greater than 20 mEq/L). Elimination of the cause is the first aim of therapy. Correction of blood volume and blood electrolyte abnormalities is tricky and requires great expertise and caution in the use of hypotonic, eutonic, or hypertonic intravenous fluids.

Some Pituitary Disorders are Caused by Suprasellar Masses

Neoplasms, cysts, and other masses located superior to the sella turcica may cause pituitary-hypothalamic dysfunction. The most common culprits are *gliomas* (tumors of brain astrocytes, Chapter 19) of the hypothalamus or optic chiasm. Vestigial remnants of *Rathke pouch*, an embryologic structure that gives rise to the anterior pituitary, may develop into a **Rathke pouch cyst**, or into **craniopharyngioma**, a benign neoplasm. In any case, these suprasellar masses make themselves known by mass effect. Diagnosis is by radiographic confirmation of a mass in the suprasellar region and pathologic proof from tissue taken at the time of surgery, which is the usual treatment.

Pop Quiz

14.6 True or false? Only 15% of the anterior pituitary must be destroyed for hormonal deficit to become symptomatic.

14.7 True or false? SIADH is characterized by low urine specific gravity and high blood osmolarity.

14.8 True or false? A prolactinoma is the most common functioning pituitary tumor.

14.9 What is the difference between Cushing disease and Cushing syndrome?

14.10 Vestigial remnants of Rathke pouch give rise to what two suprasellar masses?

Disorders of the Thyroid Gland

Disorders of the thyroid are over- and underproduction of hormones, inflammation (*thyroiditis*), and tumors, which may be functional or come to attention because of mass effect. A **goiter** is an enlarged thyroid gland (Fig. 14.9).

Blood levels of thyroid hormones in various states of thyroid function are identified in Table 14.3. Patients with severe nonthyroidal illness such as renal failure, starvation, cirrhosis, and sepsis may have abnormally low thyroid function tests but are clinically euthyroid—they do not have signs or symptoms of hypothyroidism, and, apart from their other disease, appear to have normal thyroid function. This condition is known as the **euthyroid sick syndrome**.

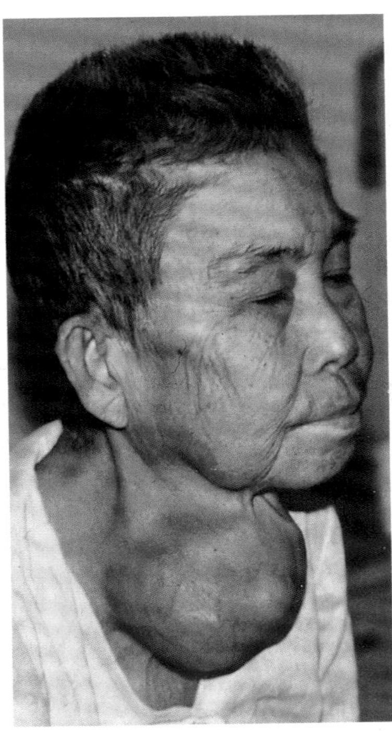

Figure 14.9 **Goiter.** The lumpy appearance of this unusually large goiter and the lack of exophthalmos suggest that it is a nodular, nontoxic goiter. (Reproduced with permission from Rubin E. *Pathology*. 4th ed. Philadelphia (PA). Lippincott Williams and Wilkins; 2005.)

Thyrotoxicosis Is a Hypermetabolic State Caused by Excess Thyroid Hormone

Thyrotoxicosis is a hypermetabolic clinical state caused by increased levels of blood T3 and/or T4, no matter the source. There are two etiologic varieties according to whether or not the gland is actively producing hormone:

1. Those caused by **hyperthyroidism**; that is, *overproduction* of T3 and/or T4 by the gland.
   - *Primary hyperthyroidism* is *intrinsic* overproduction, as with Graves disease or other conditions discussed below. This is by far the most common cause of thyrotoxicosis.
   - *Secondary hyperthyroidism* is overproduction caused by a TSH-secreting adenoma of the pituitary (rare).
2. Those not caused by hyperthyroidism. *The most common cause is overmedication*, usually an inadvertent result of treatment of hypothyroidism. Rare causes are release of stored hormone in thyroiditis and production of thyroid hormone by hyperplastic thyroid tissue in an ovarian teratoma (Chapter 17).

Remember This! There is a difference between thyrotoxicosis and hyperthyroidism—hyperthyroidism is but one cause of thyrotoxicosis.

Table 14.3 ***Laboratory Tests of Thyroid Function****

Condition	Total T4 (μg/dL)	Total T3 (ng/dL)	TSH mIU/ml	% Radioactive Iodine Uptake by Thyroid in 24 hours	Comment
Normal range	5–12	95–190	0.3–5	10–30	
THYROTOXICOSIS					
Primary hyperthyroidism, untreated	↑	↑	↓	↑	Thyroid-stimulating immunoglobulin in Graves disease
secondary hyperthyroidism, untreated	↑	↑	↑	↑	
Thyrotoxicosis from overtreatment with T4	↑	↓	↓	↓	
T3 toxicosis	↓	↑	↓	Normal to ↑	Uncommon
HYPOTHYROIDISM					
Primary, untreated	↓	↓	↑	↓	
Secondary to pituitary failure, untreated	↓	↓	↓	↓	
EUTHYROID					
Euthyroid patient treated with T4	Normal	Varies	Normal to ↓	↓	Correct dosage determined by clinical effect
Patient taking iodine	Normal	Normal	Normal	↓	
Euthyroid sick syndrome	Normal to ↓	↓	Varies	↓	No clinical evidence of hypothyroidism

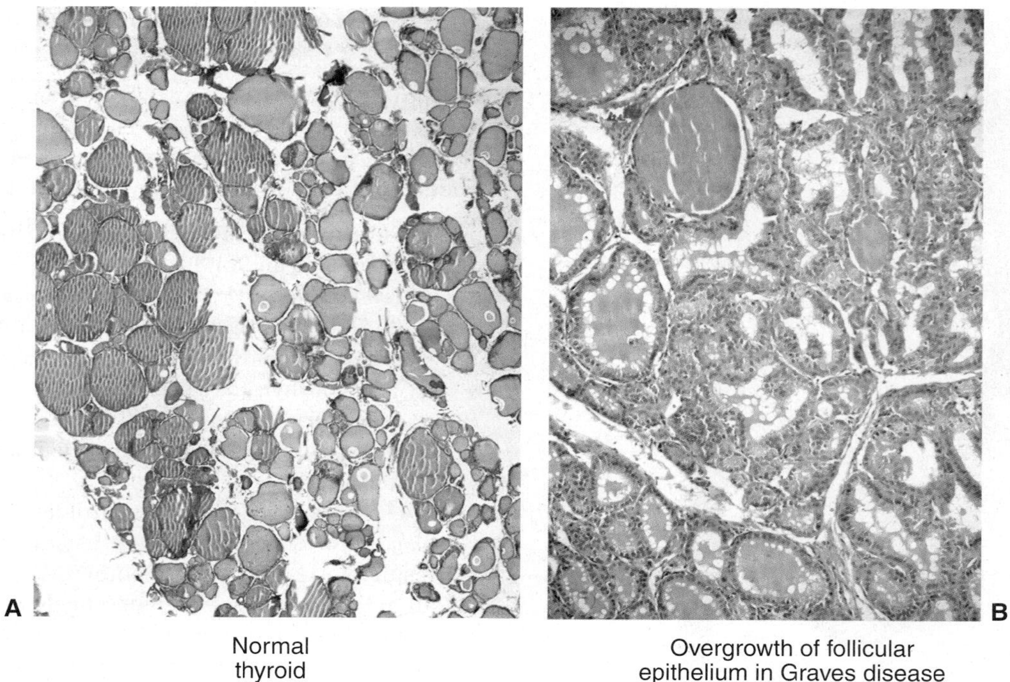

Figure 14.10 **Thyroid gland in hyperthyroidism. A.** Normal thyroid. **B.** Hyperthyroidism. Note the overgrowth (hyperplasia) of follicular epithelium.

The three most common types of thyrotoxicosis, all of which will be discussed shortly, are the following:

- *Diffuse glandular hyperplasia*, usually caused by *Graves disease*, which accounts for nearly 70–80% of cases (Fig. 14.10)
- *Multinodular goiter* with overproduction of hormones (referred to as a toxic goiter)
- *Adenoma* of the thyroid with overproduction of hormones

Each of the above hypermetabolic states is caused by a different variety of primary hyperthyroidism. About 0.1% of the U.S. population is affected by hyperthyroidism. There are no ethnic differences. Peak incidence is age 20–40 years. Women are affected much more often than men.

Signs and Symptoms of Thyrotoxicosis

The clinical evidence of thyrotoxicosis is varied and often subtle. Signs and symptoms relate to the hypermetabolic state and overactivity of the sympathetic nervous system (Fig. 14.11). If hyperthyroidism is the cause, the thyroid is usually diffusely enlarged. Other causes of thyrotoxicosis do not cause gland enlargement. The skin is soft and flushed with blood to increase heat loss. Patients are heat intolerant and may complain that room temperature is too high, or may sleep without cover while a partner sleeps under a blanket. Weight loss is typical despite an adequate diet. Cardiovascular clues include resting tachycardia, premature beats, and other arrhythmias (Chapter 9); heart failure may appear, especially in older patients. Neuromuscular evidence includes a fine tremor, muscle loss and weakness, exaggerated reflexes, insomnia, emotional instability, and an inability to concentrate. Bone calcium loss may produce osteoporosis (Chapter 18) and increased risk of fracture. The bowels may be overactive and produce diarrhea, hypermotility, and poor absorption of nutrients. The eyelids tend to retract and produce a wide-eyed, staring gaze. A characteristic eye sign of hyperthyroidism of any type is *lid lag*, a failure of the upper eyelid to retract normally when gaze moves from downward to upward. The result is a brief sleepy-eyed appearance as gaze moves upward.

Diagnosis and Treatment

Diagnosis is clinical with supporting laboratory information. Blood TSH, T3, and T4 levels vary according to the cause of thyrotoxicosis. With rare exception, blood T3 and T4 are increased. Some patients, however, may have hyperthyroidism due to selective hypersecretion of T3 (**T3-toxicosis**), in which case T4 will be low and T3 high.

When thyrotoxicosis is due to primary hyperthyroidism, TSH is low due to negative feedback from increased blood thyroid hormones. In contrast, TSH levels will be normal or high in *secondary* hyperthyroidism caused by pituitary secretion of excess TSH, or overmedication with thyroid hormone in patients being treated for hypothyroidism.

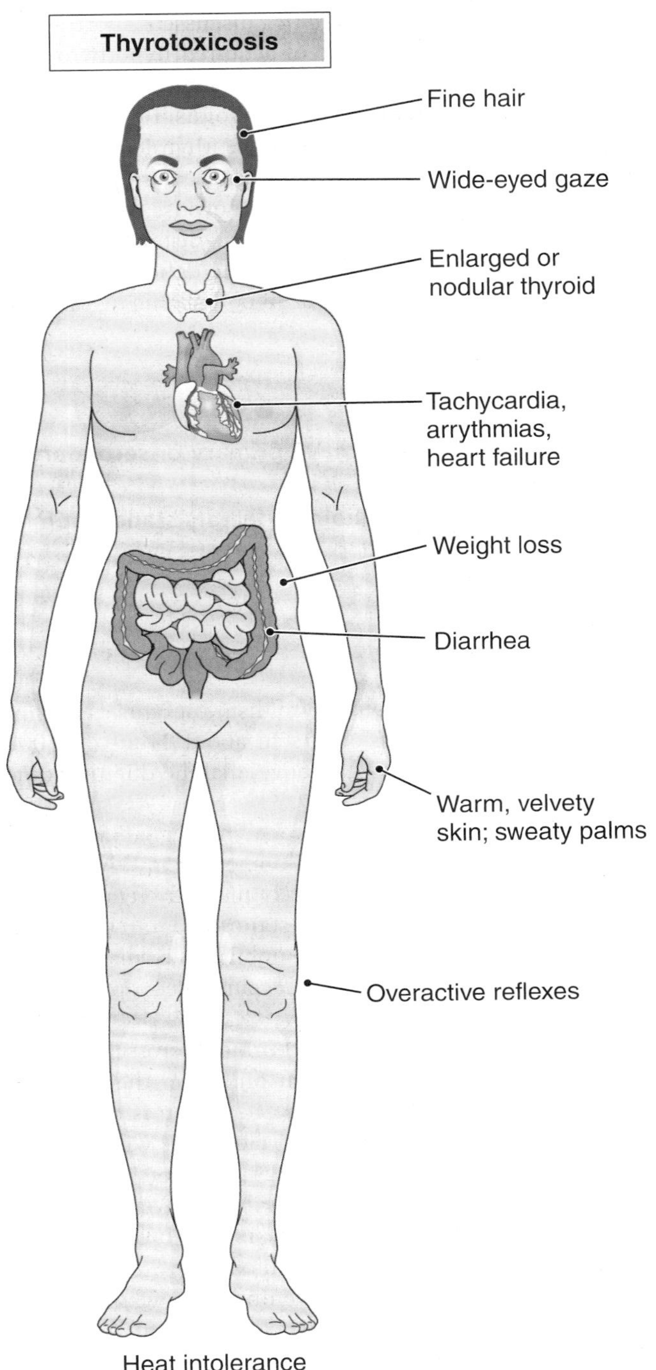

Figure 14.11 **Clinical features of thyrotoxicosis.**

Once the diagnosis of thyrotoxicosis has been established, it is useful to perform a **radioactive iodine (RAI) uptake** examination. In normal patients, the gland uses about 10–30% of the injected dose as it synthesizes hormone. Additionally, the gland can be scanned (**RAI scan**) by a camera to create an image of the distribution of the uptake in the gland. In normal patients, the uptake will be 10–30% and spread uniformly throughout the gland. In patients with hyperthyroidism, the uptake will be high and the uptake uniform. Conversely, in hypothyroidism the uptake is low. Diffuse uptake means that diffuse glandular hyperplasia is present. If a functioning thyroid adenoma is present (**toxic adenoma**), the radiation will accumulate in a single "hot spot." Low RAI uptake in a thyrotoxic patient suggests that *thyroiditis* is the cause of the thyrotoxicosis, and the gland is releasing *stored* thyroid hormone and is not rapidly synthesizing it.

Treatment varies according to the underlying cause. The most common is administration of therapeutic doses of RAI to patients with hyperthyroidism. The RAI is assimilated into T3/T4 stored in the gland. The gland is irradiated from within and shrinks; hormone output falls. An adverse effect of this therapy is that a significant number of patients later become hypothyroid because of inadvertent overradiation. Immediate clinical control can be gained by use of pharmacologic doses of iodine (non-radioactive) to block hormone release from the gland, but the effect fades in a few weeks. Antithyroid drugs are also used simultaneously for longer-term clinical control, because radiation therapy shrinks the thyroid slowly. Antithyroid drugs slow or stop synthesis of new hormone, interfere with peripheral tissue uptake of hormone, and are useful for long-term therapy. Beta-blockers are useful to counter the effects of sympathetic overactivity.

Surgical excision of all or part of the gland is indicated in patients with thyrotoxicosis that has recurred after medical treatment, and in other patients in whom medical therapy has been problematic or ineffective. Following surgery, patients usually require lifelong L-thyroxine therapy.

Case Notes

14.9 Azadeh did not have an RAI uptake test. If one had been performed, what would very likely have been the result?

Graves Disease Is the Most Common Cause of Hyperthyroidism

Graves disease is an autoimmune disease caused by the production of multiple antithyroid antibodies, the most important of which is *thyroid-stimulating immunoglobulin (TSI)*, an autoantibody that binds to the TSH receptor and mimics the effect of TSH. Graves occurs most often between ages 20 and 40. Women are affected about 10 times more often than men. Many patients will have other autoimmune disease, such as systemic lupus erythematosus (SLE). About 1–2% of women in the United States are affected. Genetic factors are important in Graves disease—the concordance rate in identical twins is 30–40%, but is <5% among nonidentical twins.

The clinical findings in Graves disease include those of thyrotoxicosis as well as the following unique signs:

- *Hyperthyroid goiter* due to diffuse thyroid hyperplasia (see Fig. 14.10B) is present in all cases.
- *Pretibial infiltrative dermopathy,* a distinctive pretibial infiltrative skin disease, is found in some patients characterized by nonpitting infiltration of proteinaceous material and which presents as scaly thickening and poorly defined, seminodular areas of induration.
- *Ophthalmopathy*, which may persist or progress despite successful treatment of thyrotoxicosis, appears to have an autoimmune origin. The lids retract as in other forms of thyrotoxicosis, but in Graves disease the globe is pushed forward, a condition called **exophthalmos**, by an accumulation of material in the orbit behind the globe. The material includes inflammatory cells, mainly T lymphocytes; edema and swelling of extraocular muscles; accumulation of extracellular matrix fluid; and increased numbers of fat cells. Lid retraction and global bulge can combine to prevent lid closure, which may result in corneal drying, inflammation, and ulceration.

Laboratory findings include increased T4 and T3 levels and low TSH. The TSI autoantibody is detectable in most patients. RAI uptake is increased, and radioiodine scans show a diffuse uptake consistent with diffuse glandular hyperplasia.

Diagnosis is clinical with laboratory confirmation. Treatment is for thyrotoxicosis as outlined above.

Hypothyroidism Is Thyroid Hormone Under-Production by the Thyroid Gland

Hypothyroidism is underproduction of thyroid hormones by the thyroid gland. It is much more common than hyperthyroidism. About 0.5% of the U.S. population is clinically affected and another 3–4% have subclinical disease. Women are affected 10 times more often than men. Prevalence increases with age.

Hypothyroidism may result from dysfunction at any point in the hypothalamic-pituitary-thyroid axis. As with hyperthyroidism, *secondary hypothyroidism* is due to pituitary or hypothalamic disease and *primary hypothyroidism* is attributable to intrinsic abnormalities of the gland. The great majority of cases are primary hypothyroidism, which can be congenital, acquired, or autoimmune.

Congenital hypothyroidism is most often due to dietary iodine deficiency, especially in developing nations; in developed nations, most table salt contains added iodine. Iodine is necessary for synthesis of T3 and T4. Much less commonly, congenital hypothyroidism is due to genetic defects that interrupt the metabolic chain of events in thyroid hormone synthesis.

Acquired hypothyroidism is disease due to nongenetic or congenital conditions. *Autoimmune hypothyroidism* is the most common form. By far, the most common variety is *Hashimoto thyroiditis*, discussed shortly. The second most common cause of acquired hypothyroidism is iatrogenic—due to surgical or radiologic ablation of the gland in the treatment of hyperthyroidism or neoplasm. A few cases can be attributed to antithyroid medication used in treatment of hyperthyroidism, or as a side effect of a drug administered for another purpose, for example, lithium in the treatment of psychiatric disorders.

Secondary hypothyroidism is due to deficiency of TSH, either as a result of pituitary or hypothalamic disease.

Case Notes

14.10 Does Azadeh have primary or secondary hypothyroidism?

14.11 What epidemiologic factors stand out in Azadeh's case?

Cretinism

In infants or children, hypothyroidism presents as **cretinism**. Congenital disease occurs in about 1 out of 4,000 live births and, as discussed above, may be due to iodine deficiency or genetic defects.

If iodine deficiency occurs early in pregnancy, infants may present with impaired development of multiple organ systems. These infants are severely mentally retarded and have spasticity, deafness, short stature, coarse facial features, protruding tongue, and umbilical hernia. On the other hand, if iodine deficiency occurs late in pregnancy, the newborn may initially show few signs or symptoms because some maternal thyroid hormone crosses the placenta. Symptoms begin to appear only after the maternal supply has been exhausted. If the condition is not recognized and treated, neurologic development will be slow, physiologic jaundice (Chapter 22) will persist, feeding will be poor, and the features described above will gradually appear. Signs and symptoms in older children are similar to those described below in adult myxedema.

Diagnosis is by routine screening of newborn blood for T4 (low) and TSH (high) before clinical signs and symptoms occur. The thyroid gland is not enlarged or in genetic cases it may be absent or only partially formed. The best treatment is prevention by assuring adequate dietary iodine for pregnant women. Treatment of the affected child is lifetime thyroid hormone replacement using L-thyroxine. Severe congenital hypothyroidism, even when promptly treated, is reversible only to a certain degree and may be associated with developmental problems and sensorineural hearing loss (Chapter 20).

Myxedema

Myxedema is hypothyroidism that develops in an older child or an adult. Figure 14.12 illustrates its clinical

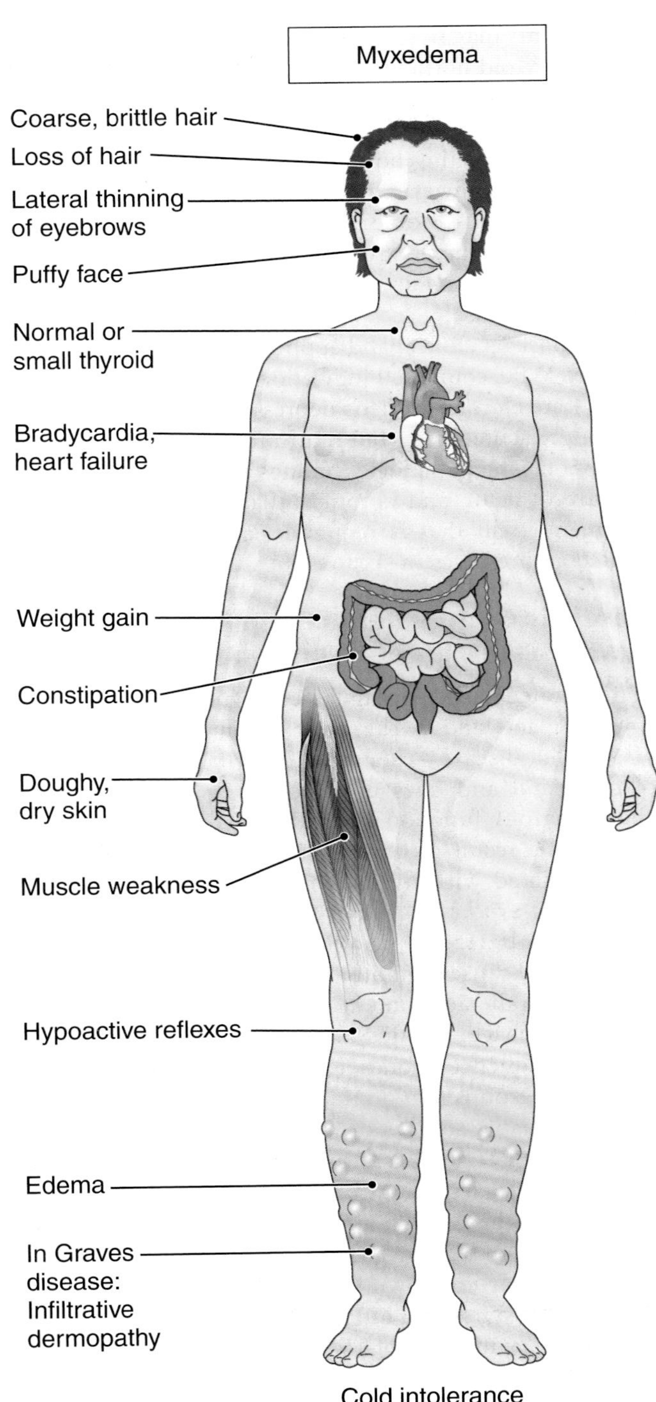

Figure 14.12 **Clinical features of myxedema.**

features. The thyroid is usually not enlarged. The clinical syndrome gains its name from accumulations of thick (myxomatous) fluid in various organs. Accumulations of this fluid produce bags under the eyes, puffy eyelids, swollen tongue, edema of the vocal cords and hoarseness, swelling of the hands and feet, pleural and pericardial effusions, and weight gain. The skin is cool and pale. Hair loss is common, especially the lateral half of the eyebrows. Patients develop mental dullness that may be misinterpreted as depression. Everything slows down: patients are weak and walk with a slow shuffle, their reflexes are slow, they are intolerant of cold, their heart rate is slow, and they are constipated.

Blood TSH is increased and is a sensitive screening test. Blood T3 and T4 are decreased. RAI uptake is low. LDL and total blood cholesterol rise, contributing to the increased cardiovascular mortality associated with hypothyroidism.

Diagnosis is clinical with laboratory confirmation. Treatment is hormone replacement using L-thyroxine.

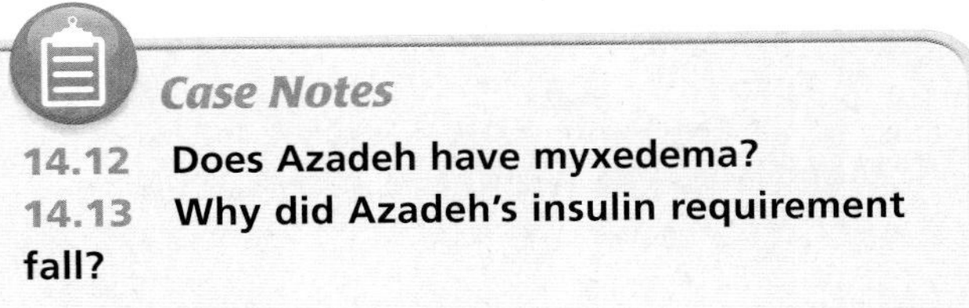

Case Notes

14.12 **Does Azadeh have myxedema?**

14.13 **Why did Azadeh's insulin requirement fall?**

Thyroiditis Is Inflammation of the Thyroid Gland

Thyroiditis is inflammation of the thyroid gland. There are several types, all uncommon and occurring mainly in women. They feature varying degrees of inflammation, scarring, and goiter. Most thyroiditis is chronic thyroiditis caused by thyroid autoimmunity. It usually presents as a painless goiter that is not associated with thyroid function abnormalities. Nevertheless, some patients may be hypothyroid if there is destruction of thyroid tissue. Alternatively, early in the disease, patients may have a brief period of gland tenderness and slight hyperthyroidism caused by inflammatory disruption of follicles with release of stored T3/T4. While the thyroid gland of most patients with thyroiditis functions normally, the cause of most hypothyroidism is thyroiditis.

Hashimoto Thyroiditis

Hashimoto thyroiditis, a chronic autoimmune disease, is by far the most common type of thyroiditis, hypothyroidism, and goiter in the United States. In the United States, the annual incidence of new cases is about 2 per 1,000, the majority of whom are women. It usually occurs as a nontoxic goiter and almost exclusively in middle-aged women (90% of cases). Antithyroid antibodies and cytotoxic T cells destroy thyroid epithelial cells. It has a distinct familial tendency—half of first-degree relatives have antithyroid antibodies in their blood and many have some other type of autoimmune disease, such as SLE. As illustrated in Figure 14.13, the gland is enlarged and overrun by masses of lymphocytes.

Hashimoto thyroiditis is usually associated with mild hypothyroidism, so mild that it may not be readily apparent. When disease first occurs, the gland may be slightly tender and the patient may be slightly thyrotoxic from

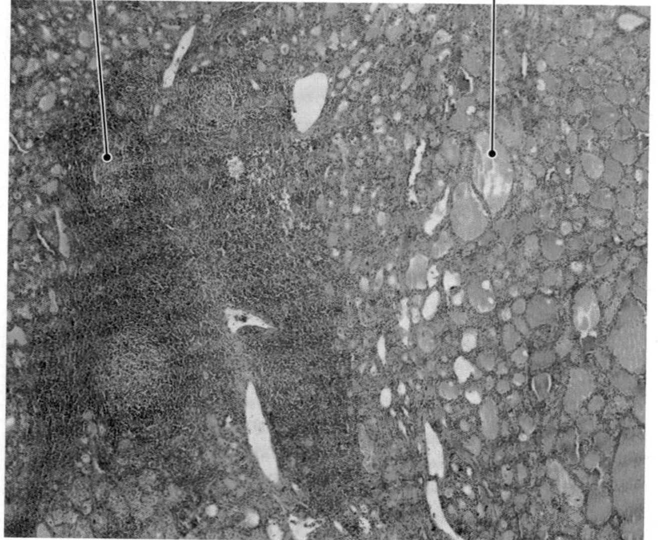

Figure 14.13 **Hashimoto thyroiditis.** Normal thyroid follicles and a collection of lymphocytes involved in the autoimmune reaction.

release of stored thyroid hormones. As disease progresses, T3 and T4 levels decline, TSH rises and thyroid autoantibodies appear in blood. Patients with Hashimoto are at risk for development of non-Hodgkin lymphoma (Chapter 7).

Diagnosis is clinical with laboratory confirmation of hypothyroidism and detection of thyroid autoantibodies. Treatment is lifetime hormone replacement therapy with L-thyroxine.

Case Notes

14.14 No biopsy was done, but is it likely that Azadeh's hypothyroidism is due to Hashimoto thyroiditis?

Subacute Granulomatous Thyroiditis

Subacute granulomatous thyroiditis (*de Quervain thyroiditis*) is much less common than Hashimoto disease. Like other forms of thyroiditis, it occurs much more commonly in women than men. The cause is unknown, but a virus is suspected—many patients have a history of recent upper respiratory infection, and some clusters of cases have been traced to measles, mumps, and other viruses.

Recall that the thyroid holds a large reserve of hormone. In subacute granulomatous thyroiditis, much of this reserve is released by the inflammatory process, such that patients may become thyrotoxic for a short period of time as thyroid hormones are washed out of the inflamed gland. Patients may then become hypothyroid for a short period of time as they replenish thyroid stores at the expense of liberating hormone into the circulation. Over the long term, however, thyroid gland anatomy and function usually return to normal. The clinical picture is one of sudden development of a painful, tender enlargement of the thyroid gland accompanied by painful swallowing, fever, and malaise.

Diagnosis is clinical and supported by laboratory data: elevated WBC count and indications of thyrotoxicosis. T3 and T4 are elevated, TSH is depressed, and RAI uptake is low in the acute phase, but return to normal with clinical resolution. The pathologic findings in the gland feature a mixture of acute and chronic inflammation. Supportive treatment is all that is required. The condition is self-limited and resolves in six to eight weeks.

Nontoxic Goiters Reflect Impaired Synthesis of Thyroid Hormone

As illustrated earlier in Figure 14.9, *goiter* is an enlarged thyroid gland and is the most common manifestation of thyroid disease—the term describes only the size of the gland and does not necessarily imply anything about thyroid function or pathology. Although goiter may be the result of hyperthyroidism, most goiters are not associated with hyperthyroidism—*they are a result of impaired synthesis of thyroid hormone* and are called **nontoxic goiters**.

The usual cause of nontoxic goiter is iodine deficiency, though high dietary content of certain staple foods (e.g., cassava, cabbage, turnips) impairs hormone synthesis. As a consequence, nontoxic goiter tends to occur in population groups that do not have access to iodized salt or other reliable sources of iodine, and those that favor these foodstuffs. Such cases are referred to as *endemic goiter*. Nevertheless, nontoxic goiter can appear in any population—these cases are termed *sporadic goiter* and usually occur in teenage girls or young adult women. The cause is usually unknown.

Impaired synthesis of thyroid hormone results in compensatory increase of TSH, which in turn stimulates hyperplasia of the glandular epithelium and enlargement of thyroid follicles in a homeostatic attempt to increase hormone production. The net result is that the gland may or may not be able to maintain normal blood hormone levels and the patient may or may not show evidence of clinical hypothyroidism (myxedema). In any case, the gland enlarges to a greater or lesser degree depending upon the severity of hormone deficiency—the size of the goiter is proportional to the degree of deficiency.

The early development of nontoxic goiter features uniform enlargement of the follicles and gland. The follicles

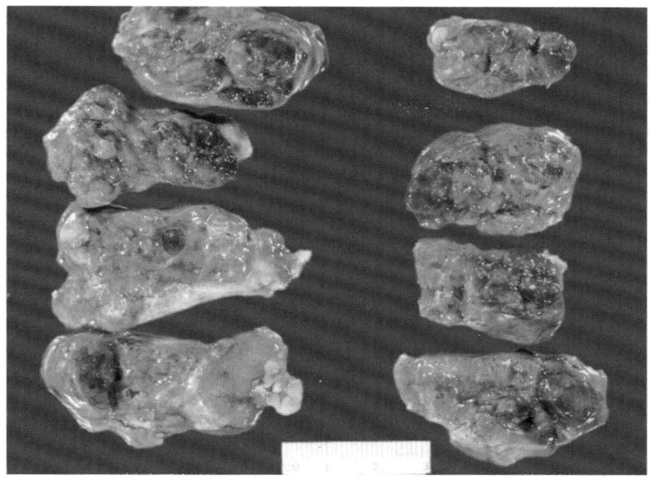

Figure 14.14 **Multinodular goiter.** Cross sections of surgically removed thyroid reveal an irregular, nodular gland.

are filled with colloid and the cut surface of the gland is smooth. These early nontoxic goiters, referred to as **colloid goiters** or **diffuse nontoxic goiters**, account for the largest goiters. Most patients are euthyroid because the increasing mass of the gland compensates for impaired hormone synthesis. Blood T3 and T4 levels tend to be in the lower range of normal and TSH near the upper end of normal.

Unless diagnosed and treated, however, with time and recurrent episodes of glandular hyperplasia and involution, diffuse goiters inevitably evolve into an irregular, lumpy form called **multinodular goiter** (Fig. 14.14). Because of their nodular nature, they are frequently suspected of being malignant. Their epidemiologic characteristics are similar to the diffuse goiters from which they arise.

The nodular nature of these goiters is believed to be due to differing local follicular responses to TSH stimulation. Some follicles appear to gain autonomy and synthesize hormone independent of TSH stimulation, while others produce little or no hormone. As a consequence, thyroid hormone output by the gland may be normal or high.

Most goiters come to attention because of mass effect—a visible mass in the lower neck, difficulty swallowing, airway narrowing, or hoarseness from pressure on laryngeal nerves. Some may obstruct blood flow of major veins in the neck.

Most patients are euthyroid, but some may have subclinical hyperthyroidism identifiable only by increased TSH. Because of the variable activity of different nodules, RAI scans may reveal one or more "hot spots," which are difficult to distinguish clinically from functional follicular neoplasms. Needle biopsy is helpful in differential diagnosis of these nodules.

Case Notes

14.15 Does Azadeh have a toxic or nontoxic goiter?

Pop Quiz

14.11 True or false? Thyrotoxicosis is one cause of hyperthyroidism.

14.12 True or false? Thyroiditis always presents with elevated levels of TSH and low levels of T3 and T4.

14.13 True or false? Graves disease is an autoimmune disease caused by thyroid-stimulating immunoglobulin, which mimics the effect of TSH on thyroid receptors.

14.14 What is the most common cause of cretinism in developing nations?

Neoplasms of the Thyroid are Common and Usually Not Aggressive

Thyroid masses are common: reported prevalence in the United States is between 1% and 10% and increases with age. About 90% of masses are non-neoplastic nodules in a nodular goiter. Of the 10% that are neoplastic, fewer than 1 in 10 is malignant. Said in other terms, <1% of thyroid masses prove to be malignant. Nevertheless, about 35,000 new cases of thyroid cancer occur each year in the United States. Fortunately, the 20-year survival rate for thyroid cancer patients is near 90%. Although these figures indicate that thyroid neoplasms are indolent and are an uncommon cause of death, a few are aggressive and all thyroid masses must be investigated. Some important points are the following:

- Solitary masses are more likely to be neoplastic than multiple ones.
- Masses that are "cold"—that do not take up RAI because they are not synthesizing thyroid hormone—are more likely to be neoplastic than are "hot" ones.
- Masses in younger patients are more likely to be neoplastic than are those in older patients.
- Masses in males are more likely to be neoplastic than are those in females.
- A history of head/neck radiation increases the likelihood that a mass is neoplastic.
- Most masses prove to be non-neoplastic lumps of nodular goiter.

Other than a few cases of genetically related thyroid carcinoma, there are no known risk factors other than radiation (see the *History of Medicine*, "Thyroid Cancer and Ionizing Radiation").

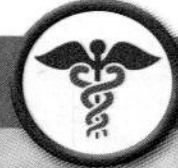

The History of Medicine

THYROID CANCER AND IONIZING RADIATION

Historically, ionizing radiation has been an important cause of thyroid cancer. In the mid-20th century, ionizing radiation was widely used to shrink enlarged tonsils and adenoids in children, and to treat acne, skin problems of the face, tuberculosis (TB) in the neck, fungus diseases of the scalp, blood vessel tumors of the face, enlarged thymus, sore throats, chronic coughs, and even excessive facial hair, and the patient's thyroid gland was not shielded during the treatment. A significant increase of thyroid cancer occurred in these patients some decades later. Moreover, the atomic bomb blasts in Hiroshima and Nagasaki (1945) and the Chernobyl nuclear plant disaster (1986) in Ukraine, which was at the time part of the Soviet Union, increased the incidence of thyroid cancer because of the direct radiation exposure and because of the subsequent increased amounts of RAI in food.

Thyroid Adenomas

Thyroid **follicular adenomas** are benign neoplasms of the epithelial cells that line thyroid follicles. They are almost always solitary, round, and discrete, and are composed of thyroid epithelium formed into follicles. Adenomas most often reveal themselves as a solitary, painless mass in an otherwise healthy woman with no evidence of thyroid hormone excess or thyroid failure. Almost all are nonfunctional. Adenomas are unlikely ever to become malignant.

Diagnosis typically begins with an RAI scan, which reveals the mass to be a cold nodule. Nevertheless, there are other causes of cold nodules, some of them malignant, so a solitary cold nodule cannot be assumed to be an adenoma. About 10% prove to be a malignancy, not an adenoma. Usually, fine-needle aspiration cytology (using a very small needle) is performed to determine if the patient is at high risk or low risk for a follicular neoplasm (i.e., adenoma or carcinoma). Needle biopsy to obtain a larger specimen is often not helpful because the microscopic appearance of adenoma and follicular carcinoma (discussed next) is very similar. A definitive diagnosis of adenoma or carcinoma is possible only by examination of the entire nodule and surrounding thyroid from a surgically resected gland. Treatment is surgical excision.

Thyroid Carcinomas

Almost all carcinomas of the thyroid gland arise from the epithelium that lines the thyroid follicles. Most are well differentiated and unlikely to cause death. Most occur in adults; females are more affected than males except in the very young or very old. The major subtypes of thyroid carcinoma are the following:

- Papillary carcinoma (~85%)
- Follicular carcinoma (~10%)
- Anaplastic carcinoma (<5%)
- Medullary carcinoma (~5%)

Papillary Carcinoma

Papillary carcinomas are the most common of thyroid carcinomas, generally occurring between ages 25 and 50. Females are affected much more often than males. Papillary carcinomas usually present as a solitary thyroid nodule that is cold by RAI scan. Sometimes they come to attention because of an enlarged cervical lymph node that contains metastatic carcinoma. Diagnosis is by microscopic study of needle biopsy or surgical specimen as mentioned above. They feature a papillary (cauliflower-like) microscopic growth pattern composed of cells with abnormal grooved nuclei that resemble coffee beans. Treatment is surgical resection, which is usually curative. Small lesions may warrant lobectomy, but larger lesions require complete thyroidectomy. They grow very slowly, and >95% of patients survive 10 years. Local invasion of nearby neck structures or distant metastases carries a poorer prognosis.

Follicular Carcinoma

Follicular carcinomas are malignant neoplasms of follicular epithelium arranged into follicles. They usually present in an older age group (compared to papillary carcinomas) as a solitary nodule that is cold by RAI scan. They account for about 10% of thyroid cancers.

Diagnosis is by pathologic examination of needle biopsy or surgically resected tissue. For the most highly differentiated tumors, it may be difficult microscopically to distinguish follicular carcinoma from follicular adenoma. Papillary growth and characteristic grooved nuclei are not present. Treatment is thyroidectomy. Most patients are offered treatment with RAI with reasoning that metastatic tumor may incorporate the element and ablate. Additionally, on the chance that a metastatic tumor may respond to pituitary output of TSH, many patients are treated with L-thyroxine to suppress TSH secretion.

When compared to papillary carcinomas, follicular carcinomas are more aggressive because they tend to invade blood vessels and metastasize widely. In contrast, papillary carcinomas preferentially spread to lymph nodes, which initially confine the tumor locally and offer hope of resection for cure. *Minimally invasive follicular carcinomas* are only marginally more dangerous than papillary carcinomas, however. Ten-year survival is 90%. Widely invasive or metastatic tumors are associated with much poorer prognosis: about 50% of patients die of their disease in 10 years.

Anaplastic Carcinoma

Anaplastic carcinoma is a highly aggressive, almost uniformly fatal malignancy of follicular epithelium that accounts for <5% of thyroid malignancies. Most present as a rapidly enlarging neck mass in patients over 65, by which time most have invaded into nearby neck structures or metastasized to the lungs. Diagnosis is by biopsy. Most therapies are palliative.

Medullary Carcinoma

Medullary carcinomas account for about 5% of thyroid cancers and arise from the specialized parafollicular epithelial cells of the thyroid, which secrete calcitonin. Most arise spontaneously, but about a third occur as a feature of one of the *multiple endocrine neoplasia syndromes (MEN)*, which are discussed later in this chapter and are a family of genetic defects associated with tumors of various endocrine organs. Medullary carcinomas usually present as a neck mass or other local effect such as coughing or hoarseness. Despite the fact that they secrete calcitonin, calcium metabolism is unaffected. A few tumors will secrete ACTH (causing Cushing syndrome) or vasoactive peptides (flushing and diarrhea) as a paraneoplastic syndrome (Chapter 5). Medullary carcinoma is a microscopically distinctive and clinically aggressive tumor that tends to metastasize via the bloodstream. The five-year survival rate is about 50%. Treatment is thyroidectomy.

Pop Quiz

14.15 True or false? The 20-year survival rate for thyroid cancer patients is near 90%.

14.16 Which thyroid carcinoma has the poorest prognosis?

Disorders of the Adrenal Cortex

Disorders of the adrenal cortex are far more common and more clinically significant than disease of the adrenal medulla. (The medulla is discussed separately below.) The importance of adrenocortical disease owes to the powerful metabolic role of adrenocortical steroid hormones, an excess or deficit of which creates serious medical conditions.

Adrenocortical Hyperfunction Features Excess Cortical Hormones

Adrenocortical hyperfunction features excess cortical hormone from any source. Just as there are three varieties of corticosteroids—glucocorticoids (mainly cortisol), mineralocorticoids (mainly aldosterone), and sex steroids (estrogens and androgens)—there are three varieties of hyperadrenocorticalism, a term that applies to excess cortical hormone from any source, endogenous or exogenous:

1. *Cushing syndrome* is created by an excess of glucocorticoid, mainly cortisol.
2. *Primary hyperaldosteronism* is a syndrome of excess aldosterone.
3. *Adrenogenital syndromes* are created by an excess of androgens.

Cushing Syndrome

Cushing syndrome is a constellation of clinical signs and symptoms that result from an excessive amount of blood glucocorticoid, usually cortisol. When caused by an ACTH-secreting adenoma, it is referred to as **Cushing disease**, after Harvey Cushing, the pioneering Canadian neurosurgeon who first described the effects of ACTH-secreting pituitary adenoma.

Cushing syndrome can have many etiologies. Cushing syndrome can be *exogenous* (from glucocorticoid therapy), or *endogenous*. There are two broad categories of *endogenous* Cushing syndrome (Fig. 14.15): *ACTH-dependent* and *ACTH-independent* (% = relative frequency):

1. In ACTH-dependent Cushing syndrome (blood ACTH is high and the cortex is thickened and nodular). There are three subtypes:
   - *Anterior pituitary ACTH adenoma* (70%).
   - *Neoplasm of nonpituitary organ* that secretes ACTH (10%): The most common cause is small cell carcinoma of the lung. Middle-aged men are most often affected. The characteristic laboratory profile is high blood ACTH and glucocorticoids.
   - *Anterior pituitary corticotroph cell hyperplasia* is rare (<1%).
2. ACTH-independent (blood ACTH is low):
   - *Adrenocortical adenoma* (10%) usually occur as a single nodule in one adrenal gland (Fig. 14.16).
   - *Adrenocortical carcinoma* (5%).
   - *Adrenocortical hyperplasia* (5%): Usually due to the pathologic response of the adrenal cortex to ACTH stimulation, it occurs rarely as primary, autonomous hyperplasia causing ACTH-independent Cushing. The cortex is thick and markedly nodular.

Nevertheless, *the most common cause of Cushing syndrome in clinical practice is exogenous—glucocorticoid medical therapy*. Exogenous glucocorticoids suppress pituitary production of ACTH and the cortex becomes thin and atrophic. Because of this atrophy, patients on long-term

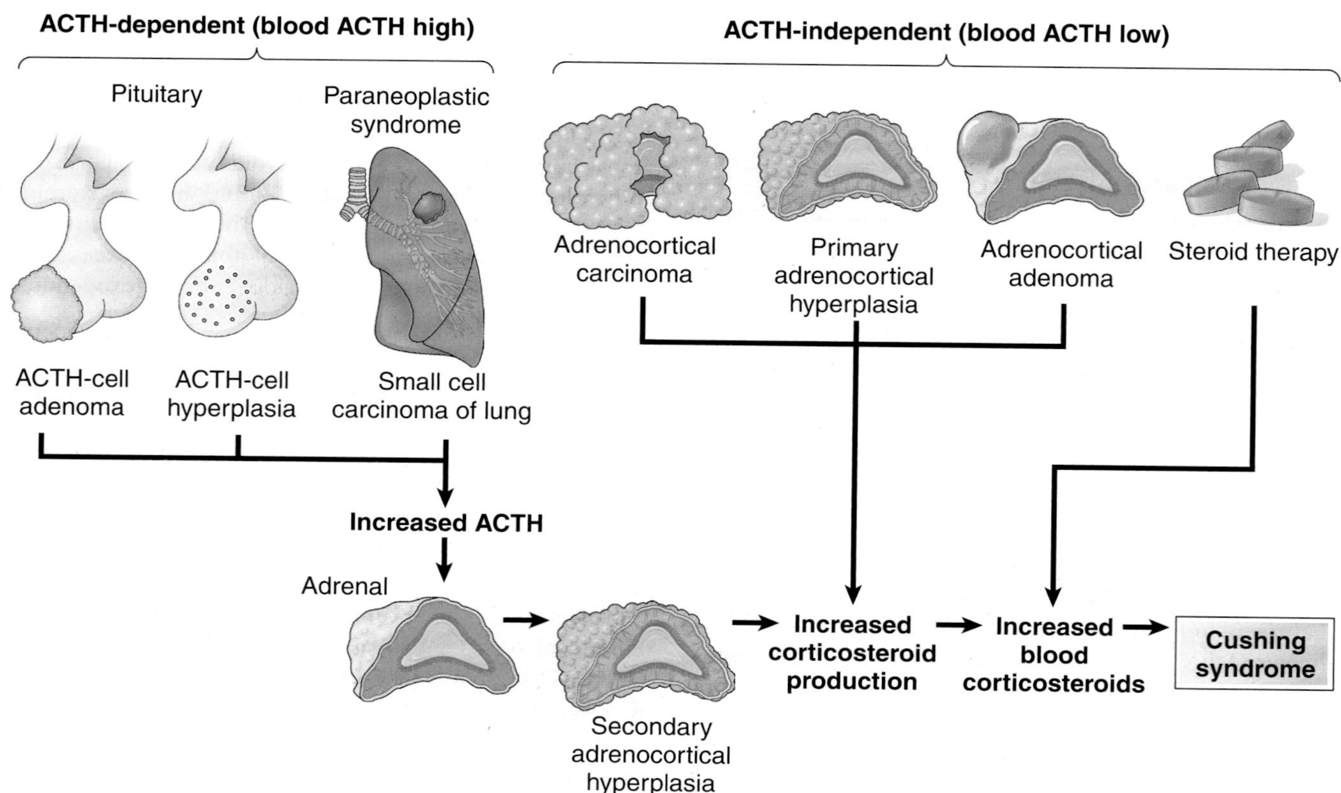

Figure 14.15 **Pathogenesis of Cushing syndrome.**

steroid therapy must be weaned off of the drug slowly to give the cortex time to recover.

Signs and Symptoms

Figure 14.17 illustrates the clinical findings in Cushing syndrome, most of which owe to the effect of cortisol, with lesser effects from other corticosteroids. It features hypertension, obesity, round (moon) facial features, diabetes, skin marks (striae), excess body and facial hair (hirsutism), and menstrual and mental abnormalities. Fluid retention promotes expanded blood volume and hypertension and weight gain, both of which often develop first and may not be recognized as pathologic until additional features occur. Truncal obesity appears, an accumulation of fat collects below the back of the neck ("buffalo hump," Fig.14.18A), and a rounded "moon facies" develops (Fig. 14.18B). The catabolic effect of corticosteroids causes skin and muscle changes. Muscle atrophy and limbs become thin and weak. The skin becomes thin and friable: it is easily bruised, and reddish-blue or brownish striae develop on the abdomen, hips, and breasts. Bones lose substance and become liable to fracture as osteoporosis develops. Secondary Type II diabetes occurs as cortisol decreases tissue sensitivity to insulin. Hyperglycemia, glycosuria, and polydipsia are the result. Increased levels of androgenic steroids cause acne and excessive hair growth, especially facial hair in women. Menstrual abnormalities and mental problems also may occur. Infections are common because cortisol suppresses immunity and the inflammatory response. Mental effects include emotional instability, depression, or outright psychosis.

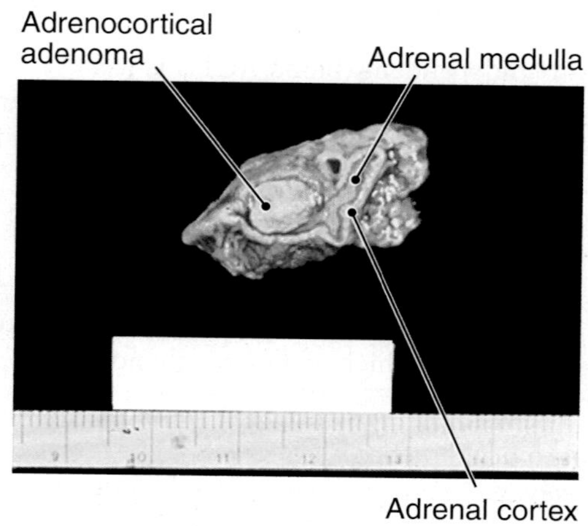

Figure 14.16 **Adrenocortical adenoma.**

Remember This! Most of the signs and symptoms of Cushing syndrome owe to the effect of excess cortisol.

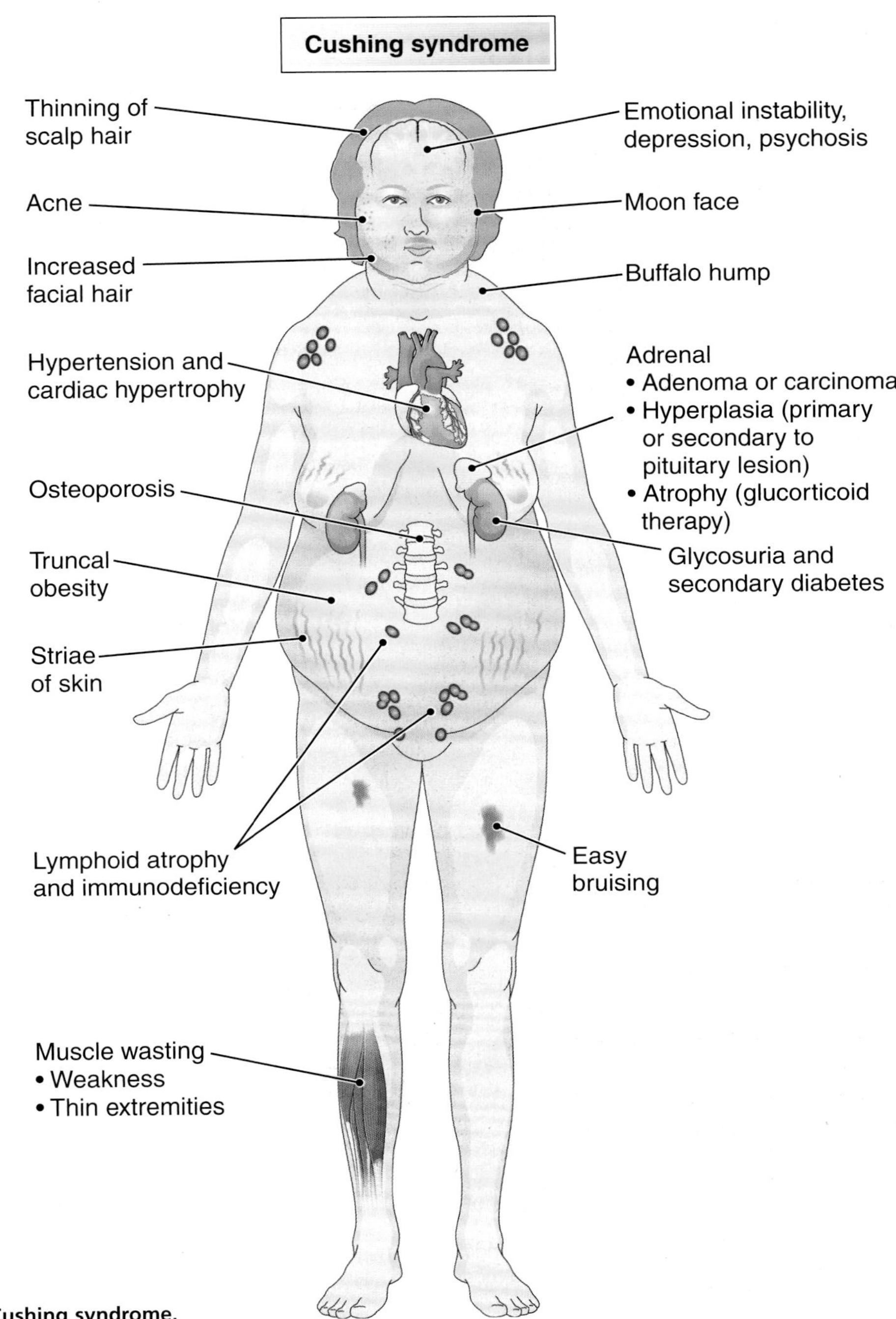

Figure 14.17 **Clinical manifestations of Cushing syndrome.**

Diagnosis and Treatment

When florid clinical signs are present, Cushing syndrome is an easy clinical diagnosis. Nevertheless, the picture is not so clear in an obese female with acne, "stretch marks," and hypertension—each of which could be of independent origin.

The laboratory is an indispensable aid in confirming clinical suspicion. The first step in diagnosing Cushing syndrome is to confirm clinical suspicion by measuring *24-hour urinary cortisol excretion*. Ninety-five percent of patients with Cushing syndrome have increased levels of urinary cortisol. Measurement of blood ACTH and cortisol is also critical. Levels of each vary according to the etiology involved.

Normal blood cortisol levels vary diurnally, peaking at 8:00 A.M. and falling to a low point at 4:00 P.M. Patients with Cushing syndrome have high blood cortisol levels, which do not vary diurnally. Nevertheless, blood cortisol levels in Cushing patients may vary erratically, making interpretation of results difficult.

Buffalo hump fat

A

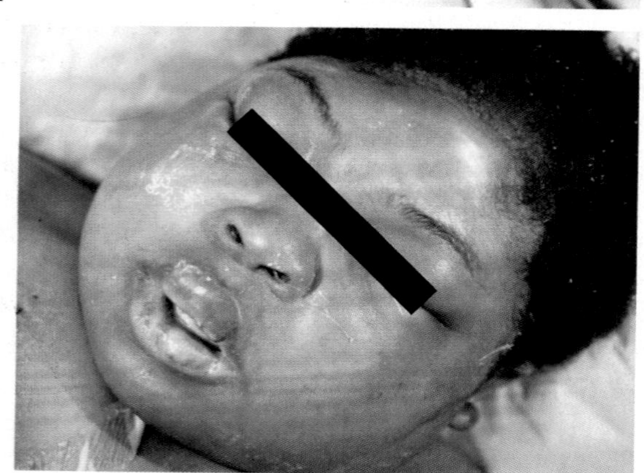

B

Figure 14.18 **Cushing syndrome. A.** Cushingoid obesity, including "buffalo hump" of dorsal fat. **B.** Cushingoid moon facies.

Of additional diagnostic importance is the **dexamethasone suppression test**. In a normal person, oral dexamethasone is a potent synthetic steroid that suppresses ACTH production by the pituitary and, therefore, cortisol production by the adrenal gland. Data is collected by measurement of blood ACTH and cortisol and 24-hour urine cortisol. Results fall into three broad categories:

1. In patients with pituitary Cushing syndrome (the most common endogenous variety), ACTH secretion and cortisol production cannot be suppressed by administration of low doses of dexamethasone. Nevertheless, high doses of dexamethasone will suppress pituitary output of ACTH and adrenal cortisol output. The dexamethasone suppression test exploits this fact for diagnostic purposes.
2. In patients with ACTH production by a nonpituitary tumor such as a lung cancer, even high doses of dexamethasone will not suppress ACTH output or cortisol secretion by the adrenals.
3. In patients with an adrenal tumor that is producing cortisol, blood ACTH levels are low, having been suppressed by tumor secretion of glucocorticoids. Tumor output of hormone cannot be suppressed by either low or high doses of dexamethasone.

Meticulous attention to test details is essential. Care should be exercised when interpreting the results, which can be influenced by many factors other than endocrine disease (e.g., 24-hour urinary cortisol can be increased because of obesity).

Cushing disease is treated according to its cause. If the cause is medical therapy, the main concern is the underlying condition for which the cortisol is being administered. For endogenous Cushing, if the clinical symptoms are severe, the effect of cortisol can be temporarily blocked by certain drugs. Tumors are treated surgically or irradiated, depending on the patient's age and general health and the type and location of tumor. Prognosis is generally good.

Primary Hyperaldosteronism

Primary hyperaldosteronism is autonomous, chronic excessive aldosterone secretion by the adrenal cortex. *Secondary hyperaldosteronism* is due to activation of the *renin-angiotensin-aldosterone system* (Chapter 6) in the regulation of blood pressure.

Primary hyperaldosteronism suppresses the renin-angiotensin system and is associated with *hypertension* and *low plasma renin*. It arises in one of the following circumstances:

- *Bilateral adrenocortical hyperplasia*, pathogenesis unknown (~60% of cases).
- *Adrenocortical neoplasm*, usually a solitary adenoma (*Conn syndrome*, ~35%). Carcinoma is rare.
- *Genetic defect* (rare).

In contrast, secondary hyperaldosteronism is associated with *increased plasma renin*. The unifying condition is low renal arterial pressure, which may be due to local or general circumstances. It is caused by conditions such as

- decreased renal blood flow and low renal pressure due to renal artery stenosis;
- arterial hypovolemia with low to normal systemic blood pressure and edema, as in heart failure, in which case renal pressure is but one aspect of systemic dysfunction.

Signs and Symptoms

The cardinal sign of primary hyperaldosteronism is hypertension. From 5% to 10% of all hypertensive patients have primary hyperaldosteronism. The prevalence rises to near 20% among patients whose hypertension cannot be controlled by medication.

The action of aldosterone on the renal tubule is to promote sodium reabsorption from tubular fluid into blood and potassium excretion from blood into tubular fluid. Retained sodium attracts water, expands blood volume, increases cardiac output, and raises blood pressure. Most, but not all, patients have low blood potassium, which can cause muscle weakness, paralysis or tetany; visual disturbances; or paresthesias.

Diagnosis and Treatment

Diagnosis of primary hyperaldosteronism requires that the patient be hypertensive. Workup includes exclusion of renal artery stenosis and other causes of secondary hyperaldosteronism. Laboratory determination of blood aldosterone, renin, sodium, and potassium are essential. A complex assortment of physiologic challenge tests is available to evaluate whether or not aldosterone production can be stimulated or suppressed by a variety of means. A requirement for the diagnosis of primary hyperaldosteronism is that aldosterone production cannot be suppressed by drug challenge.

Treatment varies according to cause. In secondary hyperaldosteronism, treatment aims at eliminating the underlying cause of activation of the renin-aldosterone mechanism. Surgery is the preferred treatment for adenoma or carcinoma. For bilateral hyperplasia aldosterone, antagonist drugs are preferred therapy. Prognosis is generally good.

Adrenogenital Syndromes

Abnormal feminization or masculinization (virilization) can be caused by drug treatment with estrogens or androgens, gonadal disease (including defects of sex determination genes, Chapter 22), or adrenal disease. Virtually any syndrome of adrenocortical hormone excess can be associated with virilization, owing to the fact that the adrenal cortex secretes *dehydroepiandrosterone* and *androstenedione*, which can be converted by other tissues into testosterone.

Congenital adrenal hyperplasia (*adrenogenital syndrome*) is a congenital disorder of sexual differentiation that arises from one of several varieties of autosomal recessive genetic defects that cause *cortical enzyme deficiency*, *androgen excess*, and *congenital adrenal hyperplasia*. The cortex is usually very thick and nodular, much more so than in any other cause of adrenal cortical hyperplasia. **21 β-hydroxylase deficiency** is the most common genetic defect, accounting for 90% of adrenogenital syndromes, and is unique in that the enzyme acts in more than one point in the production of aldosterone and cortisol. Deficiencies of 21 β-hydroxylase or the other two less commonly affected enzymes (17 α-hydroxylase or 11 β-hydroxylase) may be partial or complete, resulting in varying degrees of hormone excess or deficit. These defects interrupt the chain of events that leads to production of corticosteroid hormones, especially cortisol from precursor compounds. Precursors accumulate and are diverted into other metabolic pathways that result in excess androgen production. Too, the lack of cortisol results in increased pituitary ACTH production, which causes adrenal hyperplasia and enhances the flow of diverted precursors to feed even more androgen production. Some of these enzyme deficiencies (including 21 β-hydroxylase) are associated with aldosterone deficiency and urinary loss of sodium (**salt wasting**).

Signs and Symptoms

Deficiency of 21 β-hydroxylase results in a mix of effects that include varying degrees of virilization, ambiguous genitalia, and salt wasting. Virilization may cause ambiguous genitalia (Fig. 14.19) in females, or early virilization in males or females, some cases of which may not become evident until late childhood. Males are usually diagnosed at an older age because of precocious puberty. Older females develop an enlarged clitoris, oligomenorrhea, hirsutism, and acne. The growth of both sexes can be stunted by premature closure of the epiphyseal growth plates in long bones.

Owing to the fact that maternal renal function masks the problem in utero, salt wasting does not become apparent until birth. It is more easily recognized in females due to ambiguous genitalia, but in males it may be difficult to recognize. The clinical findings are an infant with dehydration, low blood pressure, low blood levels of sodium, and high blood levels of potassium. It can be fatal if not diagnosed and treated promptly.

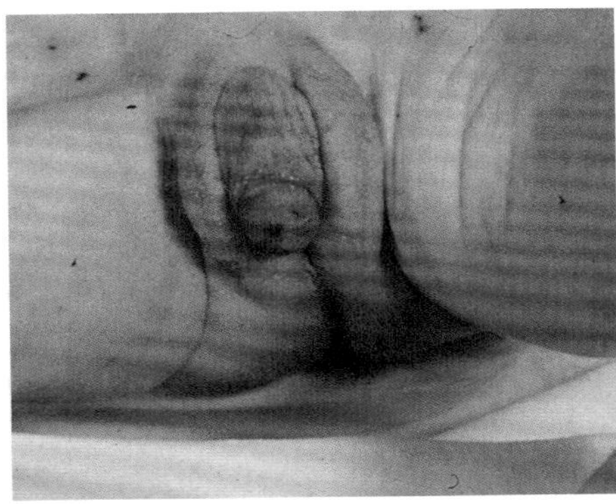

Figure 14.19 **Congenital adrenal hyperplasia (adrenogenital syndrome).** Ambiguous, masculinized (virilized) genitalia in a female infant. (Reproduced with permission from Rubin E. *Pathology*. 4th ed. Philadelphia (PA). Lippincott Williams and Wilkins; 2005.)

Diagnosis and Treatment

Diagnosis is heavily dependent on laboratory support for measurement of blood and urine hormones and is aided by routine neonatal screening for blood levels of certain steroid hormones. Genotyping may be required. Aldosterone replacement is required for salt wasting. Cortisol replacement is required to suppress virilization, but can be tricky because too much will cause Cushing syndrome, and too little will not suppress virilization. Surgical reconstruction is required for females.

Adrenocortical Failure Causes Cortisol Insufficiency

Adrenocortical insufficiency results in concurrent deficiency of all three corticosteroids, of which cortisol and aldosterone deficiency are clinically most important. Almost every cause of deficiency affects both glands equally. Primary failure may be acute or chronic; secondary failure is chronic and due to pituitary failure to secrete ACTH.

Acute Cortical Failure

Primary acute cortical failure occurs in three clinical settings and is invariably fatal without quick diagnosis and cortisol replacement.

- *Sudden withdrawal of corticosteroid therapy*. This is perhaps the most common cause of acute cortical failure. Corticosteroid therapy, usually for RA or other autoimmune disease, suppresses ACTH secretion by the pituitary gland. The result is atrophy of the adrenal cortex. Sudden withdrawal of steroid drugs leaves the patient without a replacement source for cortisol.
- *Bilateral acute hemorrhagic destruction of the adrenal glands (Waterhouse-Friderichsen syndrome)*. This syndrome is rare and rapidly fatal without prompt diagnosis and treatment by cortisol replacement and antibiotics. The classic cause is meningococcal septicemia associated with meningococcal meningitis (Chapter 4). Massive adrenal gland hemorrhage also may be associated with septicemia by other bacteria, pregnancy, disseminated intravascular coagulation, in patients on anticoagulant therapy, or in newborns as a result of birth stress or trauma.
- *Sudden worsening of chronic adrenal insufficiency*. This may occur when a patient with undiagnosed chronic adrenal insufficiency is suddenly stressed by development of an acute infection or has surgery, or it may occur in patients with known adrenal insufficiency who are on steroid therapy, if their dose is not increased during stressful illness.

Diagnosis is clinical. Treatment is cortisol replacement and management of the underlying condition.

Addison Disease

Primary chronic cortical failure is called **Addison disease**. It, too, is invariably fatal without cortisol replacement therapy. Almost all cases are attributable to one of four conditions: autoimmune adrenalitis, TB, AIDS, or metastatic carcinoma. Addison disease is rare.

Autoimmune adrenalitis (AIA) accounts for about 60–70% of Addison disease, especially in developed countries where TB and AIDS are less common than in developing nations. AIA is an acquired genetic defect that may occur in two forms. *Autoimmune polyendocrinopathy type 1 (APE1)* features Addison disease, ectodermal defects (various skin defects, oral and dental defects, and nail deformities), mucocutaneous candidiasis, and autoimmune attack on other endocrine organs, especially the parathyroids, gonads, and gastric mucosa. In the latter case, pernicious anemia (Chapter 7) may be a result. *APE2* features autoimmune attack on the pancreas, with Type I diabetes, and autoimmune thyroiditis.

Signs and Symptoms

Figure 14.20 summarizes the features of Addison disease. Onset is often insidious, but may be catastrophic if an unrecognized case is subject to stress, such as trauma or surgery. Often the first sign is weakness, easy fatigability, or syncope. Gastrointestinal complaints are common and include diarrhea, anorexia, vomiting, and weight loss. Hyperpigmentation of skin is common and tends to occur in sun-exposed skin, nipples, and genitals and over pressure points such as the neck, elbows, knuckles, and knees. The face, underarms, and groin are particularly affected (Fig. 14.21). Pigmentation owes to overproduction of pro-opiomelanocortin (POMC) in response to glucocorticoid deficiency; POMC is the precursor molecule from which both ACTH and melanocyte-stimulating hormone (MSH) are generated simultaneously. Lack of mineralocorticoid effect on the renal tubule causes potassium retention (hyperkalemia), and salt wasting (hyponatremia) with hypovolemia and hypotension. Hypoglycemia may result from failure of cortisol to stimulate glycogen conversion to glucose. Vascular collapse, shock, and death may occur without rapid diagnosis and cortisol replacement.

Diagnosis and Treatment

Diagnosis is clinical with laboratory and radiologic support. Autoimmune etiology is presumed in developed nations. A chest X-ray is useful to examine for possible TB. CT scan of the adrenals may also be useful. Blood electrolytes, cortisol, and ACTH determination are essential. Failure of a dose of ACTH to stimulate cortisol production is confirmatory.

Treatment is a lifetime of cortisol replacement. For otherwise healthy patients, the outlook is good.

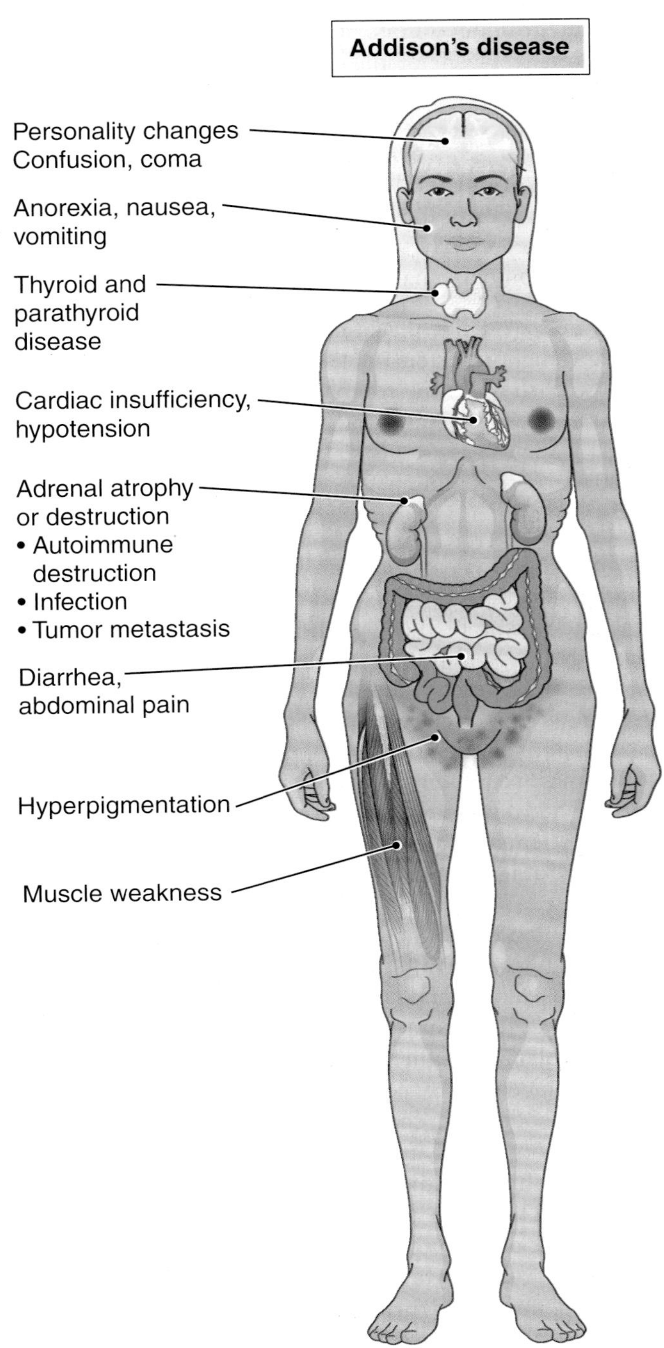

Figure 14.20 **Clinical manifestations of Addison disease.**

Remember This! Most of the danger of Addison disease is due to lack of cortisol.

Secondary Adrenocortical Insufficiency

Any disorder of the hypothalamus or anterior pituitary that reduces ACTH output—infection, infarction, hemorrhage, metastasis—may lead to low cortical hormone

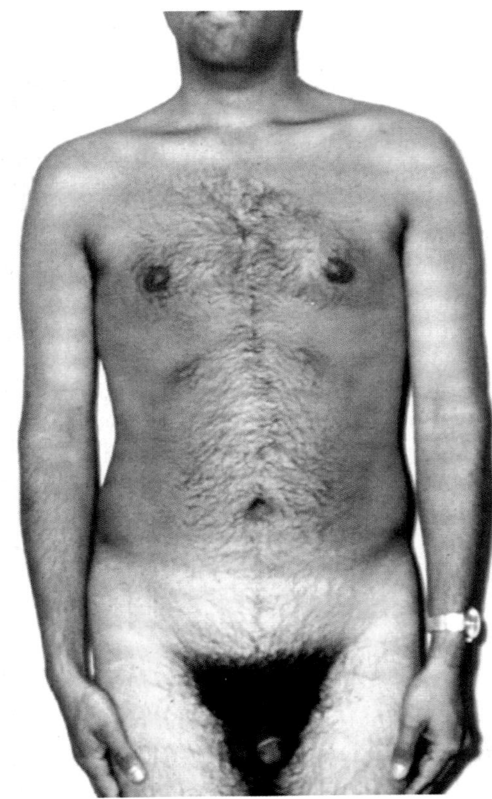

Figure 14.21 **Bronze skin pigmentation of Addison disease.**

production and clinical features somewhat similar to Addison disease. In these secondary insufficiencies, the adrenal cortex is atrophic. Nevertheless, skin hyperpigmentation is lacking because pituitary POMC production is impaired and, therefore, blood ACTH and MSH are low. Another important distinction is that mineralocorticoid production is usually not impaired, so that salt wasting does not occur. ACTH deficiency may occur as the sole manifestation of pituitary failure, but failure of other pituitary target organs may also occur (refer to the pituitary disease section above). The other clinical features of Addison disease usually appear slowly and may be compounded by symptoms of thyroid failure.

Diagnosis is clinical with laboratory and radiologic support. Skull imaging is important to look for changes to the sella turcica. Blood ACTH and cortisol are low. An ACTH challenge should stimulate cortisol production.

Treatment is correction of the underlying condition and cortisol replacement.

The Importance of Adrenocortical Neoplasms Is their Functionality

A few adrenocortical neoplasms occur as a part of a larger syndrome due to a genetic defect, but most are sporadic.

Contrary to neoplasms of most other organs, where mass effect and metastasis are most important, the main concern with adrenocortical neoplasms is their ability to make hormones. Adenomas and carcinomas occur with equal frequency in adults, but carcinomas are more common in children. Functioning adenomas usually cause Cushing syndrome or Conn syndrome (hyperaldosteronism), whereas virilization is more often caused by a cortical carcinoma. Diagnosis is by radiographic imaging and pathologic study of tissue removed at surgery. Treatment of functioning adenomas is surgical excision. Prognosis is good for adenomas, poor for carcinomas.

Notwithstanding the above, most neoplasms of the cortex are nonfunctioning adenomas discovered incidentally ("*incidentaloma*") by radiographic imaging. They are present in about 4% of the U.S. population and are clinically insignificant. They need no treatment.

Pop Quiz

14.17 True or false? The most common cause of Cushing syndrome is exogenous glucocorticoid medical therapy.

14.18 True or false? The bronze pigmentation characteristic of Addison disease is caused by overproduction of POMC, the precursor molecule from which both ACTH and MSH are made.

14.19 What hormone can be used to tell primary hyperaldosteronism apart from secondary hyperaldosteronism?

14.20 What genetic defect is the most common cause of congenital adrenal hyperplasia?

Disorders of the Adrenal Medulla

Disorders of the medulla are less important than cortical ones because the medulla is embryologically, anatomically, and functionally closely related to the autonomic nervous system, which effectively compensates for lost medullary function. Medullary failure is invariably due to destruction of the entire adrenal gland, from which every serious consequence owes to lost cortical function. Medullary hyperplasia is not known.

Pheochromocytomas, although rare, are the most common neoplasm of the adrenal medulla. Other neurogenic tumors may arise from chromaffin cells in the medulla or paraganglion system (adults, Chapter 19; children, Chapter 22) where they are known as **paragangliomas**. Most originate in the medulla, but some arise from chromaffin cells in the paraganglion system.

A convenient way to remember clinical characteristics of pheochromocytoma is the "Rule of Tens":

- 10% arise outside the adrenal as paragangliomas (in the paraganglion system).
- 10% of those in the adrenal are bilateral.
- 10% are malignant. Malignancy is more common in paragangliomas.
- 10% arise in children.
- 10% are not associated with hypertension.

As many as 25% of pheochromocytomas are part of a familial genetic syndrome featuring other tumors such as renal carcinoma or those of the multiple endocrine neoplasia (MEN) syndromes.

The most important clinical sign of pheochromocytoma is hypertension. All pheochromocytomas and paragangliomas secrete catecholamines to some degree; sometimes, secretion is high enough to produce hypertension and even very severe hypertension. About 1 in 1,000 patients with hypertension has a pheochromocytoma or paraganglioma, making them a rare but important cause of surgically curable hypertension. Most of the time blood pressure is chronically elevated and must be distinguished from essential hypertension; however, sometimes blood pressure may rise suddenly and dramatically as the result of the release of a large amount of catecholamine, which can be precipitated by exercise, stress, change in body position, or pressure on the tumor. These episodes are characterized by spasms of severe hypertension, chest and abdominal pain, palpitations, anxiety, profuse sweating, facial flushing, and nausea and vomiting. They also can cause stroke, heart attack, or fatal cardiac arrhythmia.

Laboratory procedures are required to make a positive diagnosis. Increased urinary output of catecholamines or their metabolites confirms the diagnosis. Solitary benign tumors can be removed surgically. Multifocal neoplasms require long-term medical treatment of hypertension.

Pop Quiz

14.21 What is the pheochromocytoma "Rule of Tens"?

Disorders of the Parathyroid Glands

The important disorders of the parathyroid glands are over- and underproduction of PTH (hyper- and hypoparathyroidism). The importance of parathyroid neoplasms lies entirely in their ability to cause hyperparathyroidism. Almost every parathyroid neoplasm is a functioning adenoma. Carcinomas are rare and when they occur they are usually functional. Nonfunctional tumors are very rare.

Increased blood calcium (**hypercalcemia**) is usually the finding that raises the possibility of parathyroid disease. The most common cause of hypercalcemia is *asymptomatic* hyperparathyroidism, which by definition is *incidental hypercalcemia* discovered in the course of other medical investigations. The outlook for these patients is good.

The most common cause of *symptomatic* hypercalcemia, however, is nonparathyroid malignancy, usually solid tumors of the lung or breast that are metastatic to bone, or multiple myeloma (Chapter 7) or other hematopoietic malignancy, which raises blood calcium by stimulating calcium resorption from bone near the malignant cells. Alternatively, some solid tumors, especially lung cancers, may secrete PTH-related protein (PTHrP), which produces a hyperparathyroid state as a paraneoplastic syndrome. The outlook for these patients is generally poor because of the usual nature of the underlying malignancy.

Hyperparathyroidism Is Overactivity of the Parathyroid Glands

Hyperparathyroidism is oversecretion of PTH by the parathyroid glands. High blood calcium is the cardinal laboratory finding (see *The Clinical Side*, "Hypercalcemia"). There are three varieties: primary, secondary, and tertiary. Primary overactivity is caused by parathyroid hyperplasia or adenoma; secondary and tertiary overactivity are due to chronic renal failure. Figure 14.22 illustrates the physiologic effects of excessive amounts of PTH.

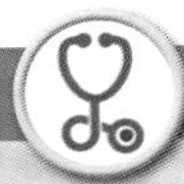

The Clinical Side

HYPERCALCEMIA

Calcium is one of the most tightly controlled of blood chemical constituents. Levels even slightly above the upper limit of normal should be taken seriously. The first step is to repeat the test to verify that calcium is, indeed, elevated. Low levels of blood phosphate confirm that an imbalance is present. If a high blood calcium level is confirmed, blood PTH level should be measured; a PTH level above normal confirms the diagnosis of hyperparathyroidism; however, remember that not all such cases are caused by parathyroid gland disease.

Of patients not in renal failure who have unexplained high blood calcium levels, the following approximations are found:

- Fifty percent (50%) have hyperparathyroidism.
- Thirty-five percent (35%) have undetected (occult) malignancy, either metastatic to bone or from paraneoplastic effect (Chapter 5), in which a nonparathyroid tumor is secreting PTH-rp (cancer of the kidney is a particular suspect).
- Ten percent (10%) have no detectable disease.

Keep in mind that hypercalcemia of any type can cause pancreatitis and renal stones.

Primary Hyperparathyroidism

Second only to diabetes mellitus, **primary hyperparathyroidism** is the most common primary endocrine disorder; that is, an endocrine disorder that is not secondary to some other condition. It is the most common cause of abnormally high blood calcium levels. Prevalence estimates vary greatly. In the U.S. population, the prevalence of symptomatic hyperparathyroidism is about 1 in 5,000 people. Nevertheless, some studies show asymptomatic hyperparathyroidism to be perhaps 10 times more prevalent, about 1 in 400 people or even higher. In any case, asymptomatic hypercalcemia due to minimal hyperparathyroidism is quite common. Most cases are postmenopausal women with a **parathyroid adenoma** (~90%, most in a single gland), while the remainder are due to hyperplasia (~10%). The majority of cases are sporadic. A few occur in conjunction with one of the multiple endocrine neoplasia syndromes (MEN).

The classic clinical findings, depicted in Figure 14.23, are easily recalled by the phrase "stones, bones, groans, with psychiatric overtones."

- "Stones" refers to kidney stones (*nephrolithiasis*, Chapter 15), which arise because of high urinary calcium concentration.
- "Bones" refers to destructive bone changes as bone calcium is mobilized into blood and leads to *osteoporosis* (Chapter 18) and increased risk of fracture. This leads to hypercalcemia, which may lead to calcium deposits in the pancreas, kidney, and aortic and mitral valves.
- "Groans" refers to the pain of peptic ulcers, pancreatitis, or gallstones that occur in some cases.
- "Psychiatric overtones" refers to the depression and fatigue that frequently accompanies the disease and is often its first and most prominent manifestation.

Typical laboratory findings are increased blood calcium level and PTH. An important diagnostic point is that

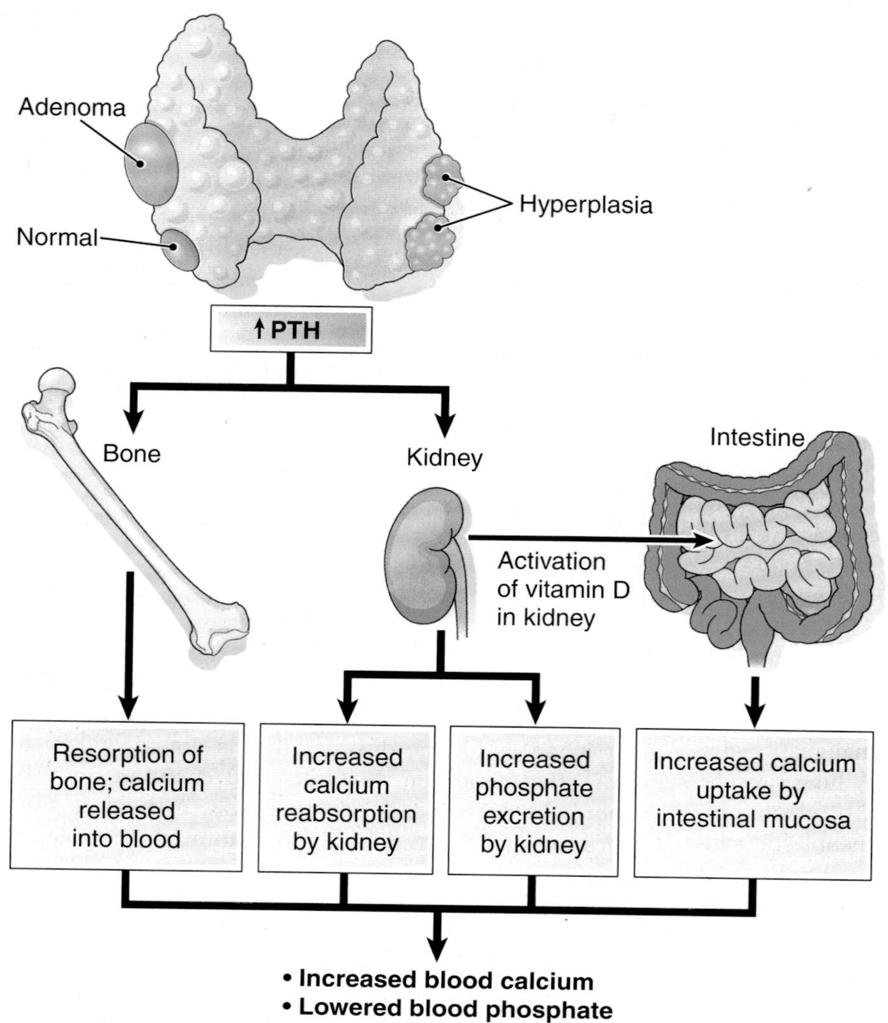

Figure 14.22 **Pathophysiology of hyperparathyroidism.**

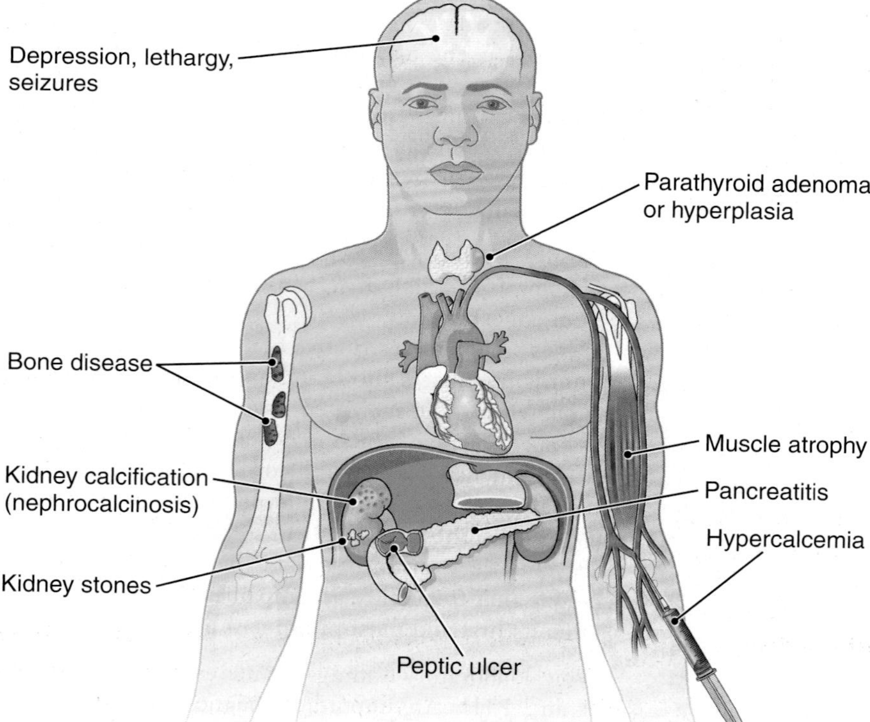

Figure 14.23 **Clinical manifestations of hyperparathyroidism.**

blood PTH levels are very low in other conditions associated with hypercalcemia.

Diagnosis is clinical with laboratory and radiologic support. Incidental hyperparathyroidism requires periodic blood calcium assays and yearly bone density surveys to check for disease progression. Nonprogressive cases are managed by a low calcium diet, exercise to stress bones and avoid the mobilization of bone calcium due to relative inactivity, and plenty of fluids to avoid renal stone formation. In progressive or symptomatic cases, treatment has two aims: controlling hypercalcemia and removal of the abnormal gland or glands. Hypercalcemia can be managed medically by oral phosphate, diuretics that increase urinary calcium secretion and drugs that suppress bone calcium mobilization. Surgery may be required in progressive cases, but the criteria for patient selection are controversial.

Secondary Hyperparathyroidism

Secondary hyperparathyroidism is a situation in which *low* blood calcium (*hypocalcemia*) is caused by a nonparathyroid condition that stimulates compensatory parathyroid *hyperplasia* and secretion of excess PTH. Because blood calcium and phosphate bear an inverse relationship to one another, the most common cause of secondary hyperparathyroidism is high blood phosphate owing to failure of phosphate secretion in chronic renal failure (Chapter 15). Other causes include hypocalcemia caused by stool calcium loss in fat malabsorption syndromes (*steatorrhea*, Chapter 11), and dietary calcium or vitamin D deficiency.

Clinical findings are dominated by chronic renal failure—high blood pressure, anemia, edema, low urine output, bleeding problems, diarrhea, and mental problems caused by accumulated metabolic waste products. The signs and symptoms of hyperparathyroidism are present, too, with the notable exception that blood calcium levels may not be increased because high blood levels of phosphate will not allow blood calcium to rise despite high blood levels of PTH.

Diagnosis is clinical with laboratory and radiologic support. Treatment is elimination of the underlying condition. In renal failure, renal transplant usually corrects the failure and cures the hyperparathyroidism.

Tertiary Hyperparathyroidism

Rarely, hyperparathyroidism persists after renal transplant because one or more of the hyperplastic parathyroid glands becomes autonomous and continues to secrete PTH despite the fact that renal function and blood phosphate levels have returned to normal. This condition is referred to as **tertiary hyperparathyroidism** and requires surgical removal of the hyperplastic parathyroid glands.

Hypoparathyroidism Is Underactivity of the Parathyroid Glands

Underactive parathyroid glands are much less common than overactive ones. Hypoparathyroidism is usually caused by inadvertent surgical removal of parathyroid glands during thyroidectomy or removal of too large a portion of aggregate parathyroid gland tissue in surgical treatment of hyperparathyroidism. Less commonly, hypoparathyroidism results from idiopathic parathyroid atrophy or genetic defect.

The major blood abnormality associated with underactive parathyroid glands is low blood calcium and PTH levels. The cardinal sign of clinically significant hypocalcemia is intermittent muscular aches and spasms (*tetany*) caused by the effect of low calcium on the electrical potential of muscle cell membrane. Other neuromuscular signs include tingling sensations of the face, lips, tongue, fingers, and feet; hyperactive reflexes; seizures; and facial and vocal cord spasms with airway obstruction.

Diagnosis is clinical with laboratory support. Short-term treatment is with intravenous calcium. Long-term treatment is with oral vitamin D and calcium supplementation.

Case Notes

14.16 The parathyroids are very close to the thyroid. Is there any reason to suspect that Azadeh's thyroid disease will affect her parathyroids?

Pop Quiz

14.22 True or false? The cardinal sign of hypocalcemia is intermittent muscular aches and tetany caused by the effect of low calcium on the electrical potential of muscle cell membrane.

14.23 What causes tertiary hyperparathyroidism?

Multiple Endocrine Neoplasia Syndromes (MEN)

The **multiple endocrine neoplasia syndromes (MEN)** are a group of heritable disorders due to gene defects that cause endocrine cell growth—hyperplasia, adenoma, or carcinoma—in various endocrine organs. Compared to sporadic individual tumors of like kind, MEN tumors tend to occur in younger patients, in multiple endocrine organs rather than a single one, tend to be multifocal in involved organs, and tend to be more aggressive.

MEN-1 syndrome (*Wermer syndrome*) is a rare heritable disorder with mutations in the MEN-1 gene (menin) that usually features abnormalities of parathyroid, pancreas, pituitary, and gastrin-secreting cells of the duodenum. Hyperparathyroidism is the main manifestation of parathyroid involvement. Pituitary involvement is usually a prolactinoma. Gastrinoma of the duodenum also may occur and can be associated with severe, refractory peptic ulcer disease (Zollinger-Ellison syndrome, Chapter 11). Some patients may also have carcinoid tumors (Chapters 11 and 14) or tumors of the thyroid or adrenal cortex. Endocrine tumors of the pancreas are the main cause of death in MEN-1. The principal clinical features of MEN-1 relate to overproduction of hormones, hypoglycemia from insulinoma, peptic ulcer disease from gastrinoma, and renal stones from hypercalcemia due to hyperparathyroidism. Diagnosis and treatment vary according to the main problem at hand.

MEN-2 syndrome may be one of three types, all of related genetic defects, generally in the RET gene. *MEN-2A* features pheochromocytoma, medullary carcinoma of the thyroid, and parathyroid hyperplasia. *MEN-2B* is similar to 2A but does not have parathyroid disease and features pheochromocytoma, more aggressive medullary thyroid cancer, widespread ganglioneuromatosis including within the gut (Chapter 19), and long, gangly limbs. The third variety attributable to MEN-2 genetic defect is familial medullary thyroid carcinoma. Diagnosis and treatment vary. Patients with familial medullary thyroid cancer syndrome should have prophylactic thyroidectomy.

Pop Quiz

14.24 Which MEN syndrome is associated with Zollinger Ellison?

Case Study Revisited

"I'm running out of gas." The case of Azadeh N.

The thyroid studies in Azadeh's case were airtight evidence of primary thyroid failure (myxedema, hypothyroidism)—T3 and T4 were low and TSH was elevated, indicating the pituitary gland was fine and working hard to stimulate the thyroid gland to produce T3 and T4, but the thyroid was not responding. The clinical picture was classic for myxedema. She had nearly all of the signs—low body temperature; slow heart rate and respirations; thinning, brittle hair; dry, flaky skin, especially over her lower legs, where it was thickened and indurated; constipation; weakness and fatigue; and dull, depressed behavior. The pedal edema and chest rales suggested fluid accumulation in her lungs and the possibility of early heart failure. Low electrocardiogram voltage also fit the picture. Adding to the evidence was the fact that her insulin requirement declined, exactly the expectation for someone who was burning less energy, a conclusion reinforced by the fact that, with thyroid hormone replacement, her insulin requirement increased to preillness levels. Similarly, low cardiac output lowered her blood pressure, which evolved into orthostatic hypotensive episodes of near fainting. Treatment of myxedema raised cardiac output and blood pressure and eliminated the orthostatic hypotension, but reestablished hypertension and necessitated upward adjustment of antihypertensive drug dosage.

Though biopsy proof was lacking, it seems highly likely that Hashimoto thyroiditis was the cause of her myxedema. She had all of the requirements: nontender goiter, antithyroid autoantibodies, autoimmune disease (type I diabetes), and a family history of autoimmune disease (an aunt with RA).

The elevated creatinine and proteinuria indicated the presence of significant diabetic and hypertensive renal disease (nephrosclerosis).

Chapter Challenge

CHAPTER RECALL

1. A 45-year-old Caucasian male presents to the clinic complaining of loss of vision. His physical exam is notable for bilateral loss of temporal (lateral) vision, a coarse facial appearance with prominent brow and chin, and large feet and hands with thick fingers. What is the likely cause of this constellation of symptoms?
   A. Gigantism
   B. Acromegaly
   C. Cushing syndrome
   D. Conn syndrome
2. Which one of the following is associated with low blood TSH?
   A. Hypothyroidism
   B. Cushing syndrome
   C. Graves disease
   D. Hashimoto thyroiditis
3. A 40-year-old Hispanic male is found to have a single thyroid nodule that is cold by RAI scan. A needle biopsy of the mass reveals a cauliflower-like microscopic growth pattern. Despite having a positive cervical lymph node, his prognosis is good. What type of thyroid cancer does he have?
   A. Anaplastic carcinoma
   B. Follicular carcinoma
   C. Medullary carcinoma
   D. Papillary carcinoma
4. Which of the following is a true statement concerning hypoparathyroidism?
   A. Underactive parathyroid glands are much more common than overactive ones.
   B. The major blood abnormality in hypoparathyroidism is low blood calcium despite elevated PTH levels.
   C. Hypoparathyroidism is usually caused by idiopathic parathyroid atrophy or a genetic defect.
   D. Hypoparathyroidism may cause seizures.
5. A 43-year-old African American male presents to the ER with chest pain, profuse sweating, nausea, and vomiting. A stat EKG rules out a heart attack, and his symptoms are attributed to severe hypertension. A urine test identifies the presence of catecholamines and their metabolites. What is the underlying etiology of the patient's hypertension?
   A. Hyperaldosteronism
   B. Cushing disease
   C. Pheochromocytoma
   D. Essential hypertension
6. Which hormone excess can cause hypokalemia?
   A. Aldosterone
   B. Cortisol
   C. Parathormone
   D. Adrenocorticotrophic hormone
7. On checkup, a 55-year-old Caucasian male with a past medical history significant for hypertension, presents with a constellation of signs and symptoms characteristic of Cushing syndrome. These symptoms include weight gain with truncal obesity, a buffalo hump, and moon facies as well as atrophic limbs and thin friable skin. A dexamethasone suppression test reveals failure of low and high doses of dexamethasone to suppress ACTH. What is the underlying etiology?
   A. ACTH secreting nonpituitary tumor
   B. ACTH secreting adrenal tumor
   C. Exogenous steroids
   D. Pituitary Cushing syndrome
8. DI is characterized by which one of the following?
   A. Destruction of the anterior pituitary
   B. Lack of antidiuretic hormone (ADH)
   C. Failure of renal tubule to reabsorb potassium
   D. All of the above
9. A 32-year-old African American mother brings her child to your clinic for a three-month checkup. Inquiring after his feeding habits, you find out that she failed to lactate. Her history is also positive for fatigue, constipation, and amenorrhea since the birth of her child. She confirms that it was a difficult birth, and that she required a large transfusion of blood. What is the likely cause of her symptoms?
   A. Sarcoidosis
   B. Pituitary apoplexy
   C. Hypothyroid
   D. Sheehan syndrome
10. Which one of the following is characteristic of secondary hyperparathyroidism?
    A. Low blood PTH level
    B. Increased blood calcium level
    C. Increased blood phosphate level
    D. All of the above
11. A 25-year-old Caucasian woman presents to her physician's office concerned that she is beginning menopause due to "hot flashes" that she describes as feeling hot all the time. She also complains of weight loss, diarrhea, and insomnia. Her physical

exam is positive for a staring gaze with lid lag, tachycardia, and scaly thickened seminodular areas of induration over her tibia. Her labs revealed elevated T3 and T4, decreased TSH, and diffusely increased uptake of RAI (in her thyroid). What is her diagnosis?
A. Toxic adenoma
B. Subacute granulomatous thyroiditis
C. Graves disease
D. Hashimoto thyroiditis

12. Which of the following cell types is responsible for milk production?
A. Somatotrophs
B. Lactotrophs
C. Corticotrophs
D. Chromaffin cells

13. An infant with ambiguous genitalia is found to have low blood pressure, hyponatremia, and hyperkalemia shortly after birth. Which of the following diseases might cause these findings?
A. Addison disease
B. Congenital adrenal hyperplasia
C. Cushing disease
D. Adrenocortical insufficiency

14. True or false? Oxytocin and ADH are the two hormones synthesized in the posterior pituitary.

15. True or false? Lab abnormalities in Addison disease include hyperkalemia, hyponatremia, hypotension, and, on occasion, hypoglycemia.

16. True or false? Pituitary adenomas are usually small, nonfunctional, and persist a lifetime without ill effect.

17. True or false? Pheochromocytomas occur only in the adrenal gland.

18. True or false? Sudden withdrawal of corticosteroid therapy is the most common cause of acute adrenal gland failure.

19. Match the following hormones with their function:
i. Prolactin
ii. Growth Hormone
iii. Oxytocin
iv. Catecholamines
v. Calcitonin
A. Promotes bone absorption of calcium and prohibits bone resorption
B. Stimulates metabolic and heart rate, dilates bronchioles and coronary arteries, and constricts peripheral blood vessels raising blood pressure
C. Stimulates liver production of insulin-like growth factor-1
D. Stimulates milk secretion
E. Stimulates milk ejection

CONCEPTUAL UNDERSTANDING

20. Name the common causes of pituitary failure.

21. Regarding masses of the thyroid, what are some characteristics that help to determine whether they are cancerous?

22. Name the MEN syndromes and their characteristic features.

APPLICATION

23. Why is cretinism rarely diagnosed in developed countries?

24. The classical clinical findings of hyperparathyroidism are easily recalled by the phrase "stones, bones, groans, and psychiatric overtones." Explain what this phrase means, and how "stones" can be prevented.

CHAPTER 15

Disorders of the Urinary Tract

Contents

Chapter Objectives

Section 1: ***Normal Anatomy and Physiology***

After studying this chapter, you should be able to complete the following tasks:

THE NORMAL URINARY TRACT

1. Discuss the relationship between the anatomy of the kidney and its five functions, including the transformation of glomerular filtrate to urine.

URINE

2. Explain the significance of some of the more important urine abnormalities such as glycosuria and others.

Section 2: ***Obstruction, Stones, and Neoplasms***

URINARY TRACT OBSTRUCTION

3. Explain the causes, manifestations, and consequences of urinary tract obstruction and reflux.

UROLITHIASIS

4. Compare and contrast the types of urinary stones capable of forming in the kidney.

NEOPLASMS OF THE URINARY TRACT

5. Name the most important malignancies of the urinary tract, and describe the findings associated with each.

Section 3: ***Disorders of the Lower Urinary Tract***

CONGENITAL ANATOMIC ABNORMALITIES

6. List the congenital abnormalities that may arise in the lower urinary tract.

INFECTION AND INFLAMMATION

7. Describe the etiology, signs and symptoms, and treatment of lower urinary tract infections.

VOIDING DISORDERS

8. List the possible causes of voiding disorders; be sure to distinguish between the various types of incontinence.

Section 4: ***Disorders of the Kidney***

CLINICAL PRESENTATIONS OF RENAL DISORDER

9. Distinguish between renal diseases and syndromes of renal disease.

INHERITED, CONGENITAL, AND DEVELOPMENTAL DISORDER

10. List the inherited, congenital, and developmental diseases that affect the kidney, and differentiate between the diseases capable of causing kidney cysts.

GLOMERULAR DISORDERS

11. Explain the difference between nephritic syndrome and nephrotic syndrome, giving examples of each; pay special attention to those that are most common.

TUBULAR AND INTERSTITIAL DISORDER

12. Describe the clinical presentation and course of acute kidney injury.
13. Discuss the etiologies, clinical features, diagnostic findings, and treatment of the various causes of tubulointerstitial nephritis.

PYELONEPHRITIS

14. Describe the signs, symptoms, and pathological features of pyelonephritis.

VASCULAR DISORDERS

15. Using examples from the text, discuss the primary mechanisms by which the kidney causes hypertension and the associated pathological changes in the kidney secondary to hypertension.

Drink, sir, is a great provoker of three things . . . nose-painting, sleep, and urine.

WILLIAM SHAKESPEARE (1564–1616), ENGLISH PLAYWRIGHT, MACBETH

Urine is the fluid excreted by the kidneys. Because it is a waste product, it gets about as much respect as feces. But the foul smell of poorly sanitized urinals derives from bacterial contamination and the products of bacterial metabolism, not from the normal constituents of urine. Most urine is clean enough to drink, or at least to taste, as English physician Thomas Willis did in 1760 in his investigation of what we now recognize as diabetes mellitus. In addition to its role as a diagnostic fluid, across the ages urine has been used for almost every conceivable purpose—ancient civilizations used it as an antiseptic; Scots soaked wool in it to prevent shrinking; and others fermented and dried it to collect potassium nitrate (saltpeter) crystals, which they used to make explosives. The *History of Medicine*, "Liquid Gold," provides some interesting details.

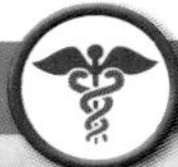

The History of Medicine

LIQUID GOLD

Clay tablets from about 4000 BCE mention the examination of urine and offer an inkling of the ancients' ideas about its importance. And it is important: patients who do not make enough of this "liquid gold" soon find themselves in deep trouble.

Urine is easy to collect and can be readily examined, features that made it a popular choice for study by early physicians, especially for the examination of women, who could not be directly examined because custom forbade it. Greek physician Hippocrates (460–377 BCE) wrote specifically about examination of urine, noting that fever changed its smell. Later, Galen (131–201 CE), a Greco-Roman physician, wrote of his belief that urine revealed the health of the liver. Galen believed that urine was a combination of the body's four "humours"—blood, phlegm, yellow bile, and black bile—and revealed if they were in or out of balance. Galen's ideas on urine, humours, and other medical matters became so entrenched in the ancient and medieval worlds that few new ideas were accepted in medicine for over 1,000 years, until the European Renaissance ~ 1500 launched a revolution in science and every other aspect of human affairs.

Nevertheless, medical advances had to compete with magicians of the time, who relied on the bubble patterns of freshly passed urine to foretell the future. Not content to peer into the darkness of a brass chamber pot, physicians and magicians developed the matula, a glass vessel shaped like the bladder, believing that urine held in a matula was more revealing because it maintained its natural shape. Apart from these well-intentioned fantasies, sometimes the practitioners were right: the ancient Greeks knew that diabetes was characterized by large volumes of urine, and English physician Thomas Willis (1621–1675) bravely tasted urine and learned that diabetic urine was unusually sweet.

Waste products in urine mainly derive from protein metabolism, which includes urea, uric acid, creatinine, and ammonia. But urine is not merely metabolic waste; it also contains water, acid, and electrolytes, each of which the kidneys adjust as they filter blood. Because 20% of cardiac output passes through the kidneys, our entire blood supply is filtered many times each hour to adjust blood osmolarity, pH, and electrolyte concentration.

Other factors—thirst, sweating, respiratory activity, and other functions—are also important in determining the composition of urine. For example, if you lose a lot of water in sweat, then the kidneys excrete less water; if you drink a glass of tart (acidic) lemonade, then the kidneys excrete more acid; if you eat a salty snack, then the kidneys up their output of sodium.

Of the organs in the urinary system, the kidneys are responsible for the critical functions. Thus, disorders involving the kidneys can have devastating effects. In 2010, about 50,000 people in the United States died of renal disease. Although this mortality rate is comparatively low—600,000 died of heart disease and nearly as many died of cancer—the morbidity of renal disease is enormous. In 2010, the National Institutes of Health estimated that over 500,000 Americans were living with chronic renal failure and another 20 million had some form of chronic kidney disease. About 350,000 are on chronic renal dialysis. Diabetes, chronic glomerulonephritis (CGN), and hypertension account for about 75% of these; the cause of the other 25% is often unknown. Approximately 90,000 are waiting for a kidney transplant, but only about 18,000 transplants are performed each year.

Discussion of renal disease focuses on the four principal anatomic components of the kidney: the glomeruli, the tubules and interstitium, and the vasculature. Each is vulnerable to a particular type of injury. Almost all glomerular disease is immunologically mediated; tubular and interstitial disease usually owes to the effect of toxins or infections; and vascular disease is usually related, either as cause or effect, to hypertension. In the early stages of renal disease, these effects tend to be anatomically isolated, but as disease progresses the damage tends to spread from one anatomic compartment to another, so that in chronic renal disease the original distinctions of etiology and anatomy are blurred.

Section 1: Normal Anatomy and Physiology

The Normal Urinary Tract

Figure 15.1 illustrates the **urinary tract**, which consists of the kidneys, renal pelvises, ureters, urinary bladder, and urethra. The kidneys and renal pelvises form the **upper urinary tract**; the ureters, bladder, and urethra form the **lower urinary tract**. The **collecting system** consists of a series of spaces that carry urine from the kidney and hold it for urination. It consists of the **renal pelvis**, the broad, funnel-shaped space that gathers urine from the kidney and channels it into the **ureter**, a muscular tube that conveys urine to the **bladder**, where it is held until elimination via the **urethra**. Normal function of the urinary tract depends on the continuous, smooth, downward flow of urine from the kidney through the collecting system. Obstruction or sluggish flow invites trouble.

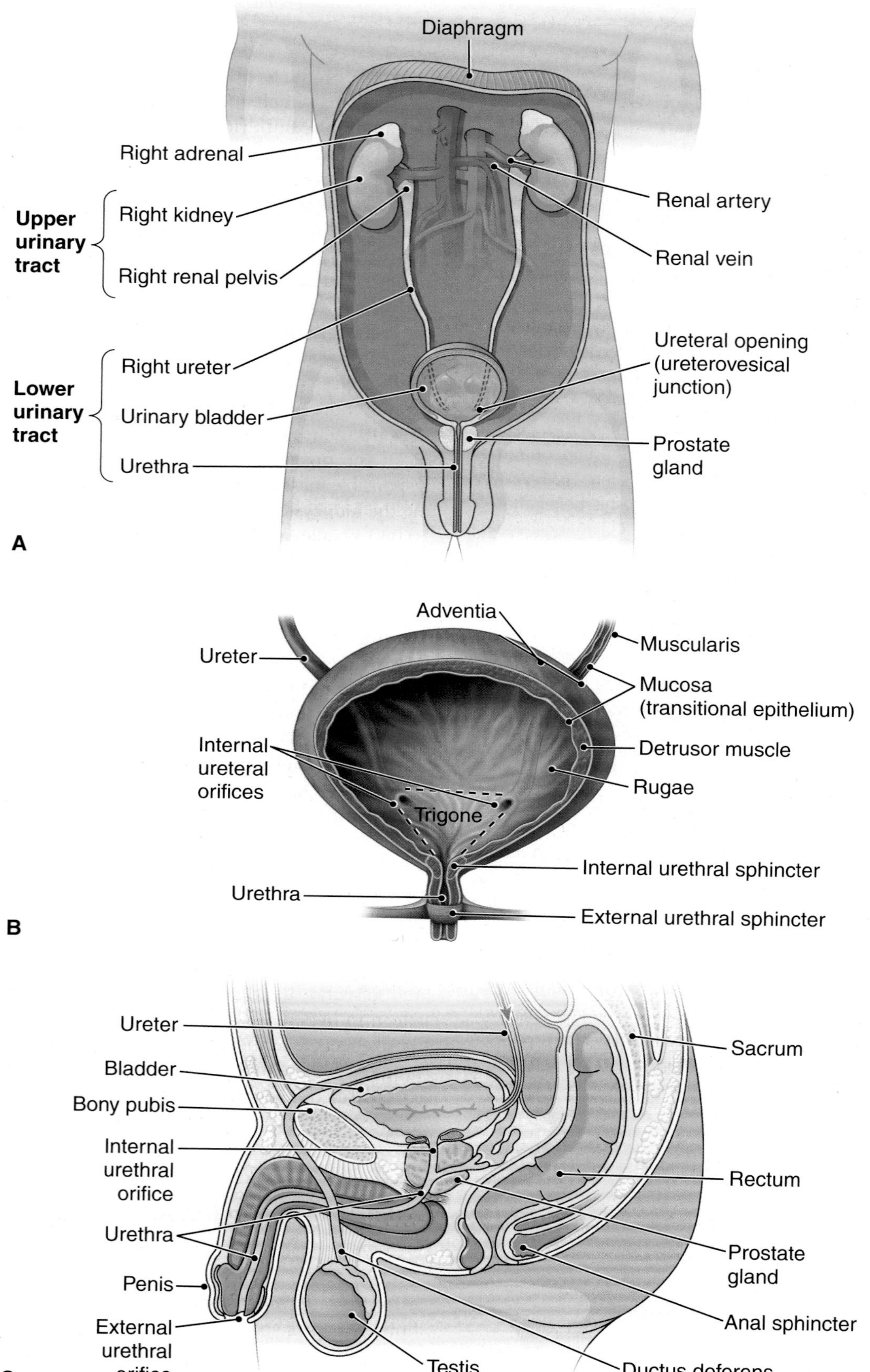

Figure 15.1 **The urinary tract (frontal view, male). A.** The urinary tract consists of the kidneys, renal pelvises, ureters, urinary bladder, and urethra. The female system is identical except for sex organs and the shorter length of the female urethra. **B.** The bladder and ureters. **C.** The lower urinary tract (lateral view, male). (B and C adapted with permission from McConnell TH, Hull KL. *Human Form Human Function: Essentials of Anatomy & Physiology.* Baltimore (MD). Wolters Kluwer Health; 2011.)

Remember This! Normal urinary tract health depends on smooth, brisk, unobstructed flow of urine.

The Collecting System Collects and Holds Urine

The *collecting system* lies in the retroperitoneum and consists of a series of tubes through which urine flows from the kidney to the bladder, where it is held until it can be emptied under voluntary control into the environment. The organs of the lower urinary tract and the internal genitalia of both sexes lie close to one another and are often involved together in disease.

With the exception of the terminal urethra, which is lined by squamous epithelium, the collecting system is lined by **urothelial cells**. The **urothelial epithelium** is sometimes called *transitional epithelium* because of its ability to transition between round and flat as the bladder mucosa stretches to accommodate increasing urine volume. The superficial layer of urothelial cells is composed of somewhat larger, flatter "umbrella cells" that resist damage by, and absorption of, the urine that constantly bathes them. The urothelium rests upon a basement membrane, beneath which is a thin lamina propria composed of loose connective tissue and blood vessels. In contrast to the GI tract, no muscularis mucosa is present. Beneath the lamina propria is the muscular wall composed of layers of smooth muscle.

The **ureters** descend in the retroperitoneum on either side of the spine and enter the bladder at a shallow angle, so that the last centimeter or so of ureter is embedded in the bladder wall. This is the **ureterovesical junction (UVJ)**, which acts as a one-way valve to prevent backflow of urine from the bladder into the ureter. The bladder meatus of each ureter and the internal meatus of the urethra form an inverted triangle of bladder mucosa called the **trigone**.

The **urinary bladder** receives and holds urine until it is expelled. It is a somewhat spherical organ with a small funnel-shaped outlet. The wall is composed of smooth muscle. The muscular wall of the bladder is called the **detrusor muscle** (Latin *detrus* = thrust down). As the bladder empties, it does not shrink like a balloon; rather the dome collapses, leaving the inferior part of the bladder unchanged. The smooth muscle wall of the ureter is innervated by the autonomic nervous system. The next layer outward is an adventitia composed of loose connective tissue. A layer of peritoneum covers the dome of the bladder. The **urethra** is the terminal conduit for urine and semen and extends from the neck of the bladder to the opening at the tip of the penis. In males it is about 20 cm long; in females about 3–4 cm. In males it is divided into three parts. The most proximal part is surrounded by the prostate and called the *prostatic urethra*. The middle section is very short and called the *membranous urethra*. The final portion is the *penile urethra*.

Urine expelled from the bladder by urination (**micturition**) is unchanged from its formation in the kidney. Gravity and ureteral peristaltic contractions (controlled by the autonomic nervous system) move urine down the ureters into the bladder. Urine is held in the bladder by two sphincters that surround the proximal opening of the urethra, the *internal urethral meatus*, where it joins the neck of the bladder. The **internal sphincter** is composed of smooth muscle and is involuntary and controlled by the autonomic nervous system. The **external sphincter** circles the urethra immediately below the internal sphincter and is composed of skeletal muscle that is under voluntary control. As urine accumulates, the bladder wall stretches and sends signals to the micturition center in the lower spinal cord, which activates reflex contractions of the bladder wall and relaxation of the internal, involuntary sphincter. At the same time, the stretched bladder sends an "I'm full" signal to the brain, which brings an increasing sense of urinary urgency, which can be relieved by voluntary relaxation of the external sphincter and urination.

Pop Quiz

15.1 True or false? The lower urinary tract is entirely lined by urothelial cells.

15.2 What are the three parts of the male urethra?

The Kidney has Five Main Functions

The functions of the kidney are the following:

1. Excretion of metabolic waste
2. Adjustment of blood pH by excretion of more or less acid
3. Adjustment of plasma salt concentration (plasma osmolality) by excretion of more or less salt and water
4. Adjustment of blood volume and blood pressure by secretion of renin (Chapter 6)
5. Stimulation of RBC production by secretion of erythropoietin (Chapter 7)

Understanding how it accomplishes these feats requires study of the microscopic anatomy.

The Anatomy of Glomeruli and Tubules

Figure 15.2 illustrates the anatomy of the kidney, which has an outer **cortex** and a central **medulla**. Glomeruli and tubules are intimately related. The cortex is a mix of glomeruli and tubules. The medulla is composed entirely of tubules. **Glomeruli** (Fig. 15.3) are the filtering apparatus of the kidney. Each is a tiny spherical network of arterial capillaries formed of a single layer of *endothelial*

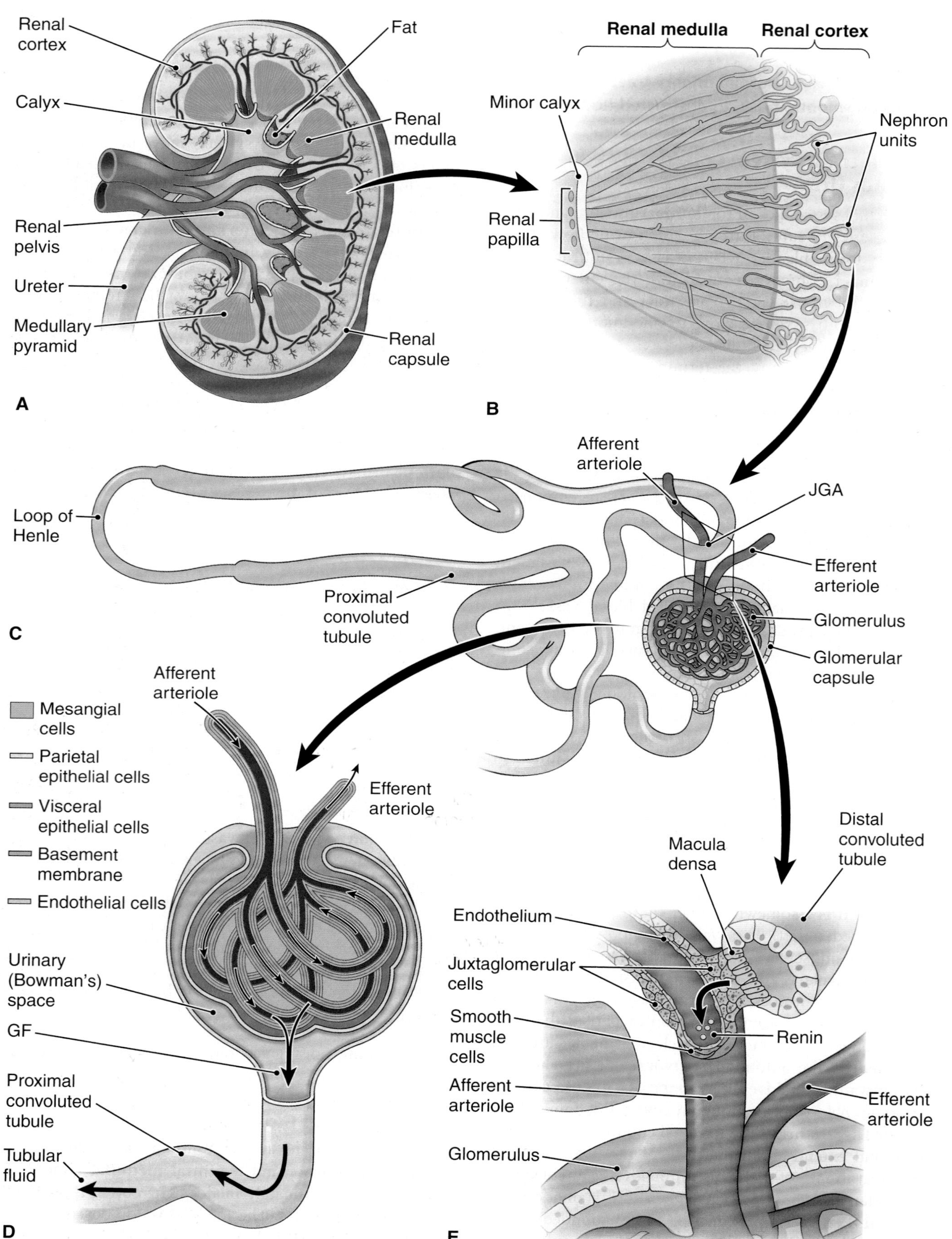

Figure 15.2 **The anatomy of the kidney. A.** Coronal section. **B.** Structure of the renal cortex and medulla. **C.** Single nephron unit (glomerulus and tubule). **D.** Anatomy of the glomerulus. **E.** The JGA.

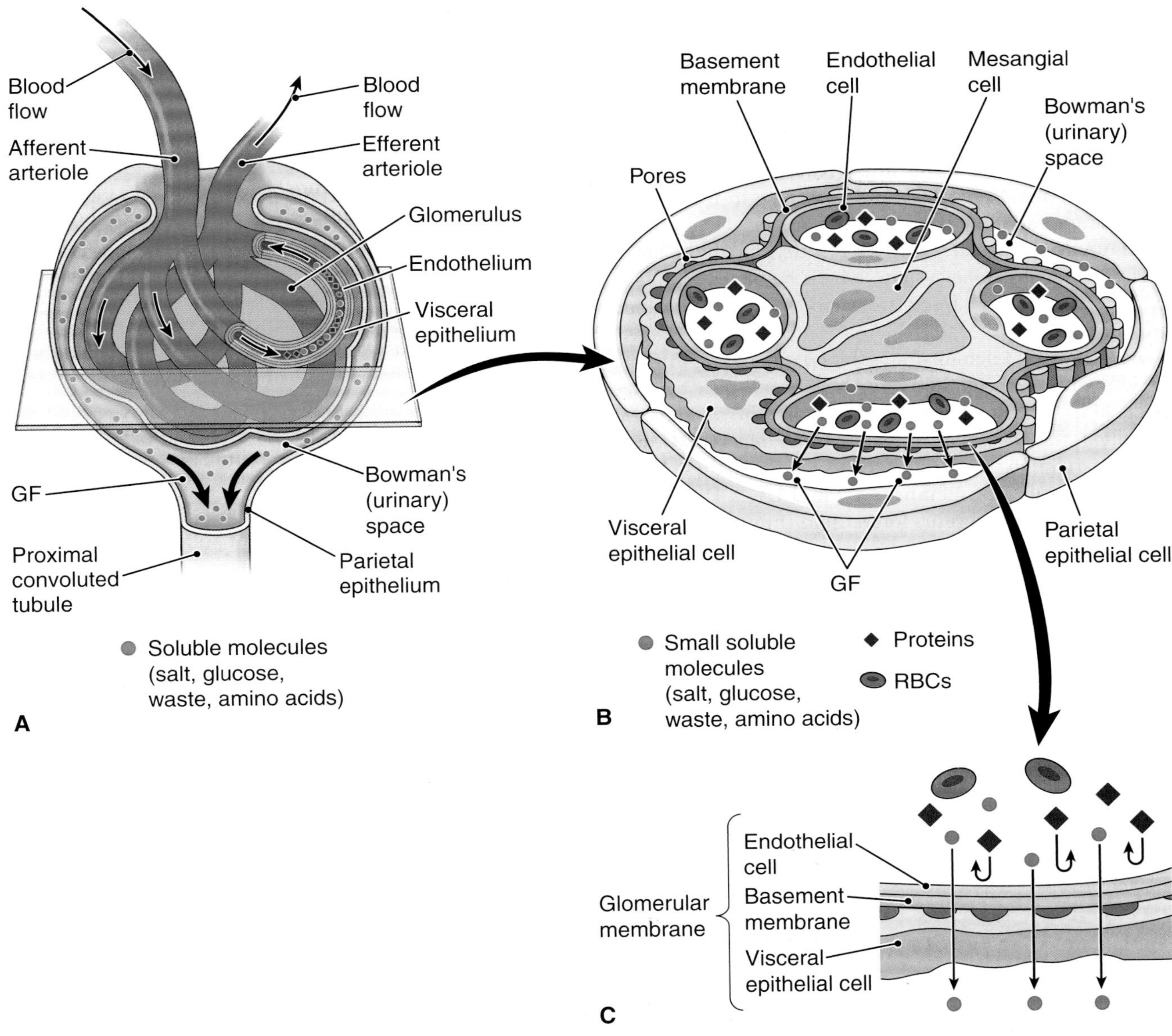

Figure 15.3 **Anatomy of the glomerulus. A.** The relationship of the glomerulus to Bowman's space. **B.** The cellular anatomy of the glomerulus (cross-section). Note the relationships among capillary endothelial cells, basement membrane, and visceral epithelial cells. **C.** The glomerular membrane is composed of capillary endothelium, basement membrane, and visceral epithelial cells. Water, salts, glucose, metabolic waste, amino acids, and other small soluble molecules cross the glomerular membrane from blood into Bowman's space as GF. Red cells, proteins and other large molecules are too large to cross.

cells. Supporting glomerular capillaries are **mesangial cells**, interstitial cells that fit between adjacent capillaries.

Each glomerulus is contiguous with the proximal end of a **renal tubule**, which together with the glomerulus forms a **nephron unit** (Fig. 15.2C). The relationship of a glomerulus and its tubule (Fig. 15.2D) can be conceived of as a fist of capillaries pressed deeply into one side of an inflated balloon, whose wall is composed of **tubular epithelial cells**. The cells of the balloon wall that touch the glomerular capillary fist are **visceral epithelial cells**; the cells of the balloon wall on the other side are the **parietal epithelial cells**. The empty space in between the epithelial walls of the balloon is **Bowman's space**. The neck of the balloon is connected to the remainder of the renal tubule, also composed of tubular epithelial cells, which receive fluid filtered by the glomerulus from blood.

Renal tubules cross from the cortex into the medulla and eventually terminate where they empty into the renal pelvis. Throughout their tortuous course, tubules are intimately associated with blood vessels, an arrangement that facilitates exchange of fluids and solutes between intratubular fluid and blood.

Blood is supplied to the glomerulus by a relatively large **afferent arteriole** and leaves through a smaller **efferent arteriole**. That the supply vessel is larger than the drainage vessel ensures that glomerular filtering pressure remains high. The afferent arteriole and a small adjacent segment of the distal convoluted tubule combine to form the **juxtaglomerular apparatus (JGA)** (Fig. 15.2E). The JGA senses blood pressure and blood flow in the afferent arteriole and sodium concentration in the distal convoluted tubule and secretes *renin* as the first step in the *renin-angiotensin-aldosterone* system, which regulates renal salt excretion as a means to control blood volume and blood pressure.

As Figure 15.3 demonstrates, blood circulating through the glomerulus is separated from the urinary space by three layers of tissue, which from inside out are: the *capillary endothelium*, the *glomerular basement membrane (GBM)*, and the *glomerular visceral epithelium*. Collectively, these layers form the **glomerular membrane** (Fig. 15.3C). High blood pressure in the glomerulus forces fluid through tiny pores in these layers like a fine mesh screen. Water and dissolved waste, salts (of sodium, potassium, calcium and others), glucose, and amino acids cross into Bowman's space, where they become the *glomerular filtrate* (GF). RBCs and proteins, however, cannot cross because they are too large to pass through the fine mesh of the glomerular layers, a function of the glomerulus known as the **barrier effect**.

Remember This! **The barrier effect of the glomerulus prevents RBCs, protein, and other large molecules from leaving blood and passing into urine.**

The Glomerular Filtrate

The tubule processes GF to create urine. The fluid initially filtered from blood is the **glomerular filtrate (GF)**, which enters Bowman's space. After leaving Bowman's space, the GF is known as **tubular fluid**. As tubular fluid moves down the tubule, water, electrolytes, acid, and other substances are exchanged between tubular fluid and blood vessels that run alongside the tubule. After exiting the tubule, the remaining fluid is **urine**.

Compared to the volume of urine, there is a much larger volume of GF. Urine output is 1.0–1.5 liters per day; by contrast, the kidney forms about 180 liters per day of GF, which means that about 99% of GF is reabsorbed by the renal tubules, leaving about 1% as urine. In healthy people, blood contains about 3.5 liters of plasma; therefore, the **glomerular filtration rate (GFR)** (the plasma cleared—cleaned—per minute) is 125 ml/min. It takes about 30 minutes for the entire plasma volume of the body to be filtered or cleared; that is to say, plasma (blood) is cleansed completely about 50 times per day.

Remember This! **Almost all of the GF is reabsorbed by renal tubules and returned to blood.**

Figure 15.4 demonstrates how the tubule adjusts the GF before it is discharged as urine. As the filtrate passes down the renal tubule, most of the water is reabsorbed into blood under the influence of antidiuretic hormone (ADH) from the posterior pituitary. As addressed in Chapter 14, the hypothalamus detects plasma osmolality (concentration of dissolved salts, mainly sodium and potassium) and commands secretion of more or less ADH to cause the renal tubules to extract more or less water from the GF and add it back to plasma to adjust the volume of plasma in which the salts are dissolved.

Final fine-tuning of plasma sodium and potassium concentration is regulated by the influence of aldosterone, the end product of the renin-angiotensin-aldosterone system. Aldosterone stimulates secretion of potassium from blood into the GF in exchange for sodium, which moves from the GF into blood. Blood sodium and potassium levels rise or fall accordingly.

The tubule also normally reabsorbs *all* glucose and amino acids; neither is present in normal urine:

- *Glucose*. Almost all blood glucose passes into the GF, so that the initial concentration in GF and in blood is nearly equal. Normally, all glucose in the GF is reabsorbed back into blood. As blood (and GF) glucose near the approximate range of 180–200 mg/dL (the renal "threshold"), however, the tubules cannot keep up with the load and some glucose passes unabsorbed all the way through the tubule and into urine (*glycosuria*), a defining characteristic in people with diabetes mellitus.
- *Amino acids*. Virtually all plasma amino acids pass into the GF, and like glucose, normally all are resorbed back into plasma by the tubules. Amino acids may appear in urine (*aminoaciduria*) if blood concentration exceeds the tubular threshold for amino acids, or if genetic disease impairs the ability of the tubules to reabsorb amino acids. Most aminoaciduria occurs in newborns and infants and is caused by inherited metabolic defects.

After all of these tubular actions on the GF, the remaining fluid is waste—urine. The principal waste products in urine are nitrogenous wastes from protein metabolism, acids from carbohydrate and fat metabolism for energy, which are normally eliminated in urine and in exhaled air. Toxins and drugs not metabolized by the liver are also eliminated in urine. The principal nitrogenous waste products in urine are **urea** and **creatinine**. *The Clinical Side*, "Blood BUN and Creatinine," discusses the importance of measuring both the amount of nitrogen in urea in blood (**blood urea nitrogen [BUN]**) and the amount of blood creatinine.

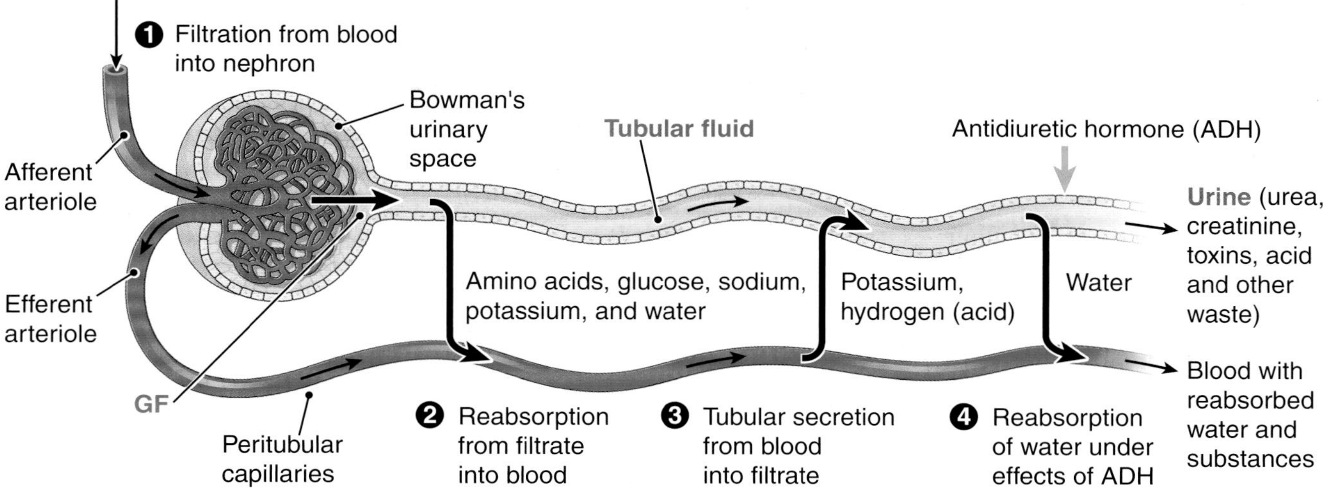

Figure 15.4 **Tubular processing of the glomerular filtrate.** Under normal circumstances, the tubule completely reabsorbs from GF all glucose and amino acids. The tubules reabsorb a variable amount of water to adjust plasma osmolarity, and secrete variable amounts of hydrogen and electrolytes to adjust plasma pH and electrolyte concentration. Toxins, creatinine, and urea pass unaltered into urine.

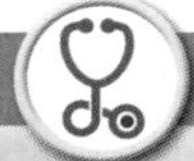

The Clinical Side

BLOOD BUN AND CREATININE

Blood urea nitrogen (BUN) and creatinine are the two most commonly ordered blood tests used to assess renal function because they are indexes of the waste disposal activity of the kidney.

Urea is produced by the liver from products of protein metabolism. Its level in blood is determined by measuring the nitrogen content of urea (BUN). Normally, urea passes freely from the glomerulus into the GF. Blood urea levels rise with declining renal function. Patients with large muscle mass or who consume a diet especially high in protein, however, may have BUN measurements that are near the upper end of normal because they are breaking down more protein, though usually not enough to produce abnormally high levels.

Creatinine is also a product of protein breakdown and also passes freely into the GF, but it does not depend on liver metabolism. Blood creatinine level is, therefore, directly related to glomerular function and is a more reliable indicator of renal performance. Blood creatinine level rises as renal function declines—in general every doubling of blood creatinine level indicates a halving of glomerular function.

Normal urine contains varying amounts of sodium, potassium, and other electrolytes that vary according to diet, exercise, hydration, metabolism, and kidney function. Finally, urine concentration (specific gravity, osmolality) varies according to the body's need to conserve or excrete water to maintain normal blood osmolality.

Pop Quiz

15.3 True or false? The presence of protein in urine is an abnormal finding.

15.4 True or false? The majority of GF leaves the body as urine.

15.5 What two blood tests are used to measure kidney health?

Urine

Normal urine is odorless, sterile, crystal clear, and pale yellow. The pH is slightly acidic (metabolism produces excess acid) and varies from about 4.5 to 8.0, and in the first-morning void is typically about 6.0. Urine may become slightly alkaline (pH >7.0) after meals as secretion of gastric acid produces an "alkaline tide" in blood and urine. Normal specific gravity of a first-morning urine is 1.016–1.022, which will fall during the day with fluid intake. Urine contains no RBCs or WBCs but may contain a few uroepithelial cells shed from the lining of the urinary tract. It contains no protein or glucose.

Descriptions of illness caused by urinary disease depend in part upon special terms that define urinary abnormalities, most of which end in "uria." Following is a list of useful terms:

- *Aminoaciduria*: a disorder of protein metabolism in which excessive amounts of amino acids are excreted in the urine
- *Anuria*: little or no urine output
- *Bacteriuria*: bacteria in urine
- *Diuresis*: increased urine output, especially in response to therapy or change in physiologic condition
- *Dysuria*: painful urination
- *Glycosuria*: glucose in urine
- *Hematuria*: intact RBCs in urine
- *Hemoglobinuria*: free hemoglobin in urine (hemoglobin not contained within RBCs)
- *Lipiduria*: fat in urine
- *Nocturia*: urination at night—getting up once is normal; twice is abnormal
- *Oliguria*: less than normal urine output
- *Polyuria*: more than normal urine output
- *Proteinuria*: protein in urine
- *Pyuria*: WBCs (pus) in urine

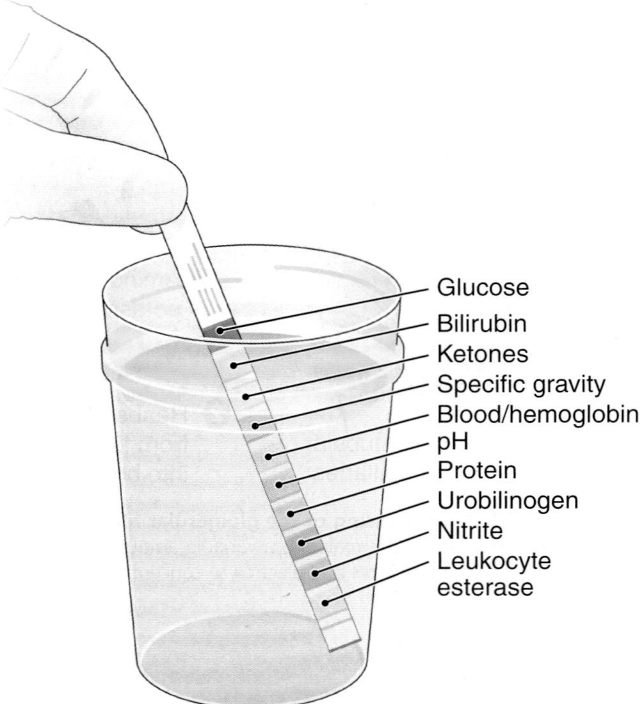

Figure 15.5 **Urinalysis.** Fresh or refrigerated urine tested by dipstick method. The intensity of color change is proportional to concentration. Microscopic examination of urinary sediment is a separate task.

Urinalysis Is Laboratory Analysis of Urine

The best specimen for urinalysis is obtained by catheterization. Otherwise, the first urine voided upon arising is best because it is the most condensed (highest specific gravity) and gives an indication of the concentrating power of the kidneys. A midstream specimen is best and is obtained by having the patient pass a small amount of urine into the toilet before collecting the urine specimen. This technique ensures that mucus, semen, or bacteria from the urethra is washed away, leaving the urine specimen representative of bladder urine. Specimen collection technique in females is especially important because the urethra in females is much shorter than in males, and the specimen can easily be contaminated by vaginal blood, mucus, or inflammatory exudate.

Specimens should be collected in special-purpose, clean, disposable containers that should never be reused. Specimens for culture should be collected in a sterile container. All specimens should be tested quickly, refrigerated, or preserved by a special additive. If left standing at room temperature for more than a short time, all urine characteristics begin to change. Bacteria proliferate, adding to the change by their metabolism; for example, urine glucose can be decreased as bacteria use glucose for fuel.

Urine Is a Diagnostically Useful Fluid

Typically, urine is tested in large laboratories by automated analyzers, or in the office or at the bedside with a strip of stiff paper (**dipstick**) containing bands of chemicals that test for various urine characteristics and substances (Fig. 15.5) indicated by color changes in the band. The density of color change corresponds to the degree of abnormality. Results are semiquantitative: negative, trace, 1+, 2+, 3+, and 4+. The specimen is then centrifuged and the sediment studied microscopically for cells, crystals, bacteria, and other formed elements (Fig. 15.6). Below is a brief description of some of the more important urine abnormalities:

- *Bacteria*: Urinary tract sterility is maintained by the flushing action of urine flow and antimicrobial properties of the urinary epithelium. Dipstick tests can reveal evidence of bacterial infection by testing for urine *nitrite*, which is produced by gram-negative bacterial metabolism. The detection of *leukocyte esterase* suggests high numbers of leukocytes (WBC), also an indicator of infection. Urine positive for either must be examined microscopically for bacteria and inflammatory cells or other formed elements, and cultured if necessary. Urine culture should be performed if laboratory and clinical findings suggest infection.
- *Bilirubin and bile pigments*: Bilirubin is not normally present in urine. Most types of jaundice (Chapter 12) are associated with bilirubin in urine (**bilirubinuria**). *Urobilinogen* is produced in the intestine by bacterial digestion of bilirubin secreted by the liver. Some of it is reabsorbed and excreted normally in urine. Jaundice due to biliary obstruction is associated with decreased amounts of bilirubin reaching the intestine, which causes urine urobilinogen to decrease or disappear. Urobilinogen is usually increased in other types of jaundice.

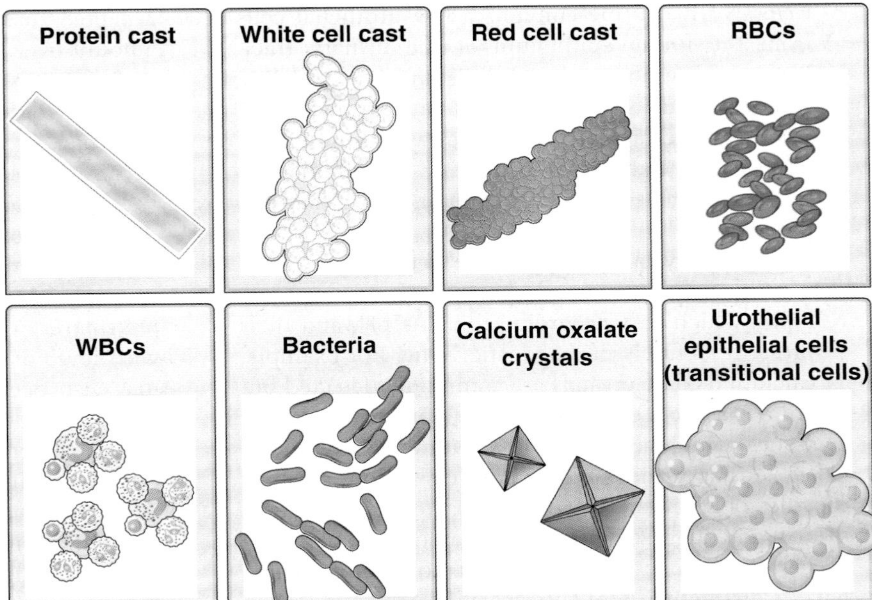

Figure 15.6 **Microscopic examination of urinary sediment.** Some of the more common formed elements found in urine are shown here.

- *Color and clarity*: The most common cause of abnormal urine color is medication. Increased urine bilirubin occurs in jaundice and imparts a dark yellow–brown color. A large volume of intact red cells turns urine dark red and opaque (depending on the number of red cells). In contrast, urine that contains hemoglobin from lysed (destroyed) red cells is red and clear. Cloudy urine is abnormal and usually caused by precipitated chemicals or cells. All cloudy urine should be examined microscopically.
- *Glucose*: Normal urine contains no glucose. By far the most common cause of *glycosuria* is diabetes mellitus; however, many other relatively uncommon conditions are capable of causing glycosuria. Sometimes other sugars can cause a false-positive test for glucose; for example, congenital galactosemia, a treatable genetic disease, may give a false-positive.
- *Blood*: Blood in urine occurs in two forms:
  - **Hematuria** is intact red cells in urine. It is not unusual to find an occasional RBC by careful microscopic examination of centrifuged urinary sediment, but there is disagreement about the number required for concern. Hematuria can be caused by renal disease or by disease elsewhere in the urinary tract. There are two types of hematuria: **gross hematuria** is blood in urine visible to the naked eye. **Occult hematuria** (asymptomatic microscopic hematuria) is grossly normal-appearing urine that contains *intact* red cells. It is usually found incidentally on microscopic study during routine urinalysis. Perhaps the most common cause is contamination of urine by menstrual blood in females. The cause of occult hematuria is not always demonstrable. In uncontaminated specimens for which a cause is found, the most common causes are *thin basement membrane disease (TBMD)* and *IgA nephropathy*, both discussed below.
  - **Hemoglobinuria**: Normal urine contains no *free* hemoglobin (hemoglobin apart from intact red cells). Dipstick testing will register positive for hemoglobin in the presence of either intact RBC or free hemoglobin. Any amount detected is abnormal. Free hemoglobin is determined to be present if the dipstick registers positive for blood but no RBC are present by microscopic study. The presence of free hemoglobin in urine may reflect free hemoglobin in blood secondary to hemolytic anemia (Chapter 7), or it may be due to hemolysis of red cells in urine. Hemoglobin in urine, whether hematuria or hemoglobinuria, is often dark due to metabolic alteration of hemoglobin by urine.
- *Ketones:* Normal urine contains no ketones. Any amount detected by dipstick is abnormal. The most important cause of ketonuria is diabetic ketoacidosis, which occurs because people with diabetes must burn fat instead of glucose. Patients who are fasting or on a low carbohydrate diet can develop ketonuria because they must burn fat instead of glucose.
- *Microscopic study of centrifuged urinary sediment:* Microscopic study identifies formed elements (Fig. 15.6).
  - *Casts:* Casts are cylindrical formations of compacted protein, red or white cells, or epithelial cells in the lumen of renal tubules, and always indicate renal disease (i.e., they are pathologic). Protein casts indicate severe proteinuria of the type seen with nephrotic syndrome (discussed below). Red cell casts indicate glomerular bleeding into the GF, a strong suggestion of glomerular disease as opposed to blood arising in the collecting system. White cell casts indicate inflammation in the kidney as opposed to inflammation in the collecting system.

- *Cells*: Normal urine contains a few urothelial cells from the lining epithelium of the urinary tract. Increased numbers of red cells indicate bleeding somewhere in the urinary tract or contamination, usually from vaginal blood. Increased numbers of white cells indicate infection or contamination, which in females is usually from vaginal inflammatory exudate.
- *Crystals*: Crystals in the urine sediment are not usually an indication of disease. There are many types, which vary according to urine pH, and their presence is rarely of diagnostic value. For example, calcium oxalate crystals are commonly detected but are not associated with the development of urinary stones, which often contain calcium oxalate.

- *Odor*: Normal urine is nearly odorless. A foul smell or the odor of ammonia is caused by bacterial metabolism of urea and suggests bacterial contamination of a stale specimen. Ketones in urine (diabetic ketoacidosis) have a distinctive odor, which smells somewhat like acetone in fingernail polish remover.
- *pH*: Both strict vegetarian and high-protein diets tend to produce alkaline urine because both diets are high in protein. Also, alkaline urine is often caused by bacterial contamination in a stale, unrefrigerated specimen. In generalized acidosis (e.g., the acidosis of respiratory failure and CO_2 retention) the kidneys excrete acid, and urine pH can be very acidic (pH <4.5).
- *Protein*: The kidneys normally keep proteins from being excreted, with only a very small amount lost in the urine, usually too little to be detected by dipstick. Protein in urine is referred to as *proteinuria*. Some regard dipstick detection of a trace of protein as abnormal; others require a 1+ positive result before considering the result abnormal. A more definitive assessment of proteinuria is quantitative assay of the amount of protein excreted in 24 hours. The most commonly accepted quantitative definitions of proteinuria are any amount over 150 mg/day or 5 mg/dL.

  Intermittent (transient) proteinuria is normal in about 5% of people. *Occult* proteinuria, only detectable by urinalysis, is protein in urine without clinical signs or symptoms. Like occult hematuria, it is discovered incidentally and may have serious or not-so-serious implications. Some people spill plasma protein into urine only when erect and not when lying down (*orthostatic* or *postural proteinuria*); others develop *physiologic proteinuria* with vigorous exercise or in association with fever or other temporary conditions. Proteinuria may also occur with a urinary tract infection (UTI). *Persistent proteinuria*, however, indicates renal disease. The most serious implication of occult proteinuria is glomerular disease or renal damage from hypertension.
- *Specific gravity*: Specific gravity is a measure of the concentration of dissolved substances (solutes), mainly urea and sodium. The specific gravity of water is 1.000. A first-morning specimen with specific gravity >1.022 indicates normal renal concentrating capacity. Otherwise, increased specific gravity is usually caused by dehydration, but increased amounts of solute (e.g., glucose or protein) can also be responsible. Low specific gravity is often caused by excessive fluid intake, and by the ethanol in alcoholic beverages (ethanol inhibits the action of pituitary antidiuretic hormone, Chapter 19).

Pop Quiz

15.6 True or false? Hemoglobinuria is the presence of hemoglobin within intact RBCs in the urine.

15.7 Define proteinuria.

Section 2: Obstruction, Stones, and Neoplasms

Case Study

"My personal plumbing is a mess." The case of Earl C.

Chief Complaint: Unable to urinate

Clinical History: Earl C. was a 61-year-old African American man who presented to the emergency room because he was unable to urinate. After catheterization delivered 300 ml of urine, the physician obtained a medical history. "My personal plumbing is a mess," Earl said. "It began with that bladder cancer." He said 15 years earlier in another city he'd had blood in his urine and "surgery through my

"My personal plumbing is a mess." The case of Earl C. (continued)

penis" to remove a "small cancer" and had been examined for tumor recurrence the next two years. "We moved here not long after that and I just never found the time to hook up with a new urologist."

Further questioning revealed he had "a bladder infection" after surgery, which had cleared with antibiotics. He said "I was doing okay until a few years ago when the bladder infection came back." He'd been treated with antibiotics on three occasions and felt fine until the last year when he began to have difficulty starting his urine stream and maintaining it. "I stand there at the urinal starting and stopping and dribbling away. I wish I could dribble as well on the basketball court! But it's not so funny anymore. I stand there in the locker room for what seems like an hour while the guys razz me that my pee time is going to cause us to miss our tea time. But bad as that is, it isn't the worst. A few weeks ago I was at a picnic and needed to go, but it took a long time to find the toilet and I lost control. I've never been so embarrassed." He went on to say that he'd been getting up at night to empty his bladder. "It's up to two or three times now. I've been intending to see someone about it, but I never got around to it. Now this."

Review of medical systems revealed his health had been good except for his urinary problems. He smoked "about half a pack a day" and had been doing so since he was in college.

Physical Examination and Other Data: He was a stocky, muscular man who appeared a bit overweight and was irritated at having to wear a catheter. Vital signs were normal except for blood pressure: 138/88. Abnormalities were confined to the urinary tract. Digital rectal exam revealed an enlarged, firm and slightly tender prostate. Blood was collected for routine tests and prostate specific antigen (PSA). Urine was submitted for urinalysis and culture. Two days later, the culture grew a few colonies of *E. coli* and the PSA was 5.6 ng/ml (normal <2.5). Complete blood count (CBC) and other blood chemistries were normal except for creatinine 1.4 mg/dL (normal <1.2).

Clinical Course: Concluding that Earl had benign prostatic hyperplasia (BPH), prostatitis, and urinary infection, the physician gave him drugs to relax prostate and bladder tension and a loading dose of oral broad-spectrum antibiotic for prostatitis and UTI. The catheter was withdrawn and Earl was sent home on antibiotics after demonstrating that he could urinate. He returned a week later for post void catheterization to measure the extent of urine retention. After voiding, he still had 145 ml of urine in his bladder. He returned home but was readmitted two days later with a second episode of acute urinary obstruction. He was recatheterized and scheduled for surgery. Preoperative prostate imaging revealed his prostate to be about 76 grams with no evidence of carcinoma. Transurethral prostatectomy was performed. Intraoperative examination of the bladder revealed no evidence of bladder cancer recurrence. He was discharged on the third hospital day and recovered well except for expected incontinence for several weeks.

Pathologic study of the prostate chips removed at surgery revealed prostatic hyperplasia and moderate-to-severe chronic inflammation. No prostatic carcinoma was present. The pathology report from his bladder cancer was obtained. The final diagnosis was low-grade papillary urothelial carcinoma; no evidence of invasion.

He was scheduled to return for a discussion with his physician about follow-up and treatment options for his various urologic problems.

Case Notes

15.1 What was the name of the muscle that contracted to expel Earl's urine?

15.2 Which sphincter did Earl C. relax voluntarily to urinate?

15.3 Did Earl have nocturia?

Urinary Obstruction

Just as a healthy nephron unit requires normal flow of blood through the glomerulus and normal flow of GF through the tubule, a healthy urinary system requires normal flow of urine. Normal urine flow depends on an unobstructed collecting system, on waves of peristalsis in the ureters to massage urine downward, and on normal function of the UVJ, which prevents urine in the bladder from regurgitating up the ureters.

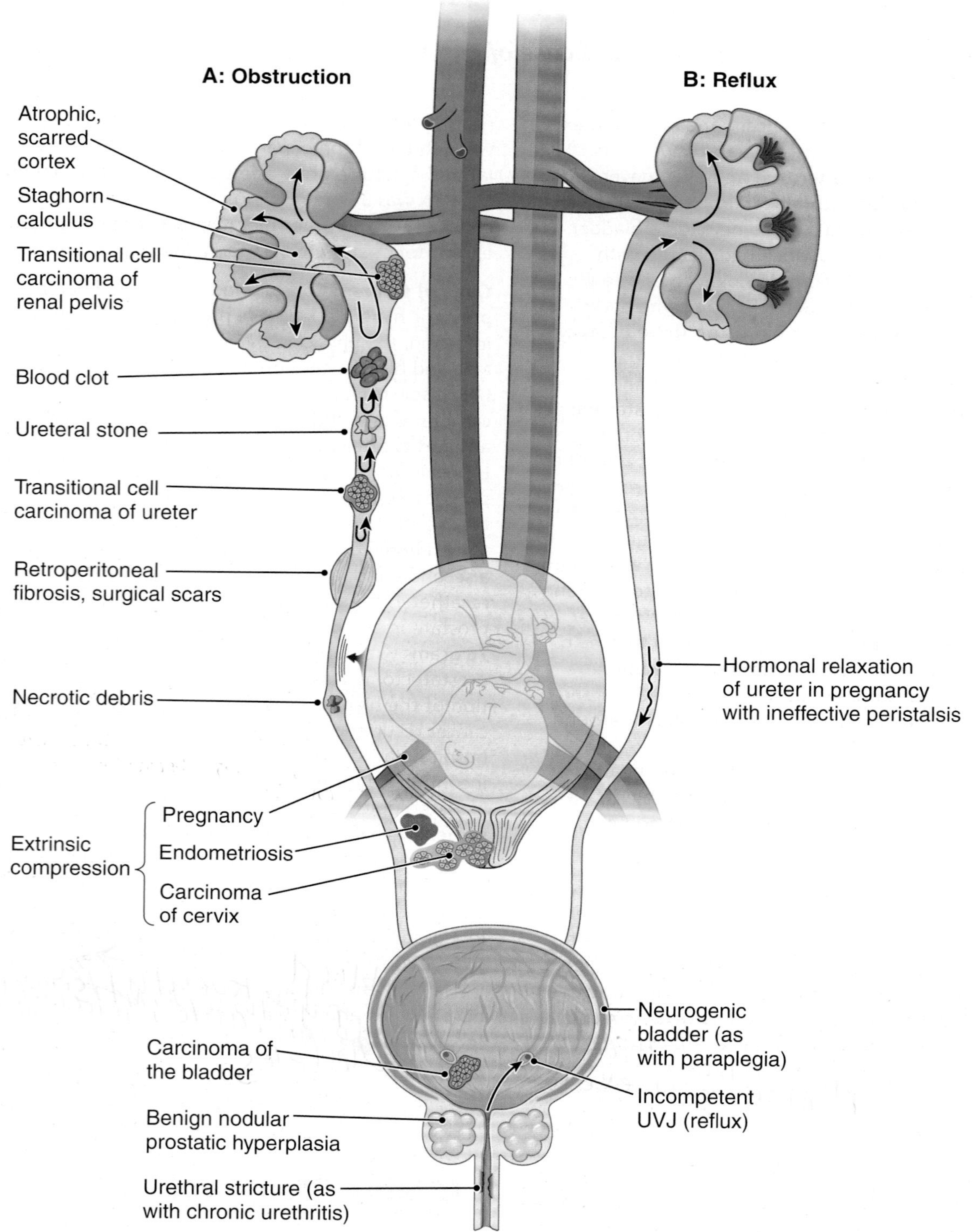

Figure 15.7 **Urinary obstruction and reflux. A.** Causes of urinary obstruction. **B.** Causes of reflux.

Urinary obstruction (Fig. 15.7A) can be unilateral or bilateral, partial or complete, sudden or insidious, arise at any level of the urinary tract, and can owe to events intrinsic to the urinary tract (e.g., ureteral obstruction by a urinary stone) or extrinsic (e.g., pressure from abdominal tumor). The causes are the following:

- Congenital anomalies that obstruct flow or allow for ureterovesical reflux
- Urinary stones (calculi)
- Benign prostatic hyperplasia (Chapter 16)
- Neoplasms (e.g., carcinoma of the bladder or prostate, carcinoma of the cervix)

- Inflammation (e.g., prostatitis, urethral strictures, surgical scars, retroperitoneal fibrosis)
- Blood clots or necrotic debris from necrosis of the tips of renal pyramids
- Pregnancy (external ureteral pressure)
- Uterine prolapse and cystocele (Chapter 17)

Acute obstruction is likely to cause flank pain due to stretching of the renal capsule of the affected kidney if the obstruction is above the bladder (e.g., a stone at the outlet of the renal pelvis). Acute obstruction below the bladder (e.g., acute prostatitis with severe edema) invariably presents as intense urinary urgency with an inability to void.

Chronic unilateral obstruction (e.g., ureteral) may be silent even as backpressure causes pathological changes. The unaffected kidney is able to maintain waste elimination and tubular water resorption, so that azotemia and lack of concentrating power do not appear. When symptoms appear, they are usually associated with hypertension, stone formation, or infection associated with the affected kidney. Chronic *bilateral partial* obstruction (e.g., in the prostate or urethra) may be manifested only by hypertension, and loss of concentrating power with polyuria and nocturia unless symptoms of complications occur. Effects on the kidney from chronic bilateral partial obstruction are similar to urinary reflux (Fig. 15.7B) discussed earlier. *Bilateral complete* obstruction is incompatible with life unless obstruction is relieved. The usual site at the neck of the bladder or the prostate—for example, obstruction caused by urethral stricture or prostatic enlargement—usually produces a painfully full bladder that prompts quick attention. If obstruction is diagnosed and relieved promptly, full renal function usually returns.

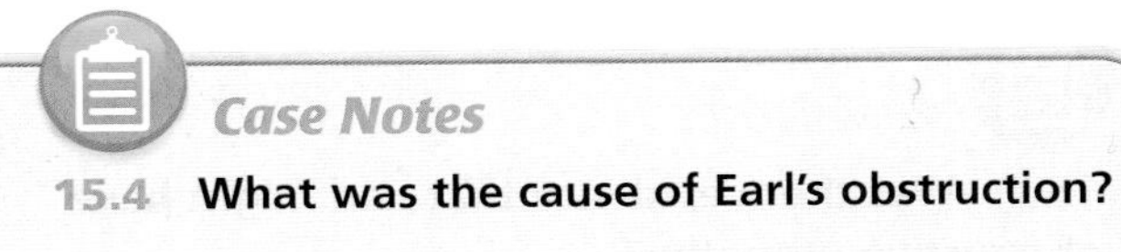

15.4 **What was the cause of Earl's obstruction?**

In older men, the most common causes of obstruction are pathologic enlargement of the prostate. In younger men, the cause is usually urethral scars (strictures) caused by infection with sexually transmitted disease. Typically, prostate or urethral obstruction prevents the bladder from emptying completely, which in turn causes urinary stasis and frequent urination (because a partially emptied bladder refills quickly). Complete obstruction of urine flow is a very uncomfortable medical emergency that requires immediate catheterization. Treatment for prostatic obstruction is **transurethral resection (TUR)** of periurethral prostate. Urethral strictures are harder to treat definitively. Dilation is effective. Other options include a flexible stent or a relaxing incision of the scar to release the constriction. In any case, permanent success occurs in less than half of cases and repeated treatment becomes necessary.

Obstructive uropathy is the effect of urinary tract obstruction on the kidney. Persistent obstruction causes chronic renal TIN, scarring, and atrophy with dilation of the renal pelvis and blunting of the renal pyramids. This anatomic condition is commonly referred to as **hydronephrosis** (Fig. 15.8), which is synonymous with *obstructive uropathy*. Importantly, obstruction encourages UTI and urinary stone formation (discussed below). It is not unusual to see the three together.

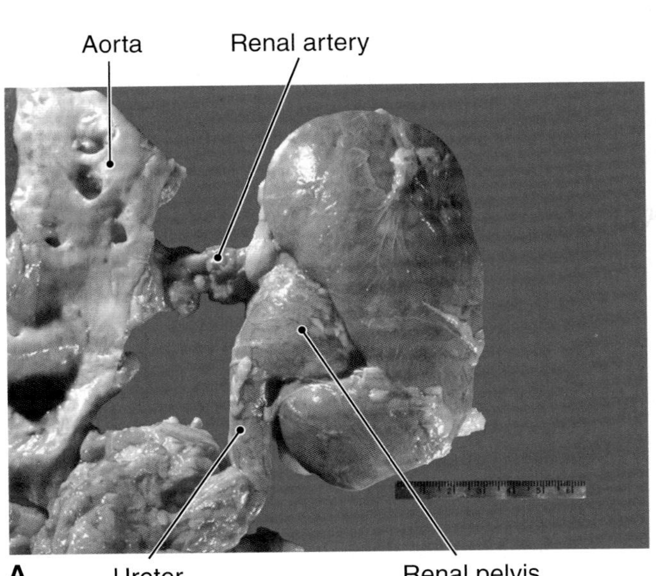

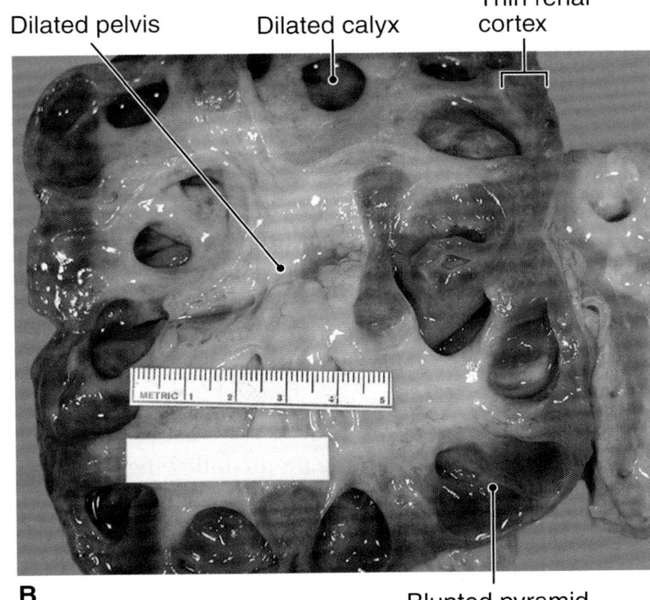

Figure 15.8 **Unilateral urinary obstruction with hydronephrosis. A.** The renal pelvis and ureter are dilated and tense with obstructed urine. **B.** The pelvis and calyces are markedly dilated and the cortex is thin, reflecting loss of functional tissue.

Case Notes

15.5 Was there evidence that Earl might have obstructive uropathy?

Diagnosis depends on presence of the clinical picture, urinalysis, blood BUN and creatinine, catheterization, or other urologic investigation of the collecting system, and imaging. Treatment is relief of obstruction.

An uncommon cause of obstruction is **sclerosing retroperitoneal** fibrosis, an inflammatory condition usually of unknown cause that occurs in conjunction with certain drugs, autoimmune disorders, and lymphomas. It features proliferation of scarlike tissue in the retroperitoneum. It tightly encases the ureters, impairs peristalsis, obstructs urine flow, and causes urinary stasis. Treatment is surgical mobilization of the ureters.

Pop Quiz

15.8 True or false? The most frequent cause of urinary obstruction in young men is urethral stricture, usually caused by sexually transmitted disease.

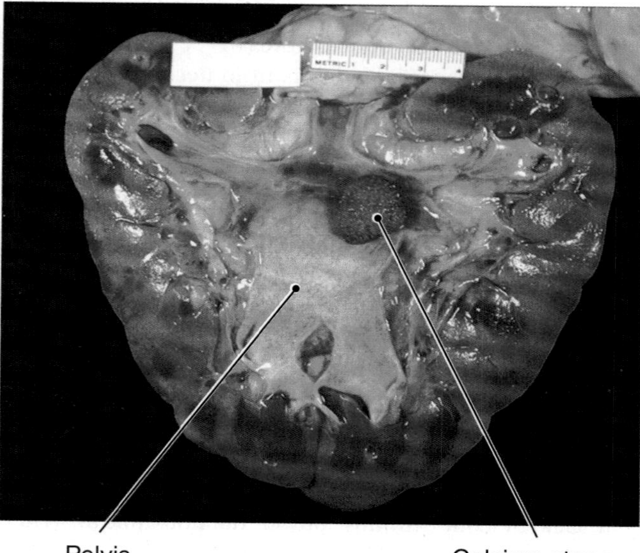

Figure 15.9 **Nephrolithiasis: calcium stone in the renal pelvis.** Dark brown coloration of the stone is a result of absorbed, discolored blood from hematuria induced by the stone.

Urolithiasis

Urolithiasis is the condition of having stones (*calculi*) in the urinary tract. It is a common condition, affecting 5–10% of Americans at some point in their lives. Most stones form in the kidney, a condition termed **nephrolithiasis**. Men are more often affected than women. Peak incidence is ages 20–30. Hereditary predisposition is a strong factor, and patients with some genetic metabolic diseases (e.g., gout, aminoaciduria) excrete in urine very large amounts of metabolic products that may crystallize into stones. The stones may be numerous and as small as grains of sand, or they may grow large enough to completely fill the renal pelvis. About 80% are unilateral.

There are Four Main Types of Stones

The four main types of stones are the following:

1. *Calcium stones* (Fig. 15.9): About 75% of stones are composed mainly of *calcium*. Typically, these stones are hard and dark because blood has accumulated in tiny crevasses of the stone surface, where sharp edges of the stone have gouged urinary epithelium. Most patients have increased levels of *urinary* calcium, but *blood* calcium levels are increased only in about 40%—a minority of these patients have hyperparathyroidism or other causes of hypercalcemia. Whatever the cause, urine becomes supersaturated with calcium, which precipitates and slowly accumulates to form a stone.
2. *Magnesium stones*: About 20% of stones are composed mainly of *magnesium*. Typically, these stones are softer and more breakable (friable) than calcium stones. Bacterial infection changes urine pH from acidic to alkaline, which causes the formation of magnesium stones. Stones and infection are especially problematic because the combination encourages a vicious circle of obstruction and stasis, stone formation, and further obstruction and stasis.
3. *Uric acid stones*: About 5% of stones are composed mainly of uric acid. About 25% of patients with gout (Chapter 18) develop uric acid stones; however, most patients with uric acid stones do not have gout or high levels of blood uric acid.
4. *Cystine stones:* About 1% of stones are composed of cystine (rarely other amino acids) excreted in urine in high concentration in certain genetic metabolic diseases (the *aminoacidurias*).

Certain conditions encourage stone formation:

- Stasis, obstruction, infection
- Increased concentration of stone constituents in urine, such as hypercalciuria in hypercalcemia (of any cause), or aminoaciduria
- Decreased urine volume with dehydration, which concentrates urine and raises the concentration of stone-forming substances
- Changed pH

Nevertheless, about half of urinary calculi form in the absence of these conditions. Conversely, some patients with high urine concentration or calcium or other stone-forming substances do not develop stones.

Signs and Symptoms Include Pain, Bleeding, and Obstruction

The clinical significance of stones derives from their ability to cause pain, bleeding, and urinary obstruction, or as a clue to an underlying condition such as hypercalcemia, infection, or aminoaciduria. Usually the first sign of a renal stone is hematuria or flank pain. As a stone or fragment passes down the ureter, it causes a distinctive and extremely painful syndrome of cramping and flank pain known as **renal colic**. A renal stone too large to pass will remain in the renal pelvis, where it may grow very large and mold itself into the shape of the calyces—called a **staghorn calculus** (Fig. 15.10), which is always associated with hydronephrosis and chronic infection. In other cases, stones are asymptomatic; some are found incidentally by X-ray or routine urinalysis that detects occult hematuria. Large stones may remain silent for a long time.

Diagnosis depends on clinical circumstances, blood calcium, urinalysis, imaging studies, and stone analysis.

Most Stones Require Treatment

Small stones may be allowed to pass with analgesic support. Some stones require transurethral endoscopic removal while others can be pulverized by ultrasound and retrieved by utereoendoscopy or allowed to pass as small stones. A few stones must be removed by ureteroendoscopy.

Prevention of repeat stone formation is worthwhile in patients with calcium stones because they are likely to develop another: 15% do so in the year following the initial episode, 40% before the end of the fifth year, and 80% by the end of the eighth year. The usual treatment is thiazide diuretics, increased fluid intake, and dietary modification to decrease sodium and increase potassium.

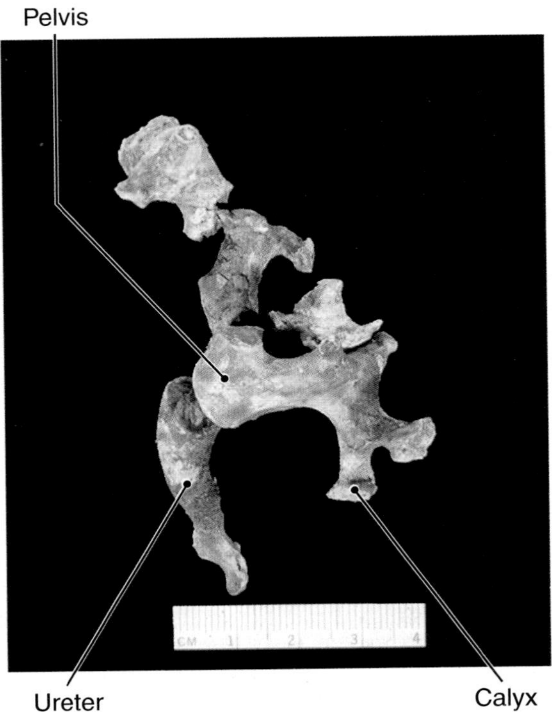

Figure 15.10 **Staghorn calculus.** The stone forms a nearly perfect image of upper ureter, renal pelvis, and calyces.

Neoplasms of the Urinary Tract

Tumors may occur at any point in the urinary tract (Fig. 15.11). Benign tumors are common and rarely cause clinical problems. They are fairly common incidental findings in medical imaging and at autopsy. Malignant tumors are much more clinically important.

Renal Cell Carcinoma Is the Most Significant Renal Neoplasm

Most tumors of the kidney are malignant, a sharp contrast to most other organ systems. Most occur in mature or older adults; men are affected more often than women.

The most significant *benign* tumor of the kidney is **oncocytoma**, which accounts for about 10–15% of renal tumors removed by surgery. Oncocytomas are rarely symptomatic and as a consequence may grow very large. Most are found incidentally and removed because they usually cannot be distinguished from malignant tumors by ordinary clinical workup. Pathologically, they are a tumor of renal tubular epithelial cells containing very large numbers of mitochondria, which swells the cytoplasm and imparts a distinctive microscopic appearance.

Renal cell carcinoma (*renal adenocarcinoma*) is a malignant neoplasm of renal tubular epithelium that accounts for about 90% of renal malignancies. In 2011, the CDC expected about 13,000 deaths and 61,000 new cases of renal cell carcinoma in the United States. Most occur in older adults. Cigarette smokers have twice the risk of nonsmokers—about one-third of renal cell carcinomas are linked to tobacco use. Many are silent for a long time and grow quite large (up to 15 cm) by the time of diagnosis. Hematuria, either gross or microscopic (occult), is often the presenting symptom, but some tumors may be large enough to find by palpating the flank of a patient presenting with flank pain. A sinister aspect of renal cell carcinoma is its tendency to invade renal veins, sometimes extending far into the inferior vena cava as illustrated in Figure 15.12, and to give rise to hematologic metastases before becoming locally symptomatic. A significant number are detected initially because of lung or bone metastasis.

Renal cell carcinomas display a variety of paraneoplastic syndromes (Chapter 5) including, but not limited to, fever of unknown origin, polycythemia, hypertension,

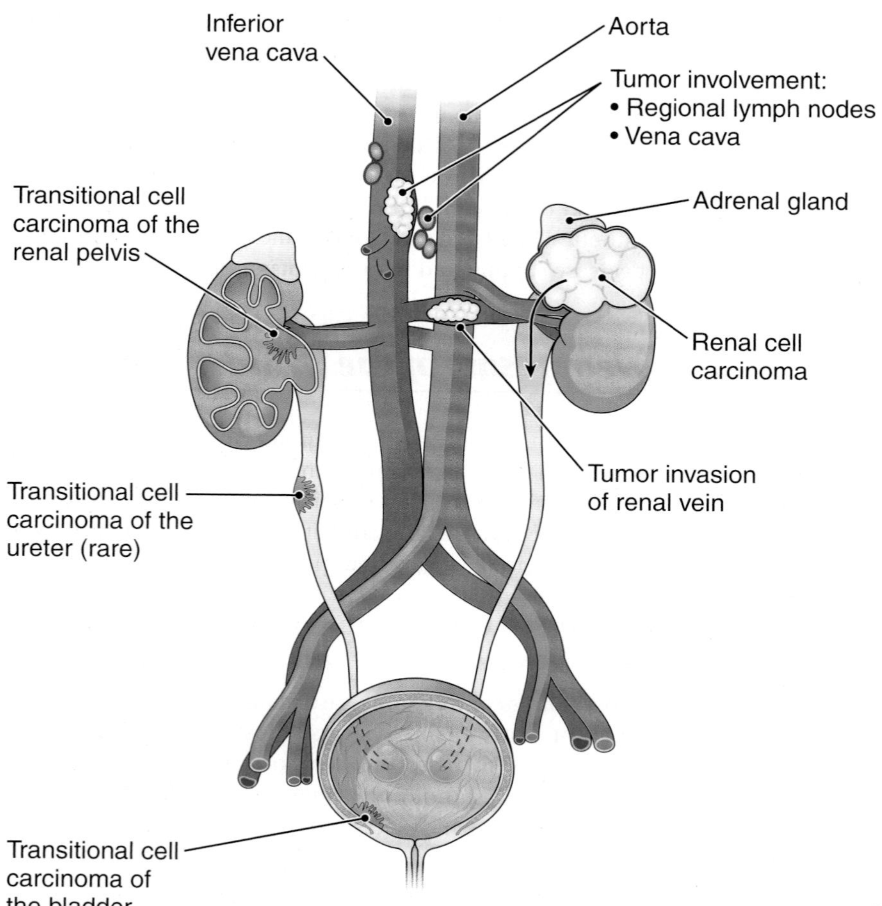

Figure 15.11 **Neoplasms of the urinary tract.**

Cushing syndrome, hypercalcemia, amyloidosis, and feminization of males or virilization of females.

Diagnosis is by medical imaging. Nephrectomy is preferred treatment for tumors without detectable metastases.

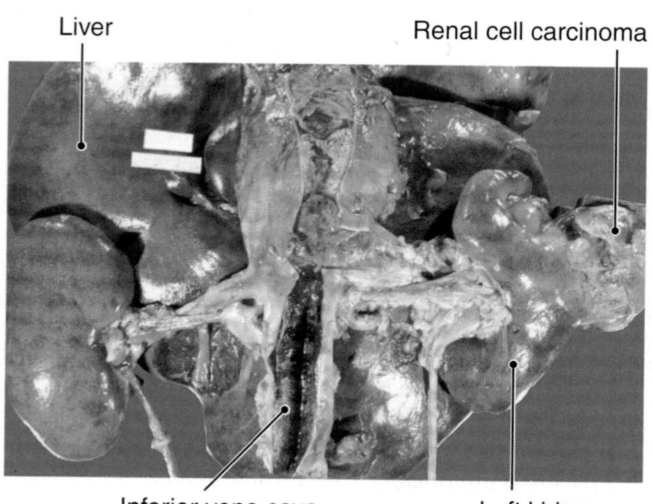

Figure 15.12 **Renal cell carcinoma.** Renal vein and vena cava are filled with invasive tumor.

Five-year survival is about 75% in patients without metastasis, about 50% in those with metastasis, and about 15% in those with grossly evident renal vein invasion.

Carcinoma of the renal pelvis arises from the lining urothelium (transitional epithelium) of the renal pelvis. It accounts for about 10% of renal malignancies. These malignancies are called *urothelial carcinoma* or *transitional cell carcinoma*. They tend to occur at multiple points in the urinary tract—about half of urothelial carcinomas of the renal pelvis are accompanied by a concurrent urothelial carcinoma of the bladder or a history of one. Urothelial carcinomas of the renal pelvis are usually papillary and fragile. They tend to fragment and bleed early—hematuria or flank pain is often the presenting symptom.

Diagnosis is by medical imaging supplemented by cytologic study of urine for malignant cells. Radical nephrectomy, including the ureter and the UVJ, is the treatment of choice. The survival rate for small, well-differentiated tumors is nearly 100%. Nevertheless, these tumors tend to invade early and the overall five-year survival rate is only about 65%. Long-term follow-up by cystoscopy is necessary because of the tendency of these patients to generate an independent carcinoma of the bladder.

Urothelial Carcinomas Occur in the Collecting System

Tumors of the collecting system almost always arise from the lining epithelium (urothelium). About 95% of tumors of the lower urinary tract are urothelial, and 95% of these occur in the bladder; the remainder occur in the ureter, renal pelvis, or renal calyces. A few adenocarcinomas, sarcomas, and other nonurothelial malignancies occur but will not be mentioned further.

The National Cancer Institute estimated that in 2012 there were about 74,000 new cases of bladder cancer and 15,000 deaths. The median age is 65, with men much more often affected than women, and Caucasians more often than African Americans, though African Americans have a worse prognosis. Incidence is highest in Egypt and nearby nations owing to schistosomiasis of the bladder. In the United States, *the most important risk factor is smoking*—smokers are about five times more likely to develop bladder cancer than nonsmokers. Urothelial tumors tend to develop simultaneously, or nearly so, at multiple sites in the same patient. Removal of one lesion does not guarantee another will not erupt fairly soon at a different location.

Case Notes

15.6 Was there any genetic or environmental factor that seems likely to have played an important role in the development of Earl's bladder cancer?

Most urothelial tumors are papillary (Figs. 15.13 and 15.14), but some are flat. The four types of papillary lesions, in order of severity, are the following:

1. **Urothelial papilloma** is a benign tumor that accounts for about 1% of urothelial neoplasms. It usually occurs in young to middle-aged adults. It is formed of unremarkable urothelium and is not precancerous (Fig. 15.13A).

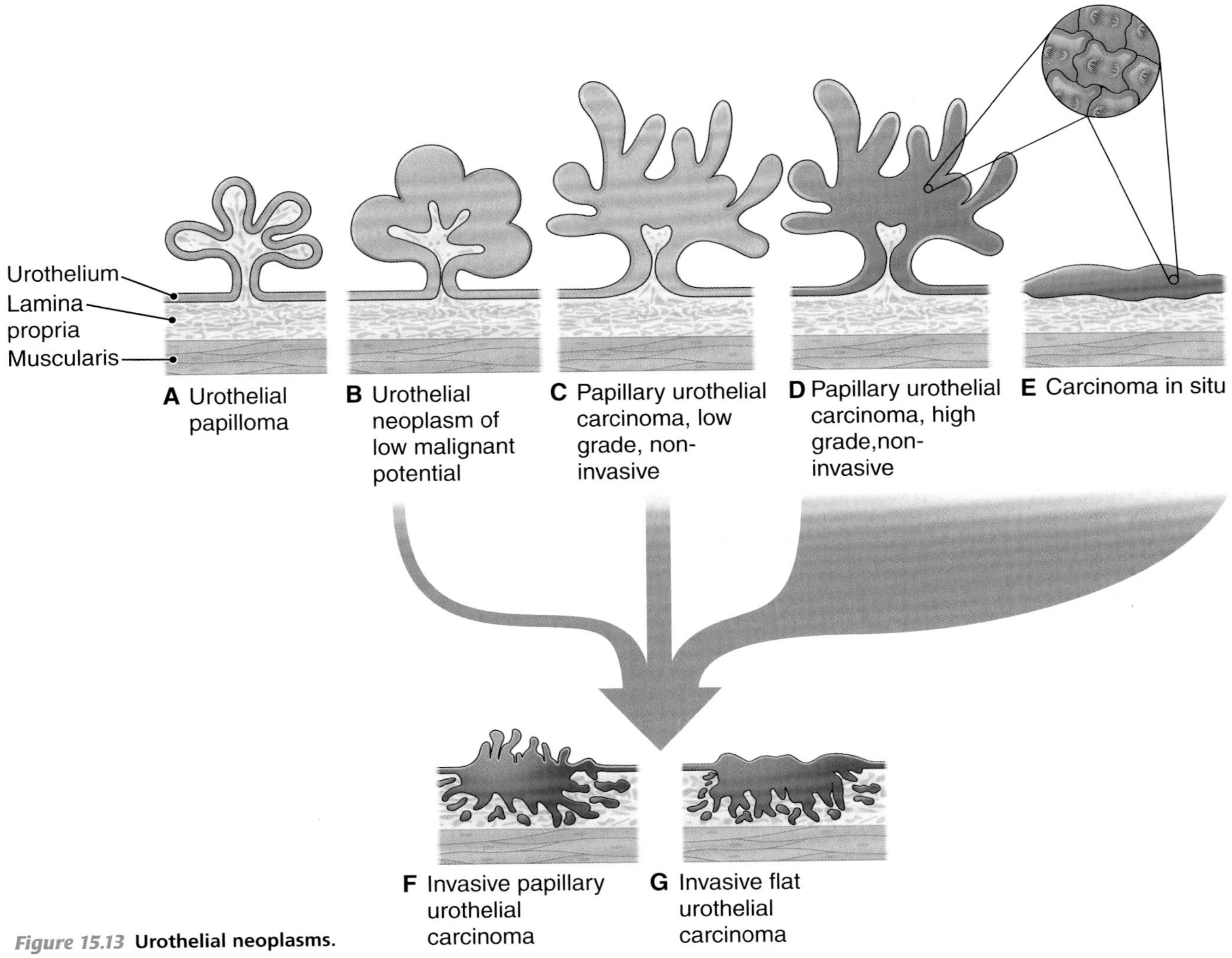

Urothelium
Lamina propria
Muscularis
A Urothelial papilloma
B Urothelial neoplasm of low malignant potential
C Papillary urothelial carcinoma, low grade, non-invasive
D Papillary urothelial carcinoma, high grade,non-invasive
E Carcinoma in situ
F Invasive papillary urothelial carcinoma
G Invasive flat urothelial carcinoma

Figure 15.13 **Urothelial neoplasms.**

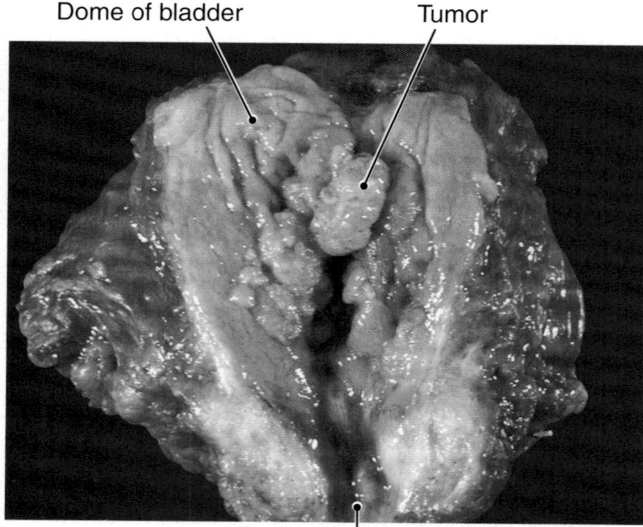

Figure 15.14 **Papillary carcinoma of the urinary bladder.**

2. **Papillary urothelial neoplasm of low malignant potential (PUNLMP)** is similar to and somewhat larger than urothelial papilloma; the urothelial cells show a limited degree of atypia (Fig. 15.13B).
3. **Low-grade papillary urothelial carcinoma** shows clear low-grade nuclear atypism, more so than PUNLMP; however, these tumors do not regularly progress to invasive carcinoma (Fig. 15.13C).
4. **High-grade papillary urothelial carcinomas** have clearly malignant, high-grade atypical cells; they frequently progress to *invasive* carcinoma (Fig. 15.13D).

Flat malignant lesions are **urothelial carcinoma in situ** (Fig. 15.13E). In most cases of invasive carcinoma, it is not clear whether the precursor lesion was a papillary or flat carcinoma in situ. Some have papillary features (Fig. 15.13F); others do not (Fig. 15.13G). Both of these precursor types lead to invasive urothelial carcinoma, but experience suggests the most common precursor is high-grade papillary carcinoma.

The fine points of pathologic diagnosis and tumor behavior are beyond the scope of this textbook, but key points are the following:

- Low-grade papillary carcinomas are usually *not* invasive at time of discovery; <10% progress to invasion. The 10-year survival rate is about 98%.
- Of high-grade papillary carcinomas, about 25% of cases are associated with invasion and death. About 80% of high-grade tumors are invasive at time of discovery.
- Of patients in whom the original lesion is carcinoma in situ, about 30% proceed to invasive carcinoma.
- Aggressive tumors invade nearby pelvic structures and metastasize widely.

Case Notes

15.7 Was Earl's urothelial tumor type unusual or common?

15.8 What was the likelihood that Earl would survive 10 years with his urothelial cancer?

Signs and Symptoms

Grossly visible painless hematuria is the most common—and often the only—symptom. All patients with gross hematuria should be considered to have a urothelial tumor in the collecting system until proven otherwise. Patients with irritative symptoms such as dysuria, urgency, and frequency occur in about one-third of cases. Carcinoma in situ (CIS) is especially likely to cause irritative symptoms without hematuria. CIS should be high on the list of possibilities in any patient with otherwise unexplainable irritative symptoms.

Remember This! Grossly visible painless hematuria should be considered a sign of urinary tract cancer until proven otherwise.

Diagnosis and Treatment

Diagnosis is by urine cystoscopic inspection with transurethral biopsy and urine cytology. Flat lesions are difficult to see by cystoscopic inspection. CIS and superficially invasive tumors are treated with TUR. After surgery the risk of recurrence can be reduced by serial intravesical instillation of chemotherapeutic agents or immunotherapy. Immunotherapy consists of installation of antigen derived from *Bacillus Calmette-Guerin* (BCG), a protein modified from the bovine tuberculosis bacterium, which stimulates a brisk immune response. Most invasive cancers are treated by complete cystectomy with urine diversion into the abdominal wall or into an ileal pouch connected to the urethra. A few invasive cancers can be treated by partial cystectomy and chemotherapy.

Tumors are staged according to the usual TNM system for tumor size, node involvement, and distant metastasis. Prognosis varies accordingly. The five-year survival rate for tumors invading the lamina propria is about 80%. For tumors invading the muscular wall, the figure is 60%; for extension beyond the bladder, about 40%; and for distant metastasis, <20%.

Case Notes

15.9 What was the cardinal symptom of Earl's bladder tumor?

Pop Quiz 

15.9 True or false? Renal cell carcinoma accounts for 90% of renal malignancies.

15.10 True or false? Precursor lesions are usually not demonstrable in high-grade urothelial malignancies.

15.11 What is the single most important risk factor in bladder cancer?

15.12 True or false? Magnesium stones are the most common type of urinary stone.

15.13 True or false? Infection is more often associated with calcium stones than with magnesium stones.

15.14 True or false? The peak incidence of stones is between ages 50 and 70.

15.15 True or false? Most patients who form a stone will never form another one.

Section 3: Disorders of the Lower Urinary Tract

These facts guide understanding of lower urinary tract disease:

- The lower urinary tract is sensitive to bacterial infection, especially infection ascending through the urethra.
- Urinary obstruction, stasis, and infection frequently occur together.
- Most tumors arise in the bladder. Bladder urothelium is more prone to develop malignancy than other urinary sites because 1) the lining urothelium is mitotically active, constantly shedding old cells and generating new ones; 2) the kidney preferentially excretes many potentially carcinogenic toxins and chemicals that bathe the epithelium; and 3) the carcinogenic effect is potentiated by the fact that urine lingers in the bladder.
- Disease usually presents with local symptoms such as urgency, dysuria, hematuria, urinary retention, and/or incontinence.

Congenital Anatomic Abnormalities

Urinary obstruction, reflux, stasis, and infection are often linked. In the lower urinary tract, congenital deformities may be the cause. **Exstrophy** of the bladder is a rare but serious congenital anomaly in which the low anterior abdominal wall and the anterior wall of the bladder fail to develop, leaving the bladder open to the environment. Surgical correction is effective, but patients usually have ureteral reflux and are at increased risk for bladder carcinoma later in life.

Normal function of the ureterovesical junction (UVJ) prevents urine in the bladder from reflux into the ureter. Sometimes the UVJ allows reflux and **vesicoureteral reflux** is the result (Fig. 15.15). Reflux creates stasis, and stagnant, high-pressure urine accumulates in the collecting system, which damages the kidney (*reflux nephropathy*, discussed later). Sometimes **congenital UVJ obstruction** is the problem. The cause is unclear. Agenesis of the opposite kidney may also be present, probably from obstruction during embryogenesis. Treatment is surgical.

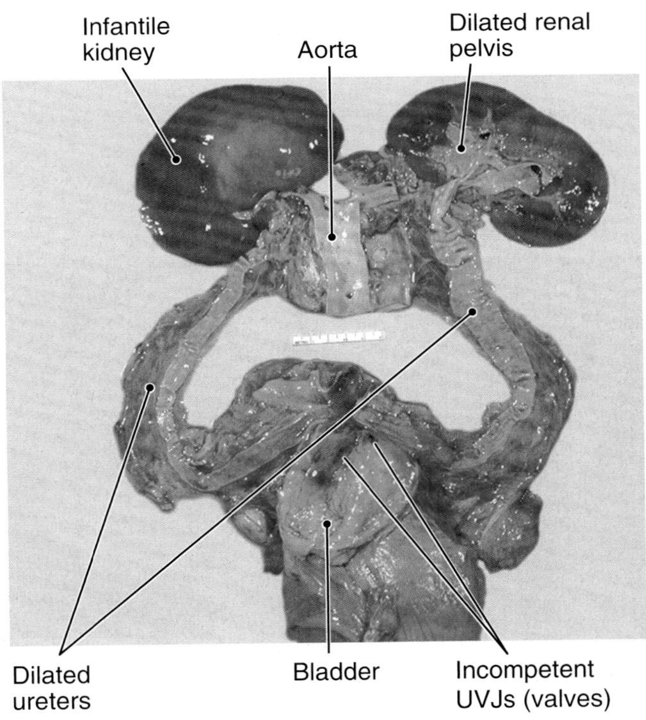

Figure 15.15 **Congenital incompetent ureterovesical junctions with bilateral hydroureter and hydronephrosis.**

Pop Quiz

15.16 Dysfunction of what anatomic structure in the collecting system predisposes a patient to infection?

Infection and Inflammation

Cystitis (Fig. 15.16) is inflammation of the bladder and is a very common problem. **Bacterial cystitis** is the most common form of **urinary tract infection (UTI)**, and is usually attributable to infection by gram-negative fecal organisms (*coliforms*) such as *Escherichia coli*. Coliforms gain access to the bladder via the urethra. Females are more often infected than males because the urethra is short and opens onto the labial mucosa, which is easily populated by bacteria from perineal skin. Infection is encouraged by sexual intercourse (*honeymoon cystitis*), urinary stasis, reflux, insertion of instruments into the bladder for diagnostic examination (*cystoscopy*), or surgery. Once the bladder is infected, infection of the kidney (pyelonephritis, discussed above) or prostate (prostatitis, discussed in Chapter 16) may follow.

Case Notes

15.10 Did Earl have a UTI?

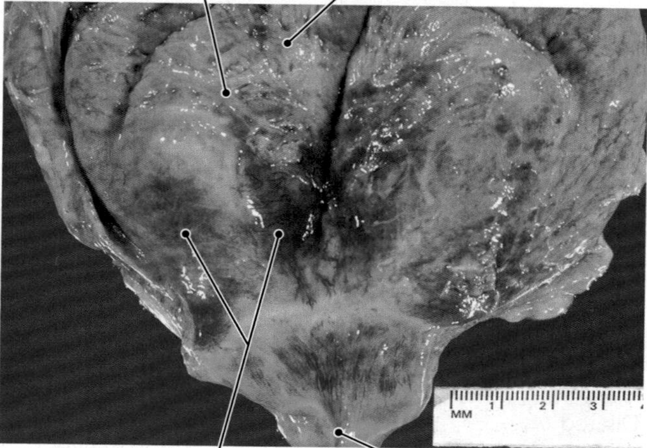

Figure 15.16 **Acute cystitis.**

Schistosomiasis is a parasitic disease that commonly causes cystitis in Egypt and nearby nations. The microorganism infects the bladder wall.

Nonbacterial cystitis is bladder inflammation without infection. A particularly severe, disabling type is **interstitial cystitis**, an especially painful chronic cystitis involving all layers of the bladder wall. It usually occurs in women and features intense chronic inflammation and mucosal ulcers (*Hunner ulcers*). The cause is unknown, but autoimmunity is suspected because it is sometimes associated with systemic lupus erythematosus (SLE) or other autoimmune diseases. Mucosal biopsy is recommended to rule out urothelial carcinoma. Therapy is supportive, experimental, and usually fruitless.

All types of cystitis feature 1) frequency and urgency (urination every 15–20 minutes in acute cases); 2) painful urination (dysuria); and 3) dull lower abdominal pain, usually immediately above the pubis. Bacterial pyelonephritis can be a complication. Diagnosis is by recognition of the clinical syndrome and urine culture. Treatment is by relief of associated conditions such as enlarged prostate or cystocele and administration of antibiotics. Women who suffer three or more UTIs per year can reduce the frequency of infection by voiding immediately after intercourse; avoiding use of IUDs, diaphragms, and spermicides; and drinking 300 ml (50 ml of concentrate) of cranberry juice daily, which acidifies the urine and reduces the rate of infection.

A less common UTI is **urethritis**, inflammation of the urethra. Sexually transmitted diseases including gonorrhea and *Chlamydia* (Chapter 4) are the most common causes. Usually urethritis is clinically symptomatic (dysuria, purulent discharge) in men because their urethra is long enough to cultivate infection; in women, the shorter urethra may be equally infected but associated infection of the female genitalia (Chapter 17) is the usual presenting complaint.

Pop Quiz

15.17 True or false? The most common cause of urethritis is a sexually transmitted disease.

15.18 Bacterial cystitis is usually caused by which type of bacteria?

Voiding Disorders

Urination (voiding) is a complex neuromuscular act with voluntary and involuntary elements. Voiding disorders are common, and although they are only rarely life threatening (rupture of the bladder), they are very serious matters to those who suffer from them.

Urinary Retention Is Incomplete Voiding or Cessation of Urination

Urinary retention is incomplete emptying of the bladder or cessation of urination. It may be acute or chronic. Causes include impaired contractility associated with neurologic conditions, bladder outlet obstruction due to enlarged prostate, inability to coordinate detrusor contraction with relaxation of the external sphincter, and drug side effects (especially drugs with anticholinergic effect). Symptoms include frequency, urgency, and overflow incontinence. Slow retention may not be painful, but acute retention is usually very uncomfortable or painful.

Diagnosis is obvious in patients who cannot void. In those who can, diagnosis is made by postvoid catheterization that recovers >100 ml of urine. Relief of acute urinary retention requires catheterization. Subsequent treatment depends on cause. In men with BPH, medications (usually α-adrenergic blockers or 5α-reductase inhibitors) or surgery may relieve bladder outlet resistance. No treatment is effective for impaired bladder contractility or neurogenic bladder—periodic self-catheterization or an indwelling catheter is required. Surgical urinary diversion may be required in some cases.

Case Notes

15.11 What was the proof that Earl had chronic urinary retention?

Urinary Incontinence Is Loss of Voluntary Control

Urinary incontinence is involuntary loss of urine. It is an embarrassing and largely hidden problem because patients often do not seek help and healthcare professionals often do not inquire about it. It may occur at any age but is more common in the elderly. About one-third of elderly women and one-sixth of elderly men are affected. It is frequently a cause for institutionalization because of the burden it imposes on caregivers. Moreover, in bedfast patients, urine irritates and macerates skin and contributes to pressure ulcers (bedsores).

Clinical patterns of incontinence vary, but there are several general types, some of which may overlap:

- *Urge incontinence* is uncontrolled leakage of moderate to large urine volume after a quick-developing and uncontrollable urge to void. Nocturia and nocturnal incontinence are usually present. It is the most common type in the elderly, but may occur at any age; for example, after use of a diuretic.
- *Stress incontinence* is urine leakage due to an abrupt increase of intra-abdominal pressure, as for example with sneezing, coughing, lifting, or laughing. It is the second most common form in women because of childbirth complications or in elderly postmenopausal women with urethral atrophy secondary to lack of estrogen support. The urethra shortens and loses closing pressure and the suppleness to ensure a tight mucosal seal.
- *Overflow incontinence* is dribbling from an overly full bladder. Loss is constant and small on each occasion but a large volume may be lost in total. It is the second most common form in men.
- *Functional incontinence* is urine loss due to cognitive or physical impairment such as dementia or stroke. Delirium, depression, and psychosis may also interfere with voluntary control or perception of need.

Case Notes

15.12 Earl reported "losing control." Which type of incontinence did he have?

Case Study Revisited

"My personal plumbing is a mess." The case of Earl C.

Earl C. presented to the emergency room unable to urinate. The diagnosis was acute urinary retention, a common but not readily explainable complication of chronic urinary obstruction due to benign prostatic hyperplasia (BPH). Earl's medical history revealed nocturia two to three times each night, a symptom suggesting chronic urinary retention from obstruction. He also reported difficulty starting his stream and had trouble maintaining it, which further suggested chronic prostatic obstruction. Digital rectal palpation confirmed that his prostate was enlarged. His prostate was also tender, which suggested the possibility of prostatitis. It was likely chronic bacterial prostatitis because he had no

(continued)

"My personal plumbing is a mess." The case of Earl C. (continued)

history of fever or pain to suggest acute prostatitis. His history of "bladder infection" after cystoscopy and bladder surgery 15 years earlier could have been cystitis or prostatitis or both. Such infections often occur after bladder instrumentation. One of the diagnoses on tissue removed by his TUR prostatectomy was "chronic prostatitis," confirming the clinical history. Further validation of infection came with the finding of a few *E. coli* in urine submitted for culture.

The pathology specimen also confirmed the presence of clinically suspected BPH.

Before beginning to resect tissue through the cystoscope, the bladder was inspected for the possible recurrence of low-grade papillary urothelial bladder cancer from 15 years earlier. No evidence of recurrence was noted, an important finding because urothelial cancers are prone to regrow even after complete removal. This precaution was especially warranted because the most important risk factor is smoking (Earl was a smoker), most urothelial neoplasms occur in middle age to older adults (Earl was 61), men are much more often affected than women, and the prognosis is worse for African Americans.

Transient incontinence is temporary and treatable. Bladder infection or irritation may cause dysuria and irresistible urgency. Excess urine production (e.g., diuretics or diabetic osmotic diuresis, Chapter 13) may also be the culprit. The list of drugs with effects on voiding is much too long to reproduce. For example, anticholinergics may impair detrusor contraction and cause overflow incontinence, and other drugs may relax the internal sphincter to cause stress incontinence.

Established incontinence is persistent and due to nerve or muscular problems. The list is long, but a few examples will convey the gist of the problem. Incontinence is a common side effect of complete prostatectomy for prostatic carcinoma. Spinal cord damage may also interfere with coordination of detrusor contraction and relaxation of urinary sphincters. Finally, diabetic neuropathy may interfere with autonomic innervation.

Diagnosis requires a very careful history and physical examination including neurologic evaluation, pelvic examination, urinalysis, urine culture, measurement of postvoid urine volume, and blood BUN and creatinine. Treatment plans can be complex and extensive. Training to change voiding habits and timing of fluid intake is generally helpful. Pelvic muscle exercise (Kegel exercise) is often effective for stress incontinence. Absorbent undergarments may be necessary. Drugs are often useful but must be used judiciously, especially in the elderly.

Case Notes

15.13 Was Earl's incontinence transient or established?

Case Notes

15.14 What was the likely initial cause of Earl's UTI?

Pop Quiz

15.19 True or false? Urge incontinence is the most common type of incontinence in the elderly.

15.20 What two categories of drugs are useful in the treatment of urinary retention in men with BPH?

15.21 True or false? The most common cause of urethritis is a sexually transmitted disease.

15.22 Bacterial cystitis is usually caused by which type of bacteria?

Section 4: Disorders of the Kidney

Case Study

"His water looks like Coca-Cola." The case of Jesus S.

Chief Complaint: Dark urine

Clinical History: Jesus S. was a 10-year-old Hispanic boy who was brought by his mother to a community health clinic in a remote part of west Texas. The nearest physician was 80 miles away. When the physician assistant (PA) asked the reason for the visit, Jesus's mother said, referring to his urine, "His water looks like Coca-Cola." She went on to say that she thought it might have been discolored the night before, but the light was poor and she couldn't be sure. This morning she noticed the toilet water was discolored after he urinated. She gave him juice and water and waited to observe for herself on his next bathroom trip about two hours later. "He's not making much water," she added.

The PA asked the usual systems review questions. Specific questioning about drug abuse, over-the-counter medicines, and exposure to toxins revealed nothing suspicious. Jesus was not taking any prescribed or over-the-counter medicines. When asked about any recent health problems, his mother revealed that he had been a picture of good health and vigor except for "a cold and a bad sore throat" a few weeks earlier.

Physical Examination and Other Data: Vital signs were: Temperature 98.5°F, heart rate 88, respirations 16, blood pressure 145/92. Jesus was quiet and not in distress and appeared to be of average height and weight. He did not appear anemic or jaundiced but his face looked round and puffy. When asked about his face, his mother said she'd noticed it but thought it was because he was tired from staying up too late the last few nights with his father branding cattle on the ranch where they lived. "I thought it was all that dust; he was sneezing a lot," she said. The remainder of the physical examination was unremarkable. He had no rash, enlarged lymph nodes, or abdominal masses.

The PA gave Jesus a big glass of water and collected some blood for the few basic tests that could be done by the office assistant on clinic equipment. Hematocrit and blood glucose were normal. Sodium and potassium were normal. BUN and creatinine were slightly increased. After two hours, Jesus passed a small amount of dark brown transparent urine, which tested strongly positive for both protein and hemoglobin by routine dipstick tests. Urinary sediment was concentrated by centrifugation. A moderate number of RBCs and a few red cell casts were noted, but they didn't seem enough to account for the strongly positive hemoglobin. No crystals or WBCs were present.

Clinical Course: The PA was puzzled. The pieces didn't seem to fit together, so she called the hospital that managed the clinic and spoke to a pediatrician, who said, "This is a classic case of acute glomerulonephritis. I haven't seen one in several years." The pediatrician outlined a treatment plan of salt restriction and therapy with diuretics and antihypertensive medication with careful monitoring of urine output. The PA dispensed the drugs from the limited supply on hand and gave Jesus's mother a calibrated, disposable urine cup, instructed her to measure Jesus's urine output and call daily with the results. His urine output was low initially but began to improve on the third day. Mother and son returned a week later. His daily urine volume had returned nearly to normal; urine hemoglobin and protein were less positive; and most of his facial swelling has disappeared. On the follow-up visit a week later, his blood pressure was near normal. A blood specimen was collected and sent to the hospital to be tested for antistreptococcal antibodies, which were detected in high concentration.

Case Notes

15.15 Other than water and waste, name some important substances Jesus excreted in his urine.
15.16 Were Jesus's kidneys part of his upper or lower urinary tract?
15.17 Jesus's blood pressure was elevated. What structure in his kidney played a role in increasing his blood pressure?
15.18 Each of Jesus's glomeruli was paired with a tubule to form a(n) ______.
15.19 Name, from inside the glomerular capillary outward, the layers of Jesus's glomerular membrane.
15.20 In Jesus's kidneys, what is the name of the first fluid that entered the renal tubules?
15.21 About what percent of Jesus's GF (1%, 9%, 19%, or 99%) was reabsorbed back into blood by the renal tubules of his nephron units?
15.22 What were the principal nitrogenous waste compounds in Jesus's urine?

Clinical Presentations of Renal Disorder

Renal disease may present as a single abnormality or as a cluster of signs and symptoms that make up one of several clinical syndromes that are typical for certain renal conditions. Some are unique to primary renal disease; others are secondary to nonrenal diseases that affect the kidney. An understanding of these syndromes requires further definition of terms.

Azotemia Is Renal Failure Manifested Only by Abnormal Laboratory Tests

Azotemia is renal failure that is manifested only by abnormal laboratory tests; no clinical signs of kidney failure are present. The root *azote-* is from the French word for nitrogen, and the most commonly detected abnormalities are increased BUN and blood creatinine. Almost any type of underlying renal disease can cause azotemia. It may be discovered in workup of urinary tract disease, but may also be discovered incidentally during examination for some other medical problem or on a routine exam, such as an employment physical. Correction of the underlying problem resolves the azotemia.

Prerenal azotemia is due to renal hypoperfusion from shock, hemorrhage, dehydration, heart failure, or any other condition in which renal blood flow is reduced as part of a broader systemic condition. Postrenal azotemia is caused by obstruction to the free flow of urine from the kidney. Relief of obstruction corrects the azotemia.

Uremia Is Renal Failure with Clinical Signs and Symptoms

Uremia (literally, "urine in blood") is renal failure that is manifested not only with increased nitrogenous wastes in the blood, but also with clinical signs and symptoms. Some of these signs and symptoms are caused by accumulation in the blood of waste products that should have been excreted by the kidneys. Others are caused by failure of other kidney functions. Uremia can be prompted by almost any type of underlying renal disease. Patients with uremia typically have the following:

- *Hypertension*, owing to increased renal output of renin due to restriction of glomerular blood flow and retention of salt and water
- *Anemia*, caused by low output of erythropoietin
- *Edema*, owing to retention of salt and water
- *Oliguria*, caused by low GFR
- Other signs and symptoms caused by accumulation of toxic metabolic waste products:
  - *Pericarditis* and *gastroenteritis* caused by the irritant effect of toxic products
  - *Bleeding/coagulation defects* caused by platelet malfunction
- Peripheral nerve disease (neuropathy) or brain dysfunction (encephalopathy)

Case Notes

15.23 What is the name for the brownish condition of Jesus's urine?
15.24 Did Jesus have proteinuria?
15.25 Jesus did not complain of dysuria. Did this suggest his bleeding was from the lower or upper urinary tract?
15.26 Jesus's urine contained RBC casts. Of what importance was this finding?
15.27 Renal stones cause hematuria. Why couldn't Jesus's hematuria be explained by a stone?
15.28 What was the name for Jesus's decreased urine output?

Acute Renal Failure Develops in Days or Weeks

Acute renal failure is uncommon and features rapid onset of azotemia and oliguria or anuria with urine output of about 400 ml/day or less. It often results from trauma or acute illness but is sometimes caused by a rapidly progressive renal disease. Clinical features include anorexia, nausea, and vomiting, and it may progress to seizures and coma if the condition is untreated. Fluid, electrolyte, and acid-base imbalances develop quickly. Diagnosis is based on laboratory tests of renal function, including serum creatinine. Treatment is directed at the cause. Fluid and electrolyte management is a major clinical challenge. Dialysis may be necessary.

Chronic Renal Failure Is a Shared Endpoint for Chronic Renal Disease

Chronic renal failure is characterized by long-standing, unremitting deterioration of renal function. It is a shared endpoint for many chronic kidney diseases. It is common and features slowly developing anorexia, nausea, vomiting, oral inflammation (stomatitis), nocturia, fatigue, pruritus (itching), loss of mental acuity, muscle cramps, water retention, tissue wasting, GI bleeding, peripheral neuropathy, and seizures.

Chronic renal failure evolves through several stages.

1. *Diminished renal reserve* is an early stage of chronic kidney disease in which the glomerular filtration rate (GFR) is about half of normal. Blood BUN and creatinine are normal.
2. *Renal insufficiency* is a more advanced stage of chronic renal disease in which the GFR is in the range of 20–50% of normal. Most patients have azotemia, anemia (from low erythropoietin output), and hypertension (due to increased renin production as a result of low glomerular blood flow). Because of decreased concentrating power, urine specific gravity is low and urine output high. Nocturia and polyuria may occur.
3. In *chronic renal failure,* GFR is <20–25% of normal. Renal regulation of blood pH and fluid and electrolyte balance is poor and patients are prone to develop edema, metabolic acidosis, and hyperkalemia. Uremia may ensue.
4. *End-stage kidney* is the final "burned out" stage of failure in most chronic renal disease. GFR is usually <5% of normal, and the patient is frankly uremic.

Some of the effects of chronic renal disease/failure on various bodily systems are the following:

- *Fluid and electrolyte balance:* dehydration, edema, hyperkalemia, metabolic acidosis
- *Bone and calcium metabolism:* hypercalcemia, hyperphosphatemia, secondary hyperparathyroidism, osteoporosis
- *Blood and bone marrow:* anemia, hemorrhagic diathesis
- *Cardiopulmonary:* hypertension, heart failure, cardiomyopathy, pulmonary edema, uremic pericarditis
- *Gastrointestinal (GI):* nausea and vomiting, bleeding, esophagitis, gastritis, colitis
- *Neuromuscular:* myopathy, peripheral neuropathy, encephalopathy
- *Skin:* pruritus, dermatitis

The pathophysiology of the development of these effects is complex and beyond the scope of this textbook.

Diagnosis is based on laboratory testing of renal function. Renal biopsy may be necessary. Treatment is primarily directed at the underlying condition. Fluid and electrolyte management is important. Many patients require erythropoietin for anemia (Chapter 7). Dialysis or transplantation may be necessary.

Case Notes

15.29 Did Jesus have azotemia or uremia?

15.30 Did Jesus have acute or chronic renal failure?

Pop Quiz

15.23 True or false? Uremia is renal failure that manifests only by laboratory tests.

15.24 True or false? Acute renal failure features rapid onset of azotemia and oliguria or anuria with urine output of about 400 ml/day.

Inherited, Congenital, and Developmental Disorder

One or both kidneys may fail to develop (**renal agenesis**). Bilateral agenesis is incompatible with life; infants are stillborn and usually have multiple other abnormalities. Unilateral agenesis is not serious; the sole kidney enlarges to maintain normal renal function.

Horseshoe kidney is a single, fused kidney. As a result of abnormal embryogenesis, the two kidneys are joined inferiorly by a thick bridge of normal, functioning renal tissue. This abnormality is often seen in patients with Turner syndrome (Chapter 22). There are usually no clinical consequences.

Cystic disease of the kidney is rather common. **Multicystic renal dysplasia** is a sporadic developmental disorder in which the fetal kidney develops as a small mass of cysts accompanied by islands of primitive cartilage and other immature tissue. It is usually unilateral. **Simple cysts** of the kidney are so commonly found at autopsy that they can be considered a normal variation

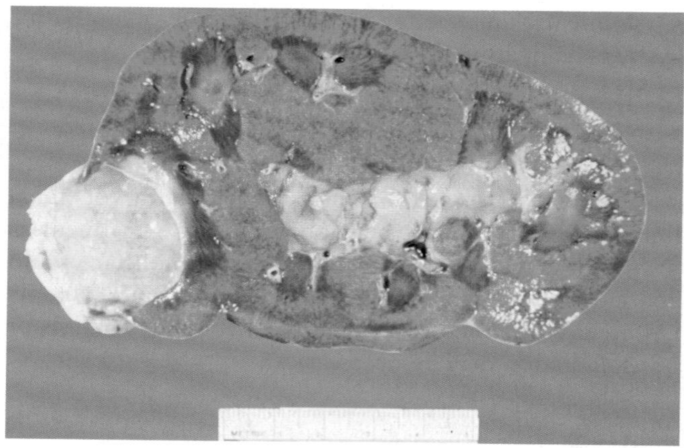

Figure 15.17 **Simple cyst of the kidney.**

(Fig. 15.17). Most are just a few millimeters in diameter, filled with clear fluid. Larger ones may be discovered incidentally in the course of radiographic exams and can pose a diagnostic problem because they appear as a kidney mass, which demands investigation.

Several types of genetic renal disease are characterized by multiple renal cysts. The most common is **polycystic kidney disease**, depicted in Figure 15.18. The two types are both caused by genetic defects. *Autosomal dominant polycystic kidney disease (ADPKD)* often is not symptomatic until adulthood. It was formerly called *adult polycystic kidney disease*. In addition to renal cysts, some patients have berry aneurysms of the circle of Willis (Chapter 19) and mitral valve prolapse. It is fairly common, accounting for about 10% of patients with chronic renal failure. Unfortunately, it usually does not become symptomatic until after age 30, by which time many patients, unaware, have passed the genetic defect to their children. It is characterized by very large kidneys riddled with thousands of expanding cysts that injure the intervening renal parenchyma and produce severe chronic TIN. Most patients come to medical attention because of hematuria, chronic UTI, or hypertension. Diagnosis is by medical imaging. Treatment is symptomatic before renal failure and transplantation afterward. About half of patients die of coronary artery disease or hypertensive heart disease. Some die of ruptured berry aneurysms.

On the other hand, *autosomal recessive polycystic kidney disease (ARPKD)* is caused by one of several autosomal recessive genetic defects and usually appears at birth as massively enlarged kidneys and a variety of other defects. It was formerly called *childhood polycystic kidney disease*. It is often associated with liver cysts and biliary ductal hyperplasia that leads to a cirrhosis-like scarring of the liver in patients who survive infancy. Most affected infants die in the perinatal period. Treatment is supportive.

Pop Quiz

15.25 True or false? The cause of death of patients with adult polycystic kidney disease is invariably renal failure.

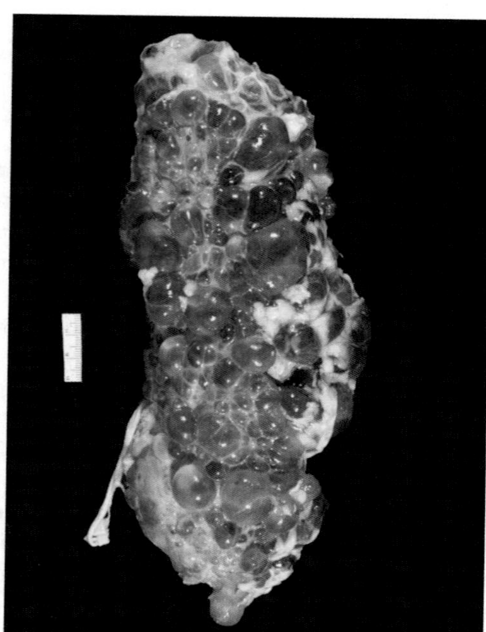

Figure 15.18 **Hereditary polycystic kidney disease.** Specimen from a 33-year-old man.

Glomerular Disorders

Glomerular diseases, especially chronic glomerulonephritis (CGN), are among the most common causes of chronic kidney disease. *Virtually all primary glomerular disease is caused by an autoimmune inflammatory reaction*, and is called **glomerulonephritis**, typically abbreviated **GN**. Conditions without an inflammatory component are called **glomerulopathy**.

Immune mechanisms cause most primary and much secondary glomerular disease. There are two varieties: injury and inflammation caused by 1) direct immune attack on the glomerulus, and 2) deposition of circulating immune complexes (Type III hypersensitivity reaction, Chapter 3). Direct attack may be of B or T cell origin and directed against antigens native to the glomerulus or deposited there from plasma. Figure 15.19 illustrates these reactions. In most instances, immunoglobulins can be demonstrated in the walls of glomerular capillaries (Fig. 15.20).

The several varieties of glomerular injury feature one of four types of tissue reaction:

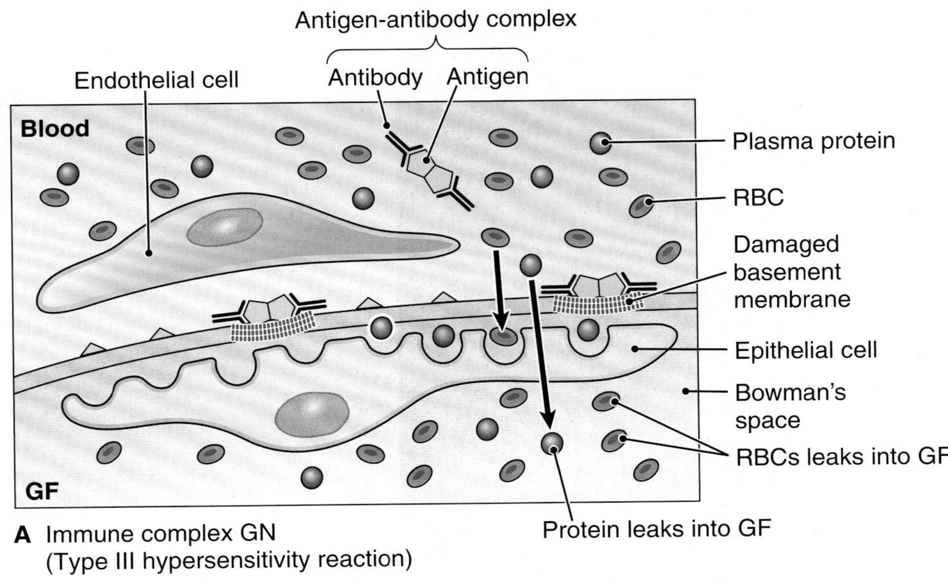

A Immune complex GN
(Type III hypersensitivity reaction)

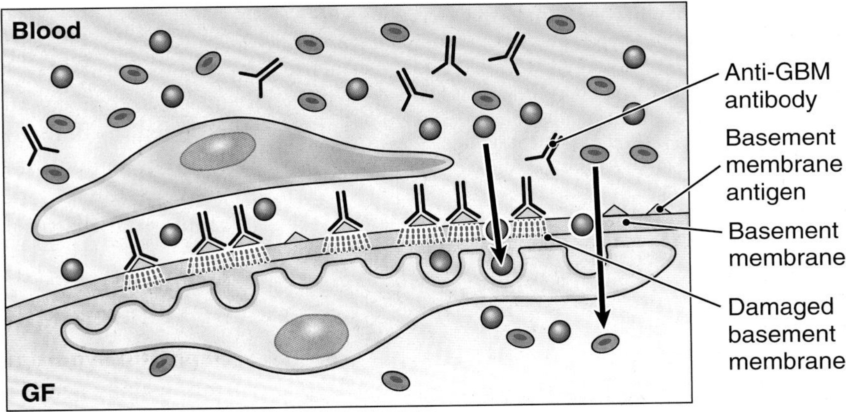

B Anti-GBM GN
(Type II hypersensitivity reaction)

Figure 15.19 **Autoimmune reactions in glomerulonephritis. A.** Immune complexes formed elsewhere circulate in blood and are deposited on the glomerular basement membrane (GBM). **B.** Antibodies circulating in blood attach to native antigens in the GBM.

1. *Thickening of the basement membrane* (Fig. 15.21) derives from deposition of immune complexes or internal synthesis of new basement membrane material, as in diabetic glomerulopathy.
2. *Hypercellularity* of the glomerulus derives from the influx of inflammatory cells and an increase in the number of mesangial, endothelial, or epithelial cells. Epithelial cell proliferation leads to formation of *crescents* (Fig. 15.22) of cells that bind the glomerulus to the parietal epithelium.
3. *Hyalinosis* refers to the accumulation of homogeneous, smooth proteinaceous extracellular material deposited from plasma into the glomerulus. It may occlude glomerular capillaries and typically is a final end-stage change in chronic glomerular disease that reduces glomeruli to nonfunctional hyaline balls.
4. *Sclerosis* is the accumulation of collagenous scar tissue in the glomerulus.

These changes may accumulate in part or all of an individual glomerulus. Changes may be confined to capillary loops, or involve a single focus, a segment, or the entire glomerulus, but all glomeruli in the kidney are involved to one degree or another.

It is worth noting that because the etiology of much chronic glomerular disease is unknown, *it is common to refer to cases of unknown cause according to the pathology found in the glomerulus* (e.g., *crescentic GN*, *membranous GN*). By contrast, *glomerular disease of known etiology is referred to according to its etiology or clinical syndrome* (e.g., *poststreptococcal GN*). Confusion is often the result among those who are not experts in renal disease.

Remember This! Almost all primary glomerular disease is autoimmune.

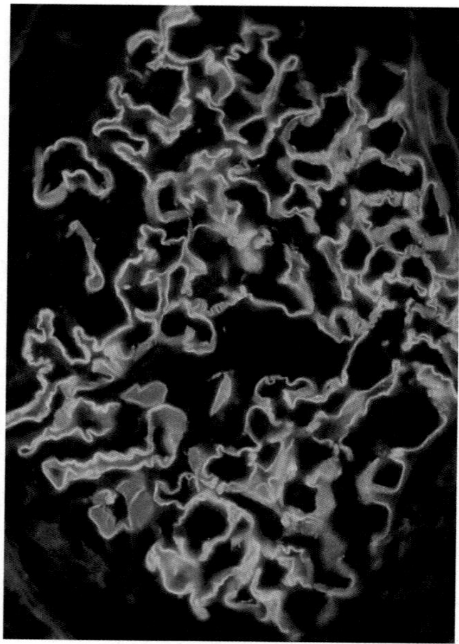

Figure 15.20 **Demonstration of immunoglobulin deposition on glomerular basement membrane (fluorescent technique).** By special technique, fluorescein has been attached to the immunoglobulin antibody molecules that have attached themselves to the basement membrane in a case of MGN. The fluorescein glows when illuminated by florescent light. The basement membrane is thickened due to the coating of immunoglobulin. Refer also to Figure 15.21. (Reprinted with permission from Rubin E. *Pathology*. 4th ed. Philadelphia (PA). Lippincott Williams and Wilkins.)

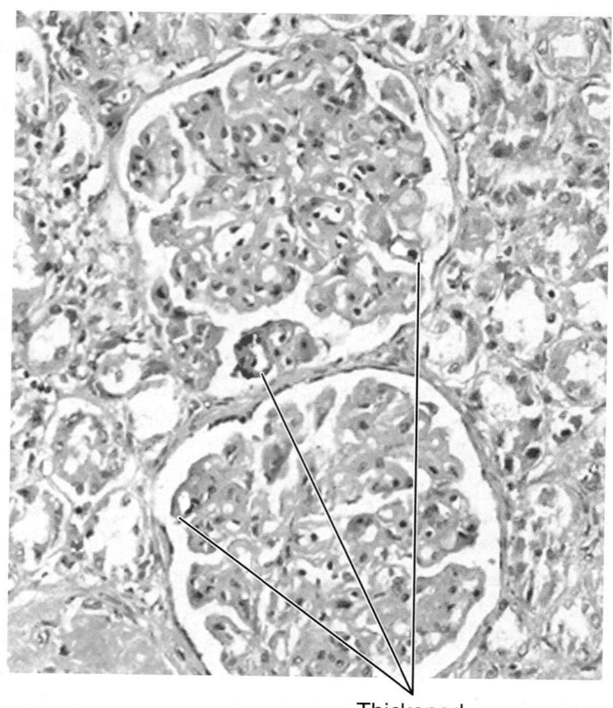

Figure 15.21 **Membranous glomerulonephritis (light microscopy).** The basement membrane is thickened by immunoglobulin deposits. See also Figure 15.20.

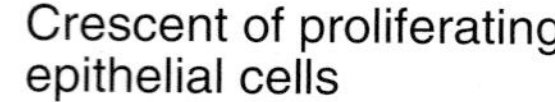

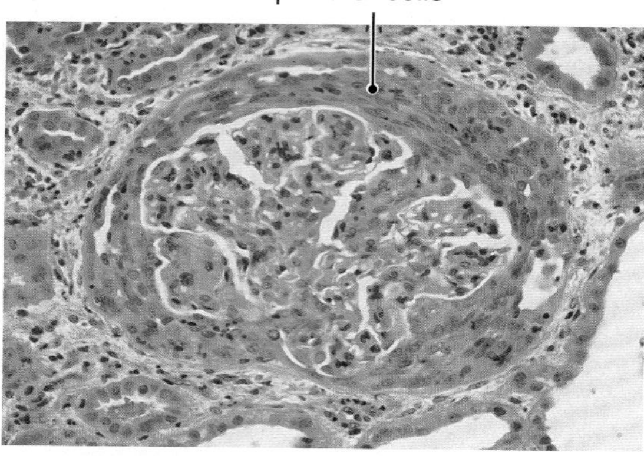

Figure 15.22 **Crescentic glomerulonephritis.** Crescent of epithelial cells proliferates along the parietal rim of the glomerular space and obliterates the glomerulus. Crescentic GN is an anatomic finding in progressively worsening GN. (Reproduced with permission from Rubin E. *Pathology*. 4th ed. Philadelphia (PA). Lippincott Williams and Wilkins; 2005.)

Table 15.1 identifies the most common syndromes of glomerular disease. Glomerular disease may be primary or be secondary to systemic disease such as SLE, hypertension, diabetes mellitus, amyloidosis, and dozens of others, including hereditary conditions. The clinical presentation and glomerular pathology can be similar for glomerular diseases of differing etiologies.

Nephritic Syndrome Is Caused by Glomerular Inflammation

Nephritic syndrome is caused by glomerular inflammation, usually acute, and is characterized by the following:

- *Hematuria* (either gross or microscopic) occurs when red cells "leak" through damaged glomerular membrane into the GF.

Table 15.1 Syndromes of Glomerular Disease

Syndrome	Signs and Symptoms
Nephritic syndrome	Hematuria, azotemia, proteinuria, oliguria, edema, hypertension
Rapidly progressive GN	Nephritic syndrome and/or renal failure
Nephrotic syndrome (called nephrosis in children)	Proteinuria >3.5 gm/day, edema, hypoalbuminemia, hyperlipidemia, lipiduria
Chronic renal failure	Azotemia progressing to uremia over months or years
Other glomerular conditions	Hematuria and/or proteinuria

- *Proteinuria* also occurs from "leaks" through the glomerular membrane, which allow protein to escape blood into the GF.
- *RBC casts in urine*, also due to "leaks" of RBC through the glomerular membrane into the GF. As RBC pass down the renal tubule they become compacted into casts.
- *Hypertension* occurs due to the fluid and salt retention that occur with falling urine output. The result is expanded blood volume and hypertension.
- Edema accumulates as fluid and salt are retained with falling urine output.
- *Azotemia* occurs as the GFR falls and less volume of blood is clear of metabolic waste and waste products accumulate in blood.
- *Oliguria* is caused by diminished glomerular blood flow and low GFR.

Nephritic syndrome is almost invariably caused by autoimmunity. The two basic types are acute and hereditary.

Acute Nephritic Syndrome

Acute nephritic syndrome (anatomically = *acute proliferative GN*) is the most common variety of nephritic syndrome and typically occurs after streptococcal infection (**acute poststreptococcal glomerulonephritis [APSGN]**) of the throat or skin (e.g., *impetigo*, Chapter 21). Less commonly, it develops after other infections, either bacterial (e.g., staphylococcal endocarditis, meningococcal meningitis), viral (e.g., hepatitis B, mumps, HIV, infectious mononucleosis), or parasitic (e.g., malaria).

APSGN usually appears within a few weeks after infection. Most cases occur in children ages 6–10, but adults may be affected. Epidemics may occur, especially in crowded or unsanitary conditions. Only certain strains of group A beta-hemolytic streptococci are nephritogenic. Rising titers of antistreptococcal antibody appear in blood and deposit as immune complexes in glomeruli. The immune reaction consumes complement and blood complement levels fall.

The classic presentation is a youngster taken with fever, malaise, nausea, oliguria, and hematuria a couple of weeks after recovering from a sore throat. Examination usually reveals hematuria, red cell casts in urine, periorbital edema, and hypertension. Blood BUN or creatinine may be elevated. In excess of 95% of children recover completely clinically, but hematuria and proteinuria may persist for months. A few recover from the acute illness but undergo slow progression to chronic GN. A very few progress to *rapidly progressive GN* (see below). Adults usually recover, too, but a larger percentage develops chronic GN or rapidly progressive GN.

Diagnosis is suggested by history and urinalysis and confirmed by low complement or antistreptococcal antibody testing. Treatment is supportive in mild cases, but some patients require treatment of hypertension and fluid and electrolyte management.

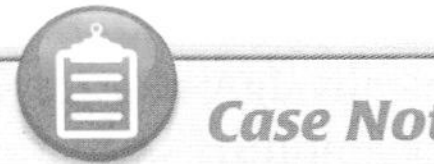

Case Notes

15.31 Did Jesus have GN or glomerulopathy?

Hereditary Nephritis

Hereditary nephritis can be caused by several genetic defects. The most common is **Alport syndrome**. Alport syndrome is due to a well-documented defect in the formation of Type IV collagen, which is critical in the formation of the glomerulus, as well as the lens and cornea of the eye, and the cochlea of the inner ear. Features vary but typically include hematuria, impaired renal function, sensorineural deafness, and ocular abnormalities (cataracts, displaced lenses, and misshaped corneas). Most Alport and other varieties of hereditary nephritis are inherited as X-linked recessive defects and thus mainly affect males. Symptoms and signs are those of nephritic syndrome that usually occurs in children or teenagers and progresses to chronic renal failure by ages 4–50. Diagnosis is by personal and family history, urinalysis, and renal biopsy. Treatment is typical for chronic kidney disease and renal failure.

Though not inflammatory, **thin basement membrane disease (TBMD)** (*benign familial hematuria*) is another hereditary glomerular condition. It typically prompts no symptoms. It usually comes to attention because of incidentally discovered hematuria: *TBMD and IgA nephropathy are the most common causes of asymptomatic hematuria.* Mild proteinuria may occur. Renal function is normal. Diagnosis is by careful family history and urinalysis of the patient and other family members. Renal biopsy may be necessary. No treatment is required. Patients have normal renal function and normal life expectancy.

Immunoglobulin A nephropathy (*Berger disease*) is a surprisingly common autoimmune glomerular disease. It is the diagnosis in 5% of renal biopsies in the United States, and the incidence is much higher in Europe and Asia. It is probably the most common variety of chronic glomerular disease worldwide.

The pathogenesis is unclear but seems to relate to increased IgA production by MALT lymphoid tissue (Chapter 3) in the respiratory or GI tract in response to infection, with glomerular deposition in genetically susceptible persons.

IgA nephropathy occurs mainly in young white men ages 20–30 years and is characterized by recurrent bouts of hematuria appearing a few days after an acute upper respiratory or, less often, GI infection. Proteinuria may also be present. It is to be suspected in young adults with recurrent hematuria for which no other cause can be found.

Diagnosis requires compatible clinical picture and hematuria. Confirmation is by renal biopsy with demonstration of IgA deposits in the mesangial cells of the glomerulus.

Treatment includes drug therapy for hypertension, steroids, and immunosuppressants. Typically, IgA nephropathy resolves spontaneously for a few months and then recurs. Most children have a benign course and recover completely; however, about half of adults develop chronic renal failure and require dialysis or renal transplant.

Case Notes

15.32 By which syndrome did Jesus's renal disease present?

15.33 What was the cause of Jesus's hypertension?

15.34 No renal biopsy was done on Jesus. If one were done, however, would it likely or not likely show immunoglobulin deposits on the GBM?

Some Glomerular Diseases Evolve into Rapidly Progressive Glomerulonephritis (GN)

Rapidly progressive glomerulonephritis (RPGN) is a form of GN that represents a common pathway toward chronic GN for many glomerular diseases, either primary or secondary. It usually affects patients ages 20–50 and progresses to renal failure in a matter of weeks or months. It features swiftly deteriorating renal function associated with oliguria and signs of nephritis. RPGN may arise from unknown cause or may be secondary to poststreptococcal GN or other specific disease affecting the glomerulus. No single mechanism can explain all cases, but most appear to be autoimmune. About half of patients report an influenza-like illness in the recent past.

Signs and Symptoms

Signs and symptoms for all types of RPGN include hematuria, red cell casts in urine, proteinuria that may reach nephrotic syndrome severity (see below), and variable degrees of hypertension and edema. Onset may be insidious, with fatigue, weakness, fever, nausea and vomiting, anorexia, and other constitutional symptoms, or it may follow acute nephritis with rapidly developing renal failure.

Diagnosis and Treatment

Early renal biopsy is essential for quick diagnosis and initiation of therapy. Half of RPGN cases have no demonstrable immune antibody in the glomerulus. In the other half, clear evidence of autoimmune disease (Chapter 3) is present: about 40% show *immune complex deposition* on the glomerular membrane and 10% are caused by direct antibody attack on the GBM by *antiglomerular basement membrane antibody (anti-GBM)*. Regardless of cause, the pathologic picture is characterized by arcs (crescents) of cells that proliferate in Bowman's space and account for its anatomic name, *crescentic GN* (Fig. 15.22). In addition, lab tests reveal anemia and elevated blood BUN and creatinine.

Treatment must begin quickly to have any hope of success, as spontaneous remission is rare and most untreated cases progress to chronic renal failure within six months. Corticosteroids and cytotoxic drugs are mainstays of therapy. Plasmapheresis to remove antibodies is very helpful in patients with anti-GBM antibody. Despite therapy, a majority of patients progress to renal failure and require dialysis and renal transplant.

Any Glomerular Disease May Produce Nephrotic Syndrome

Nephrotic syndrome is marked proteinuria and severe generalized osmotic edema due to low plasma albumin secondary to protein loss. It is characterized by the following:

- *Marked proteinuria* (>3.5 gm/day) caused by glomerular damage that allows leakage of plasma protein (albumin) across the glomerular membrane from blood into the GF (Fig. 15.23).

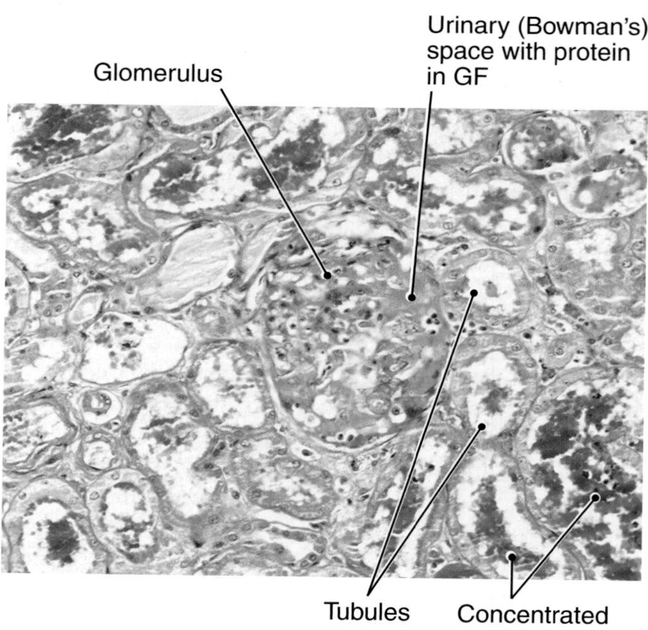

Figure 15.23 **The glomerulus in nephrotic syndrome.** Bowman's space, normally filled with unstainable, clear GF, contains a large amount of pink protein. The tubules contain dense deposits of similar, denser pink material—protein that has condensed into protein casts, which will be flushed out as a diagnostic clue in the urine sediment (Fig. 15.6).

- *Marked hypoalbuminemia* owing to loss of albumin into urine. Some patients also lose other proteins, notably immunoglobulins and endogenous anticoagulants.
- *Marked generalized edema* associated with loss of plasma osmotic pressure caused by low plasma albumin. Loss of water from the vascular space stimulates aldosterone production, which in turn commands the kidney to conserve additional water.
- *Hyperlipidemia and lipiduria* because of low plasma albumin. Low albumin stimulates the liver to increase production of albumin and other proteins, including apoproteins (Chapter 8), which soak up additional lipid to form increased lipoprotein. The result is *hyperlipidemia*, some of which spills into the urine (*lipiduria*).

Nephrotic syndrome can be the consequence of almost any glomerular disease. Among children, most cases are caused by a small number of primary glomerular diseases that are nearly certain to cause nephrotic syndrome. In adults, however, most nephrotic syndrome is usually caused by disease in which the glomerulus is secondarily involved—diabetes, amyloidosis, and SLE.

Case Notes

15.35 Did Jesus develop nephrotic syndrome?

Membranous Glomerulonephritis

Membranous glomerulonephritis (MG), an autoimmune disease, is the most common cause of nephrotic syndrome in adults. Nearly 90% of cases are idiopathic. The remainder can be linked to medications such as NSAIDS, malignant neoplasms of the lung or colon, SLE and other autoimmune disease, and infections (e.g., hepatitis B or C, malaria, syphilis).

The course of MG is often slow and unpredictable and usually begins with modest proteinuria. Progression is marked by increasing glomerular sclerosis and proteinuria, edema, rising creatinine, and hypertension. Diagnosis requires presence of the clinical syndrome with confirmation by renal biopsy, which demonstrates thickening of the GBM (Fig. 15.21) owing to antibody deposits related to basement membrane antigen (Fig. 15.20). It is critical to rule out secondary causes mentioned above, since elimination of the infection, medication, or malignancy can reverse the process.

Steroids and other immunosuppressives do not appear to offer much promise. The main thrust of treatment is management of hypertension and edema. Statins may be necessary for severe hyperlipidemia. To control severe hypoalbuminemia, a few patients require nephrectomy and dialysis or transplant. About 25% recover completely and spontaneously with little consequence. Only about 40% progress to renal failure, usually after 10 or more years.

Minimal Change Disease

Minimal change disease (MCD) is the most common cause of nephrotic syndrome in children, typically occurring between two and six years of age. It is often called **lipoid nephrosis** in children because of the hyperlipemia and lipiduria associated with nephrotic syndrome. Among adults, MCD often occurs in conjunction with lymphoma, leukemia, and use of NSAIDS. It is characterized by sudden appearance of proteinuria and edema without hypertension or laboratory evidence of renal failure. It affects glomerular epithelial cells with very subtle changes that are not visible by conventional microscopy; however, on electron microscopy, characteristic lesions are identifiable in the visceral epithelial cells. Research suggests autoimmune damage, but immune deposits are not demonstrable. Clinical association with immunizations, allergic disease, and its nearly uniform good response to steroid therapy (a distinctive clinical characteristic) add to the impression of immune pathogenesis. Most patients recover fully, but a few go on to chronic renal disease over the next few decades. Therefore, despite the fact that nearly half of cases will recover without treatment, most are treated as a precaution.

Other Causes of Nephrotic Syndrome

As mentioned above, nephrotic syndrome is often secondary. Nevertheless, there are two varieties of nephrotic syndrome that may be primary or secondary and are characterized by specific pathological changes in the glomerulus.

Focal segmental glomerulosclerosis (FSGS) is usually idiopathic but may be secondary to intravenous drug abuse, HIV infection, obesity, sickle cell disease, or loss of nephron units from other glomerular disease (see *renal ablation nephropathy* below) or subtotal nephrectomy. It manifests mainly in adolescents. Onset of nephrosis, hypertension, and azotemia is insidious. Symptoms are not distinctive. Diagnosis is confirmed by renal biopsy, which features scattered mesangial sclerosis in portions of some, but not all glomeruli and immune deposits. Treatment is with angiotensin inhibitors, corticosteroids, and cytotoxic drugs. Prognosis is poor. About 10% undergo spontaneous remission, but the majority develop chronic renal failure within 10 years.

Membranoproliferative glomerulonephritis (MPGN) is a common cause of nephrotic syndrome in children and young adults. Pathogenesis is autoimmune. In children, MPGN is usually a primary glomerular disease; in adults, it is usually secondary to other autoimmune disorders, HIV or other chronic infection, lymphoma or leukemia, or an inherited genetic defect. Clinical features are a mix of nephritic and nephrotic syndromes. MPGN is characterized pathologically by thickening and splitting of the GBM, glomerular hypercellularity, and infiltration of the glomerulus by leukocytes. Steroids and other immunosuppressives are not especially helpful. Many need renal transplant. About half develop chronic renal failure within 10 years.

Chronic Glomerulonephritis Is End-Stage Chronic Glomerular Disease

Chronic glomerulonephritis (CGN) (Fig. 15.24) is the diagnosis applied to long-standing, end-stage, "burned out" chronic glomerular disease. About half of patients have been diagnosed previously with a particular type of GN; in the other half, the diagnosis is applied to patients with chronic glomerular disease of unknown cause who presumably have had long-standing asymptomatic glomerular disease. These cases usually come to medical attention because of the incidental discovery of occult proteinuria or hypertension, or because weakness and anemia develop as a result of chronic renal failure. In the United States, about half of patients on chronic renal dialysis carry a diagnosis of CGN. On renal biopsy, some patients show residual microscopic evidence of a particular type of antecedent glomerular disease. In most, however, the glomeruli are shriveled and scarred and the tubulointerstitial framework is obliterated by inflammation and scar that erases every trace of pathogenesis. Chronic GN becomes a default diagnosis.

The development of glomerular disease has a tendency to become self-perpetuating due to **renal ablation glomerulopathy**, a vicious circle of renal destruction that begins to appear by the time one-third to one-half of glomeruli are destroyed by any renal disease. As glomerular disease progresses, the remaining kidney is strained and undergoes further damage, which accelerates the loss of kidney function. Remaining healthy nephron units are progressively destroyed in a spiral of destruction that leads to the final stage of most renal failure—a shrunken, "burned out," **end-stage contracted kidney**, which is indistinguishable from idiopathic CGN.

Diagnostic workup reveals chronic renal failure. The clinical course is progressive but variable. Hypertension and cardiovascular disease are common complications. Some patients may go on for many years before dialysis is required; others will have complete renal failure shortly after diagnosis. Dialysis and transplant are treatments of choice (see *The Clinical Side*, "Therapeutic Dialysis for Renal Failure").

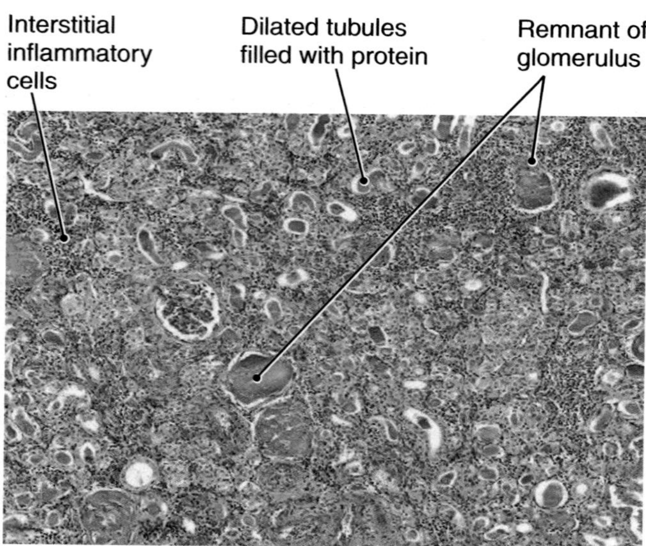

Figure 15.24 **Chronic glomerulonephritis.** Glomeruli are shriveled and scarred and the tubulointerstitial framework is obliterated by inflammation and scar that erases every trace of pathogenesis. (Reproduced with permission from Kumar V, Abbas AK, Fausto N, Aster J. *Robbins and Cotran Pathologic Basis of Disease, Professional Edition.* 8th ed. Philadelphia (PA). Saunders/Elsevier; 2009.)

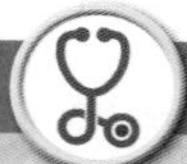

The Clinical Side

THERAPEUTIC DIALYSIS FOR RENAL FAILURE

Patients in acute or chronic renal failure can be sustained by therapeutic dialysis. The two types of dialysis are hemodialysis and peritoneal dialysis.

Hemodialysis involves creating a circuit of blood that passes from the body through a dialysis apparatus (the dialyzer) and back into the body again. In a dialyzer, blood passes through tubes with thin walls made of a unique (semipermeable) membrane that allows only certain substances to cross into and out of blood. The tubes are immersed in the dialysate, which consists of water that contains sodium, potassium, chloride, calcium, and bicarbonate, the concentration of which are varied according to patient needs. Blood cells and protein cannot cross the membrane into the dialysate, but urea, creatinine, acid, and other waste molecules diffuse easily from blood and are washed away.

Peritoneal dialysis involves infusion of dialysate into the peritoneal cavity, where the peritoneal lining acts as the semipermeable dialysis membrane. Dialysate is instilled into the abdomen so that waste can diffuse into it from blood vessels that line the peritoneum. After a suitable interval, usually 6–24 hours, the dialysate is withdrawn and replaced with fresh fluid.

Glomerular Disease Can Be Secondary to Systemic Disease

Diabetic glomerulosclerosis is a leading cause of secondary glomerular disease and a common cause of renal failure in the United States. Those most likely to develop glomerular disease are long-standing insulin-dependent diabetics, about 40% of whom develop advanced renal disease. The condition appears to develop as an effect of hyperglycemia on the GBM. Compounding the problem are diabetic microangiopathy (Chapter 13) and hyaline arteriolar nephrosclerosis (Chapters 8 and 15), which impair glomerular blood flow and contribute to glomerulosclerosis. Diabetics also tend to develop ischemic necrosis of the tips of the renal medullae, bacterial pyelonephritis, and glomerulosclerosis, which are collectively termed **diabetic nephropathy**.

Other causes of secondary glomerular disease include the following:

- *Lupus nephritis* is nephritic syndrome secondary to SLE. Circulating immune complexes deposit in glomeruli and incite inflammation.
- *Amyloidosis* (Chapter 3) is often associated with glomerular amyloid deposits. Nephrotic syndrome and uremia may be the result.
- *Bacterial endocarditis* (Chapter 9) may cause nephritic syndrome or other manifestations of glomerular disease due to deposition of immune complexes in the glomerulus.
- Finally, virtually any disease in which vasculitis is a component may affect glomerular capillaries and cause GN.

Case Notes

15.36 Did Jesus have any medical condition other than strep throat that might have explained his kidney problem?

Pop Quiz

15.26 True or false? Almost all primary glomerular disease is autoimmune.

15.27 True or false? MG is the most common cause of nephrotic syndrome in children, and responds well to steroids.

15.28 True or false? About 40% of long-standing insulin-dependent diabetics develop advanced renal disease.

15.29 What laboratory abnormalities accompany nephritic syndrome?

15.30 What is another name for RPGN, and from where does it derive its name?

15.31 Name the three components of diabetic nephropathy.

Tubular and Interstitial Disorders

Tubular and interstitial injury tend to go together. **Tubulointerstitial nephritis (TIN)** (Fig. 15.25) features pathologic changes to tubules and interstitium. Infections are an important cause of TIN because they are common and tend to recur. *Acute* TIN is uncommon and usually due to acute infection or allergic drug reaction. *Chronic* TIN is much more common and usually owes to chronic bacterial infection or urinary tract obstruction or stasis (discussed separately below because of their clinical importance and their tendency to occur together). In *primary* TIN, tubulointerstitial injury is the initial event. *Secondary* TIN occurs as a consequence of some other condition.

Primary TIN Is Due to Direct Tubulointerstitial Injury

The two main pathological groups of *primary TIN* are 1) ischemic or toxic injury to tubules; and 2) inflammatory conditions that directly injure tubules and interstitium jointly.

Acute Tubular Injury

Acute tubular injury (ATI) is a clinical and pathologic syndrome characterized by sudden decrease of renal function that is often, but not uniformly, accompanied by evidence of tubular injury or tubular necrosis. *Acute tubular necrosis (ATN)* and *acute kidney injury* are synonymous terms. Because they consume so much energy processing the GF, renal tubular epithelial cells are especially vulnerable if renal blood flow falls or toxin interferes with metabolic

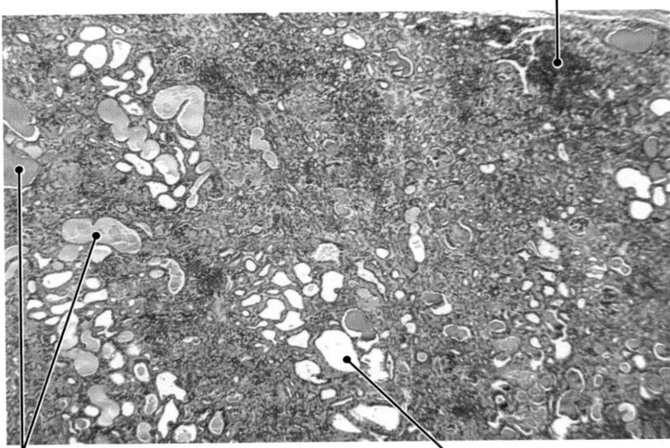

Figure 15.25 **Chronic tubulointerstitial nephritis.** The interstitium is filled with chronic inflammatory cells (lymphocytes). Tubules are dilated and filled with protein casts; tubular epithelium is atrophic. (Reprinted with permission from Rubin E. *Pathology*. 4th ed. Philadelphia (PA). Lippincott Williams and Wilkins; 2005.)

processes. After insult, renal function rapidly deteriorates and oliguria <400 ml/day develops within 24 hours.

ATI is the most common cause of acute renal failure. The most common etiology is *ischemia*, which may occur as a consequence of shock, malignant hypertension, arteritis, disseminated intravascular coagulation, or other conditions. Direct *toxic injury* can be caused by heavy metals, drugs, X-ray contrast material, hemoglobinuria (e.g., in hemolytic disease), **myoglobinuria** (e.g., myoglobin protein liberated from injured skeletal muscle due to heat stroke, crush injury), or other conditions. Regardless of the cause, the pathogenesis seems to be come from a combination of tubular injury and diminished renal blood flow.

Signs and Symptoms

Patients who survive ATI progress through three clinical phases. The first 24–48 hours (the *initiating phase*) is dominated by the main clinical event, such as hemorrhage or poisoning. Urine output falls dramatically and creatinine rises. (Note: In some patients urine volume does not fall despite the injury.) The *maintenance phase* begins usually within the first few days as patients are given supportive care and dialysis if necessary to tide them over until the tubular epithelium regrows. The *recovery phase* begins with increasing renal output that often rises to a flood of dilute urine as tubular function returns but has not regained its full ability to resorb most of the huge volume of normal GF. Urine output returns to normal as epithelium recovers.

As illustrated in Figure 15.26, the renal cortex is pale and the medullae are congested. Microscopic study typically shows signs of tubular epithelial cell injury (Chapter 2) with or without necrosis. Glomeruli, however, are spared.

Diagnosis and Treatment

Diagnosis is clinical with laboratory support. In treatment, maintaining blood volume and proper electrolyte balance are important clinical considerations. Temporary dialysis may be necessary. For nephrotoxic injury, if the patient survives damage to other organs and receives supporting care, 95% will recover normal renal function. For ischemic injury, only 50% will.

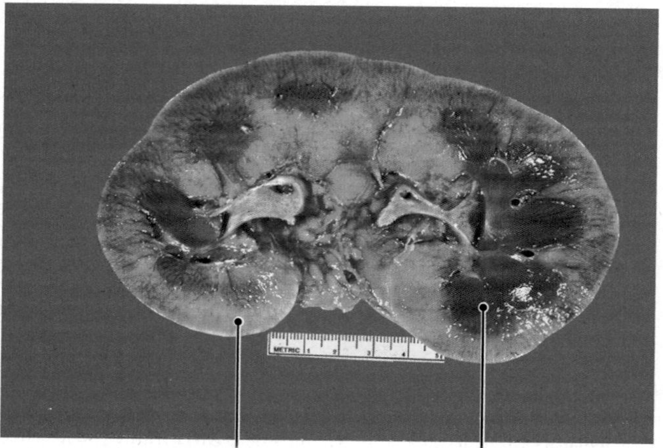

Figure 15.26 **Acute tubular injury.** The paleness of the renal cortex is caused by necrotic tubular epithelium. The medullary pyramids are congested.

Drug and Toxic Injury

Renal damage occasioned by drugs or toxins occurs in three forms: 1) *ATI*; 2) acute hypersensitivity reaction; or 3) chronic injury.

Acute drug-induced interstitial nephritis involves acute inflammation of the interstitium that evolves over a few days or months. About two-thirds can be traced to allergic drug reaction. The reaction is idiosyncratic and not dose related. Pathogenesis appears to be Type I or Type IV hypersensitivity reaction that typically appears about two weeks after drug exposure. Antibiotics, ibuprofen and other NSAIDS, and diuretics are the most common offenders. The clinical syndrome includes fever, skin rash, and peripheral blood eosinophilia associated with hematuria, proteinuria, and leukocytes in the urine. About one-quarter of patients have a skin rash, and acute renal failure occurs in about half. Withdrawal of the offending drug usually results in recovery.

Chronic analgesic nephropathy is a form of chronic TIN caused by excessive use of analgesic that contain a mixture of: *aspirin or other NSAIDS; phenacetin* or *acetaminophen* (acetaminophen is a metabolite of phenacetin); *caffeine* or *codeine*. At one time it was one of the most common causes of chronic renal failure in Australia and South Africa, but recognition and restriction of over-the-counter drug availability has reduced the problem. It accounts for about 5% of end-stage renal disease in the United States. By some unknown mechanism, these drug combinations induce necrosis of the tips of renal papillae, which restricts the flow of tubular fluid out of the medulla into the renal pelvis. Chronic tubulointerstitial damage, hypertension, and chronic renal failure may follow. Typically, the patient is an older woman who has ingested large daily doses of analgesics for more than three years seeking relief for headache, joint, or muscle symptoms. Treatment is cessation of drug use, which usually stabilizes renal function and may improve it.

Case Notes

15.37 Was there anything in Jesus's history to suggest that his illness might have been caused by drug or toxic effect?

Other Causes of Primary TIN

A variety of other compounds may cause tubulointerstitial damage. Patients with *gout* (Chapter 18) have high blood uric acid and suffer from arthritis caused by deposition of urate crystal in joints and periarticular tissue. Deposition of crystals in renal tubules causes **urate nephropathy**, which is characterized by tubulointerstitial inflammation and impaired renal function.

In some patients with multiple myeloma (Chapter 7), the metabolism of immunoglobulins liberates immunoglobulin light chain molecules (Bence-Jones proteins) that are small enough to pass across the glomerular membrane and collect into tubular casts, which impede flow of tubular fluid, damage tubular epithelium, and cause chronic tubulointerstitial inflammation and impaired renal function.

Secondary TIN Is a Consequence of Some Other Condition

Infection and urinary tract obstruction/stasis are leading causes of secondary TIN and are discussed separately below because they tend to occur together. The kidney is usually affected by bacteria that first infect the lower urinary tract and then ascend the ureters to infect the kidneys. Other causes include chronic glomerular disease, cystic diseases of the kidney, diabetes, and vascular disorders (e.g., hypertension, nephrosclerosis, vasculitis).

Pop Quiz

15.32 What is the most common cause of ATI?

15.33 Chronic analgesic nephropathy is caused by excessive use of analgesics that contain ______________.

15.34 Gout can cause tubulointerstitial inflammation due to deposition of __________ crystals.

Pyelonephritis

Pyelonephritis is an inflammatory disorder of renal tubules, interstitium, calyces, and pelvis caused by infection or some combination of infection, stasis, obstruction, or vesicoureteral reflux. Infection is common but not always present.

Pyelonephritis is a common complication of lower UTIs. In the majority of cases, the infecting bacteria are from the patient's own fecal flora. The first step of infection is colonization of the distal urethra. Organisms then often, but not necessarily, gain access to the bladder by catheterization or instrumentation. Bacterial infection of the bladder (*cystitis*) may be asymptomatic and usually does not ascend to the kidneys. Nevertheless, the presence of urinary obstruction, stasis, or ureterovesical reflux encourages bacterial proliferation and upward spread of infection. In some patients the cause of infection is not clear.

Among adults under age 50, women are more often infected than men—their urethra is short and open to bacteria that populate the labia and vaginal mucosa, and vaginal childbirth may alter pelvic anatomy to cause urinary incontinence or other problems that require surgery or instrumentation. Pregnant women are especially vulnerable due to estrogen-induced relaxation of ureteral muscular tone and associated urinary stasis. Among older adults, men are more vulnerable because of prostatic disease and associated urinary obstruction. Diabetics and patients with immune deficiency are also vulnerable.

Uncommonly, pyelonephritis may be due to hematogenous seeding of the kidney from a focus of infection away from the urinary tract.

Acute Pyelonephritis Is Acute Pyogenic Infection of the Kidney

Acute pyelonephritis is acute pyogenic infection of the kidney. It is almost always bacterial, though other types of organisms also may infect the kidney. Most cases are due to ascending infection from the lower urinary tract. The most common bacterial offenders are *E. coli* and other fecal flora.

Uncomplicated acute pyelonephritis usually presents as sudden onset of flank pain associated with fever, high peripheral WBC count, WBC in urine, and other signs and symptoms of acute infection. Bladder infection is usually present and associated with frequency, urgency, and with painful urination. The pathologic picture is acute interstitial nephritis.

Diagnosis depends on the presence of appropriate clinical picture, urinalysis, and urine culture. The microscopic picture is acute suppurative inflammation of the tubulointerstitial framework. Figure 15.27 illustrates a severe case with multiple small abscesses.

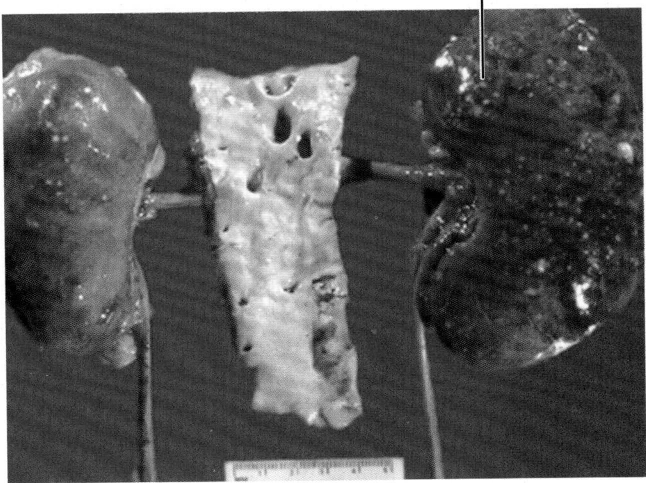

Figure 15.27 **Acute pyelonephritis.** Multiple small bacterial abscesses are present. The ureters are normal.

Treatment is with antibiotics and relief of obstruction if present. Prognosis is excellent in uncomplicated cases. Overwhelming sepsis and renal failure can occur in debilitated patients or in neglected cases.

Case Notes

15.38 Why couldn't the diagnosis for Jesus have been acute pyelonephritis?

Chronic Pyelonephritis Occurs in Two Forms

Chronic pyelonephritis is chronic tubulointerstitial inflammation and scarring of the kidney associated with pathologic involvement of the renal calyces and pelvis. It is usually associated with chronic infection, but not necessarily so—the pathologic picture can also be produced by chronic stasis caused by reflux or obstruction. Chronic pyelonephritis has two defining pathological features: 1) chronic tubulointerstitial inflammation and scarring, and 2) dilation of the calyces and blunting of the tips of renal pyramids.

Chronic pyelonephritis occurs in two anatomic forms: 1) reflux associated, and 2) chronic-obstruction associated. Renal infection is almost universal. The incidence of chronic pyelonephritis has been steadily declining due to better understanding and recognition of urinary obstruction and reflux; however, it remains an important cause of kidney disease in children with congenital urologic problems.

Reflux Nephropathy

Reflux nephropathy is the most frequent form of chronic pyelonephritis and usually occurs in children with congenital reflux due to failure of the one-way direction of downward urine flow. Infection is usually present. The problem often lies at the ureterovesical junction (UVJ) (Fig. 15.28), which normally acts as a one-way valve that prevents reflux from the bladder into the ureters at time of urination. Normally the ureters enter the bladder

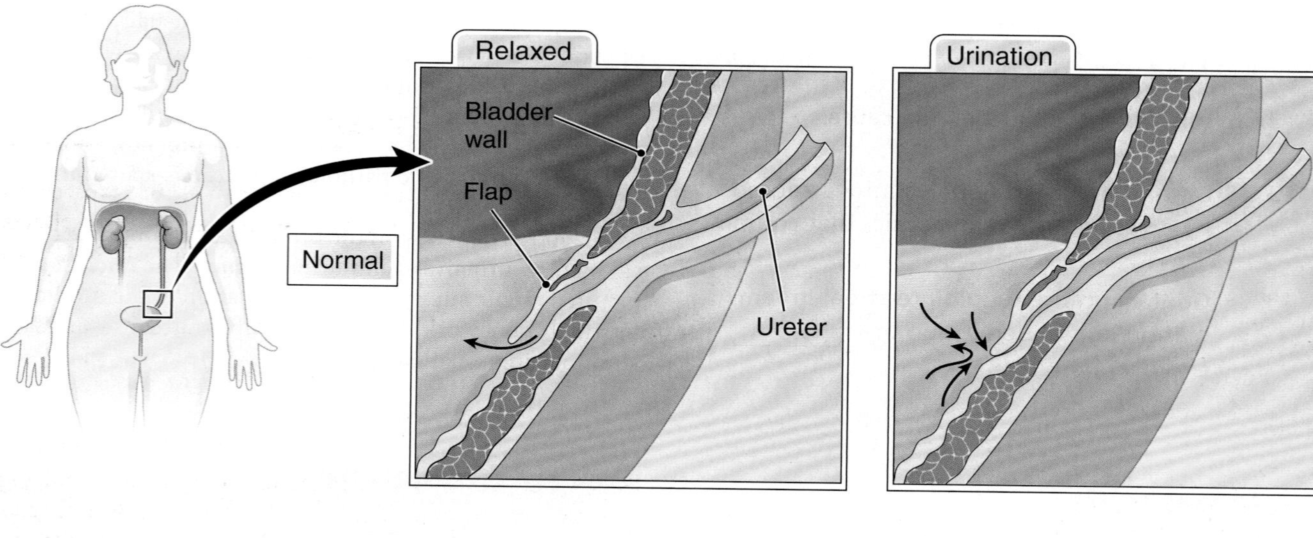

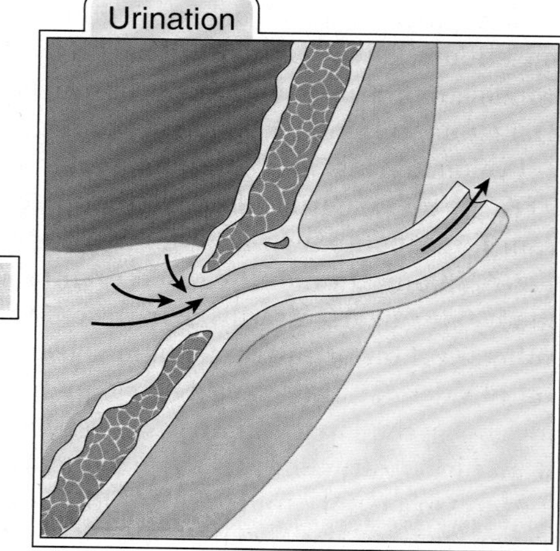

Figure 15.28 **The ureterovesical junction: normal and in reflux.**

obliquely, which creates a long intramural segment that is key to the one-way valve function of the UVJ. If the ureters enter perpendicularly, however, the intramural segment is short and one-way function is impaired. In clinical practice, most patients with bacteriuria have infection of the lower urinary tract, not of the kidney, because the ureterovesical valve prevents reflux and upward spread of infection. Reflux nephropathy without infection is especially silent and may be discovered in a workup for hypertension, especially in children.

Reflux backpressure causes chronic TIN and dilation of the renal pelvis and calyces. Calyceal dilation and renal scarring and cortical atrophy are most notable in the superior and inferior *poles* of the kidney. The tips of polar pyramids are flat or slightly concave and more readily admit reflux backpressure and reverse flow than the more sharply pointed central pyramids.

Chronic Obstructive Pyelonephritis

Chronic obstructive pyelonephritis is a consequence of chronic urinary tract obstruction. Like reflux, obstruction encourages backpressure, chronic TIN, and infection (which may or may not arise). Infection may account for episodes of acute pyelonephritis and persistent bacteriuria, and make it difficult to distinguish the effect of infection from inflammation.

Obstruction and/or infection also cause chronic TIN and dilation of the renal pelvis and calyces. In contrast to reflux nephropathy, calyceal dilation, renal scarring, and cortical atrophy tend to be widely distributed and not concentrated at the poles.

Remember This! Chronic TIN, urinary obstruction, stasis, infection, and stone formation are intimately related and may occur together.

Signs and Symptoms

Clinical presentation of chronic pyelonephritis is often insidious and may or may not feature recurrent episodes of moderate back pain, fever, dysuria, and other urinary tract symptoms. Most patients are not diagnosed until late in the course of their disease, because chronic pyelonephritis is often asymptomatic and the kidneys have a large functional reserve; that is, most renal capacity must be destroyed before clinical signs or symptoms occur. As concentrating power is lost, polyuria and nocturia may be the first signs.

Diagnosis and Treatment

Over time, pyelonephritis dilates the collecting system (the pelvis and calyces), thins the cortex by atrophy, and scars the parenchyma. Radiographic studies typically show small kidneys with dilated pelvis and irregular, broad renal scars. Microscopic study reveals extensive tubulointerstitial inflammation. Bacteriuria may be present, but often is not.

The first goal of treatment is to correct reflux or obstruction. Depending on circumstances, antibiotic therapy may be required, sometimes indefinitely. Some patients will require renal transplantation. Progression to chronic renal failure may occur, especially if the disease has been subclinical for many years.

Pop Quiz

15.35 True or false? Infection is always present in acute pyelonephritis.

15.36 True or false? *E. coli* and other fecal flora are the most common causes of acute pyelonephritis.

15.37 True or false? Infection is not necessary to produce chronic pyelonephritis.

15.38 True or false? Obstructive nephropathy tends to cause scarring at the poles of the kidney.

Vascular Disorder

Renal vasculature is very often secondarily involved in kidney disease, and systemic vascular disease often affects renal blood vessels. Hypertension is intimately linked to the kidney: renal disease can cause hypertension, and hypertension can damage the kidney.

Benign Nephrosclerosis Is Related to Age and Blood Pressure

Benign nephrosclerosis (Chapter 8) is a "wear and tear" pathologic change in the kidney that is related to advancing age and to blood pressure; some degree of nephrosclerosis is an incidental finding in all elderly persons coming to autopsy, and is so common that it scarcely warrants diagnosis. Importantly, it is more common in African Americans than Caucasians and African Americans tend to suffer more damage from it. *Identical renal changes occur at a much earlier age in patients with hypertension*; the higher the blood pressure, the earlier the change appears. Nevertheless, nephrosclerosis continues to develop without hypertension.

Case Notes

15.39 Was it likely that Jesus also had benign nephrosclerosis?

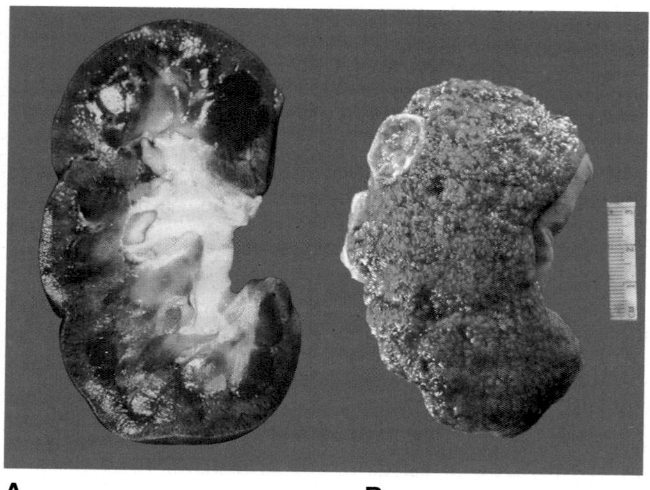

Figure 15.29 **Benign nephrosclerosis. A.** Normal kidney. **B.** Benign nephrosclerosis. The kidney is contracted and granular due to innumerable small cortical scars. This example also shows a benign simple cyst.

Benign nephrosclerosis features sclerosis of small renal arteries and arterioles, which thickens the wall and narrows the lumen. The consequence is focal ischemia, glomerular sclerosis, and tubulointerstitial inflammation. As depicted in Figure 15.29, nephrosclerotic kidneys are atrophic and have a granular, finely pebbled surface due to innumerable tiny scars. The microscopic lesion is smooth, glassy change (hyaline arteriolosclerosis, Chapter 8, Fig. 8.7) in the walls of glomerular afferent arterioles, which slowly chokes off glomerular blood supply and reduces the glomerulus to a small ball of fibrous scar tissue. Functional impairment is mild in most patients. Mild proteinuria may occur. Diagnosis is presumptive depending on age, ethnicity, and blood pressure. Renal biopsy may be necessary in a few patients to separate nephrosclerosis from other renal disease.

The best therapy is prevention by prompt diagnosis and treatment of early hypertension. Blood pressure control is especially important in African Americans and diabetics, in whom renal failure may develop.

Malignant Nephrosclerosis Is Associated with Accelerated Hypertension

Malignant nephrosclerosis (MN) is a much more severe form of nephrosclerosis seen in patients with Stage 2 hypertension (BP >160/100 mm Hg, Chapter 8), often referred to as *malignant hypertension*. MN accounts for a small percentage of patients with hypertension. MN may occur in previously normotensive people, but the great majority of cases represent acceleration of a lesser degree of pre-existing hypertension that may be essential hypertension or hypertension secondary to renal disease. It is more common and tends to be more severe in males and African Americans. The mechanism of damage to renal blood vessels and glomeruli is similar to the mechanism in benign nephrosclerosis, but it is exaggerated and happens more quickly. A sinister aspect of malignant hypertension is the tendency to develop a positive feedback loop involving blood pressure and renal damage. Hypertension damages the afferent arteriole and strangles blood supply to the glomerulus. This activates the renin-aldosterone mechanism (Chapter 8), which in turn raises blood pressure even more—a perfect vicious circle of high blood pressure, renal ischemia, renin secretion, and even higher blood pressure.

The clinical picture of malignant nephrosclerosis includes 1) renal failure; 2) vascular stress that may present as myocardial infarct, congestive heart failure, or stroke; and 3) increased intracranial pressure, which often produces the symptoms that bring the patient to attention: seizures, headache, nausea and vomiting, visual impairments, coma, or mental aberration. Physical exam typically reveals blood pressure >160/110 mg Hg (sometimes as high as 200/120 mg Hg), pounding heartbeat, and bulging optical discs (papilledema) on retinal exam, as the edematous brain pushes the optic nerves forward.

The relentless pounding of blood pressure causes pressure necrosis (*fibrinoid necrosis*) of the afferent arteriole and onionskin hyperplasia of cells in the walls of small arterioles (Fig. 15.30)—a pathologic hallmark of malignant hypertension that is visible on biopsy. Laboratory abnormalities include markedly increased blood. Initially, proteinuria and hematuria may also be present without

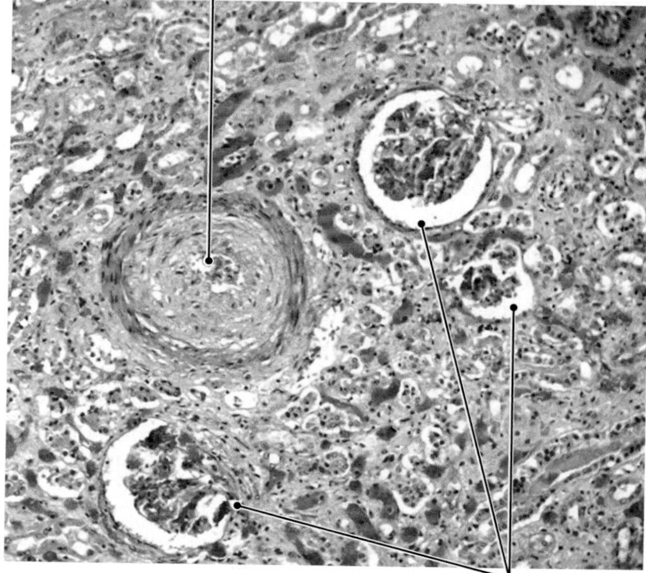

Figure 15.30 **Malignant nephrosclerosis.** The hallmark lesion is onionskin hyperplasia in the walls of renal arterioles.

much other evidence of renal impairment. Nevertheless, renal failure will develop rapidly without prompt and vigorous treatment.

Malignant hypertension is a medical emergency requiring vigorous and prompt treatment with antihypertensive drugs. Without treatment it is uniformly fatal. Among properly treated patients, 75% survive five years, the majority of whom recover their renal function.

Extrarenal Disease May Affect Renal Vasculature

Unilateral renal artery stenosis is a surgically curable cause of hypertension that accounts for a small percentage of patients with hypertension. Impaired renal blood flow lowers intrarenal blood pressure, which invokes the renin-angiotensin-aldosterone mechanism, which in turn raises blood pressure. The most common cause is atherosclerotic narrowing. Almost every man diagnosed with unilateral renal artery stenosis will have atherosclerotic narrowing, while up to 10% of women will have *fibromuscular dysplasia* of a renal artery. The latter is a family of conditions with unusual thickening of the arterial wall and narrowing of the lumen. In almost every respect, these patients resemble patients with essential hypertension, which puts a premium on looking for stenosis in the diagnostic workup of patients with hypertension. Almost all patients have increased blood renin. Diagnosis requires constant suspicion and arteriography.

Over half of patients are cured by restoration of full blood flow or excision of the affected kidney. Nevertheless, in some patients, long-standing hypertension has caused so much renal damage that restoration of normal blood flow has limited effect.

Large renal vessels may be involved with *bilateral* atherosclerotic stenosis of the renal arteries, which can account for renal insufficiency with or without accompanying hypertension, especially in the elderly. Acute atherosclerotic thrombosis or large vessel vasculitis may produce large renal infarcts or infarction of an entire kidney.

Smaller renal blood vessels may be affected by *embolization of atherosclerotic material* during aortic surgery, which can produce multiple small ischemic infarcts of no clinical significance, but can also precipitate renal failure in patients with previously compromised renal function. In somewhat similar fashion, *sickle cell disease* may cause ongoing small renal infarcts and diminished renal function. Small renal vessels may also be involved by any one of several syndromes known as the *thrombotic microangiopathies* (Chapter 6), which feature hemolytic anemia, thrombocytopenia, hemorrhage, and renal failure.

Pop Quiz

15.39 True or false? Unilateral renal artery stenosis is the most common cause of hypertension.

15.40 Malignant nephrosclerosis is characterized by hyaline arteriosclerosis.

Case Study Revisited

"His water looks like Coca-Cola." The case of Jesus S.

Jesus presented a classic case of acute nephritic syndrome secondary to infection. The history of a "cold and sore throat" earlier was significant—although culture proof is lacking that his earlier sore throat was caused by β-streptococcus, the high concentration in his blood of antistreptococcal antibody made it virtually certain.

Keys to the diagnosis were hypertension, puffy face, oliguria, hematuria, red cell casts, and proteinuria, each of which was a striking abnormality in a previously healthy child. The puffy face suggested fluid retention. Oliguria also suggested renal disease with fluid retention. Red cell casts were a sign of bleeding high in the urinary tract, not from the collecting system. Proteinuria strongly suggests glomerular leaking of protein into the GF. The dark brown color of Jesus's urine came from altered free hemoglobin liberated from degenerated RBCs in his urine. Bleeding from lower sites, such as the bladder, would have produced fresher RBCs and red hematuria. The only other cause of dark urine that might have been considered would have been hemoglobinuria from hemolytic anemia. Jesus's hematocrit was normal, however, and he was not jaundiced (the liver metabolizes hemoglobin into bilirubin).

The final clue was hypertension. GN restricted renal blood flow and invoked the renin-angiotensin-aldosterone cascade, which increased blood pressure. Pediatric hypertension is rare and most cases are caused by some form of renal disease.

Chapter Challenge

CHAPTER RECALL

1. An 18-year-old African American male presents to his family physician concerned about the presence of blood in his urine. He is concerned because a maternal uncle died of renal failure. A urinalysis confirms hematuria, and blood labs reveal an elevated BUN and creatinine. On reviewing the chart, a nursing note concerning his most recent hearing test the physician's eye: "patient appears to have bilateral hearing loss in the 2,000–8,000 Hz range, follow-up testing in 3 months recommended." What is likely the underlying cause of this patient's hematuria?
   A. TBMD
   B. Acute proliferative GN
   C. Alport syndrome
   D. Polycystic kidney disease

2. A 55-year-old African American male with a past medical history significant for irritable bowel disease and multiple UTIs (cultures negative to date) presents to the clinic with dysuria and urgency despite several courses of antibiotics. His physical exam reveals abdominal discomfort above the pubis. A cystoscopy reveals inflammation and *Hunner ulcers*. Although it rarely occurs in men, it appears that the patient has what disease?
   A. Bacterial cystitis
   B. Urethritis
   C. Chronic bacterial prostatitis
   D. Nonbacterial cystitis

3. The barrier function of the glomerulus prevents which one of the following from entering the GF?
   A. Glucose
   B. Protein
   C. Amino acids
   D. Creatinine

4. A four-year-old Caucasian female is brought to the clinic by her mother, who is concerned over her daughter's "puffiness." She reports that it began shortly after her daughter received her four-year immunizations. A urinalysis reveals marked proteinuria and lipiduria. You prescribe a month course of steroids. Her follow-up urinalysis after steroid completion is completely normal. What was the likely cause of the child's symptoms?
   A. MCD
   B. MG
   C. MPGN
   D. FSGS

5. Which of the following findings suggests a bacterial infection?
   A. Presence of leukocyte esterase and nitrite in the urine
   B. Alkaline urine pH
   C. A staghorn calculus
   D. All of the above

6. A 57-year-old Caucasian male with a past medical history significant for uncontrolled hypertension presents to the hospital with a two-week history of progressive fever, polyuria, polydipsia, and a rash. His medications include an ACE inhibitor and the recent addition of a diuretic (one month ago). His urinalysis is positive for hematuria, proteinuria, and leukocytes (previously normal) and his blood work reveals peripheral eosinophilia. From what kidney disease does he suffer?
   A. Acute kidney injury
   B. Chronic analgesic nephropathy
   C. Acute drug-induced interstitial nephritis
   D. CGN

7. Which of the following statements about the opening of the male urethra is true?
   A. The internal sphincter is composed of skeletal muscle and is under voluntary control.
   B. The internal sphincter is composed of smooth muscle and is controlled by the autonomic nervous system.
   C. The external sphincter encircles the urethra immediately above the internal sphincter.
   D. The external sphincter is composed of smooth muscle and under voluntary control.

8. Azotemia is most aptly described as which of the following?
   A. GN
   B. Lab findings
   C. Proteinuria
   D. Urinary obstruction

9. A 35-year-old Hispanic female presents to the clinic with fever, fatigue, nausea, and vomiting. Her physical exam is pertinent for both hypertension and edema, and her urinalysis reveals hematuria with red cell casts as well as proteinuria. She confirms that two weeks ago she had an influenza-like illness, but indicates that she took no medications, prescribed or over the counter. You order additional labs, including a test for anti-GBM, which is positive. You tell the patient that the best treatment for her disease is plasmapheresis: the removal of plasma, treatment of it to remove antibodies, and return of it to her circulation. Which of the below is the most likely diagnosis?
   A. Acute proliferative GN
   B. IgA nephropathy
   C. Tubulointerstitial disease
   D. RPGN

10. Which of the following statements regarding proteinuria is true?
    A. The kidney excretes <150 grams of protein a day, too small to be detected by routine tests.
    B. Intermittent (transient) proteinuria is a normal finding, and occurs in 5% of the population.
    C. Orthostatic proteinuria occurs when patients are erect, but not when lying down.
    D. All of the above statements are true.

11. A 25-year-old Caucasian female presents to the ER complaining of unilateral pain in her lower back. She describes the pain as constant and 10 out of 10. She also reports a fever of 102.5°F and a two-week history of painful, frequent urination. What is her diagnosis?
    A. Chronic pyelonephritis
    B. Nephrolithiasis
    C. Acute pyelonephritis
    D. Renal carcinoma

12. MPGN is characterized by what pathological findings?
    A. Scattered mesangial sclerosis in portions of some, but not all glomeruli and immune deposits
    B. Thickening of the GBM owing to antibody deposits
    C. Arcs (crescents) of cells that proliferate in Bowman's space
    D. Thickening and splitting of the basement membrane, glomerular hypercellularity, and infiltration of the glomerulus by leukocytes

13. A 32-year-old African American male with a past medical history significant for hypertension presents to the clinic complaining of blood in his urine. Imaging demonstrates large kidneys bilaterally with hundreds to thousands of cysts. What is likely to be the underlying etiology?
    A. Multicystic renal dysplasia
    B. ADPKD
    C. ARPKD
    D. Simple cysts

14. Which of the following statements regarding malignant nephrosclerosis is correct?
    A. The signs and symptoms of malignant nephrosclerosis include seizures, headache, nausea and vomiting, and papilledema.
    B. Malignant nephrosclerosis causes fibrinoid necrosis of the afferent arteriole and onion-skin hyperplasia of cells in the walls of small arterioles.
    C. Malignant hypertension is a medical emergency requiring vigorous and prompt treatment with antihypertensive drugs.
    D. All of the above are correct.

15. True or false? Glomeruli are only found in the cortex of the kidney.

16. True or false? Urobilinogen and bilirubin are normal urine components.

17. True or false? The innermost layer of the glomerulus is capillary endothelium.

18. True or false? The male urethra is the same length as the female urethra.

19. True or false? Atherosclerosis is the most common cause of hypertension.

20. Match the following tumors to their clinical features; choices may be used more than once and each feature may have more than one answer:
    i. Oncocytoma
    ii. Renal cell carcinoma
    iii. Transitional cell carcinoma
    A. Malignant
    B. Benign
    C. Invades renal veins, sometimes extending into the inferior vena cava
    D. May grow very large before it is found
    E. May occur at multiple points in the urinary tract
    F. Smokers have twice the risk of nonsmokers
    G. Tumor of renal tubular epithelial cells
    H. Characterized by increased numbers of mitochondria and enlarged cytoplasm
    I. May be accompanied by paraneoplastic syndromes
    J. May regrow a second primary at a new site after removal of original
    K. Lung or bone metastasis
    L. Papillary and fragile
    M. Diagnosed by cytologic study of urine revealing malignant cells

CONCEPTUAL UNDERSTANDING

21. Name the features of each stage of chronic kidney disease.

22. What is the importance of the UVJ?

23. What are the three clinical phases of acute kidney injury?

24. How is blood pressure regulated?

APPLICATION

25. How does the location of bleeding in the urinary tract change the morphology of blood in the urine?

26. A physician, having recently attended a symposium on chronic analgesic nephropathy, asks his staff to contact all his patients and recommend that they switch from acetaminophen and aspirin, to the NSAID ibuprofen, which has no association with kidney damage. Has he forgotten something?

CHAPTER

16

Disorders of the Male Genitalia

Contents

Chapter Objectives

After studying this chapter, you should be able to complete the following tasks:

THE NORMAL MALE GENITAL SYSTEM

1. Explain the function(s) of each part of the male genital system.

DISORDERS OF REPRODUCTIVE FUNCTION

2. Briefly explain the causes of erectile dysfunction.
3. Discuss the various male factors taken into consideration when diagnosing the underlying etiology of infertility.

DISORDERS OF THE PENIS, SCROTUM, AND GROIN

4. Describe the etiology, signs and symptoms, pathological findings, treatment, and consequences of penile diseases, as applicable.
5. Name the diseases affecting the scrotum and groin.

DISORDERS OF THE TESTIS AND EPIDIDYMIS

6. Discuss the etiology, presentation, diagnosis, and treatment of the following disease of the testis and epididymis: epididymitis, orchitis, torsion.
7. Explain the role of cryptorchidism in malignancy, and differentiate between germ and nongerm cell tumors.

DISORDERS OF THE PROSTATE

8. Characterize the types of prostatitis according to etiology, signs and symptoms, diagnostic findings, and treatment.
9. Compare and contrast the clinical and diagnostic features of benign prostatic hyperplasia and prostate cancer.

Case Study

"We keep testing and biopsying and still there's no cancer." The case of Marshall P.

Chief Complaint: Abnormally high PSA

Clinical History: Marshall P. was a 72-year-old Anglo man who had been in the care of a urologist for many years. His initial urologic visit was about 25 years earlier because he had not been circumcised. His erections became painful because his foreskin would not retract. He was circumcised successfully.

After turning 50, Marshall began having a blood prostate specific antigen (PSA) test with his regular annual medical checkup. His first few PSAs were normal but each year they crept higher. When he was 63, he had an elevated PSA (5.2 ng/ml; normal <4.0 ng/ml) for the first time. He returned to his urologist, who did a prostatic sonogram, which showed his prostate to be enlarged (about 42 ml). A 12-core transrectal needle biopsy under local anesthesia showed nodular hyperplasia but no cancer.

He continued to have PSAs every six months. Three years later, at age 66, his PSA had climbed to 9.1 ng/ml and another 12-core transrectal biopsy revealed only nodular hyperplasia. Continued semiannual PSA tests over the next three years showed one surprisingly big jump in PSA to 16.7 ng/ml, but a repeat study was 10.8 ng/ml and the high value was dismissed as a statistical outlier. By age 69, his PSA had reached 12.2 ng/ml, and a 32-core "saturation" transrectal biopsy under anesthesia revealed a single focus of high-grade prostatic intraepithelial neoplasia (PIN) and prostatic hyperplasia. No carcinoma was present. PSA testing continued. His most recent PSA was 14.5 ng/ml. The urologist recommended a second 32-core saturation biopsy, to which Marshall complained, "This testing may be the end of me. We keep testing and biopsying and still there's no cancer. Why don't we just stop doing PSAs and biopsies? I'm 72 years old and I hear prostate cancer isn't so bad anyway."

Further urologic history revealed that he did not have nocturia, frequency, urgency, or other complaint that suggested urine retention. He did, however, admit that it took longer to get his stream going, longer to empty his bladder, flow was frequently interrupted, and he dribbled with every void.

Review of other medical history revealed he had never smoked, exercised regularly, and had no first-degree relatives with prostate cancer.

After further discussion with his urologist, he agreed to have another 32-core biopsy.

Physical Examination and Other Data: Marshall was a trim, fit 72-year-old man with normal vital signs and blood pressure. Digital rectal exam (DRE) revealed that his prostate was moderately enlarged and of normal consistency. No areas of firmness were present to suggest prostatic carcinoma. A slight tremor was present in his left hand. He was taking statins for high cholesterol, antihypertensives for mild hypertension, and rasagiline and L-DOPA for recently discovered early Parkinson disease.

Clinical Course: Marshall was anesthetized and 32 cores of prostate were collected by transrectal biopsy. Intraoperative sonography demonstrated no evidence of carcinoma. The size of his prostate was determined to be 46 ml. He recovered uneventfully. Pathological examination of the biopsy specimens revealed prostatic epithelial hyperplasia, two small foci of high grade PIN, and two small foci of Gleason grade 7 prostatic carcinoma in samples taken from the left superior peripheral zone.

Male, n. A member of the unconsidered, or negligible sex. The male of the human race is commonly known (to the female) as Mere Man. The genus has two varieties: good providers and bad providers.

AMBROSE BIERCE (1842–1913?), AMERICAN SATIRIST, JOURNALIST, AND SHORT-STORY WRITER, IN THE DEVIL'S DICTIONARY

The Normal Male Genital System

As illustrated in Figure 16.1, the male genital system consists of the *testes*, *epididymis*, *vas deferens*, *prostate*, *seminal vesicles*, and *penis*. The main function of the male genital system is reproduction.

The **penis** is a copulatory organ that consists of two main parts: the *shaft* and the *glans* (head). At the tip of the penis is an opening, the *external urethral meatus*. The shaft is covered by skin, which folds over the head to form a retractable collar, the **prepuce** (foreskin). The penis contains three spongy cylindrical vascular compartments, two large dorsolateral ones and a single centerline ventral one. Each of the two dorsal cylinders is a **corpus cavernosum**. During sexual arousal, signals from the parasympathetic nervous system relax arterial smooth muscle tone and they are flooded with blood. At the same time, venous smooth muscles contract, obstructing blood outflow. An erection occurs as the corpora cavernosa become engorged and tense with blood. The third, smaller vascular cylinder, the **corpus spongiosum**, lies in the ventral midline. The urethra runs in its center.

In uncircumcised males, the glans is covered by moist squamous mucosa, which is protected by the *prepuce*. **Circumcision**, a common practice in many cultures for thousands of years, is removal of the prepuce. In circumcised males, the squamous mucosa is unprotected and becomes the anatomic and functional equivalent of the skin covering the shaft of the penis.

The **scrotum** is a sac of skin that holds the testis, epididymis, and proximal vas deferens. The scrotum hangs outside the body to keep testicular temperature about 5°F below the temperature of the rest of the body, because sperm will not be produced if testicular temperature is too high. Much like the heart lies in the pericardial sac, the testis is contained in a smooth serosal sac, the **tunica vaginalis**, which contains a small amount of lubricant fluid that allows free movement of the testicle in the scrotal sac.

The **testis** is a gonad and consists of two compartments: 1) **seminiferous tubules** (90% of testicular mass), where sperm are produced; and 2) **interstitial tissue** that fills the space between the tubules and produces testosterone, the primary male hormone, which is responsible for the development and maintenance of male secondary sex characteristics. The seminiferous tubules are lined by *spermatogonia*, reproductive germ cells, which divide to form sperm, and specialized partner cells, *Sertoli cells*. Sertoli cells regulate and sustain sperm production. Figure 16.1B illustrates details of normal scrotal and testicular anatomy.

As Figure 16.2 illustrates, sperm are formed from spermatogonia by *meiosis* (reduction division), a process that halves the number of chromosomes from 46 to 23: each sperm (spermatozoon) carries 22 somatic chromosomes plus one sex chromosome, either X or Y, for which the shorthand is 23,X or 23,Y. In like manner, each ovum contains 22 somatic chromosomes and an X chromosome. When joined together, the combination produces a normal complement of 44 somatic chromosomes plus two sex chromosomes (written as 46,XX for the female genotype, or 46,XY for the male genotype).

Testosterone is produced by **Leydig cells** in the testicular interstitium in response to stimulation by luteinizing hormone (LH) from the anterior pituitary. The adrenal cortex also produces some testosterone. In conjunction with follicle-stimulating hormone (FSH) from the anterior pituitary, testosterone stimulates testicular germ cells to mature into sperm and accounts for features such as facial hair, deep voice, increased muscle mass, and other masculine features.

On the posterior side of the testis, the seminiferous tubules empty into the **epididymis**, a very long coiled tube that forms an elongated, spongy mass that connects the testis to the vas deferens. As sperm migrate through the epididymis, they mature and are stored. The **vas deferens** is a narrow, stiff, heavily muscled tube that travels upward over the pelvic brim and descends into the pelvis, where it merges with the duct from the seminal vesicle shortly before emptying into the urethra. The **seminal vesicles**, glands that lie beside the prostate and bladder, are each small, elongated glands about 4 cm × 1 cm that excrete a nutrient fluid into semen. Seminal fluid contains *vesiculase*, an enzyme that causes semen to clot after ejaculation. As the vas deferens ascends from the testis in the groin, it is joined by blood vessels, nerves, and supporting tissue and is known as the **spermatic cord**.

Case Notes

16.1 Where and by what cell was most of Marshall's testosterone made?

The **prostate gland** (Fig. 16.3) encircles the urethra at the neck of the bladder. It sits immediately in front of the lower rectum and can be easily examined by palpation with a finger in the anus. In young men, it is about the size of a walnut and has a volume of about 15–20 ml. It enlarges with age. An abnormally large gland is usually defined as >30 ml. The prostate gland is wrapped by a thin capsule of fibromuscular tissue. The prostate proper is composed of glands, ducts, and fibromuscular stroma. Four *zones* are recognized according to their location, the relative amount of glandular tissue they contain and their proclivity to develop into prostatic cancer. The *peripheral zone* is largest and contains about 70% of prostatic glandular tissue. It forms the posterior part of the superior half of the gland and surrounds the inferior, distal prostatic urethra. The *central zone* contains about 25% of prostatic glands and ducts and sits high in the gland posterior to the upper part of the prostatic urethra. The *transitional zone* surrounds the

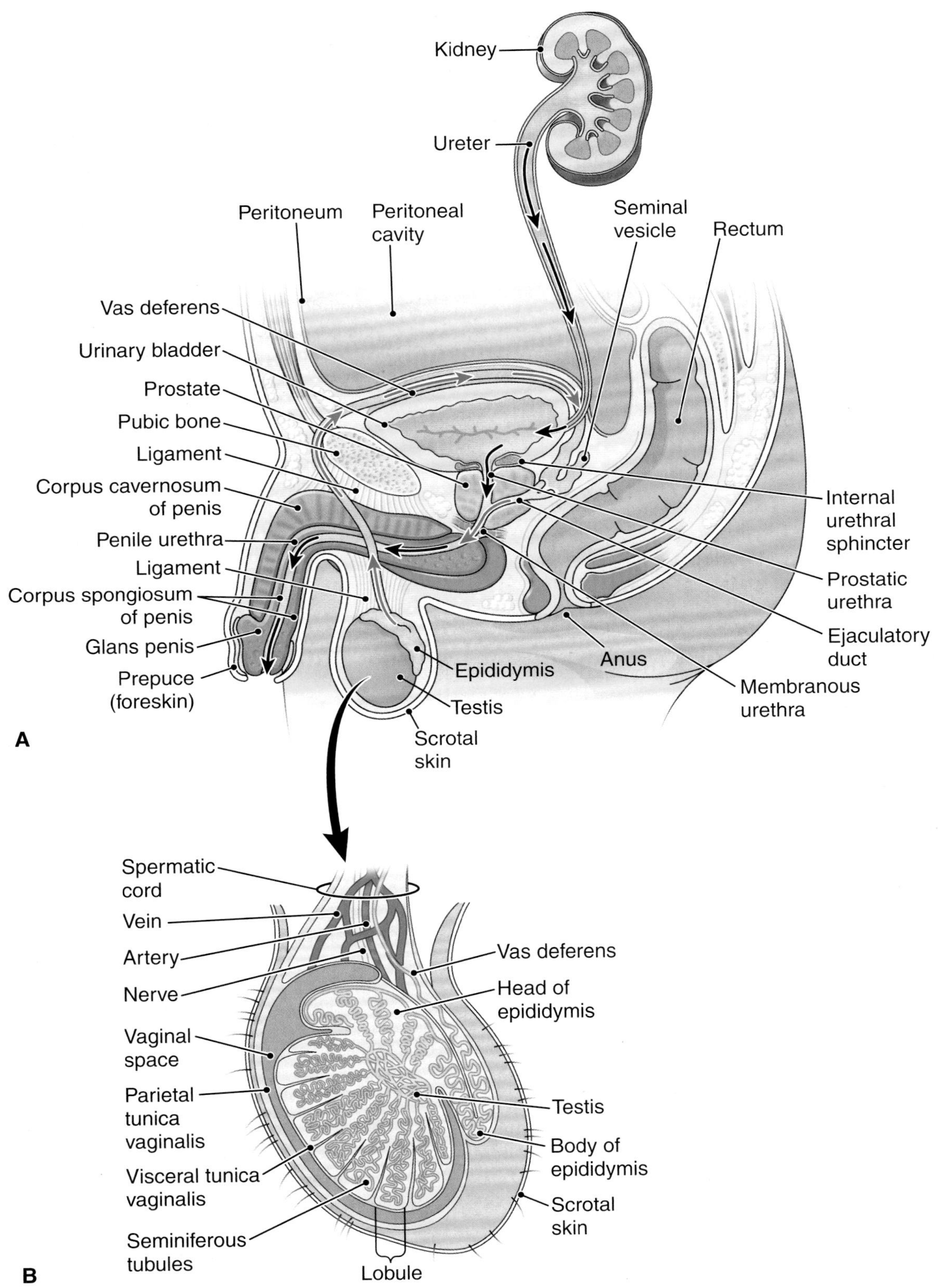

Figure 16.1 **A.** The male genital system. **B.** The scrotum, testis, epididymis, and spermatic cord.

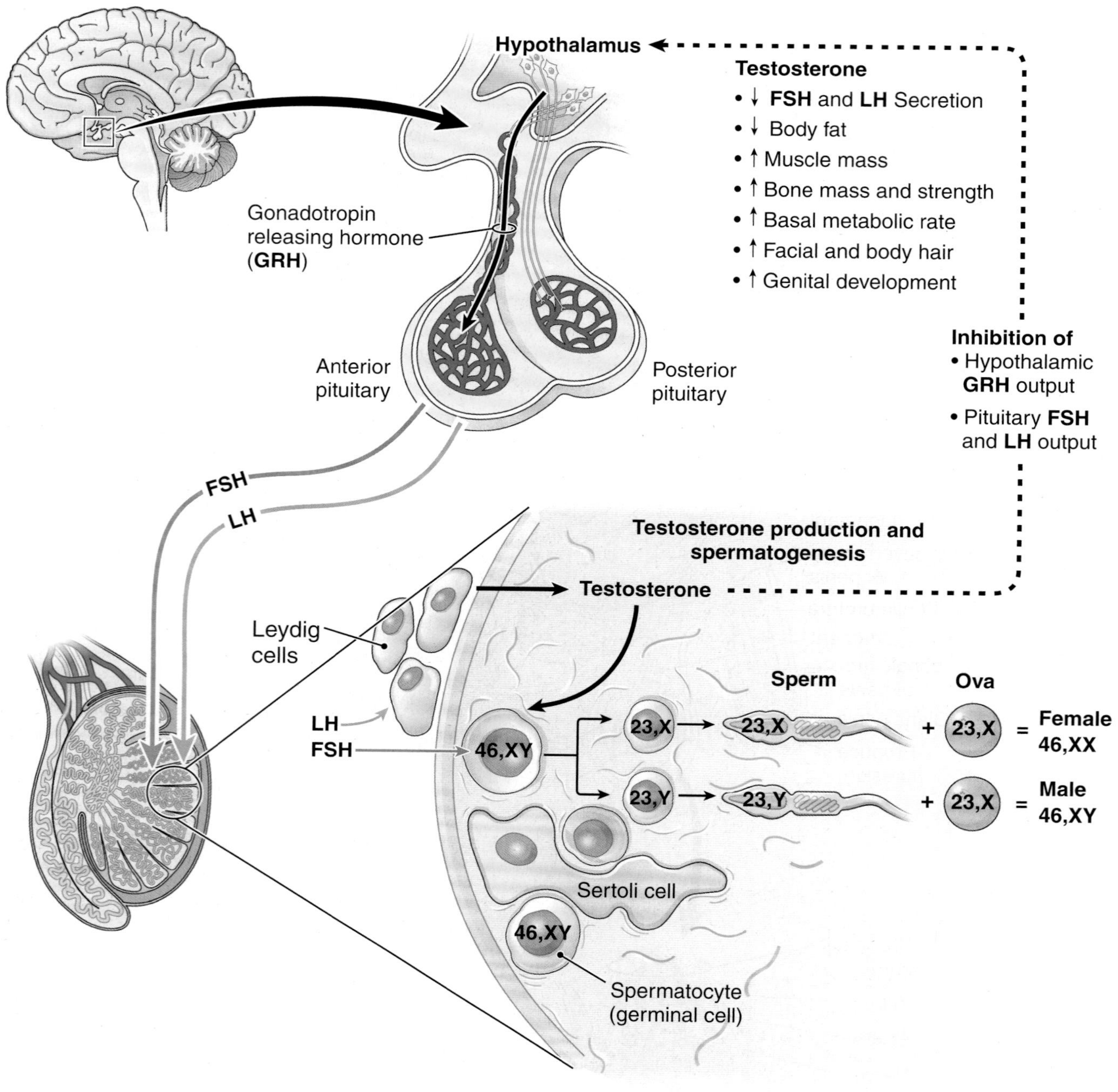

Figure 16.2 **Normal spermatogenesis.**

proximal half of the prostatic urethra and contains about 5% of prostatic glandular tissue. The anterior zone forms the anterior part of the gland and is composed entirely of fibromuscular stroma without glandular tissue.

Normal prostate function depends upon testicular androgens, mainly testosterone. The prostate gland normally increases in size during adult life, and in pathologic conditions it may become exceptionally large. It secretes nutrient fluid into semen. Prostatic fluid contains **prostate specific antigen**, an enzyme that dissolves clotted semen and allows sperm to migrate upward into the female genital tract.

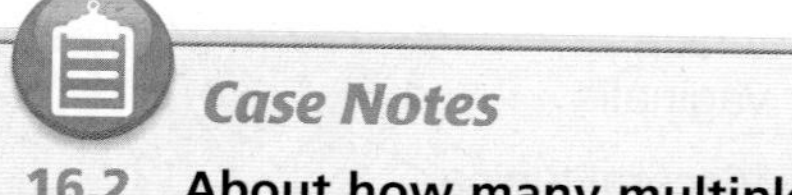

Case Notes

16.2 About how many multiples of normal was the size of Marshall's prostate gland?

Semen is formed of mature sperm from the epididymis mixed with fluids from the seminal vesicles and prostate. **Erection** is enlargement and stiffening of the penis in response to sensory signals that are mediated by the

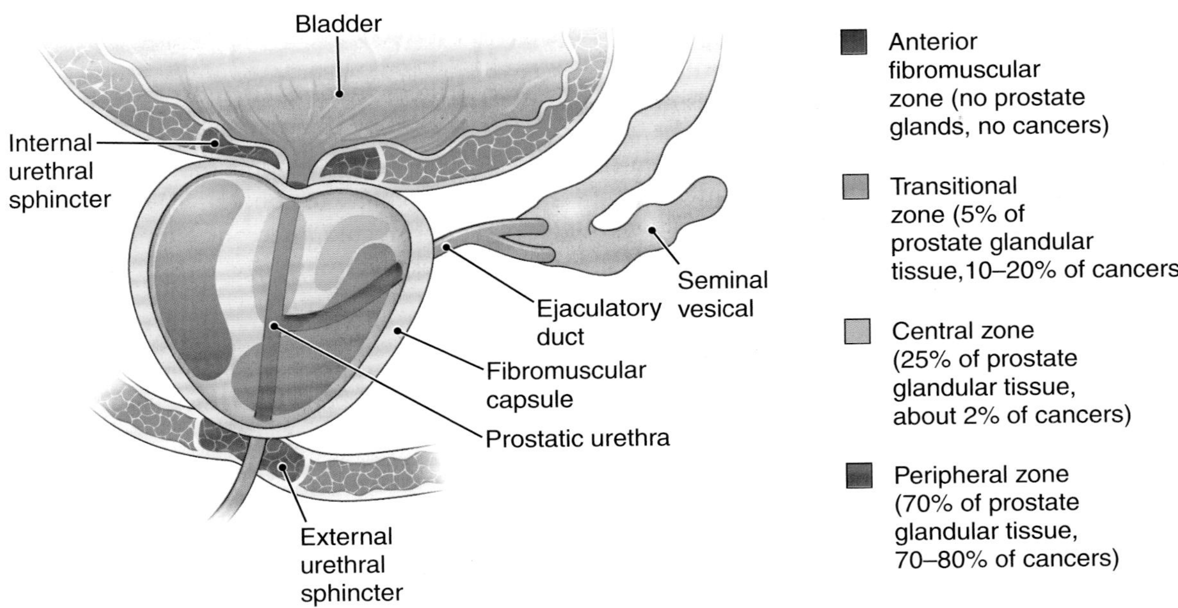

Figure 16.3 **The prostate and adjacent structures.** (Adapted with permission from Anatomical Chart Company.)

parasympathetic nervous system. **Ejaculation** is ejection of semen from the tip of the penis in response to sensory signals mediated by the *sympathetic* nervous system. It is the apex of male sexual reward mediated by waves of exquisitely pleasurable muscular contractions of the epididymis, vas deferens, seminal vesicles, and prostate.

Pop Quiz

16.1 True or false? Testicular temperature is approximately 5°F below the temperature of the rest of the body.

16.2 Seminal fluid contains ____________, an enzyme that causes semen to clot after ejaculation. Prostatic fluid contains ______________, an enzyme that dissolves clotted semen.

16.3 Normal sperm have what chromosome set?

16.4 In males, most testosterone is produced by the __________ cells of the testis.

Disorders of Reproductive Function

Compared to diseases of the female genitalia, diseases of the male reproductive system receive little attention. Most women regularly see an obstetrician/gynecologist, but most men will not visit a urologist in their lifetime. Nevertheless, public awareness of male genital conditions has improved with the public advertising campaigns for treatment of erectile dysfunction (ED), one of the most important male conditions along with infertility, infection, and prostate cancer.

Erectile Dysfunction Is Inability to Achieve a Functional Erection

About half of men over age 50 at some time experience **erectile dysfunction (ED)**, an inability to attain or sustain an erection firm enough for satisfactory intercourse. Achieving an erection is a complex physical and mental process that relies on parasympathetic nerve impulses; however, no matter the cause, ED ultimately owes to slow arterial inflow into the penis or venous drainage that is too fast. Among men who have lost their ability to have satisfactory erections, over 90% of cases are associated with physical factors such as atherosclerotic impairment of arterial inflow, disease or injury to nerves controlling penile blood flow, hormone imbalances, or therapeutic drugs. These organic problems often lead to partner discord, performance anxiety, or other psychological problems that compound the problem.

Therapeutic drugs, especially antihypertensives, account for about 25% of ED. Lesions of the brain, spinal cord, or peripheral nerves may be responsible by interfering with neural control of vascular smooth muscle tone and the flow of blood into and out of the penis. About 40% of men undergoing a prostatectomy develop some degree of ED, caused by surgical damage to nerves that regulate vascular flow in the penis. Testosterone plays an important physical and mental role, which becomes evident in older men as testosterone levels gradually decline with age. Depression may also be the cause, but is often difficult to detect without a high index of suspicion.

Diagnosis requires careful clinical evaluation, screening for depression, and blood testosterone measurement. If an underlying cause can be identified, elimination of that cause is the first step in treatment. Testosterone replacement may be useful if testosterone levels are low. Oral phosphodiesterase inhibitor drugs are now widely available and are preferred by most men. A venous constrictor snugged around the genitals can be effective by slowing venous outflow. Other treatments include intracavernous self-injection of vasodilators, intraurethral instillation of prostaglandin, application of an external vacuum pump, or surgical insertion of an internal inflatable implant.

Infertility Is the Inability to Contribute Effectively to Conception

Infertility is the inability of a partner to contribute effectively to conception. Because it is imperative to evaluate both partners, a broader and more specific definition is the inability of a couple to conceive after one year of regular unprotected intercourse. About one in five couples in the United States is affected. Factors include sperm disorders (about 35% of couples), ovulatory dysfunction (20%), fallopian tube dysfunction (30%), and abnormal cervical mucus (5%). In about 10% of couples, the etiology cannot be identified. Female aspects of infertility are discussed in Chapter 17.

Impaired spermatogenesis results in low sperm count, which directly affects the chance to fertilize an ovum. Impaired spermatogenesis can be caused by 1) hypothyroidism and other endocrine disorders; 2) infections of the testis or epididymis; 3) undescended testis (Chapter 22); 4) varicocele; and 5) drugs, including estrogen, steroids, illicit drugs, and many others.

Impaired sperm emission can be caused by 1) diabetic neuropathy and other neurologic conditions that interfere with peristalsis of the vas deferens; 2) prostatectomy; 3) obstruction of the vas deferens; 4) genetic conditions (e.g., most men with cystic fibrosis have bilateral agenesis of the vas deferens); and 5) retrograde ejaculation into the bladder.

Other problems include autoimmune antisperm antibodies and sperm with impaired motility.

Diagnosis requires semen analysis, including volume, liquefaction time, appearance, pH, sperm count, sperm motility, percent of sperm with normal morphology, and fructose (the primary sugar in semen). Endocrine evaluation may be necessary. Apart from treatment of an underlying cause, if one can be identified, clomiphene (an antiestrogen) may increase sperm count. Assisted reproduction can be offered if clomiphene fails.

Pop Quiz

16.5 True or false? ED in most men is caused by psychological factors.

16.6 What length of time must pass with an inability to conceive despite regular unprotected intercourse before a couple is termed infertile?

Disorders of the Penis, Scrotum, and Groin

The penis, scrotum, and testes constitute the physical essence of maleness. Apart from its essential role in reproduction, the penis provides males with unrivaled pleasure, and the testes produce abundant testosterone, a hormone that builds muscular strength while at the same time influencing the brain toward dominance, sexual conquest, and aggression. No wonder, then, that to deprive a male of his penis and testicles is to render him placid and uninterested in women. The *History of Medicine*, "Eunuchs," discusses the practice of amputating the testicles (and sometimes the penis) to produce *eunuchs* (literally "bedroom guard") and offers an interesting historical insight into certain aspects of male physiology and behavior.

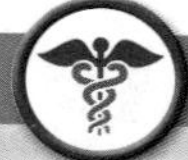

The History of Medicine

EUNUCHS

A eunuch is a castrated man, a man whose testicles have been removed. The word derives from Greek *eun*, for bed, and *oksein*, meaning to keep; thus a bed keeper or bedchamber guard or attendant.

The creation of eunuchs was practiced in ancient Egypt, China, India, and part of the eastern Mediterranean until a few hundred years ago. Castration before puberty ensured that certain male characteristics would not develop: the penis, if it was not removed with the testicles, ceased to grow, sexual desire never appeared, muscle mass did not develop, the voice remained high, and facial and body hair did not develop.

The practice was most widespread in ancient royal courts, where eunuchs were employed as keepers of royal female bedchambers, a practice that reached its peak in Constantinople (modern Istanbul, Turkey) during the Ottoman Empire (1250–1918). The last royal Chinese eunuch was born in 1903 and castrated at age eight for the royal court during the last years of the Manchu Dynasty. He died at age 93 in 1996.

This custom was not universally a practice of royalty. Beginning around 1650 in Italy, young boys wanting to sing in the opera were castrated (becoming a *castrato*) to maintain a pure, high voice. The last Italian castrato lived long enough to be recorded in 1904 and died in 1922.

The Carib Indians (for whom the Caribbean Islands are named and from which the word cannibal is derived) made a habit of castrating young male captives, well aware that early castration kept their flesh fattier and prevented the muscles from becoming tough and wiry. The Caribs fed the captives richly until they were to be sacrificed and eaten.

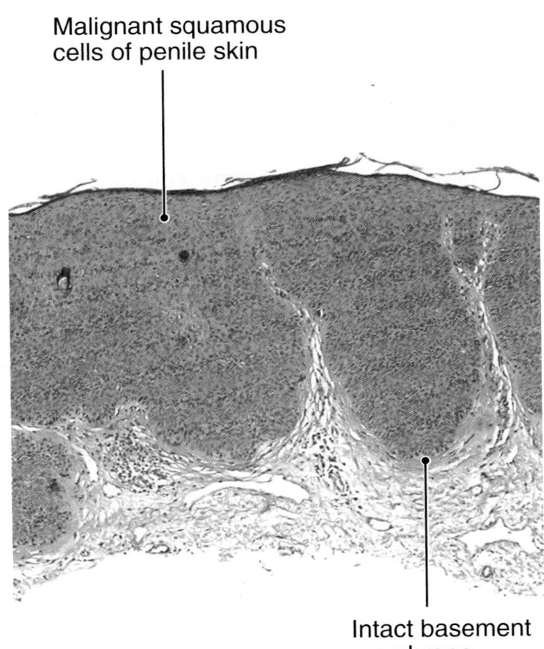

Figure 16.4 **Bowen disease of the penis (squamous carcinoma in situ).** The epithelium is composed entirely of malignant cells, none of which have invaded across the basement membrane.

Congenital abnormalities of the external urethral meatus occur in about 1 in 300 male infants. **Hypospadias** is an elongated slit on the distal ventrum; **epispadias** is a similar defect on the dorsum. Either may be associated with incontinence, infection, obstruction, or other congenital abnormalities such as *undescended testis* or *inguinal hernia*.

Phimosis is an inability to retract the foreskin over the glans. It may be congenital or acquired. It is important because an unretractable prepuce promotes poor hygiene, infection, inflammation, and scarring and may encourage the development of squamous carcinoma. If an affected prepuce is forcibly retracted, it may become trapped, a condition called **paraphimosis** that produces severe glans congestion, edema, pain, and acute urinary obstruction.

Inflammation of the glans is **balanitis**, and although many cases are caused by sexually transmitted infections (STI, discussed below), most result from poor personal hygiene in uncircumcised males. **Balanitis xerotica obliterans** is an inflammatory disease of unknown cause associated with a white, sclerotic patch of skin at the tip of the glans, which may constrict the urethral opening.

Neoplasms of the penis are uncommon. The most common is **condyloma acuminatum**, a benign sexually transmitted cauliflower-like growth caused by human papilloma virus (HPV, Chapter 4). A vaccine is available.

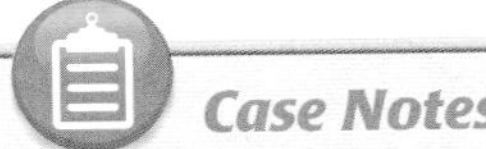

Case Notes

16.3 What was the name of Marshall's foreskin problem?

Bowen disease (Fig. 16.4) is a squamous carcinoma in situ that forms a grayish or reddish plaque on the glans and has a distinctive clinical and microscopic appearance identical to Bowen disease of the nipple, vulva, and oral cavity. Untreated, about 10% of cases progress to invasive carcinoma.

The most common invasive malignancy is **squamous carcinoma** that arises in the squamous epithelium of the glans in uncircumcised males over age 40 or in the penile urethra. Poor personal hygiene and HPV infection plays a role. Bowen disease and squamous carcinoma require microscopic diagnosis and surgical treatment.

Peyronie disease is a fibrosing condition of the corpus cavernosum or its fibrous sheath, the tunica albuginea. It may distort the erect penis to the point that erection is painful and intercourse difficult. Treatment is challenging because surgical scarring after excision may be worse than the original problem. Steroid injections have been tried with variable results.

Priapism (from *Priapus*, the Greek god of male procreative power) is a painful, persistent erection in the absence of sexual desire. Severe cases may lead to penile gangrene. Most cases are failure to fade of an otherwise normal erection owing to impaired venous outflow. In a child with sickle cell disease or leukemia, trapped RBCs or WBCs may be the cause. Some cases are caused by prescription or recreational drugs or cavernosal injection for ED. It is a medical emergency that requires urologic care. Injection of vasodilator drugs is usually effective.

There are two general types of *urethritis*, both sexually transmitted infections (STIs): *gonococcal urethritis* caused by the bacterium *Neisseria gonorrhoeae*, and *nongonococcal urethritis*, which is most often caused by *Chlamydia* or *Mycoplasma*. *Trichomonas* and *Ureaplasma* play a lesser role. Both are discussed with other STIs in Chapter 4. Gram stain, culture, and other tests for gonococci are cheap, fast, and readily available, but similar tests for *Chlamydia* and *Mycoplasma* are more expensive, troublesome, and slow. Hence, testing is usually done only for gonococci. If positive, the diagnosis is *gonococcal urethritis*. If negative, the term *nongonococcal urethritis* is used by default. All can be treated effectively by antibiotics.

Infection may spread to involve the prostate (prostatitis) or epididymis (epididymitis). Recurrent urethritis in men can produce urethral scarring (strictures) with acute or chronic urinary obstruction, topics discussed in Chapter 15.

Inguinal hernia is discussed in detail in Chapter 11. It is a protrusion of bowel into the inguinal canal or scrotum, which occurs as normal intra-abdominal pressure forces open a canal into the scrotum. Treatment is surgical.

Tinea cruris ("jock itch") is an inflammation of the scrotum or inguinal skin caused by one of the varieties of *Tinea* species, a dermatophyte fungus similar to fungi that cause scalp ringworm and athlete's foot (Chapter 4). Transmission is by personal contact or unclean athletic wear. Treatment is with a topical antifungal drug.

Varicocele is scrotal varicose veins, which may cause scrotal enlargement and infertility. **Hydrocele** is accumulation of fluid in the sac of the tunica vaginalis that surrounds the testis.

Pop Quiz

16.7 True or false? All cases of nongonococcal urethritis are caused by *Chlamydia trachomatis*.

16.8 True or false? Balanitis xerotica obliterans is an inflammatory disease of unknown cause associated with a white, sclerotic patch of skin at the tip of the glans.

16.9 What is the cause of jock itch?

16.10 Hypospadias is an elongated slit on the ________ of the penis while epispadias is a similar defect on the ________ of the penis.

Disorders of the Epididymis and Testis

The testis is a complex gland of tubes and stroma formed of germ cells, supporting cells, and hormone-producing cells that cooperate to produce sperm. Immature sperm migrate from the testis into the epididymis to mature. The epididymis is a very long, coiled tube on the posterior of the testis through which sperm migrate slowly, maturing as they go. Mature sperm are stored in the distal part of the epididymis until they are ejaculated from the epididymis into the vas deferens in the production of semen.

Cryptorchidism Is Failure of the Fetal Testis to Descend into the Scrotum

During the fetal period, the testes descend from the abdomen through the inguinal canal into the scrotum. The most important congenital abnormality of male genitalia is **cryptorchidism** (undescended testis) (Fig. 16.5). Normally during fetal development, the testes descend from the pelvis through the inguinal canal and into the scrotum, pulling with them the vas deferens and associated neurovascular supply. In cryptorchidism, one testis fails to complete this fetal journey and remains in the abdomen or comes to rest in the inguinal canal. Rarely, both testes fail to descend. Early discovery of the problem and surgical correction is necessary—an undescended testis that remains in the abdomen confers at least a 10-fold risk for testicular malignancy. Even with surgical correction, testicular malignancy risk is increased for both the corrected testes and for the one that descended properly. Because normal scrotal temperature is about 5°F cooler than body core temperature, the added warmth of the abdomen causes testicular atrophy and infertility if the testes are not surgically relocated and anchored in the scrotum.

Epididymitis Is Much More Common than Orchitis

Inflammation of the testis (**orchitis**) is much less common than inflammation of the epididymis (**epididymitis**). *Orchitis* occurs with mumps (Chapter 4) in about

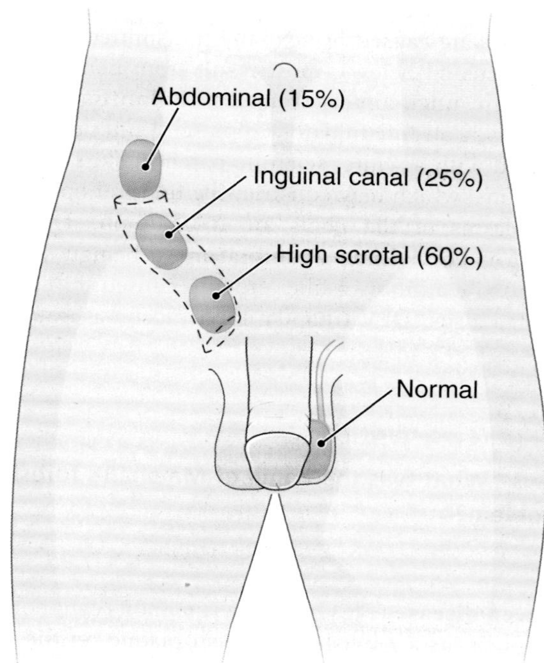

Figure 16.5 **Undescended testis (cryptorchidism).** An undescended testis may be found in the abdomen, in the inguinal canal, or high in the scrotum. Percent figures indicate the proportion of cases diagnosed at each location.

one-fourth of infected postpubertal males. Swelling and pain are treated supportively.

Most cases of epididymitis owe to retrograde infection up the vas deferens from cystitis, urethritis, or prostatitis. In men under age 35, the cause is usually a STI—*Chlamydia trachomatis* or *Neisseria gonorrhoeae*. In men over age 35, the cause is usually one of the more common urinary pathogens such as *E. coli*. Nonbacterial epididymitis is fairly common. Often the cause remains unknown, but some cases are autoimmune. Swelling and local pain are typical and may be severe. Diagnosis is clinical. Antibiotic therapy is usually effective for infection.

Spermatocele is a cyst of the epididymis that contains sperm and is formed by dilation of the epididymal tubule. It enlarges gradually with continued sperm production. Diagnosis is clinical and aided by sonographic imaging. Treatment is surgical.

Testicular Torsion Is an Emergency

Twisting of the spermatic cord (**torsion**) typically interrupts venous drainage but not arterial inflow. Severe congestion and hemorrhagic infarction of the testis may follow. Neonatal torsion may occur just before or after birth and lacks anatomic explanation. Most cases, however, arise in teenage boys who have unusual anatomic mobility of the testis in the scrotum. Torsion of one testis reveals the risk that torsion of the opposite side might occur.

Symptoms of testicular torsion include pain, swelling, nausea, and vomiting. Diagnosis is clinical. Immediate surgical exploration and unwinding is necessary, along with surgical fixation (*orchiopexy*) of both testicles in the scrotal sac.

Most Testicular Neoplasms Are Malignant

Testicular neoplasms, the majority of which are malignant, occur most commonly between the ages of 15 and 40. *The Clinical Side*, "Cyclist Lance Armstrong and Testicular Cancer," offers more information about a prominent case. Testicular neoplasms should be suspected in any male with painless enlargement of the testis. These neoplasms fall into two main groups:

- *Tumors of germ (sperm-producing) cells* (95%). Virtually all are malignant.
- *Tumors of sex-chord/stroma cells* (5%). They are named from their presumed origin from cells originating in the *embryonic sex-cord*, a primitive structure from which Sertoli and Leydig cells originate. Virtually all are benign.

Figure 16.6 illustrates the cells of origin and their types.

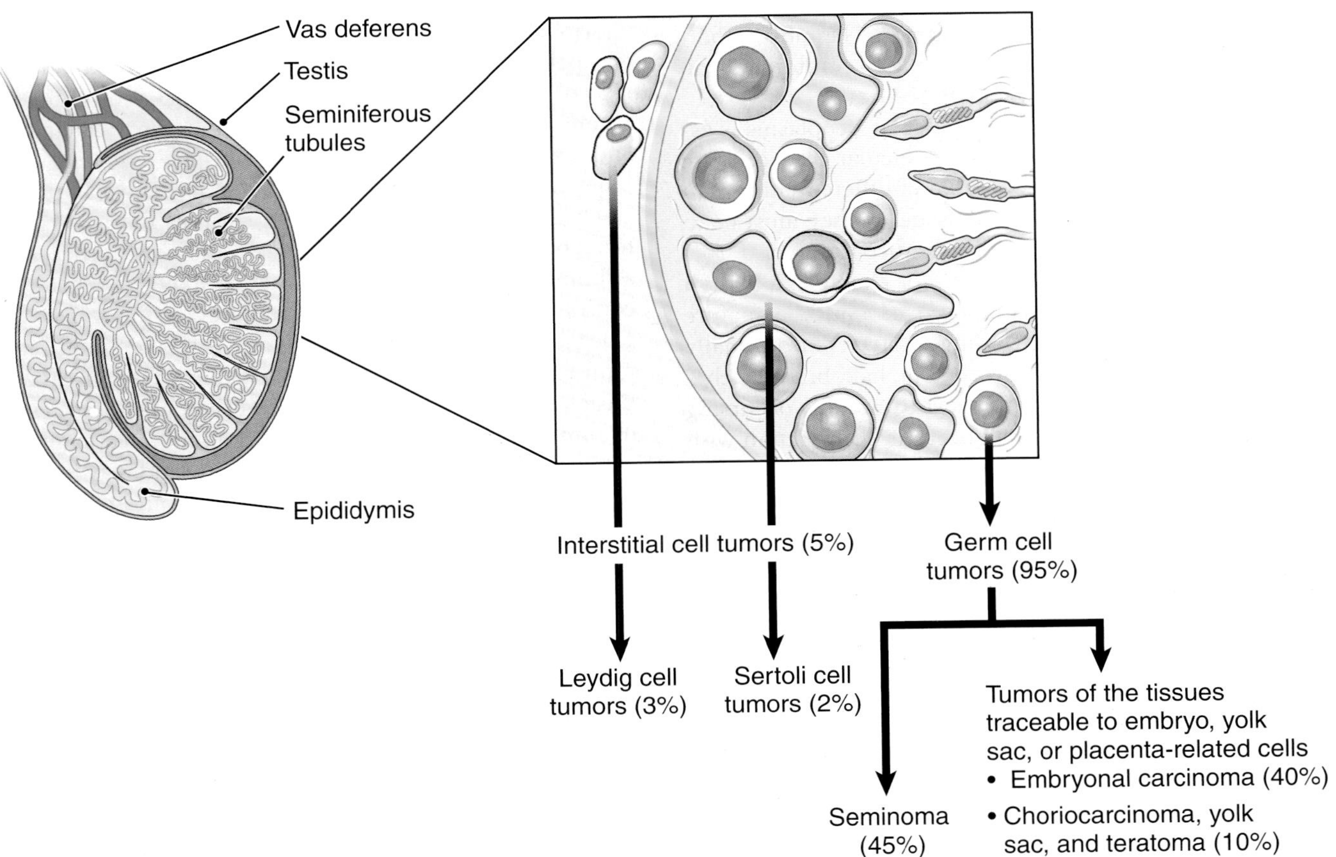

Figure 16.6 **The origin of testicular neoplasms.** There are two major groups: germ cell and interstitial cell tumors.

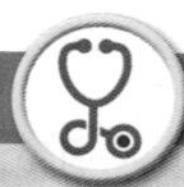

The Clinical Side

CYCLIST LANCE ARMSTRONG AND TESTICULAR CANCER

American cyclist Lance Armstrong gained fame as a seven-time winner of the grueling Tour de France, a distinction later turned into infamy by admission that he used drugs and blood doping to win. What many do not know is that before he gained worldwide notice, Armstrong was diagnosed with testicular carcinoma—in his case a mixture of embryonal and choriocarcinoma that had spread to the lungs and the brain. Armstrong had experienced painless enlargement of one testicle for three years before the diagnosis, an object lesson about testicular enlargements: all must be investigated promptly. Fortunately, Armstrong's tumor was completely eradicated by chemotherapy. Once almost universally fatal, most testicular malignancies are now curable.

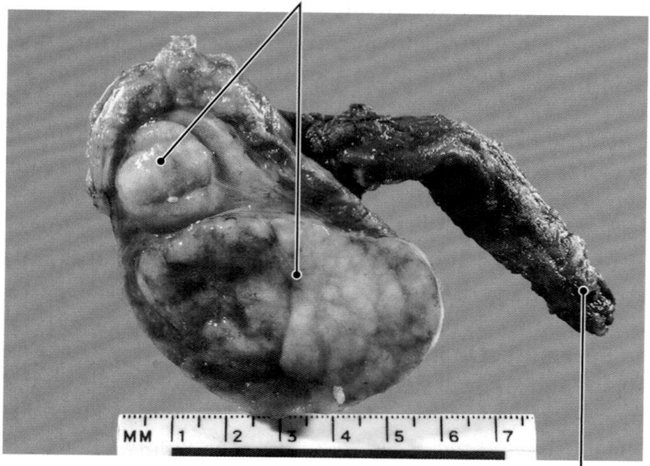

Figure 16.7 **Seminoma of the testis.** This tumor occupies the entire testis.

Remember This! A testicular mass is to be considered malignant until proven otherwise.

Germ Cell Tumors

Germ cell tumors are most common between ages 15 and 40, and about 85% occur in Caucasians. The most important risk factor for a germ cell tumor is cryptorchidism. There is also a strong family predisposition.

The variety and behavior of testicular neoplasms is astonishing and owes to the fact that testicular germ cells are totipotent; that is, they are capable of differentiating into any kind of mature or primitive tissue, as they must be to form a normal embryo. Tumors can arise from germ cells at any stage of their development. For example, a **benign teratoma** is a neoplasm composed of multiple mature (differentiated) tissues, including tissues not normally found in the testis such as normal skin, hair, brain, or thyroid tissue. Teratomas are rare, most commonly occurring in prepubertal boys. About half occur in conjunction with another variety of germ cell tumor.

Seminomas are tumors that retain features of primitive spermatocytes, hence their name (an identical ovarian tumor is the *dysgerminoma*, Chapter 17). They are the most common germ cell tumor and the most common of all testicular tumors (Fig. 16.7). Seminomas grow more slowly and metastasize later than other germ cell malignancies. One reason for their slow growth is that they are held in check by the immune system—they incite a brisk immune response and are characterized microscopically by dense accumulations of lymphocytes among the tumor cells. Treatment is surgery or radiation or both, depending on the staging and other clinical details. Nearly all patients with early stage disease are curable. Chemotherapy may be effective for metastatic disease.

Other types of germ cell tumors are **embryonal carcinoma** (composed of very primitive cells), **yolk sac carcinoma** (named for its content of embryonic yolk sac cells; it occurs almost exclusively in young boys), and **choriocarcinoma** (named for its content of placental chorionic-type cells).

About half of germ cell tumors contain more than one type of tumor and are called **mixed tumors**. For example, a common pattern is a mixture of embryonal carcinoma and teratoma (sometimes called *malignant teratoma*). Another combination is embryonal carcinoma and seminoma.

Diagnosis of testicular tumors requires that the entire testis be removed for microscopic evaluation (rather than a simple biopsy). In this rare instance, a biopsy is actually contraindicated. The inherent anatomy of the testis provides a barrier (the tunica albuginea—the membrane surrounding each testis) that prevents the spread of cancer. Breach of this barrier can seed the needle tract and result in a much poorer prognosis for the patient. Treatment depends on tumor type and surgical staging and may include a mix of surgery, radiation, chemotherapy, and hormones.

Several decades ago, testicular malignancies were usually fatal. Now, however, for patients with a germ cell malignancy that is localized to the testis or with limited metastasis to retroperitoneal lymph nodes, the five-year survival rate is over 95%. For extensive metastasis, the five-year survival rate ranges from 50% to 80% depending on tumor type and staging details. Some patients with seemingly hopeless metastatic disease may be cured.

Sex Cord-Stromal Tumors

Nongerm cell tumors have a distinctive microscopic appearance different from germ cell tumors and are presumably derived from cells of the primitive embryologic sex cord from which Sertoli and Leydig cells arise. Sex cord-stromal tumors are uncommon and almost always benign. They usually present as a painless testicular mass, but some may cause symptoms due to overproduction of steroids. Leydig cells, which produce testosterone, lie in the interstitium between testicular seminiferous tubules. **Leydig cell tumors** arise from Leydig progenitor cells in the testicular stroma. Likewise, **Sertoli cell tumors** arise from progenitor Sertoli cells, which exist in seminiferous tubules among the germ cells. Virtually all are benign. Treatment is surgical.

Pop Quiz

16.11 True or false? Torsion of the testis is due to a unilateral flaw, and the other testis is at no increased risk for torsion.

16.12 What is the most common cause of epididymitis under the age of 35?

16.13 What is the most common testicular tumor?

Disorders of the Prostate

Knowledge of prostate anatomy, illustrated in Figure 16.8 (see also Fig. 16.3), is important in understanding prostatic diagnosis and treatment. Recall that the prostate encircles the urethra where it joins the neck of the bladder. It is immediately anterior to the rectum, so that the gland is palpable by **digital rectal exam (DRE)**. Benign enlargement owes to glandular hyperplasia, mainly in the central area. On the other hand, prostate cancer usually develops in the posterior and peripheral parts, a fact that makes some prostatic cancers palpable by DRE and recognizable because they are much firmer than normal prostate.

Prostatitis Is a Common and Difficult Problem

Prostatitis is a common affliction of men. The two varieties are *bacterial prostatitis* and *chronic nonbacterial prostatitis*.

Bacterial prostatitis is usually caused by *E. coli* or other fecal bacteria of the type that typically cause urinary tract infections. Organisms seed the prostate by reflux from infected urine or following instrumentation or catheterization of the lower urinary tract.

Acute bacterial prostatitis is associated with fever, chills, dysuria, and pelvic discomfort or pain. The prostate is swollen, boggy, and very tender by DRE. Diagnosis is by clinical features and urine culture. Antibiotic therapy is usually successful in the short term, but complete eradication of organisms is difficult and often the infection recurs.

Chronic bacterial prostatitis is a more difficult matter. Patients may be nearly asymptomatic or they may present with low back pain, suprapubic or pelvic pain or discomfort, and perineal pain or discomfort. Fever is absent. In most instances, there is no history of previous acute prostatitis, though patients frequently have a history of recurrent lower urinary tract infection. Diagnosis is by clinical features, positive culture of urine or prostatic secretions, and demonstration of inflammatory cells in prostatic secretions. Organisms are the same as those responsible for lower urinary tract infections and acute bacterial prostatitis. Antibiotic therapy is usually helpful in cases with positive cultures, but antibiotics have a difficult time penetrating the prostate and sometimes the gland continues to harbor a reservoir of microbes that causes recurrent prostatitis and reseeds the lower urinary tract.

Chronic nonbacterial prostatitis is now the most common form of prostatitis. It is clinically similar to chronic bacterial prostatitis, including inflammatory cells in prostatic secretions, but cultures are negative and there is no history of urinary tract infection. The cause is unknown. Treatment is usually unrewarding. Psychoactive medications, prostatic massage, sacral nerve stimulation, and many other forms of therapy have been tried without consistent results. Pain management usually becomes the main goal.

Prostatic Hyperplasia Is Almost Universal in Elderly Men

Nearly all men, if they live long enough, develop **benign prostatic hyperplasia (BPH)**. This enlargement is caused by nodular hyperplasia of the prostate gland and the fibromuscular supporting tissue around the gland (see Fig. 16.8). BPH is very common. It is present in about 20% of 40-year-old men and 90% of those age 70 or older. Of men with an enlarged prostate, only 50% will have symptoms. The result is that about one-third of men over age 50 will have symptoms, though many of them will not seek care.

The cause is not clear. It appears that abnormal testosterone metabolism plays a major role and both gland tissue and stroma participate. It is not precancerous.

Figure 16.9 illustrates that in nodular hyperplasia the prostate gland is enlarged, sometimes greatly. In a typical case, the gland is enlarged three- to fivefold or more (sometimes up to 100 ml, or 100 grams by weight). Often the enlargement may protrude into the bladder. The gland is tense and rubbery, and the cut surface exhibits multiple bulging nodules of hyperplastic glands, as illustrated by Figure 16.10.

Obstruction often prevents complete emptying of the bladder (Fig. 16.11) and often causes problems with bladder control (Chapter 15). For unknown reasons,

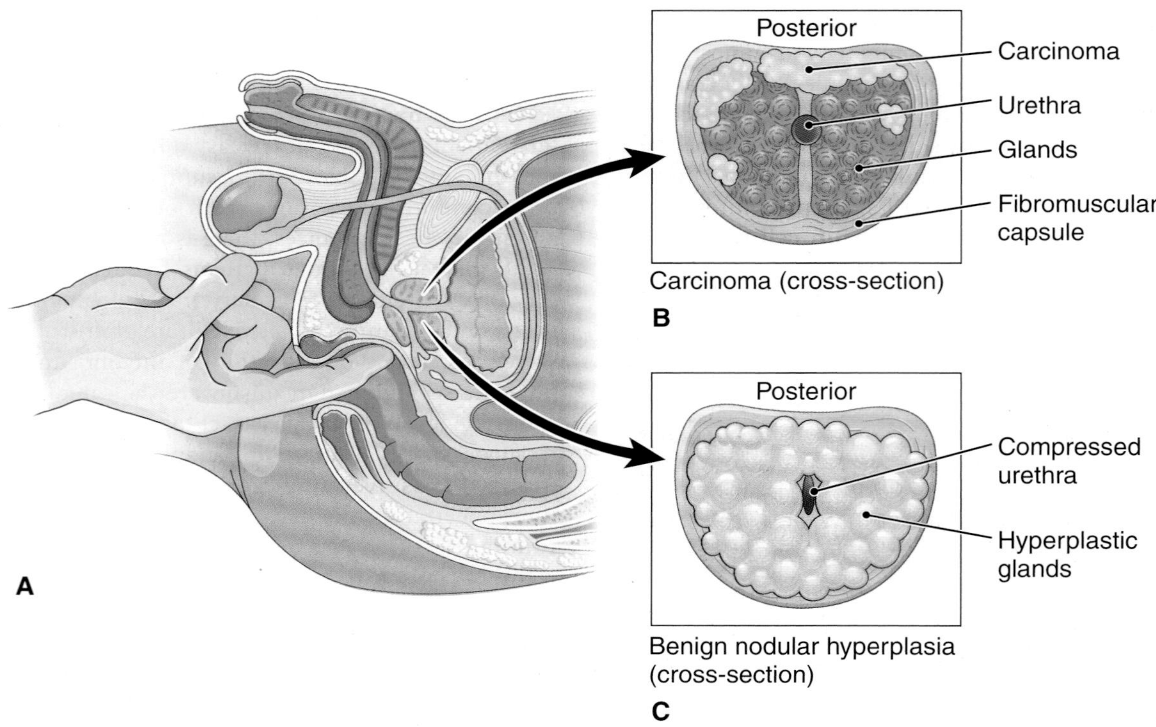

Figure 16.8 **A**. The prostate in relation to the rectum. **B.** Carcinoma of the prostate usually occurs in the posterior aspect of the gland and may be detectable by DRE. **C**. Benign nodular hyperplasia mainly involves the center of the gland.

acute urinary retention often occurs and requires emergency catheterization. Retained urine promotes frequency, urgency, and nocturia. Other signs are difficulty starting the stream (hesitancy), intermittent interruption of the stream while voiding, dribbling, and a narrow stream. Retention promotes stasis, infection, hydronephrosis, pyelonephritis, and other conditions (Chapter 15).

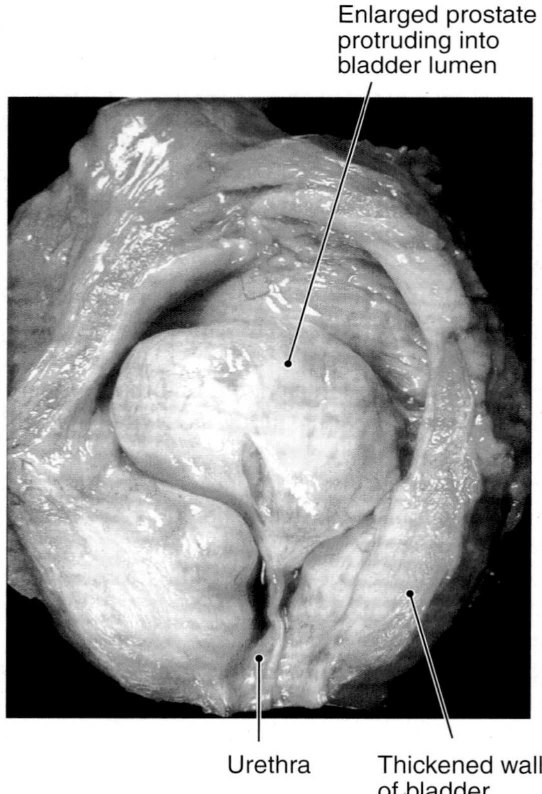

Figure 16.9 **Massive nodular hyperplasia of the prostate**. The middle part of the gland protrudes into the bladder. Note the hypertrophied bladder wall, which is caused by chronic urinary obstruction.

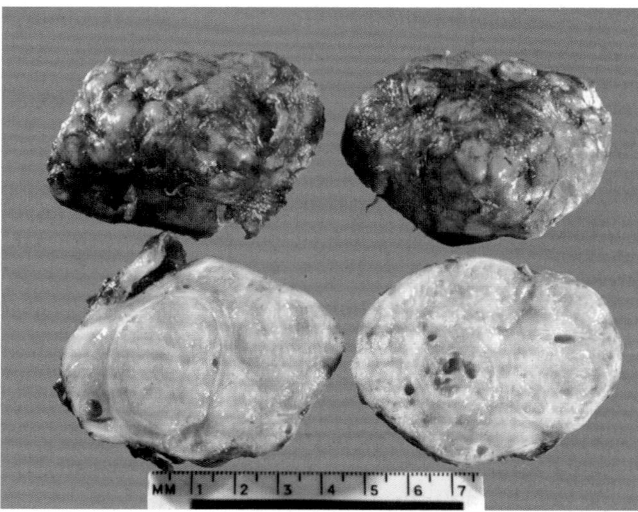

Figure 16.10 **Nodular hyperplasia of the prostate, surgical specimen.** This gland was excised for marked prostatic hyperplasia and urinary obstruction. Note the irregular nodules of hyperplastic prostatic tissue.

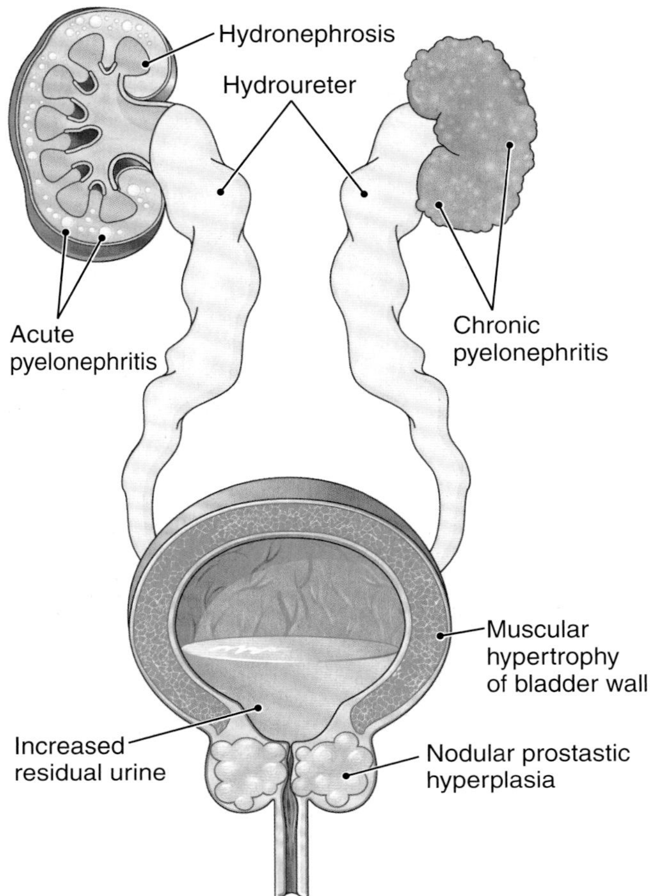

Figure 16.11 **Consequences of prostatic chronic obstruction of the lower urinary tract.** Incomplete emptying of the bladder causes nocturia, urgency, frequency, and loss of control. Ureteral reflux may cause infection and chronic kidney disease.

Mild cases can be treated by avoiding bedtime fluids and judicious management of alcohol and caffeine intake. Drugs can be effective for cases with more severe symptoms. Alpha-blockers decrease the tone of fibromuscular stroma, and other drugs inhibit prostate testosterone metabolism. The definitive therapy is surgical: either a "boring out" of prostatic tissue through the urethra (transurethral resection, or TUR prostatectomy), or other therapy to decrease the mass of tissue surrounding the urethra—ultrasound, laser therapy, radiofrequency ablation, or electrocauterization.

Case Notes

16.4 Which of Marshall's symptoms were consistent with prostatic obstruction?

16.5 Was Marshall's prostatic hyperplasia the cause of his cancer?

Prostatic Carcinoma Is the Most Common Malignancy of Humans

Prostatic adenocarcinoma (typically called "prostate cancer" or "prostate carcinoma"), a malignancy of prostate gland epithelial cells, accounts for all but a tiny fraction of prostatic malignancies. The National Institutes of Health estimated that in 2012 there were 242,000 new cases of prostate cancer, more than the number of new cases of breast or lung cancer. Nevertheless, prostate cancer is far less lethal than lung and breast cancer. In 2012, an estimated 15,000 deaths were attributed to prostate cancer, as opposed to 160,000 deaths from lung cancer and 40,000 from breast cancer. The incidence of prostate cancer found at autopsy is 20% in men in their 50 and 70% in men in their 70s and 80s, but only about 10% of these develop symptoms.

Etiology and Pathogenesis

The etiology and pathogenesis of prostate cancer are multifactorial. It is uncommon in Asians and more common in African Americans than Caucasians. Men with one first-degree relative with prostate cancer have a twofold increased risk; those with two first-degree relatives have a fivefold increased risk. The environment also plays a role: immigrants who move to the United States (where there is a high incidence of prostate cancer) from nations with low incidence of prostate cancer soon develop higher, U.S.-like, rates.

Androgens play an important role. Most established prostate cancers are androgen-dependent—castration or antiandrogen therapy therefore usually produces significant regression of metastatic or locally invasive disease, though in most cases the tumor ultimately escapes the palliative effect of treatment. Whether or not androgens play a role in the *causation* of prostate cancer, however, is another matter. There is some evidence that men with low blood testosterone develop prostate cancer more frequently than those with higher levels, but the research is inconclusive.

Another important pathogenetic topic is the importance of **prostatic intraepithelial neoplasia (PIN)**. PIN is characterized by atypical prostatic epithelial cells that contain some of the molecular changes found in prostatic carcinoma, and is present in 80% of prostates containing cancer. High-grade PIN is considered to be carcinoma in situ, and therefore a precursor to invasive prostatic adenocarcinoma. Nevertheless, it is difficult to prove this assertion because prostatic adenocarcinoma is no more likely to develop in a man with high-grade PIN than in a man without PIN.

Case Notes

16.6 Which risk factors did Marshall have for prostate cancer?

16.7 Is it unusual for PIN and cancer to occur in the same gland?

Signs and Symptoms

Cancers arise in the periphery of the gland (Fig. 16.12), away from the urethra, and rarely cause obstructive symptoms. Most tumors arise in and remain confined to the gland, are not symptomatic, and are discovered by routine blood tests that reveal increased PSA. Less commonly they are detected by DRE. Tumors that have spread locally may cause obstructive symptoms, hematuria, or other lower urinary complaint. Distant metastases are usually to bone, especially the spine, pelvis, and ribs, and may be discovered in the course of a pain workup. The metastases induce local osteoblastic bone growth with increased bone density (Fig. 16.13). Osteoblastic bone metastases in a man over age 50 are virtually certain to be metastatic prostate cancer. Patients with bone metastases usually succumb to their disease.

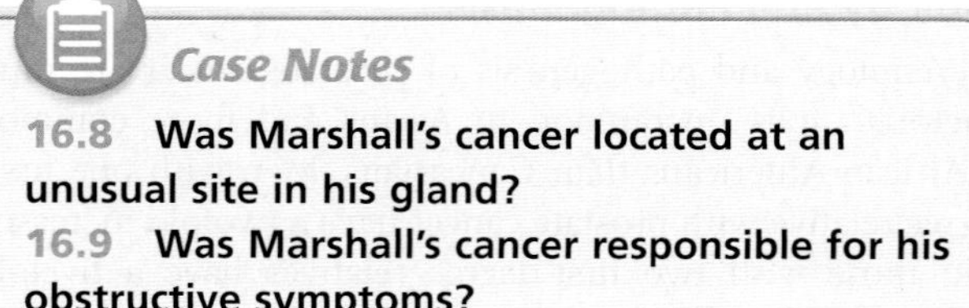

Case Notes

16.8 Was Marshall's cancer located at an unusual site in his gland?

16.9 Was Marshall's cancer responsible for his obstructive symptoms?

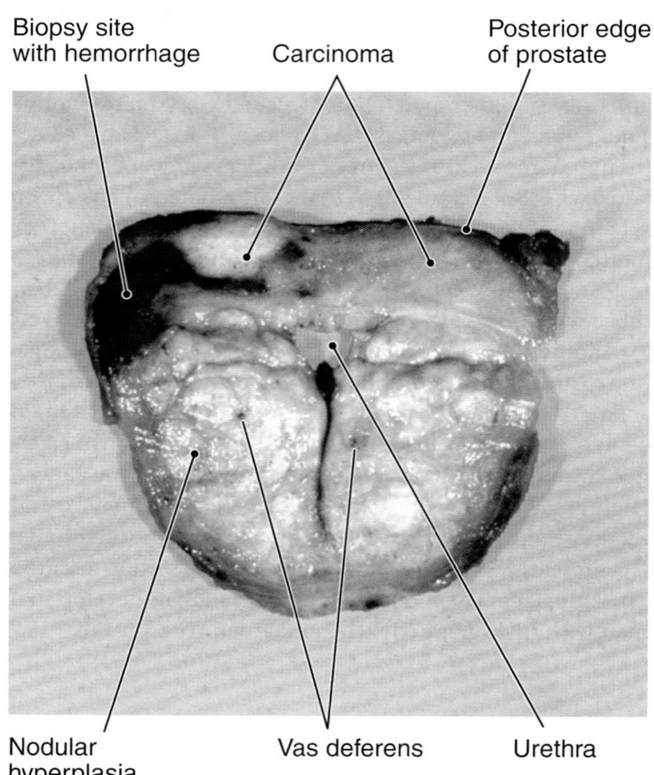

Figure 16.12 **Total prostatectomy for carcinoma of the prostate.** Most of the gland is occupied by nodular hyperplasia, as it is in most patients who have prostatic carcinoma. Note the uniform, non-nodular nature of the posterior aspect of gland, which is involved by prostatic carcinoma. Hemorrhage is at the site of a needle biopsy performed two days earlier.

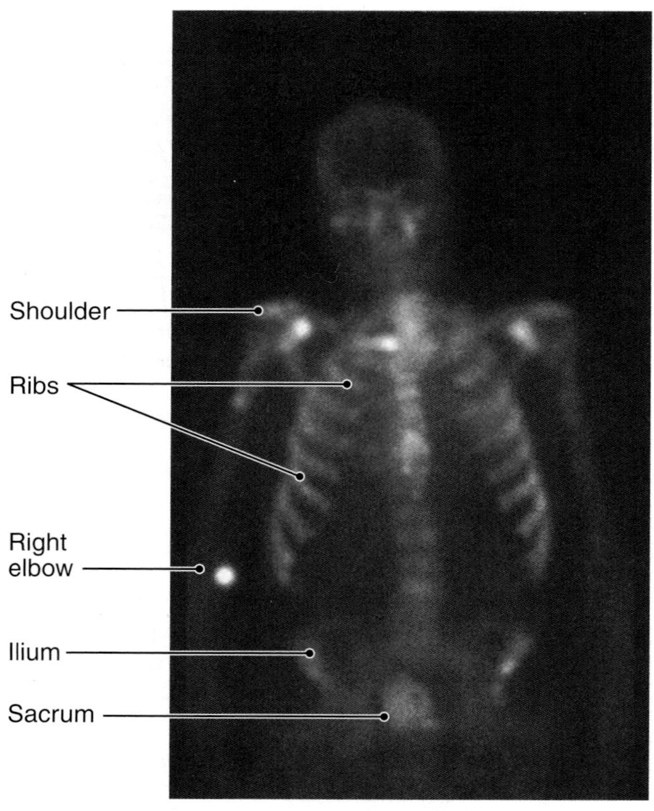

Figure 16.13 **Radioactive bone scan.** Metastatic prostate cancer is often found in bones. The cancer captures radioactive material injected intravenously and reveals its location by emitted radiation. In this patient the cancer, which appears white to the camera, is detected in the shoulder, ribs, right elbow, ilium, and sacrum.

Screening for Prostate Cancer

PSA is the most important test used in the diagnosis of prostate cancer. PSA is prostate specific, but not cancer specific, and increased PSA is, therefore, neither a very sensitive nor a very specific test for prostate cancer. The topic of prostate cancer diagnosis and treatment is currently one of the most controversial topics in medicine.

Men who have annual prostate cancer screening have a higher incidence of prostate cancer than men who are not screened. Nevertheless, *screened and unscreened groups have the same number of deaths from prostate cancer.* This suggests that many men were treated for prostate cancers that would not have been detected and would not have harmed them during their lifetime. The screened group, however, was exposed to the hazards of treatment.

Other data shows that men who are screened have a somewhat lower death rate from prostate cancer. One implication of this and the above data is that lives saved from prostatic cancer are being taken by something else, so that the overall death rate is unchanged.

The final conclusions of a metastudy of other studies issued in 2012 by the U.S. Preventive Services Task Force estimated that, for every 1,000 men ages 55–69 years who are screened every one to four years for a decade:

- About 1 death from prostate cancer would be avoided.
- About 100 men would have false positive results that lead to a biopsy.
- About 100 men would be found to have prostate cancer. About 50 of these men would have a serious complication from treatment, including ED, urinary incontinence, serious cardiovascular event, deep vein thrombosis or pulmonary embolism, or death.

Data is abundant and some of it conflicting, but the following seem safe to say:

- Whether PSA screening saves lives is uncertain. It appears to detect cancers early. Data is conflicting about whether or not it saves lives. It appears to lower the prostate cancer death. Nevertheless, patients who have PSA screening do not live longer than those who do not, which raises the question: Is a life saved from prostate cancer by PSA screening offset by a life lost to some other, nonprostate cause?
- The 10-year survival rate for tumor confined to the gland is nearly 100%, including untreated cases.
- Approximately 48 men must be subjected to treatment and associated morbidity (incontinence, ED) to save one man from dying of prostate cancer (if, as stated above, any lives are saved at all).

Based upon new data, in 2012 the American Cancer Society issued new screening guidelines, which are roughly summarized here:

- Men should have a discussion with their physician at age 50 (45 for African American men or men with a first-degree relative with prostate cancer) about the pros and cons of screening and treatment.
- Asymptomatic men with actuarial life expectancy <10 years (those about age 75) should not be offered screening.
- It is acceptable for men to choose not to be screened. Men choosing to be screened should have a PSA and digital rectal exam.
- Depending on screening results, a prostate biopsy should be offered.
- If cancer is not found, those with PSA <2.5 ng/ml should be rescreened in two years. Those with higher PSA should be screened again in one year.

Outside of its role in screening, PSA has an important role in assessing patients for prostate cancer recurrence after they have had total prostatectomy. In such patients, blood PSA should be zero. The reappearance of PSA suggests probable recurrence and a need for additional treatment.

Case Notes

16.10 If Marshall chose to have treatment for prostate cancer, was it likely to be lifesaving?

Grading and Staging

Microscopic grading of prostatic carcinoma is standardized and offers valuable prognostic and therapeutic information. Pathologists examine microscopic slides of tissue taken from the gland by biopsy or surgical excision and formulate a **Gleason score** based on histologic grading of the tumor, which can vary from one part of the tumor to another. Tumors are graded on a 1–5 scale, where 1 indicates a very well differentiated mass and 5 indicates a very poorly differentiated mass. The dominant pattern is assigned one score, the second most prevalent pattern another. The scores are summed, so that the best possible score is 2, and the worst is 10. For example, if the dominant pattern is grade 3 and the secondary pattern is grade 4, the tumor would be Gleason grade 7. Gleason scores 2–4 are considered *low grade* and typically found incidentally in prostate tissue removed to relieve obstruction by BPH. Most potentially treatable cancers identified by clinical investigation and biopsy are grade 5–7 and are considered *intermediate grade*. Tumors grade 8–10 are *high grade* and usually advanced cancers that are unlikely to be cured. Scores tend to be stable over time.

Clinical staging is based on a TNM system (Chapter 5), which accounts for tumor (T) size and extent, lymph node (N) spread, and distant metastasis (M). Important staging boundaries are as follows:

- T1: the tumor is (T1) not palpable or visible by imaging and is discovered incidentally or by PSA test and biopsy.
- T2: The tumor is palpable or visible but confined to the prostate.
- T3: The tumor has extended minimally beyond the prostate.
- T4: The tumor has invaded widely into other pelvic structures.

Lymph node involvement, distant metastasis, high PSA, and high Gleason score are associated with poorer prognosis.

Case Notes

16.11 Was Marshall's tumor low, intermediate, or high grade?

16.12 What was the clinical stage of Marshall's tumor?

Treatment and Prognosis

A debate is underway about what, if anything, should be done about some small, early tumors. Young age, high Gleason score (7–10), and high PSA argue for treatment. Otherwise, a "watchful waiting" strategy may be adopted based on the arguable point that in very early cases in elderly men, no treatment is available that is capable of extending life or of doing more good than harm.

For patients with early prostate cancer *who choose to be treated*, treatment is usually prostatectomy or radiation (of which there are many varieties). Survival rates are nearly identical for surgery and radiation the first 10 years, but by 20 years surgery shows a slight advantage. Regardless of the mode of therapy, the main complications are incontinence and ED. Complications vary somewhat according to treatment type. Personal feelings about complications, fear of surgery, fear of radiation, and the idea of living with cancer are usually deciding factors. A well-informed patient is the best decision maker.

The overall five-year survival rate for Caucasians is 99.9%; for African Americans it is 97%. For both races for tumor confined to the gland, the survival rate, treated or untreated, is very near 100%. Nevertheless, the five-year survival rate for distant metastasis is 33%. For cancer that has spread beyond the gland, treatment is palliative surgery, hormone, radiation, and/or chemotherapy.

Remember This! It is not necessary to treat all prostatic carcinomas.

Case Notes

16.13 Which facts argue for or against treatment?

16.14 How likely was it that Marshall would die from his cancer within five years?

Pop Quiz

16.14 True or false? BPH is not precancerous.

16.15 True or false? Cancer of the prostate and nodular hyperplasia do not occur together in the prostate at the same time.

16.16 True or false? The majority of men 70 or older have BPH.

16.17 Carcinoma of the prostate mainly affects which portion of the gland?

16.18 True or false? The main complications of treatment of prostatic cancer are hemorrhage and infection.

16.19 True or false? About 10% of men will die of their prostate cancer within five years.

Case Study Revisited

"We keep testing and biopsying and still there's no cancer." The case of Marshall P.

Marshall was 74 at the time of the fourth prostate biopsy, which discovered an intermediate grade (Gleason 7), small tumor confined to the gland. His life expectancy was about 10 years. Data strongly suggest his cancer would not be life threatening.

Marshall and his urologist had a discussion about what to do next. Marshall opted, and his urologist agreed, that no treatment was indicated. Their mutual rationale was that Marshall's anticipated life span was about 10 years and that prostate cancer was very unlikely to claim his life in that time span or even if he lived substantially longer. The prospect of ED or incontinence, which affects about 30–40% of men regardless of mode of treatment, was more misery and risk than either of them could justify, especially considering that Marshall might also be debilitated by advancing Parkinson disease. Marshall and his urologist disagreed on the need for further PSA monitoring. The urologist favored further testing; Marshall thought otherwise but agreed to keep an open mind as new research revealed additional information.

Chapter Challenge

CHAPTER RECALL

1. A 60-year-old African American male presents to the clinic with nocturia, occasional urgency, and a mild increase in frequency. He also reports difficulty starting his stream. Which of the following treatments is recommended?
   A. Avoiding bedtime fluids and judicious management of alcohol and caffeine intake
   B. Alpha-blockers
   C. TUR prostatectomy
   D. All of the above

2. For men with prostate cancer, which of the following statements is true?
   A. Most men who have prostate cancer die of it.
   B. About 1 man in 30 develops prostate cancer.
   C. The peak incidence of prostate cancer is in men 40–60 years old.
   D. Prostate cancer in men is more common than breast cancer in women.

3. A 32-year-old Caucasian male with a past medical history significant for asthma presents to the emergency room complaining of inability to urinate. His physical exam is remarkable for mild wheezing, which he reports as unimproved despite exceeding the recommended dose of his anticholinergic rescue inhaler. His DRE reveals a smooth unenlarged prostate with no palpable masses. What is the likely etiology for this patient's urinary retention?
   A. Drug side effect
   B. Chronic prostatitis
   C. Prostatic carcinoma
   D. BPH

4. Which of the following statements regarding the testis is correct?
   A. The seminiferous tubules make up 90% of testicular mass.
   B. Interstitial testicular tissue produces testosterone.
   C. Spermatocytes divide to form sperm and Sertoli cells in seminiferous tubules.
   D. All of the above

5. A 65-year-old Caucasian male, after undergoing a routine physical in his physician's office, is diagnosed with Bowen disease. Which of the following pathological findings is consistent with this diagnosis?
   A. A reddish plaque
   B. A cauliflower-like growth
   C. A white, sclerotic patch
   D. Distortion of the penis secondary to fibrotic tissue

6. A 16-year-old African American male is noted to have what appeared to be a painless cystic mass at the head of his epididymis. It is clearly differentiated from the testicle and transilluminated on exam. What is the most likely diagnosis?
   A. Cystocele
   B. Varicocele
   C. Hydrocele
   D. Spermatocele

7. Impaired spermatogenesis can be caused by which of the following?
   A. Hypothyroidism
   B. Diabetic neuropathy
   C. Cystic fibrosis
   D. Prostatectomy

8. A 63-year-old Caucasian male presents to his physician complaining of frequent urination. He reports a constant dribbling and denies feeling the urge to urinate prior to these occurrences. He is embarrassed as the problem has become significantly worse over the last five years since his diagnosis with advanced diabetes, and he has had to resort to wearing adult diapers. What type of incontinence is he describing?
   A. Urge incontinence
   B. Stress incontinence
   C. Overflow incontinence
   D. Functional incontinence

9. A 22-year-old Caucasian male is brought to the ER in excruciating pain that he describes as diffuse and localized to his testicles. The patient is sent to the OR immediately, as delay could result in testicular infarct. What was the diagnosis?
   A. Epididymitis
   B. Orchitis
   C. Urolithiasis
   D. Torsion

10. A 34-year-old Hispanic male presents to clinic complaining of fever, chills, and pain with urination. His physical exam is positive for a swollen boggy prostate, which is markedly tender on DRE. A urine culture is positive. What is his diagnosis?
    A. Urinary tract infection
    B. Acute bacterial prostatitis
    C. Chronic bacterial prostatitis
    D. Chronic nonbacterial prostatitis

11. True or false? Most cases of epididymitis are caused by cystitis, urethritis, or prostatitis.

12. True or false? Untreated cryptorchidism will result in testicular atrophy.

13. True or false? Therapeutic drugs account for the majority of ED.

14. Match the following tumors to their clinical features. Choices may be used more than once and each feature may have more than one answer:

i. Teratoma
ii. Choriocarcinoma
iii. Seminoma
iv. Leydig cell tumor
v. Sertoli cell tumor
vi. Embryonal carcinoma
vii. Yolk sac tumor
viii. Choriocarcinoma
ix. Mixed tumor

A. Derived from germ cells
B. Derived from nongerm cells
C. Usually Benign
D. Usually Malignant
E. Occurs almost exclusively in young boys
F. Contains multiple mature differentiated tissues
G. May cause early masculinization
H. Metastasize later as they are held in check by the immune system
I. Contain dense accumulations of lymphocytes among the tumor cells
J. Contain more than one type of tumor
K. May produce steroids or estrogen

CONCEPTUAL UNDERSTANDING

15. What are the guidelines for prostate cancer screening?

APPLICATION

16. Explain the system for grading prostate cancer as well as its importance in prognosis and its effect on treatment.

17. A 75-year-old Caucasian male presents to the clinic with back pain following a fall. His X-rays reveal no fractures or breaks, but are positive for osteoblastic lesions on several vertebrae. What do you suspect, and how do you proceed with treatment?

CHAPTER 17

Disorders of the Female Genitalia and Breast

Contents

Chapter Objectives

After studying this chapter, you should be able to complete the following tasks:

Section 1: Disorders of the Female Genital Tract

THE NORMAL FEMALE GENITALIA

1. Name and describe the components of the female genitalia.

THE PITUITARY-OVARIAN-ENDOMETRIAL CYCLE

2. Discuss the hormonal and accompanying physiological changes that occur during each stage of the menstrual cycle.
3. Discuss the advantages and disadvantages of hormone replacement therapy in women with menopause.

PREGNANCY

4. Describe the hormonal and resulting physiological changes, including complications, that (may) occur with pregnancy.

INFERTILITY

5. List the causes and treatment of female infertility.

VULVAR DISORDER AND VAGINITIS

6. Compare and contrast the causes of leukoplakia.
7. Differentiate between the various etiologies of vaginitis; include treatment where applicable.

DISORDERS OF THE CERVIX

8. Describe the conditions affecting the cervix; pay particular attention to the progression and prevention of HPV-induced carcinoma.

DISORDERS OF THE ENDOMETRIUM AND MYOMETRIUM

9. Discuss the clinical presentation, diagnostic findings, and treatment as applicable for the etiologies responsible for pathological and functional uterine bleeding and endometritis.

DISORDERS OF THE OVARY

10. Use imaging and pathological findings to differentiate between the possible etiologies of an ovarian mass.

Section 2: Disorders of the Breast

THE NORMAL BREAST

11. Describe the anatomy of the breast.

EVALUATION OF BREAST DISORDERS

12. Discuss the factors one should consider when evaluating a patient for breast cancer.

BENIGN BREAST CONDITIONS

13. Compare and contrast the clinical findings of mastitis, subareolar abscess, and fat necrosis.
14. Name the key difference between nonproliferative and proliferative fibrocystic change of the breast, and explain why the difference is important.
15. List the benign tumors of the breast, including fibroadenoma, phyllodes, and intraductal papilloma, and discuss their hallmark features.

BREAST CANCER

16. Discuss the differential diagnosis of a malignant breast mass, and describe the signs, symptoms, and pathological findings that aid in the diagnosis as well as the risk factors that affect patient prognosis.

Section 1: Disorders of the Female Genital Tract

Female, n. One of the opposing, or unfair, sex.

AMBROSE BIERCE (1842–1914?), AMERICAN SATIRIST, JOURNALIST, AND SHORT-STORY WRITER, THE DEVIL'S DICTIONARY

Case Study

"I can't get pregnant." The case of Susan A.

Chief Complaint: "I can't get pregnant."

Clinical History: Susan A. was a 34-year-old Caucasian woman, a television news reporter who was referred to a fertility specialist. When asked why she was seeking care, she offered a folder containing medical records from the referring physician's office and said, "It's all in there. The gist of it is that I can't get pregnant." She said she and her husband of three years had been trying to conceive without results. "It must be me," she said, adding that her husband had a child by a previous marriage. When asked about her sexual history, she said, "I was pretty wild in high school and college." First intercourse was at age 16 and she admitted to sex with "about a dozen" different sexual partners, most of it without condoms. "I got pregnant in college and had a first trimester abortion. My parents never found out. This is so distressing," she continued, "I always had irregular periods when I was younger and was forever afraid I was pregnant when I didn't start on time because the abortion proved I could get pregnant. Now, I'd love to be late and find I'm pregnant, but wouldn't you know it, I'm regular as clockwork."

The physician reviewed the records, which revealed no noteworthy medical problems other than the fertility complaint. A systems and general health review were unremarkable. Susan exercised regularly, and had never smoked. She had taken birth control pills in college and afterward until marrying and deciding to have children. Recent menstrual history was unremarkable.

The referral note said, "Pelvic and Pap smear not done; for fertility clinic to do."

"When did you have your last Pap smear?" the physician asked.

"Oh," she said, "it's been nearly 10 years, I imagine; I've moved around so much in this TV job I never seem to get around to it."

Using charts and diagrams, the physician explained to her the details of internal female anatomy, the menstrual cycle, conception, the role of the pituitary gland, and so on, pointing out how things can go wrong at each step of the process and bracing her for a lengthy and time-consuming workup to establish the cause, if one could be found. "Sometimes we just can't figure it out," the physician said.

Physical Examination and Other Data: Vital signs and nongynecologic exam were unremarkable. Initial laboratory blood tests revealed nothing remarkable. The vulva was unremarkable. On vaginal speculum exam, the cervix appeared to be inflamed around the os and bled easily when scraped to collect a Pap smear. On bimanual pelvic examination, she had a slightly tender left adnexal mass estimated to be about 6–8 cm in diameter. Ultrasound imagining confirmed the presence of an irregular mass on the left side of the uterus.

She was referred to another specialist for radiographic imaging to check the patency of her fallopian tubes and rescheduled for follow-up in two weeks. The consultant's report revealed "bilateral complete tubal obstruction." A laboratory test of cervical mucus was positive for *Chlamydia trachomatis*. The Pap smear report was a surprise: "High-Grade Squamous Intraepithelial Lesion. HPV detected."

Clinical Course: Colposcopy and cervical conization biopsy revealed HPV-positive squamous carcinoma in situ (CIN-III). Several weeks later, Susan had exploratory pelvic surgery. A left tuboovarian abscess was found. The right fallopian tube was bound by numerous scars. The right ovary was largely free of scar tissue and showed evidence of recent ovulatory activity. Left salpingo-oophorectomy and right salpingectomy was performed. The right ovary and uterus were left intact so that Susan could try to become pregnant by in vitro fertilization using eggs from her remaining right ovary. The pathology report described the left ovary and fallopian tube as welded into a single inflammatory mass. The left ovary showed follicle cysts and a recent corpus luteum. The left fallopian tube was dilated and filled with pus. The right fallopian tube was twisted, scarred, and obstructed.

Susan later became pregnant by IVF and gave birth to a healthy, full-term infant by vaginal delivery. She continued to have Pap smear evidence of cervical dysplasia and later had a hysterectomy. The cervix showed CIN II.

Using her public position and personal story, she became an outspoken advocate for women's health issues, especially Pap smear screening.

Arguably, the most common type of physician office visit is a woman seeking care for a gynecologic or breast complaint. Normal female reproductive physiology is burdensome. Pregnancy is an especially stressful physiologic event. Monthly ovulatory cycles, hormonal tides, and menstrual irregularities are a part of daily life. The vagina, labia minora, and urethra are open to the environment and comparatively easily infected. Sexually transmitted diseases are common. Though overshadowed in the public mind by breast cancer, cervical and ovarian malignancies are roughly twice as likely to cause death.

The Normal Female Genitalia

The **external genitalia** (the **vulva**) are illustrated in Figure 17.1 and consist of the *mons pubis, labia majora, labia minora, clitoris, external urethral orifice,* and the vaginal opening, the *introitus*. The mons pubis and labia majora are the most directly exposed to the environment and are covered by *skin*. The labia minora, clitoris, and vagina are more protected and are covered by delicate nonkeratinizing *squamous mucosa* moisturized by lubricating mucous glands (**Bartholin glands**).

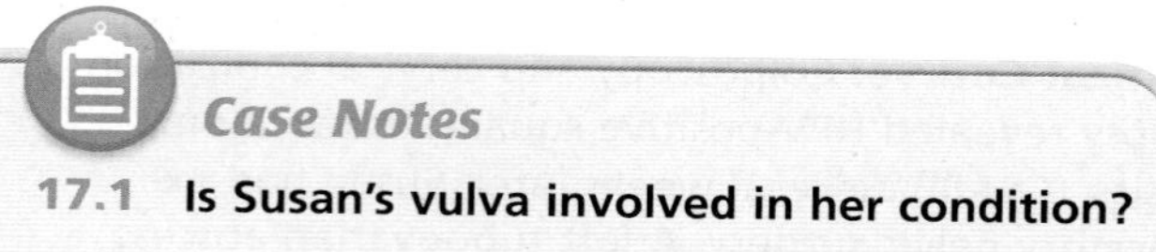

Case Notes

17.1 Is Susan's vulva involved in her condition?

Figure 17.2 and Figure 17.3 illustrate the **internal genitalia**. The **uterus** is composed of smooth muscle and consists of an upper **body**, which lies in the pelvis, and a lower **cervix**. The **fundus** is the upper end of the body. The uterus, tubes, and ovaries are stabilized by bilateral thick folds of peritoneum (the **broad ligaments**) and other ligaments. Normally the uterus sits immediately behind the pubic bone and tilts slightly forward. When not in this position, the uterus is said by some to be "malpositioned." It may be displaced to the rear or tilted (flexed) backward or forward, so called "retroversion" or "anteversion" respectively. These abnormal positions are sometimes proposed as causes of painful menstruation, painful intercourse, and infertility. Evidence supporting this idea is lacking, however.

The **vagina** is lined by squamous mucosa and connects the vaginal opening (the introitus) to the cervix. The portion of cervix that protrudes into the upper vagina is the **ectocervix**. The central opening of the cervix is the **cervical os** (mouth). The os leads upward into the *endocervical canal*, which is lined by columnar (glandular) epithelium that secretes mucus to form a plug that protects the endometrium from vaginal organisms; sperm are specially equipped to penetrate this mucus barrier.

The ectocervix and vagina are covered by squamous epithelium. The endocervix, endometrium, and fallopian tubes, on the other hand, are lined by columnar (glandular) epithelium. Glandular and squamous epithelium meet in the os at the *squamocolumnar junction*, an important anatomic landmark in the development of cervical cancer.

The endometrial cavity connects to the endocervical canal directly below. The endometrial cavity is lined by **endometrium**, which grows, dies, and sloughs away with each menstrual period. The endometrium is composed of two types of tissue—supportive *stromal cells* and *glands* formed of columnar epithelium.

The **fallopian tubes** lead from each corner of the uterus outward to the ovaries. The *fimbriated extremity* of each tube flares widely over each ovary with numerous finger-like folds lined by undulating cilia that sweep ova into the fallopian tube. Ciliated cells in the fallopian tube sweep the ovum into the endometrial cavity. Conception

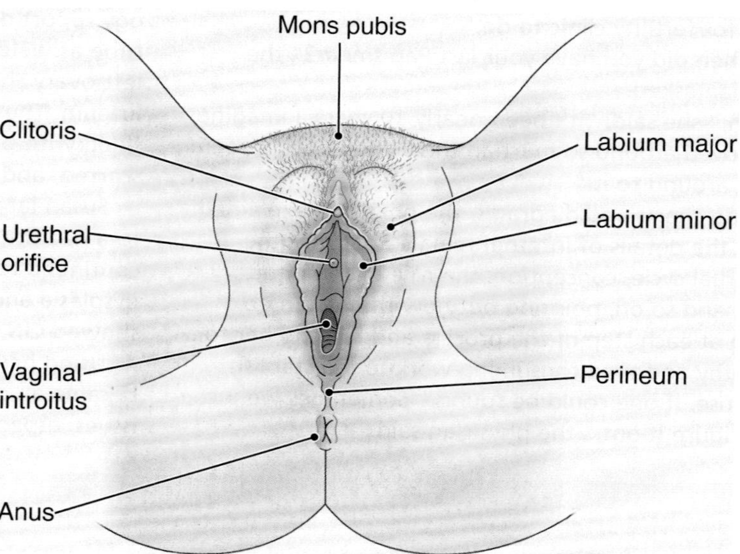

Figure 17.1 **The external female genitalia.**

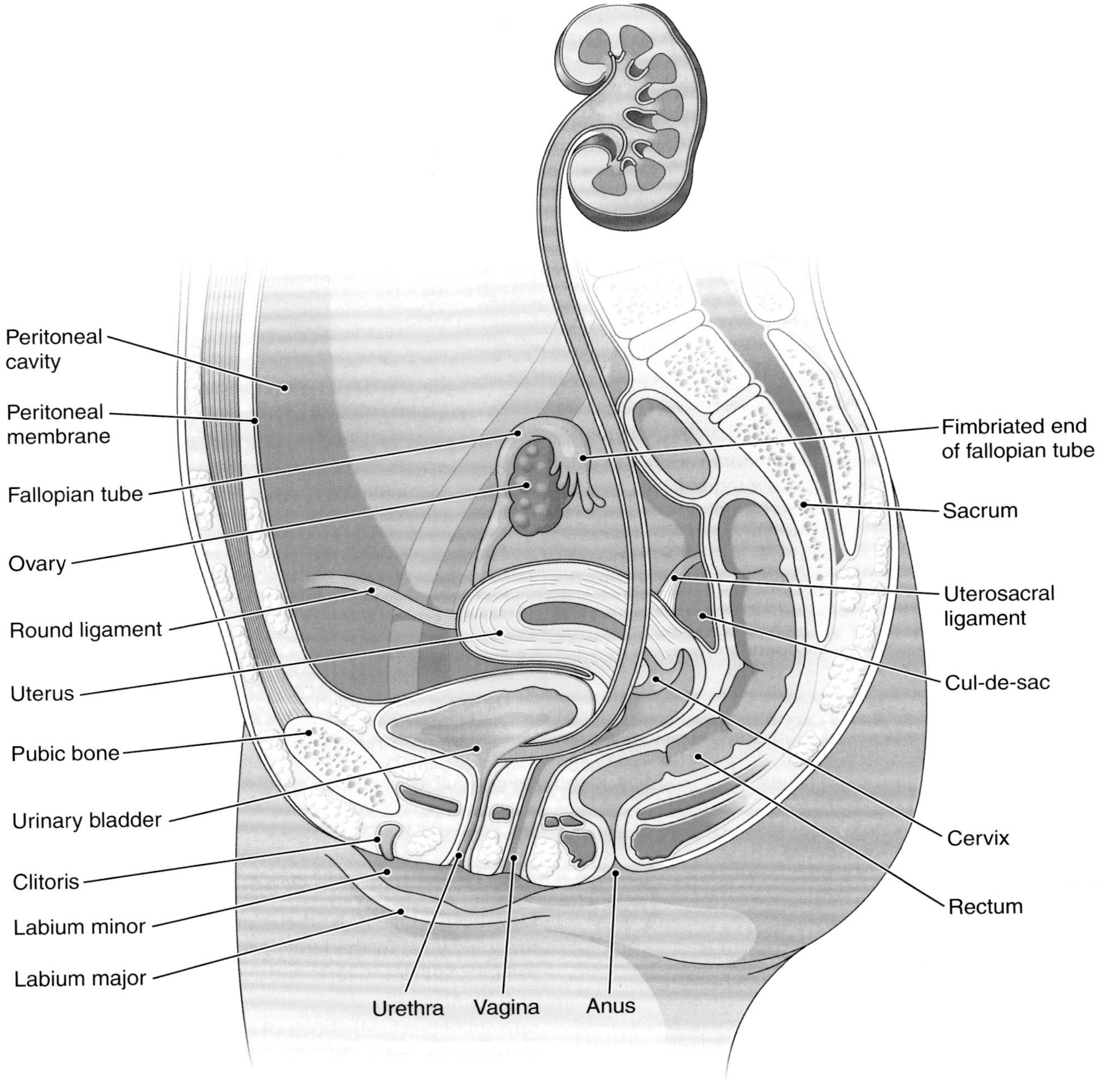

Figure 17.2 **The internal female genitalia.**

usually occurs in the abdominal cavity near the ovary or in the distal part of the fallopian tube and the conceptus is swept into the endometrium for implantation.

The **ovaries** lie within the broad ligament close to the fimbriated end of each fallopian tube. A layer of altered peritoneal cells, *surface epithelial cells,* covers the surface of the ovary. The ovary proper is composed of **oocytes** (*germ cells*), supporting connective tissue produced by *stromal cells*, and specialized *granulosa cells* and *theca cells*, which secrete hormones and support ovulation. Each oocyte is nested in the center of a small group of granulosa cells. The oocyte and its rim of granulosa cells is the **primary follicle** (see Fig. 17.4).

The ovaries and fallopian tubes are together called the *adnexa*.

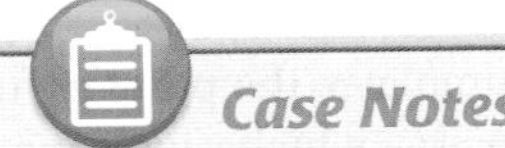

Case Notes

17.2 Were Susan's uterine adnexa involved in her condition?

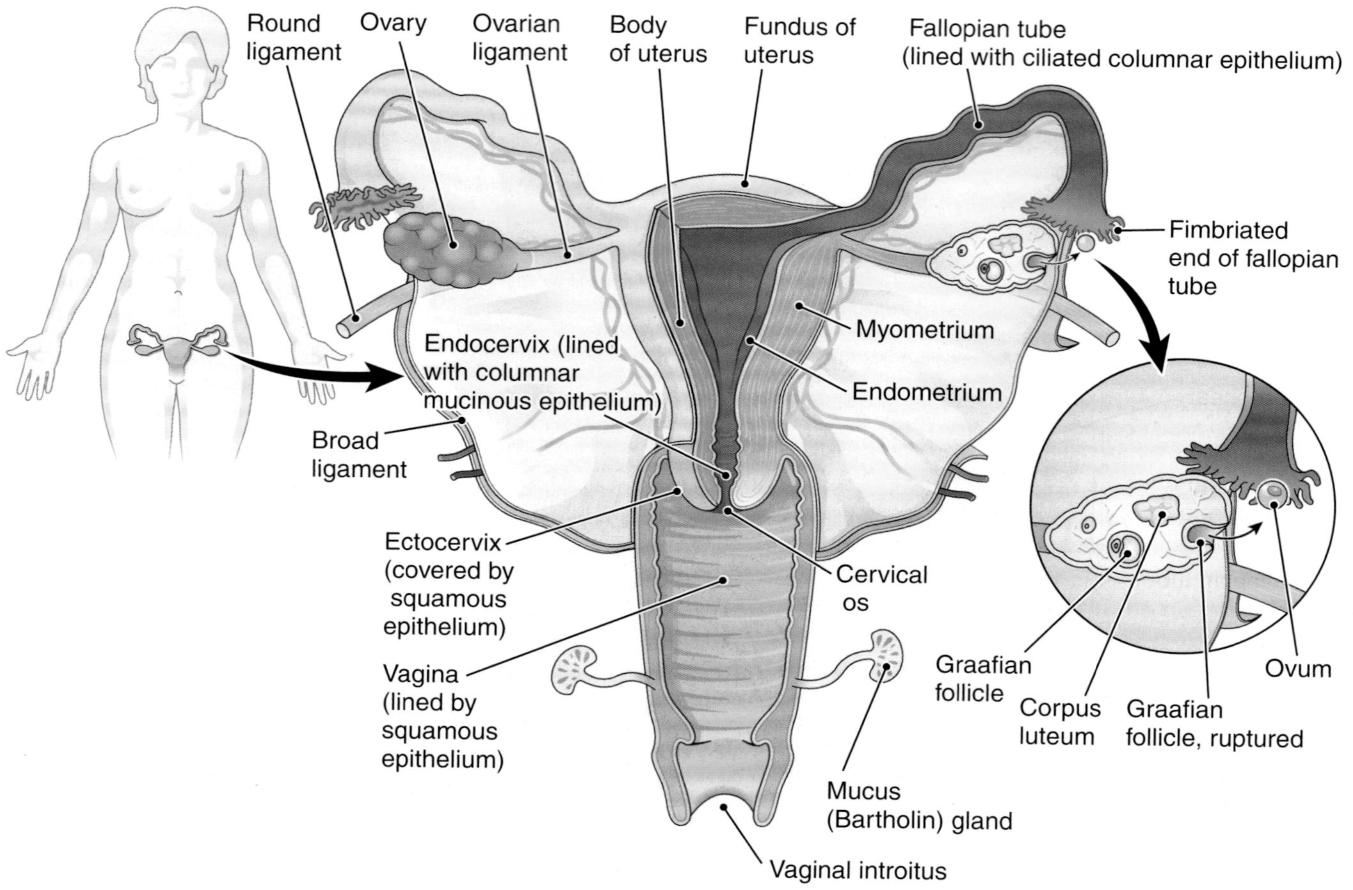

Figure 17.3 **The vagina, uterus, fallopian tubes, and ovaries.**

Pop Quiz

17.1 True or false? A primary follicle is composed of an oocyte surrounded by granulosa cells.

17.2 Name the layer of cells on the surface of the ovary.

The Pituitary-Ovarian-Endometrial Cycle

During reproductive years, the ovaries convert oocytes into ova under hormonal control of the hypothalamus (Chapter 14). The hypothalamus secretes *gonadotropin-releasing hormone* (GRH or GnRH), which stimulates the pituitary to release *follicle-stimulating hormone* (FSH), which causes ovulation, and *luteinizing hormone* (LH), which stimulates ovarian progesterone production. The regular cyclic phases of these hormones are responsible for the menstrual cycle.

The Ovarian Cycle Produces Ova

Oogenesis (Fig. 17.4) is the production of ova from primary oocytes. In the fetus, primary oocytes develop into *primary follicles*, which consist of an oocyte with a halo of follicular cells. After puberty, primary follicles mature into small cysts called **Graafian follicles**, which contain a maturing ovum in the center. At the edge of this expanding cyst, a rim of granulosa cells and theca cells secrete follicular fluid and estrogens, hormones that promote growth of the endometrium and the development and maintenance of the genitalia and breasts. Sometimes the ovaries develop more than one Graafian follicle at a time, and the additional follicles persist as unruptured *follicle cysts* that are usually small but may be several centimeters in diameter.

Each oocyte in a primary follicle contains a full set of maternal and paternal chromosomes (46,XX) derived from the future mother's own mother and father. As the primary follicle matures into a Graafian follicle, the oocyte undergoes reduction division (**meiosis**), in which the 46 chromosomes in each primary oocyte are reduced to form a *secondary* oocyte containing 23 chromosomes (23,X).

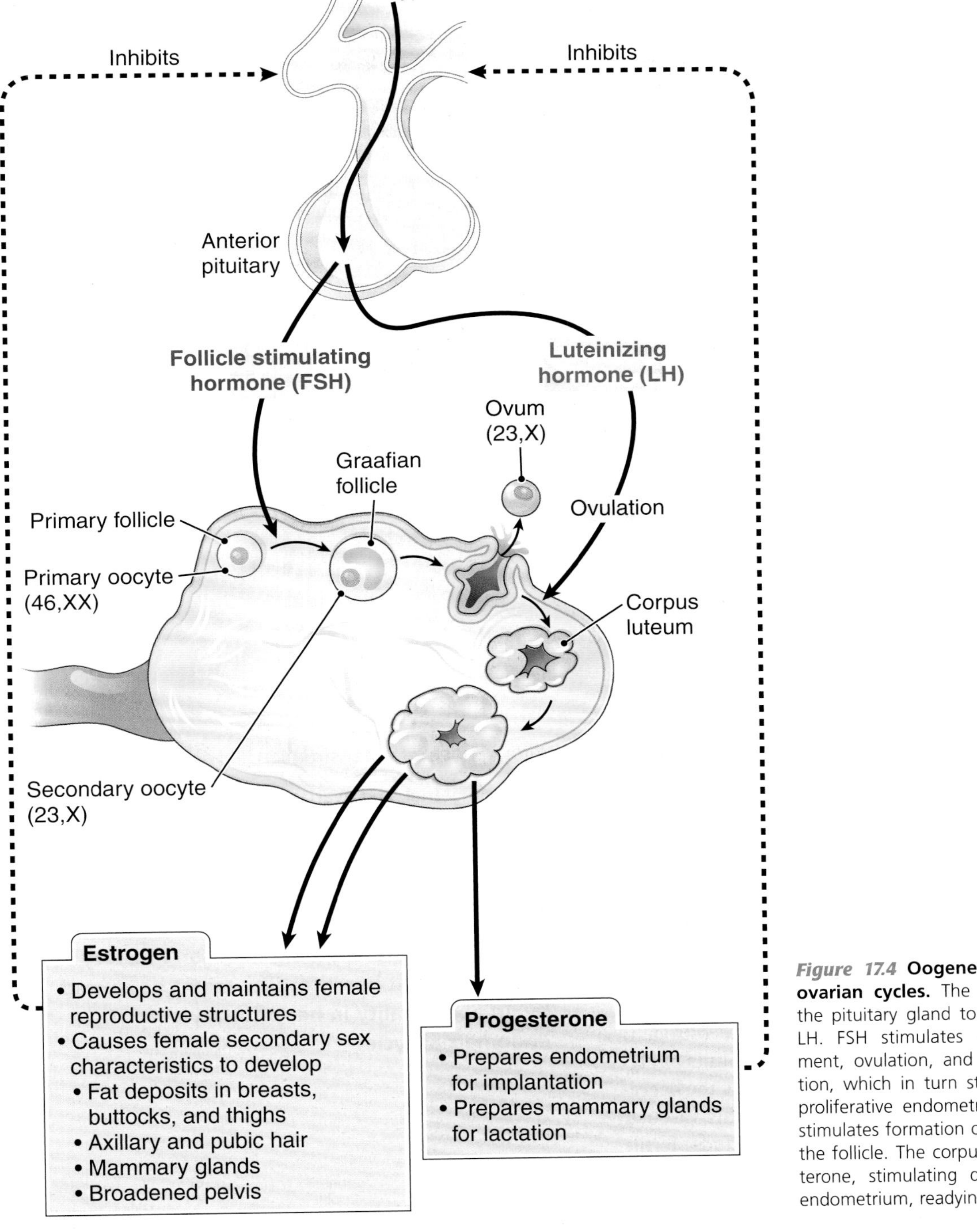

Figure 17.4 **Oogenesis: the pituitary and ovarian cycles.** The hypothalamus stimulates the pituitary gland to release FSH followed by LH. FSH stimulates ovarian follicle development, ovulation, and follicular estrogen secretion, which in turn stimulates development of proliferative endometrium. After ovulation, LH stimulates formation of the corpus luteum from the follicle. The corpus luteum secretes progesterone, stimulating development of secretory endometrium, readying for implantation.

Under continued FSH stimulation, the Graafian follicle enlarges until it ruptures and releases its **ovum** into the peritoneal cavity. This event is called **ovulation**. Under the influence of LH, the ruptured follicle develops into a **corpus luteum**, a yellow endocrine body that secretes progesterone and small amounts of estrogen to prepare the endometrium for implantation of a fertilized ovum. If pregnancy does not occur, pituitary LH production falls and the corpus luteum involutes. If pregnancy occurs, however, the corpus luteum persists.

The Uterine Cycle Parallels the Ovarian Cycle

The *uterine cycle (or menstrual cycle)* proceeds in parallel with the ovarian cycle. (Fig. 17.5). At the end of menstrual flow (*menses*, **menstruation**), only a thin layer of

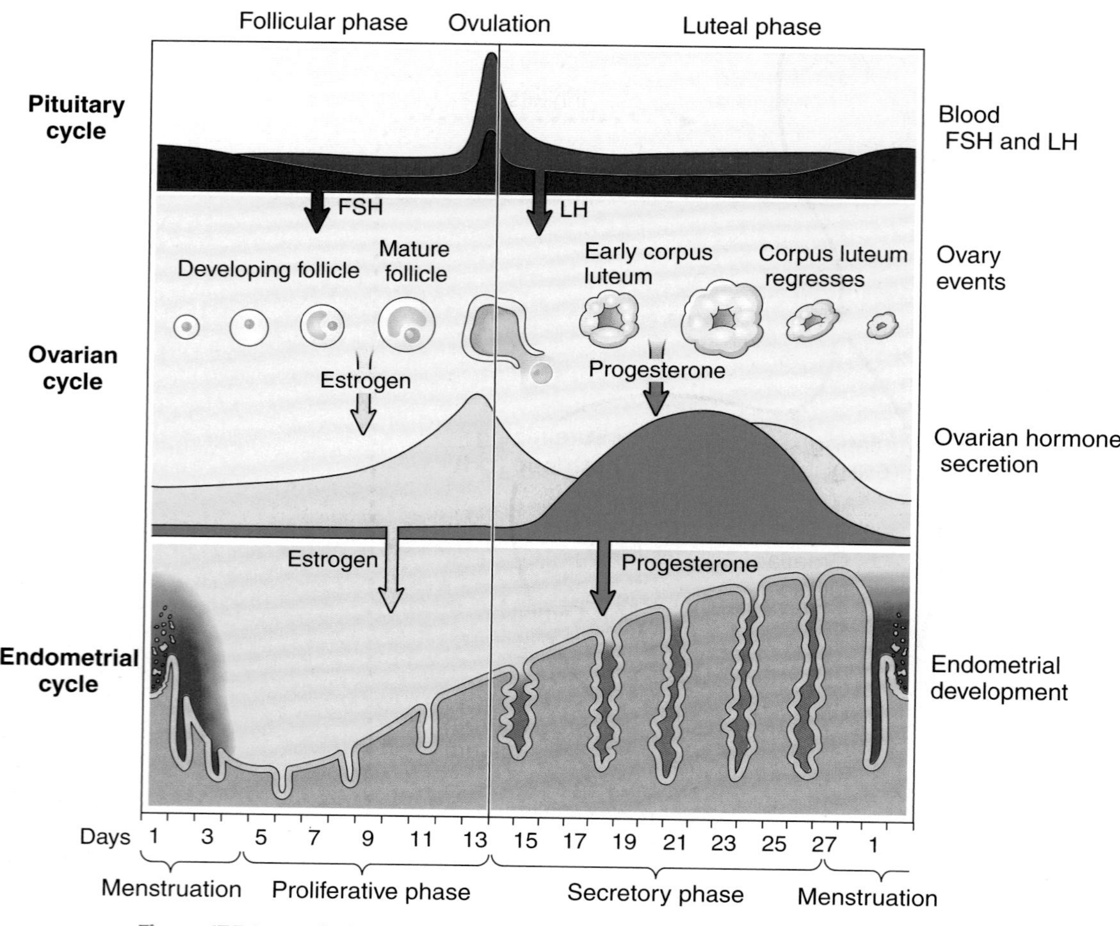

Figure 17.5 **Interrelationships among the pituitary, endometrial, and ovarian cycles.**

endometrium remains. The new menstrual cycle begins as pituitary FSH stimulates follicle growth and estrogen secretion. Estrogen in turn stimulates proliferation of endometrial stroma, a period of endometrial growth known as the **proliferative phase**. After ovulation, LH stimulates conversion of the ruptured follicle into the corpus luteum, which secretes progesterone. In turn, progesterone (aided by estrogen) stimulates the endometrium to secrete large amounts of glycogen, a period of endometrial growth known as the **secretory phase**. The endometrium is now lush—richly vascular and packed with energy-rich glycogen-filled glands; fertile soil ready for seed.

If implantation does not occur, the corpus luteum degenerates into a *corpus albicans* (white body) and the endometrium dies. Menstrual bleeding follows, as necrotic endometrium and blood are shed into the vagina. If implantation occurs, however, the conceptus begins secreting human chorionic gonadotropin (hCG)—a hormone that has the same effect as LH—thus maintaining the ovarian corpus luteum throughout pregnancy and ensuring a continued supply of estrogen and progesterone to support the pregnancy.

Case Notes

17.3 Was there anything in Susan's history to suggest that her infertility might be caused by an abnormality in her pituitary-ovarian-endometrial cycle?

Pop Quiz

17.3 True or false? The ovaries produce only one Graafian follicle at a time.

17.4 What hormone, secreted by the conceptus, is responsible for maintaining a pregnancy?

Menopause Is Cessation of Ovulation and Menstruation

Menopause is physiologic or iatrogenic cessation of menses due to decreasing ovarian function. It normally occurs about age 50, resulting from failure of the ovaries to respond to FSH and LH from the pituitary. Ovulation stops, menstruation ends, and levels of blood estrogen and progesterone decline. Some women experience no unpleasant consequences, but most suffer hot flushes (flashes) and other symptoms.

Hot flashes are episodes of vasomotor instability that affect most women going through menopause. The cause is not clear. They usually appear before complete cessation of menses and tend to persist for a year or more in most women. They are characterized by a few minutes of skin blood-vessel dilation, especially in the head and neck, and a feeling of warmth. Some women perspire profusely; others have night sweats. Other symptoms include fatigue, irritability, headache, nervousness, depression, and decline of sexual drive. Symptoms are mild in some women and debilitating in others.

The menopausal reduction of estrogen has a profound effect on the lower genital tract. The covering epidermis and squamous epithelium of the labia and vagina thins, and all parts decrease in size. Cervical, vaginal, and labial mucous production decline, and vaginal pH becomes alkaline, which encourages infection. Pelvic muscle tone relaxes and urinary incontinence may occur.

Estrogen is necessary for healthy, strong bones. Reduced estrogen is important in the development of *osteoporosis* (Chapter 18), a thinning and brittleness of bones, which occurs with age. It is a major health concern for postmenopausal women because it increases their risk of bone fractures. Estrogen also provides significant protection against cardiovascular disease in premenopausal women. The postmenopausal decline of estrogen renders women as susceptible as men to cardiovascular risk factors such as an unhealthy diet, obesity, lack of exercise, and smoking.

Until recently, it was common practice to treat women with postmenopausal symptoms—especially women at increased risk for osteoporosis—with supplemental oral estrogen or, more commonly, a combination of estrogen and progesterone. These preparations are generally referred to as *hormone replacement therapy* (HRT). This practice has declined significantly, however, as a result of research suggesting that HRT slightly increases a woman's risk for breast cancer, gallbladder disease, dementia, urinary incontinence, pulmonary embolism, thrombophlebitis, heart attack, and stroke. Though the issue remains unsettled in some respects, HRT is generally recommended for use only for menopausal women with severe hot flashes or vaginal dryness. Topical estrogen cream is effective in treating vulvar atrophy.

Pop Quiz

17.5 True or false? Hormone replacement therapy is recommended for all women experiencing the symptoms of menopause.

Pregnancy

Birth, n. The first and direst of all disasters.

AMBROSE BIERCE (1842–1914?), AMERICAN SATIRIST, JOURNALIST, AND SHORT-STORY WRITER, THE DEVIL'S DICTIONARY

Pregnancy begins with fertilization. Normally it lasts for nine calendar months (280 days, 40 weeks, 10 lunar months) as measured from the date of the onset of the *last menstrual period (LMP)*. The *expected date of delivery (EDD, due date)* is 280 days from the LMP date. The nine months are divided into three three-month **trimesters**, each of which encompasses certain fetal and maternal developments. When referring to fetal age, the term **gestational age** is used; however, keep in mind that because ovulation and fertilization do not occur until about the second week of the menstrual cycle, the actual age of the fetus is two weeks less than gestational age.

The process of labor and birth is called **parturition**. **Gravidity** refers to the number of pregnancies a woman has had; **parity** refers to the number of pregnancies in which the fetus was carried for 22 weeks (the age of presumed fetal ability to survive outside the uterus), which usually equals the number of pregnancies with a live birth. Thus, a woman pregnant for the second time, with one prior pregnancy that endured for a minimum of 22 weeks, would be referred to as "G2/P1" in typical medical chart shorthand. Sometimes a note is also made about the number of *abortions*. These distinctions are important. For example, **multiparous** (having birthed more than one child) women frequently have shorter, easier labor than **primigravid** (first pregnancy) ones; and women who have had one abortion are more likely to abort a subsequent pregnancy.

Case Notes

17.4 What was Susan's gravidity and parity after her college pregnancy? After her second pregnancy?

Pregnancy Features Marked Hormonal Changes

Though it may be a normal physiologic state, pregnancy is a hormonal storm, most of it owing to the placenta, which becomes an endocrine powerhouse. Other than those due to the physical presence of the fetus, virtually every change in pregnancy owes to hormonal influences induced by the placenta and by increased pituitary output of LH, FSH, ACTH, and TSH. Among other hormones, the placenta secretes estrogen, progesterone, and pituitary-like hormones. These pituitary analogues stimulate the thyroid and adrenal cortex to secrete thyroxine and cortisol, and prepare the breasts for lactation. The placenta also secretes human chorionic gonadotropin (hCG), the equivalent of pituitary LH, which appears in urine about one week after conception. The basis for urine tests to diagnose pregnancy depends on detection of urinary hCG.

Under the influence of these hormones, the uterus, which weighs about 50 gm initially, balloons to more than 1000 gm; breast volume may double; the vaginal introitus becomes more spacious; and the labia swell with blood. Skin may be dramatically affected: acne may blossom, tiny benign *spider angiomas* (Chapter 12) sometimes sprout on the face or upper chest; stretch marks may mar the thighs and abdomen; and the skin of the face may darken, a condition called *chloasma* or *the mask of pregnancy*.

Healthy weight gain depends on body mass index (BMI). Underweight women (BMI <18.5) should gain 28–40 lb; normal women (BMI 18.5–24.9), 25–35 lb; overweight women (BMI 25–29.9), 15–25 lb; and obese women (BMI ≥30), 11–20 lb. Most of the weight is acquired in the last two trimesters. The fetus accounts for about 7 lb; the placenta, amniotic fluid, and enlarged uterus and breasts contribute about 8 lb; increased blood and tissue fluid volume adds another 6 lb; and extra fat adds the final 3 lb. Hormonal changes also stimulate increased appetite; after all, the woman is eating for two. Failure to control appetite, however, may cause excess weight gain, sometimes as much as 75 lb, which can create problems of its own, from high blood pressure to temporary (gestational) diabetes.

During pregnancy, blood volume and cardiac output also increase. At term, blood volume is about 30% higher (an extra liter or two) than at conception and cardiac output is 30–40% greater.

Metabolic and circulatory changes are equally dramatic. The increased output of thyroid and adrenocortical hormones increases the basal metabolic rate and heart rate, which with expanded blood volume causes blood pressure to rise. Pregnant women frequently complain of being overheated, and with justification: they are constantly at work carrying an extra 24 lb and their baseline rate of energy metabolism has been boosted into overdrive.

This metabolic environment rapidly consumes calories and nutrients. Even in a normal pregnancy, the mother cannot absorb enough dietary protein, calcium, and iron in the third trimester to keep up with total demand: the fetus has priority. The deficit is taken from the mother's stores: her tissues contribute protein; her bone marrow and spleen contribute iron; and her bones surrender calcium. Iron balance is particularly sensitive. The fetus must synthesize its hemoglobin and the mother must make additional hemoglobin for her own expanded blood volume.

Increased blood volume and cardiac output also increase renal blood flow and glomerular filtration rate. Much of the extra tubular fluid produced, however, is resorbed in response to the action of steroid hormones. The net result is that, in a normal pregnancy, maternal urine output is moderately increased, which eliminates much of the fluid retained. Even so, the average fluid gain is about 6 lb.

After birth, hormone levels quickly return to normal: the placenta is expelled and adrenal output slows. The uterus shrinks to near normal size in a month or two. The breasts will remain enlarged as long as the mother is breast feeding. Renal physiology also returns to normal and excess fluid disappears. Hemorrhage associated with delivery will shrink blood volume by about 25% but the remainder persists for a few weeks, evidence of a built-in safety factor.

Case Notes

17.5 When Susan was pregnant in college, did her urine have high or low amounts of hCG?

Complications Can Affect Any System

The discussion above dealt not with complications but with the normal but somewhat exaggerated physiology of pregnancy. Thankfully, most pregnancies are uncomplicated—such is the grand design of nature. But when complications do occur, they can affect any system. The list is long, so our discussion will necessarily be confined to some of the most common and serious conditions.

Remember This! Pregnancy is a stressful physiologic state that is vulnerable to complications.

Hypertensive Disorders of Pregnancy

Hypertensive disorders of pregnancy (or *gestational hypertension*) refers to persistently increased blood pressure (systolic >140, or diastolic >90) in pregnancy. With the additional presence of significant *proteinuria*, an indicator of renal damage, and *fluid accumulation (edema)*, the triad becomes known as **preeclampsia** or **toxemia of pregnancy**. If seizures occur, preeclampsia becomes **eclampsia**. Preeclampsia affects about 5% of pregnancies in the United States and can occur any time after the 20th week and up to the 6th week postpartum, but most often appears about the 37th week. Primigravidas are most often affected. The basic cause is not known, but for some reason placental ischemia occurs, which damages the endothelial cells of placental blood vessels. Not only does placental ischemia threaten the fetus, it induces fetal vessels to release factors into blood that damage maternal endothelial cells and make maternal arterioles more sensitive to epinephrine and other factors that act to raise blood pressure.

Signs of severe pre-eclampsia include rising blood pressure, greater proteinuria, and weight gain from accumulating edema fluid. Escalating hypertension further damages the kidneys and maternal vascular endothelial cells, which increases the risk of the development of thrombocytopenia, liver hemorrhage, or disseminated intravascular coagulation.

For pregnancies of 36 weeks or more, treatment of pre-eclampsia is delivery despite the risks of fetal immaturity. Prior to 36 weeks, for mild pre-eclampsia the goal is prolongation of pregnancy to allow for fetal lung maturation (Chapter 22). Antihypertensive drugs are a mainstay of treatment. For BP control and seizure prophylaxis in severe preeclampsia, intravenous magnesium sulphate is required.

Vascular and Coagulation Disorders

Disseminated intravascular coagulation during pregnancy (Chapter 6) is rare. Nevertheless, other less dangerous vascular problems are more common.

Many pregnant women develop varicose veins. The pregnant uterus presses on the inferior vena cava, causing increased pressure and sluggish blood flow in the veins of the pelvis and legs. This combination predisposes to varicosities and to thrombus formation (Chapter 6). The risk can be significant: thrombi can embolize to the lungs. Small pulmonary thromboemboli may be asymptomatic, larger ones can cause pulmonary infarction, and very large ones may prove fatal.

Gestational Diabetes

Every pregnancy is associated with some increased resistance to insulin, which causes blood glucose, insulin, and triglycerides to rise. Gestational diabetes is a state of glucose intolerance arising during pregnancy and affecting a small percentage of patients. Exact diagnostic criteria vary and tend to depend on blood glucose response to an oral glucose tolerance test (Chapter 13). It is not clear if gestational diabetes is due solely to pregnancy or if pregnancy unmasks a previously undetected problem with glucose metabolism. In any case, complications and their management are similar to nonpregnant patients—the goal is control of blood glucose. Diabetes in pregnancy, whether gestational or in patients diabetic before pregnancy, is associated with increased risk of pregnancy-induced hypertension, abortion, infections, premature birth, and other complications. Strict glucose control lessens these risks. Infants born to diabetic mothers tend to be large for gestational age (Chapter 22). Knowing the birth weight of a prior infant may provide a clue to possible glucose intolerance in future pregnancies.

Abortion

The medical and lay definitions of "abortion" vary considerably. The public generally uses the term *miscarriage* to describe spontaneous early termination of pregnancy with death of the fetus, and reserves the term "abortion" for deliberate termination of pregnancy. Miscarriage is not a medical term. The medical definition of **abortion** is *any* interruption of pregnancy—incidental, accidental, or intentional—with death of the fetus before the end of 22 full weeks of gestation, or if the fetus weighs less than 500 grams. A pregnancy that ends between 22 and 38 full weeks of gestation and with a living infant is known as a "premature birth." A pregnancy that ends after 22 weeks with death of the fetus spontaneously in the uterus or during birth is called a **stillbirth**.

A *spontaneous abortion* is one that occurs without deliberate provocation. About 20% of known pregnancies end in spontaneous abortion, the majority of them occurring before the 16th week. About 60% of spontaneous abortions are due to chromosomal defects. Another 15% can be traced to maternal factors such as trauma, diabetes, thyroid disease, substance abuse, or dietary deficiency. No cause can be found for the remaining 25%. Contrary to popular opinion, there is no evidence that grief, fright, anxiety, anger, or mental illness can cause spontaneous abortion.

A *threatened abortion* is bleeding through an undilated cervix. An *inevitable abortion* is similar but with cramps and cervical dilation, with which abortion is sure to follow. An *incomplete abortion* is one in which some of the products of conception (POC), usually the placenta, remain in the uterus. A *complete abortion* is when all of the POC have been expelled. A related term is *missed abortion*, which describes a nonviable intrauterine pregnancy. Typically, no symptoms occur except amenorrhea. The diagnosis is usually made when the patient notices her pregnancy has stopped developing or fetal heartbeats and movements cannot be detected.

Some patients have recurrent spontaneous abortions. Despite this unhappy circumstance, there is a bright side: even with as many as three consecutive abortions, there is a 70–80% chance the next pregnancy will go to term.

Incompetent cervix is a clinical condition that may lead to abortion. In these patients, the cervix dilates early in pregnancy. The cervix may be sutured shut, but bed rest, sometimes for months, is often required.

Many early abortions go unnoticed. Perhaps half of all conceptions do not end with implantation; and, since pregnancy begins at conception, failure of implantation qualifies as an abortion. Even when implantation occurs, perhaps 50% or more abort without the patient knowing she was pregnant.

Case Notes

17.6 Susan's college pregnancy ended in the first trimester. Was her use of the term "abortion" correct?

Implantation of the Fertilized Ovum outside the Uterine Cavity

Fertilization usually occurs in the distal half of the fallopian tube, but may occur in the abdominal cavity near the ovary. The fertilized ovum is swept down the fallopian tube for implantation in the endometrium. Mechanical obstruction of this process by inflammation, scarring, or endometriosis may cause the conceptus to implant outside the uterus, producing an **ectopic pregnancy** (Fig. 17.6). In about half of cases, some mechanical obstruction can be identified; the culprit is often scar tissue from a previous bacterial infection with gonorrhea or chlamydia. In the other half of cases, the cause is unknown. About 90% of ectopic pregnancies occur in the fallopian tube; the remainder occur on the surface of the ovary or in the pelvis or abdominal peritoneum.

Early development of the embryo and placenta is normal in most ectopic pregnancies, so that an early ectopic pregnancy may be physiologically and medically indistinguishable from a normal one: menses stop, the patient gains weight, her breasts enlarge, and so on. The diagnosis can be readily confirmed by ultrasound imaging of the pelvis in a patient with high blood levels of blood hCG.

Some ectopic pregnancies announce themselves by spontaneous rupture with pain and intraperitoneal hemorrhage. More often, however, they are discovered by routine ultrasound imaging in early pregnancy, just one of the many benefits of good prenatal care. If not found, ectopic pregnancy can become dangerous: it is the leading cause of maternal mortality during the first trimester and accounts for 9% of all maternal deaths. Treatment is surgical or by injection of methotrexate or misoprostol, which induce medical abortion.

Abnormal Location or Development of the Placenta within the Uterine Cavity

Normal implantation of the fertilized ovum takes place in the upper part of the uterine cavity where there is ample capacity for growth of the uterus and fetus. When the placenta implants in the lower segment of the uterus the condition is known as **placenta previa**. The placenta may cover the internal cervical os, through which the fetus must eventually pass. Placenta previa is prone to hemorrhage because the lower uterine segment does not expand naturally with fetal growth, and, when stretched in late pregnancy or during labor, the placenta tears and severe hemorrhage can occur. Treatment is birth by caesarian section.

The placenta is naturally invasive—it must burrow into the endometrium and superficial myometrium to establish close contact with maternal blood vessels for exchange of gases and nutrients. Sometimes the placenta invades too deeply into the myometrium and does not separate spontaneously from the uterine wall after birth, a condition known as **placenta accreta**. Deeper invasions are called **placenta increta**, and, if they perforate through the uterine wall into

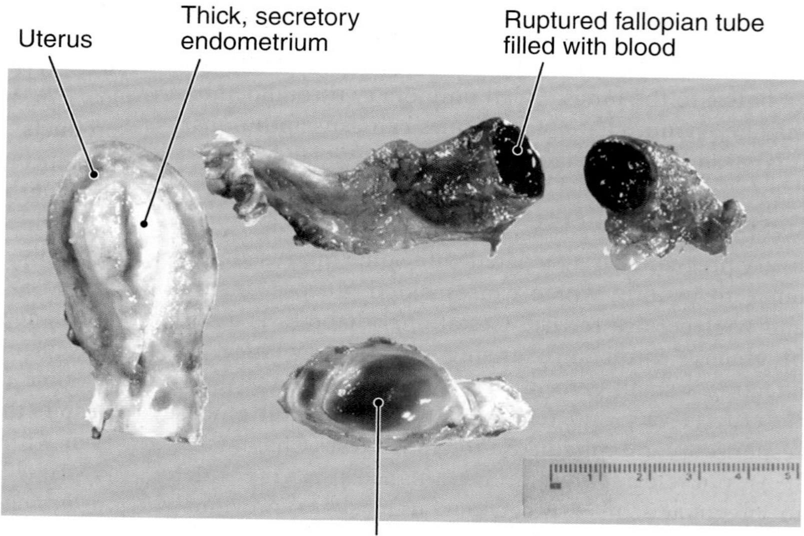

Figure 17.6 **Ectopic pregnancy in a fallopian tube.** The uterus is small and lined by thick, secretory endometrium ready for implantation of the conceptus, which has implanted in the fallopian tube. As the conceptus grew, it ruptured the wall of the tube and was expelled, causing sudden hemorrhage.

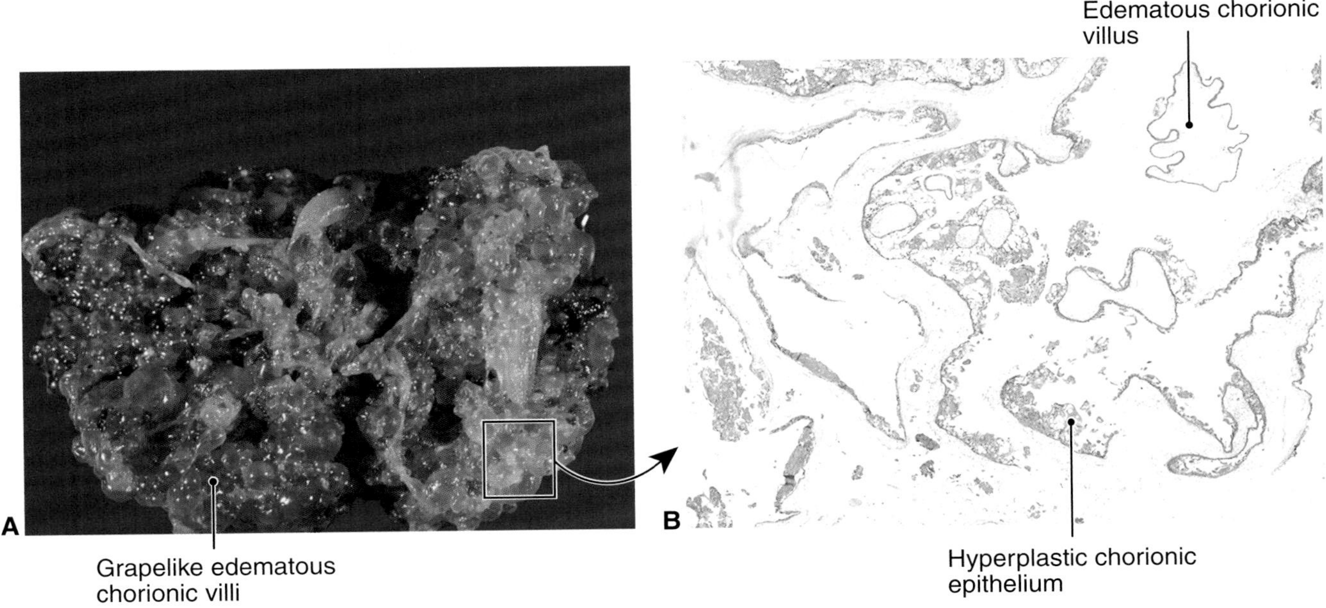

Figure 17.7 **Hydatidiform mole. A.** Note the grape-like, edematous chorionic villi. **B.** Microscopic study: note the hyperplastic chorionic epithelium.

adjacent tissues, are known as **placenta percreta**. If the placenta has not been expelled within 30 minutes of birth, serious bleeding may occur and manual extraction of the placenta is required. Manual extraction is usually successful; however, if it is not, a hysterectomy may be necessary.

Tumors and Tumor-Like Conditions of the Placenta

Abnormal fertilization may induce semi-neoplastic or neoplastic change in the chorionic epithelium, which covers placental villi. **Molar pregnancy** (Latin *mole* = mass) is a pregnancy in which a nonviable fertilized egg implants in the uterus and grows into an abnormal mass with or without recognizable fetal parts.

Hydatidiform mole (Fig. 17.7) is a benign tumor-like overgrowth of placental cells that takes its name from the Greek *hydatis*, meaning watery; thus, a watery mass. The typical hydatidiform mole is a watery mass of swollen, grapelike chorionic villi that microscopically are covered by hyperplastic chorionic epithelium. Limited embryologic development may occur in a few cases. They are rare in the United States but common in the Far East.

There are two varieties according to their chromosomal makeup. A **complete mole** contains only paternal chromosomes and is formed when one or two normal sperm fertilize an ovum without a nucleus. A **partial mole** contains both maternal and paternal chromosomes and occurs when two or more sperm fertilize a normal ovum. About 10% of partial moles may be locally aggressive (**invasive mole**). The mole invades deeply into the myometrium, and may invade nearby pelvic structures. Hydropic villi may metastasize to distant organs, but do not grow further and are not evidence of true malignancy.

About 2–3% of moles will develop **choriocarcinoma**, a malignant proliferation of trophoblastic cells that invades and metastasizes widely. Nevertheless, it responds spectacularly well to chemotherapy: virtually all patients achieve remission and most are cured. Choriocarcinomas rarely may arise from the ovary or testis. These tumors are not as responsive to treatment.

All moles secrete hCG. Increasing levels of blood hCG parallel tumor aggressiveness. The *History of Medicine*, "Right and Wrong in the Battle to Cure Cancer," offers additional insight into the role of molar lesions and cancer chemotherapy.

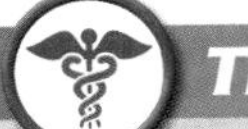

The History of Medicine

RIGHT AND WRONG IN THE BATTLE TO CURE CANCER

Sometimes being right is wrong . . . in the opinion of others.

Min Chiu Li, a Chinese physician, immigrated to the United States in 1947. After further study, he joined the National Cancer Institute (NCI) in 1955 to pursue his interest in cancer chemotherapy.

In 1956, Li's duties brought him into contact with Ethel Longoria, a young woman suffering from metastatic choriocarcinoma to her lungs, bleeding severely, and sure to die soon. Li proposed treating her with methotrexate, a drug proven to have antineoplastic effects in leukemia but never before tried for choriocarcinoma. She was given methotrexate and to everyone's surprise she survived the night. Several days later, after further methotrexate, chest X-rays, which previously showed her lungs filled with tumor, were. . . completely normal! No one had ever seen such a thing.

Despite this unbelievably good news, Li was not satisfied. Longoria's blood hCG levels had fallen dramatically, but low levels of hCG persisted. Li theorized, correctly as events would prove, that, despite clear X-rays, some viable tumor must still be present, and he insisted on continuing methotrexate therapy, in opposition to his superiors, who doubted the validity of his work. What happened next is disputed, but in any case Li was fired and left the NCI amid upset about his insistence on continuing chemotherapy until no signs of tumor activity remained. It would take years for the NCI to realize that Li was right: the patients receiving methotrexate until hCG disappeared achieved a lasting cure, while those whose treatments were cut short inevitably relapsed and died.

Li never returned to the NCI. Finally, in 1972, Li was awarded the prestigious Lasker Prize for having achieved the first chemotherapy cure of cancer. Ironically, he was forced to share his prize with one of his superiors who had been responsible for firing him.

Moles tend to occur in pregnant women who are younger than age 20 or over age 40. They present with painless vaginal bleeding about three months after conception. Examination of a patient with a mole usually reveals a uterus that is too large for the stage of the pregnancy. No fetal heartbeat can be detected, and there is no ultrasound image of a fetus in the uterus. Abnormally high levels of hCG are present in blood and urine because there is a large excess of placental tissue in the uterus. Hydatidiform mole is treated first by endometrial curettage. Persistent high blood chorionic gonadotropin after curettage suggests possible invasive mole or choriocarcinoma.

Other Conditions of Pregnancy

Infection can ascend the birth canal from the vagina and invade the amniotic fluid through a break in the amniotic membrane. The result may be fetal pneumonia (the fetus breathes amniotic fluid), sepsis, or other infection. Premature rupture of the amniotic membrane is a common cause of early labor, premature birth, and fetal pneumonia. The microbe of most concern is group B streptococcus. Preterm transplacental fetal infection is rare and is usually one of the TORCH infections discussed in Chapter 22.

Women are more prone to urinary tract infection than men because their urethra is short and opens onto a mucosal surface that harbors bacteria. This vulnerability to infection is enhanced by pregnancy. The hormonal environment causes relaxation of ureteral smooth muscle, which diminishes the downward peristalsis that assists urine down the ureter. Pressure from the enlarged uterus on the ureters adds to the problem. Urinary stagnation and infection may follow.

After full term pregnancy with vaginal delivery, especially after several vaginal deliveries, some women may develop **pelvic relaxation syndrome**. Pelvic ligaments may become so relaxed by age and multiple vaginal deliveries that the uterus may slide downward into the vagina (**uterine prolapse**), sometimes so far that the cervix protrudes from the vaginal introitus. Alternatively, when straining at stool, the rectum may bulge forward into the vagina (a protrusion called **rectocele**), which may interfere with bowel movements. The bladder also may bulge downward into the anterior aspect of the vagina (a protrusion called **cystocele**), which interferes with urination. Diagnosis is clinical. Treatment is surgical.

Case Notes

17.7 Was Susan likely to develop pelvic relaxation syndrome as a result of her pregnancies?

Pop Quiz

17.6 True or false? Choriocarcinoma secretes hCG while hydatiform moles do not.

17.7 True or false? Both blood volume and cardiac output increase approximately 30% with pregnancy.

17.8 True or false? Nearly all ectopic pregnancies are caused by mechanical obstruction.

17.9 True or false? The diagnosis of preeclampsia is made when the triad of elevated blood pressure, proteinuria, and seizures is manifested.

17.10 A(n) ____________ abortion is bleeding through an undilated cervix, while a(n) ____________ abortion includes cramps and cervical dilation.

17.11 Placenta ____________ occurs when the placenta invades too deeply into the myometrium and does not separate spontaneously from the uterine wall after delivery.

Infertility

The male aspects of infertility are discussed in Chapter 16. The causes of infertility in women include the following:

- Fallopian tube obstruction may be caused by scar tissue from chronic sexually transmitted infection (*chronic salpingitis* or *pelvic inflammatory disease*).
- Deposits of endometriosis may obstruct the fallopian tubes.
- Large uterine leiomyomas may distort the endometrial cavity so that implantation cannot occur.
- Abnormal cervical mucus can be "toxic" to sperm.
- Some ova are resistant to conception, especially those in older women.
- Irregular or infrequent ovulation significantly decreases the opportunity for fertilization.
- Hypothalamic or pituitary disease may cause a lack of hormonal support for implantation and fetal development (often an inadequate luteal phase).

Systemic factors, too, are clearly important. For example, immune reactions may interfere with conception, implantation, and fetal development.

Pelvic inflammatory disease (PID) is chronic infection of the fallopian tubes (and often the ovary and nearby peritoneum and ligaments) by sexually transmitted infections. Nongonococcal infections such as *Chlamydia* and *Mycoplasma* are the most common causes. PID is the most common preventable cause of infertility in the United States. Scarring can obstruct the tube so that sperm and ova cannot combine, or a fertilized ovum cannot reach the endometrium for implantation. The result can be infertility or ectopic pregnancy. Repeated infections may produce severe inflammation and scarring that may incorporate the ovary into a single inflammatory mass called a **tuboovarian abscess** (Fig. 17.8).

Lower abdominal pain is the primary symptom of PID. Fever and elevated WBC count are common with acute infection but may be absent with chronic disease. Tenderness on pelvic exam is common, and pus may drain from the cervical os. Acute cases respond well to antibiotics, but inflammation and scarring may be so severe in recurrent or chronic infections that only surgical removal of the tubes and ovaries can provide relief. In some cases, enough normal anatomy remains that the scars may be opened or the affected segment of tube can be excised and the ends anastomosed to reestablish patency.

Treatment of infertility may include assisted reproduction. **In vitro fertilization (IVF)** is now a common practice that usually involves the five steps listed below, but there are many variations:

1. Stimulation of ovulation by administration of clomiphene and/or hCG;
2. Collection of ova by needle puncture of the Graafian follicle;

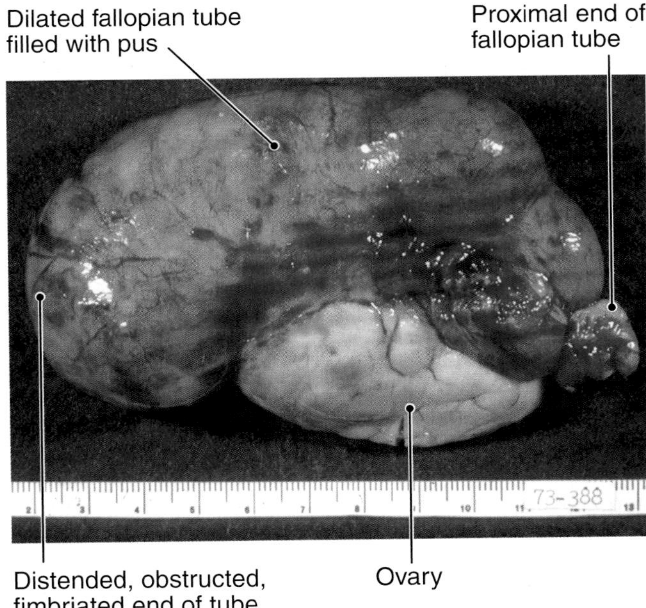

Figure 17.8 **Tuboovarian abscess.** The tube and ovary are welded into a single inflammatory mass.

3. Fertilization by mixing ova with sperm;
4. Embryo culture for two to five days;
5. Embryo transfer. One or more embryos are transferred into the endometrium. The number transferred varies according to the woman's age and clinical judgment about the chances of success. Multifetal pregnancy is a hazard, and may prompt the ethical dilemma of selective abortion to increase the viability of the remaining fetus or fetuses.

Obtaining a surrogate mother to impregnate by embryo transfer may be an option if the female cannot carry the pregnancy (e.g., because of a prior hysterectomy). Ethical issues abound, including rightful parentage should the surrogate mother refuse to relinquish the newborn.

Case Notes

17.8 What was the most likely cause of Susan's PID?

17.9 Why was Susan's right ovary left in place?

17.10 What was the main hazard in Susan's IVF procedure?

Pop Quiz

17.12 True or false? PID is the most common preventable cause of infertility in the United States.

Vulvar Disorder and Vaginitis

For the most part, diseases of the vulva and vagina are minor illnesses that cause discomfort, but not much lasting debility.

Vulvar Diseases Are Skin Diseases

Diseases of the vulva are relatively uncommon. The most common conditions are diseases of skin that are much the same as the same disease of skin elsewhere. Many are associated with white, flat, scaly lesions called **leukoplakia** (literally, "white patch"). The epithelial cells beneath these lesions, however, can be benign, dysplastic, or frankly malignant.

The most common cause of leukoplakia is a benign, hyperplastic overgrowth of surface squamous epithelium caused by chronic itching and scratching called **lichen simplex chronicus** (Chapter 21). Treatment is topical antihistamines or topical or locally injected corticosteroids.

Lichen sclerosus (*chronic atrophic vulvitis*, Fig. 17.9) is a nonneoplastic disease of unknown cause affecting the skin of the anogenital region. It features chronic atrophy, scarring, and contractures. It is characterized by atrophic, whitish, parchment-like skin dotted with patches of leukoplakia. Lichen sclerosus occurs in all age groups, but it is most common in postmenopausal women. Treatment is topical corticosteroids.

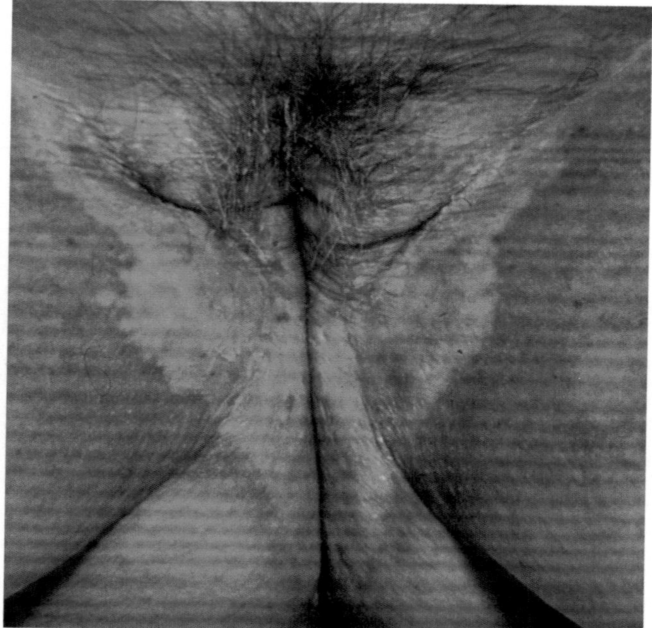

Figure 17.9 **Lichen sclerosus.** Labial skin is atrophic, fragile, and white. (Reproduced with permission from Rubin E, Farber JL. *Pathology*. 3rd ed. Philadelphia (PA): Lippincott Williams & Wilkins; 1999.)

Neoplasia is the most important disease of the vulva. *Condyloma acuminatum* is a benign growth caused by HPV infection (Chapter 4).

Vulvar carcinoma is uncommon. Squamous **vulvar intraepithelial neoplasia (VIN)** is a variety of dysplasia/carcinoma in situ (CIS) that owes to infection with certain strains of HPV and is analogous to similar lesions of the cervix (*squamous intraepithelial lesion [SIL]*). Invasive squamous carcinoma may arise. In 30% of cases, these invasive carcinomas are HPV positive. They arise mainly in women in their reproductive years. The remaining 70% of invasive squamous carcinomas are not HPV related, and instead arise in elderly women with long-standing lichen sclerosus.

Early diagnosis and surgery are effective: the five-year survival for invasive squamous carcinoma of the vulva is about 70% for patients whose lesions are treated while less than 2 cm in diameter. If diagnosis and treatment are delayed until the tumor is greater than 2 cm in diameter, only 10% survive five years.

Malignant melanomas (Chapter 21) may arise on the vulva. They are rare and tend to occur in elderly women. Their biology and microscopic characteristics are similar to skin melanomas elsewhere.

Paget disease is a peculiar variety of CIS similar to Paget disease of the nipple. It rarely invades but tends to recur after local excision.

Vaginitis Is a Common Problem

The normal vagina is populated by lactobacilli, which keep pH low (acidic) and prevent growth of other bacteria. **Vaginitis** is a common, transient superficial mucosal inflammation that is uncomfortable but typically not serious. Sometimes the vulva is involved (*vulvovaginitis*). Etiology depends on age. The most common sign of vaginitis is **leukorrhea**, an inflammatory discharge. In children, fecal flora, chemicals (e.g., bubble bath), and poor hygiene are usually responsible. Infection is the usual cause in women of reproductive age. In postmenopausal women, a lack of estrogen produces atrophic mucosa, which are fragile and subject to injury and inflammation (**atrophic vaginitis**).

Bacterial vaginosis is a form of vaginitis due to alteration of normal flora in which lactobacilli decrease and anaerobic bacteria overgrow. Symptoms include itching and a gray, thin, fishy-smelling discharge. Diagnosis is confirmed by testing vaginal secretions. The odor is characteristic, pH is >4.5, and microscopic study reveals swarms of bacteria clinging to squamous cells ("clue cells"). Treatment is with oral or topical antibiotics.

A common cause of vaginitis is **trichomoniasis** (Fig. 17.10A). It is often caused by microbes normally residing in the vagina, which become pathogenic under certain conditions that cause a change of the vaginal environment, such as diabetes or antibiotic therapy that alter the normal microbial flora, AIDS and other immunodeficient states, and pregnancy. Inflammation may be severe

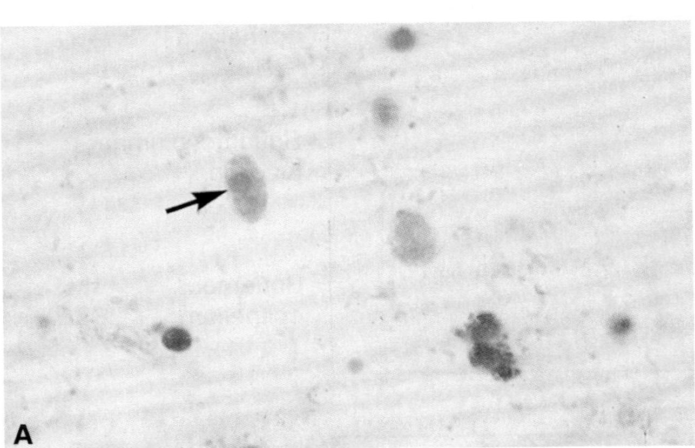

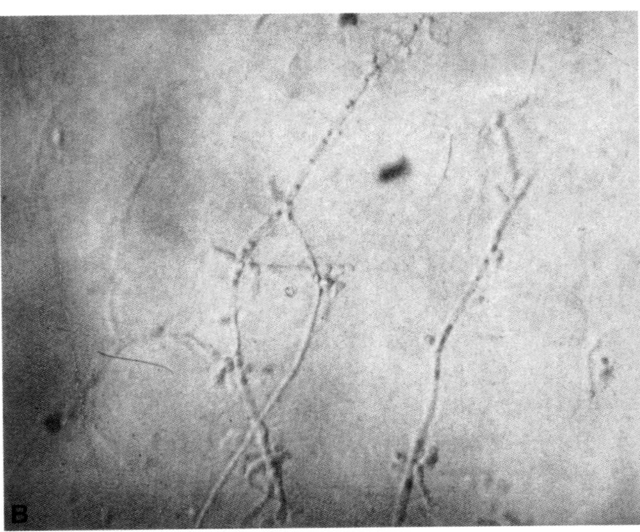

Figure 17.10 Vaginal smears of common vaginitis pathogens. A. *Trichomonas vaginalis*. **B.** *Candida albicans*. (**A.** Reproduced with permission from Sun T. *Parasitic Disorders: Pathology, Diagnosis, and Management*. 2nd ed. Baltimore (MD): Lippincott Williams & Wilkins; 1999; **B.** Reproduced with permission from Fleisher GR, Ludwig S, Baskin MN. *Atlas of Pediatric Emergency Medicine*. Philadelphia (PA): Lippincott Williams & Wilkins; 2004.)

and include dysuria. Vaginal discharge is often copious, malodorous, and greenish. Diagnosis is by microscopic finding of mobile organisms on a vaginal smear. Antibiotic therapy is effective.

One of the most common agents of vaginitis is the fungus *Candida albicans* (Fig. 17.10B). Asymptomatic *Candida* is found in the vagina of about 15–20% of non-pregnant women and 20–40% of pregnant women. Rates are higher in women who are also obese or diabetic. Development of symptoms—when *colonization* becomes *infection*—presumes some change to the patient's normal vaginal environment. Infection is called **moniliasis** or **candidiasis**. The discharge may be thin and watery or thick and chunky, and is white, and the woman may report painful urination, painful intercourse, and/or vaginal itching and burning. There may be cracks on the vulva. Laboratory analysis of a vaginal smear usually reveals an acidic pH (<4.5), and visible organisms with microscopic study. Over-the-counter antifungal creams and suppositories are effective. Moniliasis that does not respond to treatment or recurs immediately after treatment may be an early sign of HIV infection.

Pop Quiz

17.13 True or false? The majority of invasive vulvar carcinoma is owing to HPV infections.

17.14 In children, fecal flora, chemicals (e.g., bubble bath), and poor hygiene are usually responsible for vaginitis.

17.15 What is the treatment for moniliasis?

Disorders of the Cervix

Figure 17.11 illustrates the maturation of the cervix, knowledge of which is critical in the understanding of cervical disease. Recall from above that in the normal adult the *squamocolumnar junction* (Fig. 17.12) is in the cervical os. During puberty, however, the epithelium covering the ectocervix undergoes metaplasia (Chapter 2) from flat squamous cells into tall, columnar, glandular cells. The result is that the squamocolumnar junction is displaced outward. With sexual maturity the glandular epithelium reverts to squamous, and the squamocolumnar junction is restored to its original location. The area of temporarily transformed ectocervical epithelium is known as the **transformation zone**. *Virtually all dysplasia and carcinoma of the cervix arise in the transformation zone.*

Case Notes

17.11 Where exactly in the cervix was Susan's dysplasia most likely to be?

Ectropion, Polyps, and Cervicitis Are Benign Conditions

Ectropion (literally, "turning outward") of the cervix is the presence of endocervical glandular mucosa on the ectocervix. Ectropion is normal in young women and is easily visible on speculum examination of the cervix as a cuff of red, rough epithelium around the cervix (Fig. 17.13). Ectropion is normal in pregnancy, may remain postpartum,

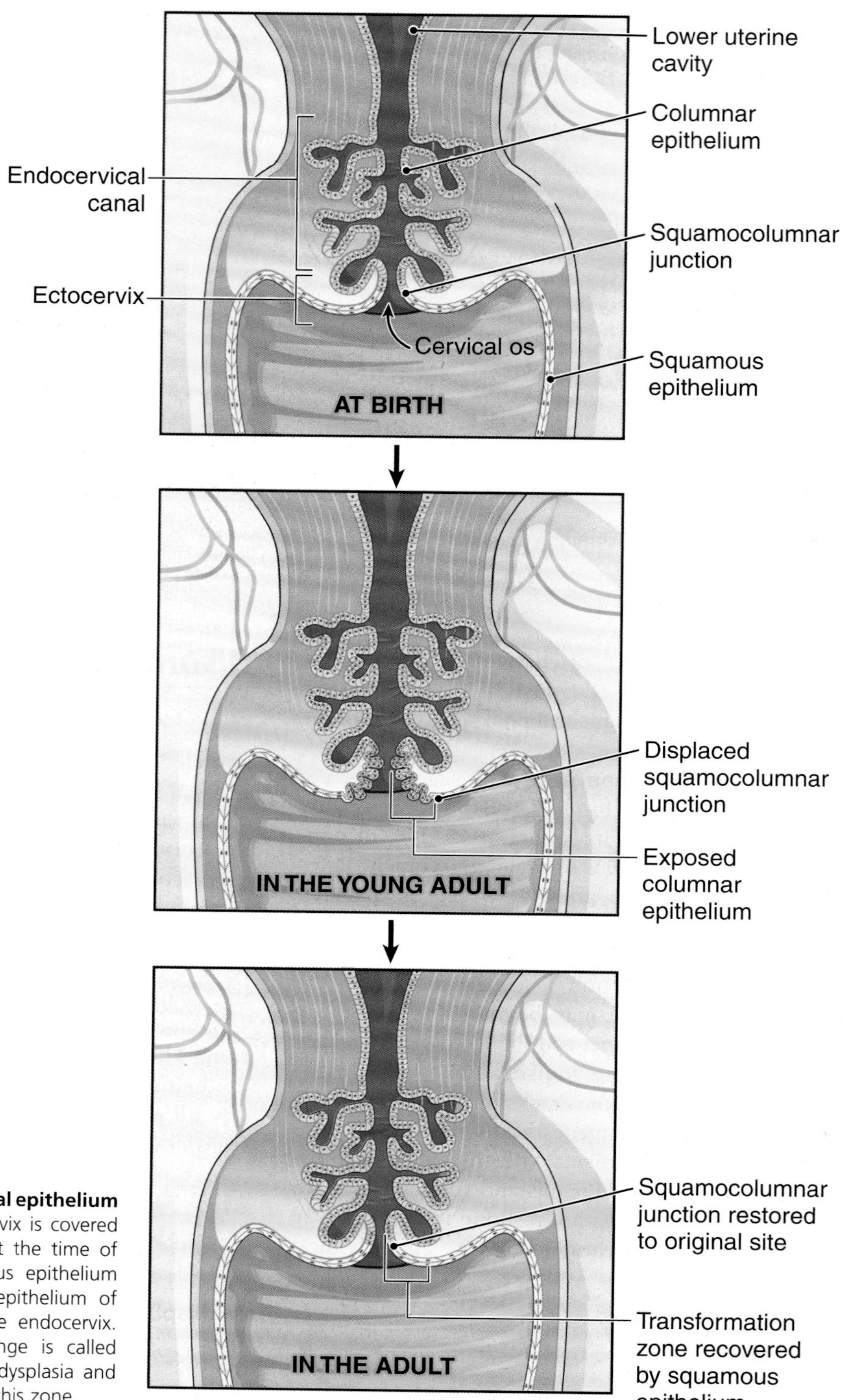

Figure 17.11 **Changes in cervical epithelium with age.** At birth, the ectocervix is covered by squamous epithelium. About the time of puberty, some of the squamous epithelium is transformed into glandular epithelium of the type normally found in the endocervix. The area undergoing this change is called the transformation zone. Most dysplasia and cancer of the cervix originate in this zone.

and may also occur in women taking birth control pills. Because ectropion resembles ulcerated (eroded) and inflamed mucosa, early physicians presumed the covering epithelium had been denuded—hence the common clinical term for it is *cervical erosion*. Ectropion is best considered a normal variant; however, it may cause spotting after intercourse. It is easily treated by applications of weak acid, which destroys the glandular epithelium and encourages return of squamous cells. Erosion plays no role in the development of cervical cancer or dysplasia.

Endocervical polyps (Fig. 17.14) are not neoplasms. Instead, they are protrusions of endocervical mucosa into

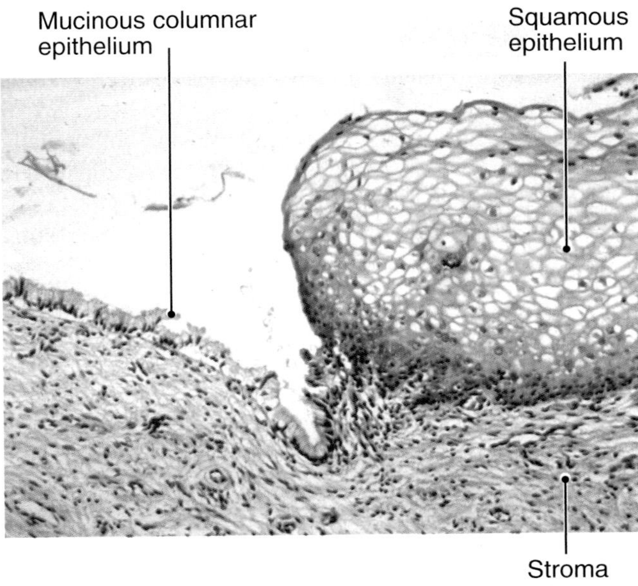

Figure 17.12 **The squamocolumnar junction of the cervix.** Columnar, mucinous endocervical epithelium (left) meets ectocervical-type squamous epithelium (right). (Reproduced with permission from Rubin E. *Pathology*. 4th ed. Philadelphia (PA). Lippincott Williams and Wilkins; 2005.)

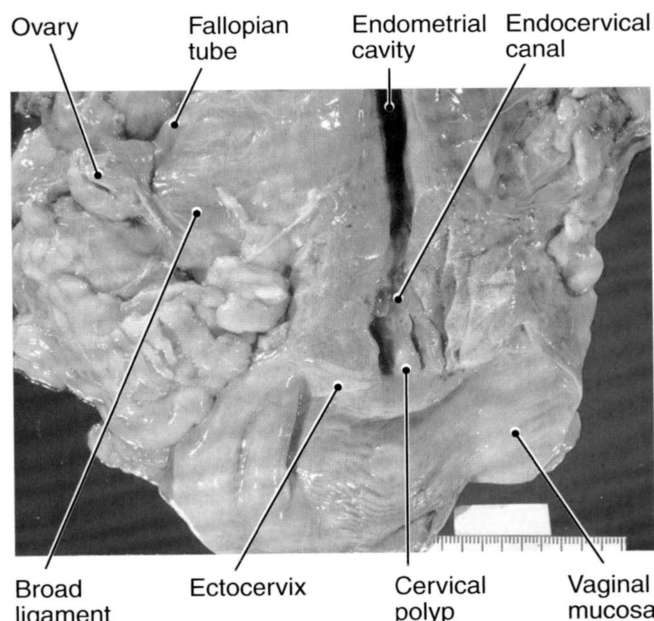

Figure 17.14 **Endocervical polyp.** A small polyp sits in the endocervical canal of this hysterectomy specimen.

the endocervical canal and are often visible on speculum examination. They are usually less than 2 cm, and tend to occur in chronically inflamed cervices. They are not premalignant. Treatment is local extirpation by surgery, caustic, laser, or similar destruction.

Cervicitis and vaginitis often occur together and may herald more serious infection (PID, discussed below). **Chronic cervicitis** is common and usually asymptomatic.

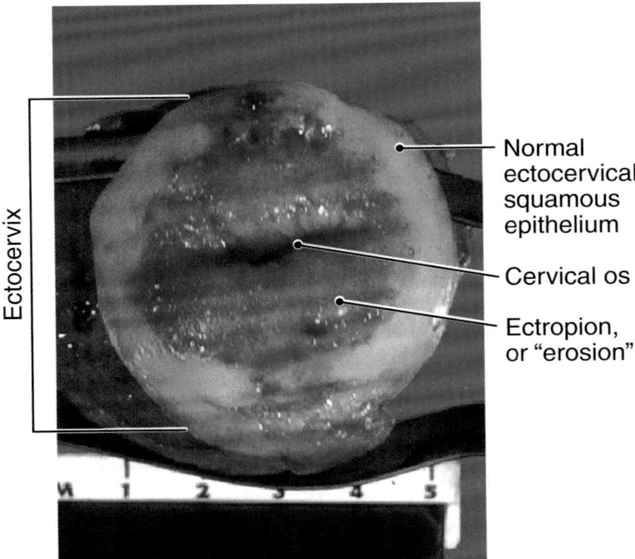

Figure 17.13 **Ectropion ("erosion") of the cervix.** Endocervical glandular epithelium has reappeared in the transformation zone in an adult woman. The rough, red appearance led early observers to believe the red, rough appearance represented epithelial ulceration (erosion).

It is a near universal finding in biopsies done for other purposes, especially in older women. It is noninfectious and may be due to local trauma from intercourse, tampons, or radiation, for example. Signs and symptoms of acute and chronic cervicitis are similar and differ only by degree.

Acute cervicitis usually occurs in young women and is usually infectious. The most common offenders are gonococci, *Chlamydia*, herpes, or other sexually transmitted infection in young women. Postpartum cervicitis is usually due to staphylococci or streptococci. Repeated douching may upset the vaginal environment and lead to infection.

Cervicitis symptoms include leukorrhea, dysuria, frequency, and postcoital spotting. The cervix may be erythematous and a film of purulent material may be present in the os, on the ectocervix, or in the vagina, and the cervix may bleed easily to touch. Laboratory study of cervicovaginal discharge is warranted if infection is suspected. Cultures are no longer routinely performed because molecular techniques (DNA probe, polymerase chain reaction, immunofluorescence) are quicker, cheaper, and more widely available. Antibiotics are the treatment of choice.

Cervicitis also may cause mildly abnormal (but benign) cells to appear on Pap smears.

Dysplasia and Carcinoma of the Cervix Are Related to HPV Infection

In 1950, invasive cancer of the cervix was the leading cause of cancer death for women in the United States. Worldwide it remains very common, but, in the United States, the number of deaths has been reduced by 70%.

This dramatic decline occurred largely because of widespread adoption of regular cervical cytology (Pap smear) exams. The *History of Medicine*, "How the Pap Smear Got Its Name," provides a look at how the Pap smear came to occupy its important role in modern medicine.

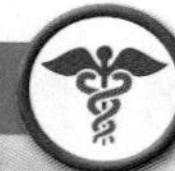

The History of Medicine

HOW THE PAP SMEAR GOT ITS NAME

The Pap smear is named after George Papanicolaôu, affectionately called "Doctor Pap" by colleagues because of his jawbreaker name. He was born in Greece, received his medical training there, and later earned a PhD in Germany before coming to New York in 1913, where he passed through Ellis Island as an almost penniless immigrant among the flood of those fleeing Europe in advance of World War I. His first job in the United States was as a rug salesman. He played the violin in restaurants before landing a job as an assistant anatomist at Cornell University, where he remained until a few years before his death in 1962.

His achievement is a powerful example of the unexpected benefits of basic research that initially may seem to have little practical application. Dr. "Pap" was studying the reproductive physiology of guinea pigs when he noticed cyclical changes of cells in the vaginal discharge. Applying his observations to humans, he found similar cellular changes. Purely by coincidence, he also noticed abnormal cells in women with uterine cancer, an insight that he instantly foresaw as having far-reaching consequences, which he later described as one of the most thrilling experiences of his life. He presented his findings in 1923, but they met with little interest in the medical community, which considered his method an unnecessary addition to existing diagnostic technique.

Dr. "Pap" persisted for 20 years and, in 1943, he published his famous paper showing how cervical cancers, the most deadly cancer of women at the time, could be easily detected earlier by his simple technique. Thus was born the "Pap" smear. Nevertheless, the natural resistance to change inherent in medical practice and the primitive manner of professional scientific communication in those days resulted in slow adoption of the Pap smear, which did not become common in medical practice until the 1950s. The rapid decline in deaths from invasive cervical cancer coincides with the widespread adoption of the Pap smear as a screening tool.

Etiology and Pathogenesis

The single most important factor in the development of cervical dysplasia and carcinoma is the infectious spread of high-risk subtypes (types 16 and 18) of human papilloma virus (HPV), which damage DNA and induce cells to proliferate. Persistent HPV infection can induce dysplasia or, ultimately, invasive cervical cancer. HPV is a sexually transmitted disease and is often detected in patients who have other evidence or history of sexually transmitted infection. An anti-HPV vaccine is now widely available. The *History of Medicine*, "Did 'Evita' Get Cervical Cancer from Her Husband?", discusses an interesting historical case of cervical carcinoma.

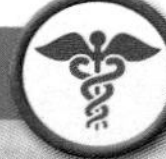

The History Of Medicine

DID "EVITA" GET CERVICAL CANCER FROM HER HUSBAND?

Eva Peron (1919–1952), wife of post–World War II Argentine strongman Juan Peron, and a charismatic woman in her own right, was the subject of the Broadway musical *Evita* and its iconic song "Don't Cry for Me Argentina." Evita died of cervical carcinoma when she was 33. Of further interest is that Peron's first wife also died of cervical carcinoma. Did he transmit human papillomavirus and (indirectly) the cancer from his first wife to Eva? No one can say for sure, but it seems likely.

Nevertheless, HPV infection is not the only factor. A high percentage of young women are infected—about one million new cases are detected annually by Pap smears—but only a few develop dysplasia or cancer. Other factors influence whether the HPV infection will regress, persist, or progress to dysplasia or cancer, and at what rate. These factors are the following:

- Young age at first intercourse
- Multiple sexual partners
- A male partner with multiple female sexual partners
- Persistent infection with high-risk HPV (e.g., types 16 or 18)
- Immunodeficient state (e.g., HIV)
- Certain HLA genotypes
- Oral contraceptive use
- Smoking

Peak prevalence of HPV infection and squamous dysplasia occurs among women in their 20s and is related to initiation of sexual activity and the acquisition of multiple partners. Most infections are transient and eliminated by the immune system over a period of 12–24 months. Reinfection may occur and reestablish the development of dysplasia. Prevalence falls as monogamous relationships and immunity develop. By contrast, peak prevalence for invasive squamous carcinoma is in the mid-40s, which emphasizes that invasive carcinoma develops only after many years of persistent infection.

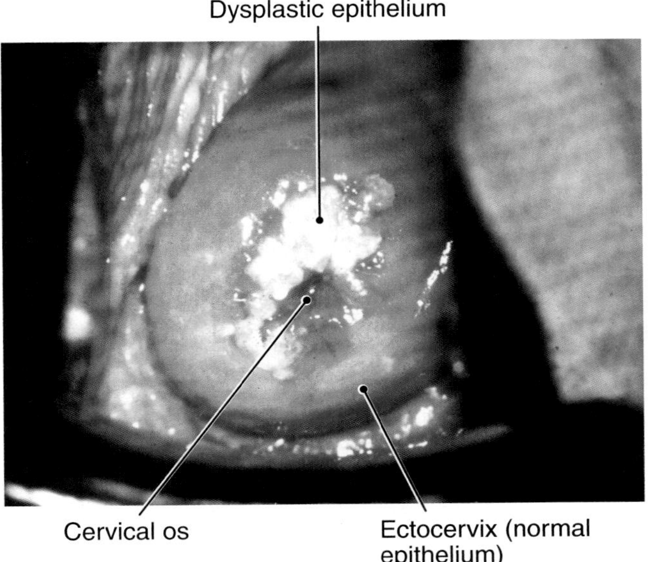

Figure 17.15 **Dysplasia of the cervix (vaginal speculum view).** Dysplastic epithelium turns white when washed by weak acid.

HPV-related changes are usually confined to the transformation zone of the cervix, which is easily visualized (Fig. 17.15) by speculum exam for biopsy or Pap smear examination.

As Figures 17.16, 17.17, and 17.18 illustrate, HPV induces changes in infected squamous cells—the nuclei become large, dark, and angular, and a clear cytoplasmic "halo" surrounds the nucleus. If infection persists, these changes become more pronounced until the entire thickness is occupied by severely atypical cells. These changes are the equivalent of carcinoma in situ (Chapter 5), the final stage before the lesion breaks through the basement membrane to become invasive carcinoma.

Remember This! Carcinoma of the cervix is caused by long-term infection by high-risk strains of HPV.

Infected cervical epithelium is not static; change is constant. Low-grade lesions usually regress and the epithelium returns to normal; high-grade lesions often progress to more severe dysplasia and some become invasive cancers. Table 17.1 displays the natural history of low- and high-grade lesions and carcinoma. It is important to note that 90% of HPV infections clear within two years, but reinfection is common, which accounts for the persistence of some cervical lesions.

Nevertheless, the process is not necessarily a smooth transition from one degree of abnormality to another. For

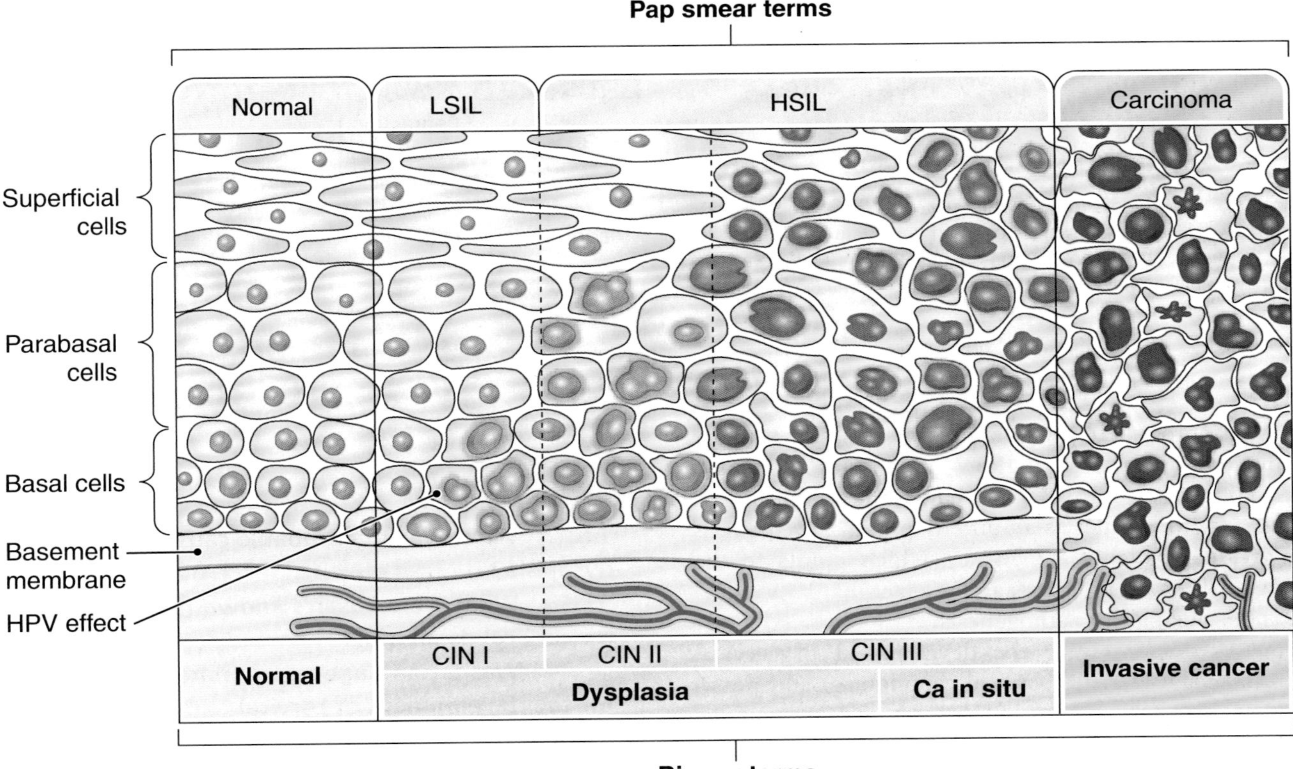

Figure 17.16 **Development of dysplasia and carcinoma of the cervix.** Repeated human papillomavirus (HPV) infections convert normal epithelium (left) into increasingly severe dysplasia until malignant epithelium breaks through the basement membrane to become invasive cancer, capable of metastasis by invasion of blood vessels and lymphatics.

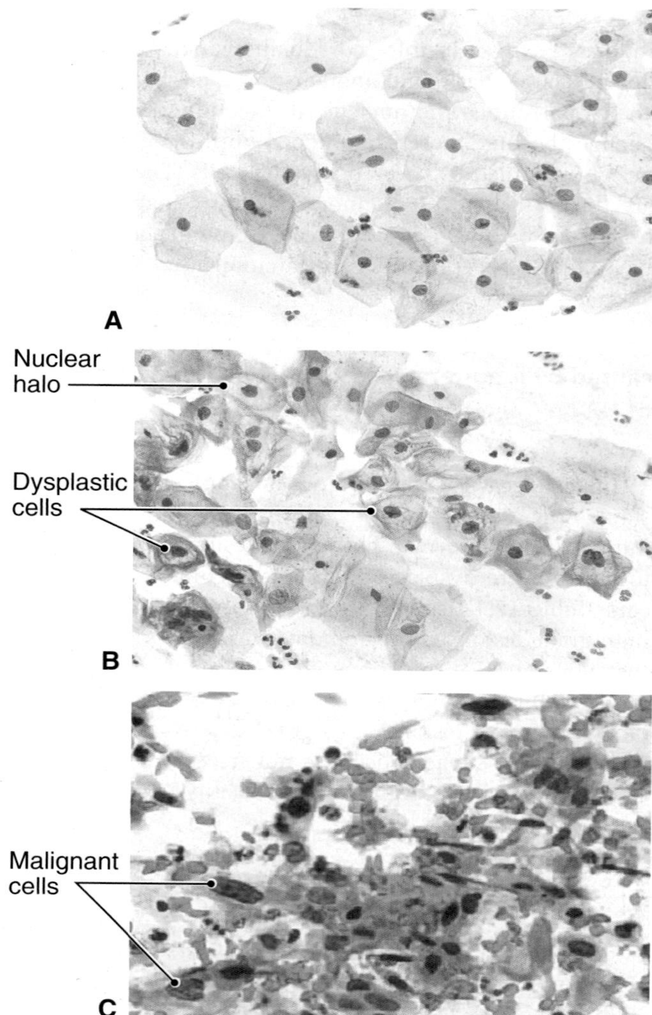

Figure 17.17 **Pap smears (diagnostic terms are from the Bethesda System). A.** Negative (normal, large, thin cells with small, uniform nuclei). **B.** High grade squamous intraepithelial lesion (nuclei are large and dark and have a halo of HPV effect). **C.** Carcinoma (larger, darker, irregular, malformed nuclei).

example, approximately 20% of high-grade lesions appear de novo, with no preexisting low-grade lesion. Although it is convenient to think of changes from one degree of abnormality to another as an orderly process, predictions in individual patients are chancy, which points to the influence of the other factors and the fact that HPV infection is but one part of pathogenesis.

HPV can also induce the development of cervical *adenocarcinoma* (10% of cervical carcinomas) and possibly other types (a small percentage). These nonsquamous tumors usually arise in the endocervical canal and are much less likely to yield cells to Pap smear specimen collection. These tumors are typically discovered only in older women when they have reached an advanced stage and cause bleeding, pain, or urinary obstruction.

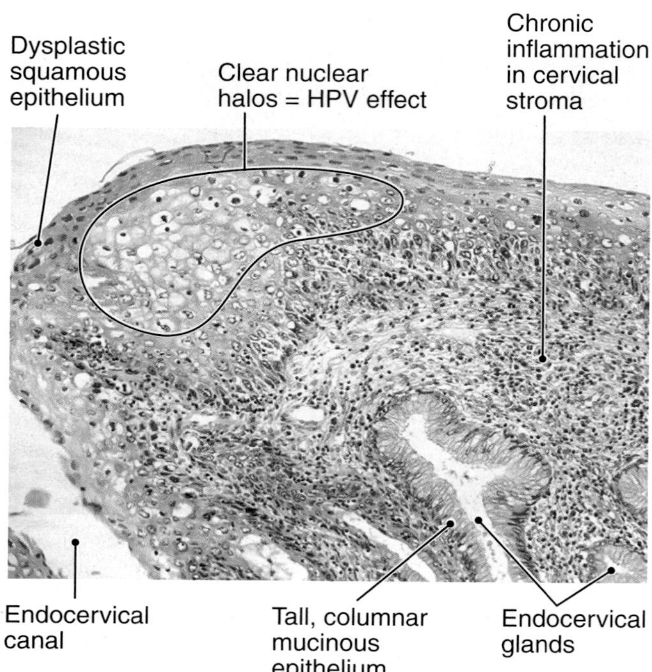

Figure 17.18 **CIN I dysplasia of the cervix (biopsy specimen).** The presence of cells with enlarged, irregular, dark nuclei indicates DNA damage. Clear nuclear halos in some cells are evidence of human papillomavirus infection.

Table 17.1 Two-Year Natural History of Dysplasia (Squamous Intraepithelial Lesion)

Diagnosis	Regression to Lesser Degree of dysplasia or Normal Epithelium	Dysplasia persists Unchanged	Progression to More Severe Degree of dysplasia
Low grade dysplasia (SIL)	60%	30%	10% to high grade SIL
High grade dysplasia (SIL)	30%	60%	10% to carcinoma

Case Notes

17.12 **What was the probable cause of Susan's dysplasia?**

17.13 **What were Susan's *known* risk factors for cervical dysplasia?**

17.14 **Was Susan's age appropriate for the development of cervical dysplasia?**

17.15 **Was it unusual for Susan to have evidence of HPV infection and other sexually transmitted disease?**

Diagnostic Terminology

Recall from Chapter 5 that *dysplasia* is a premalignant state of epithelium, that *carcinoma in situ* (CIS) is the final and most severe form of dysplasia, and that *invasive* carcinoma arises from CIS. These terms remain widely used for other anatomic sites, but not for cervical lesions. New terms were coined to bring greater precision of diagnosis and better correlation between tissue biopsy findings and Pap smear reports.

In an attempt to standardize diagnostic criteria and improve uniformity of diagnosis, the World Health Organization implemented a new terminology for classification of cervical dysplasia, renaming dysplasias of the cervix as **cervical intraepithelial neoplasia (CIN)**. Three grades were recognized: CIN I, II, and III. Be careful not to confuse these CIN tissue diagnosis terms with the *Bethesda System* terms for Pap smear (cytopathology) results (discussed next).

Pap smear reporting was similarly reformed. Pap smears should reliably *predict* biopsy findings and serve as a guide to postsmear steps in diagnosis and treatment—Pap smears are not diagnostic. Formerly, Pap smear reports used broad generalities such as "moderately atypical cells" or standard tissue diagnosis terms such as "dysplasia" or "CIN." Over the last several decades, however, consensus developed about the significance of lesions and the treatment required, and the language of Pap smears was changed to a new terminology called the **Bethesda System**, named for the Maryland town where the initial naming conference was held in 1988. At its core, the Bethesda Pap smear reporting system is a *two-tiered* classification that relies on the differing behavior of 1) low-grade dysplasia versus 2) high-grade dysplasia of the cervical epithelium.

The Bethesda reporting system uses the term **low-grade squamous intraepithelial lesion (LSIL)** to *predict* that low-grade dysplasia is present in the cervix. The term **high-grade squamous intraepithelial lesion (HSIL)** is used to *predict* high-grade dysplasia. Table 17.2 compares biopsy and Bethesda Pap smear terminologies.

The most important aspects (substantially abridged) of the standard Bethesda report are as follows:

- Negative for Intraepithelial Lesion or Malignancy
- Atypical Squamous Cells of Undetermined Significance (ASCUS)
- LSIL
- HSIL
- Carcinoma

The Bethesda System has many other specifications, too many to detail here. An example of a typical Bethesda System smear is seen in Figure 17.19.

Pap smears are collected using a spatula to scrape cells from the ectocervix and a narrow brush to collect cells from the endocervix. The cells are then smeared on a small glass slide and quickly treated with alcohol to preserve them until they reach the laboratory, where they are processed and examined.

An alternative to direct smear and examination is to place cells in a special solution to dissolve RBCs and inflammatory cells. A portion of the solution is mechanically spread onto a slide in a uniform layer that is easier to examine microscopically than a direct smear. The slide may be examined directly, but commonly it is first scanned by computer and suspicious areas are inked for further study by a laboratory professional (pathologist or cytologist).

Remember This! Pap smears are predictive, not diagnostic.

Case Notes

17.16 **Was Susan's biopsy diagnosis consistent with her Pap smear report?**

17.17 **Was Susan's HSIL Pap smear likely to regress to LSIL without treatment?**

Signs and Symptoms

The great majority of cervical carcinomas are asymptomatic at time of discovery because they are small, early, and detected initially by Pap smear. On the other hand, advanced lesions can be symptomatic. Adenocarcinomas

Table 17.2 Classification Systems for Premalignant Changes in Cervical Squamous Epithelium

Nomenclature for Biopsy Reports		Nomenclature for Pap Smear Reports	
Conventional microscopic terminology	World Health Organization classification	Bethesda system interpretation of Pap smear findings	Usual implications for treatment
Dysplasia/CIS	CIN	SIL	
Mild dysplasia	CIN I	LSIL	Watch-and-wait, resmear
Moderate dysplasia	CIN II		
Severe dysplasia CIS	CIN III	HSIL	Biopsy and treatment

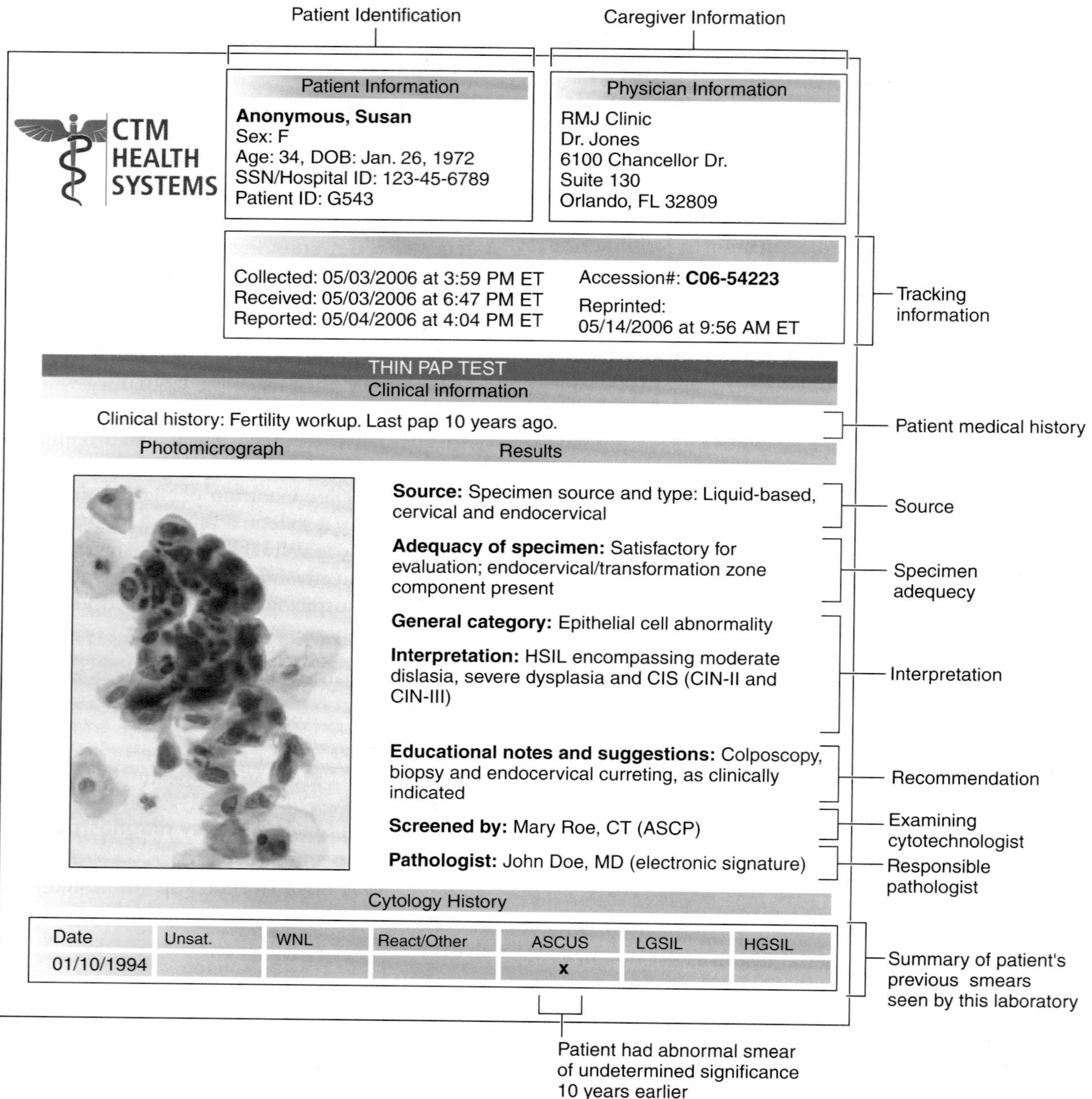
CTM HEALTH SYSTEMS

Patient Information

Anonymous, Susan
Sex: F
Age: 34, DOB: Jan. 26, 1972
SSN/Hospital ID: 123-45-6789
Patient ID: G543

Physician Information

RMJ Clinic
Dr. Jones
6100 Chancellor Dr.
Suite 130
Orlando, FL 32809

Collected: 05/03/2006 at 3:59 PM ET
Received: 05/03/2006 at 6:47 PM ET
Reported: 05/04/2006 at 4:04 PM ET

Accession#: **C06-54223**
Reprinted: 05/14/2006 at 9:56 AM ET

THIN PAP TEST

Clinical information

Clinical history: Fertility workup. Last pap 10 years ago.

Photomicrograph

Results

Source: Specimen source and type: Liquid-based, cervical and endocervical

Adequacy of specimen: Satisfactory for evaluation; endocervical/transformation zone component present

General category: Epithelial cell abnormality

Interpretation: HSIL encompassing moderate dislasia, severe dysplasia and CIS (CIN-II and CIN-III)

Educational notes and suggestions: Colposcopy, biopsy and endocervical curreting, as clinically indicated

Screened by: Mary Roe, CT (ASCP)

Pathologist: John Doe, MD (electronic signature)

Cytology History

Date	Unsat.	WNL	React/Other	ASCUS	LGSIL	HGSIL
01/10/1994				x		

Figure 17.19 **Typical Bethesda System Pap smear report.** In the "Interpretation," note the relationship between the Pap smear findings (HSIL) and the findings that the smear predicts will be present on biopsy (CIN II or III).

are overrepresented among advanced lesions because they originate in the endocervical canal and are usually missed by Pap smear. Symptoms include the following:

- Vaginal bleeding after intercourse, between periods, or after menopause
- Watery, bloody vaginal discharge that may be heavy and have a foul odor
- Low pelvic pain or pain during intercourse

Diagnosis and Treatment

Some Pap smears are ambiguous: the cytologist or pathologist cannot be certain of the implications of what is being seen on the slide. The Bethesda category for these smears is *atypical cells of undetermined significance* (ACUS). In such cases, infection or other clinical problem should be treated and the patient should return for resmear in a few months. HPV testing is an alternative. About 10–20% of these will be found at some future time to have CIN II or III (high grade dysplasia).

Patients with a Pap smear finding of LSIL constitute 90% of SIL diagnoses and are not treated as if the lesion is precancerous. Most lesions associated with LSIL smears regress without treatment and none proceed directly to invasive cancer without first progressing to HSIL, usually over a period of many years, which offers ample time for discovery. Follow-up varies considerably. Women under 20 should return in one year for resmear. Women 21 or older should be examined with a **colposcope** (a short telescope) to search for any cervical abnormality worthy of biopsy. No treatment is necessary if a lesion is not found.

For patients with a pap smear of LSIL and a lesion biopsy of CIN I, there is currently a trend toward a watch-and-wait approach. Patients may be left untreated and resmeared regularly. If CIN I persists on follow-up, additional intervention may be required.

Patients with a Pap smear finding of HSIL also require colposcopic examination and biopsy. Lesions identified as CIN I are treated as above. Lesions discovered to be CIN II may sometimes be treated by superficial excision of the affected epithelium or by freezing, laser vaporization, electrocautery, chemical peeling, or other means of destroying superficial tissue. CIN III lesions are usually treated by a surgical "coring out" of a cone of cervix (**cone biopsy** or "conization") so that a pathologist can examine the tissue to be sure all of the malignant epithelium has been removed and that no areas of invasion are present.

If, however, the lesion has penetrated the basement membrane, it becomes *invasive* carcinoma (Fig. 17.20). One of the earliest and most frequent signs of invasive carcinoma is vaginal bleeding, one of the many reasons intermenstrual or postmenopausal vaginal bleeding deserves careful investigation in every instance. Invasive carcinoma becomes progressively more symptomatic as it invades vagina, pelvis, and bladder, producing pain, dysuria, and other symptoms. Invasive tumors of any variety must be clinically staged (Chapter 5).

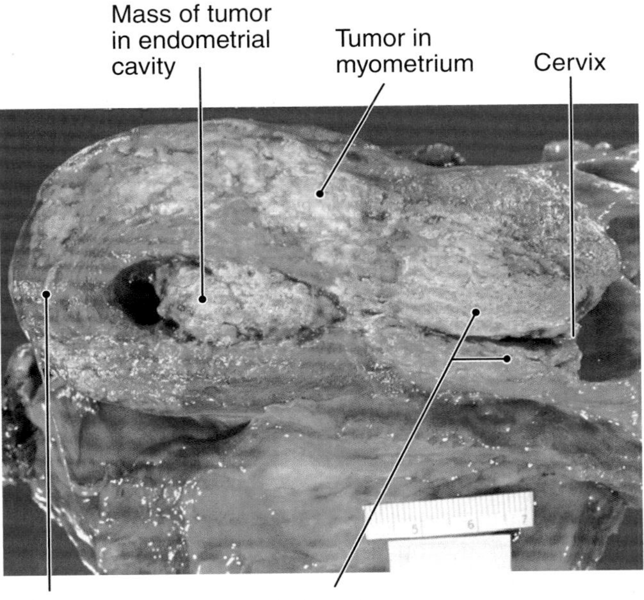

Figure 17.20 **Invasive carcinoma of the cervix.** Extensive involvement of the cervix, endometrium, and uterus.

Table 17.3 Clinical Staging of Cervical Carcinoma

Stage	Description	5-year Survival
0	CIS	100%
1	Tumor confined to the cervix (several substages)	80–90%
II	Tumor extending beyond the cervix but not to the pelvic wall	60–75%
III	Tumor extending to but not beyond the pelvic wall	30–40%
IV	Tumor extending beyond pelvic wall or involvement of rectum or bladder or metastasis	0–15%

Radical hysterectomy (removal of uterus, tubes, and ovaries), radiation, and/or chemotherapy is the treatment for invasive carcinoma. The type and extent of each depends on careful clinical staging. Table 17.3 presents the clinical stages of cervical carcinoma and the approximate five-year survival rates.

Screening for Cervical Cancer

Precancerous lesions of the cervix are asymptomatic and detectable only by screening. Screening is effective because the majority of invasive carcinomas are preceded by many years of precancerous changes. The Pap smear has been the mainstay of cervical cancer screening for 60 years. Nevertheless, new techniques such as polymerase chain reaction (PCR, Chapter 4) can detect the presence of HPV in cervical smears. PCR testing seems poised to become the primary screening test, with the Pap smear assuming a secondary or confirmatory role. Authorities disagree, however, about when to begin screening, how often it should be repeated, the age at which to stop, and whether or not both Pap smear and HPV testing should be done alone or together.

All authorities recommend screening begin at age 21 for *all* women. With some exceptions, authorities agree that women whose prior screen was negative should be rescreened once every three years. Some authorities recommend HPV cotesting every third year with a Pap smear. Others disagree or recommend use of HPV testing only in women over 30. Most recommend screening stop at age 65 after regular screening in the previous 3–10 years.

Case Notes

17.18 Looking back, what lessons might Susan draw from her experience?

Pop Quiz

17.16 True or false? Patients with HSIL should be treated with a watch-and-wait approach.

17.17 True or false? The presence of abnormal cells on a Pap smear is diagnostic of cervical dysplasia and infection with HPV.

17.18 What is the site of most cervical cancer?

17.19 What are the causes of ectropion?

Disorders of the Endometrium and Myometrium

Understanding the physiology of the menstrual cycle is critical to an understanding of endometrial conditions. The simple fact that the endometrium sheds monthly during reproductive years and is atrophic thereafter is a very important fact: it makes the endometrium unusually resistant to infection and especially susceptible to hormonal abnormalities.

Dysfunctional Uterine Bleeding Is Very Common

Menstrual problems and abnormal vaginal bleeding are the most common reasons women seek gynecologic care. Abnormal vaginal bleeding is a serious matter because it may indicate endometrial, vaginal, or cervical carcinoma, or other grave problems.

Most women feel some discomfort with menstruation, and occasionally it interferes with normal activity. In most instances, it is not associated with anatomic disease. There are several *clinical terms* useful in describing abnormal bleeding or menstruation:

- **Amenorrhea**: absence of menstruation
- **Dysmenorrhea**: painful menstruation
- **Menorrhagia**: excessive bleeding at the time of regular menstrual flow
- **Metrorrhagia**: irregular bleeding between periods
- **Polymenorrhea**: frequent, short cycles, less than three weeks
- **Oligomenorrhea**: few, long cycles, longer than six weeks

Abnormal bleeding falls into two categories. **Pathologic bleeding** is relatively uncommon and due to well-defined anatomic abnormalities such as complications of pregnancy (abortion, ectopic pregnancy, retained POC), tumors of the myometrium, or by endometrial polyps, hyperplasia, or tumors. **Dysfunctional uterine bleeding (DUB)** is any bleeding not due to identified anatomic abnormality.

DUB is caused by the following:

- *Anovulatory cycle*. If ovulation does not occur, no corpus luteum forms and no progesterone is produced. Therefore, the proliferative endometrium that grew between menstruation and ovulation does not receive the expected support from a corpus luteum, and it sloughs away as a bloody drainage at an unexpectedly early time in the cycle (about midway, immediately after ovulation should have occurred). Anovulatory cycles are most common near *menarche* (onset of menstruation) and menopause. Other causes include failure by the pituitary to secrete LH, adrenal or thyroid hormonal abnormalities, malnutrition, severe psychological or physical stress, or marked obesity.
- *Inadequate luteal phase* is due to failure of the corpus luteum to function normally. Low progesterone production does not properly support secretory phase endometrium and menstruation occurs early. It is a cause of infertility.
- *Oral contraceptives* induce a variety of changes in the endometrium that may cause irregular bleeding. New, low-dose formulations largely avoid this problem.
- *Amenorrhea* is another dysfunctional disorder. **Primary amenorrhea** is failure of girls to begin menstruation by age 14 if they have not gone through puberty (growth spurt, breast development) or by age 16 or two years after puberty. Sometimes it is due to an underlying endocrine or genetic defect (e.g., Turner syndrome, Chapter 22). **Secondary amenorrhea** is cessation of menses after they have begun. The most common cause of secondary amenorrhea is pregnancy. Other causes are delayed puberty, excessive exercise, eating disorders, stress, drug abuse, breastfeeding, and polycystic ovary syndrome.

Case Notes

17.19 Did Susan have DUB?

Endometritis Is Uncommon

The endometrium is especially resistant to infection because the cervix provides an effective barrier, it is shed regularly during reproductive years, and its atrophic state in menopause offers little nourishment to infectious agents. **Acute endometritis** is limited to bacterial infections that arise after childbirth or abortion. Retained POC are the usual culprit and become a nidus of infection for streptococci, staphylococci, or other bacteria.

The two types of **chronic endometritis** are 1) those associated with pregnancy, and 2) all others. In the obstetric population, chronic endometritis is usually associated with retained POC after delivery or abortion. In nonobstetric patients, chronic endometritis may be associated with PID, intrauterine contraceptive devices, or vaginitis.

Signs and symptoms are those ordinarily expected: fever, malaise, pelvic pain, malodorous vaginal discharge, and pelvic tenderness. Complications include peritonitis, pelvic infection, and pelvic thrombophlebitis (Chapter 6).

Antibiotics are the mainstay of treatment. Retained POC or intrauterine contraceptive devices should be removed.

Endometriosis Is Deposits of Endometrium outside the Uterine Cavity

Endometriosis is deposits of endometrium outside of the uterine cavity (Fig. 17.21). It consists of accumulations of normal endometrium in abnormal places.

Endometriosis is an important clinical condition: it affects about 10% of women between ages 20 and 40 and is often the cause of infertility, pelvic pain, and dysmenorrhea. Figure 17.22 illustrates the many and sometimes surprising places endometrium can appear, most often in the ovaries (80% of cases), uterine ligaments, and cul de sac. How endometrium comes to be located in these odd places remains unknown, but likely seems to be metastasis from endometrium regurgitated through the fallopian tube.

In endometriosis, the displaced endometrium undergoes cyclic menstrual changes and bleeding in parallel with uterine endometrium. The bleeding occurs into tissues, inciting inflammation and fibrosis, which accounts for most of the symptoms and associated problems. Deposits vary from a few millimeters to several centimeters and contain a mixture of endometrium, blood, inflammatory cells, and fibrosis.

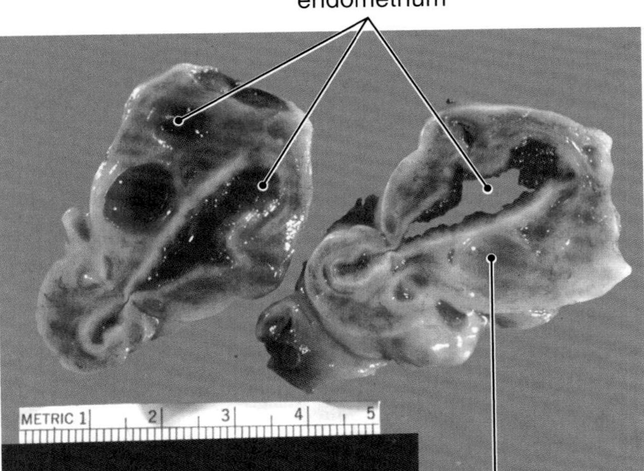

Figure 17.21 **Endometriosis of the ovary.** Hemorrhagic, cystic deposits of endometrium are visible in this ovary. Note the small follicle cyst.

Clinical symptoms depend on the anatomic sites involved—painful defecation may reflect deposits low in the posterior pelvic peritoneum; dysuria may result from deposits in the dome of the bladder; infertility may reflect blocked fallopian tubes; dyspareunia may occur from any site low in the pelvis. Half of all women with dysmenorrhea (painful menstruation) have endometriosis; in one-third of infertile couples, the woman has endometriosis.

Diagnosis requires biopsy. Treatment includes NSAIDs for pain, drugs to suppress ovarian cycling, and surgery, which may be limited to local resection or ablation. In such cases, infertile patients often regain their fertility. Total hysterectomy may be recommended for severe cases. Prognosis is good.

Endometrium also may be found deep in the wall of the uterus. This condition, called **adenomyosis**, represents an extension of endometrium (both glands and stroma) deep into the myometrium, as is illustrated in Figure 17.23. Small foci of adenomyosis occur in 20% of uteri. It may account for modest enlargement of the body of the uterus. It is usually a curiosity encountered as a pathologic diagnosis in a uterus removed for other reasons. Nevertheless, it is sometimes blamed for dysmenorrhea and abnormal uterine bleeding. It is difficult to diagnose without hysterectomy.

Endometrial Polyps and Hyperplasia Are Benign

Adenomas of the endometrial epithelium are not known. There are, however, other benign growths of the endometrium. Most common is the benign **endometrial polyp**, a neoplasm of endometrial stroma (supporting, nonglandular cells). These have abundant stroma and are populated with benign cystic glands. Endometrial polyps are not premalignant, they may occur at any age, but they are most common near menopause. They make themselves known by causing abnormal uterine bleeding.

Endometrial hyperplasia (Fig. 17.24) is an overgrowth of endometrial glandular epithelium that can proceed to endometrial adenocarcinoma. Hyperplasia and carcinoma are more common in women with conditions that tend to result in high levels of blood estrogen. Causes of excessive estrogen production include the following:

- *Obesity*: The most significant risk factor is estrogen synthesized in fat cells. Women who are 50 lb overweight have 10 times the risk of women who are not overweight.
- *Estrogen replacement therapy* in postmenopausal women.
- Anovulatory cycles, which are associated with a prolonged estrogen effect.
- *Estrogen-secreting tumors* of the ovary. These are rare.

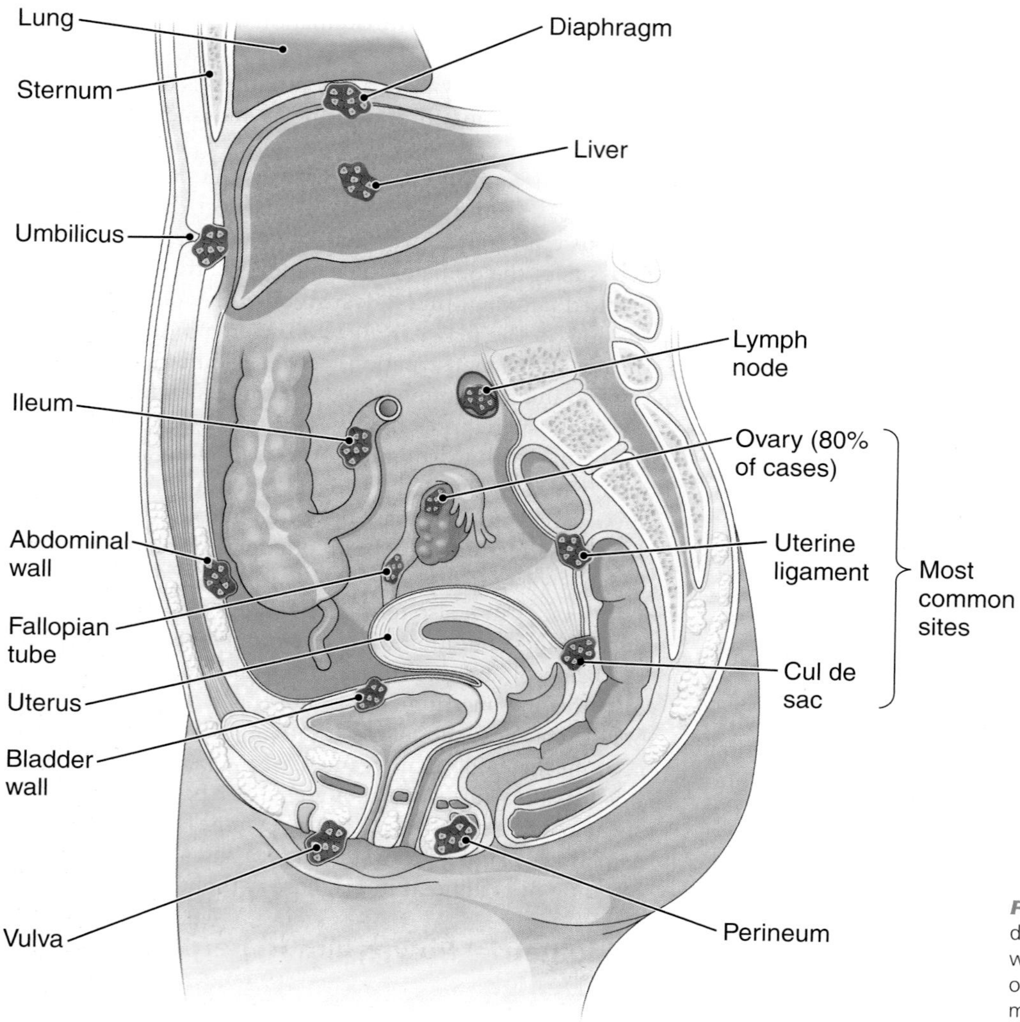

Figure 17.22 **Endometriosis.** The drawing shows some of the sites where endometrial deposits can occur. Red text highlights the three most common sites: ovary, uterine ligaments, and cul de sac.

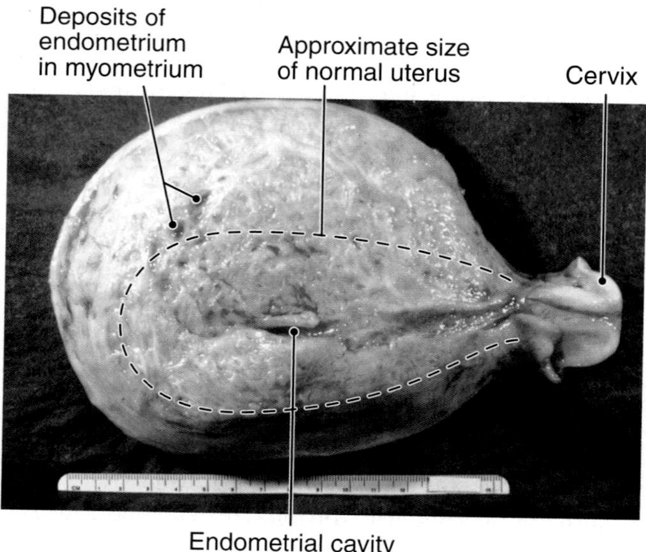

Figure 17.23 **Adenomyosis.** The enlargement of this uterus is caused by endometrial implants in the myometrium. Dotted lines indicate the normal size of the uterus.

Diabetes and hypertension are additional risk factors for endometrial hyperplasia that are unrelated to estrogen effects.

There are two types of hyperplasia. A minority of each may show some nuclear atypia:

- **Simple hyperplasia** (cystic hyperplasia). The glands are simple tubes that are often cystically dilated. The majority of cases show no nuclear atypism. If no atypism is present, the 10-year risk of endometrial carcinoma is about 1%. If nuclear atypism is present, the risk is about 8%.
- **Complex hyperplasia**. The glands are tightly packed and tortuous, and epithelium is abundant. Cases can be categorized as *complex hyperplasia without atypia* or *complex atypical hyperplasia*. If no atypical features are present, the 10-year risk for endometrial carcinoma is 3%. If atypical features are present (e.g., atypical enlarged hyperchromatic nuclei), the risk for endometrial carcinoma is high. Indeed, it is sometimes difficult to distinguish between atypical complex hyperplasia

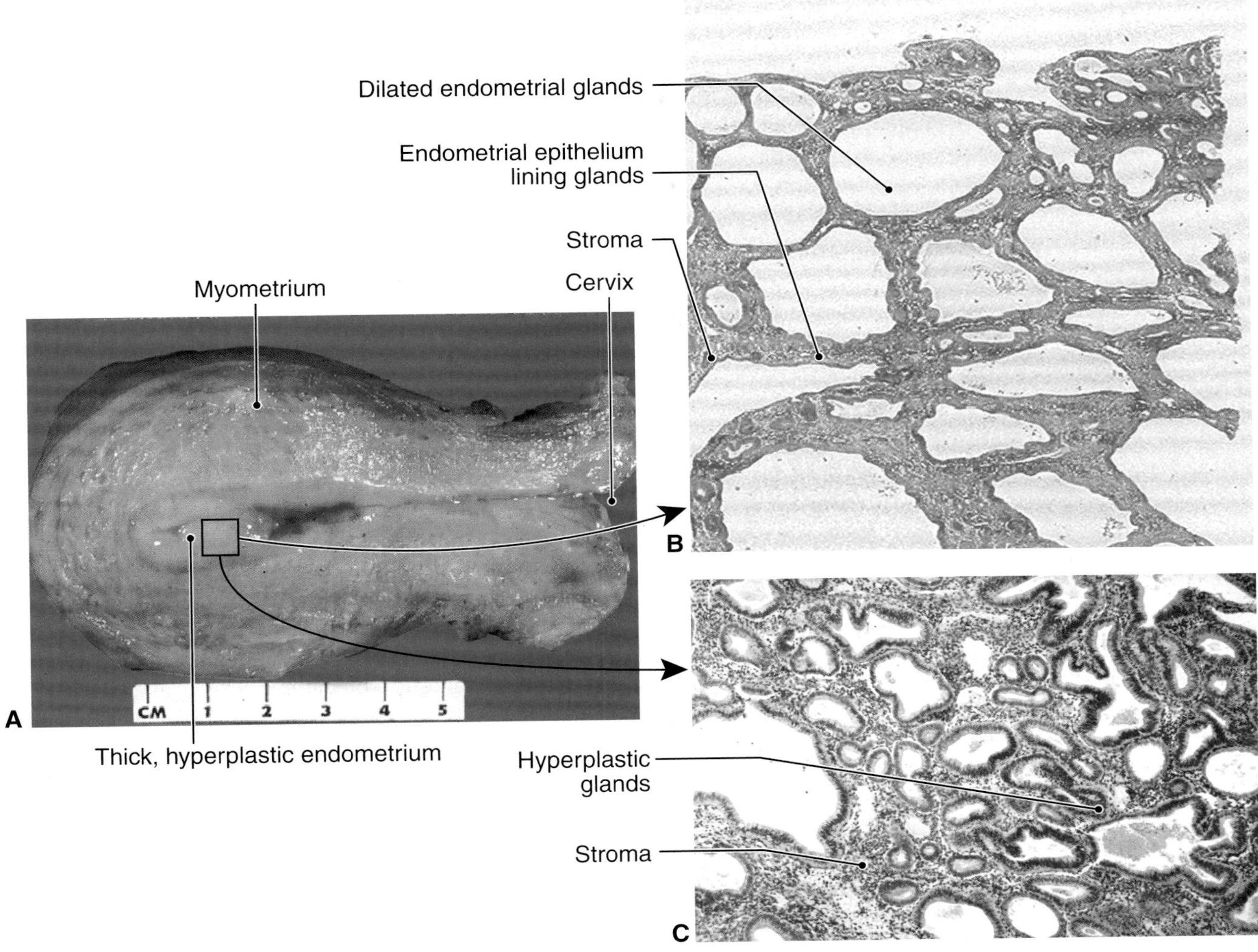

Figure 17.24 **Endometrial hyperplasia. A.** Thickened endometrium. Callouts **B.** and **C.** show two types of hyperplasia that could account for the thickened endometrium. **B.** Simple, cystic hyperplasia. Glands are dilated and the endometrial epithelium is not hyperplastic. **C.** Complex hyperplasia; no nuclear atypic is present. (**C.** Reproduced with permission from Rubin E, Farber JL. *Pathology*. 3rd ed. Philadelphia (PA): Lippincott Williams & Wilkins; 1999.)

and carcinoma, especially on small biopsy or curettage specimens. Because of the diagnostic uncertainties involved, it is difficult to know the risk for progression to frank malignancy.

Diagnosis is by endometrial curettage. For women whose hyperplasia shows no atypia, progestin therapy or oral contraceptives induce regression in virtually everyone in a few months. For women with complex atypical hyperplasia, hysterectomy is recommended. Nevertheless, in young women who want to remain able to bear children, progesterone therapy with very close follow-up is an alternative.

Endometrial Carcinoma Is the Most Common Invasive Malignancy of the Female Reproductive Tract

Effective use of Pap smears has reduced the incidence of cervical cancer such that endometrial carcinoma (Fig. 17.25) is now the most common cancer of the female reproductive tract. In 2012, there were an estimated 47,000 new cases and 8,000 deaths in the United States. Unfortunately, no useful screening test is available for endometrial carcinoma: Pap smears are not useful because malignant endometrial cells are rarely shed in sufficient numbers to be detectable. There are two common types of endometrial carcinoma (Tab. 17.4). Each has mutations in the malignant cells that distinguish them from one another.

Endometrioid carcinoma (Type I carcinoma) accounts for about 85% of cases. They are variably differentiated (many are well-differentiated) and the glands can somewhat resemble proliferative or secretory endometrium. They often arise in settings of unopposed estrogen stimulation (i.e., without progesterone) such as obesity and anovulatory cycles. They generally grow slowly and metastasize by lymphatics.

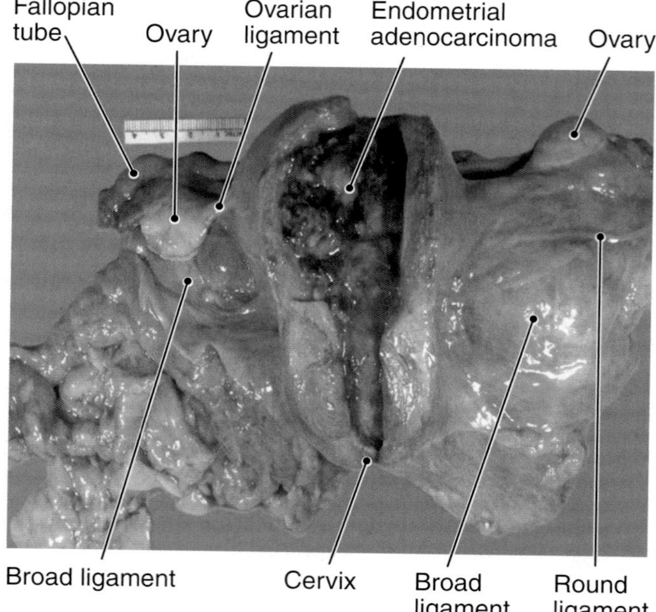

Figure 17.25 **Endometrial carcinoma.** Hysterectomy specimen. The opened uterus reveals a ragged mass of cancer filling the endometrial cavity.

Papillary serous carcinoma (Type II carcinoma) accounts for about 15% of cases. They are poorly differentiated and the glands have a papillary pattern and other microscopic features that bear no resemblance to normal endometrium. They tend to arise about a decade later than Type I and occur in a setting of endometrial atrophy: thin physique, no hypertension or diabetes, and no features associated with unopposed estrogen. They are more aggressive than Type I and tend to metastasize earlier. They spread via lymphatics and through the fallopian tube into the peritoneal cavity.

Clear cell carcinoma is a rare, high-grade carcinoma that generally occurs in older women, often in a setting of long-standing endometriosis. Other rare types of uterine carcinoma exist including squamous cell carcinoma, small cell carcinoma, and others.

Endometrial carcinoma occurs most frequently in women around 60 years old. Usually first among clinical signs is abnormal vaginal bleeding. Vaginal bleeding in a postmenopausal woman must always be thoroughly investigated because about 20% will prove to have a malignancy. There are few other clinical signs of endometrial cancer—the uterus may be slightly enlarged, but this is scarcely a reliable sign of cancer when so many other more common conditions could be responsible.

The only effective screening technique for endometrial cancer is an annual pelvic examination to search for uterine enlargement, pelvic masses, or induration. Endometrial biopsy is a reliable diagnostic tool, but it is invasive and expensive.

Treatment is a combination of radical hysterectomy, radiation, and chemotherapy depending on tumor stage. Very low-grade endometrioid carcinoma may be treated by endometrial curettage only. Clinical stages and approximate five-year survival percentages are illustrated in Figure 17.26.

Table 17.4 ***Endometrial Carcinoma***

Clinical Features	Endometrioid (85% of cases)	Papillary Serous (15% of cases)
Age	~60	~70
Clinical setting	Obesity Hypertension Diabetes Unopposed estrogen/endometrial hyperplasia	Thin physique Normotensive No diabetes Relatively low estrogen/endometrial atrophy
Microscopic appearance	Well differentiated. Malignant glands somewhat resemble normal endometrium	Poorly differentiated. Malignant glands have papillary epithelial growth pattern
Precursor	Endometrial hyperplasia	Atrophic endometrium with development of CIS
Behavior	Indolent. Spreads by lymphatics	Aggressive. Lymphatic and intraperitoneal spread
Prognosis	Good	Poor

Smooth Muscle Tumors of the Myometrium Are Common

Leiomyomas (commonly called *fibroids*) are benign tumors of smooth muscle. They do not become malignant. They may occur anywhere in the body, but in women they are particularly common in the myometrium. They occur in one-third to one-half of all women. Genetic influence is important—they are much more common in African American women than in others. They grow larger under the influence of estrogen and oral contraceptives and shrink after menopause. They are often detected at routine pelvic exam but may become symptomatic initially by causing abnormal uterine bleeding, pain, or a sensation of pelvic heaviness. Multiple tumors are often present (Fig. 17.27) and may occur in such numbers and grow to such size that they cause abnormal uterine bleeding or infertility by distorting the endometrial cavity. Large ones can interfere with pregnancy and delivery.

Diagnosis is by pelvic examination and ultrasonography. Treatment depends on the patient's desire for fertility and may include oral contraceptives, additional hormone therapy to shrink fibroids, or hysterectomy, myomectomy, or transendometrial ablation.

Leiomyosarcoma is a rare, malignant smooth muscle tumor that can arise from smooth muscle anywhere in

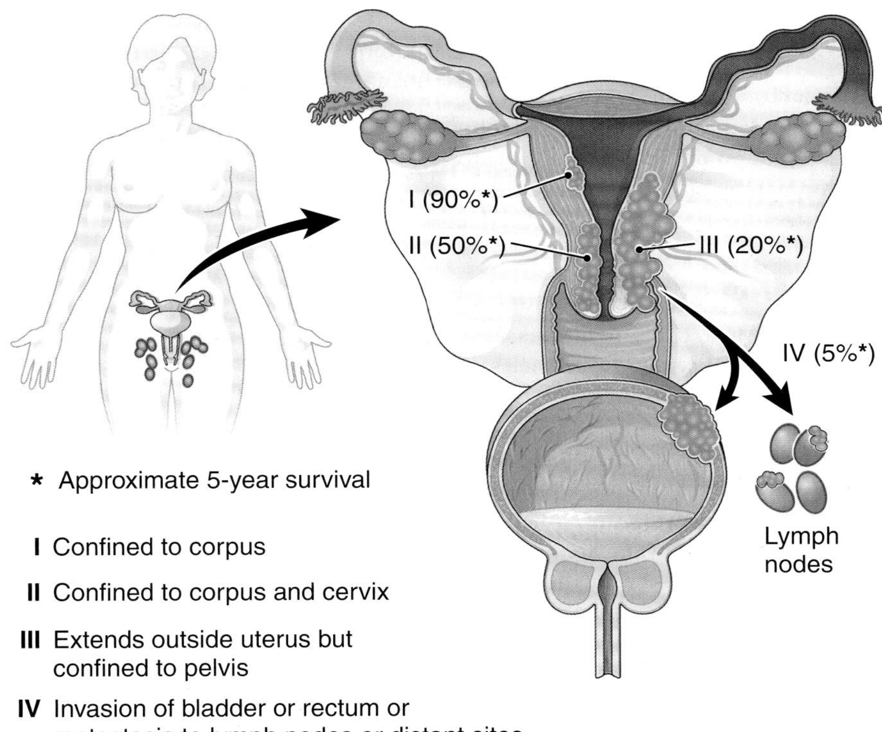

Figure 17.26 **Staging of endometrial carcinoma.** Approximate five-year survival percentage is (%) shown for various stages.

the body. In the uterus, it arises directly from uterine smooth muscle cells, not from a preexisting leiomyoma. Leiomyosarcoma is usually quite large and advanced when discovered, and it is usually fatal. It tends to recur after removal, to spread within the abdominal cavity, and to metastasize through blood to bone, lungs, and other distant sites.

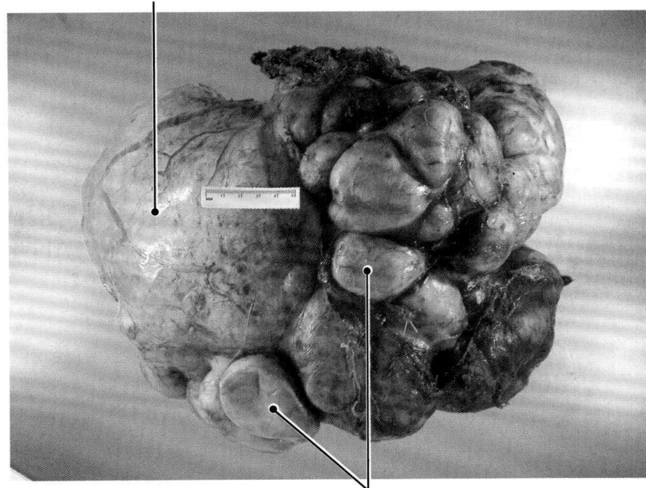

Figure 17.27 **Multiple leiomyomas of the uterus.**

Pop Quiz

17.20 True or false? Endometriosis is the extension of endometrium deep into the myometrtium.

17.21 True or false? Primary amenorrhea is defined as failure of girls to begin menstruation by age 14 if they have not gone through puberty or by 16 two years after puberty.

17.22 True or false? Leiomyosarcoma arises directly from a preexisting leiomyoma.

17.23 True or false? Type II (endometrioid carcinoma) arises in settings favoring endometrial hyperplasia.

17.24 What two bacteria are the usual culprits of acute endometritis?

17.25 Put the following in order of likelihood to progression of endometrial carcinoma: (1) Complex hyperplasia with atypia, (2) simple hyperplasia with atypia, (3) simple hyperplasia without atypia, (4) complex hyperplasia without atypia.

Disorders of the Ovary

The most common abnormalities of the ovary are nonneoplastic cysts and benign neoplasms, most of which also tend to be cystic. Inflammation of the ovary is almost always secondary to inflammation of the fallopian tube caused by sexually transmitted disease.

Most Ovarian Cysts Are Not Neoplastic

Ovarian masses are common. Most ovarian masses are cysts, and most cysts are nonneoplastic. Nevertheless, because some cysts are malignant neoplasms, all must be investigated.

The most common nonneoplastic cysts are *follicle* and *luteal* cysts, which are so common they might as well be considered normal variants. **Follicle cysts** are enlarged, unruptured Graafian follicles. **Luteal cysts** are formed of Graafian follicles that rupture and reseal in the luteal phase and accumulate fluid to become cystic. They are smooth walled and filled with thin, clear (serous) fluid. They are small, usually less than a centimeter, but may grow to 4–5 cm, and they may account for pelvic pain or a palpable mass discovered on pelvic examination. Diagnosis is by ultrasonography. Cysts <8 cm usually resolve spontaneously. Large, symptomatic, persistent cysts may require surgery.

Case Notes

17.20 What evidence in the pathology specimen provided evidence about Susan's pituitary-ovarian-menstrual cycles?

Polycystic ovary syndrome (*Stein-Leventhal syndrome*) occurs in about 5% of women in their reproductive years and features obesity, anovulatory cycles (with menstrual irregularities or amenorrhea), and signs of androgen excess (e.g., hirsutism, acne). The ovaries usually contain multiple follicle cysts (most <1 cm) beneath a thickened rind of ovarian stroma. The syndrome is defined by clinical and hormonal abnormalities, not the presence of ovarian cysts. Blood estrogen is usually increased and may be accompanied by endometrial hyperplasia. Blood testosterone is increased. The cause is unknown. Symptoms usually begin near puberty and become worse with time. Some patients are insulin resistant and others may develop Type II diabetes.

The typical patient is an overweight, infertile young woman with oligomenorrhea, hirsutism, and infertility. Diagnosis requires presence of the clinical syndrome, increased testosterone, and ultrasonographic demonstration of multiple small ovarian cysts.

Treatment is complex and in part depends on the patient's desire to become pregnant. Progestins and oral contraceptives reduce the effect of androgen excess. Wedge resections of a portion of each ovary may help restore fertility. Diabetes management techniques such as weight reduction and the administration of oral hypoglycemic agents can reverse the hormone abnormalities and infertility associated with polycystic ovary syndrome and can improve glucose and insulin metabolism and reverse blood lipid abnormalities, too.

Most Ovarian Malignancies Are Tumors of Surface Epithelium

Malignant neoplasms of the ovary are silent, lethal neoplasms that are usually discovered only after metastasizing. Although carcinoma of the endometrium is the most common cancer of the female reproductive tract, carcinoma of the ovary causes more deaths.

The ovary contains three kinds of cells: 1) germ cells for reproduction; 2) hormone-producing stromal cells, and 3) surface epithelial cells derived from peritoneum. Each type of cell produces several distinctive neoplasms (Fig. 17.28). Although the WHO classification lists 37 types and subtypes, we will focus only on the most common, basic types.

The following are some general rules about ovarian masses and neoplasms:

- Most ovarian *masses* are benign cysts.
- About half of ovarian *neoplasms* are bilateral.
- About 90% of ovarian *malignancies* are carcinomas of the surface epithelium.

The surface epithelium of the ovary is a thin membrane of flat cells derived from peritoneum. When neoplastic, however, they are transformed into tall columnar cells that may secrete fluid. Tumors of the surface epithelium comprise about 65% of all ovarian tumors. About 5% are associated with inheritance of the BRCA gene (which is also related to breast cancer). They are usually cystic and bilateral. Many secrete markers (Chapter 5) such as hCG, alpha-fetoprotein, or CA-125, which can be detected in blood and are useful for monitoring extent of disease and treatment, but are useless as screening tests.

Remember This! About half of ovarian neoplasms are bilateral.

Ovarian neoplasms are classified according to their *ability to spread* and their *cell type*. According to their potential to spread, they are classified as follows:

- *Benign*. These usually occur in women age 20–45.
- *Borderline*. These usually occur in women somewhat older than age 20–45.
- *Malignant (carcinoma)*. These occur in older women, age 50–65.

According to cell type, they are classified as follows:

- **Serous**, which resemble the epithelium lining the fallopian tube, secrete a watery fluid, and are usually

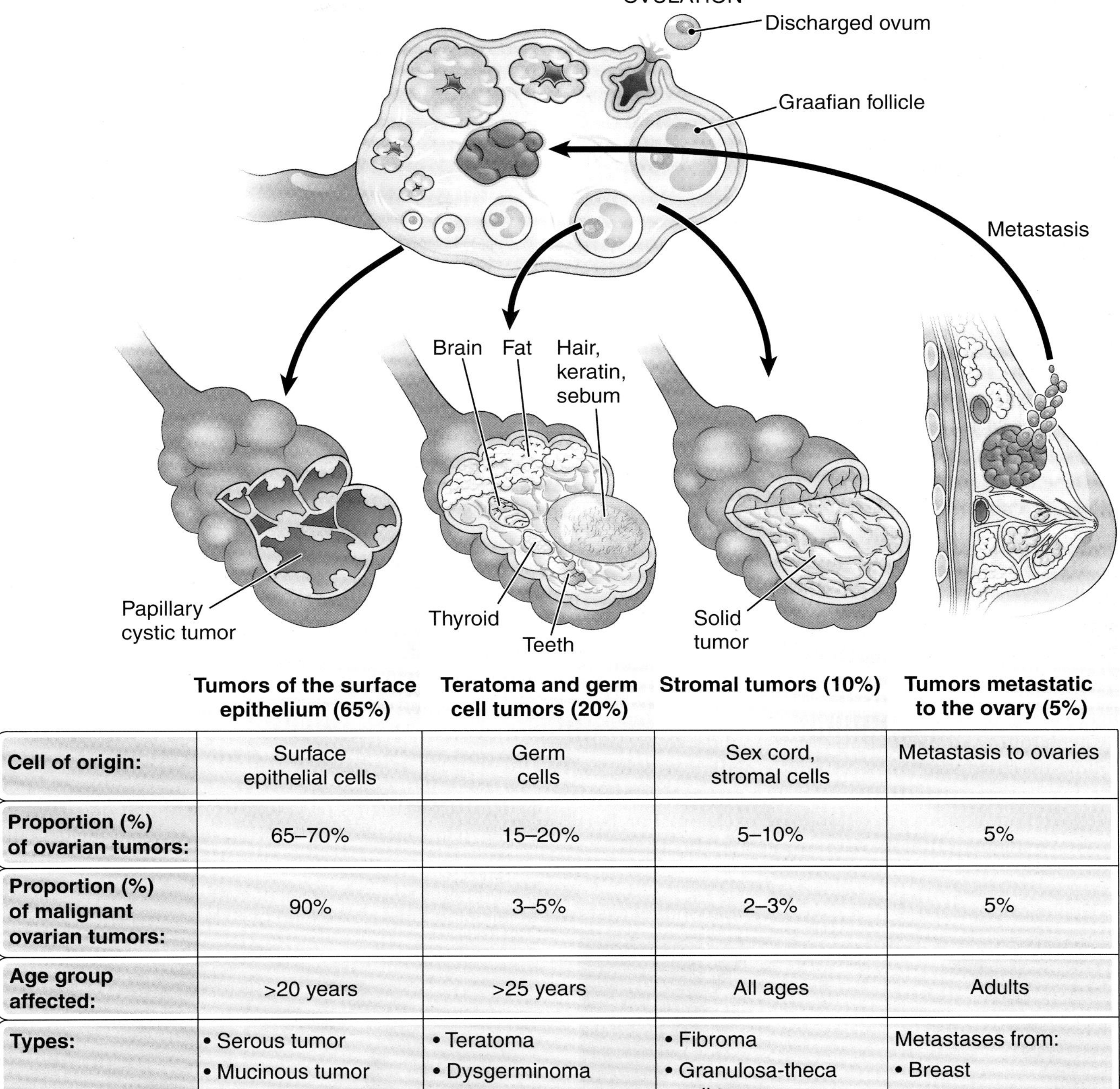

	Tumors of the surface epithelium (65%)	Teratoma and germ cell tumors (20%)	Stromal tumors (10%)	Tumors metastatic to the ovary (5%)
Cell of origin:	Surface epithelial cells	Germ cells	Sex cord, stromal cells	Metastasis to ovaries
Proportion (%) of ovarian tumors:	65–70%	15–20%	5–10%	5%
Proportion (%) of malignant ovarian tumors:	90%	3–5%	2–3%	5%
Age group affected:	>20 years	>25 years	All ages	Adults
Types:	• Serous tumor • Mucinous tumor • Endometrioid tumor • Uncommon types	• Teratoma • Dysgerminoma • Uncommon types	• Fibroma • Granulosa-theca cell tumor • Sertoli-Leydig cell tumor	Metastases from: • Breast • Lung • Colon • Other sites

Figure 17.28 **The origin and types of ovarian tumors.** The table summarizes important facts about frequency and age ranges.

cystic (Figs. 17.29 and 17.30). Two-thirds are benign or borderline. One-third are malignant and tend to be cystic and bilateral. *Malignant serous carcinomas are the most common ovarian malignancy.*

- **Endometrioid**, which resemble endometrial epithelium, tend to be solid rather than cystic. About half are bilateral. Three-fourths are malignant. They are the second most common ovarian malignancy. About 20% are accompanied by simultaneous endometrial carcinoma and/or endometriosis.
- **Mucinous**, which resemble the epithelium lining the endocervix, secrete thick mucin, are usually cystic, and have a papillary growth pattern (Fig. 17.31). They are usually not bilateral. About 15% are malignant.

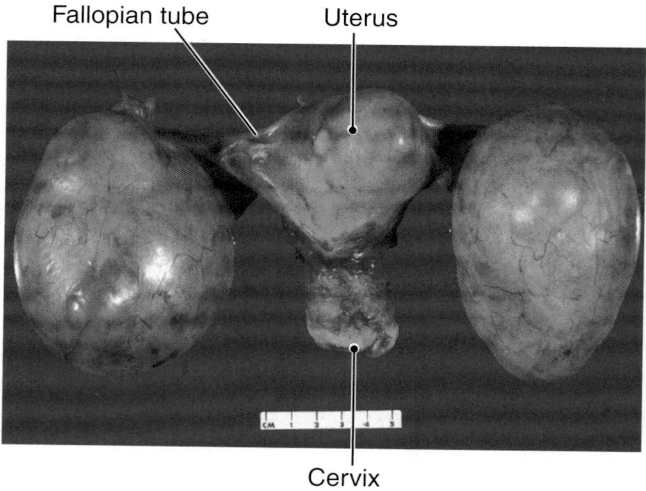

Figure 17.29 **Bilateral serous cystadenocarcinoma of the ovaries.** Ovarian tumors are often bilateral.

Depending on characteristics, they are named according to a combination of their characteristics, for example, *serous cystadenoma of borderline malignancy*.

Regardless of type, ovarian neoplasms rarely cause symptoms (pain, vaginal bleeding, or pelvic fullness) until they become large. Diagnosis is by ultrasonography, tumor markers, and biopsy at time of staging. At the time of diagnosis, more than half of malignant tumors have invaded adjacent organs or spread to the peritoneal cavity and are beyond hope of cure. Treatment is hysterectomy and bilateral salpingo-oophorectomy with follow-up chemotherapy. For frankly malignant tumors, the five-year survival is 35%; ten-year survival is about 10%. Benign tumors are curable by excision. For borderline malignant tumors with no capsular invasion, the five-year survival rate is near 100%.

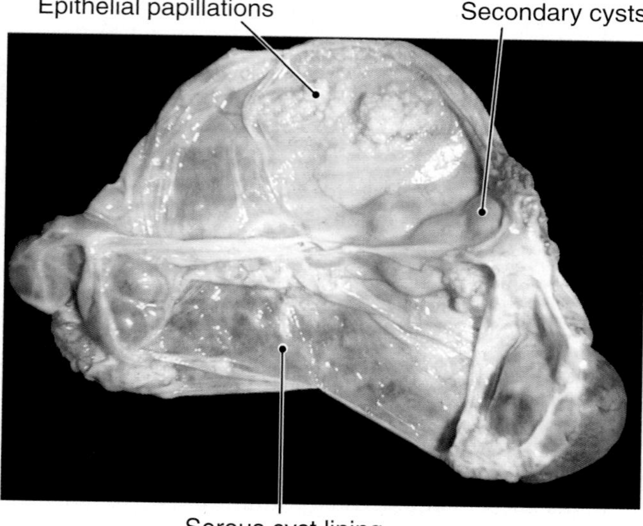

Figure 17.30 **Cystic serous tumor of the ovary, borderline malignant (collapsed cyst).** Nearly 100% of these patients survive if papillary growth does not reach the external surface.

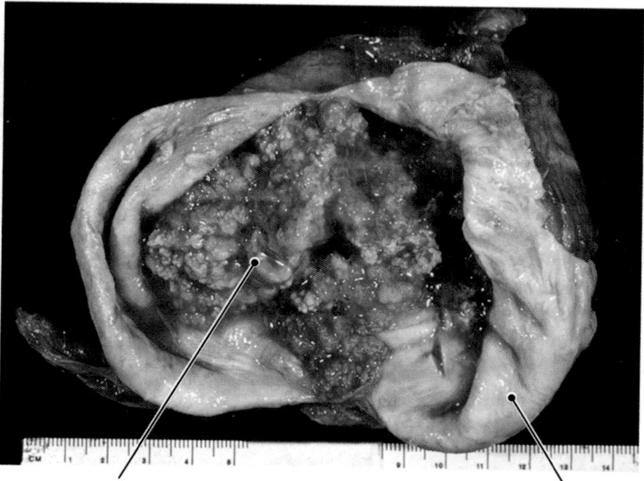

Figure 17.31 **Mucinous cystadenocarcinoma of the ovary.** Papillary epithelial growth fills the cyst cavity. Note the glistening of mucous secretions.

Teratomas Are Tumors of Germ Cells

A **teratoma** (Chapter 5) is a tumor that contains tissues not normally found in the organ from which it arises. Ovarian teratomas arise from germ cells and comprise about 20% of all ovarian neoplasms. Almost all are benign and cystic and occur in women ages 20–45. About 15% are bilateral. The most common variety contains skin and hair and are called **mature cystic teratoma** or *dermoid cyst* (skin-like cyst, Fig. 17.32). Most are unilateral and benign, arise in girls or young women, and do not grow larger than softball size. Some are discovered incidentally

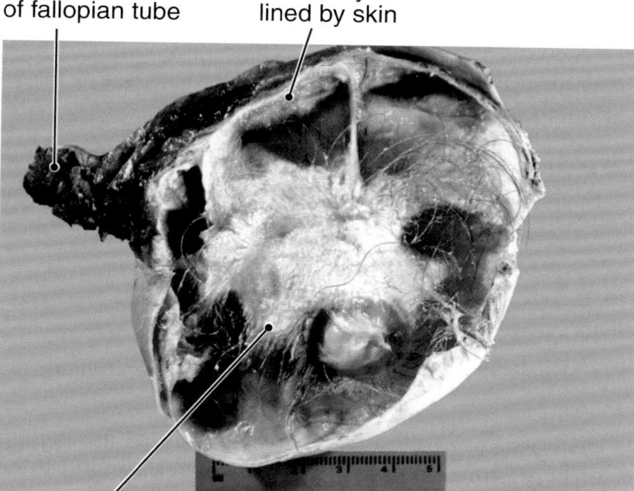

Figure 17.32 **Benign ovarian cystic teratoma (dermoid cyst).** Note hair and sebaceous material.

during pelvic exam or on radiographs that disclose odd images in the pelvis (e.g., teeth). A few may cause paraneoplastic syndrome (e.g., thyroid tissue secreting excess hormone). Malignant teratomas are rare and composed of poorly differentiated embryonal cells.

Pathologically, dermoid cysts are lined by skin and filled with pasty sebaceous material and matted long hair. Because of the totipotent nature of germ cells, literally any type of tissue can be found—teeth, bone, cartilage, brain, retina, thyroid, and/or stomach. If predominantly thyroid, it has a special name, *struma ovarii*. Some secrete hCG, which may cause a false-positive test for pregnancy.

Diagnosis is by ultrasonography and radiography, which may demonstrate teeth or bone. Treatment is surgical.

Among other germ cell tumors are *dysgerminoma*, the ovarian counterpart to testicular seminoma, and *choriocarcinoma*, a malignant tumor identical to the placental tumor of the same name.

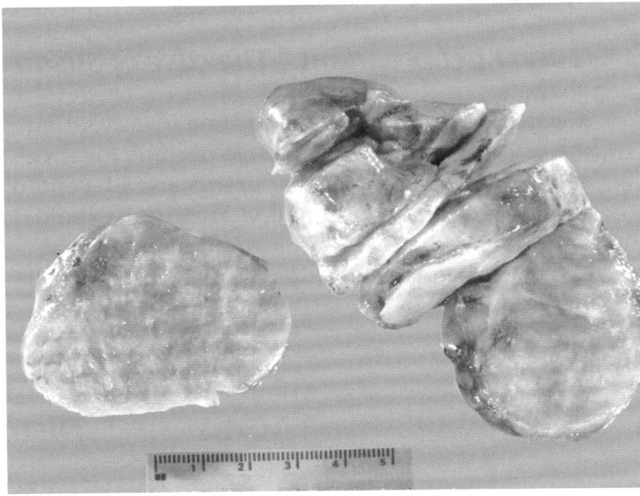

Figure 17.33 **Ovarian fibroma.** A fibroma is a solid, white tumor of ovarian stroma.

Ovarian Stromal Tumors Are Uncommon

Ovarian stromal cell tumors comprise about 10% of ovarian tumors. Most are ovarian **fibromas** (Fig. 17.33) and are composed of fibrocyte-like, spindle cells; they are solid, white, unilateral, and benign. Some are composed of plump thecal cells that secrete estrogen or androgen and are called *thecomas*. **Granulosa cell tumor** is a tumor of granulosa cells. The origin of granulosa cells is unclear, but, because of their appearance and behavior, they are categorized as stromal tumors. They are usually unilateral. Some have a significant component of thecal cells and are called *granulosa-theca* tumors. They are yellow and solid, and most secrete estrogen and are accompanied by endometrial hyperplasia. Most are benign but they may recur after excision or be frankly malignant. Diagnosis of stromal tumors is by imaging and blood hormone assay. Treatment is surgical.

Tumor metastatic to the ovarian stroma from cancer in another organ comprises about 5% of ovarian tumors. The ovary is more often the site of metastasis than its size and vascular supply would imply, suggesting that the hormonal environment is especially conducive to implantation of malignant cells circulating in blood. Of tumors large enough to be discovered clinically and mimic primary ovarian tumor, the most common site of origin is colon cancer. Other common origins are breast, lung, and stomach. Metastatic stomach carcinoma often has a distinctive microscopic appearance and is called a *Krukenberg tumor*.

Pop Quiz

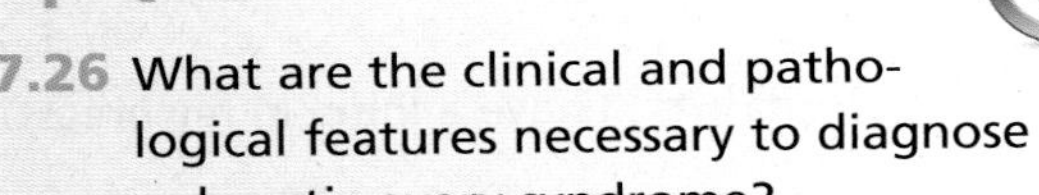

17.26 What are the clinical and pathological features necessary to diagnose polycystic ovary syndrome?

17.27 True or false? Metastatic stomach carcinoma is called a *Krukenberg tumor*.

17.28 True or false? Follicle cysts are formed of Graafian follicles that rupture and reseal in the luteal phase and accumulate fluid to become cystic.

17.29 Most ovarian malignancies are tumors of the surface epithelium.

Case Study Revisited

"I can't get pregnant." The case of Susan A.

Susan's case is an object lesson about the value of safe sex practices and of preventive medicine. Her sexual habits were virtually certain to result in her obtaining a sexually transmitted disease. She actually contracted at least two: PID and HPV infection, each of which had serious consequences. She was both fortunate and unfortunate. She was fortunate that her cervical cancer was found while

(continued)

"I can't get pregnant." The case of Susan A. (continued)

it was still in situ, before it became invasive. Had she waited longer, it could have become invasive and at the least claimed her uterus and prevented any hope of an IVF pregnancy; at worst, it could have claimed her life. She was unfortunate that early and frequent unprotected sex with multiple partners produced sexually transmitted PID and HPV infection. The former developed into the chronic tuboovarian abscesses that rendered her infertile, and the latter produced cervical dysplasia/CIS, which ultimately led to hysterectomy but not before a successful IVF pregnancy.

Section 2: *Disorders of the Breast*

I think it's about time we voted for senators with breasts. After all, we've been voting for boobs long enough.

CLAIRE SARGENT (B. 1934), 1992 CANDIDATE FOR THE UNITED STATES SENATE (ARIZONA)

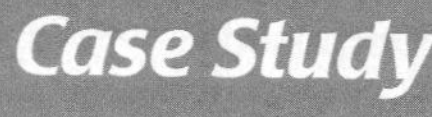

"I have a lump in my breast." The case of Anne H.

Chief Complaint: "I have a lump in my breast."

Clinical History: Anne H. was a 38-year-old pediatrician who came to her gynecologist's office because of a lump in her breast. "I have a lump in my breast," she said, pointing to her left breast with a trembling finger. "I'm really worried because it seems so big—it's like it appeared out of nowhere. I do regular breast self-examination. I've never felt a thing until I was showering yesterday."

The gynecologist knew Anne as a regular patient. She was in apparent excellent health. She was trim and fit, ate right, did not smoke, drank only socially, and otherwise did everything good health practices required. She had one child, a five-year-old son. Her parents and two sisters were living and in good health. All of her grandparents were deceased, none from cancer. There was no family history of breast cancer. She used oral contraceptives.

Physical Examination and Other Data: The gynecologist found a mobile, nontender mass about 2 cm in diameter in the upper outer quadrant. Careful palpation of the right breast was normal, and there were no palpable axillary lymph nodes on either side. "Don't worry," the gynecologist said, "it's probably benign."

Clinical Course: A mammogram showed a 2 cm mass suspicious for carcinoma. Anne was referred to a breast surgeon for needle biopsy, which revealed "poorly differentiated invasive carcinoma, no special type." A lumpectomy with sentinel lymph node (SLN) biopsy was performed the next week.

The tumor was 2.2 cm in maximum dimension. A 1 cm margin of normal tissue was present around the tumor. A mild degree of nonproliferative fibrocystic change (FCC) was present. The original pathologic diagnosis was confirmed. Tumor cells were negative for estrogen and progesterone receptors and positive for HER2/neu protein. In the SLN specimen, two of three lymph nodes contained metastatic tumor. Bone scan and chest X-ray revealed no evidence of distant metastasis. Blood calcium and liver enzymes were also normal. Anne was tested for BRCA1 and BRCA2 genes. Both were negative.

Anne was treated with radiation, chemotherapy, and anti-HER2/neu monoclonal antibody. She returned to her medical practice within three months. Quarterly checkups were unremarkable until year three when increased blood alkaline phosphatase was found. A bone scan revealed osteolytic metastases in her spine and skull. She died in a coma from liver and brain metastases five years to the day from discovery of the tumor.

The Normal Breast

The breast (Fig. 17.34) is a modified sweat gland composed of *ducts* and *glands* organized into branching networks. The breast contains several networks of ducts and glands, each somewhat similar to the stems and grapes in a bunch of grapes. These ductal networks gather into large **lactiferous ducts** at the nipple.

Two types of cells line ducts. Innermost are **luminal epithelial cells**, which overlay **myoepithelial cells** that rest directly on the basement membrane. Luminal cells in the lobules produce milk. Myoepithelial cells contract during lactation to move milk to the nipple.

Breast stroma is a mixture of fibrous tissue and fat.

Terminal ducts in the prepubertal breast terminate in undeveloped, primitive lobules. Lobules develop with the onset of puberty and cycle with each menstrual period. After ovulation, rising progesterone stimulates lobular growth and breast stroma becomes edematous. With menstruation, lobules involute and edema subsides.

The breast has a rich lymphatic network, most of which drains upward and outward to the axilla; lymphatics from the medial aspect of the breasts (between the nipples) drain into lymph nodes inside the chest on either side of the sternum (the internal mammary nodes).

With pregnancy, lobules continue to enlarge and become more numerous. After delivery, lobular luminal epithelial cells produce secretions (**lactation**). For the first 10 days, the secretion is **colostrum**, which is high in protein and maternal antibodies that the infant can absorb and deploy until its immune system becomes fully active. As progesterone levels fall after delivery, these secretions become **milk**, which is higher in fat and calories. Breast milk provides

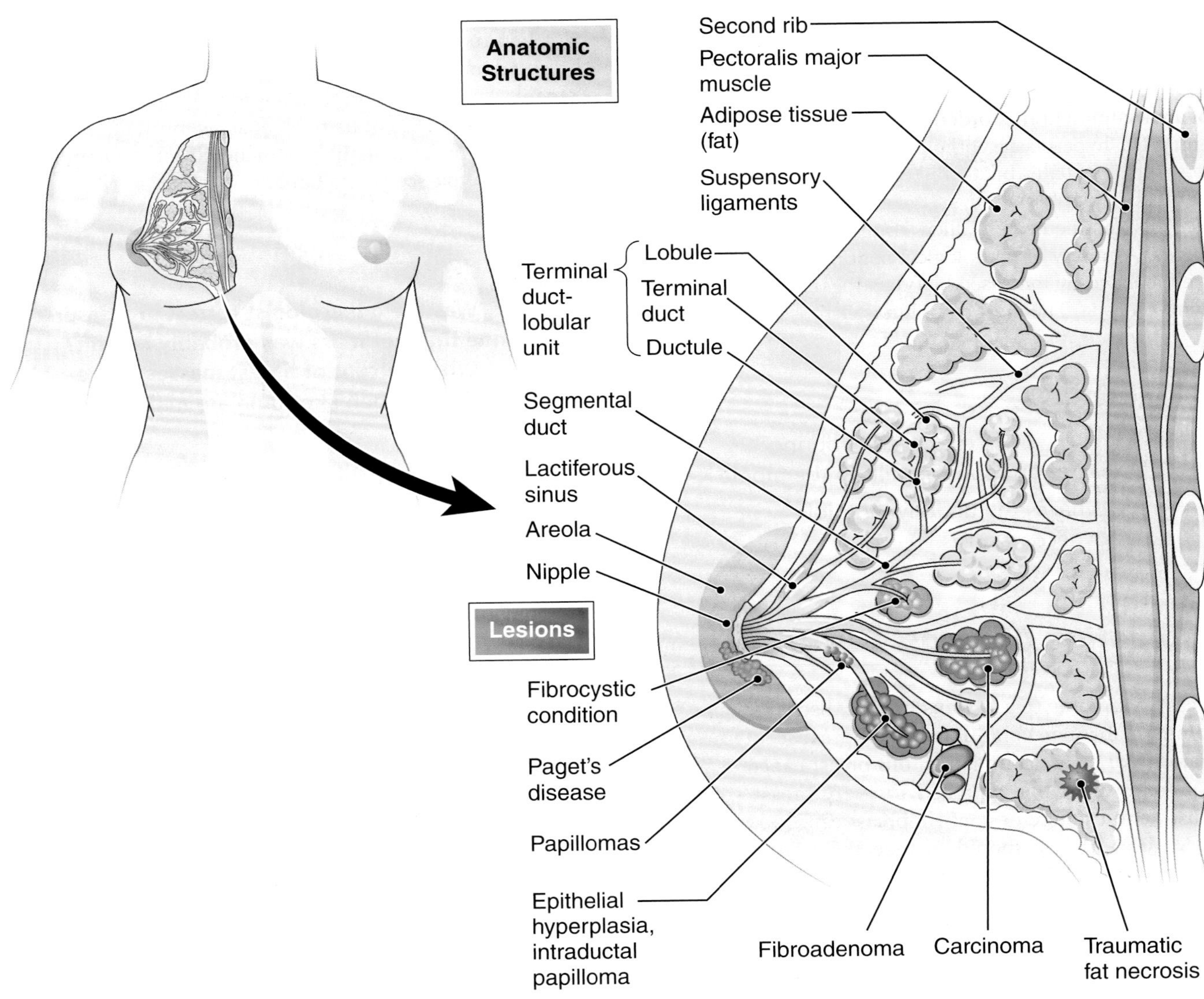

Figure 17.34 **Normal breast anatomy and sites of disease.**

complete nutrition sufficient to sustain a child's growth for several years. It also provides maternal IgA (Chapter 3) for protection against infection and allergy, and is rich in vitamins and minerals, enzymes, antioxidants, and other mediators that supplement the child's developing immune system. When lactation ends, the lobules atrophy and breast size diminishes, but not to prepregnancy size because the number of lobules is increased. By about age 30, lobules and fibrous stroma begin a slow, long involution and in postmenopausal women are gradually replaced by fat.

The sensitivity of the breast to estrogen and progesterone explains the fact that almost all breast disease occurs in women, that different diseases predominate at different phases of a woman's life as hormonal influence accumulates or changes, and that carcinoma is 100 times more common in women than men. Breast cancers in males usually occur later in life than in women. In most respects, they resemble and behave like tumors in women and are treated similarly.

Men also develop a breast disorder called **gynecomastia,** a term which literally means "female breast." It is an enlargement of the male breast resulting from an increased amount of breast-gland tissue. It presents as a small disc of firm tissue beneath the areola. Microscopically, it consists of an accumulation of orderly breast stroma and ducts with epithelial hyperplasia without atypia. It is not precancerous and is usually bilateral. It may occur physiologically in infants or pubertal boys. It can also be caused by a very long list of medicines, illicit drugs, and dietary supplements. A variety of pathological conditions, most of which are mediated by increased blood estrogen, can also prompt gynecomastia. The most common is cirrhosis (Chapter 12).

Pop Quiz

17.30 _________ cells contract during lactation to move milk to the nipple.

17.31 What is the underlying etiology of gynecomastia?

Evaluation of Breast Disorders

Breast symptoms (e.g., lumps, nipple discharge, pain) are common. Benign conditions are the cause of the great majority of breast complaints, but breast cancer is always a possibility, so the approach to every breast complaint must be to exclude or confirm breast cancer.

Medical history should include the relation of symptoms to menses and pregnancy, drug or hormone therapy, family history of breast cancer, and mammogram results, if any. The breasts should be inspected for symmetry, nipple inversion, discharge, dimpling, or bulging. Any mass detected should be measured, located by quadrant, and described carefully, for example, tenderness, mobility. Testing should include a diagnostic mammogram.

The most common breast complaints are pain, nipple discharge, lumpiness, and discrete mass. The most common pain is diffuse and cyclic with menses. It is not associated with a pathologic condition. Localized noncyclic pain can be due to unrecalled injury, ruptured cyst, or infection, but most often no lesion can be identified. *Almost all painful masses are benign*, but a few breast cancers are painful.

Nipple discharge is an uncommon event and never to be disregarded. It is most alarming when unilateral, spontaneous, and bloody; signs that usually indicate tumor near the nipple. **Galactorrhea** is lactation in a nonpregnant female or male. It is not associated with malignancy. It can be caused by pituitary conditions (Chapter 14) and other endocrine syndromes, oral contraceptives, certain drugs, and repeated nipple stimulation.

A certain degree of lumpiness in the breasts is normal; however, discrete masses are always pathologic. The most common causes of a discrete mass are fibrocystic condition, fibroadenoma, and carcinoma. Masses become palpable when they reach about 2 cm. Crossing the palpability threshold makes them appear to have arisen suddenly. Palpable masses are most common in premenopausal women. About 10% of palpable masses in premenopausal women are malignant. In postmenopausal women, over half of such masses are malignant.

Case Notes

17.21 Was the gynecologist correct in reassuring Anne that her mass was probably benign?

17.22 What percent of breast masses in premenopausal women like Anne are malignant?

Mammography is an especially useful tool in evaluating breast masses. Sensitivity and specificity (Chapter 1) improve with patient age as the dense breast tissue of younger women is replaced by fat in older women. At age 40, about 10% of suspicious lesions prove to be malignant. By age 50, however, the percentage jumps to 25%.

The principal mammographic signs of breast cancer are densities and calcifications. The main value of mammography is its ability to detect densities (masses) that are not palpable. Calcifications are common in breast cancers but are also caused by fat necrosis, cysts, benign tumors, and other breast diseases.

Pop Quiz

17.32 True or false? Every breast lump should be investigated as if it is cancer.

Benign Breast Conditions

Benign conditions of the breast usually are either inflammatory, epithelial proliferation, or both.

Mastitis Is Inflammation of the Breast

Acute mastitis is uncommon, and almost all cases are caused by infection in lactating women. Typically acute mastitis is bacterial and caused by staphylococcus or streptococcus that gains access through dilated breast ducts plugged with mammary secretions. Staph infection usually produces an abscess; strep infection tends to be more diffuse and produces generalized swelling, tenderness, and pain. Diagnosis is clinical. Treatment is antibiotics.

Subareolar abscess is a local inflammatory condition near the nipple that appears as a painful, inflamed mass. It often occurs in women with an inverted nipple and in most instances it is not an abscess, but an inflamed fistula filled with cellular debris that has accumulated in the wall of a lactiferous duct. Curiously, almost every patient is a smoker. Treatment is surgical excision.

Chronic breast inflammation and tenderness is usually associated with *FCC*, a very common condition.

Fat necrosis is a type of necrosis that occurs only in adipose tissue. It is associated with inflammation and is especially likely to cause local calcium deposits. The cause of fat necrosis is often unknown, but many cases can be traced to trauma. Fat necrosis heals by scarring and is often stippled with calcium, features that give it a hard, gritty character and an irregular outline that can suggest breast cancer on mammogram. It is most often found in women with large, fatty breasts, most of whom cannot recall any trauma. Diagnosis is by mammography. Treatment is supportive.

Diabetic mastopathy is an inflammatory disorder of the breast that may form a mass lesion. It occurs mainly in diabetic patients or sometimes in patients with autoimmune disorders. Breast lobules are involved by a severe chronic inflammatory reaction. Treatment is surgical excision.

Fibrocystic Change Is a Common Benign Condition

Fibrocystic change (FCC) (Fig. 17.35) is a common breast condition that accounts for lumpy breasts that often require mammography to rule out a breast mass. The change is characterized by cystic dilation of terminal ducts, inflammation, and increased fibrous stroma. Cysts vary from a few mm to several cm and are filled with thin, cloudy fluid. Cysts often rupture and incite inflammation (which may be painful) and fibrosis (which adds nodularity and firmness). *Proliferative changes* of the type described below may or may not occur in conjunction with FCC but are not part of FCC. FCC is present in three-fourths of premenopausal women, but symptomatic (with lumpiness and pain) in only about 10%. It appears to be caused by the repeated changes that occur as part of the menstrual cycle. FCC usually comes to attention because

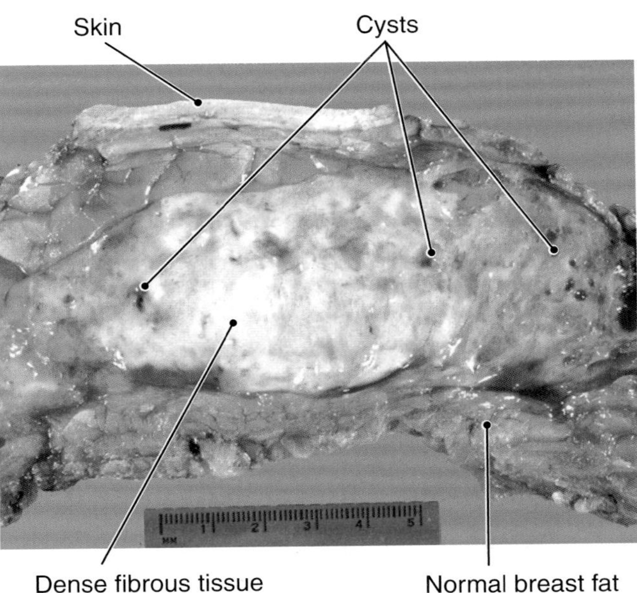

Figure 17.35 **Fibrocystic change.** This gross study shows that most of the abnormal tissue is fibrous. Cysts are small in this example.

it produces pain, tenderness, or a possible palpable mass. The presence of FCC alone *does not increase* the risk of breast cancer. Nevertheless, proliferative changes are often present, which do increase breast cancer risk. Biopsy is required for diagnosis. General treatment is supportive. Large cysts can be aspirated to reduce size and symptoms.

Proliferative Changes Increase Breast Cancer Risk

A second variety of benign change in the breast is *proliferative changes*. Unlike FCC, proliferative changes are accompanied by increased breast cancer risk, which extends to both breasts. These changes ordinarily do not produce physical or mammographic abnormalities and are typically found in conjunction with biopsy for unrelated mammographic abnormalities or as incidental findings in breast biopsies done for any reason. There are two types:

- **Proliferative change without atypia** (Fig. 17.36) is characterized by proliferation of ductal epithelium and the absence of cellular atypia. FCC may or may not be present. Changes include 1) *simple epithelial hyperplasia* featuring piled-up layers of unremarkable epithelial cells (Fig. 17.36 A); 2) intraductal *papillomas*; and 3) *sclerosing adenosis* (Fig. 17.36 B), a variety of proliferative change in which there is an increase in the number of acini in lobules, some of which may be disorganized and disrupted by fibrosis. For women with *proliferative change without atypia*, the relative breast cancer risk is about twice that of women without any risk factors and the lifetime risk is about 6%. These patients are usually followed by periodic breast exams and mammography.
- **Proliferative change with atypia** includes *atypical ductal hyperplasia* and *atypical lobular hyperplasia*.

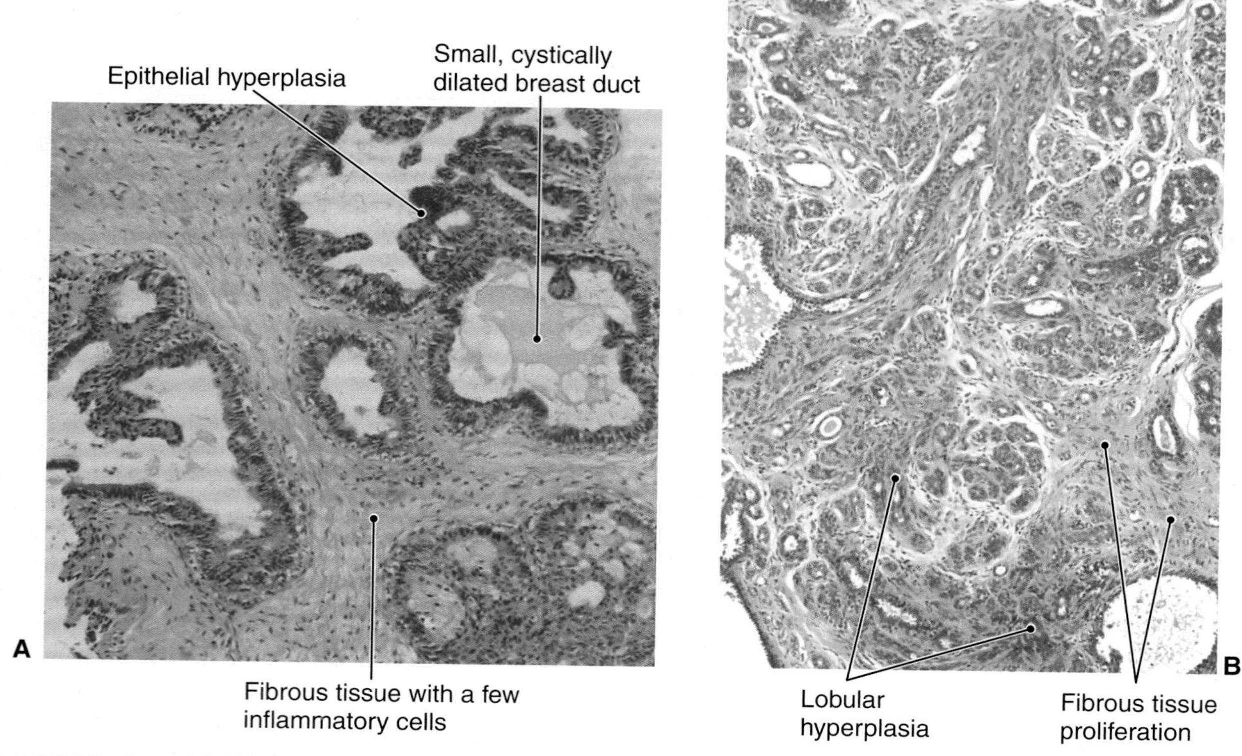

Figure 17.36 **Benign epithelial changes. A.** Proliferative change without atypia. **B.** Proliferative change with sclerosing adenosis. (**B.** Reproduced with permission from Rubin R, Strayer DS. *Rubin's Pathology: Clinicopathologic Foundations of Medicine*. 5th ed. Philadelphia (PA): Lippincott Williams & Wilkins; 2008.)

These lesions resemble ductal or lobular CIS but lack enough atypism to warrant a diagnosis of either ductal or lobular CIS. For women with proliferative change with atypia, the relative breast cancer risk is about five times greater than the risk for women without any risk factors and the lifetime risk is about 15%. Some patients with atypical epithelial changes elect to have prophylactic subcutaneous mastectomy and reconstruction. Others prefer close follow-up.

By comparison, for women with ductal or lobular CIS, the relative breast cancer risk is about 10 times greater than the risk for women without any risk factors and the lifetime risk is about 30%.

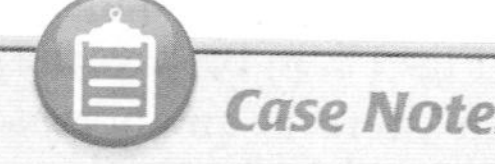

Case Notes

17.23 Was the FCC in Anne's breast related to her development of cancer?

Most Neoplasms of the Breast Are Benign

Fibroadenoma is a benign tumor of breast stroma. It is the most common tumor of the female breast, occurring most often in women in their 20s as a solitary, round mass about 1–5 cm in diameter and composed of dense fibrous tissue interspersed with compressed breast ducts. It is not premalignant, and simple surgical removal is curative. **Phyllodes tumor** is an uncommon, much larger, somewhat aggressive version of fibroadenoma. It may be sluggishly malignant; some recur locally after excision, but metastasis is rare. Rarely, they can be malignant and behave like sarcomas (malignant phyllodes tumor).

Solitary **intraductal papilloma** is a benign neoplasm that most often occurs in the large milk ducts near the nipple. It may call attention because it is palpable, bleeds, or causes a nipple discharge, or because the nipple becomes inverted (retracted). Solitary papillomas, by far the most common papilloma, are not premalignant, but multiple papillomas (**intraductal papillomatosis**) are a variety of proliferative breast disease and as such carry an increased risk for breast carcinoma.

Pop Quiz

17.33 True or false? Almost every patient diagnosed with a subareolar abscess is a smoker.

17.34 True or false? The identification of calcium deposits on a mammogram is diagnostic for carcinoma.

17.35 Is FCC associated with increased breast cancer risk?

17.36 True or false? Proliferative changes usually cause physical or mammographic abnormalities.

17.37 True or false? Intraductal papillomas carry no increased risk of breast cancer.

Breast Cancer

The phrase "breast cancer" implies carcinoma of the breast—a malignancy of the breast ducts or glands. Carcinoma of the breast is arguably the most feared of all cancers—it threatens life, appearance, self-esteem, and relationships to a degree unmatched by any other tumor. More than 95% of breast malignancies are adenocarcinomas of breast epithelium.

Apart from skin cancers (Chapter 21), most of which are innocuous, breast cancer is the most common malignancy in women. The cumulative risk by age 90 is that one in eight women will develop the disease. Breast cancer is second to lung cancer as a cause of cancer death in the United States. The Centers for Disease Control estimated that, in the United States in 2012, there were 227,000 new cases of breast cancer and 40,000 deaths.

Despite improvements in diagnosis and treatment, about 20% of women who develop breast cancer die of the disease. By comparison, 40% of women who develop colorectal cancer and 75% of women who develop lung cancer die of their disease. A comparison of these statistics is deceptive, however, because carcinoma in situ (CIS, discussed below) is routinely included in breast cancer statistics, but not in those for colorectal or lung cancer. Because CIS in any organ has a very favorable prognosis, breast cancer appears to be much less lethal. Nevertheless, if statistics for *invasive* breast cancer are compared with colorectal and lung cancer, breast cancers are nearly as lethal as colorectal, though neither is nearly as deadly as lung cancer.

All breast carcinomas arise from cells in the **terminal duct-lobular unit (TDLU)**. Before this fact was established, breast cancers were divided into two main groups, *lobular carcinoma* and *ductal carcinoma,* because of differing microscopic appearance. With the understanding that all arise from the same population of TDLU cells, however, this distinction has lost much of its meaning. Nevertheless, the terms are still used and serve to highlight some differences in tumor discovery and behavior.

Case Notes

17.24 What percent of breast cancers are like Anne's type?

17.25 From what part of the breast anatomy did Anne's tumor arise?

17.26 Which is most lethal: lung cancer, colorectal cancer, or breast cancer?

Remember This! All breast carcinomas arise from cells in the TDLU.

Multiple Factors Influence the Risk of Developing Breast Cancer

The major risk categories for development of breast cancer are hormonal (90% of cases) and genetic (10%). The hormones affecting breast cancer risk are estrogen, which promotes cancer, and progesterone, which limits the effect of estrogen.

Gender is the most important *hormone-related factor* (99% of breast cancers occur in women). Other hormone-related factors are less important. Increased estrogen exposure is associated with early onset of menses and causes longer lifetime estrogen exposure. Childlessness and first childbearing after age 30 limit the estrogen-opposing effect of progesterone, and postmenopausal estrogen replacement therapy (ERT) increases risk about 50%. Oral contraceptives have no influence on breast cancer risk, but are associated with slightly increased risk for endometrial and ovarian carcinoma. As estrogen exposure endures, risk increases with age, peaking between ages 70 and 80. Breast cancer is relatively uncommon under age 30.

A woman having cancer in one breast is 10 times more likely than average to develop a cancer in the opposite breast because the hormonal environment and other factors affect both breasts equally. Because endometrial and breast cancers share risk factors, women with endometrial carcinoma are at higher-than-average risk of developing breast cancer.

Genetic factors are important, too. Breast cancer in family members, especially first-degree relatives (mother, sister, or daughter), increases risk two- or threefold. *Molecular Medicine*, "Inheritable Breast Cancer," provides additional detail on this. Caucasian (Anglo, white) women have the greatest risk. On average, African American and Hispanic women have more aggressive tumors and develop breast cancer 15 years earlier than white women.

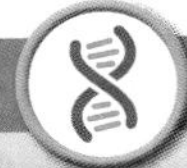

Molecular Medicine

INHERITABLE BREAST CANCER

Not every gene related to the development of breast cancer has been identified. In fact, three-quarters of women with a family history of breast cancer do not have an *identifiable* abnormal gene. **BRCA1** and **BRCA2**, however, are tumor suppressor genes that have been identified as having harmful mutations that increase breast cancer risk. BRCA mutations are present in about 1 of every 300 people in the general population. Harmful BRCA1 mutations confer an approximate 70% lifetime risk for the development of breast cancer (and 20–30% risk for ovarian cancer) and account for about 2% of breast cancers. Harmful mutations of BRCA2 occur about half as often, confer an approximate 60% lifetime risk for breast cancer (and 15% for ovarian cancer), and account for about 1% of breast cancers. Because identifiable genetic mutations cause so few breast cancers, screening is advisable only in women who have close relatives with breast cancer or a family member with a known BRCA1 or BRCA2 mutation.

Diet appears to have little effect. Heavy consumption of alcohol increases risk slightly. Obesity causes a small increase of risk. Exercise is mildly protective. Breastfeeding reduces risk.

The presence of breast epithelial hyperplasia increases risk.

Case Notes

17.27 What major and minor risk factors were in Anne's favor/disfavor?

Carcinoma in situ Has a Favorable Prognosis

About one-quarter of all breast cancers are in situ at time of diagnosis (*carcinoma in situ*, CIS). The remaining 75% are invasive. As screening techniques improve, more tumors will be discovered in the CIS stage.

The term **carcinoma in situ** has the same meaning in the breast as elsewhere: the malignant epithelium has not penetrated the basement membrane. The prognosis is good: the five-year survival is 93%. The 7% of women who die typically have undiagnosed invasive ductal cancer elsewhere or develop it soon after discovery. *CIS usually does not produce a palpable mass*; most cases are discovered by mammography or as an incidental finding in breast tissue removed for other reasons.

CIS arises in the TDLU and extends through nearby ducts, filling them with intraluminal cancer. Because CIS is a microscopic distinction, it is not possible to be certain during surgery that the entire tumor has been excised. As a result, mastectomy is a common alternative treatment instead of lumpectomy. Nevertheless, some women prefer close follow-up and regular mammography because of the relatively low rate of progression to invasion—of women with ductal CIS who get no treatment, about 30% will later develop invasive carcinoma.

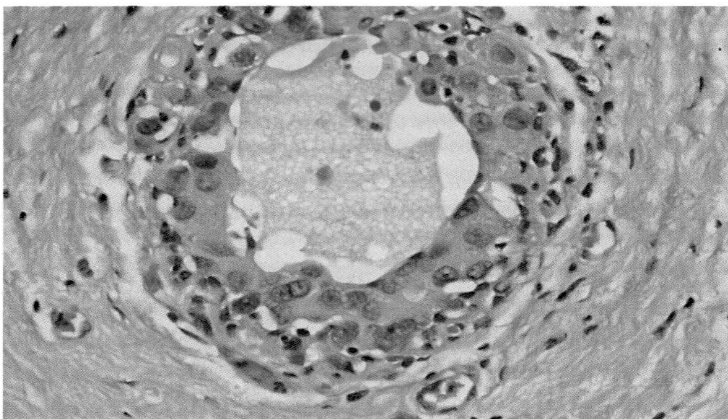

Figure 17.37 **Ductal carcinoma in situ.** The duct is partially filled with malignant cells. The surrounding stroma shows no evidence of invasion. (Reproduced with permission from Mulholland MW, Maier, RV et al. *Greenfield's Surgery Scientific Principles and Practice.* 4th ed. Philadelphia (PA): Lippincott Williams & Wilkins; 2006.)

There are two microscopic types of breast CIS: *ductal* and *lobular*. About 80% of CIS cases are **ductal CIS (DCIS)** (Fig. 17.37). Ductal CIS accounts for half of cancers found by mammography because it is associated with calcifications or nodular density. It is bilateral in 10–20% of cases. Microscopically, ducts are filled with malignant cells and no stromal invasion is detectable. Some cases may have a focus of microinvasion, but it does not alter therapy or prognosis. Surgery followed by radiation and/or chemotherapy is curative in 95% of cases. Breast reconstruction is possible. Recurrence or death is rare and attributable to invasive cancer arising in DCIS in subcutaneous tissue not removed at surgery.

The remaining 20% of CIS cases are **lobular CIS (LCIS).** Lobular CIS is not associated with mammographic calcifications or densities and is therefore always an incidental finding in breast tissue excised for other reasons, such as benign tumors or cysts. It tends to occur at an earlier age than DCIS and is more often bilateral (20–40%) than DCIS. LCIS features lobules composed of atypical cells; ducts are not involved. Therapy is the same as for DCIS.

Paget disease is a special variety of in situ carcinoma that occurs in the skin of the nipple in women who have a breast carcinoma immediately beneath the nipple. In situ tumor cells migrate into the epithelium of lactiferous ducts and then into the basal layer of skin. The nipple and nearby areola are involved by an inflamed, tender, red, cracked, oozing, crusted lesion that looks like eczema, an inflammatory skin disease (Chapter 21). The underlying tumor may be in situ or invasive.

Invasive Carcinoma Is the Most Common Form of Breast Cancer

About 75% of breast cancers have progressed to invasion by time of diagnosis. *Progression from CIS to invasion is the*

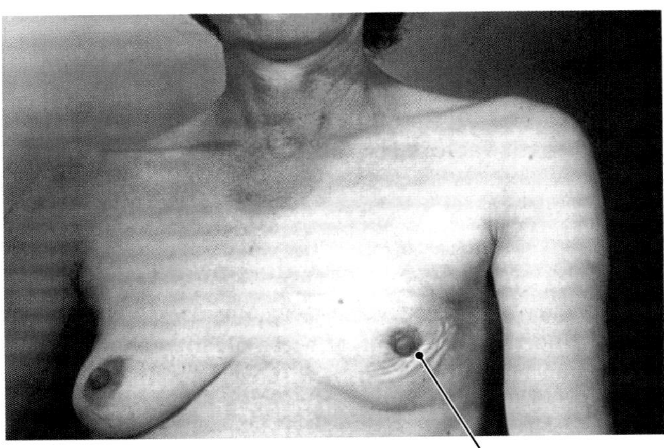

Figure 17.38 **Carcinoma of the breast.** An advanced case that has invaded the skin, causing retraction of the skin, areola, and nipple.

most important step in the development of breast cancer: the tumor gains access to lymphatics and blood vessels and can metastasize.

Some invasive carcinomas are discovered by mammography, but many are discovered as a palpable mass. *If a palpable mass is an invasive breast cancer, half of patients will have axillary lymph node metastases at the time of diagnosis.* Those discovered by mammography are about half the size of those discovered as a palpable mass; only about 20% of these will have positive axillary nodes.

Some large tumors may be fixed to skin or chest wall (Fig. 17.38). Those near the areola may cause nipple inversion. Breast lymphatics may become engorged with tumor cells, which causes thickening of the skin and lymphedema (Chapter 6). As tissue swells and strains against breast ligaments, the skin may take on an orange-peel dimpling referred to with the French phrase *peau d'orange*. Widespread lymphatic invasion may cause marked swelling and erythema of the entire breast, a condition referred to as **inflammatory carcinoma**. The prognosis for these cases is poor. Treatment is radiation and chemotherapy followed by mastectomy after the tumor shrinks.

Case Notes

17.28 **Does it make much difference that Anne's tumor was discovered by palpation rather than mammography?**

Invasive Ductal Carcinoma

There are several types of invasive carcinoma. The most common is **invasive ductal carcinoma (IDC)**, which comprises about three-quarters of all breast cancers (invasive or in situ). About 80% of *invasive* breast cancers are a single variety: **invasive ductal carcinoma, no special type (IDC-NST)** (Fig. 17.39). *Invasive lobular carcinoma* accounts for about 10% of invasive breast cancers. Other types of invasive cancer are even less common.

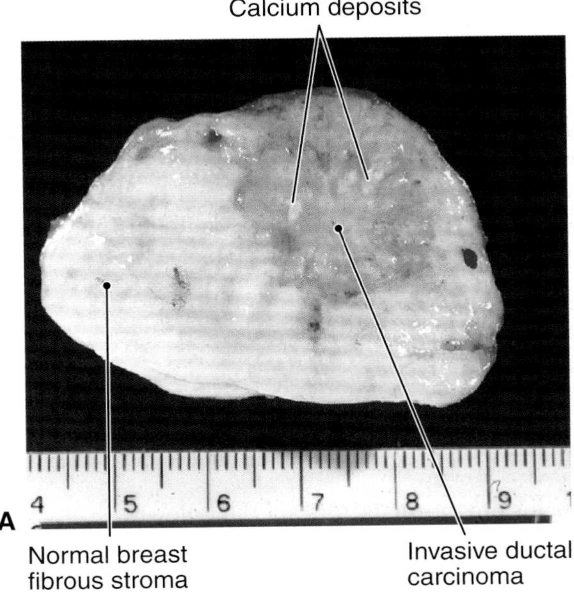

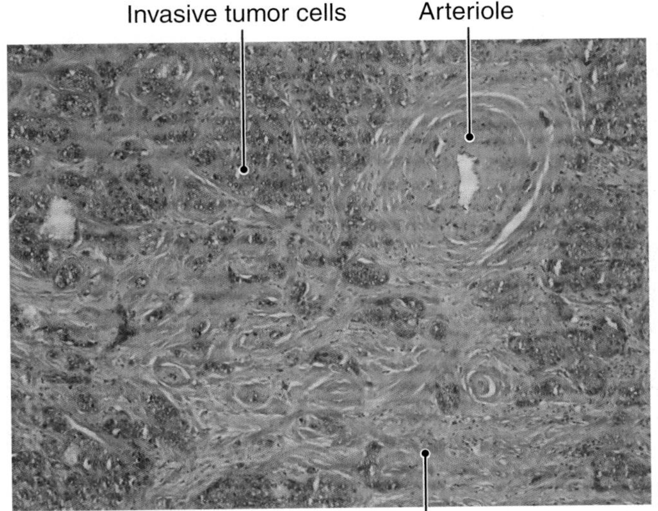

Figure 17.39 **Invasive carcinoma, no special type (NST). A.** Gross specimen. Note the irregular, stellate shape and calcium deposits. **B.** Microscopic study. Ragged cords of malignant cells embedded in dense fibrous stroma.

IDC-NST cancers stimulate growth of dense fibrous stromal tissue and calcification, which makes them gritty and hard and accounts for the density and calcium deposits seen on mammography (Fig. 17.40). They are usually poorly circumscribed and send fingers of invasive tumor into nearby tissue.

Molecular characterization of tumor DNA, RNA, and proteins has identified several subtypes of invasive carcinoma according to the presence or absence of *estrogen receptors (ER), progesterone receptors (PR), HER2/neu protein* and others, the presence or absence of which affects therapy and prognosis. The presence of ER and PR are favorable; the presence of HER2/neu is unfavorable.

Treatment and prognosis of IDC and other carcinomas are discussed below.

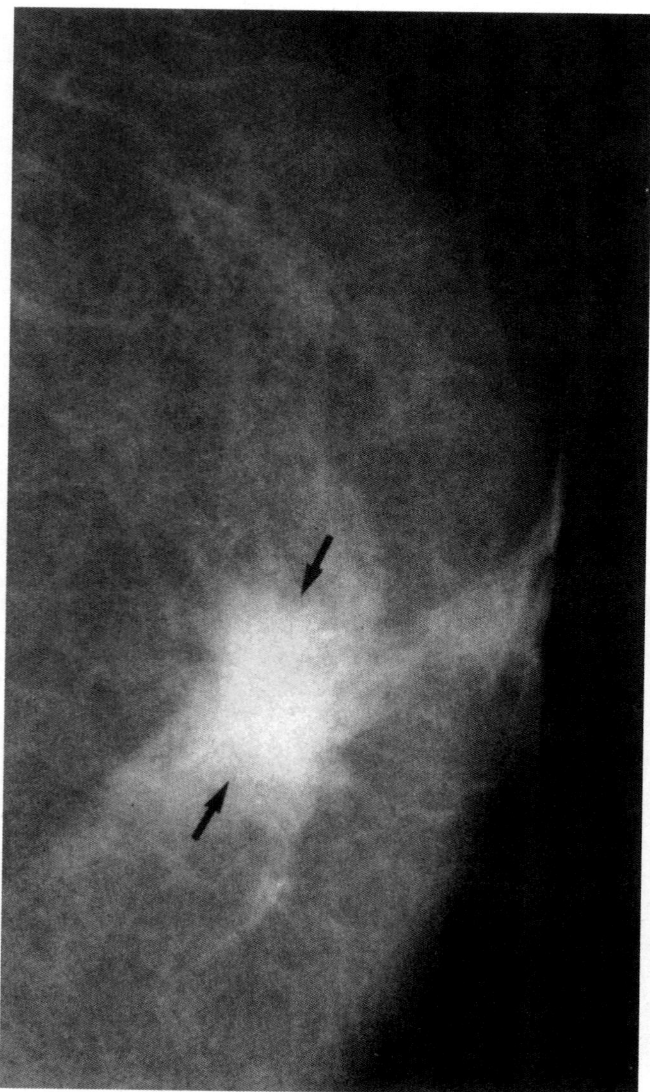

Figure 17.40 **Mammogram, invasive carcinoma, no special type (NST).** (Reproduced with permission from Rubin E, Farber JL. *Pathology*. 3rd ed. Philadelphia (PA): Lippincott Williams & Wilkins; 1999.)

Case Notes

17.29 **List the favorable and unfavorable prognostic factors for Anne's tumor.**

Other Varieties of Invasive Carcinoma

Other varieties of invasive cancer comprise about 20% of breast cancers. About half of these are **invasive lobular carcinoma (ILC).** ILC can be discovered either by mammography or as a palpable mass. It differs in some ways from IDC. ILC tends to be somewhat less dense and more difficult to palpate and to spot on a mammogram because it is less densely fibrotic than IDC and grows more diffusely. It is graded and staged similar to IDC and, if matched by grade and stage, has a similar prognosis. Nevertheless, its pattern of metastasis is different from IDC. It more often metastasizes to meninges, peritoneum, GI tract, and internal genitalia and is less likely to spread to bone and lungs.

Medullary carcinoma, mucinous (colloid) carcinoma, and *tubular carcinoma* are other subtypes of invasive carcinoma. They tend to have a somewhat better prognosis than IDC or lobular carcinoma.

Sarcomas of the breast are rare, malignant tumors of breast stroma (fibrous tissue, blood vessels, nerves, and fat) similar to malignant tumors of those tissues that occur elsewhere in the body. Most common is **angiosarcoma**, a malignant tumor of small blood vessels, which arises in a very small percent of women receiving radiation therapy for breast cancer.

Multiple Factors Affect Prognosis

The five-year survival rate for women with breast cancer varies from 100% to near 10% depending on multiple factors. The two gravest prognostic signs are clinical: women who present with distant metastasis or with inflammatory carcinoma. Very few patients in either category survive five years. With the exception of these two clinical presentations, general prognosis is determined by staging based on clinical findings and pathologic study of the primary tumor and axillary lymph nodes (Tab. 17.5).

Case Notes

17.30 **What was the stage of Anne's tumor?**

The major prognostic factors are the following:

- *Carcinoma in situ or invasive carcinoma*: This is the most important of all pathologic distinctions. The vast majority of women treated for CIS are cured. Conversely, half of all invasive cancers are metastatic at time of diagnosis.

Table 17.5 Staging of Breast Cancer*

Stage	Primary Tumor (T)	Positive Axillary Lymph Nodes (N)	Distant Metastasis (M)	5-Year Survival
0	DCIS, LCIS	None	None	93%
I	Invasive, ≤2 cm	None	None	88%
II	Invasive, >2 cm Invasive, <5 cm	None 1–3 nodes	None	74–81%
III	Invasive, >5 cm Invasive, any size Invasive, attached to skin or chest wall or inflammatory carcinoma	1–3 nodes ≥4 nodes 0–>10 nodes	None None None	41–67%
IV	Any invasive carcinoma	Any lymph node status	Present	15%

*Abridged from American Joint Committee on Cancer

Remember This! The two most important of all pathologic distinctions in breast cancer are whether the tumor is in situ or invasive and whether or not lymph node metastasis has occurred.

- *Distant metastasis* (Fig. 17.42): Cure is highly unlikely.
- *Lymph node metastasis*: In the absence of distant metastasis, this is the most important of all pathologic risk factors. Eighty percent (80%) of invasive cancers occur in the central/subareolar area or the two lateral quadrants. These invasive tumors metastasize first to axillary lymph nodes; those in the medial half spread first to internal mammary nodes (Fig. 17.42).

  If no nodes are involved, the 10-year survival rate is near 80%. It falls to near 15% if 10 or more lymph nodes are involved. Nodal metastasis occurs first in one or two **sentinel lymph nodes**. If sentinel nodes biopsy is negative, it is unlikely other nodes are involved and further axillary exploration is not necessary. Nevertheless, about 10–20% of women with negative nodes will later have spread of tumor, presumably through internal mammary nodes.
- *Tumor size*: After metastasis, this is the second most important factor for invasive cancers. For women with invasive cancers <1 cm in diameter the five-year survival rate is >90%. For tumors >2 cm, the rate is about 75%.
- *Locally advanced disease*: Invasion of skin or chest wall or inflammatory carcinoma have a very poor prognosis.

Minor prognostic factors are the following:

- *Histologic type*: The 30-year survival rate for ILC and other special types is near 60%; for IDC cancers it is near 20%.
- *The histologic grade*: Well-differentiated cancers have a better prognosis than poorly differentiated ones.
- *Estrogen (ER) and progesterone receptors (PR)*: The presence of both ER and PR indicates an 80% chance the tumor will respond to hormonal manipulation. If only one is present, the response rate is 40%. If neither is present, only 10% respond. Absence of ER or PR suggests the tumor is less likely to respond to chemotherapy.
- *HER2/neu receptor*: HER2/neu is a protein coded by the ERBB2 gene, a proto-oncogene (Chapter 5), which promotes cell growth. Overactivity (overexpression or amplification) of this gene is reflected by the amount of HER2/neu detected in the tumor. Detection of HER2/neu is prognostically unfavorable. Its main importance, however, is as a predictor of favorable response to monoclonal antibody therapy aimed at HER2/neu.

Diagnosis Is Standardized; Treatment Is Individualized

Diagnosis depends on mammography screening, physical examination, biopsy, and molecular profiling of the tumor. Mammographic detection of early breast cancer has resulted in a 25% decline in the death rate from breast cancer in the United States since 1990. Nevertheless, mammography does not replace careful breast examination by a professional: 10–20% of breast cancers detected by physical examination were missed by an earlier mammogram.

Biopsy is required for conclusive diagnosis. Radiographically guided needle biopsy is widely used and effective, but open surgical biopsy may be required if needle biopsy is inconclusive. Tissue from the initial biopsy or later surgery should be assayed for the presence or absence of molecular markers. Treatment can be delayed for a few weeks to accomplish a thorough workup for distant metastases, which at a minimum should include physical examination for enlarged lymph nodes or liver; radiographic imaging of chest, liver, bones, and brain; and blood assays for liver and bone enzymes that might indicate distant metastasis.

Treatment of breast carcinoma depends on pathologic classification, staging (Tab. 17.5), and molecular profiling. Lumpectomy, mastectomy, and axillary lymph node dissection is aimed at *local control*. Radiation and chemotherapy

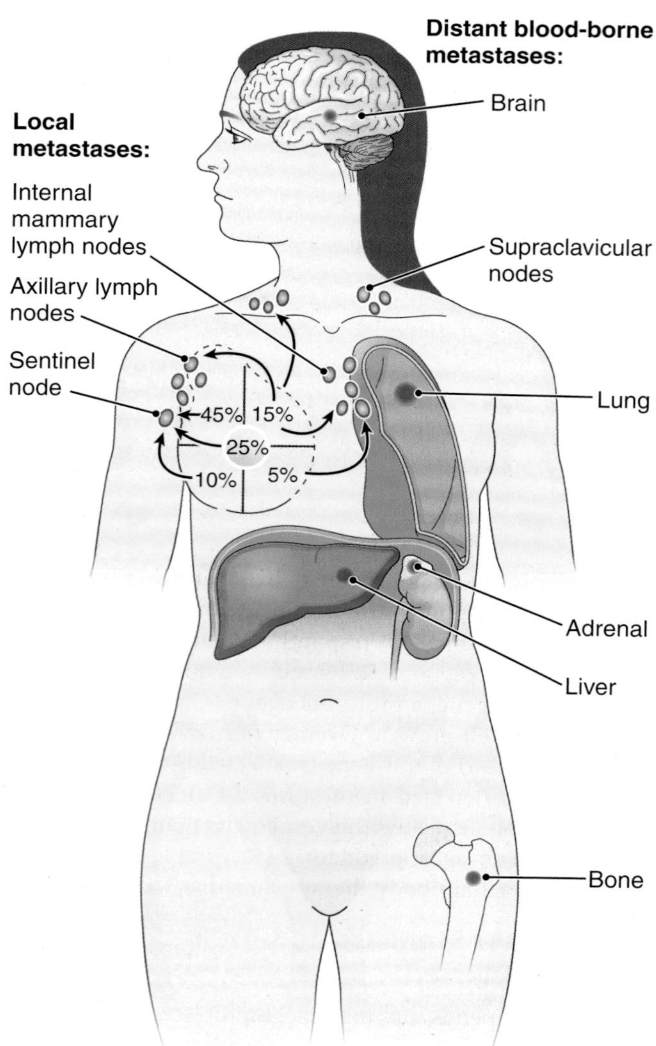

Figure 17.41 Sites of breast cancer origin and metastasis.

are aimed at *systemic control* and presuppose that the tumor has metastasized, even though proof of metastasis may be lacking. History has shown that radical or extensive surgery is no more effective at promoting survival than lumpectomy or simple mastectomy. How to treat breast cancer is a complex and evolving question. As more breast cancers (NST and others) are being discovered early by mammography and as molecular profiling and other insights accumulate, treatment is becoming sharply individualized and features aspects of both local and systemic control.

Breast cancers usually metastasize first to the nearest lymph nodes, but occasionally some spread to lymph nodes in the lower neck just above the clavicle (supraclavicular nodes) (Fig. 17.41). Ultimately, however, blood-borne metastasis may occur. The most common sites are to lung, bone, and liver, but no site is exempt. One of the most threatening and depressing features of breast cancer is that sometimes a decade or more after an apparent cure, tumor may suddenly emerge in a distant site.

Case Notes

17.31 Did Anne's lymph node metastases conform to usual tumor behavior?

17.32 Was lumpectomy the proper surgical therapy?

Pop Quiz

17.38 True or false? Breast cancer is the number one cancer killer of women.

17.39 True or false? LCIS tends to occur at an earlier age than DCIS and is more often bilateral (20–40%).

17.40 True or false? Only about 25% of women with CIS who get no treatment go on to develop invasive carcinoma.

17.41 What is the term used to refer to the edematous tissue straining against breast ligaments that takes on an orange-peel dimpling?

17.42 Invasive tumors of the upper outer quadrant of the breast spread first to the __________ lymph nodes, while those in the medial half spread first to the ____________ lymph nodes.

Case Study Revisited

"I have a lump in my breast." The Case of Anne H.

As a physician, Anne H. was far more knowledgeable than the average patient and she did everything she had learned to do: she had practiced breast self examination (BSE) and sought medical care immediately, but it was not enough to avoid a devastating outcome.

One of the important points this case makes is why BSE is now discouraged: it proved ineffective and instills a false sense of security. It has been supplanted by breast self-awareness (BSA), a program that emphasizes understanding:

1. Personal risk, (e.g., family history of breast cancer)
2. Personal breast norms, (e.g., knowing the warning signs of breast cancer)
3. Screening recommendations, (e.g., mammography)
4. Healthy lifestyle choices, (e.g., don't smoke)

By all but one major prognostic criterion, this tumor was ominous. It was invasive, NST; it was large (>2 cm) and poorly differentiated; and the sentinel lymph node biopsy was positive. The only thing in Anne's favor was no evidence of distant metastasis. Minor prognostic criteria were also unfavorable: estrogen and progesterone receptors were negative and HER2/neu was positive. The tumor's ultimate behavior—widespread metastasis in a few years—was in keeping with its initial character.

The only thing that might have made a difference is if the tumor had been discovered earlier. In retrospect, it seems probable the tumor would have been found several years earlier by routine mammography or clinical examination by a physician. Nevertheless, current recommendations call for mammography to begin at age 40 (American Cancer Society) or 50 (U.S. Preventive Services Task Force) unless there is some family history or genetic indication for beginning earlier. Anne had no risk factors favoring beginning mammography before age 40.

Within two years of Anne's death, however, her mother underwent a bilateral mastectomy with reconstruction after she was found to have ductal CIS after a suspicious mammogram. No genetic studies were done on Anne before her death, but studies of her mother, her two surviving sisters, and one aunt revealed that none of them carried a BRCA gene. Five years after Anne's death, one of her surviving sisters elected to have a bilateral prophylactic mastectomy. Lobular CIS was found in one breast. Shortly thereafter, her other sister had a prophylactic mastectomy. Ductal CIS was found in one breast.

Case Notes

17.33 **Were genetic influences important in the development of Anne's cancer?**

Chapter Challenge

CHAPTER RECALL

1. A 35-year-old African American female presents to her primary physician's office for evaluation of a female problem. She reports being very itchy and says she finds herself constantly scratching her "female area." A biopsy of the white patch found on her vulva identifies hyperplastic overgrowth of surface squamous epithelium. What treatment is advised?
   A. Topical antihistamines
   B. Topical steroids
   C. Locally injected steroids
   D. Any of the above

2. Which of the following secretes progesterone?
   A. Pituitary
   B. Corpus luteum
   C. Theca cells
   D. Granulosa cells

3. Which of the following is true of breast milk?
   A. Breast milk is lower in protein than colostrum.
   B. Breast milk is lower in fat and calories than colostrum.
   C. Breast milk contains insufficient maternal IgA for protection against infections.
   D. Breast milk must be supplemented with formula, as it is deficient in vitamins and enzymes necessary for infant development.

4. An 18-year-old Hispanic female visits the free-care clinic for evaluation of vaginal bleeding. She reports her LMP as four months ago, and states that three months ago a urine pregnancy test was positive. On examination, no fetal heartbeat is detected. You suspect a hydatiform mole. If your diagnosis is correct, when examining the uterus what do you expect to find?
   A. A uterus that is large for gestational age
   B. A uterus that is small for gestational age
   C. A uterus that is normal for gestational age
   D. Any of the above
5. Which of the following is associated with proliferative-phase endometrium?
   A. Estrogen
   B. Progesterone
   C. Corpus luteum
   D. Glycogen accumulation
6. Which of the following skin findings may be observed in a pregnant woman?
   A. Acne
   B. Spider angiomas
   C. Chloasma
   D. All of the above
7. A 45-year-old Caucasian female presents to her primary care physician complaining of an itchy red rash on her right breast. She reports that the rash initially began on the nipple three months ago before spreading to the areola and then her breast. She thought it was eczema, but is seeking care today as it began to ooze and crust two days ago. What is your diagnosis?
   A. Mastitis
   B. Paget disease
   C. Phyllodes tumor
   D. Angiosarcoma
8. Which of the following is the most dangerous cervical lesion?
   A. HPV infection
   B. CIN-I
   C. Ectropion
   D. CIS
9. A 23-year-old Caucasian woman, postpartum day 14, brings her new baby daughter in for a two-week checkup. She mentions that her left breast has become diffusely painful and swollen, and this has made breastfeeding her daughter difficult. What is the most likely diagnosis?
   A. Inflammatory carcinoma
   B. Phyllodes tumor
   C. Acute mastitis
   D. Paget disease
10. Which of the following can cause an ectopic pregnancy?
   A. PID
   B. Tuboovarian abscess
   C. Endometriosis
   D. All of the above
11. A 32-year-old African American G3/P2 female, 39w6d (gestation age: 39 weeks, 6 days), is wheeled into the ER by her husband with complaints of contractions three minutes apart. Reviewing her charts, you note that she was recently diagnosed with placenta previa. How should her baby be delivered?
   A. Natural birth
   B. Induction
   C. Caesarian section
   D. None of the above
12. Which of the following is associated with endometrial hyperplasia and carcinoma?
   A. Tuboovarian abscess
   B. Leiomyoma
   C. Obesity
   D. Multiple childbirth
13. A 22-year-old African American female is seen in her OB/GYN's office for vaginal itching. Physical exam reveals a gray, thin, fishy-smelling discharge, and a microscopic study of the discharge reveals "clue cells." Which of the following diseases is most likely to have caused her symptoms?
   A. Moniliasis
   B. Bacterial vaginosis
   C. Trichomoniasis
   D. Chlamydia
14. Which of the following therapies is a treatment for polycystic ovarian syndrome?
   A. Progestins and oral contraceptives
   B. Wedge resections of a portion of each ovary
   C. Weight reduction and the administration of oral hypoglycemic agents
   D. All of the above
15. A 16-year-old Hispanic girl presents to the ER following a car accident. She is complaining of severe abdominal pain. A sonogram reveals a large right-sided mass of nonuniform density, and a follow-up MRI reveals a mass containing what appear to be teeth! What is your diagnosis?
   A. Teratoma
   B. Serous cystadenoma
   C. Mucinous adenocarcinoma
   D. Pregnancy
16. True or false? The endometrium is composed solely of glands formed of columnar epithelium.

17. True or false? The most common tumor of the breast is a fibroadenoma.

18. True or false? All painful masses are benign.

19. True or false? Infants born to diabetic mothers tend to be large for gestational age.

20. True or false? The majority of breast cancers are caused by hereditary genetic defects.

21. True or false? FCC does not increase the risk of breast cancer.

22. True or false? The most common cause of gynecomastia is cirrhosis.

CONCEPTUAL UNDERSTANDING

23. Using examples from the text, discuss some of the underlying etiologies of female infertility.

24. Explain why failure to ovulate may cause DUB.

25. Explain how the behavior of lobular carcinoma is different from that of ductal carcinoma.

APPLICATION

26. A 55-year-old Asian American woman was recently diagnosed with breast carcinoma. What treatment options are available to her?

27. Discuss the controversies associated with Pap smears, and the current recommendations.

28. As you enter your patient's room, she begins to complain loudly about how warm it is, despite the room being somewhat chilly. She tells you that she is always tired, has frequent headaches, and has been especially down for the last six months (starting shortly after her 50th birthday). A menstrual history reveals irregular menses for the last year. What is causing her symptoms and what treatments are available?

CHAPTER

18 Disorders of Bones, Joints, and Skeletal Muscle

Contents

Chapter Objectives

After studying this chapter, you should be able to complete the following tasks:

Section 1: The Normal Musculoskeletal System

THE NORMAL SKELETON

1. Explain the functions of the skeletal system in relation to its organization.

NORMAL JOINTS

2. Categorize the types of joints and describe their components.

NORMAL SKELETAL MUSCLE

3. Describe the anatomy of skeletal muscle and its connection to the nervous system.

Section 2: Disorders of Bone

DISORDERS OF BONE GROWTH, MATURATION, MODELING, AND MAINTENANCE

4. Describe the clinical presentation of bone disorders affecting growth, maturation, modeling and maintenance.
5. Distinguish between osteoporosis and osteomalacia, taking into consideration pathogenesis, clinical presentation, diagnosis, and treatment.

FRACTURES

6. List fracture types, their potential risk factors, and their phases of healing.

BONE INFARCTION AND INFECTION

7. Name the types of bone infarctions and infections.
8. Discuss the most common etiologies of bone infection, noting the clinical and diagnostic features.

BONE TUMORS AND TUMOR-LIKE LESIONS

9. Classify the tumors affecting the bone according to their composition, whether they are benign or malignant, their location, their pathological findings, and their prognosis.

Section 3: Disorders of Joints and Soft Tissues

ARTHRITIS

10. Characterize the kinds of arthritis according to etiology, signs and symptoms, diagnostic findings, and treatment.

INJURIES TO JOINTS AND PERIARTICULAR TISSUES

11. List the types of injuries to joints and periarticular tissues.

PERIARTICULAR PAIN SYNDROMES

12. Name the distinguishing features that separate fibromyalgia from arthritis and other painful musculoskeletal syndromes.

TUMORS AND TUMOR-LIKE LESIONS OF JOINTS AND SOFT TISSUES

13. Differentiate between ganglion cysts and tenosynovial giant cell tumors using location, clinical presentation, and or diagnostic findings as applicable.

Section 4: Disorders of Skeletal Muscle

PATHOLOGIC REACTIONS OF MUSCLE

14. Distinguish between neurogenic and disuse atrophy of skeletal muscle.

MYOPATHIES

15. Using examples from the text, characterize each of the dystrophies, congenital myopathies, inborn errors of metabolism, causes of myositis, and toxic myopathies according to the diagnostic and clinical findings.

MYASTHENIA GRAVIS

16. Explain the molecular pathogenesis of myasthenia gravis.

Section 1: The Normal Musculoskeletal System

The Normal Skeleton

The phrase "bred-in-the-bone" conveys the universal understanding that heredity and early childhood influences are so deeply ingrained in our being that they become part of our bones. The saying reflects the common knowledge that bones are the most enduring parts of our bodies. Indeed, most of what we know about the evolution of humankind is a tale written in the scattered bones of our apelike ancestors, bones that have endured hundreds of thousands of years. Ancient remains provide evidence of occupation, nutrition, lifespan, and many disorders—from tuberculosis and other infections, to cancer, fractures, arrow and spear injuries, and more.

The durability of bones can be deceiving. They look absolutely rigid, but in fact are slightly flexible (otherwise they would be brittle); they seem to be solid, but in fact are porous and have a hollow core; they appear inert, but in fact they are metabolically dynamic. Their stores of calcium, phosphorous, and other minerals are constantly being resorbed, renewed, and remodeled.

In the discussion that follows, remember that the word *bone* has two meanings. *Bone* can refer to an organ, such as the femur. Or it can refer to a tissue; for example, the *lamellar bone* that forms the bulk of bone tissue, or the *woven bone* that is one stage in the growth of new bone.

Bone has three functions: mechanical, metabolic, and hematopoietic. Its mechanical properties are attributable to its light weight and strength, which serve to protect internal organs and act as a framework for the force of skeletal muscle contractions. Its metabolic properties relate to its mineral content: bone is 65% mineral and 35% protein, and contains 99% of the body's calcium, 85% of the body's phosphorus, and 65% of the body's sodium, all of which are in a constant state of flux between bone, blood, and other tissues. Its hematopoietic properties are derived from its central marrow cavity, where many bones house the dynamic red marrow, production site for most blood cells.

Much of our modern knowledge of bones comes from radiographic imaging. An interesting vignette about radiographic imaging is provided in the *History of Medicine*, "The Discovery of X-Rays."

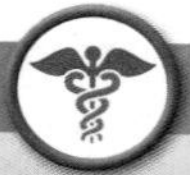

The History of Medicine

THE DISCOVERY OF X-RAYS

Confronted with crisis deep in the body, ancient physicians surely must have longed to see beneath the skin. Wilhelm Roentgen, a Dutch physicist, not a physician, made it possible to see through the skin when he discovered X-rays as he experimented with electricity by passing an electrical current from one metal pole to another in a vacuum tube. When the current was at low power, the apparatus produced ordinary light and other types of rays, which Roentgen focused into a beam and aimed at various materials to see what happened. One such material was a barium compound painted on a panel, which fluoresced (glowed) slightly if he held it very close to the vacuum tube.

On November 8, 1895, Roentgen conducted an experiment that required the vacuum tube to be covered with tinfoil and cardboard to keep all of the light and other rays from escaping. To confirm that nothing was escaping, he darkened the room and turned up the current. Sure enough, the apparatus was dark—no light or rays could be seen escaping. He was about to turn on the lights when across the room a glow caught his eye—the barium panel was glowing. Roentgen instantly recognized that some kind of ray—he later dubbed it the X-ray—was passing from the tube, through the foil and cardboard, and striking the barium panel, making it glow.

On closer inspection of the fluorescing panel, he noticed a dull black line running across it. Looking carefully in the path of the mysterious rays, he discovered a wire, which was absorbing some of the rays. Then he took a simple but profound step—he put a piece of paper in the beam and noticed no interference. Next he tried a playing card, then a book, finding that the book dimmed the beam slightly. If he had stopped at this point he would have done enough to ensure a lifetime of fame in the world of physics. But he went further and held a small lead disc in the beam, a simple act that required him to place his hand in the beam, an act that ultimately led him to the first ever Nobel Prize in physics. Lead stopped the strange rays completely, and—in a moment that literally changed impossible to possible—he noticed eerily glowing on the panel the unmistakable image of his fingers, the bones clearly visible beneath the hazy outline of his flesh.

Bones Are Composed of Bone Tissue

Beyond fetal life, all *normal* bones (Fig. 18.1) are composed of **lamellar bone**, one of the two varieties of bone tissue. It is made slowly and is highly organized (Fig. 18.1C). Lamellar bone is formed of parallel bundles of collagen that are mineralized into layers around a central vascular channel, the **Haversian canal**, to form an **osteon**. Bundles of osteons run with the long axis of bones to provide strength, in the same way that individual sticks add strength to a bundle.

The other variety of bone tissue is **woven bone**, which is formed of an irregular lattice of crossing collagen fibers and numerous osteocytes. It forms rapidly and is metabolically very active. In the fetus, it is present during normal bone development and provides temporary scaffolding for the production of lamellar bone. Woven bone also appears in the healing of fractures and bone diseases. *The presence of woven bone in an adult is always abnormal* and is certain evidence of normal healing or other bone tissue reaction to injury.

Bones Structure Is Organized for Strength and Growth

The *lamellar bone tissue* that composes all normal adult bone is organized into two anatomic types of structural bone. **Compact bone** (*cortical bone*) is dense, solid bone tissue that forms the hard outer shell of bones (the **cortex**). It comprises 80% of bone tissue. Its main function is structural support. **Spongy bone** (*cancellous* or *trabecular bone*), as the name implies, contains many small open spaces, which give it the appearance of a sponge and make it much lighter than compact bone. It is metabolically much more active than compact bone and has a high ratio of bone cells to bone mass. Spongy

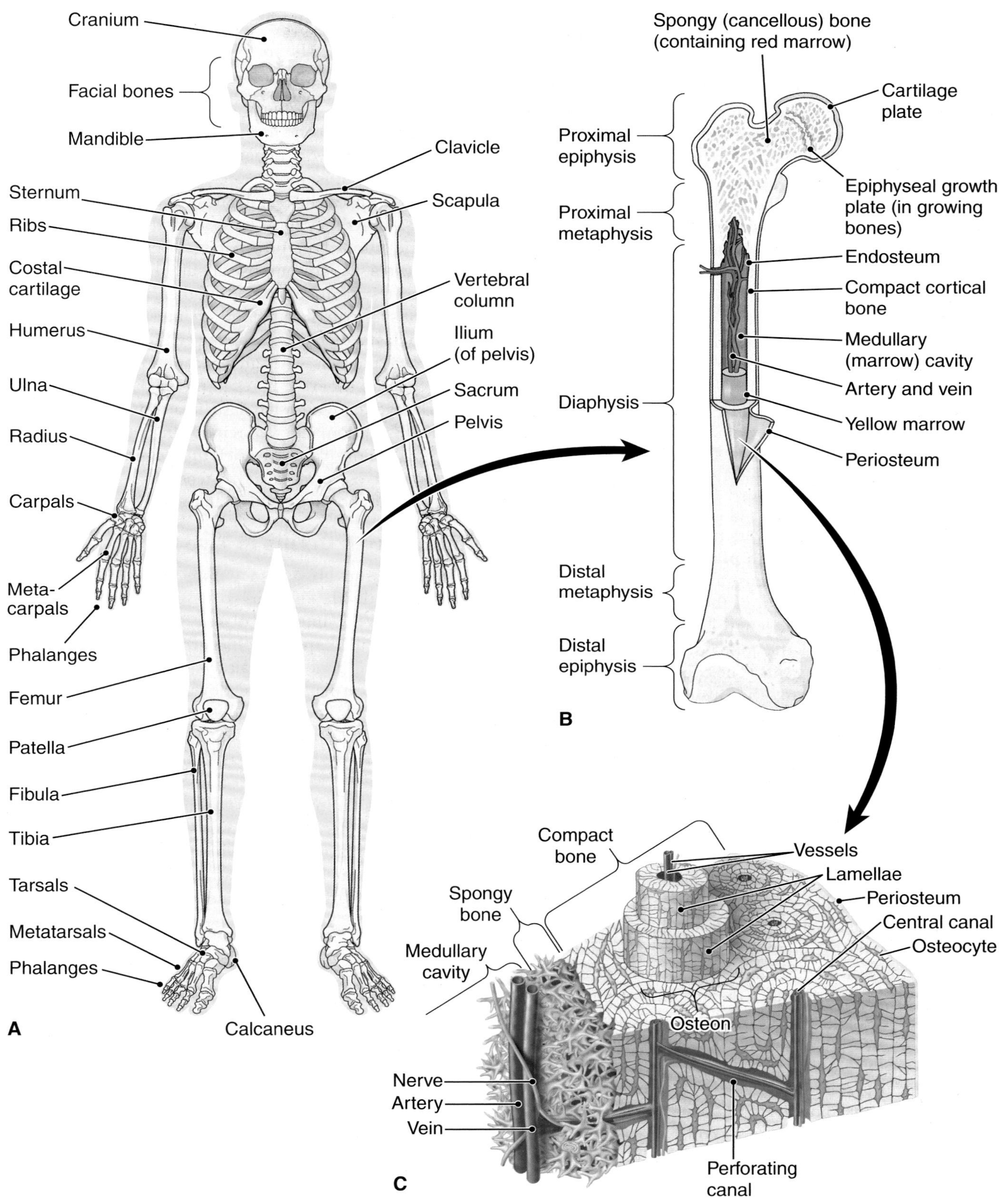

Figure 18.1 **The structure of normal bones. A.** The skeleton. **B.** The structure of long bones. **C.** Detailed structure of lamellar bone tissue. This figure illustrates a section of the diaphysis, in which a central canal is surrounded by a thin layer of spongy bone and a thick outer layer of compact bone. Compact bone is organized into osteons, each containing rings of bone tissue and bone cells surrounding a central canal. Spongy bone is organized into a latticework of bone spikes called trabeculae. (**C.** Reproduced with permission from McConnell TH, Hull KL. *Human Form Human Function: Essentials of Anatomy & Physiology*. Baltimore, (MD): Wolters Kluwer Health; 2011.)

bone is found in the central **marrow cavity** and at the ends of long bones, where it is formed into a latticework of spicules called **trabeculae**. The surface of spongy trabeculae is lined by a layer of cells, the **endosteum**, which is rich with bone cells, including stem cells. In children, the marrow cavity of all bones contains only *red marrow*; that is, marrow that is producing blood cells. As the skeleton matures, however, fat-storing *yellow marrow* displaces red marrow in the shafts of the long bones of the limbs. In adults, red marrow remains chiefly in the axial skeleton—the ribs, the vertebrae, the pelvic bones, and the skull.

All bones contain both compact and spongy bone, but proportions differ. The shaft of long bones, for example, is composed mainly of compact bone, but the expanded ends are composed mainly of spongy bone. In contrast, the skull is formed of relatively thin outer and inner tables of compact bone covering a thick layer of spongy bone.

The Anatomy of Bones Is Defined in Relation to the Growth Plate

The anatomy of bones (especially *long bones*, see below) is defined in relation to a transverse cartilage plate present in the growing child, the **growth plate** or *physis*. It is a layer of cartilage unrelated to the cushioning cartilaginous plate in the joint space at the end of the bone. The epiphyseal growth plate adds to bone length by forming cartilage on the advancing (toward the joint) side, which is turned into bone on the trailing side. The epiphyseal growth plate disappears when bone growth stops in early adult life, but leaves a distinctive line of dense bone to mark its place.

The **epiphysis** (*epi* = above) is a cap of spongy bone, usually the widest part of a bone, which extends from the growth plate to the distal (articular) end of the bone. The **metaphysis** (*meta* = behind) is funnel-shaped area of spongy bone that extends in the opposite direction—from the growth plate toward the diaphysis. The **diaphysis** (*dia* = connecting) is the long, slender, middle part of the length of the bone that joins the distal parts.

Bones are classified according to their shape. **Long bones** occur in the extremities; **short bones** and **flat bones** constitute the feet, hands, skull, ribs, pelvis, scapula, and spine. Figure 18.1B illustrates the anatomy of long bones. The place where bones meet is a **joint**, which can be very tight and allow no movement (as with the joints between the bones of the skull), or which can be loose and allow for movement of a limited degree (the vertebral joints) or a large degree (the shoulder).

Bone is covered by a tough, collagenous membrane, the **periosteum**, which contains osteoblasts, nerves, and blood vessels. The periosteum is rich in nerve endings (most of the pain from a broken bone originates in the periosteum), and its undersurface contains stem cells capable of forming new bone. Blood vessels enter bone through a **nutrient foramen** and travel through bones in the Haversian canal system.

There Are Four Types of Bone Cells

Osteoprogenitor cells are pluripotent stem cells found in bone marrow and periosteum, which differentiate into osteoblasts and osteoclasts.

- **Osteoblasts** are bone-forming cells, which form bone by depositing a network of bone matrix protein fibers called **osteoid**, which is unmineralized bone. Osteoblasts bind osteoid with calcium and phosphate to form mineralized bone. As they form bone around them, osteoblasts become trapped in tiny pores (*lacunae*) and become **osteocytes**, which comprise about 90% of all bone cells. Osteocytes are linked to one another by cytoplasmic extensions that run through tiny channels called *canaliculi*.
- **Osteoclasts** are bone-dissolving cells derived from bone marrow stem cells. They are concentrated mainly around the edges of the bone pores in the medullary cavity and work together with osteoblasts in a continual process of bone absorption, renewal, remodeling and repair, and in the regulation of blood calcium and phosphorus. The activity of osteoclasts and osteoblasts is regulated by parathyroid hormone and vitamin D (Chapter 14).

Bone Growth Occurs in Two Ways

Most body tissues grow from within. That is, cells throughout a tissue divide and add to tissue mass. Bone grows differently, at the interface of one surface with another, in a process called **appositional growth**. For example, in a growing long bone, the epiphyseal plate is the growth surface. New cartilage is laid down along the advancing (distal) edge and the trailing edge leaves behind new bone.

There are two types of appositional bone growth. **Endochondral ossification** is a manner of growth in which cartilage forms first, then is transformed into woven bone, and finally into lamellar bone. In contrast, in **intramembranous ossification**, bone growth occurs on the surface of fibrous tissue, which becomes woven bone and then lamellar bone. No cartilage phase occurs. Both methods of growth produce lamellar bone.

Pop Quiz

18.1 True or false? Compact comprises 80% of bone tissue.

18.2 True or false? Woven bone is always abnormal.

18.3 What are the two types of appositional bone growth?

18.4 What cell type is responsible for making bone?

18.5 In what layer of bone does most of the pain of a broken bone occur?

Normal Joints

Apart from the heart, joints are mechanically the busiest, hardest working parts of the body. They keep "life and limb" together and enable the movements of life. They are subject to continual and strong stress.

A **joint** is the place where two bones meet (Fig. 18.2). *Functionally*, joints are classified according to the movement they allow. A *synarthrosis* allows no movement; an *amphiarthrosis* allows limited twisting or sliding; a *diarthrosis* allows full motion. *Structurally*, joints are classified according to the nature of their anatomical union.

Types of joints
(a structural classification)

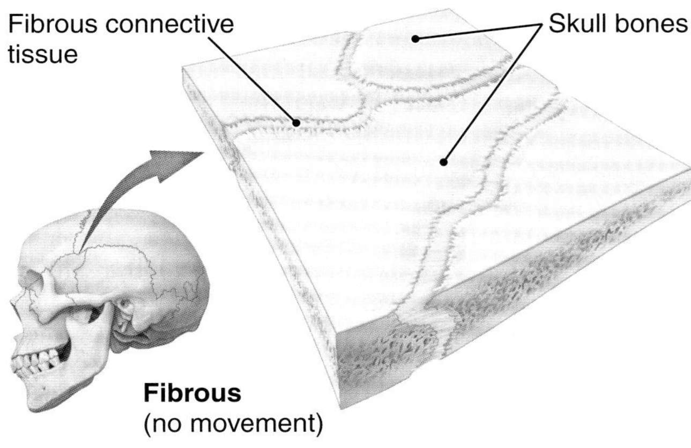

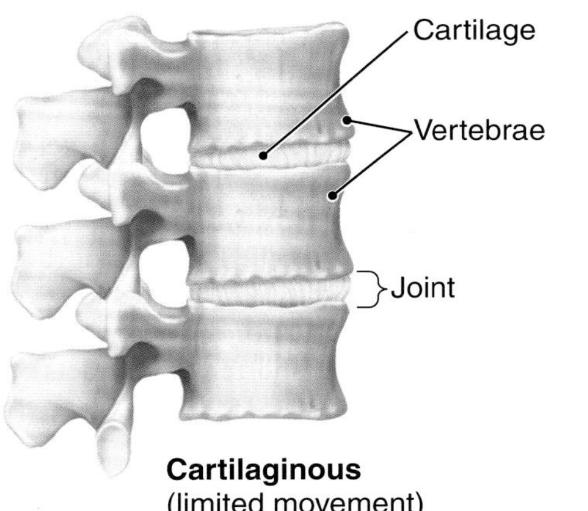

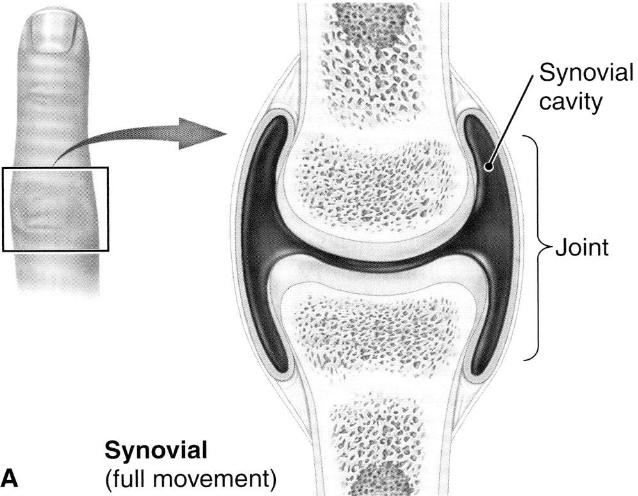

The structure of a synovial joint

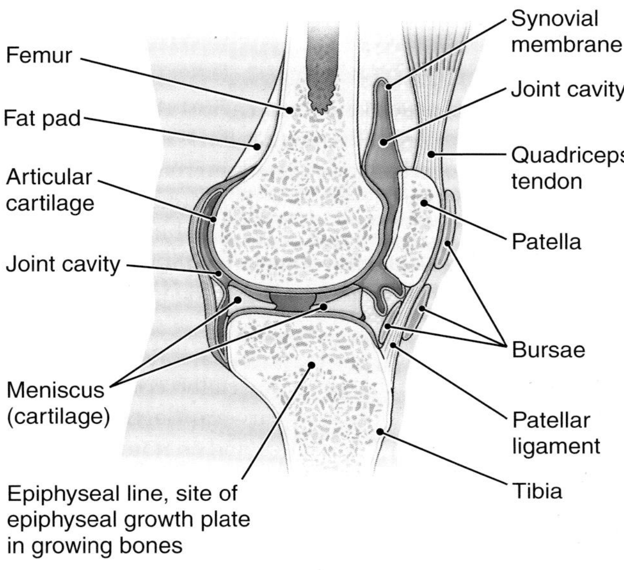

Figure 18.2 **The anatomy of joints. A.** Types of joints. **B.** The structure of a synovial joint (the knee). (**A.** Reproduced with permission from McConnell TH, Hull KL. *Human Form Human Function: Essentials of Anatomy & Physiology*. Baltimore, (MD): Wolters Kluwer Health; 2011.)

Fibrous joints are synarthroses that join bones by a heavy weld of fibrous tissue. No joint space is present and no movement occurs. The bones of the skull are fibrous joints. **Cartilaginous joints** are amphiarthroses that join bones by cartilage, have no space, and allow limited movement. The joints between vertebral bodies and the bones of the wrist are bound together into a unit by cartilaginous joints. **Synovial joints** (Fig. 18.2 B) are diarthroses that join bones by ligaments, have a joint space, and allow great range of motion. The knee, elbow, shoulder, wrist, and hip are synovial joints. Synovial joints have the following characteristics:

- *They contain a space* (the joint cavity) that is enclosed by a sheath of fibrous tissue that binds the outer edges of the bones together and is lined internally by a special membrane (the **synovium**), which is formed of special cells (**synovial cells**) that secrete a lubricating fluid (**synovial fluid**). The synovial membrane lines only the outer edges of the joint space; it does not cover the articular surface.
- *They contain a plate of cartilage* to cushion movement. This **articular cartilage** is specially constructed to painlessly buffer shock and wear—cartilage lacks blood supply, nerves, and lymphatics and is nourished with oxygen and nutrients from joint fluid.
- *The ends of the bones are usually bound together and kept in alignment by strong fibrous straps* (**ligaments**).

The movement of tissues around joints is smoothed by **bursae**—small, closed fibrous sacs lined by synovial cells, which secrete a lubricating fluid that partially fills the sac (much like a collapsed balloon containing a small amount of fluid). Bursae are positioned between tendon and bone or between skin and bony protuberances, such as the elbow, to smooth the movement where tissues rub together.

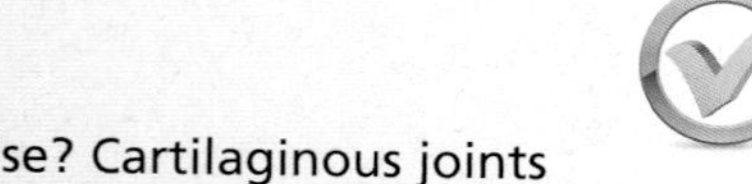

Pop Quiz

18.6 True or false? Cartilaginous joints are amphiarthroses that join bones by cartilage, have no space, and allow limited movement.

Normal Skeletal Muscle

The fundamental element of the neuromuscular system is the **motor unit** (Fig. 18.3A), which consists of the following:

- A *lower motor neuron*, which is located in the brain stem or spinal cord and extends via a long cytoplasmic extension (axon) to skeletal muscle
- A *motor end plate*, the neuromuscular junction, where nerve meets muscle
- A *skeletal muscle cell or cells*

Signals are sent from the brain by an *upper* motor neuron in the cerebral cortex that connects with the *lower* motor neuron by a long axon, which in turn relays the signal to muscle cells by attachment to them with a special nerve ending known as a **motor end plate**. Where the motor end plate and muscle cell join is the **neuromuscular junction**, which is a special kind of cell union known as a synapse. A **synapse** is a junction between two neurons or between a neuron and a muscle or gland cell; it features a very narrow space (the *synaptic space*) between the signaling nerve cell and the receiving cell (in this instance, muscle).

Signals are transmitted down nerve axons as waves of electrical disturbance (*action potential*) in the cell membrane. On arrival at the motor end plate, the signal stimulates release of **acetylcholine** (the *neurotransmitter*) into the synaptic space. Acetylcholine quickly crosses the synaptic space and interacts with skeletal muscle to cause electrical disturbance of the muscle cell membrane and contraction of muscle fibers. In the process, acetylcholine is broken down by an enzyme, **cholinesterase**, enabling the next signal to cross the synapse.

Muscle cells are elongated and have multiple nuclei, which lie at the edge of the cell out of the way of muscle fiber contractions. Compared to most other cells, cytoplasm in muscle cells is especially abundant in order to accommodate large amounts of long, thin, specialized protein molecules, **actin** and **myosin**, which lie in parallel rows running lengthwise in the cell. The slide of these molecules upon one another creates more or less molecular overlap. When electrical stimulation by acetylcholine increases the overlap, the muscle shortens (contracts); a decreased overlap relaxes the muscle.

Muscle is composed of two fiber types: **Type I fibers**, *red* or *slow twitch*; or **Type II fibers**, *white* or *fast twitch*; Table 18.1 summarizes the characteristics of each. Type I fibers are designed for sustained action; Type II for short bursts of intensity. In humans, various muscles have different percentages of Type I and II fibers, depending on their task.

The differences in Type I and Type II are exemplified in birds. Ducks and geese fly long distances. Their breast muscles are Type I fibers and are packed with energy-providing mitochondria that give them a dark, reddish color ("dark meat"). By contrast, quail and pheasants are nonmigratory birds that make short, bursting flights. Their breast muscles are Type II fibers and have fewer mitochondria, which makes them light pink ("white meat").

Human muscles differ, too, but the distinctions are less obvious. For example, the calf muscles in the lower leg that are used for walking and running are mainly Type I fibers; in contrast, the small muscles attached to

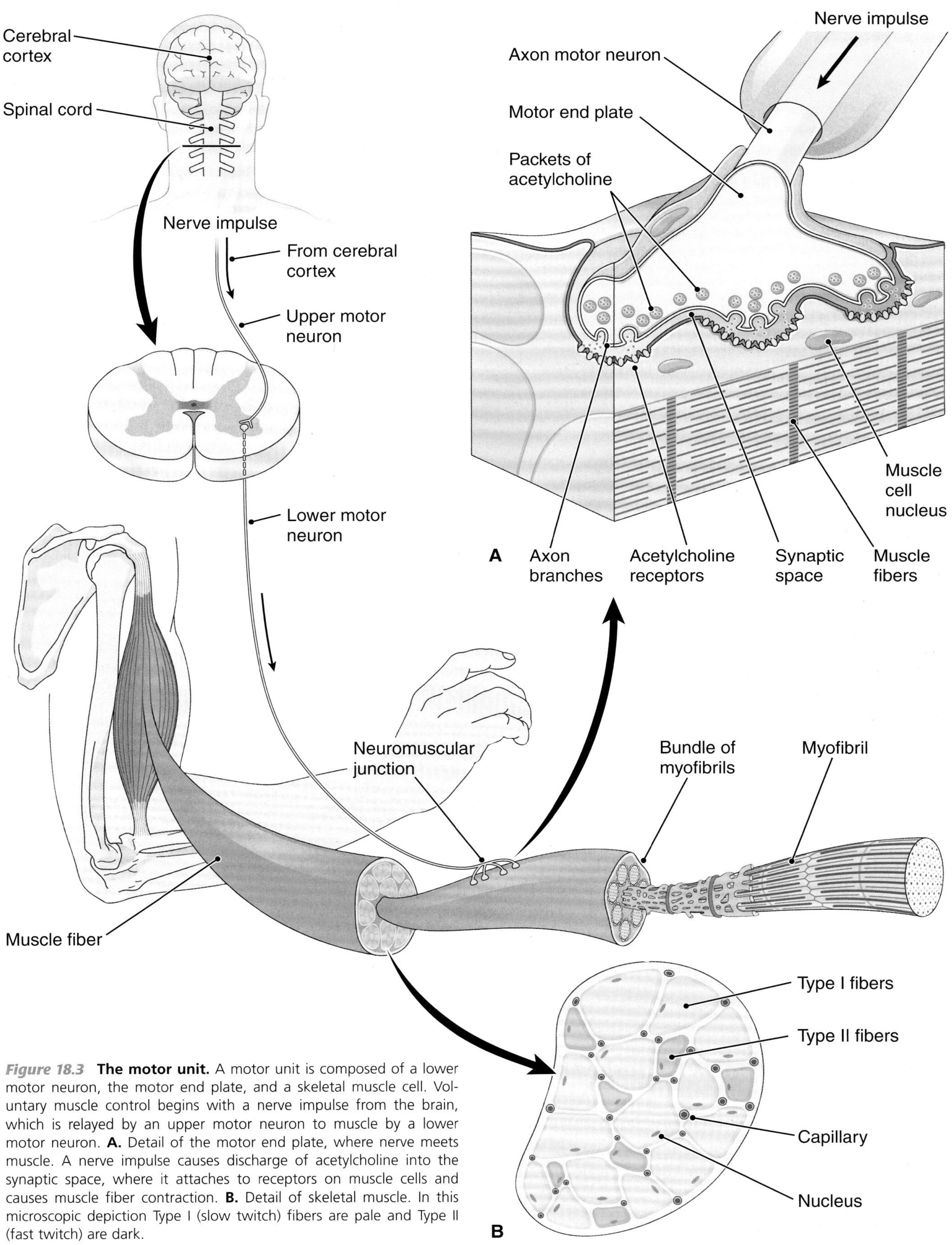

Figure 18.3 **The motor unit.** A motor unit is composed of a lower motor neuron, the motor end plate, and a skeletal muscle cell. Voluntary muscle control begins with a nerve impulse from the brain, which is relayed by an upper motor neuron to muscle by a lower motor neuron. **A.** Detail of the motor end plate, where nerve meets muscle. A nerve impulse causes discharge of acetylcholine into the synaptic space, where it attaches to receptors on muscle cells and causes muscle fiber contraction. **B.** Detail of skeletal muscle. In this microscopic depiction Type I (slow twitch) fibers are pale and Type II (fast twitch) are dark.

Table 18.1 Muscle Fiber Types

	Type I Slow Twitch	Type II Fast Twitch
Action	Sustained force or weight bearing	Sudden movement or purposeful motion
Color (due to fiber myoglobin content and vascular supply)	Red (dark)	Pale (white)
ATPase stain intensity	Dark	Light
Fat	Abundant	Scant
Glycogen	Scant	Abundant
Example of muscle with high fiber type content	Neck muscles	Eye muscles

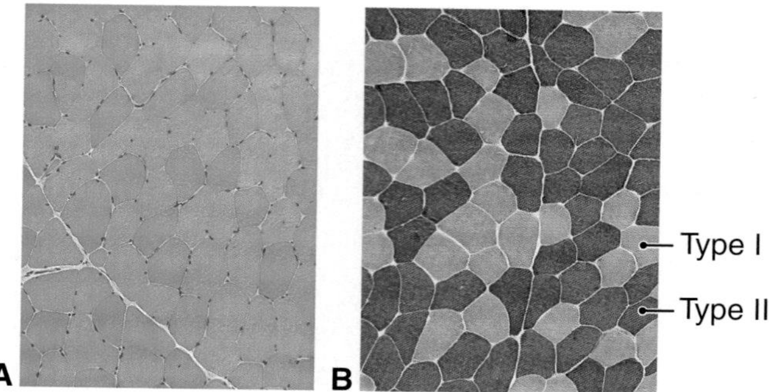

Figure 18.4 **Normal muscle. A.** Conventional microscopic study. **B.** Special stain of demonstrating Type I and Type II fibers. (Reproduced with permission from Rubin E. *Pathology*. 4th ed. Philadelphia, (PA). Lippincott Williams and Wilkins; 2005).

the eyeball, which control eye movement, are mainly Type II fibers. Type I and II fibers are easily distinguishable microscopically by special stains (Figs. 18.3B and 18.4). Some muscle conditions affect only one type of fiber.

During embryonic development, primitive muscle stem cells fuse to form a single muscle cell. Adult cells (muscle fibers), therefore, have multiple nuclei. Some muscle stem cells persist into adulthood and are called **satellite cells** because they are located in the interstitium near the edge of muscle fibers. Although mature muscle cells are fully differentiated and incapable of dividing to regenerate, satellite cells can be activated by exercise or injury to form new muscle cells. Nevertheless, the number of satellite cells is relatively small and cannot regenerate enough new cells to repair a major injury. Large muscle injuries heal by fibrosis and scarring.

Pop Quiz

18.7 True or false? Muscle cells are multinucleate.

18.8 True or false? Slow twitch is a red, Type I muscle fiber, while fast twitch is a white, Type II muscle fiber.

Section 2: Disorders of Bone

What is bred in the bone will never come out of the flesh.

FROM THE PANCHATANTRA, A COLLECTION OF ANIMAL FABLES FROM THE INDIAN SUBCONTINENT WRITTEN ABOUT 200 BCE, AND KNOWN IN THE WEST AS THE FABLES OF BIDPAI, AN INDIAN SAGE

Case Study

"You'd think I'd crashed a motorcycle!" The case of Maggie H.

Chief Complaint: Painful injury to the ankle.

Clinical History: Maggie H., a 67-year-old grandmother, was training for her 10th marathon. During a 10-mile training run, she made a misstep that caused her to catch herself awkwardly on the lateral edge of her left foot, with the sole turned inward. As she

"You'd think I'd crashed a motorcycle!" The case of Maggie H. (continued)

tumbled to the ground, she reached out to break her fall, and caught herself mainly on the heel of her left hand. "I could hear my ankle snap," she said, "but my wrist was a surprise! I thought I'd just sprained it. I can't believe such a small thing could break so many bones. Look at me!" She managed a wry smile. "You'd think I'd crashed a motorcycle! All I was trying to do was get some exercise."

Her medical history was unremarkable. She had never smoked and denied recreational drug use or alcohol abuse. She was not taking any prescription medications. She required glasses for reading and volunteered that her ophthalmologist said she probably would have to have cataract surgery soon. Her parents died of cardiovascular disease. A sister was a breast cancer survivor. She had two healthy adult children.

Physical Examination and Other Data: Vital signs were unremarkable. She was a small, slender woman who appeared her stated age. She stated her height and weight to be 5′ 4′ and 117 lb. The fracture site in her ankle was about 5 cm above the medial prominence of the left ankle. The bone remained aligned. A sizeable hematoma was present in the fracture and surrounding tissue. Her left wrist was swollen and painful, particularly over the distal radius. She also had bruises to her left hip and the left side of her face. The radiologist's report of X-rays of her skull, spine, hip, ankle, and wrist described complete fracture through the distal metaphysis of the tibia and fibula. The radius showed a simple hairline fracture extending completely across the epiphysis of the radius about 3 cm above the wrist joint. No bone displacement was present. The radiologist also noted degenerative changes in the left knee and generalized osteoporosis, which was most notable in the vertebrae, where an old fracture was noted. The final diagnosis was "1) Complete, simple, closed, nondisplaced fracture of the left tibia and fibula. 2) Complete hairline fracture of the distal left radius. 3) Generalized osteoporosis with old compression fracture of the vertebral body of T2. 4) Osteoarthritis of the left knee."

Clinical Course: The bones were realigned and the limbs were placed in casts. She was confined to a wheel chair and knee-scooter for weeks but recovered in keeping with expectations. She was advised to take up speed-walking for exercise, and she was prescribed a treatment regimen for osteoporosis that included supplemental calcium, vitamin D, and bisphosphonate. Because of her family history of breast cancer, she refused long-term estrogen replacement therapy after a discussion with her doctor.

Case Notes

18.1 **Did Maggie break lamellar or woven bone?**

18.2 **What is the name of the hard layer of outer bone in Maggie's broken tibia and fibula?**

Disorders of Bone Growth, Maturation, Modeling, and Maintenance

Bone grows in the fetus and in youth until it matures and stops growing in young adults. Nevertheless, activity does not stop. Osteoclasts are always active resorbing bone, which is continually replaced by osteoblasts making replacement bone. This ongoing renewal supports the repair and reshaping (remodeling) of bone according to the stresses placed upon it.

Disorders of Bone Growth Produce Stunted or Deformed Bone

Of the dozens of disorders of *bone growth*, only a few are mentioned here. Most are due to metabolic or inherited disease.

Reactive bone formation is the formation of new membranous bone in response to stress or injury to a bone or soft tissue. For example, new bone may appear around a site of chronic bone infection, or in a scar in soft tissue. **Heterotopic ossification** is similar but appears without injury or stress in skin, subcutaneous tissue, and soft tissue or muscle (where it is called *myositis ossificans*). It may be genetic or it may follow surgery, trauma, or other condition. Patients have normal calcium and phosphorous metabolism. The mechanism is unclear.

Cretinism (Chapter 14) is caused by fetal or infantile deficiency of iodine, which is needed for thyroid hormone synthesis. Hypothyroidism affects the epiphyseal growth plate and causes stunted growth and skeletal deformities.

Achondroplasia is a genetic syndrome of short-limbed dwarfism caused by failure of epiphyseal cartilage to form normally. The clinical picture is one of a relatively normal trunk to which are attached short arms and legs. Also, the face is small compared to the skull, giving the patient a bulbous-appearing forehead. A saddle nose, small jaw, bowed legs, and a sway-back posture (*lordosis*) complete the clinical picture. Achondroplasia is not associated with reduced mental functioning, reproductive capacity, or lifespan.

Asymmetric cartilage growth in the young can produce "bow legs" or "knock knees." When it occurs in the spine it causes abnormal curvatures (Fig. 18.5). **Scoliosis** is abnormal lateral bending of the spine; **kyphosis** is abnormal forward curvature; **lordosis** is abnormal backward curvature. In the elderly, these conditions are due to osteoporosis, intervertebral disc disease, and other bone conditions. Severe cases may be associated with cardiorespiratory compromise. Treatment includes physical therapy, braces, or surgery.

Osteochondroma (*exostosis*, Fig. 18.6) is a nonneoplastic, tumorlike growth that features a short, bony stalk covered by a cap of cartilage. It develops on the shaft of a long bone, and results from aberrant, side-directed growth of the epiphyseal growth plate. An inherited autosomal dominant gene defect is the cause of *multiple osteochondromatosis*.

Enchondromatosis (*Ollier disease*) is a bone growth defect that features multiple deforming cartilaginous masses within bone. Cartilage of the epiphyseal growth plate fails to ossify, remains cartilage, and continues to grow as tumor-like masses.

Disorders of Bone Maturation and Remodeling Produce Brittle or Deformed Bone

Osteogenesis imperfecta (*brittle bone disease*) is a disorder of bone *maturation*. It includes a spectrum of inheritable disorders caused by genetic defects in collagen formation. The basic defect in all varieties is too little bone tissue. Bones have a thin cortex and are easily fractured. Defective middle ear bones cause deafness, and defective collagen also causes abnormal tooth development, floppy heart valves, and thin sclerae, which accounts for the semi-transparent, bluish sclerae characteristic of these patients.

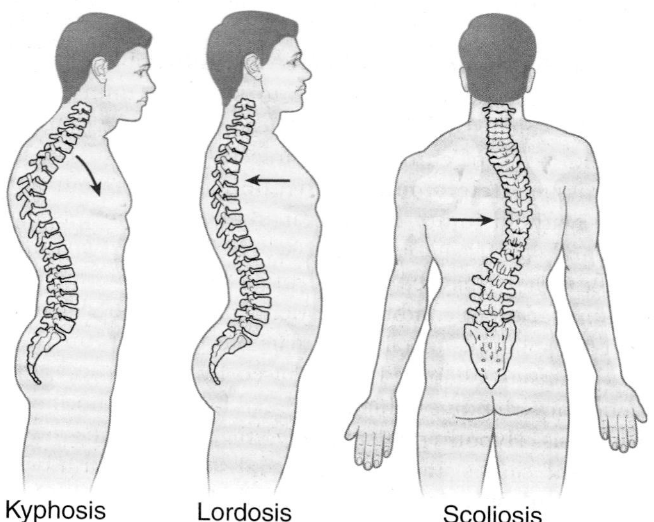

Figure 18.5 **Abnormalities of spinal curvature.**

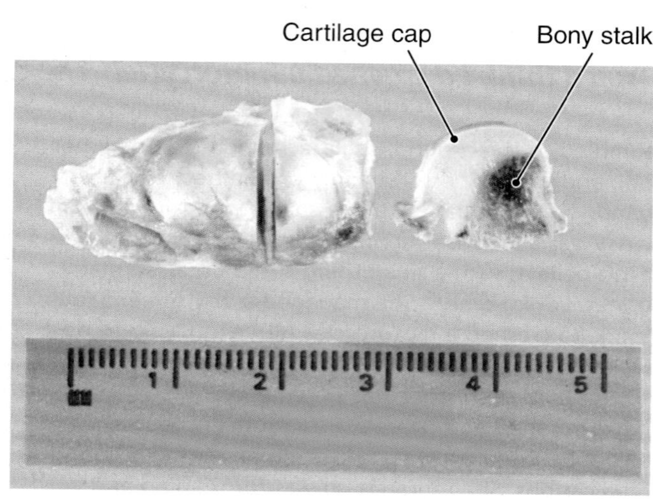

Figure 18.6 **Osteochondroma.** These small nonneoplastic growths appear on the epiphyseal surface of long bones and have a characteristic cap of cartilage.

Marble bone disease (*osteopetrosis, Albers-Schönberg disease*) is a disorder of bone *remodeling*. It is a family of inherited disorders caused by failed osteoclast formation or failure of existing osteoclasts to resorb bone during bone growth and remodeling. Osteoclasts may therefore be absent or present in abundance. The result usually is dense, sclerotic bones that fracture easily, like a piece of chalk. Cases may be mild or severe. Some patients are severely anemic because masses of osteoclasts crowd out the marrow. Failure of cranial foramina to grow (remodel) may cause hydrocephalus (Chapter 19) and cranial nerve entrapment with blindness and deafness. Because osteoclasts are derived from bone marrow stem cells, some patients benefit from bone marrow transplant.

Paget disease of bone (*osteitis deformans*)—not to be confused with Paget disease of skin—is a bone disease of unknown cause in which bone *remodeling* is defective. Evidence points to a chronic slow-virus infection that stimulates osteoclast activity. Genetics is important: it is very rare in Asian, African, and South American bloodlines. In the United States, however, it affects at least one bone in about 3% of people over 40. Increased osteoclast activity breaks down bone and stimulates new bone formation by osteoblasts. The result is formation of irregular, thick, exceptionally dense bone. Any bone may be affected, but usually more than one bone is involved; the femur, pelvis, and spine are the most common sites. Ultimately, bone resorption and regrowth burn out into a final quiet phase in which bone is deformed and densely sclerotic. About 1% of patients will develop an *osteosarcoma* or other malignant bone tumor in affected bone.

Paget disease of bone is usually asymptomatic and discovered incidentally on X-ray studies done for other purposes, or by finding an unexpected increase of blood *alkaline phosphatase (AP)*, an enzyme important in osteoblast activity. Pain, deformity, and fractures are the most common clinical problems. Bisphosphonate drugs suppress osteoclast activity and are useful in retarding disease progression, especially when bony defects create neurologic problems such as hearing loss and nerve compression.

Disorders of Bone Maintenance Produce Weak Bones

Recall that healthy bones require constant stress to remain healthy and that they are metabolically very active—they are continually being refreshed by replacement of older tissue with new. Failure to maintain normal stress and nutrition has adverse consequences.

Osteoporosis

Osteoporosis is an acquired condition of decreased mineralization of bones, increased bone porousness, and decreased bone mass to the point that bone tissue no longer provides proper mechanical support and strength. It is a *quantitative* defect: the microstructure of lamellar bone is normal but there is not enough of it (Fig. 18.7). Regardless of cause, osteoporosis represents enhanced bone resorption relative to new bone formation. *Primary* osteoporosis is the most common variety and occurs mainly in postmenopausal women. *Secondary* osteoporosis is caused by a defined condition, such as hyperparathyroidism (Chapter 14).

Primary osteoporosis is due in part to the declining blood estrogen levels that occur in postmenopausal women. Genetic factors are important: Caucasians and Asian Americans are much more frequently affected than are African Americans, and a family history of osteoporosis greatly increases the risk. About 80% of people with osteoporosis are women. Also important are lack of exercise, cigarette smoking, and inadequate intake of vitamin D and calcium.

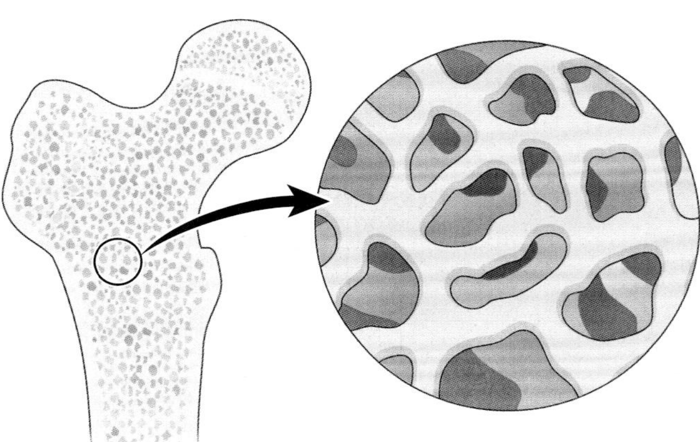

A Normal bone

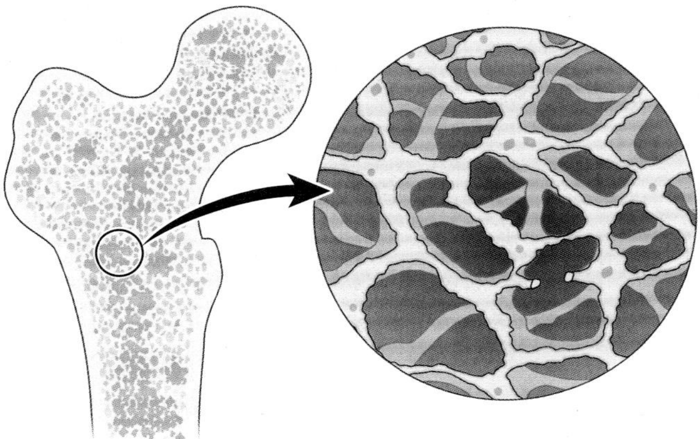

B Osteoporosis

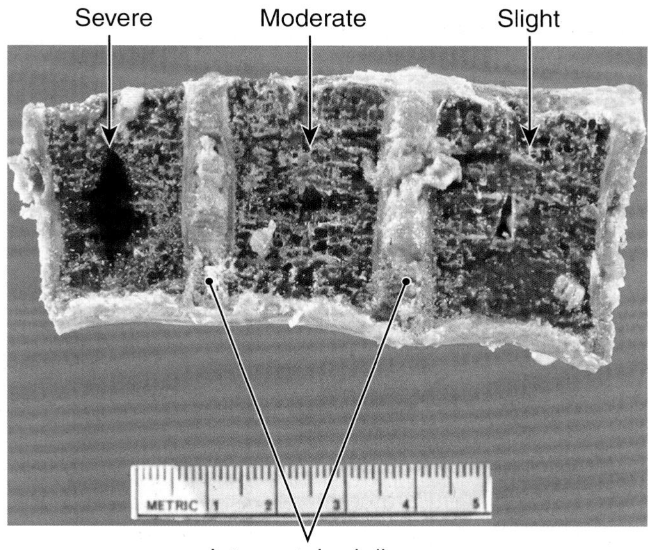

C Osteoporosis

Figure 18.7 **Osteoporosis. A.** Normal spongy bone. **B.** Osteoporotic bone. Bone organization is correct, but the lattice is thin and less bone mass is present. **C.** Osteoporosis of the vertebral column. From right to left, these vertebral bodies are progressively more severely affected.

Osteoporosis caused by some other condition is *secondary osteoporosis*. Causes include cortisone excess (*Cushing syndrome*, Chapter 14), deficiency of calcium or vitamin D due to *malabsorption syndrome* (Chapter 12), immobilization from prolonged bed rest, lack of weight-bearing exercise due to disability (such as limb paralysis or disease), anticonvulsant medication with diphenylhydantoin (Dilantin©), and anticoagulant therapy with heparin.

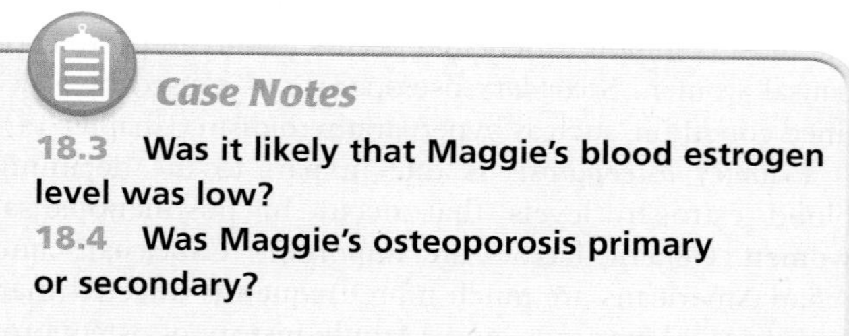

Case Notes

18.3 Was it likely that Maggie's blood estrogen level was low?

18.4 Was Maggie's osteoporosis primary or secondary?

Signs and Symptoms

Most patients are asymptomatic until a fracture occurs. Osteoporotic fractures are a major medical and social problem in the elderly, especially among postmenopausal Caucasian females. Although most of these fractures are minor, many are nevertheless seriously debilitating. The bones most often fractured are weight-bearing ones—vertebrae, femur, and pelvis—and wrist fractures from trips and falls. The immobilization required to treat a broken hip may lead to pneumonia and death. About 40,000 people die each year in the United States as a direct or indirect result of broken bones related to osteoporosis.

Remember This! One-third of women over age 65 will suffer a fracture due to osteoporosis.

As Figure 18.8 illustrates, the typical patient with osteoporosis is an elderly, thin Caucasian female. She is likely to be short and stooped: short due to collapsed vertebrae and stooped due to spinal kyphosis. Her medical history probably includes a recent fall and fracture. Spontaneous fractures may occur, especially collapse fracture of the vertebral body (Fig. 18.9), which is eight times more common in women than men.

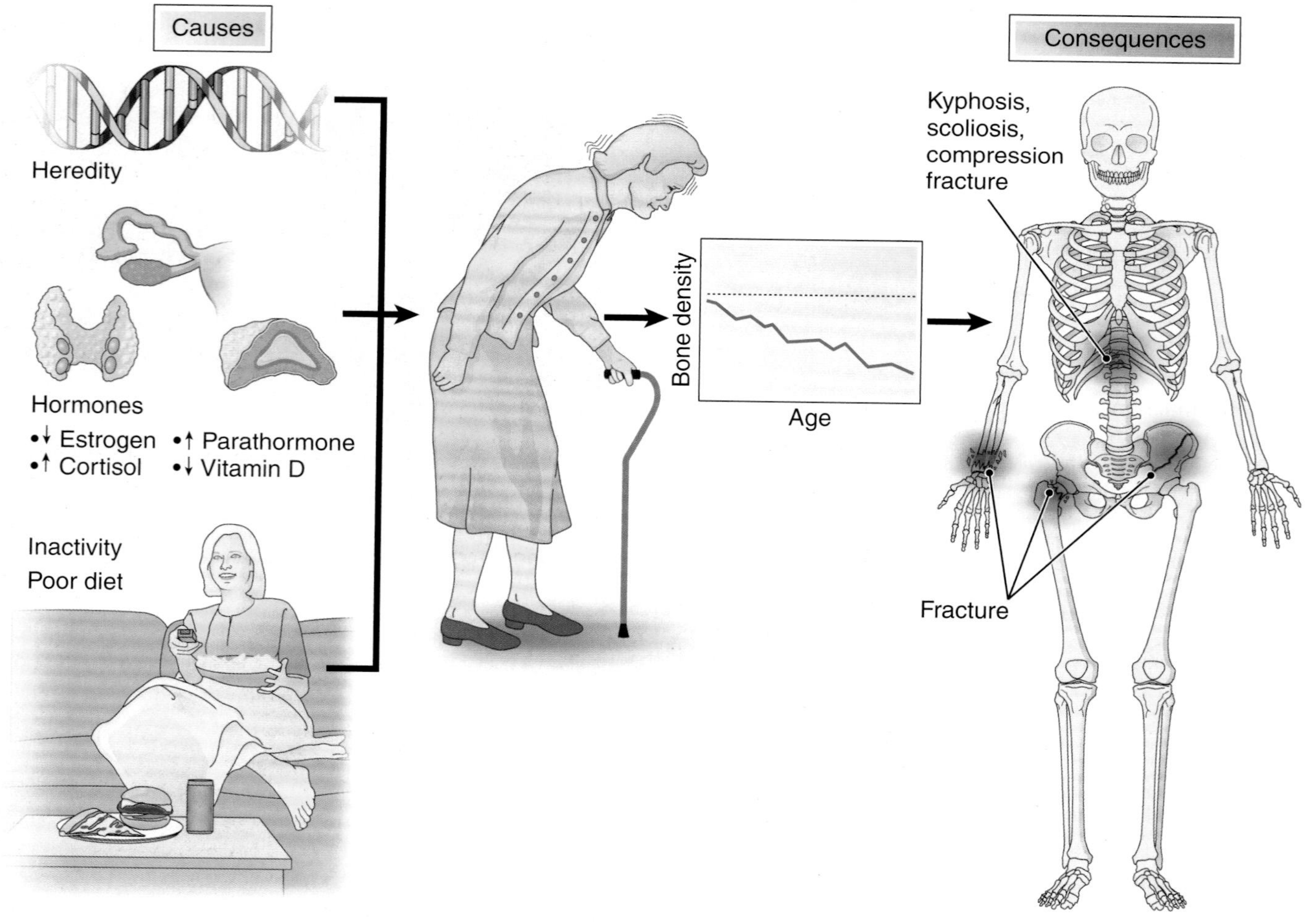

Causes

Heredity

Hormones

•↓ Estrogen •↑ Parathormone

•↑ Cortisol •↓ Vitamin D

Inactivity

Poor diet

Bone density

Age

Consequences

Kyphosis, scoliosis, compression fracture

Fracture

Figure 18.8 **The causes and consequences of osteoporosis.**

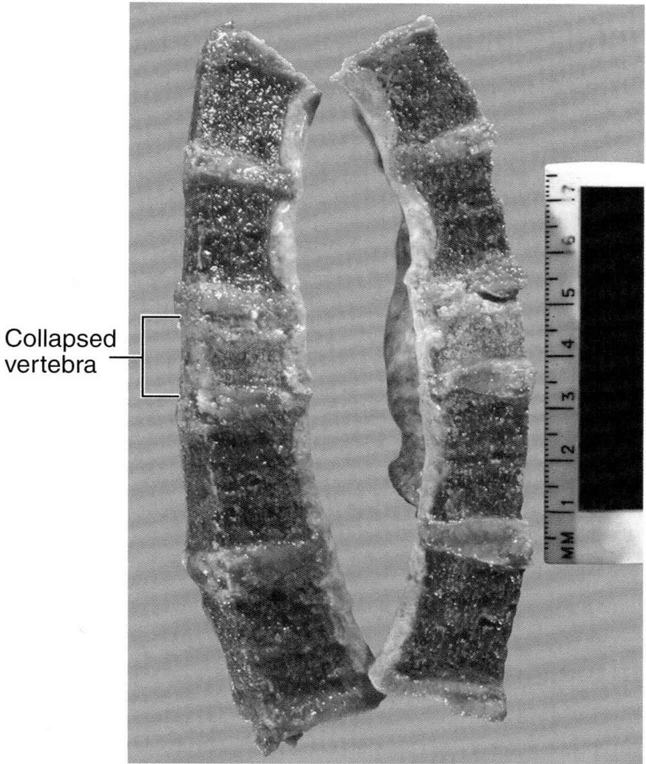

Figure 18.9 **Collapse fracture of a vertebral body.** This is a midline section of the vertebral column in a patient with osteoporosis.

Diagnosis and Treatment

Diagnosis is by X-ray imaging and specialized bone densitometry. Early osteoporosis is asymptomatic and cannot be detected by standard X-ray technique until about one-third of bone mass has disappeared; however, dual energy X-ray absorptiometry (DEXA or DXA) can detect low bone density before changes are detectable on routine X-rays.

Prevention is the best approach for primary osteoporosis, although new drugs show promise of rebuilding bone in some patients. Bisphosphonate drugs inhibit bone resorption and are first-line therapy. Treatment also aims to slow bone loss in those who are susceptible, and includes weight-bearing exercise, calcium and vitamin D supplementation, and smoking cessation. Historically, hormone replacement therapy (Chapter 17) proved effective in slowing postmenopausal bone loss, but its use has been sharply curtailed in recent years because of concerns about associated health risks. For secondary osteoporosis, correction of the underlying condition is the best therapy.

Osteomalacia

Osteomalacia (literally "soft bones") is defective mineralization (calcification) of bone protein fibers (osteoid). In contrast to osteoporosis, it is uncommon and is a *qualitative* defect: osteocytes make a normal or near normal amount of normal osteoid, but it does not mineralize properly.

Etiology

Most osteomalacia is due to disturbances in the metabolism of the dietary essentials calcium, phosphate, or vitamin D, usually from insufficient intake or poor intestinal absorption.

Meat and dairy products are the main dietary sources of the calcium and phosphate required for healthy bone mineralization. In the United States, vitamin D is routinely added to milk and milk alternatives; however, dietary deficiency is still common, especially in people in northern latitudes and those who drink mostly soft drinks and similar beverages. Additional vitamin D is synthesized in the skin as a result of sunlight exposure, so that inadequate sun exposure (polar living, for example) may be a factor. Dark-skinned people are more susceptible to vitamin D deficiency because sunlight has less effect in the synthesis of vitamin D. In underdeveloped countries, deficiency is widespread and is associated with childhood osteomalacia (*rickets*).

Small bowel disease (such as *Crohn disease*, Chapter 12) may interfere directly with calcium and vitamin D absorption. Intestinal malabsorption syndromes may sweep vitamin D away because it is fat soluble and lost in fatty stools. In either circumstance, the loss of calcium, phosphate, and vitamin D causes compensatory increased secretion of parathormone from the parathyroid glands (*hyperparathyroidism*, Chapter 14), which causes osteoclasts to increase their bone-dissolving activity.

Chronic renal failure may cause **renal osteodystrophy**, a variety of osteomalacia similar to that found in patients with hyperparathyroidism (Chapter 14). Failing kidneys do not excrete phosphate properly and blood phosphate rises, which lowers blood calcium. Low blood calcium stimulates the parathyroid glands to secrete parathyroid hormone, which in turn stimulates osteoclasts to leach calcium from bone in an effort to increase blood calcium. The result is osteomalacia due to demineralization of bone.

Signs and Symptoms

Osteomalacias bone is susceptible to deformity and fracture. Skeletal deformities are a particular characteristic of **rickets**, a form of osteomalacia due to vitamin D deficiency in growing children. Typically, children with rickets have bowlegs, delayed dentition and speckled teeth, and a highly characteristic abnormality of the anterior chest wall where the ribs join the sternum: the tips of the ribs are enlarged into nodules that produce a striking, beaded appearance called "rachitic rosary."

Diagnosis and Treatment

Apart from signs and symptoms associated with an underlying cause or rickets, most patients are asymptomatic until a fracture occurs. Radiologic findings are subtle and difficult to distinguish from osteoporosis.

Treatment is oral vitamin D, calcium and phosphate supplementation, and eliminating the cause, if any.

Pop Quiz

18.9 Scoliosis is abnormal ________ bending of the spine, while kyphosis is abnormal ________ curvature, and lordosis abnormal ________ curvature.

18.10 What is the treatment for Paget disease of bone?

18.11 True or false? Osteoporosis is a qualitative defect of bone.

18.12 How much bone loss must occur before a standard X-ray can detect it?

18.13 True or false? Most osteomalacia is due to disturbed calcium, phosphate, or vitamin D metabolism, from insufficient intake or poor intestinal absorption.

Fractures

The most common lesion of bone is **fracture**, a broken bone, which is defined as a discontinuity of the anatomy of a bone. Healthy bones require mechanical stress, such as weight-bearing exercise, which stimulates constant osteoblast and osteoclast activity to rebuild and refresh bone. Too little mechanical stress, as with space flight or prolonged bed rest, causes osteoporosis and increases susceptibility to fracture. On the other hand, too much mechanical stress causes a broken bone.

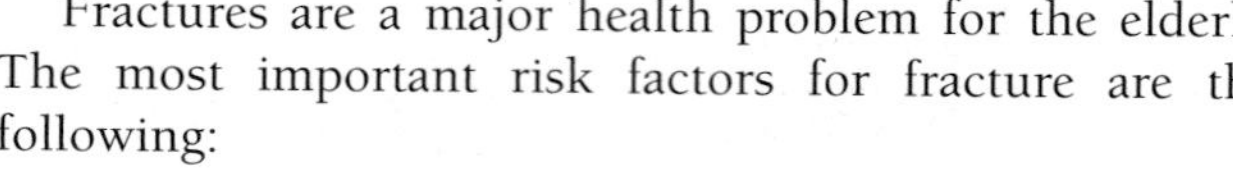

Fractures are a major health problem for the elderly. The most important risk factors for fracture are the following:

- Age over 80 years
- Weight less than 130 lb
- Long-term use of benzodiazepines (widely used sedatives)
- Little or no walking or running for exercise
- Poor vision
- Brain disease that affects physical stability or mental capacity

Case Notes

18.5 Which fracture risk factors did Maggie have?

Fractures Are Classified according to the Pattern of the Break

Figure 18.10 illustrates the clinical classification of fractures according to the pattern of the break and whether or not bone has broken through skin. A *closed* fracture is one in which bone has not broken through skin. If bone protrudes through skin, the fracture is *open* or *compound*. A single fracture line is a *simple* fracture. A simple fracture line extending all the way across the bone is a *complete* fracture; otherwise the fracture is *incomplete*. Multiple fractures in a single site form a *comminuted* fracture. Children's bones are more flexible than adults and tend to bend or break partially (incompletely), in a manner known as a *greenstick* fracture. Twisting force can cause a

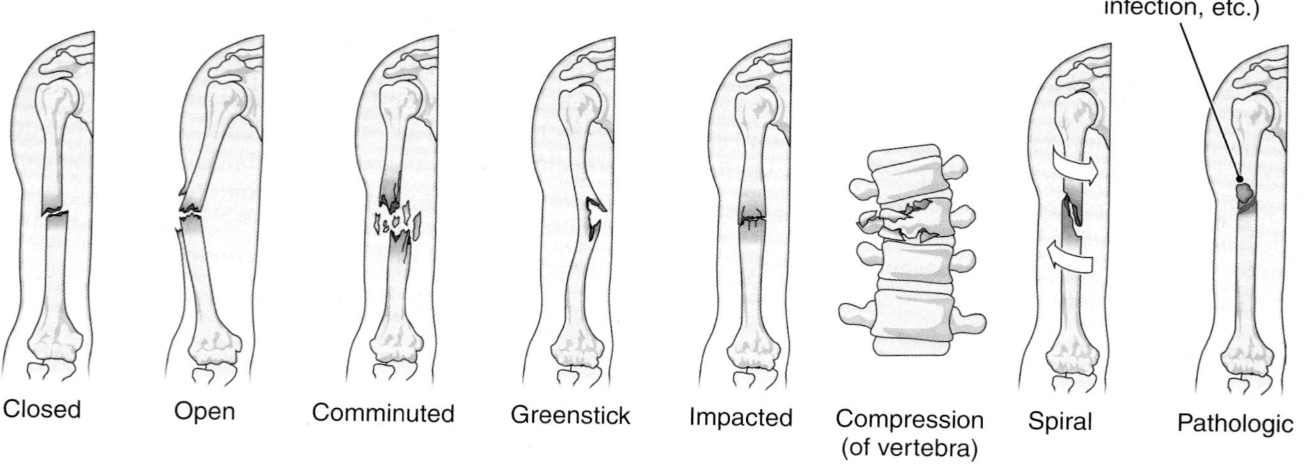

Figure 18.10 **Types of fractures.** A closed fracture is any type of fracture in which the skin is not punctured by broken bone. An open fracture is one with protruding bone. Compression fractures are most common in vertebrae.

spiral fracture. Sudden end-to-end force that causes bone to collapse upon itself is an *impacted* fracture, also called a *compression* fracture (especially in vertebrae).

A **pathologic fracture** is one that results from disease that has weakened bone locally, so that the fracture occurs with normal stress. For example, a patient with a tumor in the femur may suffer a fracture through the lesion while doing something as ordinary as getting out of bed. Most fractures occur suddenly, but *stress* fracture occurs slowly due to repeated microfractures caused by high stress; for example, in the foot of a long-distance runner. Stress fractures do not displace bone, but are painful. Highly stressed bone may become painful and develop a small reparative *callus* (see below) before the fracture occurs.

Case Notes

18.6 **Classify Maggie's fracture of the left ankle.**

Force powerful enough to break bone also can damage nearby tissue. Fractures often are accompanied by injury to muscles, blood vessels, nerves, and ligaments, so that often the amount and degree of bleeding and injury is greater than might be expected from a quick glance at an X-ray image.

Fractures Heal in a Predictable Manner

Figure 18.11 illustrates the healing of a fracture. A hematoma accumulates rapidly (Fig. 18.11A). By the end of the first few days, the repair process is in its **inflammatory phase** (Fig. 18.11B) as fibroblasts, new blood vessels, and woven bone appear. In the second week, new islands of bone appear. During the next few weeks, as new bone continues to appear, the repair process is in its early **reparative phase**. This mixture of granulation tissue (Chapter 2), fibrous tissue, and new islands of bone is called a **soft callus** (Fig. 18.11C), which unites the ends of the broken bone but is not capable of bearing weight. As the reparative phase continues, dead bone is resorbed by osteoclasts and the lesion becomes a **bony callus** (Fig. 18.11D), which forms new spongy and compact bone and is capable of limited weight bearing. As weight-bearing stress continues, the repaired fracture is in the **remodeling phase** (Fig. 18.11E). As new lamellar bone forms in the cortex, it aligns in the long axis and unstressed bone disappears, a process which continues until the healed bone regains most of its normal contour (Fig. 18.8 F).

Case Notes

18.7 **At the end of the first two to four days, in what phase of healing was Maggie's fracture?**

Diseased bone, as with *osteoporosis* or *osteomalacia*, heals poorly. Normal healing of a fracture requires good nourishment. Healing fractures of large bones like the femur can consume a great many calories, a demand that some patients cannot readily meet. For example, alcoholics are notable for fracture-prone behavior and poor diet, and thus their fractures may not heal quickly or well. Adequate intake of vitamin D, phosphate, and calcium are especially important. Impaired vascular supply, as in patients with diabetic microangiopathy, may also impair healing.

Some fractures do not unite bone normally, a condition called *nonunion*, which is characterized by continued motion across the fracture site, and can be due to lack of immobilization, poor blood supply, infection, or poor diet. If this flexible portion of bone functions as a joint, it is called a *pseudarthrosis* (literally, a false joint). If the ends of the fracture are allowed to heal in a nonanatomic alignment, at an angle, for example, the fracture is *misaligned*.

Treatment Requires Alignment, Immobilization, and Stress Relief

Immediate treatment includes analgesia and splinting for immobilization. For open fractures, treatment includes debridement of damaged or contaminated soft tissue and bone and antibiotic therapy. Proper restoration of function requires that the fractured pieces of bone heal while in normal anatomic position. If pieces are displaced or angled improperly, realignment may be necessary, a procedure called **reduction**. This requires manipulation, a painful procedure that usually requires anesthesia. *Closed reduction* (without skin incision) is preferred, but *open reduction (surgical reduction)* may be required. Some fractures require **internal fixation** with plates, pins, screws, or other apparatus. For example, internal fixation is required for fractures across a joint surface, where precise alignment is necessary, or when the prolonged immobility required for healing is not acceptable, (e.g., in hip fractures). Once in proper alignment, the break must be immobilized, usually by extending the cast to encompass the joints above and below the break, (e.g., the ankle and knee for a fractured lower tibia). Stress must also be taken off, usually by a sling, crutches, wheelchair, or other device.

Pop Quiz

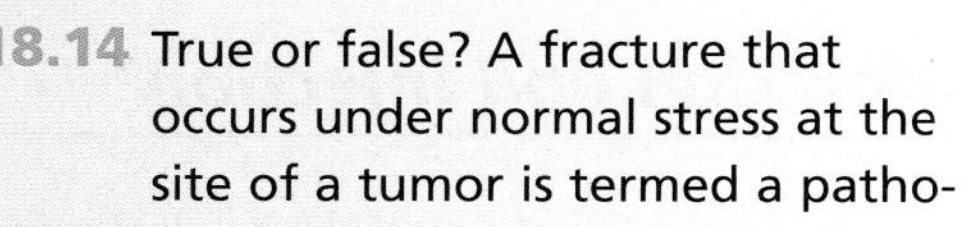

18.14 True or false? A fracture that occurs under normal stress at the site of a tumor is termed a pathologic fracture.

18.15 True or false? A soft callus is weight bearing.

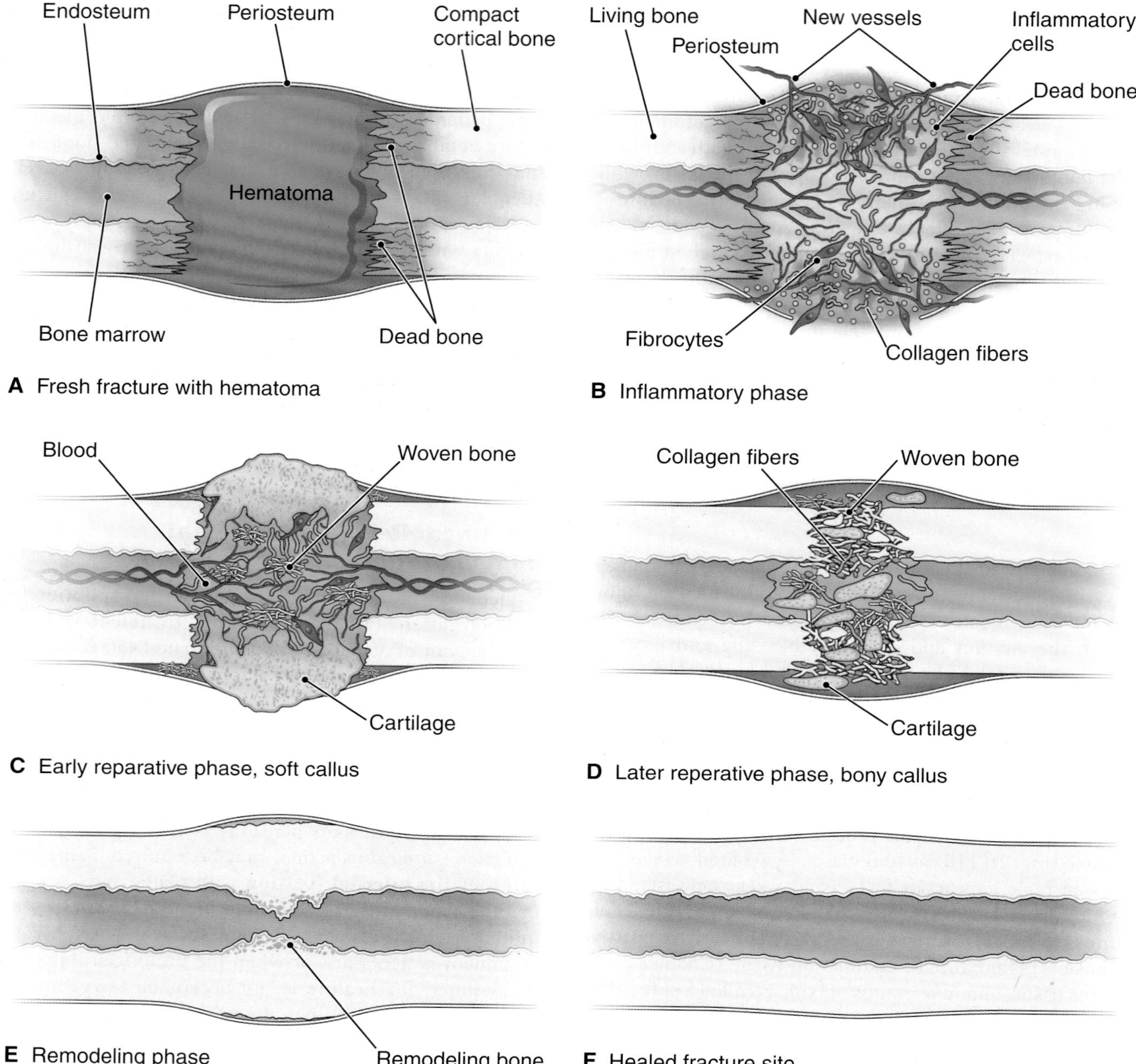

Figure 18.11 **The healing of a fracture (days/weeks/months vary). A.** Day 1, Fresh fracture. A *hematoma* forms. **B.** Days 2–7, *inflammatory phase*. Inflammation, neovascularization, early fibrosis, and initial appearance of woven bone. **C.** Weeks 2–6, *early reparative phase, soft callus*. The callus develops further as Inflammation and granulation tissue fade, woven bone becomes abundant, and cartilage appears at the periphery; **D.** A few months, *later reparative phase, bony callus*. **E.** Later months, *remodeling phase*. Linear stress causes alignment of new bone. Unstressed bone at periphery disappears. Dense lamellar compact bone appears, joining new bone to old; **F.** Years, *healed bone*.

Bone Infarction and Infection

Bone infarction (**osteonecrosis**) is bone death in the absence of infection. It is often called **aseptic necrosis**, a name retained from the preantibiotic era when most bone necrosis was due to bacterial infection, or **avascular necrosis**, which reflects the fact that many bone infarcts are caused by impaired blood flow. Therapeutic steroids are often the cause of bone infarct, but the mechanism is unclear. Other predisposing conditions include fracture with interruption of blood supply, radiation, and sickle cell disease (Chapter 7). In many instances, the cause cannot be related to any event. Some bones are more vulnerable to ischemic necrosis than others: the head of the femur and the carpal bones of the wrist (especially the navicular bone) are more often involved than other bones because of peculiarities of their vascular supply.

Whatever the cause, bone infarcts are mainly a problem of growing children (because rapid bone growth requires a lot of blood), and of the elderly (because vascular disease may impair blood flow). Necrosis of the head of the femur is a special risk in elderly persons following fracture of the femoral neck, and for chronic alcoholics (the mechanism is unclear). Infarcts that involve joints can lead to severe mechanical arthritis (osteoarthritis) as the dead bone within the joint is worn away.

Pain is the usual symptom. Diagnosis is radiographic. Treatment is surgical: debridement, bone graft, or joint replacement.

Osteomyelitis is bacterial infection of bone and bone marrow. Traumatic, direct implantation of bacteria into bone is the main cause of osteomyelitis in adults. In contrast, most children who develop bone infection do so from bloodborne bacteria from minor infections elsewhere in the body, perhaps a skin or tooth infection. Boys ages 5–15 are most often affected. Pyogenic infections are most common but bacteria are often difficult to culture and identify with certainty because many patients have been treated with antibiotics by the time culture is attempted. Nevertheless, *staphylococci* and *streptococci* account for most of the *identifiable* bacteria. The metaphysis is most often the site because it is the most vascular part of bone, especially in growing long bones (knee, ankle, hip).

Vertebral osteomyelitis affects the vertebral body. It appears to begin in the intervertebral disc and spread from one vertebra to another. Staphylococci are the most common culprit. Predisposing factors are intravenous drug abuse, urologic infection or instrumentation, and hematogenous spread from another site.

Osteomyelitis caused by the tuberculosis bacterium (*Mycobacterium tuberculosis*) remains a problem in developing countries. The AIDS epidemic and increased international travel have brought a resurgence of tuberculosis, including tuberculous bone infections, to the United States.

Acute bacterial infection of bone is accompanied by bone necrosis and inflammation. The cause is obvious when infection follows fracture, but, in children, signs and symptoms may prove subtle and diagnosis can be difficult. Pain in the affected area is accompanied by typical signs of infection: malaise, fever, chills, and increased white blood cell count. X-rays typically reveal local loss of bone density (osteolytic lesions). Although usually diagnosed clinically, sometimes acute or chronic osteomyelitis is diagnosed by pathologists on diagnostic biopsy of bone.

Acute bacterial osteomyelitis may prove difficult to treat, and requires vigorous and prolonged antibiotic therapy. Even so, about 5–10% of infections become chronic and can serve as a focus of continuing infection that can spread to other parts of the body to cause, for example, bacterial endocarditis (Chapter 9) or generalized blood stream infection (sepsis). Surgical drainage and wound debridement may be necessary.

Pop Quiz

18.16 What two bones are especially vulnerable to ischemic necrosis?

18.17 Traumatic, direct implantation of bacteria into bone is the main cause of osteomyelitis in children.

Bone Tumors and Tumor-Like Lesions

The most common tumor *in* bone is metastatic cancer. Carcinoma of the prostate, breast, and lung are the three most common malignancies in humans, and all have a predilection for bone metastasis.

Bone tumors have a distinct tendency to occur in certain anatomic sites. For example, of primary bone tumors, 80% occur in the lower femur or upper tibia and fibula near the knee.

About 40% of primary tumors in bone are hematopoietic—multiple myeloma and lymphoma (Chapter 7). Another 40% are evenly divided between bone-forming and cartilage-forming tumors. The remaining 20% are a varied group arising from fibrous, vascular, embryonal, and other cells, some of uncertain origin.

Benign tumors are much more common than malignant ones and occur mainly in patients under age 30. Bone tumors in the elderly usually are malignant. The rarity and diverse histologic appearance of primary bone tumors often makes them difficult for pathologists and radiologists to diagnose correctly.

Excluding hematopoietic tumors, bone tumors fall into four groups reflecting their composition. These are tumors that are predominantly composed of: bone (tumors whose name usually begins with "osteo..."); cartilage ("chondro..."); fibrous tissue ("fibro..."); and a miscellaneous category. As Figure 18.12 illustrates, various bone tumors have distinct affinities for certain age groups, particular bones, or parts of bones.

Clinically, bone tumors present with pain, as a slow-growing mass, or as an unexpected pathologic fracture. X-ray studies are an important part of the diagnostic assessment, but biopsy and pathologic assessment is essential for diagnosis and prognosis.

Some Bone Tumors Form Neoplastic Bone

Benign bone-forming tumors are not premalignant, and are usually small and of little consequence except that they can be painful or, in the skull, may press on nerves or other critical structures.

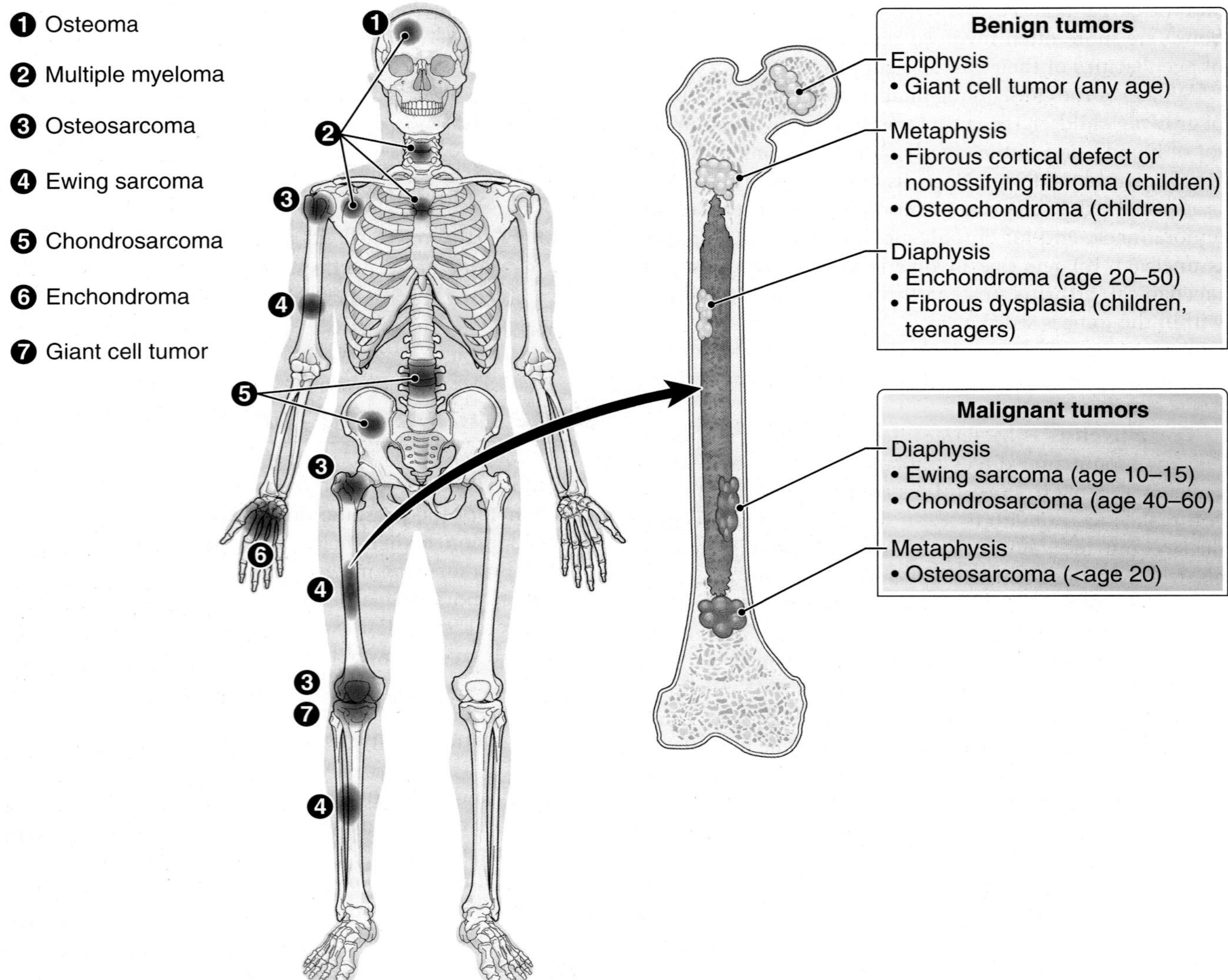

Figure 18.12 **Common sites of primary bone tumors.** The enlarged femur shows that in long bones some tumors tend to occur at particular locations and at certain ages.

Osteoma is usually a small, roundish, sessile benign tumor on the surface of a bone. It is composed of unremarkable bone and is of little consequence except in the skull. **Osteoblastoma** (>2 cm) and **osteoid osteoma** (<2 cm) have similar microscopic features and differ only in size, site, and symptoms. Diagnosis is radiologic. They may be quite painful. Aspirin is especially effective for pain relief. Treatment is radiation or surgical curettage.

Osteosarcoma (*osteogenic sarcoma*) is a malignant tumor that forms neoplastic bone. Excluding tumors of bone marrow, osteosarcoma is the most common primary tumor of bone and occurs most often in the metaphysis of long bones—about half occur in the tibia or femur near the knee—a feature probably related to the fact that the metaphysis is where bones grow and where most cell division takes place. Two age groups are most affected: 75% occur in patients under 20, and most of the remainder occur in the elderly, many of whom have some underlying condition such as Paget disease or bone irradiation received in the treatment of another condition.

Osteosarcoma usually presents as a painful, enlarging mass. Diagnosis is radiologic and pathologic. It spreads by the bloodstream and about 20% of patients have lung metastases at time of initial diagnosis. Surgery and chemotherapy cure about two-thirds of patients who do not have detectable metastases at time of diagnosis.

Some Bone Tumors Form Neoplastic Cartilage

At one time, *osteochondroma* and *enchondroma* were thought to be benign cartilaginous neoplasms, but they are now understood to be defects of bone growth.

Chondrosarcoma (Fig. 18.13) is a malignant tumor of bone that forms neoplastic cartilage. It occurs about half

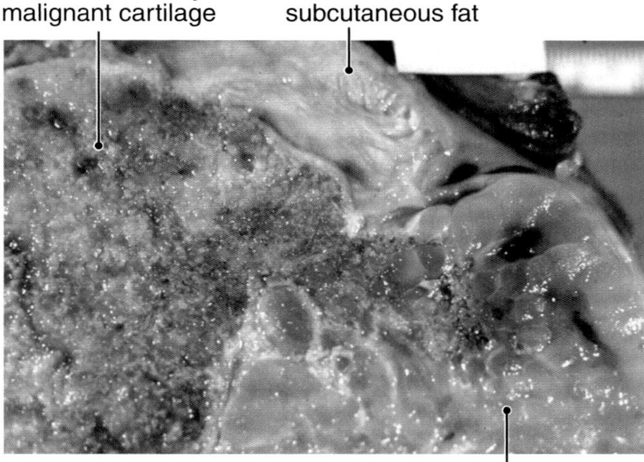

Figure 18.13 **Chondrosarcoma of the sternum.** Most chondrosarcomas arise in the central skeleton (pelvis, spine, shoulder girdle, and rib cage).

as frequently as osteosarcoma and is the second most common primary malignant tumor of bone. It favors the spine, ribs, pelvis, and vertebrae and occurs most commonly in adults ages 40–60. Like osteosarcoma, microscopic grade is of paramount importance in predicting tumor behavior. Fortunately, most are low grade (well differentiated), sluggish tumors for which the five-year survival is about 80%. For high-grade (poorly differentiated) tumors, the survival rate is about 40%. Wide excision is the treatment of choice; chemotherapy is not effective.

Some Bone Tumors Form Fibrous Tissue

Fibrous cortical defect (FCD) (small) and **nonossifying fibroma (NOF)** (large) are tumorlike developmental defects that differ only in size. FCDs are usually <1 cm and solitary and occur in the metaphysis of 30–50% of children over the age of two years. They are discovered incidentally. Diagnosis of FCD is radiologic. No therapy is required. NOF is a larger version, usually several cm in diameter. It may be discovered as a mass or because it causes pain or pathologic fracture. Diagnosis is radiologic and pathologic. Surgery is necessary to restore bone integrity and to differentiate it from bone neoplasms.

Fibrous dysplasia is a benign, nodular growth of fibrous and bone tissue that affects growing bones in children and teenagers. It is probably a developmental abnormality—all components of normal bone are present but they do not grow in a coordinated manner into mature bone. Instead, they produce tumorlike masses of bone in a fibrous matrix. The most troublesome clinical problems are disfigurement and fracture. *Monostotic* fibrous dysplasia affects a single bone and accounts for three-fourths of cases. *Polyostotic* fibrous dysplasia affects multiple bones, especially the face and skull, and may be associated with pigmented skin lesions and endocrine abnormalities. Diagnosis is radiologic and pathologic. Most patients require multiple corrective orthopedic surgeries. Bisphosphonates are useful in diminishing bone pain.

Fibrosarcoma is a malignant tumor of fibrocytes and can occur in bone or soft tissue. It usually presents as a painful mass and requires biopsy diagnosis and surgical excision.

Other Types of Tumors Arise in Bone

Aneurysmal bone cyst is not a tumor but forms tumorlike masses in the metaphysis of long bones of children and youth. The cause is unknown. It is composed of large, richly vascular cysts containing pools of blood, which expand and erode normal bone and may become quite large. Diagnosis is radiologic. Treatment is surgical.

Giant cell tumor (*osteoclastoma*) of bone derives its name from the fact that it contains large cells with multiple nuclei (giant cells), which have a microscopic appearance similar to normal osteoclasts. They are rather uncommon but are important because they can be locally aggressive. Most occur near the knee in the epiphysis of the femur or tibia. They can be locally destructive and may present as a pathologic fracture. Diagnosis is radiologic and pathologic. Surgical curettage cures about half, but others recur and require additional surgery. A few metastasize to lung.

Ewing sarcoma is a malignant tumor on a spectrum with varying degrees of primitive neuroectodermal differentiation that accounts for 5–10% of malignant bone tumors. It most often arises in the medullary cavity of the femur or pelvis in children younger than age 15. It occurs almost solely in Caucasians. Ewing sarcoma may present as a painful mass, but some patients have fever, leukocytosis, increased sedimentation rate and C-reactive protein (CRP), and other signs that initially suggest infection. Diagnosis is radiologic and pathologic. Treatment includes surgery, radiation, and chemotherapy. With proper treatment, about 75% survive five years.

Multiple myeloma (Chapter 3) and **malignant lymphoma** (Chapter 7) are hematopoietic neoplasms. They are also the most common neoplasms arising in bone. They are discussed in previous chapters.

Common laboratory tests are a useful aid in the differential diagnosis of diseases of bones, joints, muscles, and related tissues. Table 18.2 offers a short list of useful tests.

Pop Quiz

18.18 True or false? The majority of tumors affecting bone occur near the knee.

18.19 What are the Latin stems for tumors made up of bone? Cartilage? Fibrous tissue?

Table 18.2 Common Laboratory Blood Tests in Musculoskeletal Disease

Test Type	Primary Disease Association	Comments
TO DETECT INFLAMMATION		
Erythrocyte sedimentation rate (ESR)	Inflammation anywhere in the body	Increased in infection, autoimmune disease, polymyalgia rheumatica (PMR), some malignancies, anemia, pregnancy, renal failure. Low in some diseases of red blood cells. Normal in fibromyalgia.
C-reactive protein (CRP)	Inflammation anywhere in the body	Increased in same conditions as increased ESR (except for patients with anemia). Also increased in atherosclerosis. Normal in fibromyalgia.
TO DETECT BONE DISEASE		
Alkaline phosphatase (AP)	Osteomalacia, bone tumors and metastases, Paget disease of bone, hyperparathyroidism	Hepatic or biliary disease, normal bone growth, late in pregnancy (from placenta)
TO DETECT DISEASE OF JOINTS AND RELATED TISSUES		
Antinuclear antibody (ANA)	Positive in 95% of patients with systemic lupus erythematosus	Also can be positive due to rheumatoid arthritis (RA), scleroderma, Sjögren syndrome, certain therapeutic drugs
Rheumatoid factor (RF)	Positive in about 70% of patients with RA	Also can be positive due to other autoimmune diseases
TO DETECT MUSCLE DISEASE		
Creatine kinase (CK)	Myositis, myopathy, trauma	Also can be positive due to severe muscular exertion, seizures, heat stroke, myocardial infarction

Case Study Revisited

"You'd think I'd crashed a motorcycle." The case of Maggie H.

Maggie's case is representative of a large population of small-frame Caucasian, postmenopausal women who develop osteoporosis and suffer fractures. Fitness was important in her uneventful recovery. Had she been older and less fit, she might have become bedfast and been put at risk for pneumonia, thromboembolism, and other complications. Lack of estrogen was certainly a factor in her osteoporosis, but she rejected long-term hormone replacement therapy because of her family history of breast cancer. Vitamin D, calcium, and bisphosphonates should stabilize her osteoporosis but will not substantially reverse it.

Section 3: Disorders of Joints and Soft Tissues

The joint lubrication was not what it was when I was competing, and I decided that not having arthritis or rheumatism for the rest of my life was a lot more important to me than returning to the track.

EDWIN MOSES (B. 1955), LEGENDARY AMERICAN TRACK AND FIELD ATHLETE, EXPLAINING WHY HE CHOSE NOT TO RETURN TO COMPETITION AFTER RETIRING

Case Study

"I'm just a bucket of problems." The case of Raynelle C.

Chief Complaint: Aching pains of the neck, shoulders, chest, hips, and knees

Clinical History: Raynelle C. was a 43-year-old woman, a carpenter and Colorado mountain fishing guide in the summer, and a ski resort real estate saleswoman in the winter. During a lunch break while guiding her personal physician on a day of fly-fishing, she began asking questions about the pains she had been having. She related that, since the previous summer, she had been having aching pains in the back of her neck, in her upper chest and shoulders, and around her hips and knees. The pain was not related to activity and was not relieved by rest. "I hurt all the time," she said.

In response to questions, she reported numbness and increased sensitivity to touch in her extremities and added that her hands felt stiff each morning until she loosened them up, but said she had not had any weight loss, nor did she have fever or swollen joints. She confessed that she worried a lot about her husband's real estate business and their personal finances, and was not sleeping well. She also complained of being tired all the time.

"Well," the physician said, "this is not something we can solve on a fishing trip. Call the office tomorrow and we'll get to the bottom of this." They finished the trip uneventfully.

The physician saw Raynelle later in the week.

"I'm tired all the time," she sighed. "No wonder; I'm not sleeping very well. Sometimes I feel stiff as a zombie and I'm sore all over. I feel blue most of the time and sometimes I just don't want to get out of bed. I'm irritable, too. I seem to fly off the handle with my husband at the smallest things. I'm just a bucket of problems," she said.

Further questioning revealed no history of recent illness. Systems review was unremarkable. Family history revealed that her parents, aunts, uncles, and two adult children were alive and healthy. There was no history of RA, headache, or insect bites. Her grandparents on both sides lived into their 80s and 90s. She did not know how they died.

Physical Examination and Other Data: Vital signs and blood pressure were unremarkable. She was of average height and a very fit, lean woman who appeared her stated age. No lymphadenopathy was present. Her skin showed no rash or hemorrhage. Her muscle strength was normal. There were no enlarged lymph nodes, rashes, joint abnormalities, or masses. Neurological exam was normal. Her temporal artery was not painful or nodular. Despite complaining of stiff hands and other joints, her joints were normally flexible and motion caused no pain.

The most outstanding abnormality was tenderness to touch, sometimes to the point of jumpiness, in the muscles and tendons at the base of her skull and neck, shoulders, low paraspinal muscles, and around her knees and elbows. Her joints were not swollen or tender to manipulation. Upper arm, buttocks, thighs, and calf muscles were not tender to a firm squeeze.

Laboratory tests were ordered and included CBC, blood chemistries, RF, ANA, CRP, CK, hepatitis C antibody, thyroid hormones, Lyme disease antibody, and ESR.

She was referred for X-rays of her hands and spine.

Clinical Course: She returned two weeks later for follow-up. X-rays and all laboratory tests were normal.

The physician concluded she probably had *fibromyalgia* and prescribed a short, low dose course of steroids as a diagnostic test. Her failure to improve confirmed the diagnosis. The physician outlined a program of regular gym visits for moderate exercise and stretching; NSAIDs, heat and massage for pain; and antidepressants and sedatives to improve sleep.

She responded fairly well. Pain lessened but did not disappear and she continued to work. Her mood and sleep improved, and she became less "jumpy" on physical examination.

Case Notes

18.8 **Raynelle complained of pain in her neck. What type of joint is present between vertebral bodies in her neck?**

Arthritis

By its very name, *arthritis* ("itis") is a disease of joint inflammation. Nevertheless, the most common variety of arthritis (*osteoarthritis*) is not an inflammatory disease. A better definition is that **arthritis** is a painful joint condition associated with joint abnormalities.

Osteoarthritis Is Caused by Mechanical Wear-and-Tear

Osteoarthritis (*degenerative joint disease*) features progressive, noninflammatory erosion of joint cartilage (Fig. 18.14). It is the most common type of arthritis. Although the suffix "itis" implies an inflammatory condition, in fact inflammation is not present in osteoarthritic joints.

Primary osteoarthritis is osteoarthritis that cannot be attributed to some specific circumstance, such as the osteoarthritis that can occur in the hands of people operating vibrating machinery, those doing repetitive tasks that stress joints, or in the knees of the obese or those who repeatedly carry heavy loads. Although mechanical factors are important in the production of all osteoarthritis, they are not the sole factors. For example, osteoarthritis tends to occur in the last joint of the fingers near the tip (the distal interphalangeal joint), a joint that gets little mechanical stress. Indeed, in patients with arthritis of the hands, involvement of the distal interphalangeal joint of the hands is a key diagnostic point that suggests osteoarthritis instead of some other diagnosis such as RA. Primary osteoarthritis occurs with increasing frequency with each decade of life; it mainly affects weight-bearing joints, especially the hip, knee, and spine; mechanical stress is clearly the cause in most cases.

Secondary osteoarthritis can be produced by the abnormal stress on a joint—obesity is a major cause. It is also due to repeated harsh physical activity—it occurs in the knees of professional football players; from physical malformations that create abnormal joint stress, such as the osteoarthritis in the lower limbs of persons with an abnormal gait due to neuromuscular diseases; or in the joints of people with peripheral nerve disease, who cannot feel pain in their joints and traumatize their joints without realizing it (as is the case in the lower limbs of patients with diabetic peripheral neuropathy (Chapter 13).

Pathophysiology

Pathological changes in most cases of osteoarthritis are minimal: they rarely show inflammation except in advanced cases, a fact that reinforces the idea that wear and tear is the cause. Cartilage, which contains no nerves, becomes thin, frayed, or completely worn away and bone surfaces, which are rich in nerves, begin to rub painfully against each other. The irritated bone surfaces become dense and sclerotic, with a hard, ivory-like surface. Figure 18.15A illustrates that striking changes may develop in advanced disease as further stress and degeneration produces subcompact bone cysts and jagged growth of new bone (*joint spurs* or *osteophytes*) that project into adjacent soft tissue and cause inflammation, swelling, and pain.

Signs and Symptoms

The most important clinical characteristic of osteoarthritis is that *activity-related* joint pain is *relieved by a short rest*, whereas the pain of most other types of arthritis lasts an

Articular cartilage worn away
Sclerotic bone
Normal layer of articular cartilage
Normal bone

A Apex of femur head

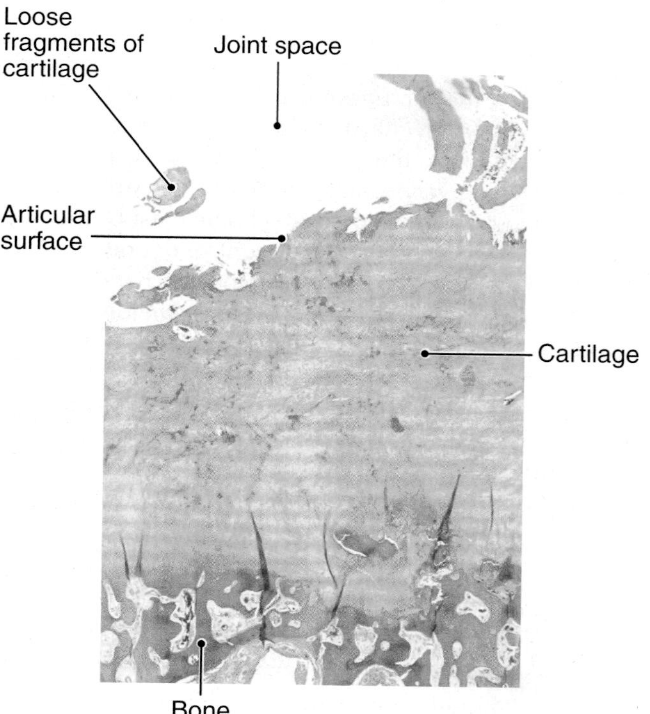

B Microscopic study

Figure 18.14 **Osteoarthritis. A.** Superior surface of the head of the femur. The normal cap of articular cartilage is worn and the underlying bone is dense and sclerotic. **B.** Cartilage damage in osteoarthritis. The articular surface is jagged and torn from mechanical force. Note that no inflammation is present.

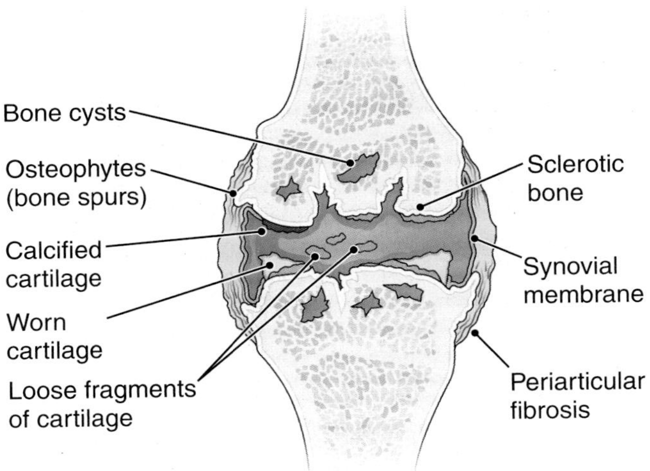

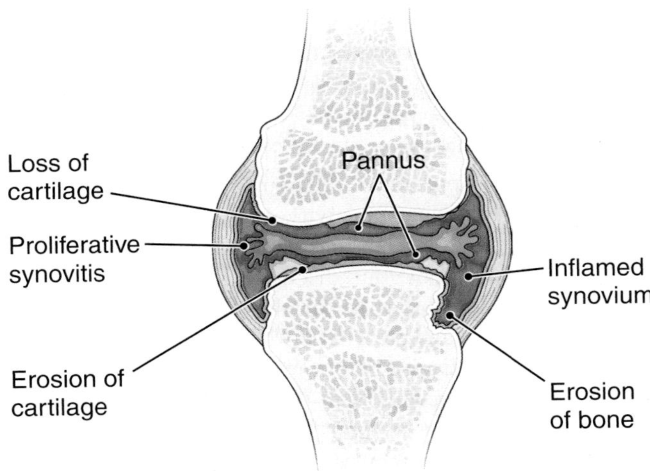

Figure 18.15 **Joint changes in arthritis. A.** Osteoarthritis. Cartilage and bone damage; no inflammation is present. **B.** RA. The joint capsule (synovial membrane) is inflamed and a pannus of inflammatory tissue has formed across the articular surface.

hour or so despite rest. In osteoarthritis, joint motion may produce a grinding effect (*crepitus*) as rough edges of bone and cartilage grate across one another. Early diagnosis is difficult and entirely based on the clinical findings discussed above; X-ray and laboratory findings are minimal. Aspirated joint fluid shows no bacteria, and very few, if any, inflammatory cells. In advanced disease, X-rays show a narrowing of the joint space due to cartilage destruction and sclerosis of bone on either side of the joint; bone cysts and spurs also may be present. The swollen distal interphalangeal joints of the hands can be quite prominent and are known as *Heberden nodes*. Joints most affected are the hip, knee, and cervical and lumbar spine. The most commonly affected joint in the foot is the joint where the big toe joins the foot (first metatarsophalangeal joint), which enlarges and forces the big toe laterally into the other toes (*bunion* deformity).

Diagnosis is clinical and radiologic. Occupational and physical therapy and NSAIDs are the mainstays of therapy. Joint surgery may be necessary to remove bone spurs or repair or remove torn cartilage, or to replace the entire joint, an option increasingly used for severe osteoarthritis of the knee.

Case Notes

18.9 Why was Raynelle's problem not likely to be osteoarthritis?

Rheumatoid Arthritis Is a Systemic Autoimmune Disease Involving Synovial Joints

Rheumatoid arthritis (RA) (Fig. 18.15 B) is a chronic, systemic autoimmune disease that involves mainly synovial joints, but which regularly affects other tissues. About 1–2% of the U.S. adult population is affected. In contrast to osteoarthritis, joints are intensely inflamed. Women are affected two to three times more often than men. The root cause of RA is unknown, but evidence suggests that a virus or other agent triggers a T lymphocyte autoimmune reaction that attacks the synovial membrane. A familial tendency is present—about 75% of RA patients have similar HLA genes (Chapter 3).

Remember This! Eighty percent of RA occurs in women.

Etiology and Pathogenesis

Again, the exact cause of the autoimmune reaction in RA is not known, but viruses are suspected and there is a definite genetic predisposition. The autoimmune reaction is mainly due to T lymphocytes. Nevertheless, B lymphocytes also play a role—about 75% of patients with RA have in their blood **rheumatoid factor (RF)**, a circulating antibody complex. Laboratory detection of RF is very helpful but not required to establish a diagnosis of RA. RF can also be found in some patients with hepatitis B infection or other autoimmune disease.

The inflammatory reaction stimulates growth of blood vessels and fibrous tissue into the synovium and joint cartilage. As a result, a highly vascular inflammatory membrane (a **pannus**, from the Hebrew word for "blanket" or "bed covering") forms over the cartilage surface (Fig. 18.15 B), and oozes destructive enzymes and other agents that dissolve the cartilaginous plate. The inflammatory reaction also stimulates a papillary overgrowth of the synovium known as *proliferative synovitis*. The end result may be complete destruction of the joint, which can undergo fibrous repair that welds together the ends of the bones to produce an immovable joint (**ankylosis**).

Signs and Symptoms

Especially characteristic of RA are two unique clinical conditions. First is deviation of the bones of the hand toward the radial side of the arm, which is accompanied by deviation of the fingers in the opposite (ulnar) direction to produce the classic **Z deformity** of the hand (Fig. 18.16). Second, about 30% of patients will ultimately develop **rheumatoid nodules** (Fig. 18.17), which are painless 1–2 cm subcutaneous inflammatory nodules not found in other forms of arthritis.

The clinical course of RA is quite variable: it waxes and wanes; it may strike young or old, and it may be mild or crippling. It is usually symmetrical and begins in small joints. It appears first in patients in their 30s and 40s, and begins subtly with low grade fever, malaise, and early morning joint pain and stiffness. The most commonly affected joints are where the fingers meet the hand (the metacarpophalangeal joint) and the next joint in the finger (the proximal interphalangeal joint), the wrist, elbow, shoulder, and ankle, but any joint may be involved. Severe disease of vertebral joints can be especially painful, stiffening, and debilitating.

RA also affects tissues other than joints. Heart (myocarditis and pericarditis), blood vessels (vasculitis and infarcts), eyes (scleritis), skin (subcutaneous rheumatoid nodules), lungs (interstitial fibrosis and pleuritis), and skeletal muscle (myositis) are notably susceptible, but no tissue is protected.

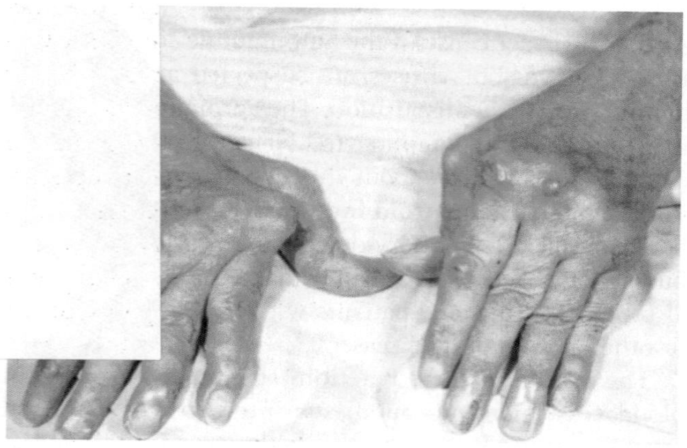

Figure 18.16 Rheumatoid arthritis. The fingers are deviated laterally (toward the ulna, away from the viewer) as part of the typical "Z" deformity of chronic RA. (Reproduced with permission from Rubin E. *Pathology*. 3rd ed. Philadelphia, (PA). Lippincott Williams and Wilkins; 1999).

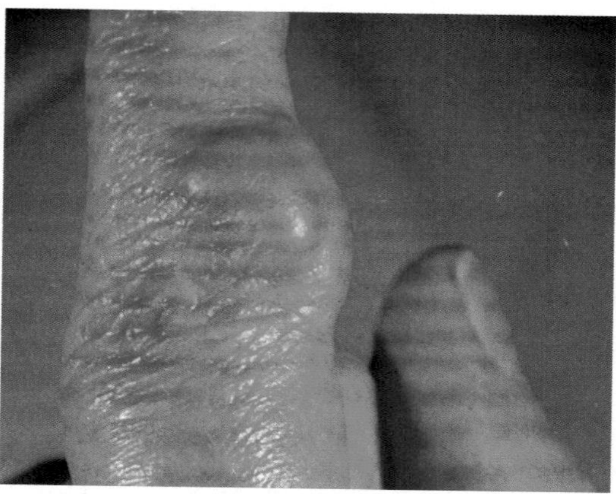

Figure 18.17 Rheumatoid nodule. Rheumatoid nodules are diagnostic of RA when found in patients with other clinical features suggesting RA. (Reproduced with permission from Rubin E. *Pathology*. 4th ed. Philadelphia, (PA). Lippincott Williams and Wilkins; 2005).

Diagnosis, Treatment, and Prognosis

Diagnosis of RA is mainly a clinical exercise that depends little on laboratory tools. Radiographic findings in joints are often distinctive. History and physical examination are of paramount importance. Joints are swollen, warm, painful, and stiff following inactivity. Joint fluid should show chronic inflammatory cells and be free of bacteria and uric acid crystals (a sign of gout, discussed below). Rheumatoid nodules and detection of RF in blood confirm the clinical diagnosis if they are present, but their absence does not exclude RA as a diagnosis in a patient with arthritis. *Anti-cyclic citrullinated peptide (anti-CCP)* is a newly discovered autoantibody present in about half of RA patients, even in the earliest stages of disease. It is more specific than RF and if detected is diagnostic.

Case Notes

18.10 Why was Raynelle's problem likely not to be RA?

Early diagnosis (less than three months from first symptoms) is especially important because immediate, vigorous drug therapy plus physical therapy pay big dividends in the long run. Treatment is aimed at pain relief, suppression of inflammation, and maintenance of joint range of motion. Historically, the most important drugs have been aspirin and other NSAIDs and steroids; recently however, pharmacologically produced antibodies (e.g., *infliximab*), which block natural inflammatory molecules, have proven effective.

The disease usually progresses to a disabling arthritis over a decade or two as pannus formation erodes joint cartilage and underlying bone. Despite sometimes crippling deformity, average life span is reduced only about five years. Fatalities can be due to treatment: GI hemorrhage from chronic administration of aspirin and nonsteroidal anti-inflammatory drugs, or infection associated with chronic steroid therapy.

Some patients with severe chronic inflammatory disease, including RA, may develop **secondary amyloidosis** (Chapter 3) due to deposition in various tissues of breakdown products of antibody immunoglobulin.

Juvenile Idiopathic Arthritis Affects Youth

Formerly known as *juvenile rheumatoid arthritis*, **juvenile idiopathic arthritis (JIA)** is any arthritis arising in someone less than 16 years old that persists for six weeks. It differs from RA in several important ways. It more often involves one or few joints; it more often features acute, systemic "toxic" onset; it more often affects large joints; rheumatoid nodules and RF are usually absent; and ANA are more often present.

Some patients have explosive onset (**Still disease**) with fever, skin rash, hepatosplenomegaly, and polyserositis (inflammation of pleura, peritoneum, and pericardium). Some young males present with tendinitis of the tendons that attach skeletal muscle to bone in the lower extremities (*enthesitis*).

The majority of patients recover fully; few develop chronic arthritis. Treatment is similar to therapy for RA.

Spondyloarthropathies Affect the Spine

The vertebrae are complex bones, each of which articulate with one another and with the ribs by several joints. The term **spondyloarthropathy** derives from Greek *spondylos*, meaning vertebra, and describes several related types of autoimmune, genetically influenced, vertebral arthritis that occur in patients who *do not have a specific antibody in their blood*; that is to say, they are *seronegative*.

They are distinct from RA in the following ways:

1. Arthritis is usually confined to the synovial joints of the vertebral articular processes and the sacroiliac joints.
2. Inflammation also involves tendons where they attach to bone.
3. RF, ANA, and other antibodies are absent from blood.
4. The cells of most patients carry HLA-B27 antigen.

The following spondyloarthropathies share overlapping clinical features: the majority of patients are young adults; males are affected much more often than females; infection seems to trigger the onset of disease; and many patients have extra-articular inflammatory conditions such as iritis (Chapter 20) or vasculitis (Chapter 8).

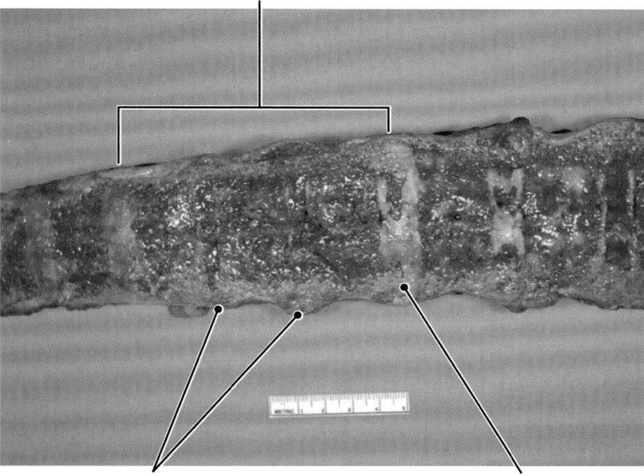

Figure 18.18 **Ankylosing spondylitis**. Two intervertebral discs have been destroyed and three vertebrae are fused into a single mass.

- **Ankylosing spondylitis** (*rheumatoid spondylitis, Marie-Strümpell disease*) is a chronic relapsing arthritis primarily affecting the joints of the vertebral processes of the spine (Fig. 18.18), and especially the sacroiliac joints. Most patients are men who suffer from spinal rigidity and chronic back pain but otherwise usually lead full lives. Almost all patients are HLA-B27 positive.
- **Reiter syndrome** is reactive arthritis, defined as a syndrome of arthritis, nongonococcal urethritis or cervicitis, and conjunctivitis. Most patients are men in their 20s or 30s. Most are HLA-B27 positive. It tends to appear in the wake of *Chlamydia* infection in the urinary tract or gastrointestinal infection by *Shigella*, *Salmonella*, *Yersinia*, or *Campylobacter*. Low back, ankles, knees, and feet are most often involved. Some patients develop extra-articular problems that may include cardiac valve disease and arrhythmias. The clinical course varies greatly.
- **Enteritis-associated arthritis** is similar to Reiter syndrome. It follows GI infection but does not feature conjunctivitis or urethritis. It usually disappears after a year. A few patients develop ankylosing spondylitis.
- **Psoriatic arthritis** is seen in about 10% of patients with psoriasis (Chapter 21). The small joints of the hands and feet are usually first affected, but the spine and sacroiliac joints are often involved later. Some patients develop iritis and conjunctivitis.

Diagnosis includes radiographic imaging of the lower back, ESR and CRP, and presence of clinical criteria. Treatment includes NSAIDs, exercise, and supportive measures. Some patients benefit from methotrexate, a cancer chemotherapy drug that inhibits cell metabolism.

There Are Many Other Types of Arthritis

Joints are affected primarily or secondarily by a great number of conditions, too many to discuss here. Below are brief discussions of several examples of other types of arthritis.

Gout

Primary **gout** is a chronic metabolic disease associated with high blood uric acid levels; joint deposits of uric acid crystals; and inflammatory, nodular subcutaneous deposits (*tophi*) of uric acid crystals. Uric acid crystals are sharp and incite intense inflammation, which causes a severe acute and chronic relapsing arthritis. The kidney excretes uric acid, which, when it causes renal deposits of urate crystals, may result in renal failure. There is a strong familial tendency but no genetic defect has been proven.

Gout can also be *secondary* to other conditions. Because the kidney excretes uric acid and under special circumstances may not be able to keep up with the load, blood uric acid may rise very high. In some instances, renal failure is to blame. In others, the cause is increased production of uric acid occasioned by metabolism of the large amounts of DNA derived from the nuclei of dead malignant cells in patients with leukemia and lymphoma.

About 80% of gout occurs in men. The great toe is affected in 90% of cases and is such a distinctive finding that it has its own name: *podagra* (from the Greek root *pod* for foot, as in *pod*iatrist, a specialist in foot diseases, and *agra*, meaning trapped or seized; thus a short way of saying "foot seizure"). Acute gouty arthritis is characterized by severe inflammation and affected joints are exquisitely tender. Other joints in the feet and hands are also affected. Chronic, deforming arthritis may occur in some patients. Uric acid stones may cause renal colic and obstruction—about 20% of those with chronic gout die of renal failure. High serum uric acid accelerates atherosclerosis; patients with gout have a high incidence of cardiovascular disease.

Diagnosis is clinical. Treatment includes drugs to increase renal uric acid excretion, and dietary modification—uric acid is derived from purines, a type of organic chemical found in high concentration in animal and fish flesh and certain other foods, consumption of which can aggravate pre-existing gout. Alcohol inhibits renal excretion and also should be avoided.

Acute Septic Arthritis

Acute septic arthritis is uncommon. In adults, the most common organism is the gonococcus, *Neisseria gonorrhoeae*—about 5% of patients with untreated genital gonorrhea will develop acute, septic gonococcal arthritis. Most patients have clear risk factors: for example, patients on corticosteroid therapy or patients with immune disease, which are associated with weakened immune resistance to infection; or intravenous drug abuse or infected intravenous lines or catheters, which introduce bacteria into the blood stream. Patients with RA are particularly at risk because they frequently are debilitated, they often are on steroid drugs, and the rich vascularity of their inflamed joints is a natural seedbed for deposits of bloodborne bacteria. Another well-defined group at risk for acute septic arthritis is children who have a bacterial infection elsewhere in the body—middle ear infection, for example—and seed a joint with bloodborne bacteria. Half are affected children who are younger than two years old, and, in most cases, only a single joint is involved.

Diagnosis is clinical. Antibiotics are the mainstay of therapy.

Lyme Disease

Arthritis is a prominent feature of late-stage **Lyme disease**, a summer and fall bacterial infection caused by *Borrelia burgdorferi*, a corkscrew-like bacterium (spirochete) that is spread from rodents to humans via the bite of a deer tick. The tick is difficult to find because it is unusually small and may burrow deeply into genital, axillary, or scalp skin (Fig. 18.19A). Most cases occur in a band of states from Massachusetts to Maryland; another cluster occurs in Wisconsin and Minnesota; another in California and Oregon.

In most cases, the tick must be attached for at least 36 hours before the spirochete can be transmitted. Transmission is followed by spread of the organism throughout the body and is accompanied by fever, enlarged lymph nodes near the bite, and an expanding, annular rash with a clear center (*erythema migrans,* Fig. 18.19B), which resembles a target and is diagnostic to a skilled observer. A majority of untreated patients develop arthritis within a month to two years. Arthritis is the dominant feature of chronic infection, but meningitis and myocarditis may also occur. Established arthritis may not respond to antibiotic treatment because of infection-induced autoimmunity.

Lyme disease is often suspected in patients with rashes, fevers, aches, pains, and fatigue that arise in the summer or autumn; however, infection is difficult to prove. Lab tests for anti-*Borrelia* antibodies may be helpful but false positives are common. Treatment is with broad-spectrum antibiotics.

Case Notes

18.11 Why was Raynelle's condition not likely to be Lyme disease?

Polymyalgia Rheumatica

Polymyalgia rheumatica (PMR) and *giant cell arteritis* (*GCA, temporal arteritis*) are probably different manifestations of the same condition, but etiology and pathogenesis are unknown. PMR is the more common of the two.

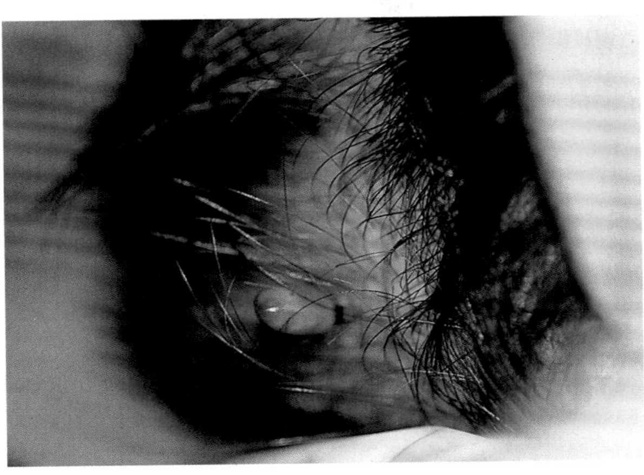

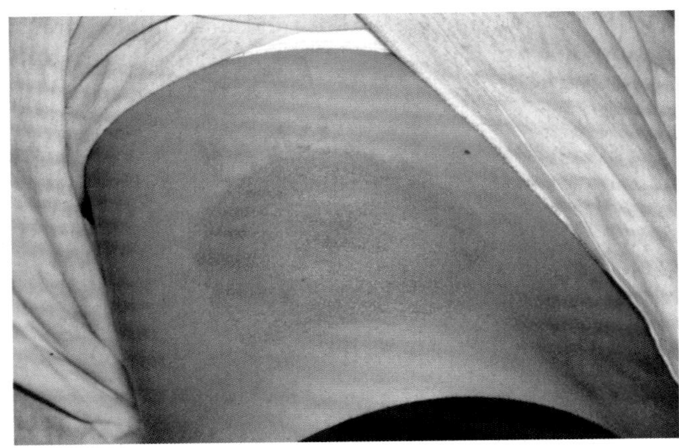

Figure 18.19 **Lyme disease. A.** Deer tick embedded in the scalp. **B.** Erythema migrans. The target-like appearance is distinctive and diagnostic. The lesion may continue to expand and become quite large. (**A.** Reproduced with permission from Fleisher GR, Ludwig S, Baskin MN. *Atlas of Pediatric Emergency Medicine*. Philadelphia, (PA): Lippincott Williams & Wilkins; 2004; **B.** Reproduced with permission from Goodheart HP. *Goodheart's Photoguide of Common Skin Disorders*. 2nd ed. Philadelphia, (PA): Lippincott Williams & Wilkins; 2003.)

A few patients with PMR develop GCA, an autoimmune vasculitis that most often affects the temporal and cranial arteries of elderly women (Chapter 8). About half of patients with GCA will develop PMR.

PMR features aching pain and stiffness in the shoulders, neck, and hips that may be associated with stiffness. Discomfort is worse in the morning. Provable arthritis—a swollen joint, for example—is absent. PMR must be distinguished from arthritis and inflammatory diseases of muscle. The diagnosis is confirmed by finding an increased CRP or ESR (clear indication that inflammation is present), and by the absence of increased muscle enzymes in blood, which, if present, would suggest inflammatory disease of muscle. PMR differs from RA by the absence of significant joint abnormalities and absence of RF.

Diagnosis is clinical. Patients with PMR respond very well to steroid therapy; failure to respond suggests another diagnosis. In patients with GCA, early diagnosis and steroid treatment is necessary to avoid possible blindness or stroke from vascular occlusion.

Case Notes

18.11 **Why was Raynelle's condition not likely PMR**

Pop Quiz

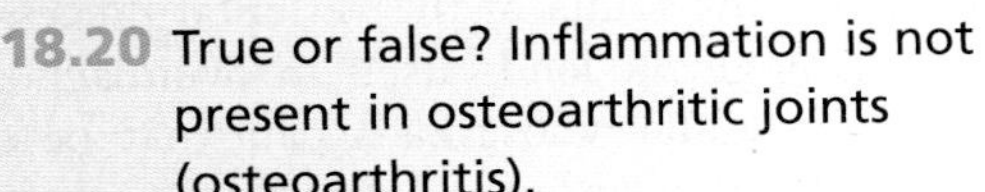

18.20 True or false? Inflammation is not present in osteoarthritic joints (osteoarthritis).

18.21 True or false? A negative test for RF rules out RA.

18.22 What new autoantibody is present in half of RA patients, and more specific than RF?

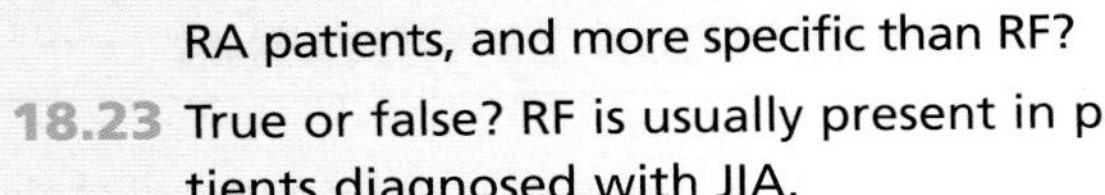

18.23 True or false? RF is usually present in patients diagnosed with JIA.

18.24 True or false? The cells of most patients with seronegative spondyloarthropathies carry HLA-B27 antigen.

18.25 True or false? The treatment of choice for seronegative spondyloarthropathies is infliximab.

18.26 True or false? Podagra is present in 90% of gout cases.

18.27 True or false? The most common cause of acute septic arthritis in adults is *Chlamydia*.

18.28 What species of bacteria is responsible for Lyme disease?

Injuries to Joints and Periarticular Tissues

Dislocation is displacement of one bone in a joint such that the articular surfaces no longer meet. **Subluxation** is a lesser degree of separation. Both usually are due to trauma and can be associated with injury to adjacent soft tissue and joint ligaments and cartilage.

Joint cartilage, ligaments, and tendons may be torn when a joint is forced to move through a greater than normal range of motion. Sports knee and ankle injuries are especially common causes of torn ligaments, tendons, and cartilage. A **sprain** is an injury to a *ligament* induced by stretching it too far. The same injury to a *tendon* is a **strain**. The injury may completely tear the ligament or tendon or pull it away from its attachment (*avulsion*) and require surgical reattachment. Severe tears are accompanied by hemorrhage and swelling. Minor sprains and strains are tender and painful but no hemorrhage or swelling occurs.

Diagnosis is clinical. RICE—rest, ice, compression, and elevation—is the mainstay of treatment. Surgery may be necessary.

Pop Quiz

18.29 A __________ is an injury to a *ligament* induced by stretching it too far; a ________ is an injury to a tendon by stretching it too far.

Figure 18.20 **Herniated intervertebral disc.** The central pulp has herniated laterally to impinge on a spinal nerve.

Periarticular Pain Syndromes

Considered here are a group of painful musculoskeletal conditions that are not arthritis, but occur in ligaments and muscles near joints.

Spinal pain is very common and often not associated with demonstrable pathologic changes. *Acute spinal pain* is usually due to acute muscle strain. On the other hand, **chronic spinal pain**, especially in the *lower spine*, is a much, much bigger and more complex matter. Chronic lower back pain *may last a lifetime and sometimes defies anatomic explanation*, the principal reason so much quackery and nonsense swarm about the problem. Nevertheless, many causes of back and neck pain are associated with clear pathologic abnormality—spinal nerve compression, RA, metastatic cancer, and vertebral fractures, for example.

Some Spinal Pain Is Due to Intervertebral Discs

Vertebrae are stacked one upon another and separated by *intervertebral discs*, which are cushions of soft, pulpy tissue (the *nucleus pulposus*) encircled by a rind of tough, fibrocartilaginous tissue. Degeneration of the rind (**degenerative disc disease**) occurs with age and can allow the nucleus pulposus to bulge or rupture (**herniated intervertebral disc**) (Fig. 18.20) outward and impinge on spinal nerve roots or on the spinal cord itself. Pressure on spinal nerves or spinal cord tracts can cause pain, numbness, tingling, or paralysis. For example, a herniated disc can press on sensory nerve roots composed of axons that travel in the sciatic nerve, the main nerve to the leg, to cause the clinical syndrome of *sciatica*—pain in the buttock, thigh or lower leg. Pressure on motor nerve roots can cause partial paralysis that is manifest as *foot drop*, a dragging of the foot due to an inability to flex the ankle. Diagnosis is by radiographic imaging and clinical syndrome. Surgery is usually effective.

Spinal Pain May Occur If Vertebrae Slide Out of Alignment

When vertebrae slide anteriorly or posteriorly out of alignment to a degree detectable by imaging studies, the condition is called **spondylolisthesis** (from Greek *spondylos* for vertebra, and *listhesis* for sliding). The stack of vertebrae that form the spinal column are interlocked and stabilized by contact at synovial joints on the arch of bone that surrounds the spinal cord (e.g., the joints that are involved by ankylosing spondylitis and idiopathic juvenile arthritis). Sometimes, however, the locking mechanism in the vertebral arch fails due to bone degeneration, chronic stress, fracture, or intervertebral disc disease, and vertebrae may slip out of alignment.

Spondylolisthesis is often asymptomatic. Indeed, most people with radiographic evidence of spondylolisthesis have no symptoms. The most common variety is forward slippage of the L5 lumbar vertebra at its junction with the sacrum. It usually occurs in the lower lumbar vertebrae and is most often seen in adolescents or young adults with low back pain associated with nerve impingement (pain, numbness, muscular weakness), vertebral stress fracture, or arthritis in the joints of the vertebral processes. Diagnosis is radiologic. It lends itself to overdiagnosis, especially in older adults whose back pain may be due to many other reasons. Conservative treatment relies on physical therapy, braces and other orthotics, chiropractic, and supportive measures. Surgery may be required in some instances but choice of patients and type of surgery are controversial.

Periarticular Structures May Become Painful

Repeated or excessive motion may cause painful syndromes of tendinitis and tenosynovitis. Infiltrates of inflammatory cells are usually not present, and the exact mechanism of the pain in these circumstances is not clear. **Tendinitis** is inflammation or pain in a tendon; **tenosynovitis** is inflammation or pain of the synovial sheath through which tendons slide in their motion. Pain and tenderness are often located at the point where tendon attaches to bone. The elbow, wrist, shoulder, and knee are most often involved. An example is **tennis elbow**, a painful condition of the ligaments that attach forearm extensor muscles to the lateral epicondyle of the humerus. A related example is **shin splints**, an affliction of runners that is characterized by pain and tenderness along the anterior aspect of the tibia where muscle attaches to bone. Diagnosis of these conditions is clinical. Treatment is rest and NSAIDS. Surgery is rarely necessary.

On the other hand, some tendinitis and tenosynovitis is accompanied by clear-cut chronic inflammation and fibrosis. An example is **carpal tunnel syndrome**, a condition of the tendons and tendon sheaths of the ventral wrist (Fig. 18.21) in persons doing tasks that require repetitive finger and wrist motions. Inflammatory scarring and strictures constrict nerves and blood vessels passing through the carpal tunnel, causing pain, swelling, numbness, and discoloration in the hand or fingers. Surgery may be required to open the tendon sheaths and release the pressure.

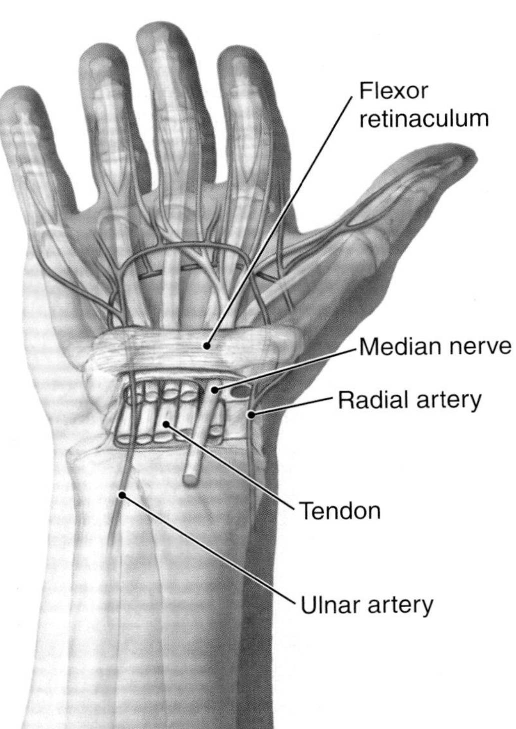

Figure 18.21 **Tendon anatomy of the wrist.** (Adapted with permission from Clay JH, Pounds DM. *Basic Clinical Massage Therapy: Integrating Anatomy and Treatment.* 2nd ed. Philadelphia, (PA): Lippincott Williams & Wilkins; 2008.)

Bursitis is inflammation of a bursa and is typically due to direct trauma or the stress of repetitive motion. The bursa fills with inflammatory fluid to become a tender, fluctuant mass. Rest and nonsteroidal anti-inflammatory drugs are usually effective.

Fibromyalgia Is a Pain Syndrome without Objective Abnormalities

Fibromyalgia is a *clinical* syndrome of fatigue, and muscle and periarticular tendon and ligament pain, tenderness, and stiffness that is *not associated with objective signs of disease*—laboratory, X-ray, and other studies are normal.

Fibromyalgia is one of the most common of all arthritis-like conditions, affecting about 5% of the general population, most often women between ages 20 and 50. Fatigue, insomnia, depression, vague feelings of numbness, and headaches are common. Patients may complain their joints are stiff and swollen, though swelling is not observable. Patients frequently have tenderness at specific "trigger points" near joints in the neck, shoulders, low back, and thighs. An important diagnostic point is that the pain is out of proportion to physical findings.

Diagnosis is by exclusion of other disorders that could account for the patient's symptoms; those disorders include various types of arthritis, PMR, and inflammatory diseases of muscle. Fibromyalgia differs from PMR in that fever, weight loss, anemia, increased ESR, and other measurable abnormalities are not present in fibromyalgia.

The lack of objective laboratory, physical, radiologic, and other objective abnormalities raise the question: Is fibromyalgia a psychological condition? Some research suggests that the fault may be in the brain's pain-processing system; other evidence points to insomnia. Regardless of the cause, the pain, stiffness, and soreness are real enough to patients and the syndrome is seen by caregivers with enough frequency and consistency that it is now a generally accepted medical diagnosis. Nevertheless, skeptics consider it a behavioral disorder. Anti-inflammatory drugs are not effective. Indeed, failure to respond to a short course of steroids is a diagnostic point in favor of fibromyalgia. Antidepressants, sedatives, improved sleep, and exercise are helpful.

Case Notes

18.13 Which clinical features favored a diagnosis of fibromyalgia in Raynelle?

Pop Quiz

18.30 True or false? Fibromyalgia is not associated with objective signs of disease, and laboratory, X-ray and other studies are normal.

18.31 ________________ is a condition in which vertebrae have slipped out of alignment.

Tumors and Tumor-Like Lesions of Joints and Soft Tissues

Soft tissue refers to nonepithelial tissue that is not bone, cartilage, brain, nerve, meninges, bone marrow, or lymphoid tissue. Neoplasms and tumor-like growths may occur in soft tissue at virtually any point in the body. By definition, this includes tendons, ligaments and other fibrous tissue, skeletal and smooth muscle, and fat. Moreover, some tumors that grow in soft tissue are composed of cells that cannot be identified as derived from a particular tissue. Soft tissue tumors may be benign, fully malignant, or somewhere in between—locally aggressive but not capable of metastasis. Nearly half occur in the lower extremity, especially the thigh.

The cause of most soft tissue tumors is unknown. Radiation-induced sarcoma, Kaposi sarcoma of AIDS, and the neurofibromas of neurofibromatosis (Chapter 22) are exceptions that have clear causes.

Some Soft Tissue Growths Are Joint-Related

Joint-related growths almost always occur in soft tissue, not actually in the joint.

Ganglion cyst (Fig. 18.22) is a small (usually <1.5 cm), smooth, fluctuant, fluid-filled, simple cyst that arises near a joint or tendon sheath; the wrist is a typical site. Ganglion cyst is a focal myxoid degeneration of connective tissue and lacks an internal lining cell layer (and therefore should be called a pseudocyst). The fluid is oily, similar to synovial fluid. Ganglion cysts are innocuous but may be surgically removed if they limit motion, are painful, or are unsightly.

Tenosynovial giant cell tumor (formerly *pigmented villonodular synovitis*) is a benign neoplasm of synovial joints, bursae and tendon sheaths, 80% of which occur in the knee that typically arises in patients 20–40 years old. It can involve an entire joint or can be a small nodule on a tendon sheath. Larger lesions may be locally aggressive and invade bone, but do not metastasize. Surgical excision is usually curative, but some tumors may recur locally.

Nonarticular Soft Tissue Growths May Occur Anywhere

Lipoma (Fig. 18.23) is a benign tumor of fat cells and is by far the most common soft tissue tumor. It may arise anywhere but is most often seen in subcutaneous fat. It resembles normal fat and is completely benign; it never becomes malignant.

Liposarcoma is a malignant tumor of fat cells that generally arises in deep tissues. It is the second most common sarcoma of adults and comprises 20% of malignant soft tissue tumors. Liposarcomas usually arise in adults older than 50 and are sluggishly malignant: they are locally aggressive and may grow very large. Several types are recognized. Survival correlates with histologic grade—five-year survival for well-differentiated tumors is 70%; it is <20% for poorly-differentiated tumors. Surgery is the mainstay of treatment. Some varieties are radiosensitive.

Neoplasms of skeletal muscle (*rhabdomyoma* and *rhabdomyosarcoma*) are rare. **Rhabdomyosarcoma** is predominantly a malignancy of infants, children, and adolescents. Several types are recognized. Treatment includes surgery, radiation, and chemotherapy. Formerly universally fatal, nowadays the cure rate is 80% for those with localized or regional disease.

Fibrocytic tumors may occur in any part of the body. They vary from tumorlike inflammatory proliferations that are benign to extremely malignant sarcomas. Pathologic

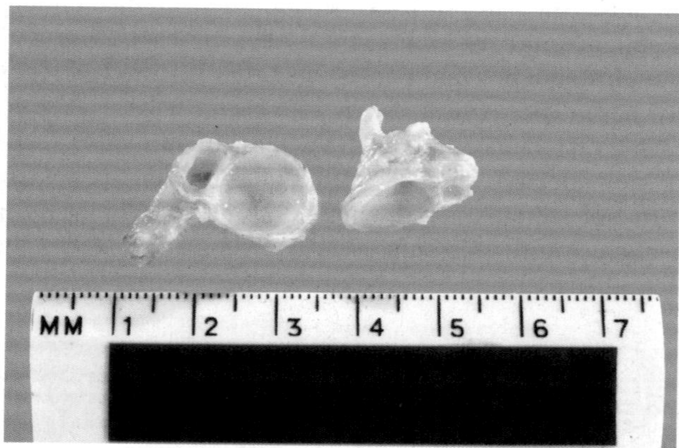

Figure 18.22 **Ganglion cyst.** These small benign cysts occur near joints, especially the wrist. This particular one was removed because it interfered with wrist motion.

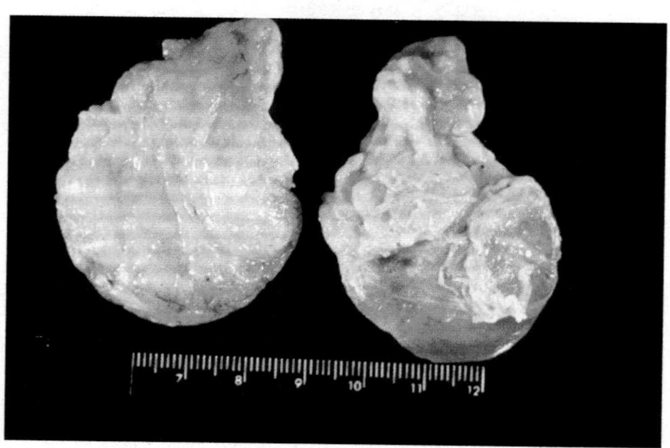

Figure 18.23 **Lipoma.** Nodular, neoplastic mass of fat excised from the forearm for cosmetic purposes.

diagnosis can be tricky because two benign conditions, nodular fasciitis and fibromatosis, can mimic sarcoma microscopically. **Nodular fasciitis** is a benign mass of inflammatory, immature scar tissue that occurs most often on the forearm, back, or trunk. It is probably a reaction to trauma. It tends to grow rapidly and the microscopic appearance can be deceptively suggestive of malignancy. Diagnosis requires biopsy. It is self-limiting and cured by excision.

A **fibromatosis** is a confined proliferation of fibrous tissue that can be locally aggressive and may recur after excision, but does not metastasize. Superficial fibromatoses usually occur in fascia of the palm or sole and present as small, hard, slowly growing nodules. Fibromatoses may occur at almost any location; for example, *Peyronie disease* is a fibromatosis of the penis that may substantially deform the erect penis. Although they may recur after simple excision, fibromatoses are not malignant. Fibromatosis in deep fascia is called **desmoid tumor** and is somewhat more aggressive but does not metastasize. An example is desmoid tumor of the abdominal wall fascia.

Sarcomas of fibrocytic cells occur in various forms:

- **Fibrosarcoma** is a malignant tumor of fibroblasts that can present as several microscopic variants, some of which were at one time thought to be other tumors (e.g., *malignant fibrous histiocytoma*). It occurs most commonly around the knee, thigh, and retroperitoneum. They tend to recur locally and metastasize to the lungs. Five-year survival is about 50%. Treatment is surgery, radiation, and chemotherapy.
- **Synovial sarcoma** is a malignant tumor of fibrocyte-like cells that arises near joints in tendons, ligaments, bursae, and joint capsule in adolescents and young adults. Behavior and treatment are similar to fibrosarcoma.

Leiomyoma is a benign tumor of smooth muscle that is most often found in the uterus, where it is often called a "fibroid" (Chapter 17). In soft tissue, however, it usually arises from the wall of a subcutaneous blood vessel. It does not become malignant. **Leiomyosarcoma** is a malignant, smooth muscle tumor; it is rare and may occur at any location in the body.

Pop Quiz

18.32 True or false? Superficial soft tissue tumors tend to be benign; deep ones tend to be malignant.

18.33 True or false? A ganglion cyst is not actually a true cyst.

Case Study Revisited

"I'm just a bucket of problems." The case of Raynelle C.

Most people, in or out of a doctor's office, have aches and pains of one kind or another, they lose sleep for a variety of reasons, they worry, and they feel tired. Complaints like those Raynelle had are often difficult to assess because they lack specificity. The diagnostic problem is to sort out the cases of those with fibromyalgia, arthritis, and other conditions from those who are "the worried well," or, in a word, hypochondriacs.

One of the easiest diagnostic points to make is the absence of laboratory, radiologic, or other concrete abnormalities, especially lack of elevation of the inflammatory markers C-reactive protein (CRP) and erythrocyte sedimentation rate (ESR). Raynelle's laboratory tests and X-rays were normal, which much favored the diagnosis of fibromyalgia. A good point to remember about CRP is that it is a sensitive test and is elevated in atherosclerosis. It can, therefore, be increased for reasons having nothing to do with fibromyalgia. ESR is a much less sensitive test; therefore, when positive, it is a more specific confirmation of inflammation. An elevated ESR would have been certain evidence that something other than fibromyalgia was the diagnosis.

Raynelle's history was also consistent with the diagnosis. She was not sleeping well, and she felt fatigued, scarcely a unique diagnostic combination but certainly one that reinforced the doctor's ultimate conclusion.

Her physical exam was helpful, too, in both a positive and negative sense. She was tender to the point of jumpiness at certain points, but her joints were not stiff, sore, or inflamed to the examiner's eye and the remainder of her physical exam was unremarkable.

The final diagnostic point was a trial course of low-dose steroids. Raynelle's failure to improve confirmed the diagnosis.

Case Notes

18.14 **Why did Raynelle not improve on steroid therapy?**

Section 4: Disorders of Skeletal Muscle

Muscles come and go; flab lasts.

BILL VAUGHAN (1915–1977), AMERICAN WRITER AND HUMORIST

Case Study

"He's had these pains all of his life." The case of Hammid S.

Chief Complaint: Muscle cramps

Clinical History: His mother brought Hammid S., a 10-year-old boy, to a pediatrician's office. The family had immigrated to the United States from Afghanistan 10 months earlier. With the aid of an interpreter, she explained that Hammid was becoming increasingly upset by his inability to keep up with the other boys on his soccer team because of painful muscle cramps that occurred in his legs with strenuous exercise. He had also been complaining that everyday activities requiring significant muscle effort, such as climbing stairs, caused him pain.

She explained further, "He's had these pains all of his life, but not so bad as now. The doctor in Herat told me he probably had liver disease because his urine is red or brown sometimes. But the dark urine always appears after the muscle cramps come. The cramps go away if he rests for a while."

Further questioning revealed that Hammid's older brother and younger sister were not affected by similar symptoms.

Physical Examination and Other Data: Hammid was of normal height and weight for his age, and his vital signs were unremarkable. Muscle size and tone were unremarkable. Mild proximal muscle weakness was present in all extremities and he had difficulty walking on his heels or toes more than 8–10 steps because cramps developed in his calf muscles.

Laboratory evaluation revealed abnormally high levels of CK in blood. Inflammatory markers (ESR, CRP), CBC, electrolytes, glucose, liver enzymes, and other tests were normal. ANA was negative.

A presumptive diagnosis of McArdle disease (Type V glycogen storage disease, due to a genetic deficiency of muscle glycogen phosphorylase) was made and he was given an appointment with a specialist in muscular diseases.

Clinical Course: At the specialty clinic, a forearm ischemia test was performed, in which a blood pressure cuff was inflated to cut off blood flow and Hammid was asked to squeeze a rubber ball for a minute or until cramps appeared. Study of blood lactic acid in a forearm vein was abnormal: the normal increase of lactic acid did not occur during the test. A muscle biopsy was performed and showed increased amounts of glycogen in the muscle fibers and a severe decrease in muscle content of glycogen phosphorylase.

Specialists at the clinic explained to Hammid's parents the way in which his genetic defect was inherited and that there was currently no treatment available.

They also reassured them that, although Hammid would have difficulty all of his life with strenuous exercise, he would be unlikely to suffer other problems.

Case Notes

18.15 When Hammid was playing soccer, what substance carried signals between his nerves and muscles?

18.16 Did Hammid's calf muscles have more Type I or Type II fibers?

Pathologic Reactions of Muscle

To remain healthy, skeletal muscle, like all other tissue, must have an adequate supply of blood, oxygen, nutrients, and other necessities. Likewise, muscle cells die by necrosis or apoptosis, or they respond to stress or injury (Chapter 2) by inflammation, atrophy, hypertrophy, fibrosis, and other reactions. Nevertheless, muscle cells differ from all others in one way: to remain healthy they must also be connected to (*innervated* by) a healthy peripheral nerve.

Denervated or Unused Muscle Atrophies

Denervation leads to muscle fiber atrophy (**neurogenic atrophy**). Both Type I and Type II fibers are affected. Nerve damage associated with diabetes (*diabetic peripheral neuropathy*, Chapter 13) is the most common cause, but peripheral nerve trauma and diseases of the peripheral nervous system also can be responsible.

Spinal muscular atrophy is an inherited autosomal recessive denervation atrophy that is associated with progressive degeneration of anterior horn cells (lower motor neurons) in the spinal cord. The *infantile* form (*Werdnig-Hoffman disease*) is usually fatal within the first year of life. The *juvenile* form (*Kugelberg-Welander disease*) appears later and is not necessarily progressively fatal.

Disuse atrophy occurs in muscles that are inactive due to some reason other than lower motor neuron denervation; for example, in bedfast patients, or in patients with stroke or other brain disease that affects upper motor neurons and renders patients unable to initiate voluntary movement. Disuse atrophy selectively affects Type II fibers only.

Rhabdomyolysis Releases Myoglobin

Rhabdomyolysis is a term used to describe sudden necrosis of skeletal muscle with release of large amounts of myoglobin into the circulation. It is always secondary to some underlying serious medical condition. Causes are burns, heat stroke, alcoholic binge drinking, crush injury, muscle contractions during seizures, drug overdose, poisoning, electrical shock, and influenza. Myoglobin is cleared from blood by the kidneys (myoglobinuria). A large load of myoglobin may cause renal failure—about 10% of acute renal failure owes to myoglobinuria. Some metabolic diseases of muscle (e.g., *glycogen storage disease*) may cause mild myoglobinuria and visibly dark urine without threat of renal failure.

Affected muscles are swollen, tender, and very weak. Pathologically, necrosis and regeneration are prominent, but inflammation is usually minimal.

Case Notes

18.17 Explain Hammid's dark urine after exercise.

Pop Quiz

18.34 True or false? Diabetic peripheral neuropathy is the most common cause of neurogenic atrophy, affecting both Type I fibers only.

18.35 Define rhabdomyolysis.

Myopathies

Myopathy literally means "disease of muscle." Nevertheless, we define it broadly as *any condition of muscle unrelated to any disorder of innervation or the neuromuscular junction*. There are hundreds of varieties, but only a few will be mentioned here. Diagnosis and treatment depend on recognition of the clinical syndrome, documentation of muscle fiber abnormalities by biopsy, and the presence of expected blood abnormalities.

Myopathies can be primary and due to intrinsic disease of muscle such as genetic conditions—muscular dystrophy is an example; or they can be secondary to some other process—steroid myopathy is an example. They also can be classified as inflammatory, metabolic, or genetic. In this discussion, we categorize *muscular dystrophy* as a myopathy, although some do not.

Case Notes

18.18 Did Hammid have a myopathy?

18.19 What enzyme did Hammid lack?

Muscular Dystrophies Are Inherited Defects of Muscle Contractility

The **muscular dystrophies** are a group of hereditary, progressive, noninflammatory diseases of striated muscle—skeletal and cardiac—associated with defective contractility, which causes muscle weakness.

Duchenne muscular dystrophy (DMD) is the most common form of muscular dystrophy. It is an X-linked inherited disease (Chapter 22) caused by the absence of *dystrophin*, a protein found in normal muscle and other tissues. A less common and milder form of the same type is **Becker muscular dystrophy (BMD)**, in which dystrophin is present but abnormal. Because they are X-linked recessive diseases, both occur almost exclusively in males. In 70% of cases, the patient's mother is a clinically normal heterozygous carrier; in 30% of cases, the mutations are spontaneous in the conceptus and the mother is not a carrier.

Pathologically, muscle fibers atrophy and die and late in the disease are replaced by fat and fibrous connective tissue.

The main clinical manifestation of both is muscle weakness, especially in pelvic and shoulder muscles (Fig. 18.24). The child is slow to take first steps, clear impairment is present by age five, and patients are confined to a wheelchair by the teenage years. Many patients have some degree of mental impairment due to lack of dystrophin in brain cells. Some patients develop cardiac muscle weakness and congestive heart failure (Fig. 18.25)

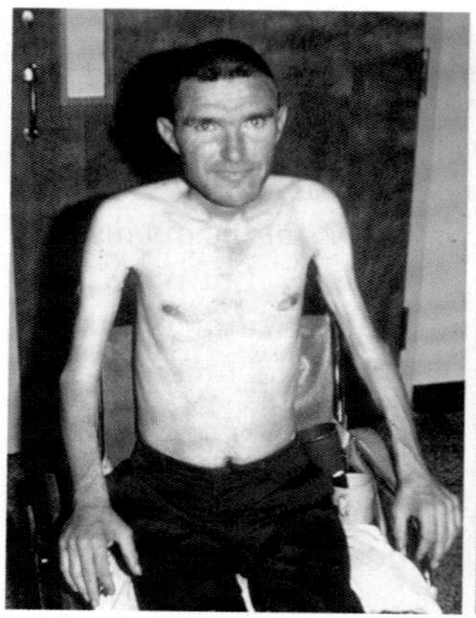
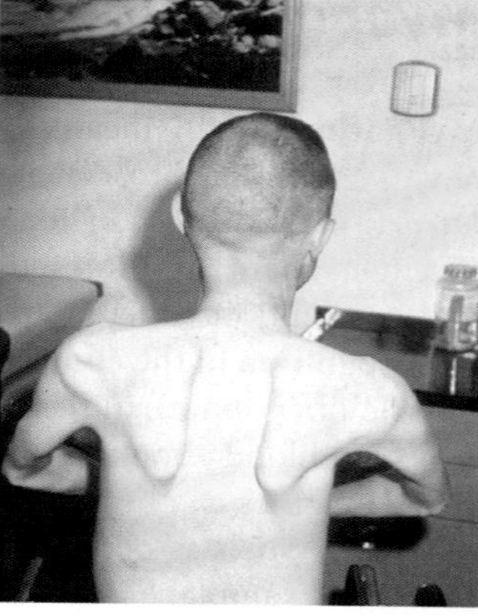

Figure 18.24 **Muscular dystrophy.** Severe muscle atrophy of shoulder girdle.

and die in their 20s of respiratory insufficiency. Becker is more variable, in general starting later and progressing more slowly. Patients with mild forms of either type of muscular dystrophy may remain ambulatory until well into adulthood.

Other forms of muscular dystrophy are recognized and rare. **Myotonic muscular dystrophy** is an example. It features impaired muscle relaxation that produces extended involuntary contraction of muscle groups and a constellation of distinctive physical findings.

Diagnosis of muscular dystrophy depends on recognition of characteristic clinical features. In DMD and BMD shoulder and hip muscle weakness, family history of muscular dystrophy, and markedly elevated serum *CK* are key diagnostic points. Special microscopic tissue stains for dystrophin are helpful in distinguishing between the two—patients with DMD have no demonstrable dystrophin; however, dystrophin is identifiable in patients with BMD. Treatment is supportive.

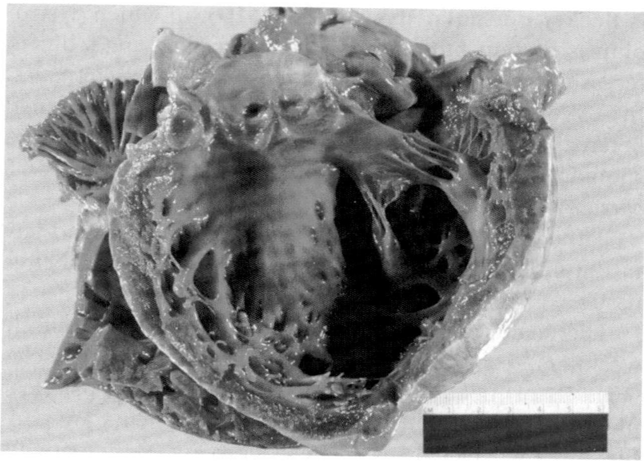

Figure 18.25 **The heart in muscular dystrophy.** Mechanical weakness of the muscle in this heart has caused congestive heart failure and cardiac dilation.

Congenital Myopathies Feature General Hypotonia

Congenital myopathies are a large and diverse group of conditions that feature *hypotonia* (below normal muscle tone) and are initially categorized as **floppy infant syndrome**. Some are known to be due to specific genetic defects; others are of unknown, but presumably genetic, defect.

Some have a benign course. Hypotonia persists throughout life but the person remains ambulatory and has a normal life span. Muscle biopsy and blood CK are normal.

Others have more severe hypotonia with decreased deep tendon reflexes, decreased muscle bulk, delayed developmental motor milestones, and joint contractures. Early respiratory distress and pulmonary complications are common. Among this group are the following:

Central core disease is an autosomal dominant condition that features decreased Type II fibers. Type I fibers have a pale central core.

Nemaline myopathy features decreased Type II fibers and rod-like intracytoplasmic inclusions. Inheritance varies.

Central nuclear myopathy features nuclei in the center of the fiber rather than at the edge. Inheritance varies.

Diagnosis requires muscle biopsy. Treatment is supportive.

Some Myopathies Are Associated with Inborn Errors of Metabolism

This group of myopathies features defective metabolic processes, some of which occur in mitochondria.

Lipid myopathies feature genetic defects that interfere with fatty acid metabolism and result in lipid droplet accumulation in muscle cells. Fatty acids are metabolized for energy after glycogen stores have been burned. The result is a syndrome of muscle weakness, pain, tightness, and myoglobinuria in the fasting state or after initial exercise consumes glycogen stores.

Glycogen storage diseases are a diverse group of myopathies associated with an inability to degrade glycogen. Effects on muscle vary and the severity of disease varies even within type. Some patients may be severely hypotonic at birth and die of respiratory or cardiac failure. Others may suffer little more than cramps and impaired exercise endurance. *Type II glycogenosis* (*Pompé disease*) is rare but distinctive for the large amounts of intracellular glycogen that accumulate in muscle cells. *Type V glycogenosis* (*McArdle disease*) is one of the most common inherited metabolic myopathies. Patients lack phosphorylase, an enzyme necessary for converting glycogen to glucose. Muscles cramp with exercise and myoglobinuria may occur, but ordinary exertion is little affected.

Familial periodic paralysis is a family of autosomal dominant disorders that features episodes of weakness or paralysis followed by quick recovery. The defect involves transmembrane transport of sodium and potassium flux into and out of cells. During an attack, muscle fibers do not transmit the action potential and contraction does not occur. Some varieties are associated with hyperkalemia, others with hypokalemia or normal blood potassium.

Myositis Is an Inflammatory Myopathy

Inflammatory myopathies are a diverse group of acquired disorders featuring weakness of proximal muscles, increased muscle enzymes in blood, and nonsuppurative inflammation of skeletal muscle.

The most common type of **myositis** is muscle infection by a virus in association with viral illness elsewhere in the body. The muscle aches of influenza, for example, are symptoms of mild viral myositis. *Trichinella spiralis* is a parasitic worm usually transmitted when someone eats undercooked pork. *Trichinella* preferentially infects muscle, causing the disease known as *trichinosis*, which is characterized by widespread muscle tenderness and marked increase of blood eosinophils.

Bacterial infection of muscle is rare unless in association with a wound, and usually occurs in deep, dirty wounds, burns, or illicit drug injection sites. Many of these infections are due to anaerobic bacteria.

Skeletal muscle can also be affected by autoimmune disease. This usually takes one of two forms: *dermatomyositis* and *polymyositis*. Both are uncommon. Proximal muscle inflammation, soreness, and weakness begin insidiously and are manifest by difficulty with ordinary tasks such as climbing stairs or combing hair. Patients may have dysphagia or trouble keeping their head erect. Blood CK and other muscle markers are high and muscles are infiltrated by lymphocytes (Fig. 18.26). **Dermatomyositis** is distinguished from other myopathies by a characteristic rash on the eyelids, face, and upper chest. It may occur in conjunction with scleroderma (Chapter 21) or other autoimmune conditions. Children and adults are affected. **Polymyositis** is similar to dermatomyositis, but there is no skin involvement and most patients are adults. Despite their similarities, the immune mechanisms (Chapter 3) are different. In dermatomyositis, muscle inflammation is due to deposition in muscle of circulating antigen-antibody complexes; in polymyositis, muscle inflammation is due to direct muscle damage by autoimmune T cells.

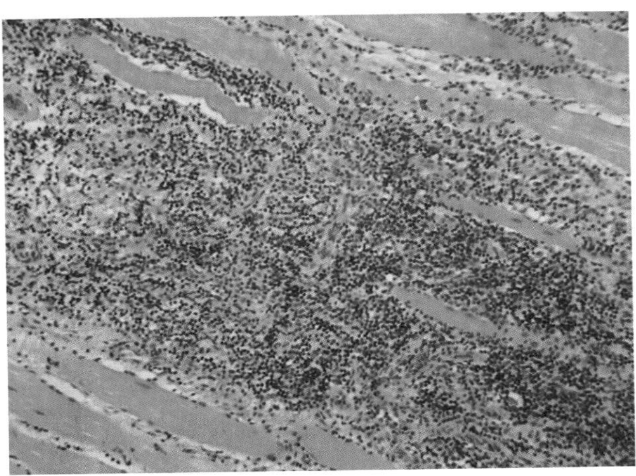

Figure 18.26 **Myositis.** Muscle biopsy in a patient with polymyositis. A dense infiltrate of inflammatory cells (lymphocytes) is present among muscle fibers (cells). (Reproduced with permission from Rubin E. *Pathology*. 4th ed. Philadelphia, (PA). Lippincott Williams and Wilkins; 2005).

Case Notes

18.20 Why was it unlikely that Hammid had an inflammatory myopathy?

Nonmuscle Conditions Cause Toxic Myopathy

Thyrotoxic myopathy may be one of the first signs of thyroid dysfunction. Hyperthyroidism may cause myopathy of eye muscles with exophthalmic ophthalmoplegia (movement paralysis). Hypothyroidism may also be associated with muscle weakness, soreness, and aches.

Binge drinking may cause **ethanol myopathy** with rhabdomyolysis, marked myoglobinuria, and renal failure.

Drug myopathies are usually manifest like others—by proximal muscle weakness, soreness, and aches. **Steroid myopathy** may occur with Cushing syndrome or drug therapy. Interestingly, the degree of myopathy is not necessarily related to blood levels or dose strength.

Statin drugs are especially widely prescribed in the United States as antiatherogenesis agents. About 1% of patients develop **statin myopathy**, which disappears with drug withdrawal. The myopathy does not depend on dose, duration of therapy, or drug type.

Pop Quiz

18.36 True or false? Nemaline myopathy features decreased Type II fibers and rod-like intracytoplasmic inclusions.

18.37 True or false? Thyrotoxic myopathy may be one of the first signs of thyroid dysfunction.

18.38 What infectious myopathy is accompanied by peripheral eosinophilia?

18.39 What presents earlier, Becker or DMD

Myasthenia Gravis

Myasthenia gravis is an uncommon, acquired autoimmune disease of the neuromuscular junction. Antibodies attach to acetylcholine receptors on the muscle side of the synapse (see Fig. 18.3A, and Chapter 3, Fig. 3.7B), blocking acetylcholine released from the motor end plate, and thus interrupting transmission of the nerve impulse. Sensory and autonomic function is not affected. Some patients also have other autoimmune disease (e.g., lupus erythematosus). The thymus is somehow involved in the development of myasthenia gravis—thymic hyperplasia is present in 65% and another 15% have a *thymoma*. Exactly how thymic abnormalities are involved in the disease, however, is not known.

Myasthenia gravis may occur at any age but usually affects women ages 20–40; affected men tend to be older. Drooping eyelids or double vision due to periorbital and eye muscle weakness are often the first symptoms. Slack facial muscles and difficulty chewing are common complaints. As the disease spreads, proximal limb muscles are next involved; ultimately any muscle may be affected. In advanced stages, respiratory failure may occur.

Diagnosis is by measurement of blood acetylcholine receptor (AChR) antibody levels and electromyography. Sometimes IV edrophonium challenge, which briefly lessens the weakness, is diagnostic.

Treatment is symptomatic; no cure is available. Removal of circulating antibody by filtering plasma (plasmapheresis) offers relief, sometimes for several years before the disease reappears. Steroids and anticholinesterase drugs may be helpful. If the thymus is abnormal, removal may be beneficial, especially in young women.

Pop Quiz

18.40 What is the underlying etiology of myasthenia gravis?

Case Study Revisited

"He's had these pains all of his life." The case of Hammid S.

Hammid's case was very straightforward. The physician in Afghanistan focused on his dark urine, thinking it was caused by bilirubinuria, which in turn led to a reasonable but erroneous presumption that something was wrong with his liver. Myoglobin also produces dark urine, just as do hemoglobin and bilirubin. The best clues were in his mother's words: the dark urine always came after cramps, and the cramps always were related to exercise and disappeared with rest. The combination pointed straight to glycogen storage disease with rhabdomyolysis and myoglobinuria. Confirmation came with the study of venous blood lactate in his forearm after forearm exercise. If he were burning glucose normally, he should have liberated lactic acid. Postexercise lactic acid was not increased, indicating impaired glucose metabolism. Muscle biopsy showed increased glycogen content of muscle fibers, finalizing the diagnosis.

Case Notes

18.23 What laboratory evidence indicated Hammid was not burning glucose properly?

Chapter Challenge

CHAPTER RECALL

1. Which of the following contains red marrow?
   A. The ribs & vertebrae
   B. The pelvic bones
   C. The skull
   D. All of the above

2. A 56-year-old Hispanic woman presents to her physician's office complaining of progressively worsening chronic pain (>5 years) in her right knee and the distal interphalangeal joint of her left little finger. Pain in both joints is relieved by a short rest. A physical exam demonstrates intact (though accompanied by crepitus) right knee range of motion, and Heberden nodes. Which of the following is likely to be seen if a pathologic examination were performed on the patient's right knee?
   A. Dense sclerotic bone, with a hard, ivory-like surface
   B. Uric acid crystals in joint fluid
   C. A pannus formed over the surface of the cartilage
   D. No changes

3. Which of the following abnormalities may accompany a diagnosis of rickets?
   A. Rachitic rosary
   B. Blue sclerae
   C. Hydrocephalus
   D. Floppy heart valves

4. A five-year-old Caucasian male is brought to the clinic for evaluation by his mother. She is concerned because he was slow to take his first steps, walks with a waddling gait, and frequently falls when ambulating. He also has difficulty standing from a seated position, brushing his teeth, and combing his hair. Family history is positive for a maternal uncle who died of respiratory failure in his early 20s. Which of the following familial disorders do you suspect?
   A. Central nuclear myopathy
   B. Becker muscular dystrophy
   C. Nemaline myopathy
   D. Duchene muscular dystrophy

5. The normal growth of long bones occurs in which part of the bone?
   A. Epiphysis
   B. Metaphysis
   C. Diaphysis
   D. Cortex

6. A 22-year old Hispanic male presents to the student health clinic with numerous complaints including fever, red eyes, burning on urination, and swelling and pain of the right knee and both ankles. His recent medical history includes a bout of diarrhea two weeks ago; he denies a history of STDs or new sexual partners. What is the likely cause of the patient's numerous symptoms?
   A. Septic arthritis
   B. Still disease
   C. Enteritis-associated arthritis
   D. Reiter syndrome

7. Which of the following is a true statement regarding polymyositis?
   A. Damage is caused by direct muscle damage by autoimmune T cells.
   B. There is a presence of rash on the eyelids, face, and upper chest.
   C. It may occur in conjunction with scleroderma and other autoimmune conditions.
   D. Damage is caused by the circulation of antigen-antibody complexes.

8. A 55-year old Caucasian female suffers from early morning joint pain and stiffness of her hands. On physical exam, you identify distinctive Z deformities of both hands (radial deviation of the hand bones, and ulnar deviation of the fingers). What is her diagnosis?
   A. Osteoarthritis
   B. Gout
   C. RA
   D. Psoriatic arthritis

9. The constellation of fever, skin rash, hepatosplenomegaly, polyserositis, and enthesitis is diagnostic of which of the following arthritic diseases?
   A. JIA
   B. RA
   C. Reiter syndrome
   D. Still disease

10. A 27-year-old Korean marathon runner presents to the first aid station at mile 18 with intense pain in her right foot. She is taken by ambulance to an ER, where an X-ray demonstrates a number of microfractures. What are these fractures called?
    A. Spiral fractures
    B. Simple fractures
    C. Greenstick fractures
    D. Stress fractures

11. Which of the following is a drug-induced myopathy?
    A. Ethanol myopathy
    B. Steroid myopathy
    C. Statin myopathy
    D. All of the above

12. Physical exam of a 43-year-old African American male with a past medical history of left middle cerebral artery stroke six months ago demonstrates markedly reduced muscle mass of his right arm and leg. This type of atrophy affects what muscle fibers?
    A. Type I fibers
    B. Type II fibers
    C. Both
    D. Neither

13. What is the treatment of choice for pain relief in a patient diagnosed with an osteoma?
    A. Aspirin
    B. Steroids
    C. Chemotherapy
    D. All of the above

14. A G1/P0 23-year-old Caucasian female is seen at the women's clinic for follow-up. Reviewing her chart, you note a growing discordance between fetal femur length and biparietal diameter. You explain to the mother-to-be that her fetus has a genetic syndrome that will result in shortened arms and legs with a normal trunk, and that, additionally, the child may have a small face to skull ratio, a saddle nose, a small jaw, and bowed legs. What is the intrauterine diagnosis?
    A. Paget disease
    B. Osteogenesis imperfecta
    C. Achondroplasia
    D. Marble bone disease

15. RF can be found in which of the following?
    A. Hepatitis B infection
    B. Ankylosing spondylitis
    C. Reactive arthritis following genitourinary or intestinal infection
    D. The arthritis of psoriasis

16. True or false? Cartilage obtains its nutrients and oxygen from a rich vascular supply.

17. True or false? Shin splints are characterized by pain and tenderness along the anterior aspect of the tibia where muscle attaches to bone.

18. True or false? Femur head necrosis is a potential complication of femoral neck fracture in an elderly patient.

19. True or false? PMR is a diagnosis of exclusion, as there are no measurable abnormalities.

20. True or false? The most common tumor in bone is metastatic cancer.

21. True or false? Central core disease affects only Type II fibers, which feature the pathognomonic pale central core.

22. True or false? Muscle is a permanent tissue, incapable of regenerating following injury.

23. Match the following tumors to their characteristics below:
    i. Fibromatosis
    ii. Fibrosarcoma
    iii. Leiomyoma
    iv. Leiomyosarcoma
    v. Lipoma
    vi. Liposarcoma
    vii. Rhabdomyoma
    viii. Rhabdomyosarcoma
    ix. Synovial sarcoma
    x. Tenosynovial giant cell tumor
    A. Benign neoplasm of synovial joints, bursae, and tendon sheaths
    B. Benign tumor of fat cells, the most common soft tissue tumor
    C. Malignant skeletal muscle tumor
    D. Benign locally aggressive confined proliferation of fibrous tissue
    E. Benign skeletal muscle tumor
    F. Malignant tumor of fibroblasts, occurs most commonly around the knee and thigh and retroperitoneum
    G. Malignant tumor of fibrocyte-like cells that arises near joints in tendons, ligaments, bursae, and joint capsule in adolescents and young adults
    H. Benign tumor of smooth muscle; most often found in the uterus
    I. Rare malignant smooth muscle tumor
    J. Locally aggressive malignant tumor of fat cells

CONCEPTUAL UNDERSTANDING

24. How do the underlying etiologies of primary osteoporosis differ from secondary osteoporosis?

25. What is the best possible treatment for a sprain or strain?

26. What treatments are available for patients suffering from myasthenia gravis?

27. What are some of the potential causes of rhabdomyolysis?

APPLICATION

28. A 45-year-old African American male is diagnosed with gout. Are there any other tests you might like to run?

29. Explain why, despite a negative culture in a child suspected to have osteomyelitis, a physician might prescribe antibiotics?

30. A five-year-old boy with X-ray evidence of multiple fractures in various stages of healing is removed by force from his mother's arms and child protective services is subsequently notified. Upon more extensive imaging, additional fractures of the ribs are noted. Were the X-rays incorrect, or was something missed?

CHAPTER 19

Disorders of the Nervous System

Contents

Chapter Objectives

After studying this chapter, you should be able to complete the following tasks:

THE NORMAL NERVOUS SYSTEM

1. Name the parenchymal and ancillary cells of the central nervous system (CNS).
2. Discuss the architecture of the brain: the difference between gray matter and white matter; the production, circulation, and absorption of cerebrospinal fluid (CSF); and the arrangement and special properties of cerebral vasculature.
3. Distinguish between the somatic and autonomic nervous systems.

INCREASED INTRACRANIAL PRESSURE

4. Explain the causes and consequences of increased intracranial pressure.

CNS CONGENITAL AND PERINATAL DISORDERS

5. List the congenital and perinatal diseases of CNS.

CNS TRAUMA

6. Describe the clinical and pathologic findings (as applicable) of concussions, contusions, and diffuse axonal injury.
7. Compare and contrast the anatomic location, the cause, and the consequences of subdural hematoma, epidural hematoma, and subarachnoid hemorrhage.

CEREBROVASCULAR DISORDER

8. Distinguish between hemorrhagic and nonhemorrhagic infarct, noting the differences between the anatomic location, causative factors and/or precursors, and pathologic findings.

CNS INFECTIONS

9. Classify the etiologies of CNS infections according to their site of infection and the population they infect.

CNS DEMYELINATING DISORDERS

10. Discuss the probable cause, the signs and symptoms, and the pathologic findings of multiple sclerosis.

CNS METABOLIC DISORDERS

11. Catalogue the metabolic disorders of the CNS according to their cause.

CNS DEGENERATIVE DISORDERS

12. Explain the clinical and diagnostic features of the various causes of dementia, as well as their underlying biochemical dysfunction (where applicable).

CNS NEOPLASMS

13. Classify the CNS neoplasms according to their cell/tissue type.

DISORDERS OF PERIPHERAL NERVES

14. Review the diseases, both neoplastic and non-neoplastic that affect peripheral nerves, giving their clinical and pathologic features.

Case Study

"Something doesn't seem right in my head." The case of Ted H.

Chief Complaint: Swollen feet

Clinical History: Ted H. was a 92-year-old man who had been in general good health until he noticed his feet were swollen. After a visit to his physician's office, he was hospitalized for heart failure.

Past medical history revealed that he hailed from a long line of octogenarians and had been in exceptionally good health except for a heart attack in his 60s, after which he gave up smoking and began walking regularly for exercise. Shortly before his 90th birthday, he developed atrial fibrillation and was placed on oral medicine to control his rapid heart rate, and anticoagulant therapy to prevent formation of atrial thrombi. He responded well and returned to his usual routines.

Physical Examination and Other Data: Vital signs were unremarkable except for an irregular tachycardia (102 beats/min.). Chest auscultation revealed a galloping cardiac rhythm and wet, crackling breath sounds suggesting heart failure. The edge of his liver was palpable, and his feet and legs were swollen with 2+ pitting edema. A chest film showed cardiac enlargement and pulmonary congestion. Laboratory data were normal except for mild elevation of

"Something doesn't seem right in my head." The case of Ted H. (continued)

liver enzymes. Cardiac enzymes and troponins were normal. An electrocardiogram showed atrial fibrillation. The admission diagnosis was arteriosclerotic heart disease with congestive heart failure and chronic atrial fibrillation.

Clinical Course: He was placed on digoxin to slow his heart rate and strengthen cardiac contractions. On the evening of the third hospital day, he rang the nursing station to say, "Something doesn't seem right in my head." A nurse examined him and noticed he was struggling to find words and was becoming frustrated about it. The nurse called a resident physician, who concluded he was having a transient ischemic attack with aphasia. Over the next few days, his language problem gradually improved and his heart failure responded to therapy. He was discharged to home on the seventh day.

The next day, he collapsed at home and was returned to the hospital. Admission diagnosis was ischemic cerebral infarct with right hemiplegia. He was alert but completely aphasic and had difficulty swallowing. He became progressively less responsive, then comatose. He died on the eighth hospital day.

An autopsy revealed a moderately enlarged, dilated heart with large mural thrombi in both atria. There was severe coronary atherosclerosis with marked narrowing of all vessels, but no fresh occlusion. The brain revealed a large, fresh, nonhemorrhagic infarct of the left cerebral hemisphere in tissue supplied by the left middle cerebral artery. The infarcted tissue was edematous. Moderate cerebellar tonsillar herniation was present with secondary pontine hemorrhage. Marked cerebral atherosclerosis was present, but no embolus or thrombus was identifiable. The lungs were congested and edematous, the liver showed moderate chronic passive congestion, and the spleen was congested and enlarged. Microscopic studies confirmed gross autopsy findings. There was no microscopic evidence of Alzheimer disease (AD).

Brain, n. An apparatus with which we think that we think.

AMBROSE BIERCE (1842–1914?), AMERICAN SATIRIST, JOURNALIST, AND SHORT-STORY WRITER, THE DEVIL'S DICTIONARY

Communication is the key to our survival. External communication, which we call language, is a tool that enables us to cooperate with one another to fend off external threats and to manage our surroundings for stability and mutual benefit. Civilization is the result. In like manner, internal communication enables our tissues and organs to respond cooperatively to external and internal environmental changes that threaten homeostasis.

The body contains two main internal communication systems. The *endocrine system*, discussed in Chapter 14, communicates by releasing chemicals into blood and other body fluids. The *nervous system*, the topic of this chapter, combines electrical and local chemical signals to move muscles at will and to organize incoming sensory signals into the unfathomable miracle we call "consciousness" so that we can organize thoughts and act.

The Normal Nervous System

The nervous system is divided into two parts. The **central nervous system (CNS)** consists of the brain and spinal cord. It receives and integrates (into consciousness) incoming sensory signals and responds with outgoing voluntary motor commands. The **peripheral nervous system (PNS)** exists mainly outside of the CNS and consists of a complex network of nerves connected to the CNS. The *somatic division* consists of cranial and spinal nerves originating from brain and spinal cord, which bring incoming sensory signals (sight, smell, etc.) to the brain and transmit *voluntary* (conscious) motor signals to muscles. The *autonomic division* is a network of nerves connected to viscera, skin, and other organs. It senses and transmits *involuntary* (unconscious) signals in the regulation of the heart, intestines, endocrine glands, and other organs.

Cells of the Nervous System

Neurons are the primary effector cells of the nervous system (Fig. 19.1). Neurons do not divide: diseased or dead neurons cannot be replaced, which limits the ability of the CNS to respond to injury. Each neuron extends one or more short **dendrites** to connect with other brain cells, and a single long (a few inches to a few feet) **axon** to connect with other neurons or with target tissue cells such as sensory receptors in skin or nose or effector cells such as those in skeletal muscle or glands. Bundles of axons are gathered into **nerve tracts** within the brain and **nerves** outside the CNS.

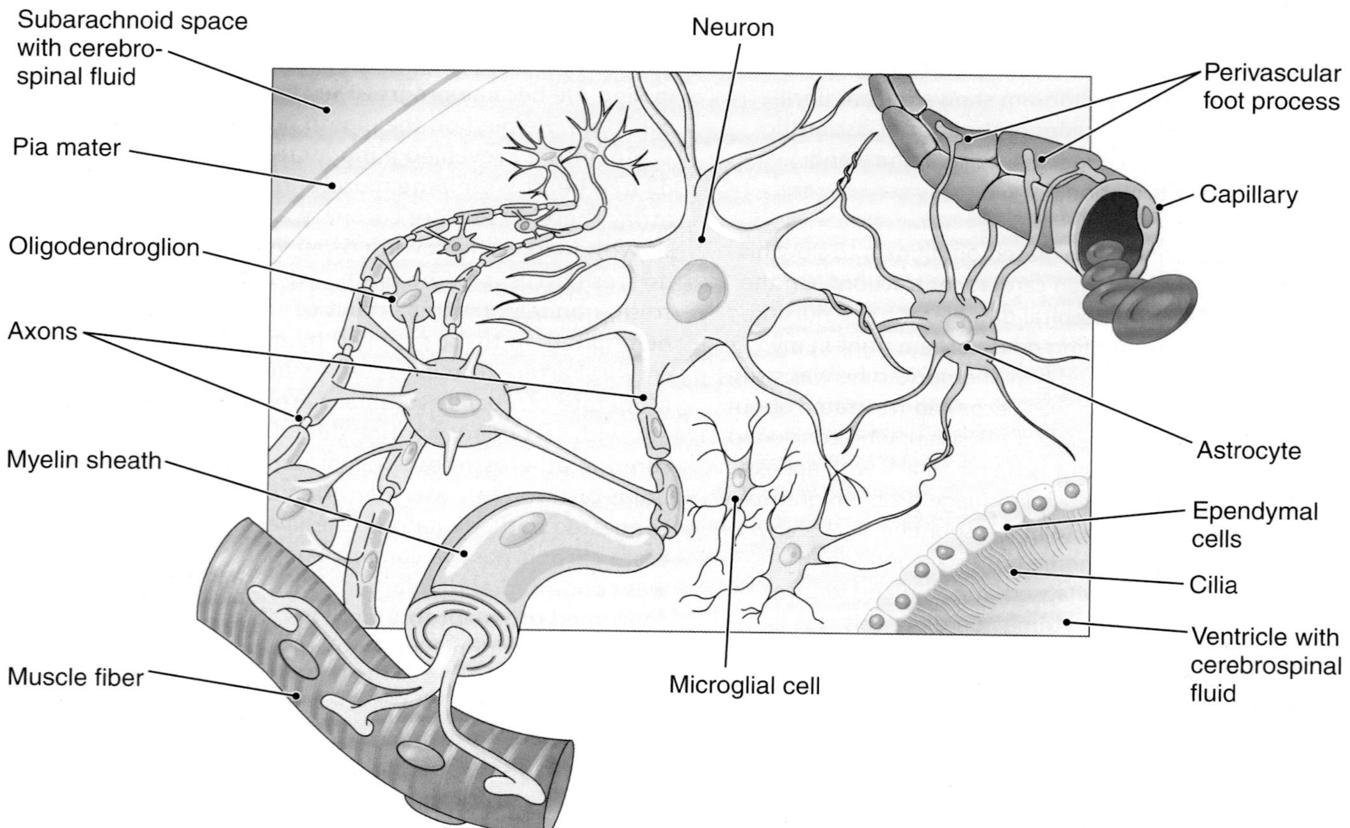

Figure 19.1 **Cells of the nervous system.** Neurons are the main functional cell of the nervous system and connect with other neurons by axons. *Glia* are cells that support neurons: *astrocytes* provide structure and functional support; *oligodendrocytes* wrap neuronal axons with a layer of myelin (myelin sheath); *microglia* are brain macrophages.

Neurons have a large cell body. When gathered together, they are grayish and are collectively referred to as **gray matter**. Neuron cell bodies form the outer layer of the brain, the cerebral cortex, and the central core of the spinal cord. Nodular collections of neuron cell bodies in the brain are called **nuclei**. Neuron cell bodies gathered together in the PNS form nodules called **ganglia**.

All other cells in the nervous system function in support of the neuron. All of the nonneuron cells in the brain form the **glia** (Greek = *glue*). **Astrocytes** are star-shaped glial cells that support neurons and promote repair. They fill a structural and supportive role similar to fibrocytes elsewhere in the body. **Oligodendrocytes** (literally, cells with few dendrites) are filled with a whitish fat, **myelin**, and wrap themselves around axons to insulate nerve signals passing down the axon; that is, they prevent "short circuits." Nerve tracts in the CNS are composed of myelinated axons, which are white due to their myelin coating. In the CNS, they are collectively referred to as **white matter**. **Ependymal cells** line the cerebral ventricles and the central canal of the spinal cord. Specialized ependymal cells form the **choroid plexuses**, small papillary organs in the ventricles that secrete **cerebrospinal fluid (CSF)**. Ependymal cells encourage CSF flow and modulate molecular exchange between CSF and CNS cells. **Microglia** are the scavenger (phagocytic) cells of the CNS and are analogous to macrophages elsewhere.

Neurons connect with one another and with effector tissues by a **synapse**. A synapse is characterized by an exceedingly narrow space (the *synaptic space*) between the signaling nerve cell or its axon and the target cell.

The membrane of an undisturbed (resting) nerve cell carries a positive electrical charge on the outside and a negative charge on the inside, a difference that creates potential electrical energy. This electrical difference, measured in millivolts, is called **membrane potential**.

Nerve signals are transmitted as a wave of electrical disturbance in the membrane potential that sweeps down the axon to the synapse. On arrival at the synapse, the signal stimulates release of a chemical **neurotransmitter** (of which there are many varieties) into the synaptic space. The neurotransmitter crosses the synaptic space and reinitiates a membrane potential on the other side, which in turn produces an effect; for example, contraction of muscle, secretion of fluid in a gland, constriction of a blood vessel. The neurotransmitter is then instantly broken down and reconstituted to be ready for the next signal to cross the synapse.

Case Notes

19.1 When Ted was unable to think of the right words, which of his CNS cells were failing?

19.2 Which cells in Ted's CNS made the CSF that was obtained by lumbar puncture?

19.3 When Ted spoke to the nurse, he used the muscles of his tongue, lips, larynx, and chest. What part of what CNS cell carried speech signals from his brain to these various muscles?

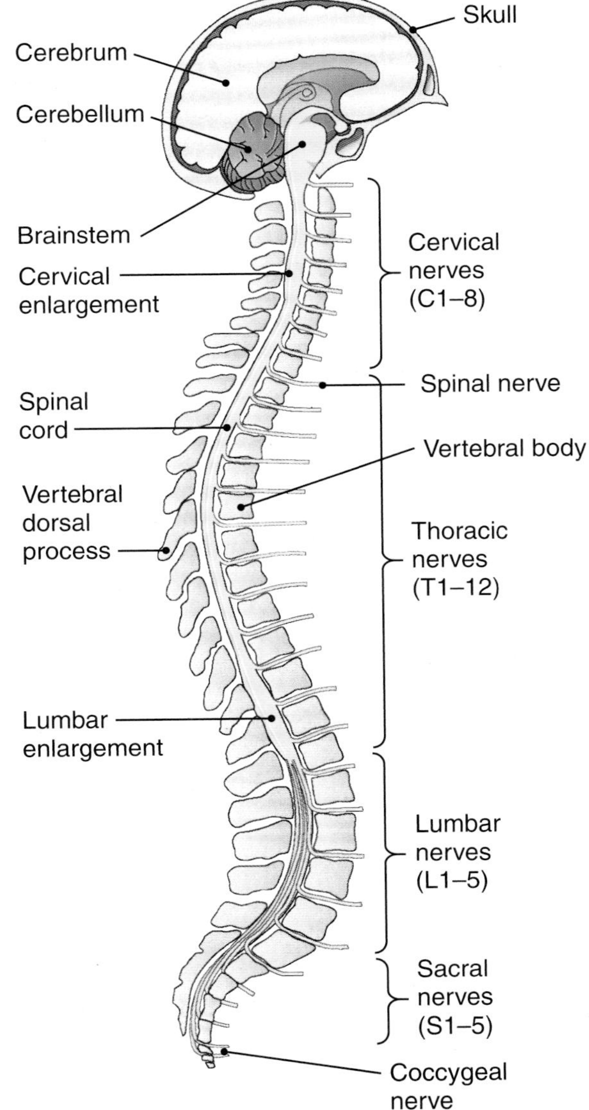

Figure 19.2 **The central nervous system.**

The Central Nervous System

The **central nervous system (CNS)** is composed of the **brain** and **spinal cord**. Figure 19.2 illustrates their relationship to the skull and vertebrae. Figure 19.3 depicts the internal anatomy of the brain.

The elements of the CNS are stacked vertically with the most complex functions located higher in the stack than the more primitive ones. The most superior and largest part of the brain is the **cerebrum**, home to the most complex functions. The cerebrum is divided into two parts, the right and left **cerebral hemispheres**, which are connected one to the other and to the spinal cord by large nerve tracts.

The outermost (top) layer of the cerebral hemisphere is the cerebral **cortex** (Latin = bark). The cortex is home to the highest brain functions—reasoning, emotion, voluntary motion, and speech. The cortex is composed of the plump cell bodies of neurons, which perform the most complex brain functions, from voluntary motor movement to abstract thinking.

Nerve tracts and nerves serve to carry electrical signals from one area of the brain to another and between brain and body. Nerve tracts form the white matter that occupies much of the central mass of each hemisphere.

The *midbrain*, *pons*, and *medulla oblongata*, collectively called the **brain stem**, sit below the cerebral hemispheres and above the spinal cord. The brainstem is the main traffic route of the brain, and most of its mass is composed of nerve tracts connecting brain and spinal cord. It is also home to numerous gray matter nuclei that control some of the most basic aspects of human physiology. The **midbrain**, the most superior part, contains nuclei important in eye and head movements and mediates some hearing functions. The **pons** (Latin = bridge) is the middle and largest part and contains nuclei important in regulating respiration. The lowest part of the brain, the **medulla oblongata**, is where nerve tracts from one side of the body cross over to connect to the opposite cerebral hemisphere. The medulla also contains nuclei that modulate heart rate, peripheral vascular tone in the regulation of blood pressure, respiratory rate, touch and vibratory sense, and reflexes for swallowing, coughing, vomiting, and sneezing.

The cerebral hemispheres and brain stem also contain nuclei that give rise to *cranial nerves (CN)*.

The **cerebellum** sits inferior to the cerebrum and posterior to the brain stem. It mediates balance, controls fine motor activity, especially rapid, complex, coordinated movements such as writing, and is home to the *proprioceptive sense*—the sense of body and body-part position (e.g., knowing where one's arms are without having to look at them).

The **spinal cord** passes out of the skull through a large opening, the **foramen magnum**, and through the vertebrae, which encircle it like a pole through the holes of a stack of donuts. It is composed of nerve tracts and a central core of gray matter, which gives rise to *spinal nerves*. The nerve tracts and nerves carry motor signals

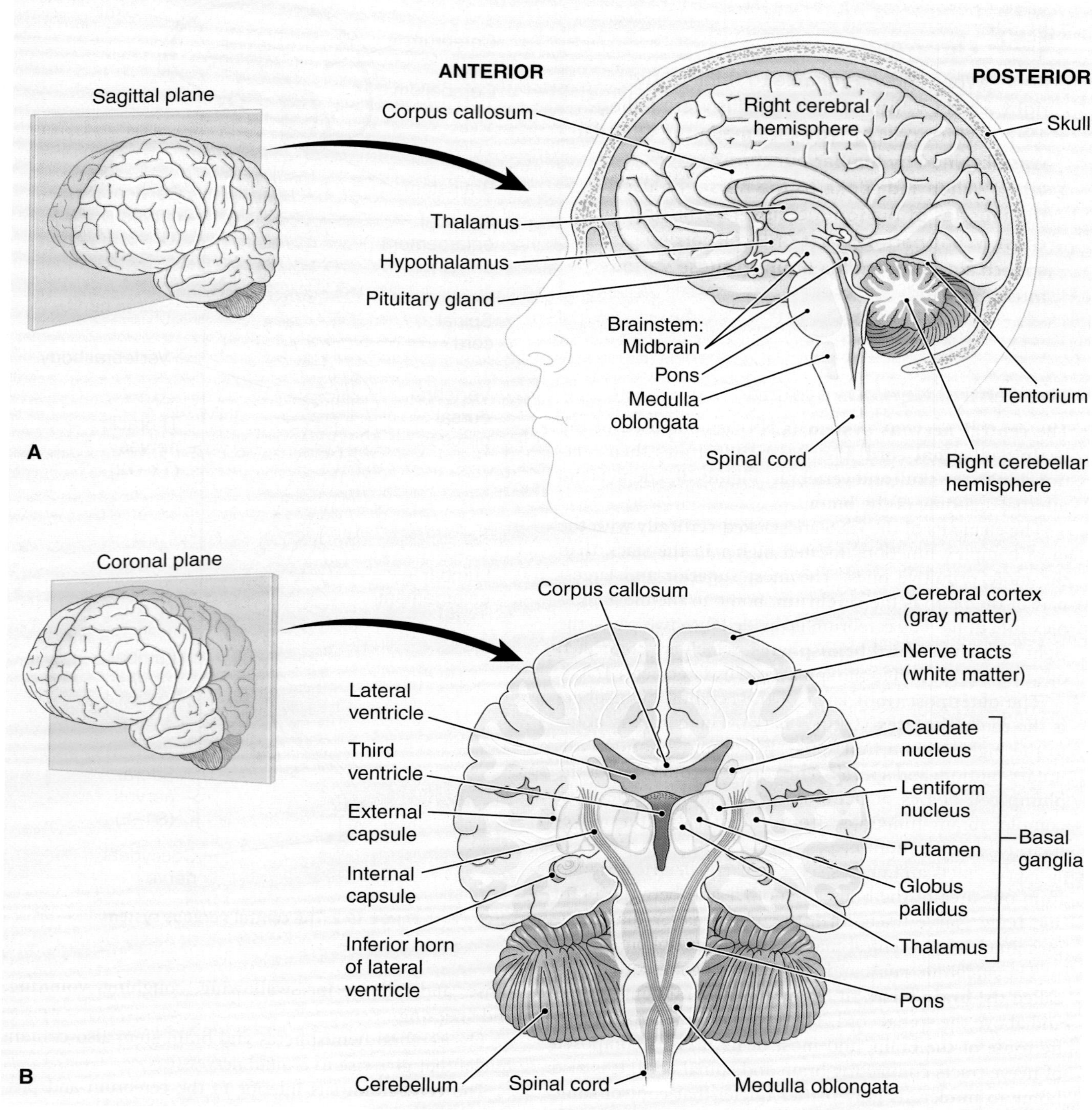

Figure 19.3 **The brain. A.** Sagittal section. **B.** Coronal section.

downward from the brain to the body and sensory signals upward from the body to the brain.

The Brain and Spinal Cord Are Enclosed by Bone and Membranes

The brain is encased by the bone of the skull. The spinal cord is encased by a flexible stack of vertebral bone—anteriorly the vertebral bodies and posteriorly the interlocking vertebral arches.

Inside this bony fortress, three membranes enclose the brain and spinal cord, protecting and stabilizing it (Fig. 19.4). The outermost is the **dura mater** (the *dura*), a tough, thick sheet of fibrous tissue that is tightly stuck to the inside of the skull and surrounds the spinal cord

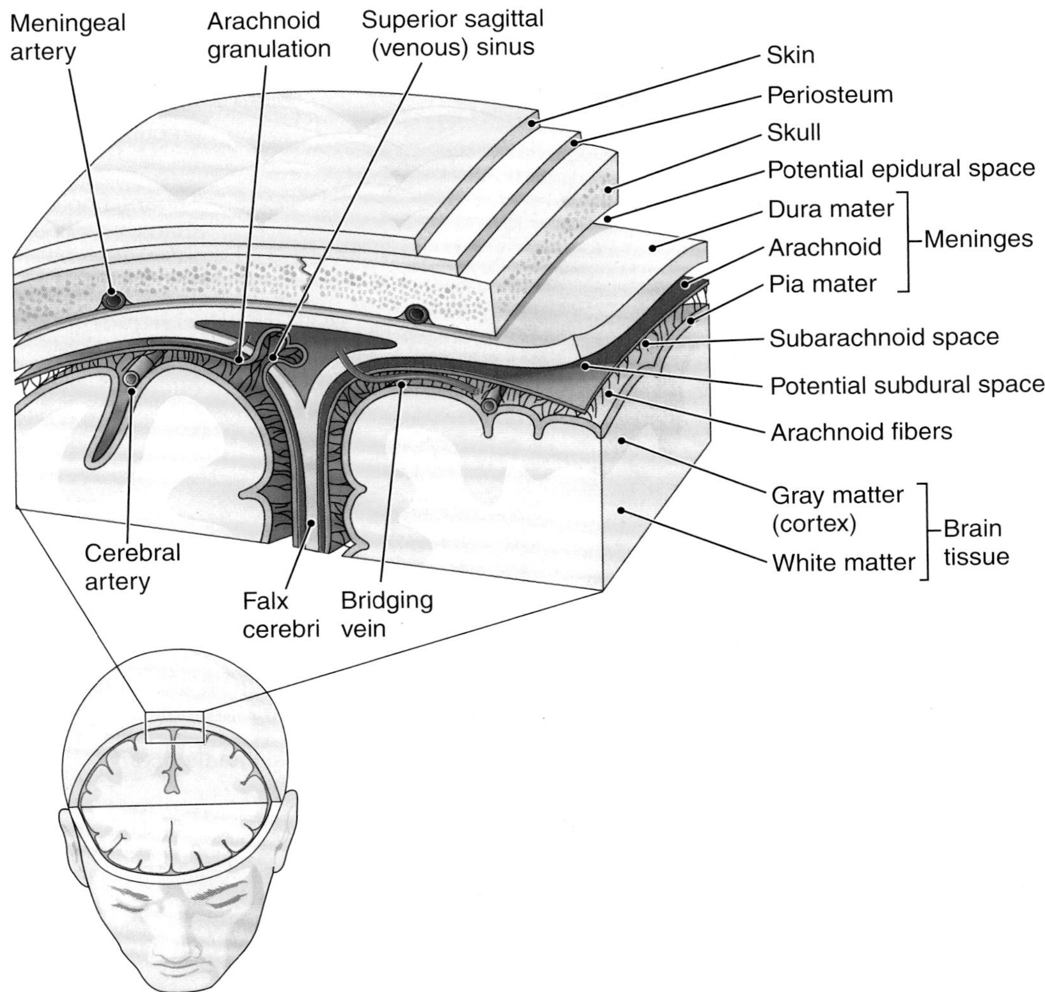

Figure 19.4 **The meninges and their relationship to the skull and brain.**

inside the spinal canal. Between the dura and the bone of the vertebrae is the **epidural space**, which is filled with a thin layer of fat. Immediately beneath the dura is the **arachnoid mater** (the *arachnoid*), a thin membrane beneath which is the **subarachnoid space**, containing the CSF. The major arteries on the surface of the brain lie in the subarachnoid space. The arachnoid gets its name from the Greek word *arachno* for cobweb, a reference to the web of thin fibers that cross the arachnoid space from the arachnoid and anchor to the **pia mater** on the surface of the brain. These fibers help limit brain movement within the skull. The innermost pia mater (the *pia*) is a very thin membrane intimately attached to the surface of the brain and spinal cord.

Two extensions of the dura mater form internal membranes to stabilize the brain. The **falx cerebri** is a vertical fold of dura mater formed into a membrane on the inside of the skull. It runs from front to rear, extends downward to separate the right and left cerebral hemispheres, and encloses the **superior sagittal sinus**, an elongated lake of venous blood that runs front to rear under the center of the skull. The **tentorium cerebelli** (Fig. 19.5) is a second, horizontal fold of dura in the back of the skull that separates the cerebral hemispheres above from the cerebellum below. It contains the **tentorial sinus**, which is continuous with the superior sagittal sinus.

The Brain and Spinal Cord Are Filled with and Immersed in Fluid

The brain and spinal cord are filled with and surrounded by **cerebrospinal fluid (CSF)**. Figure 19.5 illustrates the production, flow, and absorption of CSF. In the center of each cerebral hemisphere are hollow spaces—the **right** and **left lateral (first and second) ventricles**—filled with CSF. The CSF is a watery substance that circulates slowly and fills the ventricles and all other space in and around

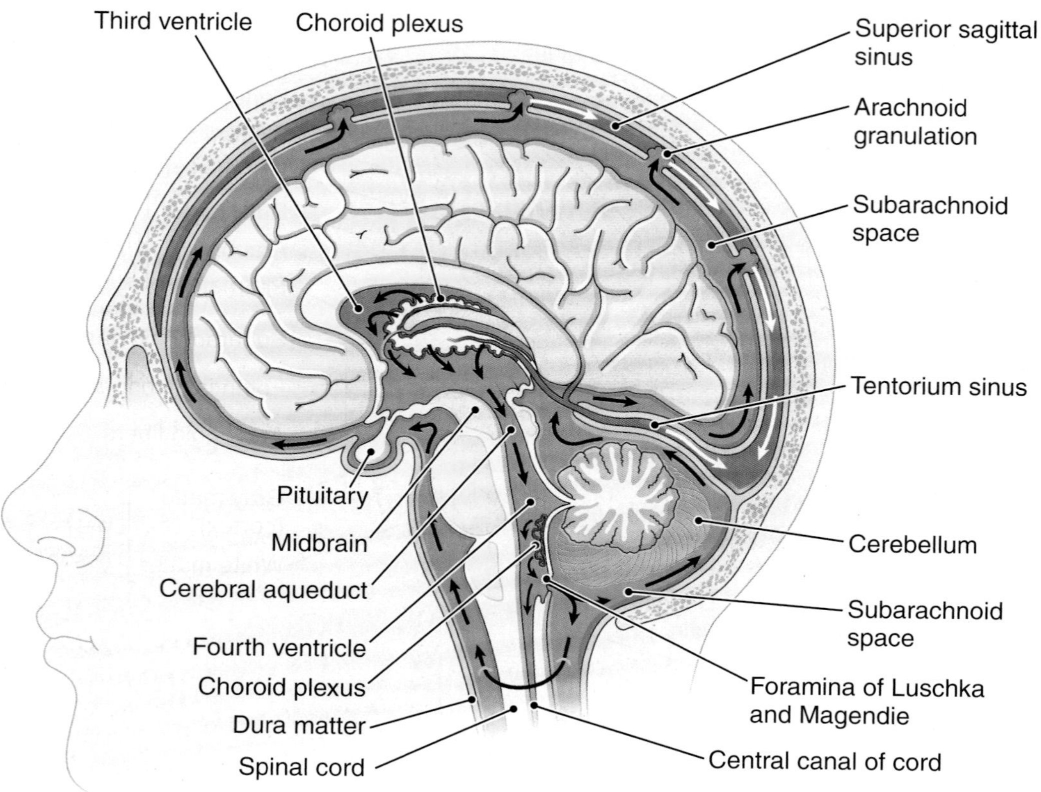

Figure 19.5 **Production, flow, and absorption of cerebrospinal fluid (CSF).** CSF fills the ventricles and all other space in and around the brain and spinal cord. CSF is made by choroid plexuses in the ventricles, which regulate CSF pressure. CSF flows through the ventricles and out of the brain through the foramina of Luschka and Magendie in the roof of the fourth ventricle. Outside the brain, the CSF fills and flows through the subarachnoid space. CSF is absorbed out of the subarachnoid space and into blood through arachnoid granulations, which project into the superior sagittal sinus.

the brain and spinal cord. CSF cushions the brain and spinal cord and mediates exchange of substances with the blood. CSF is made by choroid plexuses, which produce CSF and serve to regulate CSF pressure by the formation of more or less CSF. CSF flows through the ventricles and out of the brain into the subarachnoid space through small holes (the *foramina of Luschka and Magendie*) in the roof of the fourth ventricle. CSF is absorbed out of the arachnoid space and into blood through **arachnoid granulations**, papillary projections of arachnoid into the superior sagittal sinus.

Normal adults have about 150 ml of CSF volume and produce about 500 ml per day, a daily turnover of three to four volumes. Because of the rate of CSF production and reabsorption, obstruction of CSF flow or reabsorption causes increased intracranial pressure, which usually has serious consequences.

Study of CSF can be a valuable diagnostic tool. *The Clinical Side*, "Collection and Examination of Spinal Fluid," looks at how spinal fluid is collected and studied.

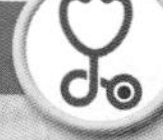

The Clinical Side

COLLECTION AND EXAMINATION OF SPINAL FLUID

Laboratory study of CSF is critical in many diseases of the CNS, especially infectious diseases.

CSF is usually collected by inserting a needle between lower lumbar vertebrae into the subarachnoid space. The lower end of the spinal cord is above this site; only the nerves of the cauda equina are present in the dural sac, so that the needle cannot injure the spinal cord.

The procedure is called a **lumbar puncture**. It is indicated in patients suspected of having meningitis and other CNS inflammations, subarachnoid hemorrhage, leukemic infiltration of the meninges, and some neoplastic disorders. If increased intracranial pressure or intracranial mass is suspected, radiographic images should be obtained for further assessment before proceeding because lowering spinal pressure by draining fluid from the spinal canal may cause downward herniation of the cerebellar tonsils, which can cause paralysis or death. Most patients tolerate lumbar puncture well, but some experience headache, and a few have minor bleeding into the CSF.

Lumbar puncture was first performed in 1891 by Heinrich Quincke, a German physician who thought drainage of CSF might help infants with hydrocephalus (a condition, usually in children, in which CSF accumulates in or around the brain and often is associated with brain damage). The technique is relatively simple (see the accompanying figure): the patient usually lies on one side in the knee-chest position and a long, thin needle is threaded between vertebrae and into the subarachnoid space. Typically 2–3 ml of fluid is collected and divided among several sterile tubes for culture, cell count, and chemical/immunologic/molecular studies. A blood specimen should always be collected at the same time: it is important to compare levels of blood glucose and protein with CSF values.

The following are some noteworthy findings in CSF (see also the summary in the accompanying table):

- Pressure: Increased pressure reflects increased intracranial pressure.
- Color: Bloody fluid followed by clear fluid after the first few drops indicates bleeding caused by the procedure. Bleeding associated with disease is characterized by uniformly colored CSF. Fresh blood is pink, but blood from bleeding four to six hours old may be orange or yellowish due to metabolism of blood into bilirubin (Chapter 12).
- Cells: A few lymphocytes are normal, but the presence of even a few (or one?) red blood cell(s) or neutrophil(s) is abnormal. Purulent meningitis is associated with very high neutrophil counts. Viral meningitis is associated with increased numbers of lymphocytes. If a tumor is present in the CNS sometimes tumor cells can be identified.
- Protein: An increased level of protein is usually a sign of infection, inflammation, degenerative disease, or hemorrhage. Low protein is a sign of CSF leakage, the most important cause being basilar skull fracture, in which CSF leaks out through the nose (CSF rhinorrhea).
- Glucose: CSF glucose is derived from blood glucose and fluctuates with it. For example, patients with diabetes who have a high blood glucose level will have high CSF glucose. Low CSF glucose level may be due to low blood glucose level, but, more importantly, it may reflect bacterial or fungal infection and metabolism of glucose by the infecting organism or inflammatory cells stimulated by the infection.
- Culture: Normal CSF is sterile.

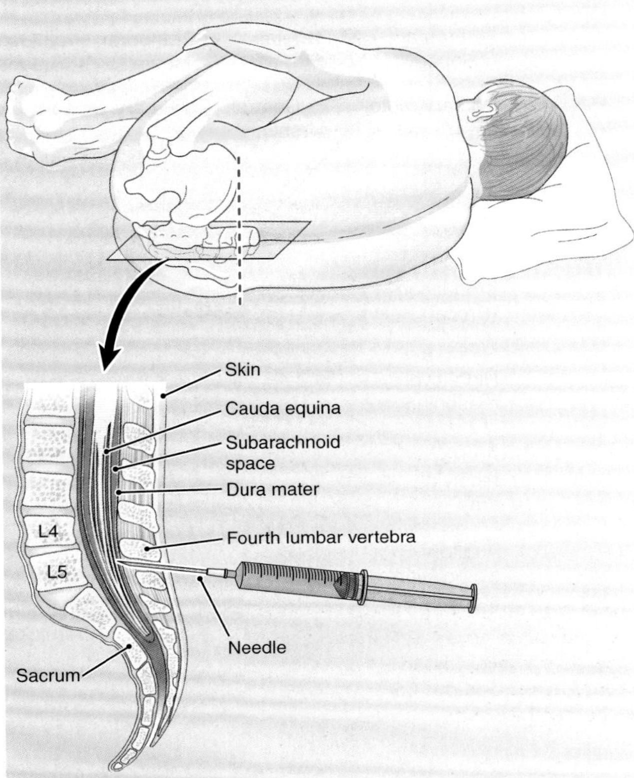

Lumbar puncture. A long, thin sterile needle is inserted between lower lumbar vertebrae in the region of the *cauda equina* of the spinal cord.

Normal Adult CSF*

Test	Findings
Pressure	70–180 mm Hg
Color	Clear
Total cell count (per µl)	0–5
Cell differential count	Mononuclear cells only—lymphocytes, macrophages, occasional meningeal cells
Protein (mg/dL)	15–45
Glucose (mg/dL)	50–80

*Newborn CSF may be substantially different

Functions of the Cerebral Cortex Are Lateralized

Figure 19.6 illustrates that, unlike other organs, because of the specific connections of nerve pathways within the brain and to and from every part of the body, *every anatomic part of the brain fulfills a function different from every other part.* For example, vision is perceived in the posterior (occipital) cerebral cortex, but high-level reasoning is controlled in the anterior (frontal) cortex. By contrast, each part of the liver functions the same as every other part.

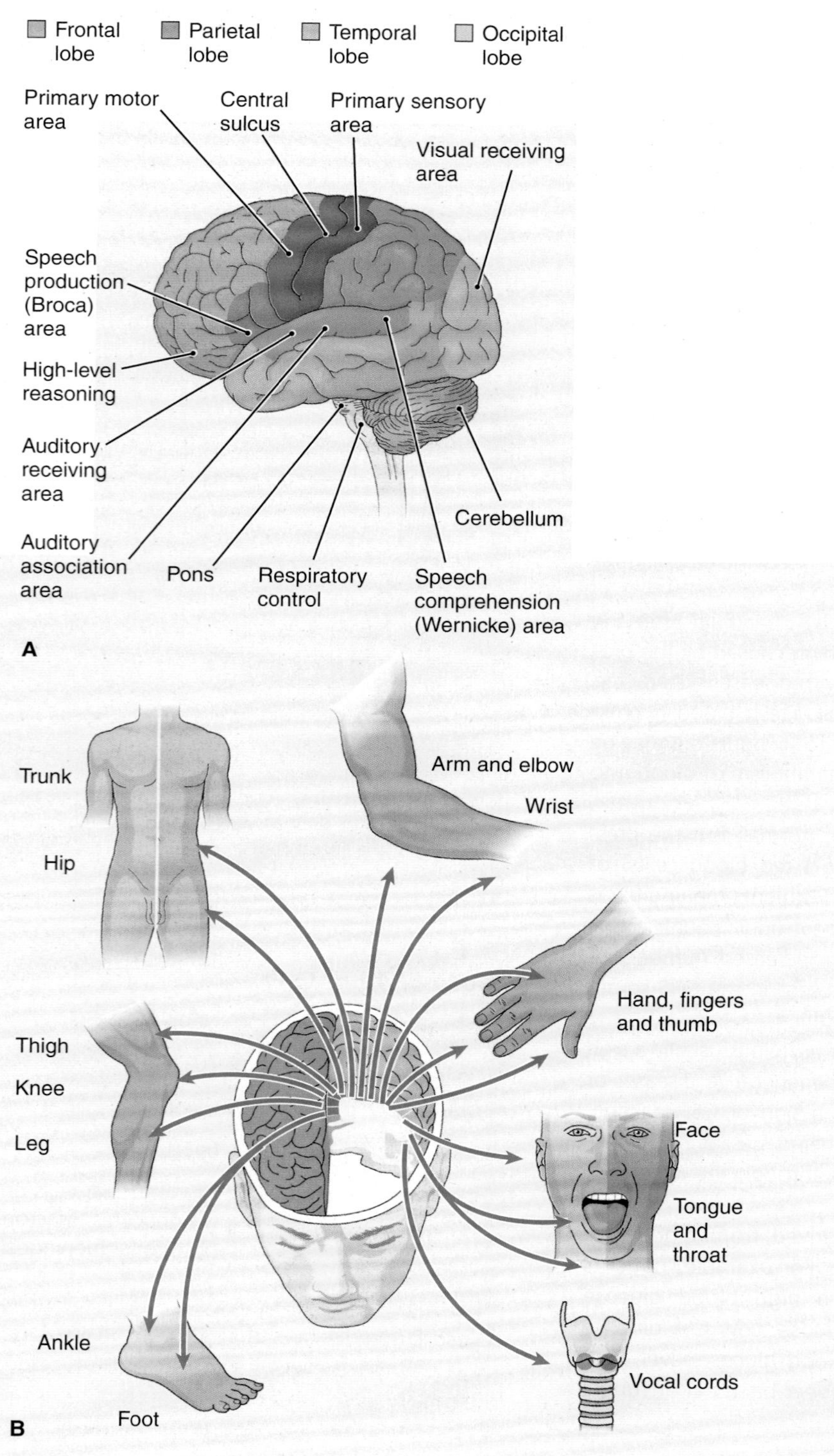

Figure 19.6 **Functional anatomy of the brain. A.** Map of cortical functions. **B.** Detailed map of motor functions, which reside in the left cerebral cortex in a right-handed person.

The cortex of each cerebral hemisphere is connected to the opposite side of the body; that is, the left cerebral cortex connects to the right side of the body. Incoming sensory signals from the right side of the body register in the left cerebral cortex, and outgoing voluntary motor signals to the right side of the body originate in the left cerebral cortex.

Furthermore, one side is dominant over the other, a feature that influences the "handedness" of the person. For example, the left cerebral hemisphere is motor dominant in right-handed people because it contains all of the brain tissue that gives the right side of the body more skill. The opposite is true in left-handed people. Also of importance, speech is modulated by the left cerebral cortex in 95% of right-handed people. In left-handed people, speech is modulated on the left in 80%. Nevertheless, even in speech, one of the most lateralized functions, the side opposite the dominant one is responsible for accent, intonation, and some grammatical functions.

The complex functions of the brain—spatial conceptualization, face recognition, visual imagery, musical ability, mathematics and logic, to name a few—require contributions from both sides. They are not necessarily the same from one person to the next. Most experts agree that the differences in right-brain versus left-brain function have been exaggerated in the popular press. In every person, the two hemispheres work together and share information through the nerve tracts that form the corpus callosum.

Case Notes

19.4 When Ted had trouble speaking, which side of his cerebrum was most likely responsible?

19.5 On his second hospital admission, Ted was paralyzed on his right side. Which side of his cerebrum was responsible?

The CNS Vascular Supply Is Unique

Figure 19.7 depicts two of the three unique aspects of the vascular supply to the brain: 1) the interconnections of vessels at the base of the brain; and 2) the relative lack of interconnections elsewhere in the cranium. The third unique feature is the structure of brain capillaries.

The vascular network of the brain is designed to allow alternative routes of flow if one route becomes obstructed. The main blood supply to the brain travels through the internal carotid arteries in the anterior neck; a second primary supply routes through the vertebral arteries in the posterior neck. Flow from the carotids and the vertebral arteries is linked into a circle by anterior and posterior communicating arteries to form a loop of interconnected vessels (the **circle of Willis**) in the subarachnoid space, which circles the brainstem on the floor of the skull and offers an alternative route for blood if one supply vessel becomes obstructed (Fig. 19.7A). For example, if one carotid is obstructed, lost flow can be replaced with blood flowing from the other carotid across the anterior communicating artery, or from the vertebral arteries via the basilar and posterior communicating arteries.

Above the circle of Willis brain arteries have few interconnections. This anatomic fact makes brain tissue at the far end of the vascular supply especially vulnerable to decreased blood flow because no alternative supply routes exist. Figures 19.7B and 19.7C illustrate that each area of the brain is supplied by distinct blood vessels. Where these areas adjoin is a long, thin strip of cortex that is at the far end of the blood supply from both sides. This area is especially vulnerable to ischemia or infarction if blood flow or oxygen level is low. Such vulnerable areas are called *'watershed'* areas, the name taken from the resemblance of brain blood vessel distribution to water drainage routes on either side of a ridgeline.

The third unique aspect of CNS vasculature is the very tight union with one another of the endothelial cells that form CNS capillaries. Adjacent cells do not have tiny slits between them as do the endothelial cells of capillaries in other tissues. The walls of capillaries in the brain are cemented together so tightly that many bloodborne substances simply cannot pass. This extremely low permeability of brain capillaries is known as the **blood–brain barrier**. Adding to this molecular barricade is the effect of the pia mater, which plays a role in keeping some molecules from diffusing into the brain from the CSF.

As a result, only small molecules—mainly gases and fat-soluble substances—can move across these barriers without assistance. Alcohol, caffeine, and nicotine are small and fat-soluble and easily diffuse into the brain. Certain small, water-soluble substances, such as glucose and amino acids, pass by active cell membrane transport. Large molecules, proteins (antigens and antibodies, in particular), and many drugs (especially some antibiotics) cannot enter brain tissue. The blood–brain barrier also prevents most bacteria from infecting delicate brain tissue.

The Peripheral Nervous System

The **peripheral nervous system (PNS)** consists of a network of nerves, which exists mainly outside of the CNS but is connected to it. It has two divisions, *somatic* (*voluntary*) and *autonomic* (*involuntary*).

The Brain and Spinal Cord Give Rise to Nerves of the Somatic Division

The **somatic division** (Figs. 19.8 and 19.9) of the PNS is composed of nerves that arise from the brain and spinal cord. These nerves carry incoming (*afferent*) sensory signals from sensors for sight, smell, taste, hearing, touch, pain, heat, and others, and outgoing (*efferent*) motor signals to skeletal muscle.

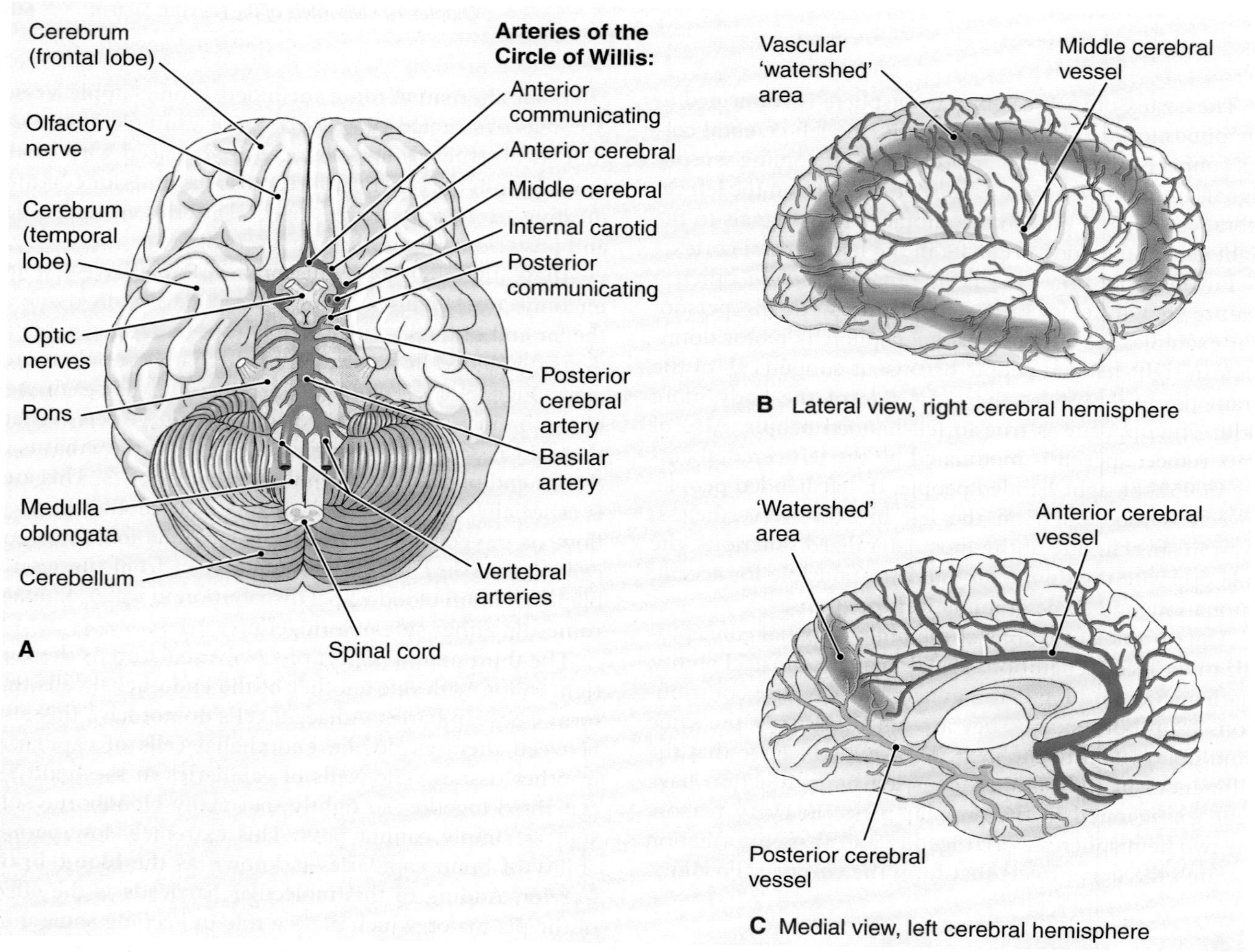

Cerebrum (frontal lobe)
Olfactory nerve
Cerebrum (temporal lobe)
Optic nerves
Pons
Medulla oblongata
Cerebellum
Spinal cord
Arteries of the Circle of Willis:
Anterior communicating
Anterior cerebral
Middle cerebral
Internal carotid
Posterior communicating
Posterior cerebral artery
Basilar artery
Vertebral arteries
A

Vascular 'watershed' area
Middle cerebral vessel
B Lateral view, right cerebral hemisphere

'Watershed' area
Anterior cerebral vessel
Posterior cerebral vessel
C Medial view, left cerebral hemisphere

Figure 19.7 **Arterial blood supply to the brain. A.** The major vessels and their interconnections in the circle of Willis. **B.** and **C.** The vascular supply to the cerebral cortex with emphasis of "watershed" areas.

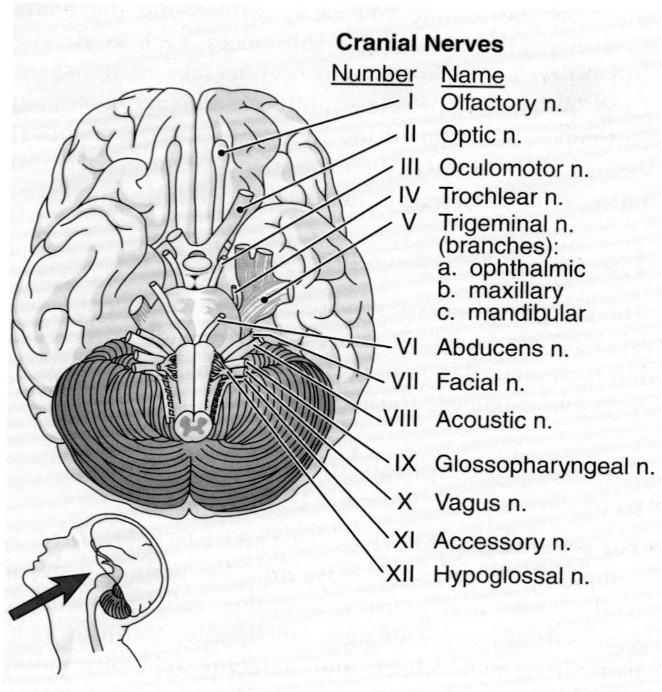

Figure 19.8 **The peripheral nervous system: cranial nerves.**

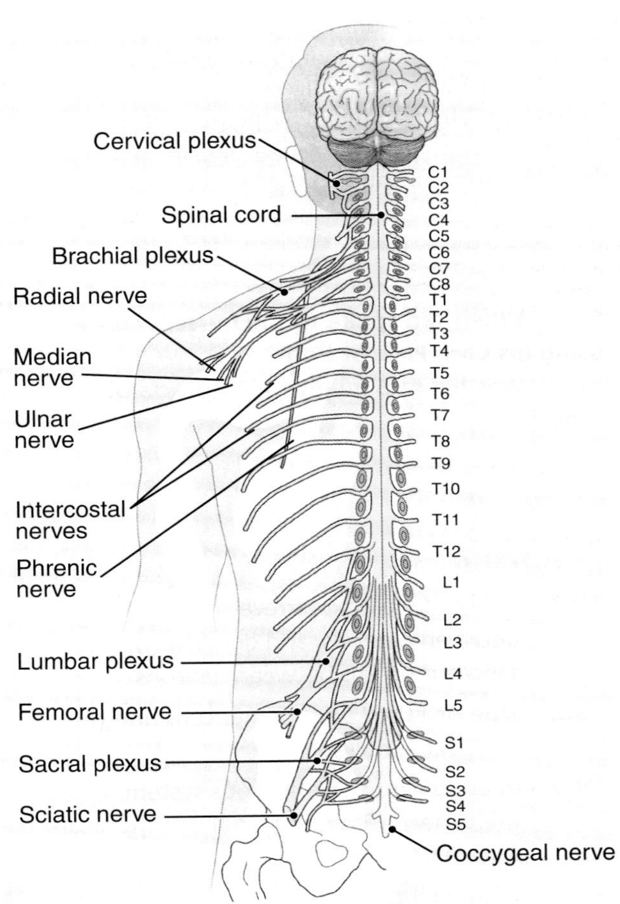

Figure 19.9 **The peripheral nervous system: spinal nerves and nerve plexuses.**

Cranial nerves (CN) arise from the brain. The cell bodies of CNS neurons are located in nuclei in the brain. They are traditionally numbered from superior to inferior by Roman numerals (Fig. 19.8). They are also named according to the most important structure they control. For example, CN I is the *olfactory nerve*; CN II is the *optic nerve*, and so on. Most carry a mix of motor and sensory signals. Some, however, are purely sensory (e.g., the olfactory, optic, and vestibulocochlear), while others are purely motor (e.g., the oculomotor and others serving eye movement).

Thirty-one pairs of **spinal nerves** arise from the sides of the spinal cord (Fig. 19.9). A cross section of the spinal cord reveals a central core of gray matter arranged roughly in the shape of a butterfly (Fig. 19.10). Each wing is called a **horn**. The ventral horns contain the cell bodies of motor neurons. The dorsal horns contain the unmyelinated (and therefore gray) axons of sensory neurons whose cell bodies are located outside the spinal cord in the dorsal root **ganglion** (a collection of neuron cell bodies outside the CNS). Fitted between and around the horns are thick bundles of myelinated nerve axons called **white columns**, which convey sensory and motor signals up and down the cord.

With the exception of the cervical nerves, the spinal nerves are named according to the vertebra superior to their point of exit from the vertebral canal. For instance, the first lumbar nerve (L1) exits inferior to the first lumbar vertebra. For cervical nerves, however, the opposite applies. Nerves 1 through 8 are named for the vertebra inferior to their point of exit because the first spinal nerve exits inferior the cranium and superior to the first cervical vertebra (the atlas).

Spinal nerves have three portions, much like the roots, trunk, and branches of a tree. Each nerve has two roots—a **ventral root** through which motor axons exit the cord carrying outgoing signals, and a **dorsal root** through which sensory axons enter the cord carrying incoming signals. Just after exiting the cord, dorsal and ventral roots join to form a short, thick combined nerve *trunk*, which exits the vertebral column as a spinal nerve and then

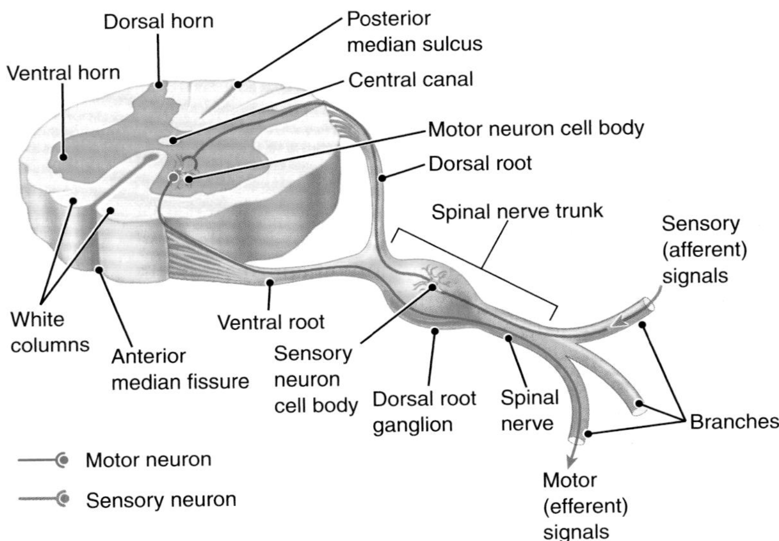

Figure 19.10 **Cross-sectional anatomy of the spinal cord.**

divides into multiple *branches* that spread outward like tree branches to connect with body structures.

Each spinal nerve serves a particular anatomic site. For example, sensory signals from the thumb travel up a nerve branch in the arm and enter the spinal cord via the dorsal (sensory) root of the sixth cervical nerve (C6). Outbound C6 motor signals to muscles and other tissues in the arm travel through the ventral motor root.

The ventral branches of thoracic nerves 2 through 12 extend directly to the structures they supply. The ventral branches of cervical, lumbar, sacral, and coccygeal spinal nerves, however, intermingle to form plexuses (Latin = braids)—webs of interlaced axons that recombine to form nerves that carry axons from multiple spinal cord segments. For example, branches of some lumbar nerves and most sacral nerves unite to form the *sacral plexus*. The axons of many of these branches recombine to form the *sciatic nerve*, the largest nerve in the body.

The Autonomic Nervous System Is Involuntary

The **autonomic nervous system (ANS)** (Fig. 19.11) is an involuntary system of nerves that carries motor and sensory signals to and from the hypothalamus. Neurons of the autonomic system send axons down cranial and spinal nerves to connect with autonomic ganglia near the spinal cord or in target tissue. The ANS acts on cardiac muscle, smooth muscle, and glands to control functions such as heart rate, blood pressure, sweating and other gland secretions, and bowel peristalsis. The ANS has two divisions: *sympathetic* and *parasympathetic*, which have opposing effects.

The **sympathetic division** (or *thoracolumbar division*) is a network of nerve fibers and ganglia that originates from neurons in the thoracic and lumbar spinal cord. They synapse in ganglia of the **sympathetic chain**, which runs vertically on either side of the thoracic and lumbar spinal column. Sympathetic fibers also connect directly to the adrenal medulla, which can be thought of functionally as a very large sympathetic ganglion.

The hypothalamus reacts to stress by initiating sympathetic signals that stimulate secretion of the neurotransmitter *norepinephrine* from nerve endings in target tissue. Because sympathetic signals have an effect like secretion of epinephrine and norepinephrine from the adrenal medulla, the action of the sympathetic system is called the **adrenergic effect**. Secretion of norepinephrine affects tissues and organs in what is typically called the "fight-or-flight" response—heart rate and blood pressure rise, the metabolic rate increases, pupils and bronchi dilate, the liver releases glucose, and sweating begins.

The **parasympathetic division** (or *craniosacral division*) is a network of fibers and ganglia that originates from neurons in the brain and lower (sacral) spinal cord. In contrast to sympathetic ganglia, which are located along the vertebral column, parasympathetic ganglia lie in or near the target tissue. Hypothalamic stimulation of the parasympathetic system causes release of the neurotransmitter *acetylcholine*, which is a "rest-and-digest" effect that is opposite of the adrenergic "fight-or-flight" response. This is called the **cholinergic** effect. Table 19.1 lists the effects of the sympathetic and parasympathetic systems on selected organs.

Case Notes

19.6 When Ted spoke to the nurse, was he using his CNS, PNS, or both?

19.7 Was his ANS involved in his acts of speech?

Pop Quiz

19.1 True or false? Axons receive signals between neurons, and dendrites send out signals between neurons.

19.2 True or false? Ependymal cells line the cerebral ventricles.

19.3 In addition to the nervous system, what is the other primary internal communication system?

19.4 What cell type is responsible for making myelin in the CNS?

19.5 True or false? Every part of the brain has the same basic function as another part of the brain.

19.6 True or false? The cerebellum lies above the tentorium cerebelli.

19.7 What structure in the brain is responsible for communication between the cerebral hemispheres?

19.8 In what layer of brain do the higher functions occur?

19.9 True or false? There are 32 pairs of spinal nerves.

19.10 True or false? The sympathetic nervous response is also called "fight-or-flight" response.

19.11 What are the two components of the ANS?

19.12 The ______ roots of the spinal nerves are responsible for motor function, while the ______ roots of the spinal nerves are responsible for sensory function.

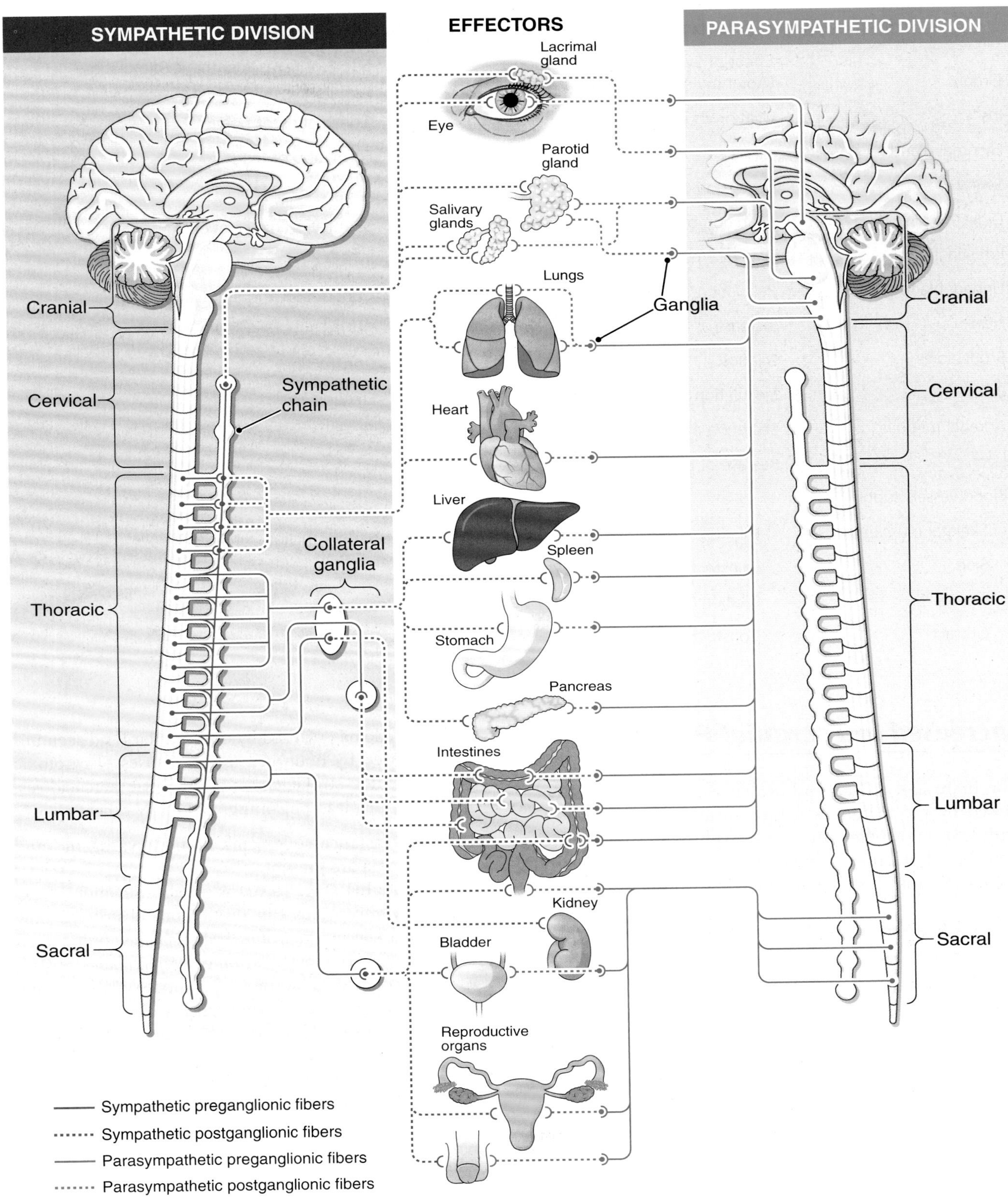

Figure 19.11 **The autonomic nervous system.** (Reproduced with permission from Cohen B. *Memmler's The Human Body in Health and Disease.* 10th ed. Baltimore, MD. Lippincott Williams and Wilkins; 2005.

Table 19.1 The Effects of Autonomic Stimulation on Selected Target Organs

Organ	Effect of Sympathetic Stimulation (Adrenergic Effect)	Effect of Parasympathetic Stimulation (Cholinergic Effect)
Iris	Dilation of pupil	Constriction of pupil
Lacrimal gland	—	Formation of tears
Sweat glands	Formation of sweat	—
Digestive glands	Inhibition of secretions	Stimulation of secretions
Intestinal motility	Decrease peristalsis	Increase peristalsis
Urinary bladder	Relaxation and expansion	Contraction and emptying
Heart	Increase in rate and power of contraction	Decrease in rate and power of contraction
Bronchioles	Dilation	Constriction
Penis	Ejaculation	Erection
Adrenal medulla	Secretion of epinephrine and norepinephrine	—
Liver	Release of glucose	—
Blood vessels supplying:		
Skeletal muscle	Dilation	Constriction
Skin	Constriction	—
Lung	Dilation	Constriction
GI tract	Constriction	Dilation

Increased Intracranial Pressure

The brain and spinal cord are encased in bone and enclosed by the meninges, which form a sealed sac filled with CSF under pressure that is slightly greater than venous blood pressure. Intracranial pressure is regulated by the production, circulation, and reabsorption of CSF.

Increased Pressure Is Due to Brain Edema, Abnormal CSF Flow, or Intracranial Mass

An abnormal increase in intracranial pressure can be caused by cerebral edema, obstruction to flow or resorption of CSF, or an intracranial mass. Increased intracranial pressure can cause herniation of brain tissue through cranial foramina or from one side of the falx or tentorium to another, or ischemia and infarction by restricting blood supply. Alternatively, it may prevent normal venous outflow, which can cause severe venous congestion and hemorrhage.

Cerebral edema is due to increased fluid in brain cells or between them. The two types are as follows:

- *Vasogenic* edema is caused by disruption of the blood-brain barrier with increased vascular permeability. Causes of vasogenic edema include malignant hypertension, altitude sickness, and brain tumors.
- *Cytotoxic* edema is caused by intracellular fluid accumulation caused by brain cell injury. Causes of cytotoxic edema include stroke, infection, diabetic ketoacidosis, hyponatremia, lead poisoning, and many others.

In many instances, elements of both vasogenic and cytotoxic edema are present.

Hydrocephalus (Fig. 19.12) is an accumulation of excess CSF. Hydrocephalus can result from obstructed flow (*obstructive* or *noncommunicating hydrocephalus*) or impaired resorption of CSF (*communicating hydrocephalus*). Most cases are accompanied by increased intracranial pressure, though normal pressure hydrocephalus (NPS) does occur. Obstruction usually occurs in the aqueduct of Sylvius between the third and fourth ventricles but may occur at any point of flow. The culprit is often congenital brain-skull base malformations or infection. Impaired resorption from the subarachnoid space is usually the result of infection or hemorrhage. In children, because skull bone sutures are not fused, increased intracranial pressure due to excess CSF is relieved by enlargement of the skull and pressure remains near normal. Later in life, however, the skull cannot expand and intracranial pressure rises without cranial enlargement. Pressure expands the ventricle and can cause atrophy of brain *parenchyma* (the functional cells of an organ, as distinct from supporting cells), a condition called *hydrocephalus ex vacuo*.

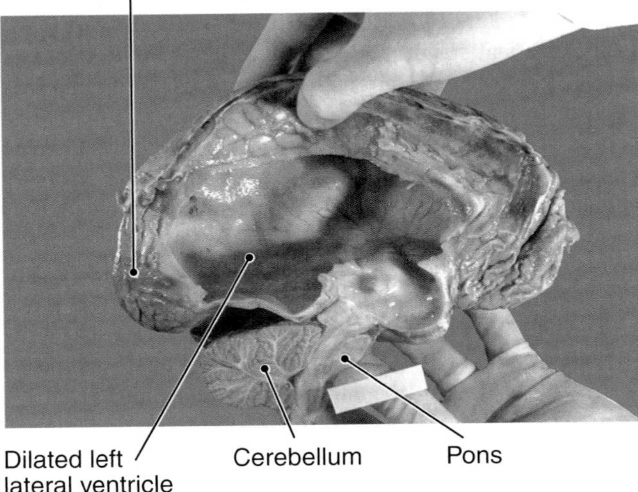

Figure 19.12 **The brain in hydrocephalus.** In this patient, flow of CSF was obstructed in the aqueduct of Sylvius (not labeled) between the third and fourth ventricles (noncommunicating hydrocephalus). Increased intraventricular pressure caused ventricular dilation and atrophy of surrounding brain tissue.

Normal pressure hydrocephalus (NPH) can occur in adults and is usually due to impaired CSF absorption. The result is expanded ventricles, cerebral atrophy, and dementia in a patient with normal CSF pressure. NPH accounts for about 5% of dementia in the United States. Symptoms include incontinence, impaired gait, and other neurologic signs and symptoms, which may mimic multiple sclerosis (MS), Parkinsonism, and other degenerative brain disease.

Increased intracranial pressure is pathologic and, like fluid under pressure in any closed space, CSF seeks natural relief by enlarging the space or escaping through any available opening. In older children and adults, however, the skull cannot enlarge. In the case of a mass such as a tumor, abscess or hemorrhage presses on other parts of the brain; if the mass expands slowly, as many brain tumors do, the result is pressure atrophy. Nevertheless, a rapid increase of mass or pressure within the strict confines of the adult skull can force the brain to herniate through internal or external openings in several ways (Fig. 19.13).

A **subfalcine herniation** is herniation of the lower medial aspect of the affected cerebral hemisphere horizontally across the lower margin of the falx cerebri, which may press on the anterior cerebral artery to produce cerebral ischemia or infarct. A **tentorial herniation** is herniation of the ipsilateral (same side) temporal lobe

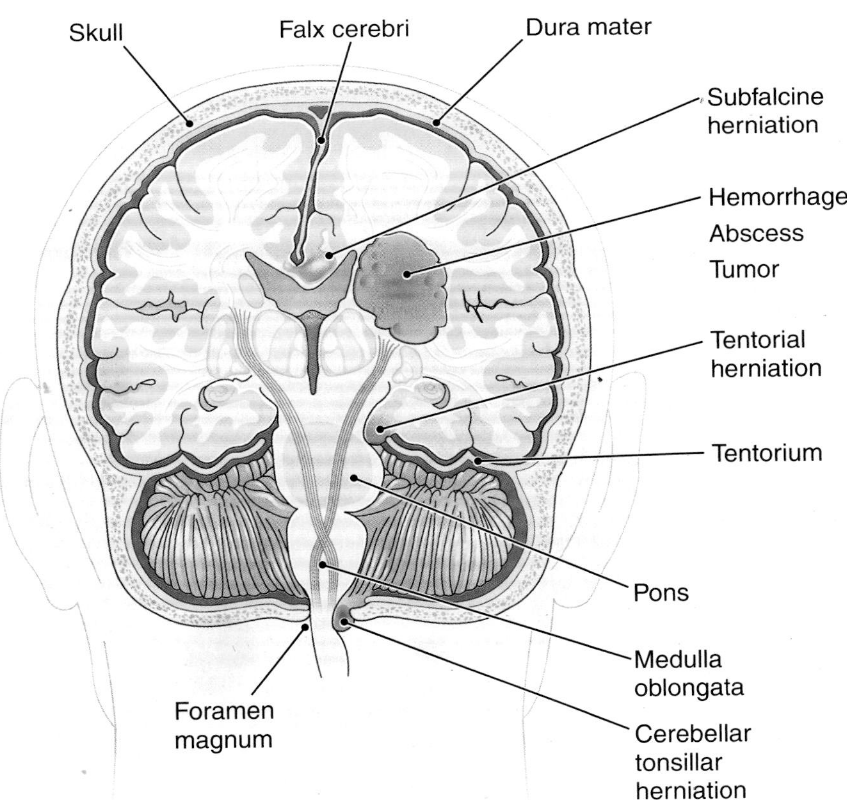

Figure 19.13 **Brain herniations.** Brain edema, intracranial tumor, and hemorrhage are the usual causes.

downward and medially through the tentorium. The herniated brain may press on the third CN, causing dilation of the pupils or impairment of eye motion, or it may press on and obstruct the posterior cerebral artery to cause brain hemorrhage or infarction. A **tonsillar herniation** is herniation of the lower cerebellum, an area known as the cerebellar tonsils, through the foramen magnum. Tonsillar herniation obstructs venous and arterial blood flow in the brainstem and can produce hemorrhage or infarction in the midbrain. Figure 19.14 illustrates a case of pontine hemorrhage, which usually occurs secondary to tonsillar herniation caused by massive intracerebral hemorrhage.

Increased intracranial pressure can also push on one or both of the optic nerves and cause bulging of the optic disc, where the optic nerve enters the eye, a condition known as **papilledema**.

Finally, diseases that cause brain atrophy—AD, for example—are accompanied by compensatory accumulations of CSF in the ventricles or over the surface of the brain (*hydrocephalus ex vacuo*) to make up for lost brain tissue.

Signs and Symptoms Are Distinctive

Evidence of increased intracranial pressure is a distinctive combination of signs and symptoms that often include papilledema, dilated pupils, increased blood pressure with bradycardia, abnormal respiratory pattern, headache, nausea, projectile vomiting, seizures, drowsiness, altered consciousness, CN palsy, and other neurologic signs and symptoms.

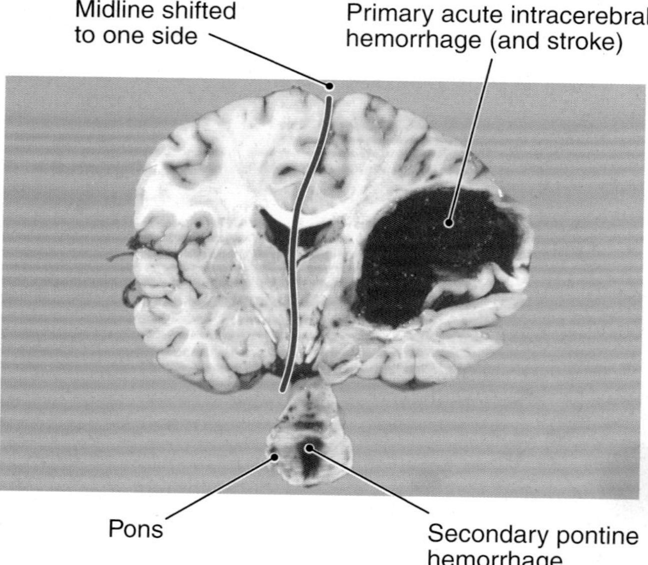

Figure 19.14 **Pontine hemorrhage secondary to cerebellar tonsillar herniation.** A massive intracerebral hemorrhage in a patient with hypertension has forced the cerebellar tonsils into the foramen magnum, which obstructed venous blood flow in the pons and caused secondary pontine hemorrhage.

Diagnosis and Treatment Are Urgent

Diagnosis and treatment are urgent because increased pressure impairs blood flow into the brain and compression of critical structures may cause permanent injury or death. Pressure measurement, neurologic examination, and imaging are the most important diagnostic tools. Pressure is usually measured by a pressure sensor attached to a needle inserted into the lumbar spinal subdural space (a spinal tap). Neurologic exam looks for eye signs such as papilledema, abnormal pupils, and abnormal eye movements, and for altered mental status and sensory or motor defects. Imaging is usually CAT or MRI scan to look for a mass, accumulations of blood, narrowed cortical sulci (which would suggest edema), or shifts of anatomic parts, (e.g., shift of the midline structures to one side).

Treatment is twofold: eliminate the cause and reduce the pressure. If the cause is hydrocephalus, a surgically inserted shunt may be used to drain CSF into the peritoneum. For cerebral edema, the treatment includes osmotic agents to increase blood osmotic power and draw fluid out of the brain. Craniotomy may relieve pressure. Steroid therapy is effective in vasogenic edema. Medically induced coma, hypothermia, and paralysis with mechanical respiration can buy time by slowing brain metabolism.

Case Notes

19.8 Ted's CSF pressure was normal by lumbar puncture measurement when he was admitted with an ischemic infarct. Though it was not measured again, was it likely to be normal, high, or low when he died?

19.9 What caused Ted's secondary pontine hemorrhage?

Pop Quiz

19.13 True or false? Hydrocephalus ex vacuo is due to decreased brain volume, rather than increased CSF pressure.

19.14 True or false? Hyponatremia causes cerebral edema.

19.15 What are the three main types of herniation of the brain?

19.16 Increased intracranial pressure can be seen during an eye exam. What is the term for this finding?

CNS Congenital and Perinatal Disorder

Most congenital brain defects result from interruptions of critical embryologic development or cytogenetic disease. Neural tube defects such a *spina bifida* and *meningomyelocele* and cytogenetic disorders such as *Down syndrome* are among the most common and are discussed in Chapter 22.

Arnold-Chiari malformation is a defect in which the brainstem and cerebellum are compacted into a shallow posterior fossa beneath a low tentorium. It is often associated with a neural tube defect.

Congenital hydrocephalus usually owes to stenosis of the aqueduct of Sylvius.

There are several varieties of cerebral gyri. **Polymicrogyria** is an excessive number of narrow gyri. **Agyria** (lissencephaly) is absence of gyri: the cerebral surface is smooth. Most of these disorders are associated with mental retardation.

Microcephaly is an unusually small skull and brain that may be caused by cytogenetic abnormalities, fetal alcohol syndrome, and congenital infection by the AIDS virus (HIV).

Cerebral palsy (Fig. 19.15) is a broad clinical term applied to permanent, nonprogressive motor problems (spasticity, paralysis) that arise owing to an insult to the brain before it reaches a certain maturity. Because brain development continues during the first two years of life, cerebral palsy can result from brain injury occurring in utero or before age two. About 75% of all cerebral palsy cases arise from unknown prenatal conditions. Some cases are associated with birth trauma. Neonatal risk factors for cerebral palsy include prematurity, low birth weight, and intrauterine growth retardation. About 15% of cases arise from injury after birth: brain or meningeal infections, hyperbilirubinemia, automobile accidents, falls, or child abuse.

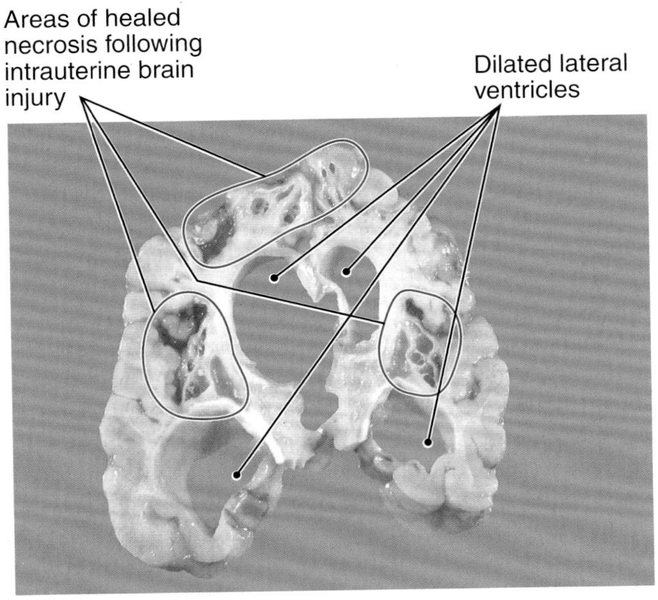

Areas of healed necrosis following intrauterine brain injury

Dilated lateral ventricles

Figure 19.15 **The brain in cerebral palsy.** Coronal section of the brain of a child showing severe tissue loss and dilated ventricles.

Epilepsy is a paroxysmal, transient disorder of brain function that is often associated with loss of consciousness, sensory or mental disturbance, and abnormal motor activity. It is caused by abnormal electrical discharge in the cerebral cortex. Newborns and infants are particularly vulnerable. About 75% of epilepsy cases are not associated with demonstrable anatomic defect. Most of the remainder are caused by arteriovenous malformations, gliosis (scarring) of any cause, or tumor. Fever may cause epileptic seizure in children. About 2% of adults will have an epileptic seizure; two-thirds will not have another.

Treatment is usually medical; however, surgery may be necessary to excise the excitatory focus.

Pop Quiz

19.17 True or false? Most cases of cerebral palsy are due to prebirth conditions.

19.18 Name two neural tube defects.

19.19 True or false? Most adults who have a seizure will have another one.

CNS Trauma

CNS injury can be caused directly by contact between an object and the brain or spinal cord, or indirectly by transmission of kinetic energy, which causes brain movement and damage within the skull. Trauma may be *penetrating* or *blunt*. The injury may be *open* or *closed* according to whether or not the skull has been fractured or penetrated. The results of trauma are *fracture*, *parenchymal injury*, and *vascular injury*; all three may coexist. The consequences of trauma depend on the location of the lesion and the limited capacity of the CNS to repair functional damage. Automobile accidents are the most common cause of injury; other causes include assaults, falls, and child abuse.

Any skull fracture may damage CN, vessels, the vestibulocochlear apparatus of the inner ear, or the pituitary (Fig. 19.16). A fracture in which the bone is displaced into the cranial cavity by more than the thickness of the bone is a *displaced skull fracture*. Displaced bone may lacerate meningeal or cerebral arteries or the sagittal or tentorial sinuses.

Parenchymal injury may cause purely functional disorder such as a concussion, or it may cause tearing, laceration, or bleeding.

Intracranial hemorrhage is a common consequence of head trauma. It is classified according to its anatomic

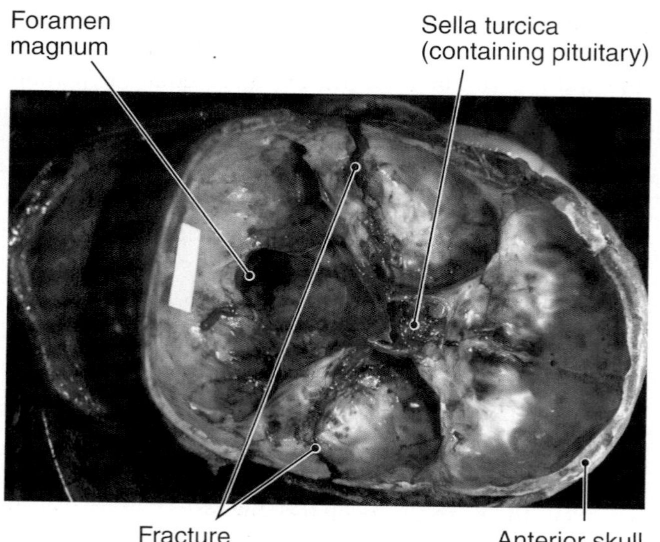

Figure 19.16 **Basilar skull fracture.** This patient developed an acute epidural hematoma, caused by bleeding from an artery torn by the fracture.

location: within the tissue of the brain (intraparenchymal) or on the surface of the brain (extraparenchymal). Extraparenchymal hemorrhage is classified according to its relationship to the skull and meningeal layers: epidural, subdural, or subarachnoid.

Spinal Cord Injury Is Usually Due to Severe Neck Extension or Flexion

Spinal cord injury usually results in paralysis. *Paraplegia* is paralysis of the lower limbs. *Quadriplegia* is paralysis of all four extremities. *Hemiplegia* is paralysis of one side of the body.

Etiology

Trauma to the spinal cord may be direct due to penetrating injury, but more often the cord is damaged by extreme forced extension or flexion. Extreme extension (e.g., shallow water–diving accidents) can tear the anterior spinal ligament. The extreme rearward tilt of the neck swings the posterior arch of a vertebral body downward and into contact with the posterior side of the cord. Extreme flexion injury usually occurs in conjunction with downward force (e.g., American football collisions to the top of the helmet), which fractures a vertebral body, allowing it to slide forward. This brings the anterior side of the cord into contact with posterior edge of the underlying vertebra.

Spinal cord *concussion* is the mildest spinal cord injury. Temporary paralysis or weakness may appear and disappear rapidly. Spinal cord *contusion* is more severe. Variable degrees of permanent flaccid paralysis occur. Spinal cord *laceration* or *transection* is most severe and causes permanent flaccid paralysis according to the degree and location of disruption.

Signs and Symptoms

The consequences of spinal cord injury vary according to the severity of the injury. Very high cord injuries may damage the respiratory center in the medulla oblongata and paralyze respiratory effort. Autonomic control of bowel and bladder function may be lost, but eventually may return. Full transverse injury at the C8-T1 level causes complete, flaccid paralysis and anesthesia of the legs. Similar injury at progressively higher levels includes more extensive paralysis of the upper extremity. Injury at C5 or above includes complete, flaccid paralysis below the neck and may include respiratory paralysis. Partial injury produces mixed sensory and motor effects depending on the particular anatomic damage. Damage to the cervical cord deprives the chest wall of motor nerve innervation and can cause respiratory impairment.

Diagnosis and Treatment

If vertebral fracture or spinal cord injury is suspected, the first step is immobilization. Diagnosis is clinical with confirmation by X-ray and CT imaging of the spine. Treatment includes respiratory and vascular support if necessary. Surgical decompression and permanent immobilization (vertebral fusion) may be necessary. Steroid therapy and other measures may limit further damage.

Nonpenetrating (Closed) Head Injury May Cause Serious Permanent Injury

A **concussion** is a clinical syndrome of temporary brain dysfunction following head injury. It is not associated with immediate anatomic brain lesions. About 10% of concussion victims are rendered unconscious, usually only for a few minutes. Minor symptoms (not necessitating emergency care) include headache, drowsiness, confusion, and amnesia for events immediately before and after the injury. Nevertheless, if these symptoms persist or worsen, emergency care is required. Major symptoms, which require emergency care, include nausea and vomiting, convulsions, muscle weakness of one side of the body or of a limb or other body part, unequal pupils, unusual eye movements, or trouble walking or standing upright.

Repeated blows to the head, with or without concussion, can cause chronic brain disorders including dementia or Parkinson syndrome (e.g., as suffered by American boxer Muhammad Ali).

Nonpenetrating trauma also may cause **contusion**, superficial (cortical) bleeding that is equivalent to a bruise in soft tissues. It is characterized by hemorrhages caused by sudden shift of the brain that brings the cortex into contact with the skull. Blunt force to an immobile head causes injury to brain tissue immediately beneath the site of the blow. This is referred to as the **coup injury** (French *coup* = blow). If the brain is injured by being propelled into the skull opposite the site of the blow, however, the injury is a **contrecoup injury**. In general, if the head is immobile at the time of injury, the contusion is coup; if

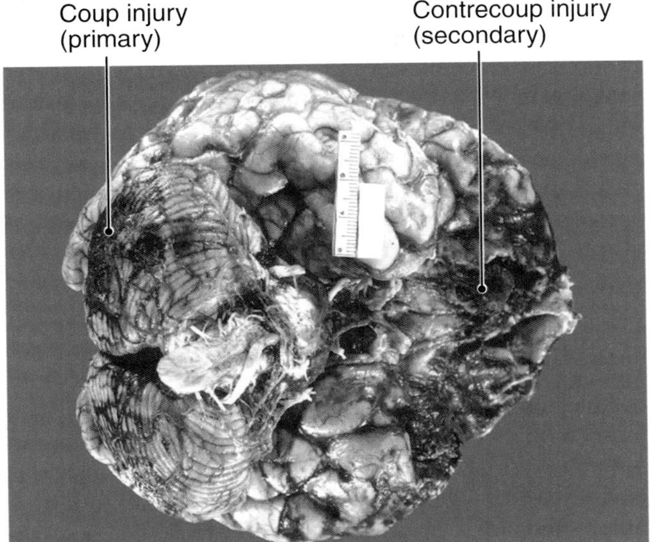

Figure 19.17 **Brain contusion: coup and contrecoup injuries.** This patient received a primary blow (the coup injury) to the posterior skull (occiput). At the opposite (frontal) side of the skull is a contusion in the frontal lobes (the contrecoup injury) caused by commotion of the brain inside the skull.

the head is mobile, both injuries may occur. Figure 19.17 illustrates the coup-contrecoup combination. The main hazards are direct damage to brain tissue at the site of hemorrhage and increased intracranial pressure.

The signs and symptoms of a mild contusion are similar to those of concussion; however, more extensive cortical hemorrhage may be associated with increased intracranial pressure, brain herniation, or focal neurologic deficit.

Diagnosis is clinical. CT imaging typically reveals areas of cortical bleeding and injury, whereas, in concussion, no imaging abnormalities are present. Treatment may require surgical decompression if intracranial pressure becomes high.

A third variety of closed head injury is **diffuse axonal injury**, which occurs when sudden, severe twisting motion of the head (as in an auto accident) can stretch brain nerve tracts (white matter) to the point of injury. Gross abnormalities may be minimal, but severe neurologic deficit (e.g., dementia or permanent coma) can occur. About half of people who become comatose shortly after head trauma are believed to have diffuse axonal injury.

Diagnosis is clinical. Imaging typically reveals extensive lesions in central white matter. Treatment is supportive.

Laceration and Blast Effect Are the Result of Penetrating Objects

Objects such as bullets and knives that penetrate the brain produce a **laceration** of tissue. In the absence of direct injury to vital brain centers (e.g., respiratory center), the immediate threat to life is hemorrhage. Bleeding may create a hematoma that presses on vital centers or creates a herniation of brain tissue. The velocity of the penetrating object, usually a bullet, contributes to an effect called **blast effect**. The object itself disrupts tissue but the blast effect may be more deadly: the blast effect of a high-velocity bullet wound can cause immediate death by herniating the cerebellar tonsils through the foramen magnum, which fatally compresses the brainstem.

Seizures are a threat to patients with a penetrating wound that has healed. They usually first occur about 6–12 months after the injury.

Treatment of penetrating trauma is surgical decompression and removal of blood.

Epidural Hematoma Is Due to Arterial Bleeding between Skull and Dura

Epidural hematoma is an accumulation of blood between the skull and the dura mater. It is almost always caused by a skull fracture that tears the middle meningeal artery; hence bleeding is rapid and the hematoma forms quickly (Fig. 19.18). Meningeal arteries are partially embedded

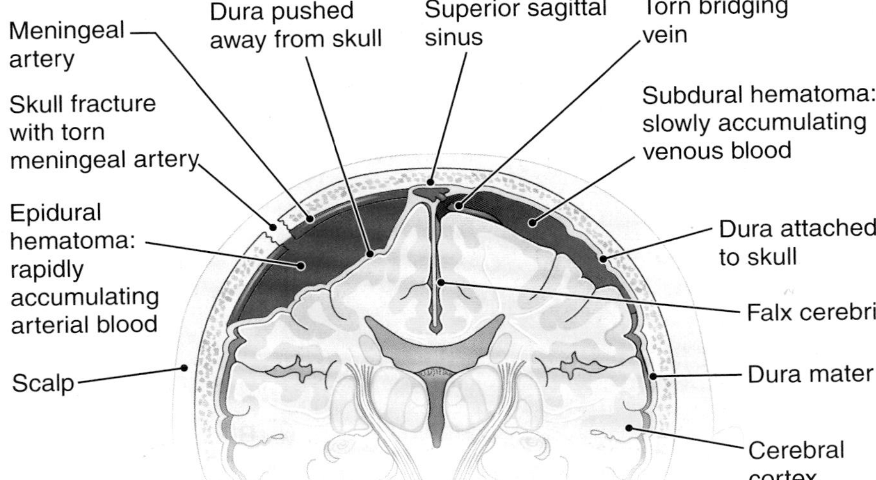

Figure 19.18 **Epidural and subdural hematomas. Left.** Epidural hematoma. Blood accumulates between dura and skull. Bleeding is arterial and rapid because the edges of a skull fracture sever a meningeal artery. **Right.** Subdural hematoma. Blood accumulates between the dura and arachnoid. Bleeding is slow and venous because shifting of the brain tears bridging veins that travel in the space between the arachnoid and dura (Fig. 19.14).

in the inner convexity of the skull and covered internally by the dura mater (see Fig. 19.4), so that they are easily torn by fracture. Because the dura is tightly bonded to the skull, the epidural space does not easily expand laterally and most of the accumulated blood bulges inward into the cerebrum. The enlarging epidural mass presses inward and downward, forcing a tentorial herniation (Fig. 19.13) of cerebral tissue that causes fatal compression of the midbrain. Epidural hematoma is almost universally fatal within 24 hours unless treated quickly by surgical hemostasis and evacuation of the hematoma.

In a significant minority of cases, subdural hematoma presents with a distinctive history. The initial trauma is a concussion severe enough to render the patient unconscious. The patient recovers consciousness for a while before becoming unconscious again, owing to accumulation of the hematoma and mounting intracranial pressure. This "lucid interval" is a key clinical diagnostic point. By contrast, patients with other types of intracranial bleeding from head injury usually show no lucid interval between episodes of unconsciousness.

Subdural Hematoma Is Due to Venous Bleeding between Dura and Arachnoid

Subdural hematoma (Figs. 19.18, 19.19, and 19.20) is an accumulation of blood between the dura and arachnoid caused by relatively slow venous bleeding. The degree of force that causes it to commence is less than that required to cause skull fracture. The trauma may be so mild that neither the patient nor anyone else can recall it, so there may be no history of head trauma. For example, patients on anticoagulant drugs bleed easily and may not recall the injury. Bleeding may be caused by almost any abrupt motion of the head resulting in significant internal shifting of the brain, including from falls, assaults, car accidents, and athletic injuries. A violently shaken infant (**shaken baby syndrome (SBS)** may develop subdural hematoma and related injuries. SBS is usually seen in infants under age two and may occur after less than five seconds of violent shaking (typically by an angry parent or caregiver), as the infant is unable to control its head. Neck and rib fractures may occur and can offer a diagnostic clue. Symptoms vary greatly and may be subtle. Seizures are obvious, but less obvious are lethargy, failure to smile, sleepiness, loss of vision, lack of appetite, irritability, and vomiting.

Subdural bleeding originates from small *bridging veins* that travel from the cerebral cortex through the subarachnoid space, cross the arachnoid, and run to the superior sagittal sinus between the arachnoid and dura. Because the bleeding in subdural hematomas is venous and low pressure, it usually stops due to local tamponade after an accumulation of 25–50 ml. The subdural space expands laterally with relative ease, so that the distribution of blood tends to be wide and not very thick. For this reason, subdural hematomas may never produce symptoms or may produce them only after a delay of days, weeks, or months. The hematoma lies outside the subarachnoid space, and no blood may be found in the CSF.

Subdural hematomas can be classified as *acute* or *chronic*:

- In **acute subdural hematoma** (Figs. 19.19 and 19.20), the history of trauma is usually clear and symptoms occur within hours or days. These patients are usually elderly and taking antiplatelet or anticoagulant drugs. Symptoms build over a period of several hours or days.
- Conversely, a clear clinical history of trauma may not be available in **chronic subdural hematoma**. After the original bleed, the hematoma may gradually resorb and leave no clinical trail, only microscopic evidence of its existence. Sometimes the hematoma remains static. These static hematomas organize and repair (Chapter 2). The hematoma becomes encapsulated

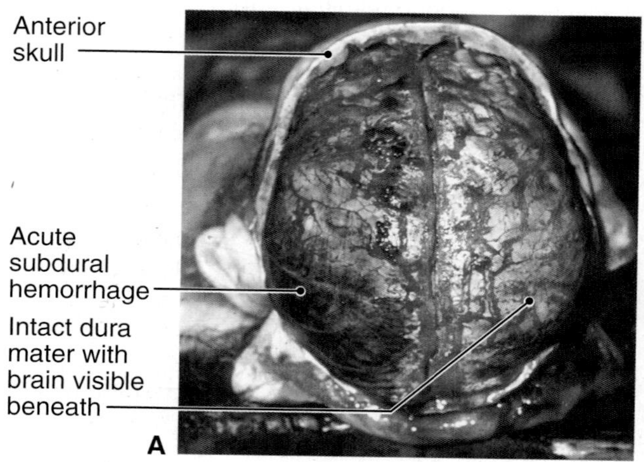

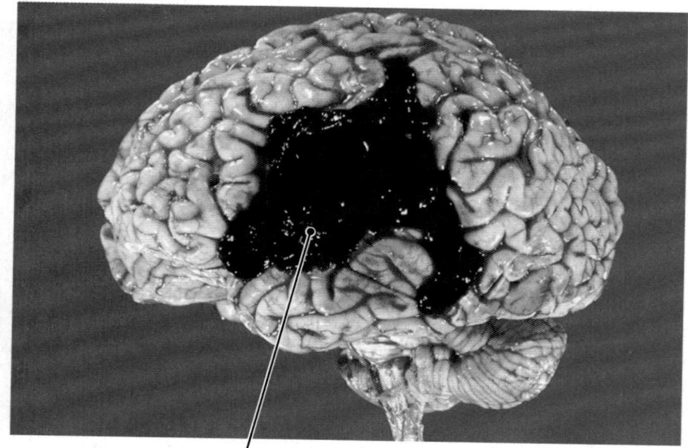

Figure 19.19 **Acute subdural hematoma.** This patient was taking anticoagulants and died of acute subdural hematoma after a mild head injury. **A.** Brain in the skull. Blood is visible through the intact dura mater. **B.** The brain with dura removed.

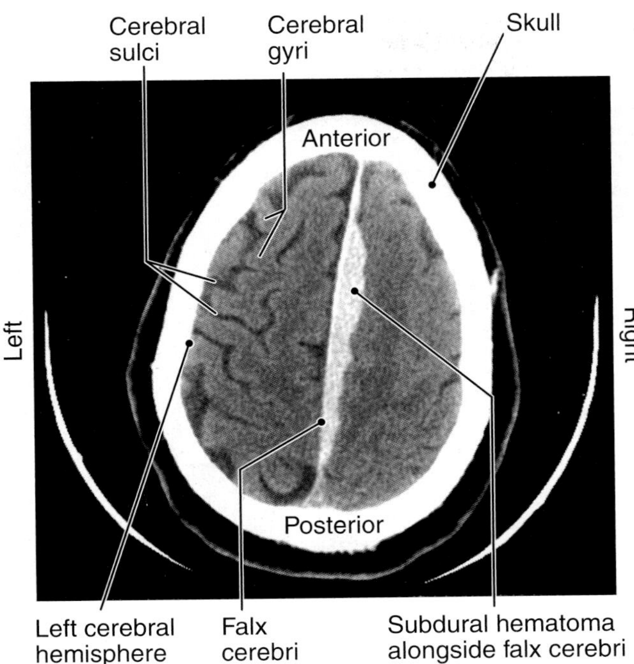

Figure 19.20 **Subdural hematoma (radiographic study).** Blood is accumulated to the right side of the falx cerebri. Note the blurring of sulci and gyri on the right owing to cerebral edema.

within a fibrous sac that sometimes contains highly vascular granulation tissue. It is postulated that rebleeding causes the hematoma to enlarge. Alternatively, some postulate that degenerating blood cells in the sac create high osmotic pressure that slowly expands the sac by attracting water.

Remember This! Epidural hematoma forms quickly; subdural hematoma forms slowly.

Subdural hematoma may be difficult to diagnose because the symptoms are so diverse. Stretching of the meninges causes headache while pressure on the motor cortex may produce contralateral weakness or seizures. Bilateral chronic subdural hematomas may impair cognition and cause dementia. Rebleeding and rapid expansion may produce fatal tentorial herniation.

Diagnosis depends on CAT or MRI imaging. Treatment is surgical evacuation of the fluid mass.

Trauma May Cause Subarachnoid Hemorrhage

Subarachnoid hemorrhage may be seen as a consequence of trauma. Nevertheless, unlike epidural and subdural hematomas, traumatic subarachnoid hemorrhage is usually not an isolated finding but occurs in conjunction with traumatic bleeding in other parts of the brain. When subarachnoid hemorrhage is an isolated finding, it is usually caused by vascular malformations, which account for about three-fourths of all subarachnoid hemorrhage.

Pop Quiz

19.20 True or false? A concussion is brain injury that lasts for a long period of time.

19.21 True or false? Contrecoup contusion occurs on the side of the brain opposite the blunt force trauma.

19.22 What are the three main types of intracranial bleeds?

Cerebrovascular Disease

Cerebrovascular disease is the fourth-leading cause of death in the United States behind heart disease, cancer, and chronic lower respiratory disease (COPD, Chapter 10). It is also the most common fatal neurologic condition. Types of cerebrovascular disease include arterial thrombosis, embolism, and hemorrhage. All cerebrovascular disease produces one or both of two basic processes:

- Ischemia, hypoxia, and infarction from impairment of blood flow
- Hemorrhage from rupture of a blood vessel

Any sudden, *spontaneous* vascular event in the brain is called a **stroke**, or **cerebrovascular accident (CVA)**. A stroke may be caused by infarction (80% of cases) or hemorrhage into the brain or subarachnoid space (20% of cases). To understand how the word "stroke" came to apply to this brain event, see the *History of Medicine*, "Stroke and Apoplexy."

The History of Medicine

STROKE AND APOPLEXY

The Oxford English Dictionary lists 26 specific meanings for the word *stroke*. Among them: to pass the hand gently over a surface; to use an oar; to have influence; to strike a blow with a sword or bat; a bolt of lightning; the ring of a clock bell, and so on. The first use to describe brain disease occurred in 1694 when an English diarist wrote that the Archbishop of Canterbury " . . . had a paralytic stroke."

Stroke is loosely used or understood by the lay public to describe any sudden, unexpected, catastrophic event in the brain. Among medical professionals, the term is used to describe a sudden vascular event in the brain: either acute hemorrhage or infarction.

A much older term with the same meaning is *apoplexy*. It is derived from the Greek word *apoplegia*, a combination of *apo* for "off" (as in "not working"), and *plegia*, "to strike a blow." So, quite literally a stroke is a blow that stops activity.

Remember This! Cerebrovascular disease is the fourth-leading cause of death in the United States.

Hypoxia, Ischemia, and Infarction Are Consequences of Low Oxygen Delivery

The brain is uniquely sensitive to oxygen deprivation. Oxygen, not metabolic fuel (e.g., glucose), is the rate-limiting substance for brain metabolism.

Infarction—tissue death due to oxygen deprivation—can result from either global hypoxia or local ischemia. **Hypoxia** is the term pathologists use to describe a *global* event caused by low oxygen partial pressure (PO_2) in blood (as with asphyxiation or drowning) or low oxygen-carrying capacity of blood (as in anemia or carbon monoxide poisoning). **Ischemia** is the word used to describe a *local* event caused by low or absent blood flow, which deprives tissue of both oxygen and nutrients.

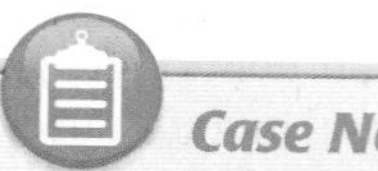

Case Notes

19.10 On his second admission, did Ted's brain suffer from global hypoxia or local ischemia?

Infarction from Global Hypoxia

Global hypoxia can be caused by severe anemia, carbon monoxide poisoning (Chapter 23), smoke inhalation, near-drowning, or pulmonary disease. It can also be caused by hypotension and low cerebral blood flow, as with cardiac arrest or severe shock. Some patients may suffer confusion with complete recovery and no lasting anatomic damage. Children tolerate global hypoxia better than adults; for example, some children may be submerged in water (usually cold water) for half an hour or longer and recover completely.

In most patients, however, irreversible damage occurs. The neurons most sensitive to oxygen deprivation are those of the superficial cerebral cortex and certain cells (*Purkinje cells*) in the cerebellum. If the hypoxia is relieved, the rest of the brain may recover, leaving in the superficial cerebral cortex a layer of necrotic neurons, a condition known as **laminar cortical necrosis** (Figs. 19.21 and 19.22). Global ischemia may produce temporary coma or other neurologic deficits, but laminar

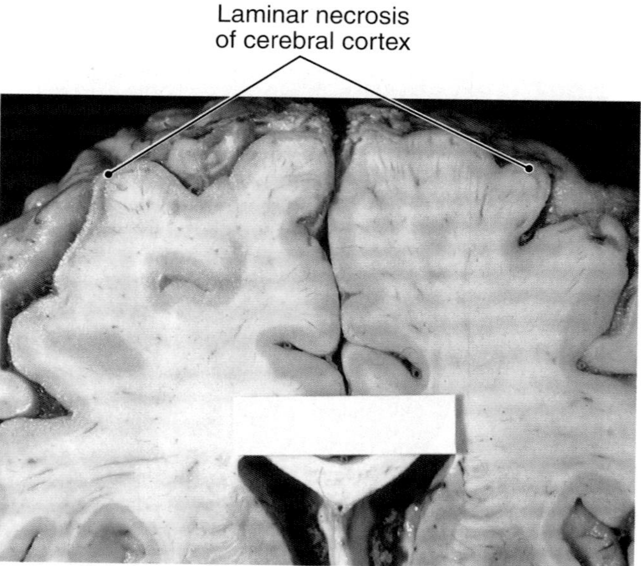

Figure 19.21 **Laminar cortical necrosis.** This patient suffered global cerebral hypoxia secondary to vascular collapse (shock) following traumatic hemorrhage.

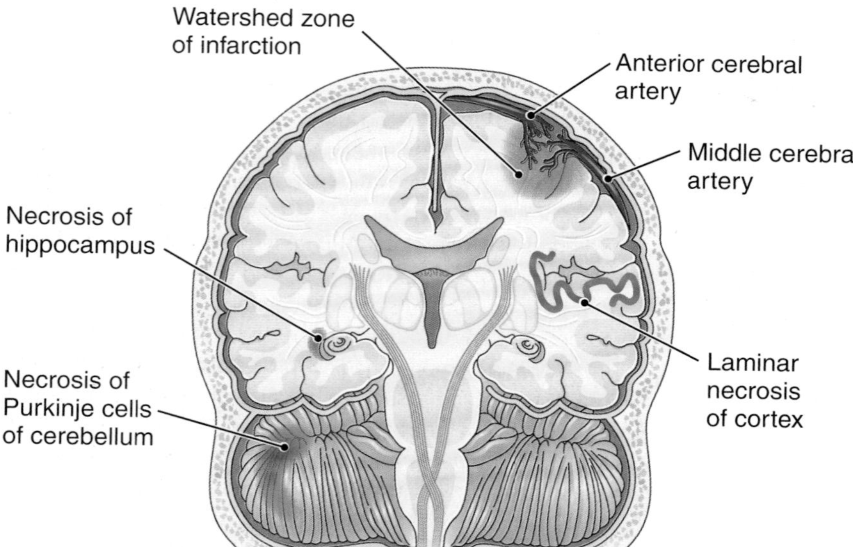

Figure 19.22. **Watershed infarcts and other consequences of global ischemia.** Patients with global hypoxia (ischemia) may develop watershed infarcts of the cerebrum, laminar cortical necrosis of other areas of the cortex, necrosis of the hippocampus, and necrosis of cerebellar Purkinje neurons.

depends largely on the speed with which correct antibiotic therapy is begun.

Diagnosis and Treatment

In acute bacterial meningitis, findings in the spinal fluid are characteristic: large numbers of neutrophils, glucose level that is lower than blood glucose (because of bacterial metabolism of glucose in spinal fluid) and high levels of protein (from inflammatory exudate). Treatment of bacterial meningitis is antibiotics.

In contrast, viral meningitis features a lymphocytic infiltrate in the arachnoid and in the CSF. CSF findings are of paramount importance: the cells are almost all lymphocytes, and CSF protein is increased owing to inflammatory exudate. Nevertheless, in contrast to bacterial meningitis, CSF glucose level is usually normal because viruses do not metabolize glucose. Treatment of viral meningitis is supportive.

Brain Abscess Is a Serious Local Infection

Brain abscess is, like abscesses elsewhere, a localized area of dead, liquefied tissue (liquefactive necrosis, Chapter 2) and acute inflammatory cell exudate caused by bacterial infection (Fig. 19.29). Infection usually occurs in patients with another serious illness and reaches the brain by spreading through the blood from another site, by direct implantation from trauma, or by extension from nearby infection (e.g., from an infected sinus). The lungs are important in the etiology of brain abscess—bloodborne spread frequently arises from lung abscess or from the pus-filled bronchioles associated with bronchiectasis. Patients with cyanotic heart disease (right-to-left shunt) are susceptible because blood bypasses the sieve of the lungs that otherwise filters out bloodborne bacteria, allowing greatly increased numbers of organisms to circulate in the blood and through the brain. Patients with bacterial endocarditis are also at risk for bacterial embolization and brain abscess.

Diagnosis is by clinical suspicion with confirmation by radiographic imaging. Treatment is antibiotics and surgical drainage.

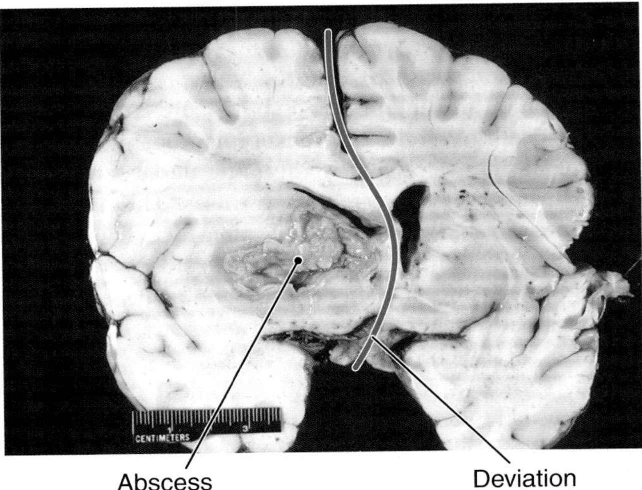

Figure 19.29 **Brain abscess.** An abscess in the basal ganglia in a patient with bacterial endocarditis. The deviation of the midline resulted from unilateral cerebral edema.

Encephalitis Is Usually Viral and Affects Particular Parts of the Brain

Most **encephalitis** is due to viral infection of the brain. Viral infections tend to involve the meninges as well, hence the common use of the term *viral meningoencephalitis*. Infections tend to affect a particular part of the brain according to the tropism of the virus. For example, *herpesvirus* tends to affect the temporal lobes and the *poliovirus* tends to infect brainstem motor neurons. As in most viral infections, the inflammatory reaction is lymphocytic, which is seen as an elevated lymphocyte count in the CSF in addition to perivascular cuffs of lymphocytes in the brain parenchyma, the pathologic hallmark of viral encephalitis. Clinical onset is usually abrupt with fever, headache, and disorientation and may be accompanied by seizures or focal neurologic deficits. Diagnosis requires CSF analysis and radiologic imaging. Treatment is supportive. Antiviral drugs may be useful in some instances.

Some types of infection are more common in immunodeficient patients. For example, *cytomegalovirus (CMV) encephalitis* is a fatal or debilitating infection that occurs predominantly in immunodeficiency. The HIV virus itself tends to infect the brain as well as the immune system and produces a progressive neurologic disease, *AIDS encephalopathy*. *Progressive multifocal leukoencephalopathy (PML)* is a form of fatal encephalitis caused by the *JC virus* (the initials of the first patient with PML proved to be due to this virus). It occurs almost exclusively in immunodeficiency. Infection destroys cerebral and cerebellar white matter.

Arbovirus encephalitis is a variety of epidemic encephalitis borne by mosquitoes and ticks, usually in late summer. Animals are reservoirs (e.g., horses for *Eastern and Western Equine encephalitis*). The multiple subtypes vary geographically and clinically. Some cases are mild, with minor fever and headache and may not be recognized as encephalitis. Others are fulminant and proceed to coma and death within a week.

Herpesvirus infection is the cause of cold sores (Chapter 4). After the initial infection, the virus lingers in neurons cell bodies in a latent state. Meningitis caused by *herpesvirus* (or other members of the herpes family of viruses: varicella-zoster, Epstein-Barr, and CMV) tend to be relatively mild and self-limited, but encephalitis caused by these viruses is usually severe. Neonates, children, and youth are most often affected. The temporal lobes are most severely involved. Diagnosis is by clinical suspicion and isolation of viral DNA from CSF. Death and permanent disability are common, but early diagnosis and antiviral agents can improve the outlook.

In most parts of the world, *poliomyelitis* has been nearly eliminated by vaccination, but it remains a problem in some areas. In unvaccinated people, *poliovirus* infection usually produces gastroenteritis, but in some it may cause meningitis or encephalitis. In its most severe form, it infects the motor neurons of the spinal cord and causes flaccid paralysis, including of the respiratory muscles.

The *measles virus* can cause a rare brain disease called *subacute sclerosing panencephalitis*. It is usually fatal within a few years and features gradual onset of subpar schoolwork, sleeplessness, and emotional instability. It progresses to seizures, speech problems, hallucinations, and dementia. The disorder usually occurs in children who became infected by the measles virus before age two. Treatment is supportive. Vaccination programs have nearly eliminated it.

Prions Cause Transmissible Spongiform Encephalopathy

The *spongiform encephalitides* are a group of universally fatal, very rare diseases that deserve mention because of the uniqueness of the infective agent and because they are related to veterinary disease—*mad cow disease*, *scrapie* in sheep, and chronic wasting disease in deer and elk. They have received wide publicity because of the fear that eating infected beef may communicate a devastating condition.

Spongiform encephalopathy is a progressive, transmissible, chronic, degenerative brain disease caused by *prions* (Chapter 4), which are proteins. Prions have no DNA or RNA and no metabolism. They are corrupted forms of a previously normal protein, *prion protein* (PrP). Infection spreads within the CNS by corrupting nearby PrP, which in turn corrupts other PrP in a vicious circle, much like a snowflake grows by adding more ice crystals.

The most common spongiform encephalopathy of humans is **Creutzfeldt-Jakob disease (CJD)**. CJD usually appears in the seventh decade. The first symptom is subtle memory impairment, but dementia and death follow quickly, usually within a year. Eighty-five percent of CJD cases are spontaneous. Most of the remaining cases are hereditary. This classic variety of CJD is *not* related to mad cow disease.

One human variety of CJD is related to mad cow disease. The human version of mad cow disease is known as **variant Creutzfeldt-Jakob disease (vCJD)**. It is transmitted by consumption of contaminated meat—in most cases low-grade ground beef or sausage that contains fragments of the animal's spinal tissue. As of 2012, England had reported 176 vCJD deaths and continental Europe another 25 or so. In the United States, three or four vCJD cases have been reported, all in people who had traveled in Europe. Although a few U.S. cows have been identified as having mad cow disease, no food transmission to humans has been known to have occurred in the United States. A few iatrogenic infections have been reported; for example, corneal transplant, meningeal transplant, or insertion of an internal appliance.

Pop Quiz

19.27 True or false? Brain abscesses can come from infected sinuses.

19.28 Viral infections can occur in the CNS; for example, the temporal lobes are infected by ____________, while the brainstem motor neurons are infected by ____________.

19.29 What two groups are especially at risk for developing meningococcal meningitis and should get a vaccine to help prevent the disease?

19.30 True or false? Prions, like viruses, have DNA or RNA.

CNS Demyelinating Diseases

Recall that nerve fibers (axons) are insulated from one another in much the same way that electrical wires are insulated, a feature that prevents signals from crossing to another neuron except at a synapse. Oligodendrocytes produce myelin and insulate axons in the CNS; in peripheral nerves it is the function of Schwann cells. Loss of the myelin sheath impairs nerve signal transmission down the axon. Because oligodendrocytes cannot multiply, lost myelin cannot be replaced. Therefore, demyelinating diseases tend to be progressive. Most demyelinating disorders are acquired; some are hereditary.

Multiple Sclerosis Is an Autoimmune Disease

Multiple sclerosis (MS) features widespread patches of demyelination in the brain and spinal cord. It affects the myelin sheath of motor and sensory neurons in the brain and spinal cord, particularly the optic nerves and white matter near the lateral cerebral ventricles. The pathological lesions are characteristic microscopic foci in white matter that show infiltrates of lymphocytes and macrophages, loss of myelin, and marked decrease of oligodendrocytes.

MS is caused by an autoimmune attack on components of the myelin sheath. As with most autoimmune disorders, there is a distinct familial tendency.

MS usually first appears in adults 18–40 years old and is famously unpredictable and subtle in its first manifestations—blurred vision or scotomata (spots), tingling, numbness, minor gait disturbances, stumbling speech, weakness, spasticity, bladder dysfunction, or mild mental impairment. Neurologic impairments tend to be multiple and variable with fluctuating length, severity, and recovery, which gradually add up to disability. Women are affected twice as often as men.

Diagnosis is by clinical suspicion with fluctuating neural deficits and white matter lesions seen on neural imaging. Finding oligoclonal bands of immunoglobulins in CSF is confirmatory. Therapy is supportive, but steroids and other anti-immune therapy may be beneficial.

Other Demyelinating Diseases Are Less Common

Other demyelinating diseases are much less common. The *leukodystrophies* are a group of autosomal recessive genetic demyelinating diseases that are discussed below with related genetic diseases.

Central pontine myelinolysis is a rare condition featuring patchy demyelination in the pons. It most commonly is due to overly rapid correction of hyponatremia in chronic alcoholics and other malnourished states or in persons with severe electrolyte disturbances. Symptoms may be mild or severe and include weakness in any or all limbs, respiratory weakness, depressed consciousness, coma, or death. Most patients retain severe neurologic deficits.

Rarely, vaccines and some viral exanthems such as measles, rubella, and chicken pox may be followed in a few days or a few weeks by **postinfectious** or **postvaccinal encephalomyelitis** that primarily affects white matter. Headache and fever may be transient and mild or may progress to paraplegia, coma, and death.

Pop Quiz

19.31 True or false? Oligodendrocytes produce myelin.

19.32 True or false? MS affects mostly men.

19.33 What is the rare demyelinating disorder caused by rapid correction of hyponatremia?

CNS Metabolic Disorders

Metabolic disorders of the CNS fall into several broad categories: *lysosomal storage disorders, metabolic disorders,* and *toxic encephalopathies.*

Lysosomal Storage Disorders Are Inherited Enzyme Deficiencies

Lysosomal storage disorders are inherited enzyme defects that cause the accumulation of upstream metabolic substrates (Chapter 22) necessary to synthesize certain complex lipids and saccharides. According to the nature of the accumulated substance, they may be referred to as *sphingolipidoses, mucopolysaccharidoses,* and so forth.

As with all genetic disease, ethnic patterns are present. Many of these conditions are most common in Jews. Diagnosis depends on the particulars of the clinical findings with confirmations by enzyme assays of tissues. Treatments are generally experimental and include bone marrow transplantation. Prenatal screening is available.

Gaucher disease is an autosomal recessive disorder that is the most common of these enzyme defects. Only 10% of patients have CNS problems. The other 90% of cases feature accumulation of glucocerebroside in tissue macrophages and present with hepatosplenomegaly, and bone and bone marrow problems from massive accumulations of macrophages. The 10% of CNS cases feature glucocerebroside accumulation in neurons. They develop dementia, ataxia, spasticity, seizures, and other neurologic problems. Most die before age two.

Tay-Sachs disease is a fatal autosomal recessive disorder caused by an inborn enzyme defect (Chapter 22) that causes an accumulation of ganglioside in CNS neurons. Affected infants appear normal at birth but die within a year or two of progressive neurologic decline: weakness, blindness, and mental impairment.

Hurler disease is an autosomal recessive disorder that features neuron accumulation of mucopolysaccharides. It is typically expressed in infancy or early childhood as dwarfism, corneal opacities, skeletal deformities, hepatosplenomegaly, and progressive mental decline.

Neiman-Pick disease features accumulation of sphingolipid in macrophages. Infants fail to thrive and develop progressive neurologic symptoms.

The **leukodystrophies** are a subset of lysosomal enzyme defects characterized by defects of myelin resulting from a DNA coding errors for enzyme proteins important in the production and maintenance of healthy myelin. Lesions occur in the white matter. The leukodystrophies are diseases of infancy and childhood and are uniformly fatal. The most common leukodystrophy is **metachromatic leukodystrophy**, which derives its name from the accumulation of cerebroside in CNS white matter. It imparts a pinkish alteration to blue dyes used in microscopic study of myelin.

Other Metabolic Neuronal Disorders May Be Inherent or Acquired

Phenylketonuria (PKU) is an autosomal recessive disorder that causes accumulation of phenylalanine in blood and tissue. In undetected cases, it becomes evident in the first few months of life and leads to seizures, mental retardation, and poor physical development. Routine neonatal screening has been effective in detection before adverse consequences occur. Treatment is lifelong phenylalanine restriction. Prognosis with treatment is excellent.

Wilson disease (Chapter 12) is an autosomal recessive disorder of copper metabolism. Defective liver excretion of copper causes copper deposition in the liver and brain. A hallmark finding is green copper deposition at the edge of the cornea, the *Kayser-Fleisher ring*. First symptoms occur between ages 5 and 40. In about half of patients, neurologic manifestations occur first and include motor problems, mental instability, tremor, dystonia, dysphagia, and other symptoms. Confirmation of clinical suspicion is by finding increased blood and urine copper.

Cretinism (Chapter 14) is severe hypothyroidism in infancy. Lack of thyroid hormones in utero or in infancy (often due to maternal dietary iodine deficiency) can cause severe motor and mental impairment. Diagnosis is by blood testing for thyroid hormones. Treatment with thyroid hormones is effective.

Hepatic encephalopathy is a common consequence of liver failure (Chapter 12). It is a brain syndrome of personality changes, confusion, and a depressed level of consciousness as a result of accumulated metabolic products, especially ammonia, that cannot be metabolized properly by the sick liver.

Vitamin B_{12} deficiency can cause anemia (Chapter 7), but can have severe and irreversible neurological defects from degeneration of the posterolateral white tracks in the spinal cord. Burning and paresthesias in the feet and legs are often the first sign, followed by weakness in all limbs, incoordination, and ataxia. If caught early, the changes are reversible with vitamin supplementation, typically by injection to circumvent lack of intrinsic factor; nevertheless, for the most part, the changes are permanent.

The most common brain disorder associated with nutritional deficiency is **thiamine (vitamin B_1)** deficiency, which may take several forms. One form is known clinically as **beriberi** (from the Sinhalese—Sri Lankan, Ceylonese—word *beri*, meaning weakness: beriberi means very weak). Beriberi (Chapter 23) is manifested by motor weakness because of peripheral neuropathy, and general weakness because of congestive heart failure.

Other manifestations of thiamine deficiency are two related brain syndromes, seen primarily in chronic alcoholics. **Wernicke encephalopathy**, a syndrome associated with cerebellar atrophy (Fig. 19.30), features ataxia, tremors, confusion, and paralysis of extraocular muscles, none of which have to do with acute drunkenness but can look a lot like it. Untreated Wernicke encephalopathy may evolve into **Korsakoff psychosis**, a permanent defect of both short- and long-term memory that leads patients to confabulate aimless, convoluted tales of explanation that never get anywhere because the patient cannot remember where the conversation should go.

Hyperglycemia is usually a product of diabetic ketoacidosis (Chapter 13). The high glucose increases blood osmolarity, which attracts water from brain cells. Confusion, stupor, or coma may occur. **Hypoglycemia** is usually seen in diabetics due to relative excess of insulin. Because the brain is dependent upon glucose, laminar cortical neuronal necrosis may occur in a pattern similar to global hypoxia (see above).

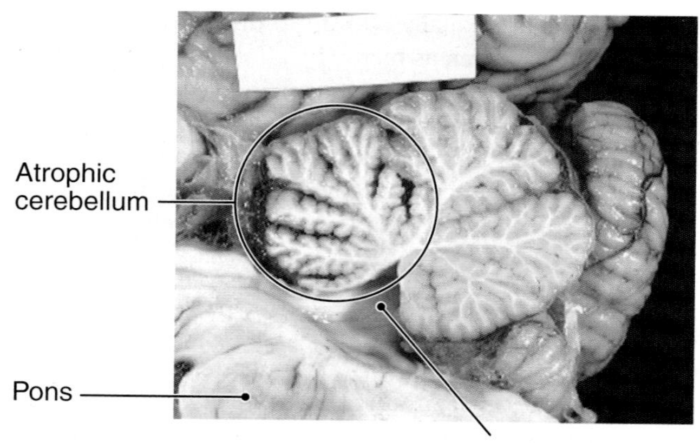

Figure 19.30 **Wernicke encephalopathy.** Cerebellar atrophy in a patient with chronic alcoholism.

The List of Brain Toxic States Is Almost Endless

The list of toxic states that affect the brain is almost endless, and includes water (*water intoxication*, Chapter 6). The most common toxic substances are *illicit drugs* and *alcohol* (Chapter 23). Chronic alcoholics tend to develop cirrhosis (Chapter 16) and liver failure, one consequence of which is hepatic encephalopathy. Apart from the nutritional effects of chronic alcoholism, **ethanol** itself can be toxic to the brain. **Methanol** is a toxic alcohol that is heavily traded and used worldwide for a multitude of industrial purposes. It is found in antifreeze, shellac, varnish, and countless other products. Toxicity causes headache, weakness, seizure, retinal blindness, and other problems.

Carbon monoxide intoxication (Chapter 23) can cause fatal global hypoxia by binding permanently to hemoglobin and displacing oxygen.

Patients with **lead poisoning** (Chapter 23) may develop peripheral neuropathy with weakness, numbness, and tingling in the limbs, or seizures brought on by brain edema and increased intracranial pressure.

Pop Quiz

19.34 What substance causes brain injury in Wilson disease?

19.35 Give two examples of lysosomal storage disorders.

19.36 True or false? PKU is treated by lifelong restriction of phenylalanine.

19.37 True or false? Hyperglycemia and ketoacidosis from diabetes can cause neurologic symptoms including coma.

CNS Degenerative Disorders

There are many degenerative diseases of gray matter, some associated with dementia, others with paralysis or movement disorders. Some involve relatively local areas of the brain; others are more widespread. *Parkinson disease, amyotrophic lateral sclerosis,* and *Huntington disease* affect particular parts of CNS anatomy. In contrast, *AD* affects the brain more widely. Degenerative diseases share in common a tendency to develop abnormal intracellular or extracellular aggregates of amyloid-like (Chapter 3) protein. These protein deposits characterize both the genetic and spontaneous variants of each disease and also occur in some other conditions (e.g., Down syndrome) in which the brain is affected. How these deposits are related to disease is not clear: they may be markers only, or they may have a role in causation. Degenerative diseases share certain characteristics. They usually

- have no known cause, though some are inheritable;
- occur in selected areas while leaving other areas unaffected;
- may feature abnormal protein deposits in affected tissue;
- may be associated with dementia.

Degeneration of Cortical Neurons Causes Dementia

Dementia is defined as a global, irreversible deterioration of cognition—mental capacities such as memory, attention span, and reasoning—due to degeneration of neurons in the cerebral cortex. Dementia is not normal, no matter the patient's age. There is usually some minimal decline of cognition with advancing years, particularly the speed of recall, but it is not dementia because it does not affect the daily functions of life. An intermediate state is **mild cognitive impairment (MCI)**, which is defined as impaired cognition that does not interfere with daily activities.

Dementia usually begins with impairment of short-term memory or language problems such as word finding. It progresses to interference with daily activities such as balancing a checkbook, finding one's way while walking or driving, or remembering where things were put. **Agnosia** (impaired ability to recognize people and things), **apraxia** (impaired ability to do previously learned motor skills), and **aphasia** (impaired comprehension and use of language) follow. Late-stage dementia patients cannot walk or feed themselves and may be incontinent. End-stage dementia results in coma and death, usually due to infection.

The many types of dementia are too numerous to cover here. Some are rare neurological conditions while others are the effect of conditions such as chronic subdural hematoma, hypothyroidism, and alcoholism. The most common is AD.

Case Notes

19.13 Though Ted showed no signs of dementia in his long life, at the end he had trouble with language. What is the name that applies to this condition?

Alzheimer Disease

Alzheimer disease (AD) is a degenerative disorder of cortical neurons that is the cause of over half of all cases of adult dementia. It affects women more often than men. About 1% of people ages 60–64 are affected, but the prevalence rises rapidly with advancing age, and AD affects up to one-third of people over the age of 85.

AD's cause is unknown; however, about 10% of cases have a familial association. The most important risk factor is advanced age. Females are at more risk than males. Other risk factors include repeated head trauma, hypertensive and atherosclerotic vascular disease, poorly controlled diabetes, smoking, and lack of exercise.

The clinical symptoms begin insidiously as memory loss and progress through the stages of dementia outlined above. Death usually occurs from infection, usually pneumonia, within about 10 years. At autopsy, pathologic findings are distinctive. The most notable is atrophy of the cerebral cortex: gyri are narrowed and sulci are broad (Fig. 19.31) due to loss of gray matter neurons. Microscopically the cerebral cortex contains pathologically characteristic tangles of abnormal protein fibrils (Fig. 19.32) and deposits (plaques) of amyloid-like protein.

The first sign of AD is usually short-term memory loss. Other cognitive defects follow and include inability to plan and perform tasks, especially new ones; confusion of time and place; inability to carry on a conversation; misplacing objects; and mood swings and depression. Some drugs show promise of slowing the progress of AD and offer temporary symptomatic improvement, but treatment is generally supportive. An experimental vaccine holds promise.

Frontotemporal Dementias

The **frontotemporal dementias** are a group of disorders that share progressive deterioration of language and personality changes. Pathologic changes include degenerative change and amyloid-like protein deposits and atrophy of the frontal and temporal lobes.

Vascular Dementia

Repeated vascular injury to the brain can cause **vascular dementia**. Etiologies include multiple microinfarcts, laminar necrosis from global hypoxia, showers of emboli, and diffuse cerebral changes associated with hypertension. Vascular changes may combine with AD to produce dementia more severe than otherwise would be present.

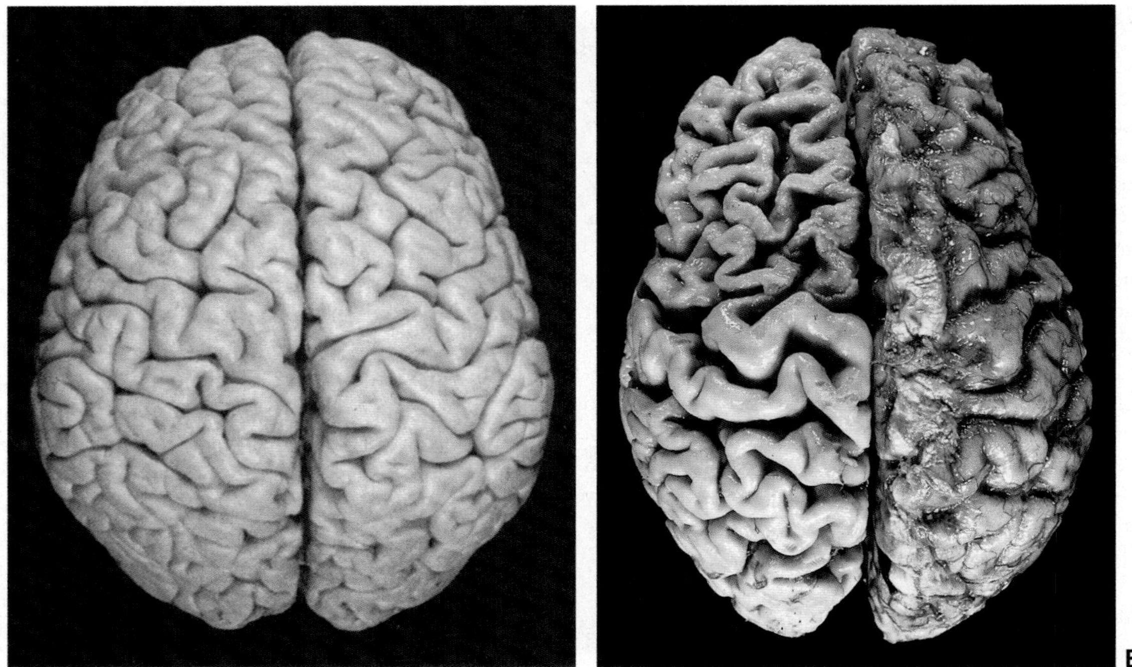

Figure 19.31 **Alzheimer disease. A.** Normal brain. **B.** AD showing severe frontal lobe atrophy. Gyri are narrow and sulci are wide, especially in the frontal lobes (top). Meninges have been removed on the left, but are in place on the right. (**A.** Reproduced with permission from Rubin E, Farber JL. *Pathology.* 3rd ed. Philadelphia, PA: Lippincott-Raven; 1999.)

Degeneration of Neurons in the Basal Ganglia and Brainstem Causes Movement Disorders

Degeneration of neurons in the basal ganglia (Fig. 19.3B) and brainstem are usually associated with movement disorders. They generally feature reduced voluntary movement or an excess of involuntary movements such as *chorea* (involuntary jerky movements, especially of the hips, shoulders, and face), rigidity, and abnormal posturing.

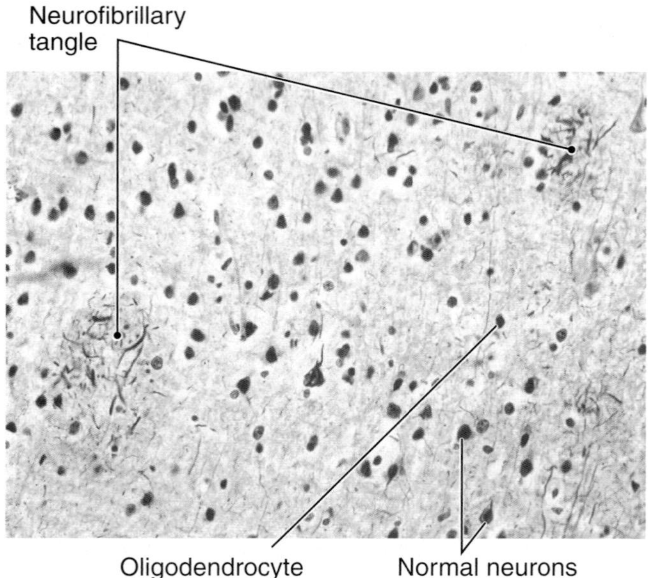

Figure 19.32 **Alzheimer disease.** Characteristic neurofibrillary tangles are visible in this microscopic study.

Parkinsonism

Parkinsonism is a clinical syndrome characterized by diminished facial animation, slowness of voluntary movements, progressively stooped posture, rigidity, gait abnormalities, and tremor. Symptoms result from a lack of sufficient dopamine, a neurotransmitter chemical. When the etiology is unknown, as it is in most people, patients are said to have **Parkinson disease**. When the cause is known, however, patients are said to have Parkinson syndrome secondary to a particular cause, such as repeated head injury (e.g., the cause of Parkinsonism suffered by American boxer Muhammad Ali). Parkinsonism may be inherited as a Mendelian genetic trait; it can also be caused by vascular disease, toxins, repeated head trauma, or viral encephalitis.

The fundamental defect in Parkinsonism is faulty nerve signal transmission in the basal ganglia, especially the substantia nigra. Pathologic findings include loss of pigment in basal ganglia, and the presence in affected neurons of *Lewy bodies* composed of the amyloid-like protein present in the dementias mentioned above. Lewy bodies, however, can also be found in other degenerative brain diseases such as *Lewy body dementia*, which may occur without Parkinsonism.

Parkinsonism is mainly a disease of the elderly, but some patients become symptomatic in their 40s. Most cases begin in people over age 60. About 10% of people over 80 are affected, men more frequently than women. There are no racial differences. Onset is usually slow, and usually begins with a slow, coarse, resting tremor in one hand. The tremor worsens with chill, tension, and fatigue. Full-blown cases are characterized by tremor of all limbs, difficulty walking, rigidity, shuffling gait and other gait abnormalities, slurred speech, and a wooden, emotionless facial expression. About 10% of patients with Parkinsonism also have dementia. Other parts of the nervous system may be involved, causing dysphagia, constipation, orthostatic hypotension, urinary hesitancy, and loss of smell.

Diagnosis is clinical. Administration of l-DOPA, a dopamine precursor, is often effective for symptomatic treatment, but it does not slow progression of the underlying disease. Other drugs currently in development show promise of slowing disease progression. There is no cure; however, implantation of stimulating electrodes is proving effective in selected cases with severe symptoms.

Huntington Disease

Huntington disease is an autosomal dominant genetic disease that causes neuron degeneration in the basal ganglia. Most cases are inherited, and it occurs in whites of northern European ancestry. Some new cases occur as spontaneous mutations. Like other degenerative neuronal diseases, it features microscopic deposits of amyloid-related protein in the basal ganglia.

Huntington disease has been traced to a gene that codes for an abnormal protein that interferes with the function of nerve cells in the cortex and midbrain. This gene is autosomal dominant; that is, only one copy is necessary for the disease to manifest. Huntington disease does not become symptomatic until adult life (typically at about ages 20–40); therefore, an adult with the defective gene often has already had children, who may or may not have inherited the gene, before the condition is recognized. Early signs may include subtle personality changes, restlessness, and uncoordinated body movements. Later stages are characterized by dementia and more dramatic involuntary, writhing movements called *chorea* from the Greek word meaning "dance." It is relentlessly progressive and fatal, usually within 10–20 years of first symptoms.

Diagnosis is by genetic analysis. Treatment is supportive. Genetic counseling of relatives is imperative.

Degeneration of Motor Neurons Causes Paralysis

Selective degeneration of motor neurons form a group of inherited or sporadic diseases that affect the lower motor neurons of the spinal cord, brainstem motor nuclei, and the upper motor neurons in the cerebral cortex. They vary greatly in age of onset, severity of symptoms, and rapidity of progression. Disease of lower motor neurons (in the spinal cord) causes weakness and flaccid paralysis. Disease of upper motor neurons (in the cerebral cortex) produces weakness, exaggerated reflexes, and spasticity.

Amyotrophic lateral sclerosis, also known as *Lou Gehrig disease* after the famed New York Yankees baseball player who died from it, is a degenerative condition of motor neurons in the gray matter of the cerebral cortex, brainstem, and spinal cord. The most striking finding is demyelination of motor axons in the dorsolateral spinal cord (Fig. 19.33).

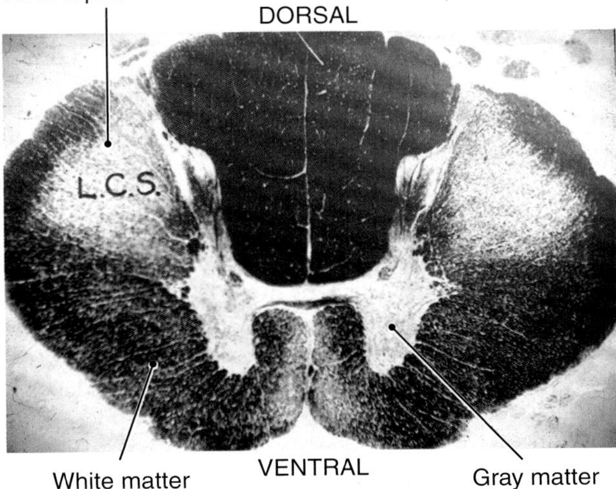

Figure 19.33 **Amyotrophic lateral sclerosis (Lou Gehrig disease).** Microscopic study of a cross-section of spinal cord. Myelin is stained black. The lateral corticospinal tracts (L.C.S. in the section) are pale due to loss of myelin.

A familial form has been identified, which accounts for about 10% of cases. Despite identification of multiple acquired gene defects, however, the precise cause remains unclear.

The average age at onset for sporadic cases is 55; for familial it is 35–45. It presents with weakness, atrophy, and muscle twitching (fasciculations) and progresses to interfere with speech, locomotion, and respiratory effort. Cognitive and sensory functions are usually unimpaired. Death usually occurs because of respiratory failure. Diagnosis is clinical. Treatment is supportive.

Bulbospinal atrophy (BSA) is an X-linked Mendelian, adult-onset disorder featuring distal limb atrophy, fasciculations of the tongue, and dysphagia. Those affected also have hormonal metabolic defects.

Spinal muscular atrophy is a group of disorders of lower motor neurons in children.

Pop Quiz

19.38 True or false? AD is the most common cause of adult dementia.

19.39 What diagnosis is generally made before the onset of AD?

19.40 True or false? Parkinson disease is caused by degeneration of neurons in the cortex.

19.41 What neurodegenerative disorder primarily affects the motor neurons?

CNS Neoplasms

The World Health Organization (WHO) classification and grading system for CNS neoplasms guides the discussion that follows. It is important to keep in mind that the WHO uses the phrase "CNS neoplasm" to refer to any primary tumor arising *intracranially*, as distinct from tumors of a certain tissue. The WHO system divides CNS neoplasms into two large groups. **Neuroepithelial tumors** are tumors of glia, neurons, ependymal cells, choroid plexus, pineal gland, and embryonal cells. The **other CNS tumors** include tumors of meninges, pituitary and CN, plus lymphomas, vascular tumors, and tumors of other tissue types.

The WHO system also sets microscopic standards for grading (Chapter 5) all CNS neoplasms. Grade I is the most innocuous and benign appearing; Grade IV is the most vicious and malignant appearing.

CNS neoplasms are neither common nor rare. The exact number of new cases occurring annually in the United States is difficult to determine because classification (benign vs. malignant, neuroepithelial vs. intracranial) has been inconsistent. A comparison with new lung cancers is helpful. The American Cancer Society estimated that, in the United States in 2012, there were 226,000 new cases of lung cancer. Based on data from the 2012 report of the Central Brain Tumor Registry of the United States, the authors estimate that in 2012 there were 61,000 *primary* intracranial neoplasms (CNS neoplasms in WHO-speak). Of these, the most common were meningiomas (35%), followed by gliomas (33%), pituitary tumors (15%), and CN tumors (8%).

Primary intracranial tumors have a tendency to occur in certain parts of the brain and associated tissues (Fig. 19.34). Primary tumors rarely occur in the spinal cord. In adults, most intracranial tumors occur above the tentorium in or around the cerebral hemispheres. By contrast, most intracranial tumors of children occur below the tentorium in and around the cerebellum and brainstem in what is referred to as the *posterior fossa* of the skull. Brain tumors in children are more likely to be malignant than those in adults and account for about 20% of childhood cancers.

About two-thirds of intracranial tumors are metastatic from other body sites (metastases are not included in the figures above). Metastases are mainly a problem in the elderly, who have more malignancies. The three most common sources are lung cancer, breast cancer, and malignant melanoma. Brain metastases rarely occur with carcinoma of the prostate or ovary or sarcomas of any kind. Lymphoma may be a primary brain neoplasm or lymphoma/leukemia may spread to the brain or meninges.

Conversely, even highly malignant primary CNS tumors rarely spread to other parts of the body: invasion of blood vessels is rare because vascular endothelial cells are so tightly joined to form the blood-brain barrier, and lymphatic spread is rare because there are few lymphatics in the brain.

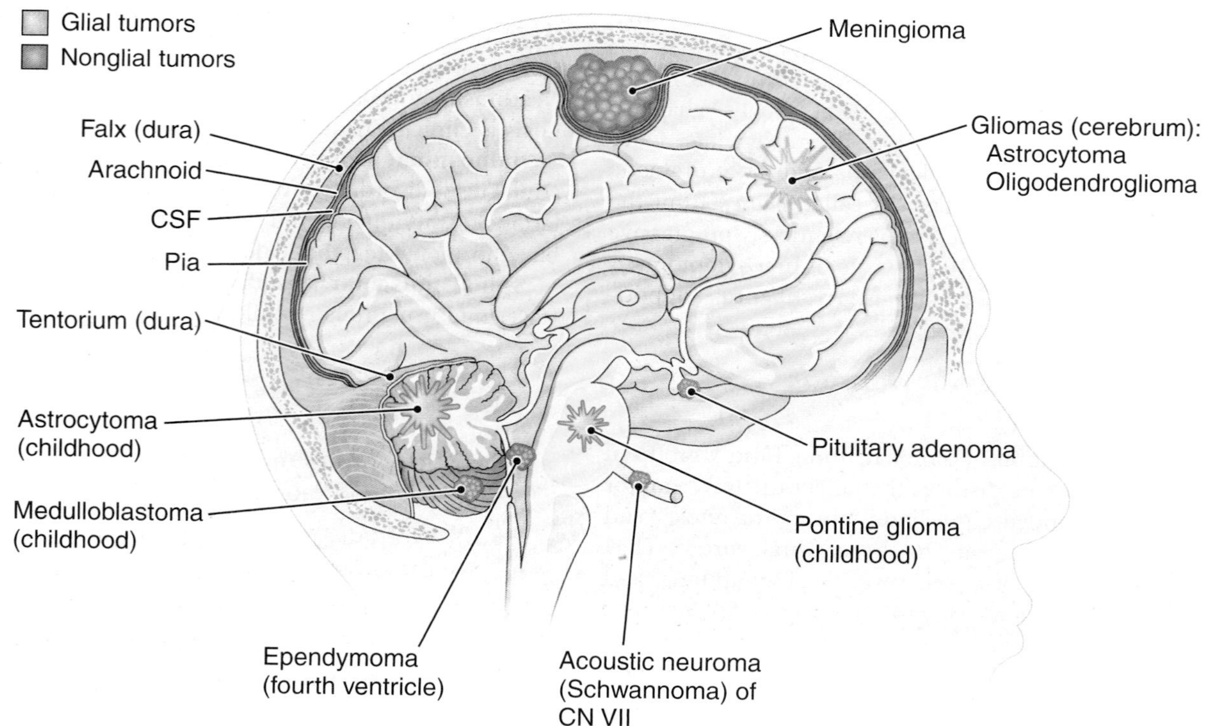

Figure 19.34 **The most common intracranial tumors.**

Gliomas Are the Most Common Neuroepithelial Tumors

Gliomas are neuroepithelial tumors of astrocytes, oligodendrocytes, or ependymal cells.

Astrocytomas

Astrocytomas are tumors of astrocytes and constitute the great majority of gliomas. They occur principally in adults but may be seen at any age. Traditionally, astrocytomas are given differing names according to WHO grade:

- Grade I: *pilocytic astrocytoma* (mean survival ~10 years)
- Grade II: *diffuse astrocytoma* (Fig. 19.35) (mean survival ~5 years)
- Grade III: *anaplastic astrocytoma* (mean survival ~ 18 months)
- Grade IV: *glioblastoma*, formerly *glioblastoma multiforme* (Fig. 19.36) (mean survival <12 months)

Astrocytomas present unique tumor management problems because of the following:

- The margins of the tumor may be indistinguishable from normal tissue (Fig. 19.35).
- They may be in a location (e.g., brainstem) that defies surgery because they are so intimately related to essential structures that surgery is out of the question.

Pilocytic astrocytomas (grade I) account for a small minority of astrocytomas, tend to occur in children and young adults, and are usually located in the cerebellum, the optic nerves, or in the brain near the third ventricle. They grow slowly and are often successfully removed by surgery. The other varieties account for the great majority astrocytomas. Most astrocytomas tend to behave more aggressively with time.

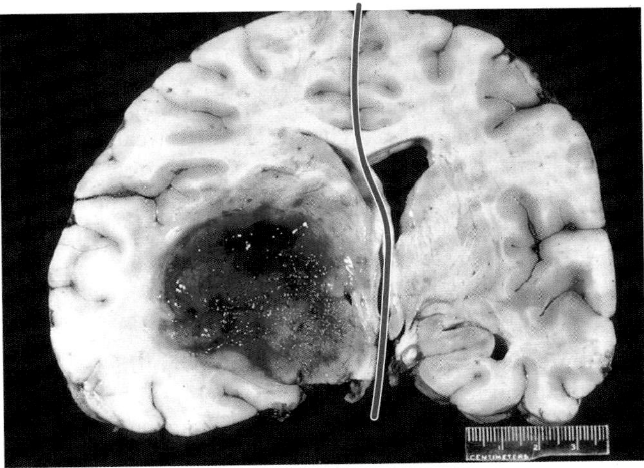

Figure 19.36 **Glioblastoma (Grade IV of IV).** This poorly differentiated tumor is easy to distinguish from surrounding normal tissue. The midline is pushed to one side by the expanding tumor mass.

Astrocytomas usually become symptomatic because of increased intracranial pressure, destruction of neural tissue with localizing signs of lost function, or bleeding. Typical signs and symptoms include headache, confusion or other deterioration of mental status, or focal signs such as weakness, paresthesias, seizures, aphasia, oculomotor problems or visual field defect, or other functional problem.

Diagnosis requires clinical suspicion and imaging. Treatment varies greatly. A few grade I tumors may be excised successfully, but more often treatment consists of radiation, chemotherapy, and surgery.

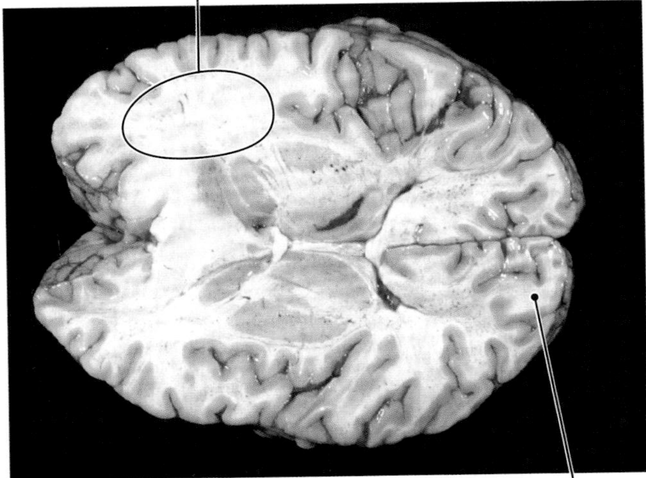

Figure 19.35 **Diffuse astrocytoma (Grade II of IV)**. Shown here is a horizontal section of a tumor in the occipital (posterior) lobe. It is difficult to distinguish the tumor from normal white matter.

Oligodendrogliomas

Oligodendrogliomas constitute about 10% of gliomas. They occur most often between the ages of 20 and 40. They usually arise in the white matter of the cerebral hemispheres and are moderately aggressive grade II or III primary brain neoplasms that usually grow more slowly and less predictably than astrocytomas. Progression from grade II to grade III usually occurs within five years. Average survival is about 5–10 years. Diagnosis and treatment are similar to astrocytoma.

Ependymomas

Ependymomas are rare tumors of ependymal cells that line the ventricles. They most often arise around the ventricles in children and teenagers. The most common site is near the fourth ventricle. They usually become symptomatic due to hydrocephalus secondary to obstruction of CSF flow. Diagnosis and treatment are similar to astrocytoma.

Other Neuroepithelial Tumors Are Rare

Neuronal tumors are uncommon and usually have a glial component. **Ganglioglioma** is usually a slow-growing tumor of neurons and glial cells that appears in the temporal lobe and often presents with seizures.

Medulloblastoma is a tumor of primitive embryologic cells that occurs almost exclusively in the cerebellum of children. It is highly malignant and, if untreated, is uniformly fatal. It is, however, peculiarly sensitive to radiation therapy. With excision and radiotherapy, the 10-year survival rate is about 50%.

Meningiomas Are the Most Common Non-Neuroepithelial Tumor

Meningiomas are tumors of arachnoid epithelium that usually attach to the dura. They are usually solitary, slow-growing, and well-differentiated, and appear over the surface of the brain, especially in the parasagittal region (Fig. 19.37). Meningiomas produce problems mainly by mass effect—they press on adjacent structures until headache, seizure, mental aberration, or localized neurologic deficit occurs. For example, a meningioma pressing on the CN VII can cause paralysis of facial muscles. They are uncommon in children. In adults, two-thirds occur in women. Some are discovered incidentally by skull imaging for another purpose (e.g., after trauma).

The intracranial portion of cranial nerves may become neoplastic. **Acoustic neuroma** is a tumor of the Schwann cells of CN VIII. It is the most common peripheral nerve tumor to occur in the cranium and can cause deafness or a ringing sound (tinnitus). Acoustic neuromas can press on other cranial nerves, such as the facial nerve, that are near to CN VIII.

Recall that *microglia* are the macrophages of the CNS. When malignant, they are called **microgliomas**, a variety of lymphoma related to histiocytic lymphoma elsewhere in the body. They are very rare.

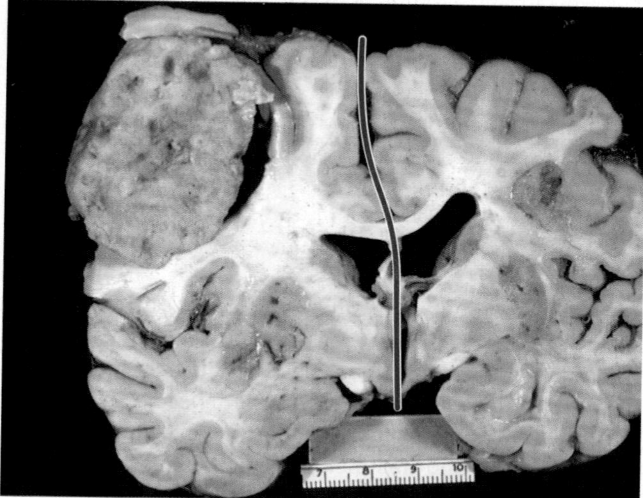

Figure 19.37 **Meningioma.** This tumor originated from arachnoid on the inner surface of the parietal bone. The underlying brain is atrophic, and the midline is pushed to one side by the expanding mass.

Primary lymphomas of the brain tend to occur in immunosuppressed patients and usually in the absence of lymphoma elsewhere in the body. Most are B cell lymphomas. They tend to be aggressive and do not respond well to radiation or chemotherapy.

Pinealomas are tumors of the pineal gland. They are rare and vary from benign to aggressive.

Pop Quiz

19.42 True or false? Most brain tumors are primary brain tumors.

19.43 What is the term for the highest grade of astrocytic tumors according to the WHO?

Diseases of Peripheral Nerves

The anatomy and connections of the PNS were detailed earlier in this chapter in Figures 19.8 through 19.11. Recall that peripheral nerves are composed of axons of neurons located in the brain or spinal cord, and that each axon is wrapped by layers of Schwann cell cytoplasm containing myelin. Peripheral nerve disease primarily affects either the axon or the Schwann cell.

Neuropathies Are Non-Neoplastic Diseases of Peripheral Nerves

A **peripheral neuropathy** is any nonneoplastic disease of peripheral nerve that is a malfunction of one or more nerves. Interrupted sensory and motor signals cause weakness, paralysis, pain, or *paresthesia* (numbness, tingling, pain, or other sensation). The etiology of neuropathies may be inflammatory, infectious, hereditary, or toxic/metabolic.

Guillain-Barre Syndrome

Guillain-Barre syndrome (GBS) is a life-threatening, T cell-mediated immune neuropathy characterized by weakness that may progress to paralysis. Mild sensory loss also may occur.

In about two-thirds of cases, the patient has experienced, about a week or two earlier, some variety of mild, acute, influenza-like syndrome, which is usually in the recovery phase when neurologic signs and symptoms appear. Microscopic examination reveals infiltration of nerves by lymphocytes. Numerous infectious agents have been documented as triggers for this immune reaction, but they are not identifiable in the nerves.

The clinical picture features *ascending paralysis* that begins in the distal limbs, progresses proximally, and may involve respiratory muscles. Diagnosis is clinical. CSF may contain increased protein but usually no inflammatory cells are present. Nerve conduction speed is slow. GBS is a medical emergency that requires close monitoring of respiratory function, usually in an intensive care unit. Treatment is supportive and may include respiratory assistance. Plasmapheresis to remove autoantibodies may be helpful. A significant minority of patients may be left with permanent disability.

Bell Palsy

Among the most common peripheral neuropathies is **Bell palsy**, a paralysis of facial muscles resulting from impairment of the facial nerve (CN VII). Etiology is unknown, but presumably owes to inflammatory/immune swelling and pressure on the nerve as it exits the skull through the stylomastoid foramen. About 35,000 people in the United States are affected each year. Bell palsy usually affects mature adults and arises suddenly. Most patients recover within a month or two; others require nearly a year. A few patients may suffer permanent paralysis. Diagnosis is clinical. The mainstay of treatment is steroids.

Other Neuropathies

Some neuropathies owe to infection. **Leprosy** (**Hansen disease**) is caused by nerve infection of Schwann cells by *Mycobacterium leprae*, which grows best in cool temperatures and therefore favors infection of fingers, toes, the tip of the nose, and the external ear. The agent of **diphtheria**, *Corynebacterium diphtheriae*, secretes an exotoxin that can produce a sensory neuropathy. Nerve infection by the *varicella-zoster virus* causes **shingles**, a painful, vesicular eruption in skin.

Some neuropathies are hereditary. They are a diverse and poorly understood group that tends to be progressive and debilitating. Most well-known is **Charcot-Marie-Tooth** disease, which is often autosomal dominant. It usually presents in childhood with weakness and atrophy of the lower legs. Orthopedic problems dominate the clinical picture but patients usually live a normal lifespan.

There are *toxic/metabolic peripheral neuropathies* too numerous to list. The most prominent associations are with diabetes, uremia, lead poisoning, and alcoholism. **Diabetic peripheral neuropathy** (Chapter 13) is the most common. It affects mainly sensory fibers and is caused by vascular disease in small blood vessels serving the affected nerves. **Alcoholic peripheral neuropathy** arises from vitamin or other nutritional deficiency.

Traumatic peripheral neuropathy can occur from laceration, crush, or stretch, or from prolonged pressure. "Saturday night palsy" may occur in persons intoxicated by alcohol or illicit drugs who sleep off a binge with their arms in an awkward position. Trauma to peripheral nerves may cause death of the axon and Schwann cells distal to the point of injury.

Axons and Schwann cells can regenerate, but they regrow very slowly, and axonal reconnection to the target organ is not always effective. Within one week of trauma, new nerve axons sprout from the proximal point of injury. If the injury is a clean, complete transection, and the ends of the separated parts are close together, the sprouting fibers stand a good chance of regrowth and reattachment to the target organ. If the ends are too far separated, the sprouting fibers and scar tissue may accumulate into a nodule, a *traumatic neuroma* (amputation neuroma), which can be quite painful. Women who regularly wear high-heeled shoes are prone to develop traumatic neuroma (*Morton neuroma*) near the distal head of the first metatarsal from repeated nerve compression.

Peripheral neuropathy also occurs as a paraneoplastic syndrome (Chapter 5) in patients with cancer.

Neoplasms of Peripheral Nerve Arise from Schwann Cells

Tumors of the PNS arise from neurons of the ANS, or from nerve sheath cells (Schwann cells or fibrocytes that reside in the nerve sheath).

Schwannomas are slow-growing, benign, usually solitary tumors that arise from Schwann cells. They are not premalignant. Schwannomas may arise in any nerve; however, schwannoma of the vestibular branch of the vestibulocochlear (acoustic nerve, CN VIII) accounts for 8% of primary intracranial neoplasms and is often called "acoustic neuroma." Spontaneous schwannomas are unilateral and present with hearing loss, tinnitus, and vestibular dysfunction (e.g., vertigo). They may become large enough to cause increased intracranial pressure and related neurologic signs. Bilateral schwannomas are a hallmark sign of *neurofibromatosis, Type* 2 (NF2), a genetic disease.

Neurofibroma is a tumor of Schwann cells, fibroblasts, and related perineural cells. Most are benign, but some may evolve into a malignant neoplasm (*neurofibrosarcoma*). Neurofibroma is microscopically somewhat similar to schwannoma but distinction is important because neurofibromas are closely related to *neurofibromatosis, Type 1* (NF1). Most neurofibromas are spontaneous and occur in skin and have no relationship to NF1.

Neurofibromatosis is an autosomal dominant disorder associated with peripheral nerve tumors. Type 1 neurofibromatosis (NF1 or *von Recklinghausen disease*, Fig. 19.38) accounts for 90% of cases and features multiple neurofibromas that may create neurologic, skin, and bone problems. It is usually apparent at birth because of multiple skin nodules (neurofibromas) and brownish skin patches (*café au lait spots*). Related bone troubles include fibrous dysplasia, bone cysts, scoliosis, and other problems. Type 2 neurofibromatosis (NF2)

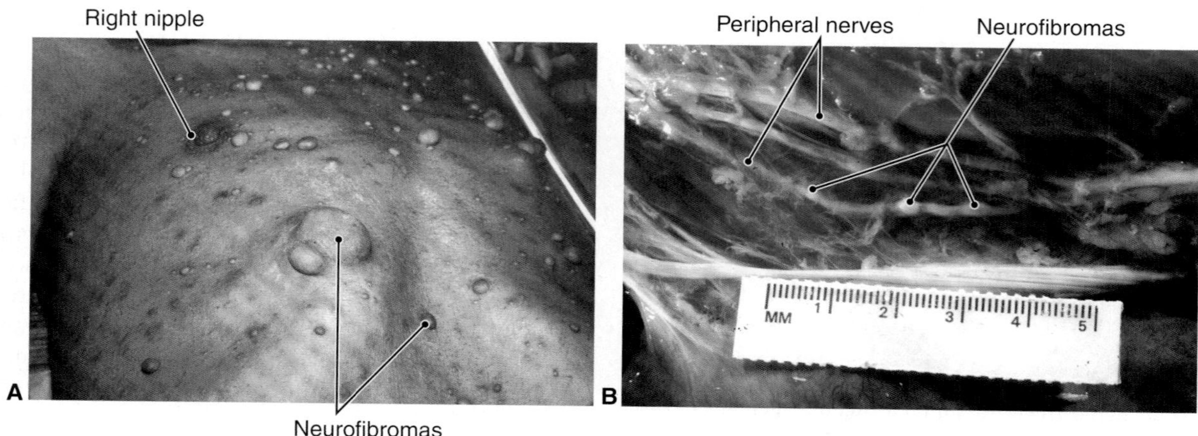

Figure 19.38 **Neurofibromatosis, Type I (von Recklinghausen disease). A.** Skin of the chest with multiple neurofibromas. **B.** Dissection of forearm showing multiple neurofibromas of peripheral nerves.

accounts for 10% of cases, and presents primarily as congenital bilateral acoustic neuromas. Diagnosis of schwannomas and neurofibromas is by biopsy. Diagnosis of neurofibromatosis is by clinical suspicion. Treatment is surgical.

Malignant peripheral nerve sheath tumor (MPNST) is a malignant tumor of peripheral nerve. Half are spontaneous; the other half arise in patients with NF1. Diagnosis is by biopsy. Treatment is surgical. Prognosis is poor.

Pop Quiz

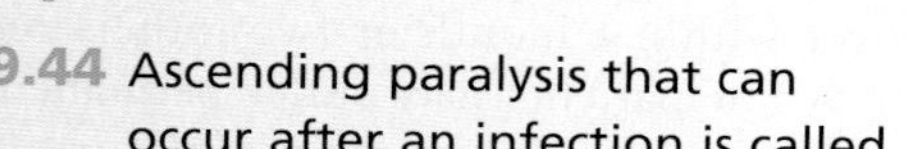

19.44 Ascending paralysis that can occur after an infection is called ________________.

19.45 True or false? Acoustic neuromas seen in neurofibromatosis, Type 2 (NF2) are actually schwannomas.

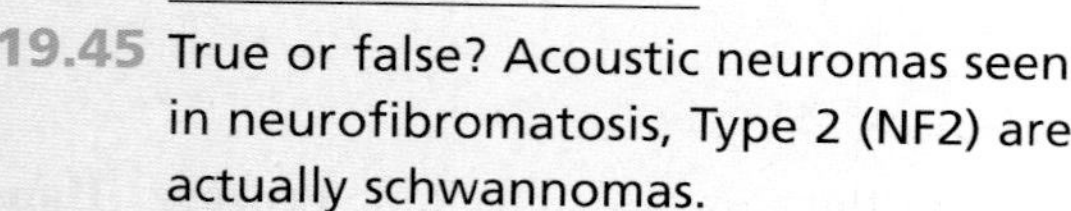

Case Study Revisited

"Something doesn't seem right in my head." The case of Ted H.

Ted's underlying problem was atherosclerosis. One of the more remarkable facts in his history was that he smoked until he was in his 60s but quit after a heart attack and began exercising and lived nearly 30 more years. Usually nature is not so forgiving, but his long-lived ancestors bequeathed him a wonderful genetic endowment.

Chronic myocardial ischemia resulting from coronary atherosclerosis eventually produced atrial fibrillation and congestive heart failure. Atrial fibrillation is well known to promote formation of atrial thrombi. Atrial thrombi are fragile, break apart easily, and embolize. Those in the right atrium embolize to the lungs and are of little consequence because they are small. Those from the left atrium, however, are a different matter. Even a small thrombotic embolus to a cerebral artery can cause a serious, even fatal, ischemic infarct, as in this case. That the thrombus was not demonstrable at autopsy is not surprising: it was dissolved by natural thrombolytics in the eight days between the event and death.

The first indication of brain trouble came from Ted's complaint that something was not right in his head. That same day, he became aphasic, an indication that blood flow to the middle cerebral artery, which serves the speech area of the cerebral cortex, had been compromised, a conclusion confirmed by autopsy findings. The initial episode was a TIA and, because he recovered, we can safely say it did not produce an infarct. The second episode, however, produced a massive, fatal infarction. Both were caused by atrial embolic thrombi.

Points to remember include the following:

- Complications of atherosclerosis affect mainly the heart and brain.
- One of the consequences of atrial fibrillation is the formation of atrial thrombi.
- Embolic arterial thrombi can cause brain infarction.

Chapter Challenge

CHAPTER RECALL

1. A 72-year-old Caucasian female is brought to her primary physician's office by her son after becoming lost in her own home. She enters the room with a marked shuffling gait. A review of systems is positive for incontinence but is otherwise unremarkable; she denies the presence of tremor. A CT shows enlarged ventricles. What is the most likely etiology for her constellation of symptoms?
   A. MS
   B. Parkinsonism
   C. Alzheimer
   D. NPH

2. Which is the most likely cause of acute purulent meningitis in a two-year-old?
   A. Escherichia coli
   B. Streptococcus pneumoniae
   C. Haemophilus influenza
   D. Neisseria meningitidis

3. A 22-year-old Hispanic male is brought to the emergency department following a motor vehicle accident in which he was an unrestrained passenger. He is conscious on exam, and complains of double vision. A quick exam reveals a dilated right pupil and impaired ocular movement. What has caused his symptoms?
   A. Herniation of the brain stem through the foramen magnum
   B. Herniation of the ipsilateral side of the temporal lobe through the tentorium
   C. Herniation of the lower medial aspect of the hemisphere under the falx cerebri
   D. None of the above

4. What type of edema is caused by diabetic ketoacidosis?
   A. Vasogenic edema
   B. Cytotoxic edema
   C. Both of the above
   D. None of the above

5. A 10-year-old Caucasian male is brought to the ER by his parents after they were unable to wake him up for dinner. Earlier in the afternoon, he'd been hit in the side of the head by a baseball. He was only unconscious for approximately 30 seconds, but when he woke up, he claimed he was fine. What vessel was damaged?
   A. Middle meningeal artery
   B. A bridging vein
   C. Carotid artery
   D. Basilar artery

6. Which of the following tumors arises from ependymal cells lining the ventricles?
   A. Ependymomas
   B. Subependymomas
   C. Glioblastomas
   D. Medulloblastomas

7. A nine-month-old African American male is seen at his pediatrician's office for failure to meet motor milestones. Physical exam reveals abnormal muscle tone and limb spasticity. His past medical history is significant for prematurity with a low birth weight and hyperbilirubinemia. What is your diagnosis?
   A. Epilepsy
   B. Cerebral palsy
   C. Arnold Chiari malformation
   D. Agyria

8. Your mother calls you concerned that your 50-year-old father may be having a stroke. She reports that he cannot close his right eye, raise his right eyebrow, or smile with the right half of his mouth. She tells you that, though his speech is garbled, he is understandable; she denies additional symptoms. From which neurological condition does he suffer?
   A. Guillain Barré
   B. Amyotrophic lateral sclerosis
   C. Bell palsy
   D. MS

9. Which hereditary disease features accumulation of glucocerebroside in macrophages and/or neurons?
   A. Tay sachs
   B. Cerebral palsy
   C. Hurler
   D. Gaucher

10. Reviewing the history of your recently deceased 45-year-old patient, you notice that his dementia, personality changes, and physical limitations progressed in a stepwise fashion, with distinct declines in function every few months. What is the most likely cause of this rapidly progressing disease?
    A. AD
    B. Frontotemporal dementia
    C. vCJD
    D. Vascular dementia

11. Which of the following cells makes cerebral spinal fluid?
    A. Astrocytes
    B. Oligodendrogliomas
    C. Ependymal cells
    D. Microglia

12. A 24-year-old female visits her campus clinic complaining of new-onset blurry vision in one eye. Six months prior, she had come to the clinic complaining of weakness and spasticity in her right leg. Oligoclonal bands of immunoglobulin were identified in her CSF, confirming your suspicions. From what disease does she suffer?
A. MS
B. Guillain Barré
C. Amyotrophic lateral sclerosis
D. TIAs

13. Autopsy on a 65-year-old Caucasian female with a past medical history of dementia reveals general atrophy of the cerebral cortex with narrowed gyri and broad sulci as well as neurofibrillary tangles and plaques of amyloid-like protein on histology. What was the cause of her dementia?
A. AD
B. Parkinson disease
C. Lewy body dementia
D. Huntington disease

14. PML is a form of fatal encephalitis caused by which of the following viruses?
A. CMV
B. Herpesvirus
C. *JC* virus
D. Arbovirus

15. A 55-year-old Hispanic female is worked up for new-onset seizures. Her MRI reveals a solitary lesion in the parasagittal region that appears to be growing on the surface of the brain. What type of tumor does she have?
A. Glioblastoma multiforme
B. Meningioma
C. Astrocytoma
D. Oligodendroglioma

16. A 43-year-old Caucasian woman is brought to the clinic by her husband. Her illness began several years earlier with increased nervousness, irritability, and depression and had progressed to include a jerky gait with strange dance-like movements of her upper and lower extremities. Her family history was significant for a mother with similar symptoms and psychosis who died at 45 shortly after being committed to an asylum. What is her diagnosis?
A. Parkinsonism
B. Parkinson disease
C. CJD
D. Huntington disease

17. A 65-year-old Caucasian male's physical exam is remarkable for an emotionless facial expression, stooped posture, a shuffling gait, and a slow, coarse, resting tremor of his right hand. Where is his lesion and what medication can be used to treat his disease?
A. Substantia nigra, L-dopa
B. Basal ganglia, supportive treatment
C. Frontal cortex, supportive treatment
D. Wernicke area, L-dopa

18. True or false? Neurons do not divide; therefore, diseased or dead neurons cannot be replaced.

19. True or false? About 25% of patients who have a TIA have a nonhemorrhagic infarct within five years.

20. True or false? Respiratory failure is the leading cause of death in a patient suffering from amyotrophic lateral sclerosis.

21. True or false? Aseptic meningitis is acute inflammation of the meninges caused by something other than an infectious agent.

22. True or false? In patients with CNS trauma caused by a penetrating object, the disruption of tissue is the leading contribution to patient morbidity and mortality.

23. True or false? The most common leukodystrophy is metachromatic leukodystrophy.

24. Match the following anatomic locations to their characteristics below:
i. Cortex
ii. Nerve tracts
iii. Brain stem
iv. Midbrain
v. Pons
vi. Medulla oblongata
vii. Cerebellum
viii. Dura
ix. Arachnoid
x. Pia
xi. Falx cerebri
xii. Tentorium cerebelli
xiii. Choroid plexus
xiv. Arachnoid granulations
A. The innermost meningeal membrane
B. Uppermost part of the brain stem, important in eye movement and hearing
C. Responsible for carrying electrical signals between the brain and body

D. Lowest part of the brainstem, modulates heart rate and blood pressure
E. Responsible for absorbing CSF
F. Composed of the midbrain, pons, and medulla oblongata
G. Dura mater that encloses the superior sagittal sinus
H. Thick sheet of fibrous tissue stuck to skull and surrounding the spinal cord
I. Home to reasoning, emotion, voluntary motion, and speech
J. The dura separating the cerebral hemisphere from the cerebellum
K. Middle and largest part of the brain stem, important in respiration
L. Mediates balance, fine motor activity, and proprioceptive sense
M. Thin membrane between dura and subarachnoid space
N. Responsible for the production of CSF

CONCEPTUAL UNDERSTANDING

25. Compare and contrast the two divisions of the ANS.
26. What are the causes/ contributing factors to the development and rupture of saccular (berry) aneurysms?
27. What are the diagnostic features of neurofibromatosis?

APPLICATION

28. In the setting of suspicion for an intracranial mass or increased intracranial pressure, what should be done prior to performing a lumbar puncture?
29. Which is worse, hypoxia or ischemia?
30. What compensatory mechanism is in place to prevent infarcts in someone with blockage/stenosis of one of their carotids?
31. Describe the various symptoms arising from thiamine deficiency.

CHAPTER

20 Disorders of the Senses

Contents

Chapter Objectives

After studying this chapter, you should be able to complete the following tasks:

Section 1: Disorders of the Eye

THE NORMAL EYE AND ORBIT

1. Describe the anterior segment (both the anterior and posterior chapters) and the posterior segment (including all layers) of the globe, and trace the flow of aqueous humor.

DISORDERS OF ALIGNMENT AND MOVEMENT

2. Discuss the causes and complications, where applicable, of strabismus and nystagmus.

TRAUMA

3. List the causes of ocular trauma.
4. Name the causes of proptosis.

DISORDERS OF REFRACTION

5. Compare and contrast myopia, hyperopia, presbyopia, and astigmatism.

DISORDERS OF THE EYELID, CONJUNCTIVA, SCLERA, AND LACRIMAL APPARATUS

6. Catalog the disorders of the eyelid, conjunctiva, sclera, and lacrimal apparatus according to their underlying etiology (whether infectious, autoimmune, both, or other) and discuss their clinical presentation and treatment.

DISORDERS OF THE CORNEA

7. Distinguish between infectious and noninfectious disorders of the cornea, and discuss the accompanying signs and symptoms.

DISORDERS OF THE LENS

8. Explain the pathophysiology of cataracts.

DISORDERS OF THE UVEAL TRACT

9. List the components of the uveal tract and discuss the types, etiologies, and complications of uveitis.

DISORDERS OF THE VITREOUS HUMOR AND RETINA

10. Discuss the differential diagnosis for someone experiencing vision loss, noting key signs and symptoms that can be used to discriminate amongst the etiologies.

DISORDERS OF THE OPTIC NERVE

11. Distinguish between primary open-angle glaucoma, primary closed-angle glaucoma, and secondary glaucoma, and discuss the relationship of intraocular pressure to glaucoma.

OCULAR NEOPLASMS

12. Compare and contrast ocular malignant melanoma and retinoblastoma.

Section 2: Disorders of the Ear

THE NORMAL EAR

13. Name the three anatomic divisions of the ear, and describe the anatomy responsible for hearing and equilibrium.

DISORDERS OF THE EXTERNAL EAR

14. Discuss the risk factors, etiology, and signs and symptoms of otitis externa.

DISORDERS OF THE MIDDLE EAR

15. Distinguish between the types of otitis media.

DISORDERS OF THE INNER EAR

16. Explain the differential diagnosis of a patient suffering with vertigo.
17. Name the three general categories of hearing loss.

Section 3: Disorders of Other Senses

NORMAL TASTE AND SMELL

18. Explain the mechanisms responsible for taste and smell, and their relationship to one another.

DISORDERS OF TASTE AND SMELL

19. List the disorders that affect taste and smell.

NORMAL SOMATIC SENSES

20. Name the receptors of sensation and their corresponding somatic sense.

DISORDERS OF SOMATIC SENSES

21. Using examples from the text, discuss the etiology and clinical findings of patients with somatosensory disorders.

Sensing and *sensation* are separate things. **Sensing** is the detection of a stimulus by a sensory receptor. It does not require conscious perception. Some sensory receptors in our bodies continually sense things of which we have no conscious awareness (e.g., blood pressure, blood pH) because their signals are not relayed upward to the cerebral cortex for integration into consciousness. **Sensation** is conscious perception of sensory signals by the cerebral cortex.

The notion of a "sixth sense,"—a hunch—springs from the classic notion that there are five human senses: vision, hearing, taste, smell, and touch. But the truth is that we have more than five. Exactly how many is a matter of definition, but it is closer to ten than five.

Consider the matter of the relative position of body parts. Normal humans know precisely the position of their head, limbs, fingers, and toes without seeing them. This position sense is called *proprioception*. Also consider the matter of *equilibrium*, our sense of balance. If we're off balance, we have mechanisms, both conscious and reflexive, to bring us back into balance. Being in equilibrium does not mean being still; it means being in control. Failed equilibrium leads to a stumble or fall.

If you add proprioception and equilibrium to the traditional five senses, then there are seven senses. But what about the sensation of *pain*, or of *temperature*? These, too, are separate senses.

It's easier to account for the body's senses if we classify them into three groups:

- The **visceral senses** are structures and mechanisms that detect changes in our internal environment, such as an increase in blood pressure, a decrease in blood glucose, and so on. They operate entirely below the level of consciousness. We shall not discuss them further.
- The **somatic senses** (Greek *soma* = body) are simple structures with uncomplicated detection mechanisms. They are widely distributed in skin, muscle, bones, joints, and other tissues, and are not clustered into a special anatomic site or organ. Touch, one of the historical "five senses," for example, is a somatic sense.
- The **special senses** are complex systems with sophisticated detection apparatus. Vision, smell, taste, and hearing, four of the historical "five senses," are special senses. Equilibrium is another special sense.

Section 1: Disorders of Vision

None so blind as those that will not see.

MATTHEW HENRY (1662–1714), NONCONFORMIST ENGLISH CLERGYMAN, WHOSE MOST FAMOUS QUOTATION IS "BETTER LATE THAN NEVER."

Case Study

"I'm having a terrible headache." The case of Madelyn Q.

Chief Complaint: Headache

Clinical History: Madelyn Q., a 50-year-old diabetic woman, environmental activist, and nonpracticing attorney, was in a large city visiting her daughter. While having dinner at a restaurant, she developed a severe, aching, dull headache. She felt nauseated and vomited in the toilet. Her daughter drove her to a local urgent care facility owned by a large community hospital.

When the emergency physician questioned her about what led her to seek care, she said, "I'm having a terrible headache." On further questioning, she revealed she was in general good health and active despite having Type II diabetes and hypertension. She developed Type II diabetes when she was 38 and began taking oral hypoglycemic agents for blood glucose control. Three years later, she was found to be hypertensive. Her BP was controlled by oral antihypertensives. She had worn glasses for reading since she was a child. She described the pain as severe, dull, and aching, and centered above her right eye. She also complained of excessive tearing and hazy vision in the right eye with "halos around all of the lights."

Physical Examination and Other Data: Madelyn was a well-groomed, poised woman who looked younger than her stated age. Vital signs were unremarkable, and physical exam revealed no

"I'm having a terrible headache." The Case of Madelyn Q. (continued)

abnormalities except for the right eye—there was mild scleral congestion, tearing, and the lids were slightly swollen. The right pupil was dilated and fixed. The left pupil reacted normally to light.

Clinical Course: Concluding that she had an eye disease, possibly acute glaucoma, but unable to make a definitive diagnosis, the emergency physician made a referral to the emergency department of the parent hospital.

A few days later, the emergency physician called the hospital, curious to know what had happened. A nurse in the ophthalmology department told him that the patient was diagnosed in the emergency room with acute closed-angle glaucoma. Records faxed from the hospital revealed that she was examined that evening by an ophthalmologist. Initial intraocular pressure in the right eye was 48 mm Hg (normal <21) and 18 in the left eye. Visual acuity was 20/60 in the right eye, 20/40 in the left eye. Slit lamp examination of the anterior segment revealed shallow anterior chambers in both eyes. Early cataract was present in the left lens. In the right eye the conjunctiva was congested, the cornea was cloudy, the pupil was dilated and fixed, and the anterior chamber angle was closed all the way around. The right retina could not be visualized because of corneal edema. Study of the left retina revealed a few hemorrhages and exudates, slight copper wire effect, and AV nicking consistent with nonproliferative diabetic retinopathy. A visual field examination for loss of peripheral vision was not performed.

She was given drugs to constrict her pupils and lower intraocular pressure and a systemic osmotic drug to increase blood osmotic pressure and thereby draw fluid from the globe. On follow-up the next afternoon, intraocular pressure was normal and inflammation had disappeared. Both optic discs were normal and showed no evidence of glaucomatous change. Laser peripheral iridotomy was performed in both eyes to give aqueous humor an alternative route to the canal of Schlemm.

The ophthalmology department arranged to transfer her care to an ophthalmologist in a city near her hometown and she was given a supply of ocular medicines to use for the next week until she could keep her appointment.

The Normal Eye and Orbit

Vision is the detection of light by the eye *and* integration into consciousness of the sensory signals produced. It is the special sense most people value above all others.

The **eye** is the organ of vision. In its entirety, it is referred to as the *eyeball*, a sphere about 24–25 mm (one inch) in diameter. The specific light-sensing cells in the eye are *photoreceptors*. The nerve connections between photoreceptors and the visual cortex of the brain is the **visual pathway**. By sensing minute variations of color, light, and dark, we perceive one aspect of the world around us—the world revealed by light. Unlike all other sensory organs, the body can manipulate the eyes: they can be aimed in a certain direction and focused near or far, an indication of their Darwinian survival value.

The **eyeball** (the *globe*, Fig. 20.1) and its accessory structures occupy a bony socket in the skull, the **orbit**, which protects the globe on all sides but the anterior. Anteriorly, the leading edge of the skull above and maxilla below protect the recessed globe between.

Accessory Structures Are Present in and around the Orbit

Around the orbit are other structures important to eye function.

- **Eyebrows** shield the eye from particulate matter and glare.
- The **eyelids** (*palpebrae*) are flaps of tissue covered externally by skin and lined internally by mucosa, called the **conjunctiva**, which is lined by a layer of epithelial cells and contains numerous mucus-secreting cells. The conjunctival mucosa extends deep under the eyelid where it connects with the outer covering of the globe, the sclera. The epithelial cells of the sclera continue across the front of the globe to form the epithelial layer of *cornea*. The lids also contain other structures:
  - The **tarsal plate**, a band of stiff, fibrous tissue that is especially dense along the lid edge and maintains the structure of the lid
  - Fibers of skeletal muscle that move the lids (blinking)
  - Eyelashes and hair follicles and their sebaceous glands

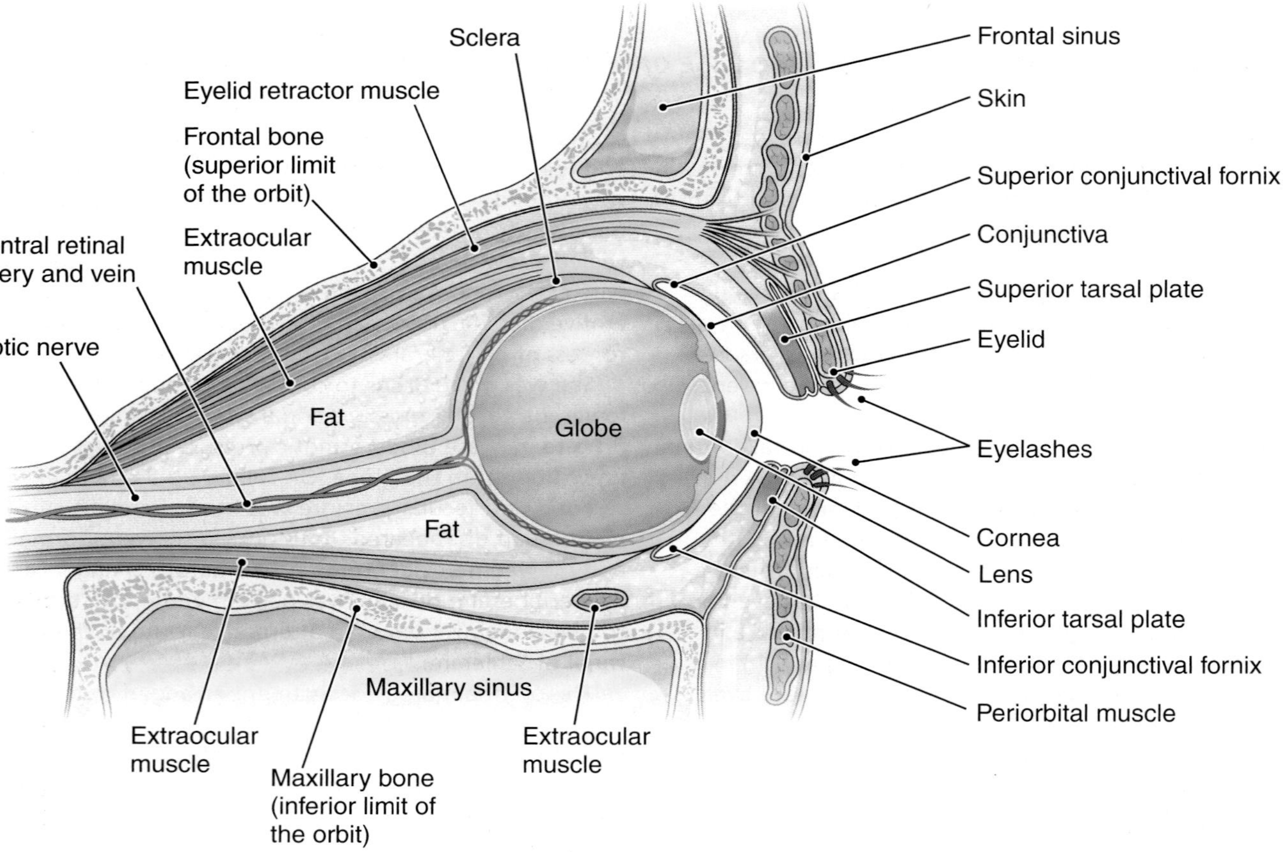

Figure 20.1 **The orbit and its contents (sagittal section).**

Within the orbit, other accessory structures are present:

- The **external muscles** of the eye: six small skeletal muscles that move the globe
- The **nasolacrimal apparatus** consisting of the **lacrimal glands**, one in the upper-outer edge of each orbit, which secrete **tears**, and the associated **tear drainage ducts** (Fig. 20.2)
- Nerves, blood vessels, fat, loose fibrous tissue, and interstitial fluid

The *nasolacrimal apparatus* keeps the eye bathed in tears produced by lacrimal glands, one under the upper lateral edge of each orbit. Tears cross the eye to drain through tiny pores in the nasal margin of the upper and lower eyelids into short ducts that lead to a lacrimal sac in the wall of the nose. From there, tears drain into the nose via the nasolacrimal duct.

The **globe** (Fig. 20.3) is divided by the posterior edge of the lens (the clear, round, pillow-shaped focusing organ) into the *anterior segment*, consisting of the lens and everything in front of it, and the *posterior segment*, which lies posterior to the lens. The wall of the globe is formed of three membranes or **tunics**.

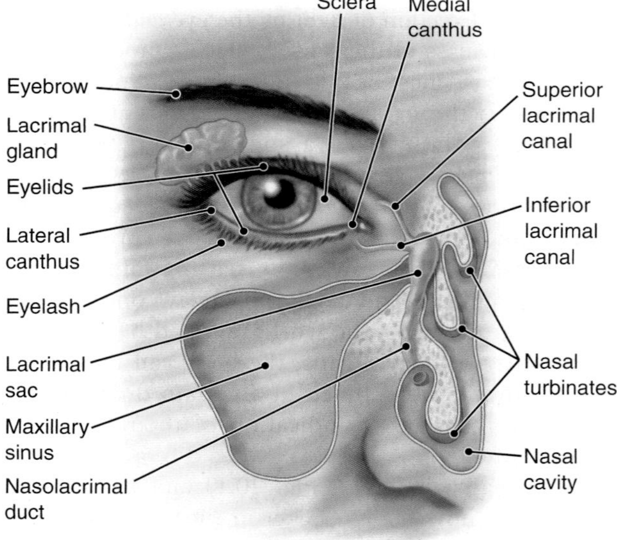

Figure 20.2 **Accessory structures of the eye.** (Reproduced with permission from McConnell TH, Hull KL. *Human Form Human Function: Essentials of Anatomy & Physiology*. Baltimore, MD: Wolters Kluwer Health; 2011.)

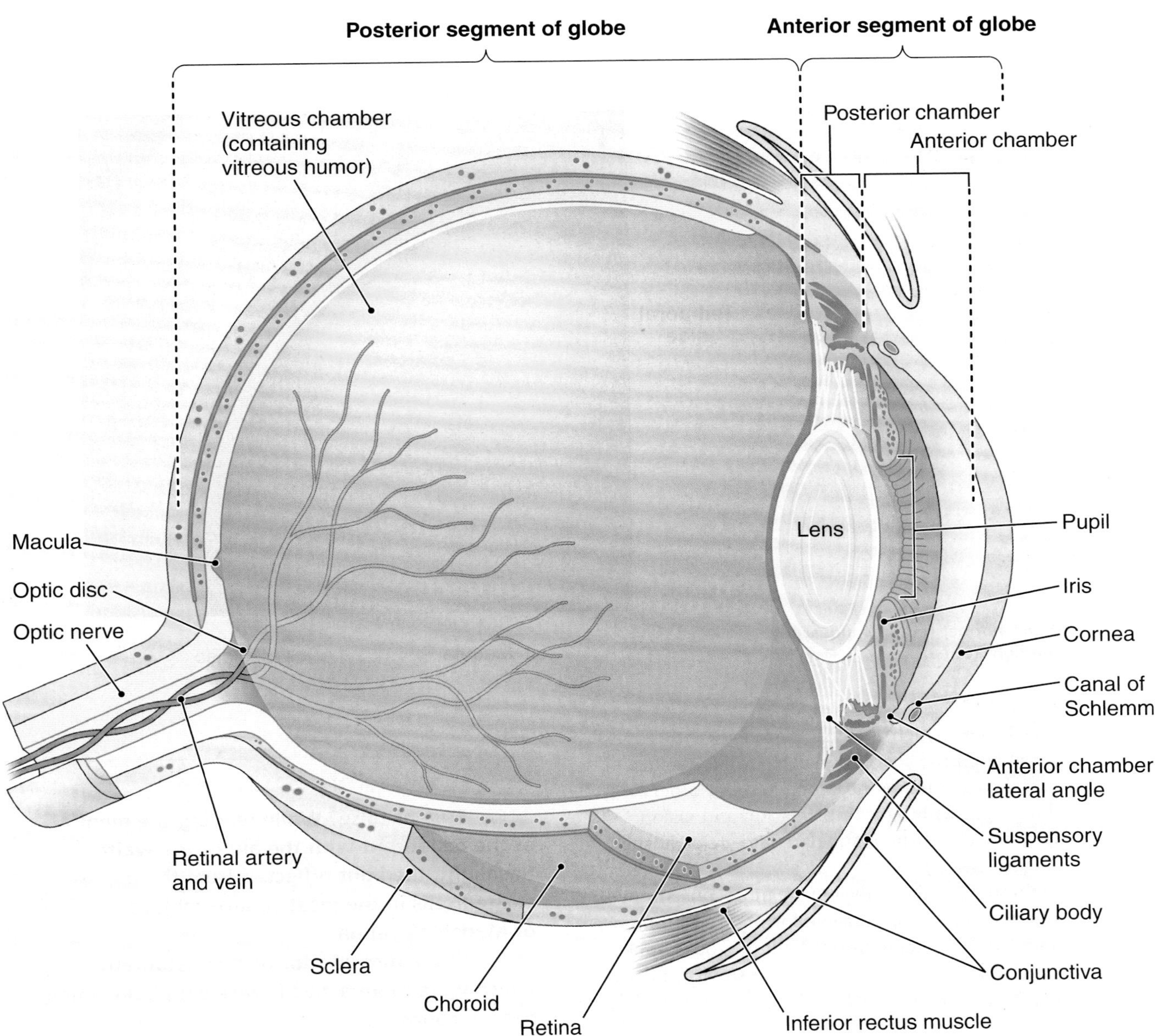

Figure 20.3 **Internal anatomy of the globe.**

The Globe Is Formed of Three Layers

Layers of the globe are called "tunics." The outermost layer of the globe is the **fibrous tunic** or **sclera**, a tough fibrous protective layer that anteriorly is visible as the white of the eye and continues anteriorly to form the cornea.

Next inward is the **vascular tunic** or **choroid**, a richly vascular, pigmented layer of the globe that also contains collagen fibers and melanocytes, which produce pigment in proportion to the degree of pigmentation of the skin. The melanin produced by these cells absorbs light and prevents reflection back to the innermost layer, the retina. The choroid continues forward into the anterior segment to form the *ciliary body* and *iris*. The choroid, ciliary body, and iris are called the **uveal tract** or **uvea**.

The innermost layer of the globe is the **neural tunic** or **retina** (Fig. 20.4), the light-sensing layer of nervous tissue. The retina contains three layers. The innermost is a transparent layer of *nerve fibers* carrying sensory signals. They converge to form the optic nerve, which carries the signals to the brain. The middle layer is *a sensory-neural layer* of specialized cells (*rods* and *cones*), which convert light into nerve signals. The deepest layer of the retina is the *retinal pigmented epithelium*, a layer of pigmented cells that absorb excess light and prevent reflection.

Dead center in the retina, straight back from the cornea, is the **macula**, a small and highly sensitive part of the retina responsible for detailed, central vision. In the center of the

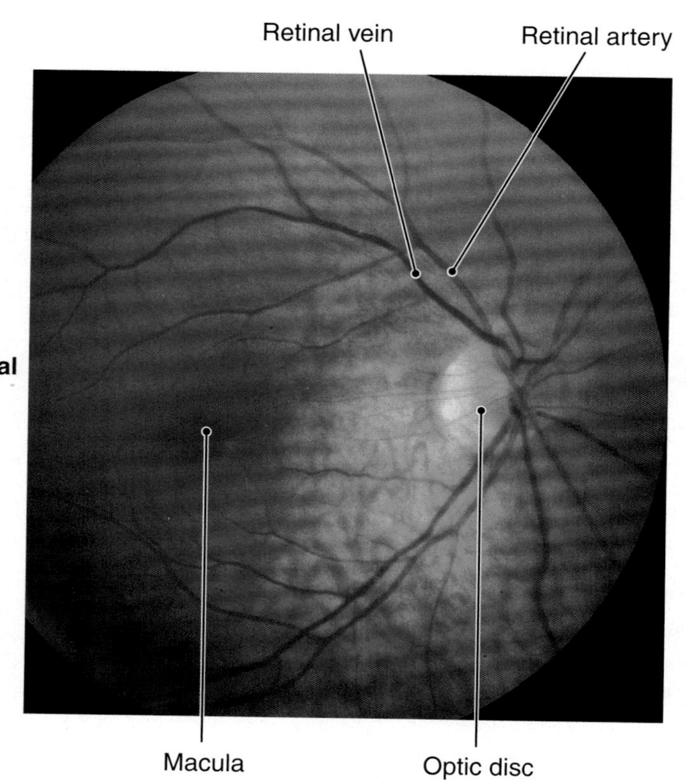

Figure 20.4 **The normal retina (funduscopic view is of the right retina).**

macula is the **fovea**, which is densely packed with cones and is responsible for the sharpest vision. Unlike the rest of the retina, the fovea contains no blood vessels; otherwise, they would interfere with light transmission and vision.

Rods discriminate only light and dark and are exquisitely sensitive to light—a single photon can stimulate a rod. They are scattered throughout the retina but are most concentrated at the periphery. They are responsible for night vision, motion detection, and peripheral vision. Multiple rods connect to a single cortical neuron. This increases sensitivity of cortical perception but at the expense of detail. It we had only rods for vision, our view of the world would be like an old black and white, low resolution television.

Cones sense color but require bright light for peak performance. They are concentrated in the center of the retina and most densely packed in the fovea. There are three varieties: one each for *blue*, *green,* and *red* light. In the fovea, each cone connects through the optic nerve to a single cortical neuron. This increases perception of detail but at the expense of sensitivity; hence the need for bright light for best color perception.

The **optic nerve** connects the retina to the brain. The retinal blood supply travels from the internal carotid artery with the optic nerve into the eye. Where the optic nerve connects with the eye, it forms the **optic disc** (Fig. 20.4), a coin-shaped white spot in the retina at which nerve fibers from the retina gather to form the optic nerve. The retinal artery and vein also enter the globe through the optic disc and radiate outward into the retina.

Case Notes

20.1 **True or false? While reading the menu at the restaurant with the aid of the waiter's flashlight, the light reflected from the menu excited cells in the most superficial layer of Madelyn's retina.**

20.2 **In the dim interior of the restaurant, which were more active in receiving light signals: rods or cones?**

20.3 **Where on Madelyn's retina were menu item images focused?**

20.4 **Madelyn developed dull aching pain at dinner. Which somatic sensors were involved and what fibers transmitted the sensation?**

20.5 **Madelyn's pain was above her eye despite the fact that the disease was in her eye. What is the name for this type of displaced pain?**

The Globe Is Divided into Anterior and Posterior Segments

The **anterior segment** of the globe (Fig. 20.5) consists of the *cornea, iris, lens,* and *ciliary body*. The anterior segment is divided into two spaces: the **anterior chamber**, a

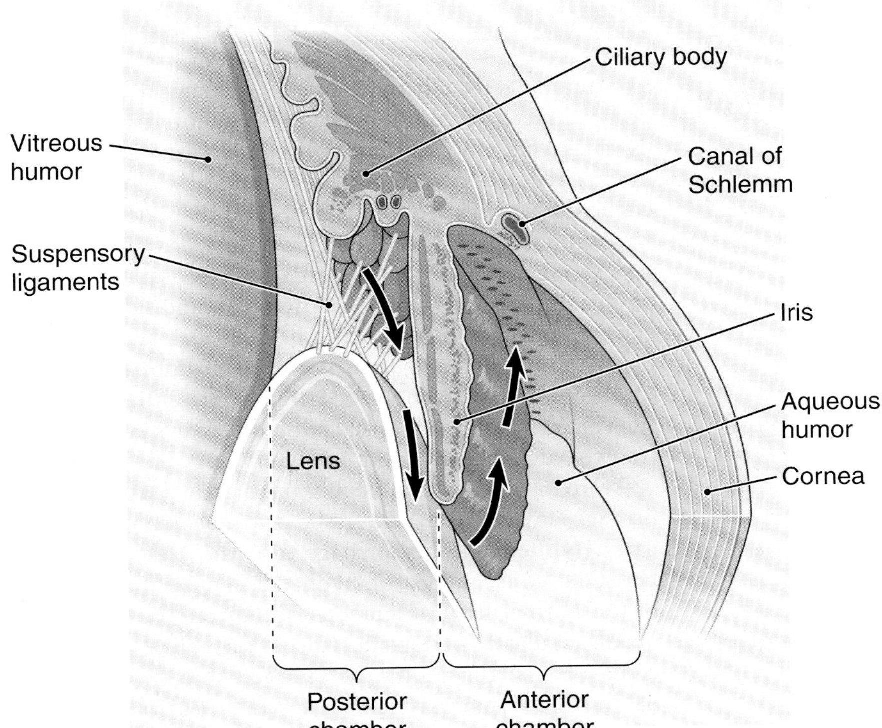

Figure 20.5 **Anatomy of the anterior segment.** Black arrows indicate the flow of aqueous humor.

fluid-filled space that lies behind the cornea and in front of the iris, and the **posterior chamber**, which lies behind the iris and in front of the lens. Note that the posterior chamber is in *front* of the lens. Light passing into the eye travels across the following structures and spaces, in order, before falling on the light-sensing layer (retina) at the back of the eye: the cornea, anterior chamber, pupil, posterior chamber, lens, and vitreous humor (the fluid that fills the posterior segment).

Remember This! The anterior and posterior chambers are in the anterior segment of the globe.

The **cornea** is the domed, clear (it lacks blood vessels and lymphatics) anterior part of the eye, which has much more light-bending (focusing) power than the lens. The cornea is covered by a layer of squamous *epithelial cells* that is an extension of the conjunctiva. Beneath this epithelium, the *stroma* of the lens is composed of fine, precisely aligned collagen fibers, which enhance transparency. A single layer of *endothelial cells* lines the inner surface of the cornea.

Encircling the anterior segment along its outer edge is the **ciliary body**, a highly vascular, doughnut-shaped organ that encircles and attaches to the iris and lens. The **iris** is a thin, pigmented membrane between the cornea and lens with a central opening (the **pupil**). It contains circular and radial smooth muscle fibers, which react to light and other stimuli by becoming larger (contraction of radial fibers) or smaller (contraction of circular fibers) to admit more or less light.

The **lens** sits immediately behind the iris. It is a flattened sphere held under constant lateral, flattening stretch by **suspensory ligaments** attached at its outer edge. The suspensory ligaments connect farther outward to a ring of circumferential smooth muscle, the **ciliary muscle**, in the ciliary body. Contraction of ciliary muscle fibers decreases the diameter of the ciliary muscle and relaxes tension on the suspensory ligaments and lens, which allows the lens to become thicker (less flattened) to focus on near objects. For distant focus the opposite occurs.

The ciliary body secretes a clear, watery fluid, **aqueous humor**, into the posterior chamber. Aqueous humor flows out of the posterior chamber through the pupil and into the anterior chamber (Fig. 20.4). It then flows outward to the edge of the anterior chamber and enters the **Canal of Schlemm**, a tirelike duct in the ciliary body that encircles the anterior chamber, and is absorbed into blood. Production of aqueous humor creates and maintains intraocular pressure, which is transmitted from the anterior segment into the posterior segment, keeping the globe inflated to a uniform pressure.

The **posterior segment** of the globe consists of the globe posterior to the lens. It consists of the globe wall, its chamber (the **vitreous chamber**), and the fluid filling it (the **vitreous humor**), which is 99% water and 1% collagen.

Case Notes

20.6 As Madelyn focused on menu items, which two eye structures focused light to make a sharp image? Of the two, which had the greater focusing power?

20.7 Where was the focusing apparatus in Madelyn's eye: the anterior segment or the posterior segment?

Pop Quiz

20.1 True or false? The optic nerve connects the retina to the brain.

20.2 True or false? The globe is divided into anterior and posterior chambers.

20.3 What are the three components of the uveal tract or uvea?

20.4 What part of the eye produces aqueous humor which flows through the canal of Schlemm?

Disorders of Alignment and Movement

Normal vision requires that the eyes be precisely aligned and move together in strict coordination. **Strabismus** is an abnormal alignment of one eye (cross-eye) that may be caused by neurologic disease or by weakness or shortening of an ocular muscle. *Diplopia* (double vision) is the result. In children, strabismus must be surgically corrected promptly or the brain will permanently suppress the signal from the affected eye, which will have dim vision (*amblyopia*) or become blind despite having no pathologic abnormality other than deviation.

Nystagmus is rapid, involuntary, rhythmic, repetitive motion of one or both eyes. Movement may be horizontal, vertical, or circular and may be caused by neurologic disease (especially of the cerebellum), disease of the inner ear, or drug toxicity. Nystagmus can interfere with vision by causing objects in the visual field to oscillate. Elimination of cause is the first goal of treatment. If the cause cannot be eliminated, oral or intraorbital drugs, or surgery may be indicated.

Pop Quiz

20.5 What is the term for misalignment of the eyes, or "cross-eyed"?

Trauma

Eye trauma is usually mechanical or chemical. Minor superficial mechanical trauma can be diagnosed and treated by caregivers who are not ophthalmologists, but serious trauma requires a specialist. A common minor injury is **corneal abrasion**, a superficial wound that does not penetrate much beyond the first few layers of corneal cells. It is associated with pain, foreign body sensation, photophobia, and tear production. The sclera and lids may become edematous or inflamed. Abrasions can be visualized by conjunctival instillation of a drop of fluorescein dye. Minor abrasions do not need treatment. Others require topical anesthetic and topical antibiotic to avoid infection. An eye patch is usually not necessary.

More serious mechanical trauma may lead to hemorrhage anywhere in the globe and necessitates expert care. **Hyphema** is hemorrhage into the anterior chamber. One consequence of hyphema can be interruption of the normal flow of aqueous humor and development of intraocular hypertension (discussed below with glaucoma). Hemorrhage into the vitreous, into the retina, or behind the retina may not be apparent until the patient complains of red discoloration of vision or partial loss of vision. It may have serious consequences, including blindness. The most serious trauma is laceration of the globe, which always requires emergency intervention by a specialist.

Chemical trauma from acids or caustics can cause severe scarring of the cornea and conjunctiva and may require corneal transplant.

Displaced fracture of the orbit, especially the floor, is fairly common with blunt facial injury, usually as a result of an assault by one male on another. The eye is often injured as well. Even if the eye is uninjured, the globe may be displaced. Forward displacement of the globe in the orbit, or bulging eyes, is **proptosis** (**exophthalmos** when both eyes are affected). The usual cause of exophthalmos is increased tissue and fluid in the orbit behind the globe caused by *Graves disease* (Chapter 14). Proptosis also occurs with orbital inflammation, infection, or mass such as hemangioma, lymphoma, or lacrimal gland adenoma. Regardless of cause, displacement of the globe is associated with double vision (diplopia) and other visual symptoms. Treatment is surgical.

Pop Quiz

20.6 True or false? Hyphema is increased anterior chamber pressure.

20.7 True or false? Proptosis is usually caused by Graves disease.

Disorders of Refraction

Normal vision requires multiple steps:

1. Light must pass uninterrupted from cornea to retina.
2. The cornea and lens must refract (bend) light to focus images precisely on the retina.
3. Retinal cells must receive the light rays and convert them into nerve signals.
4. Nerve signals must pass normally along the optic nerve and the visual tracts in the brain to the visual cortex in the occipital lobes.
5. The visual cortex must receive the image and, with other parts of the brain, assimilate it into a perception.

Refractive disorders (Fig. 20.6) are those in which images are blurred by failure of light rays to focus (converge) sharply on the retina. These abnormalities may be caused by abnormal shape of the cornea, elongation or shortening of the globe, or stiffening of the lens, which interferes with focus adjustment. There are no underlying pathological abnormalities that account for purely refractive disorders.

Remember This! All refraction errors are caused by abnormal shape of the globe or cornea, or stiffness of the lens.

If the globe is elongated, rays converge in front of the retina, and the image is blurred, a condition called myopia (Fig. 20.6B). People with myopia are said to be "nearsighted" because the lens is usually able to overcome the defect for near objects. On the other hand, if the globe is foreshortened, the retina is too close to the cornea, the focal point is behind the retina, and the image is blurred, a condition called hyperopia (Fig. 20.6C). People with hyperopia are said to be "farsighted" because the lens is often able to overcome the defect for distant objects.

For focus on distant objects, ciliary muscles tug at the edges of the lens to flatten it. For near objects, the muscles relax and allow the lens to assume a thicker, more globular shape. Focusing power is gradually lost over the years and results in a slow decrease in the ability of the eye to focus on objects nearby, a condition called **presbyopia** (from Greek *presbus* = old man, Fig. 20.6D). About age 40, the great majority of people gradually notice an inability to focus on near objects and find they need to hold reading materials further away. Presbyopia is a natural part of the aging process and affects almost everyone.

Remember This! Almost everyone >40 years old has some degree of presbyopia.

Sometimes, however, misfocused images are caused by irregularities in the curvature of the cornea. The normal cornea has the same curvature in every imaginary cross-section. For example, visualize a clock face imposed on the cornea: the curvature across the cornea in the 1 o'clock to

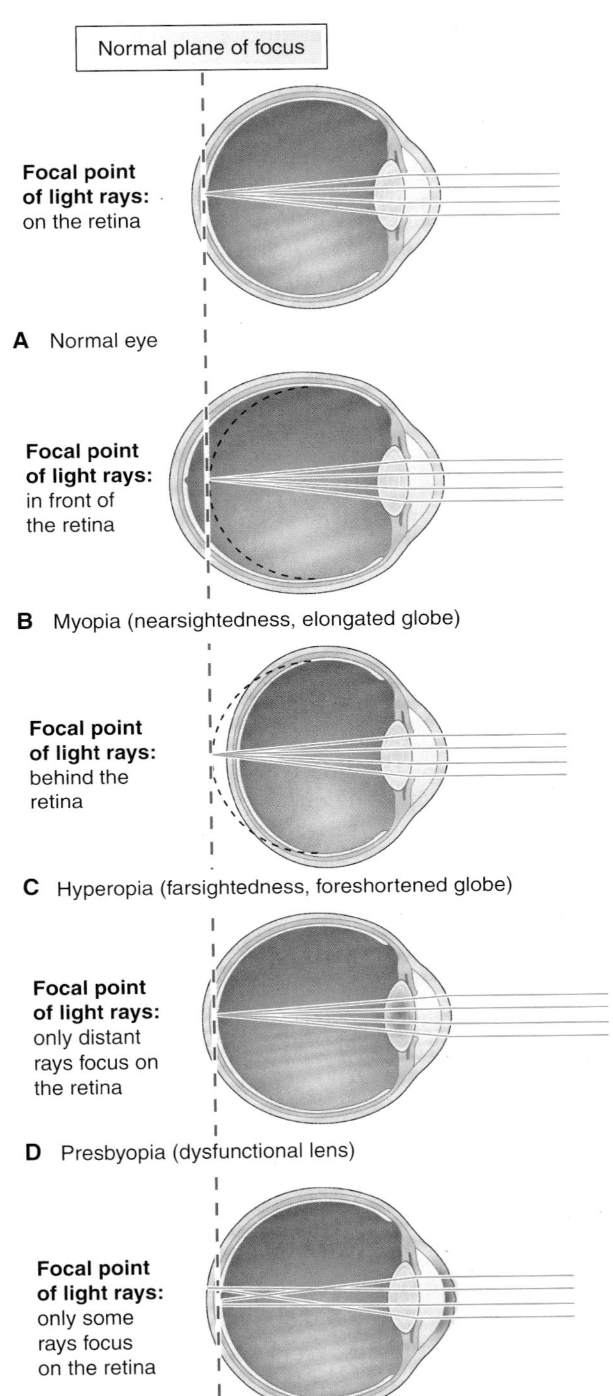

Figure 20.6 **Refractive disorders. A.** Normal. **B.** Myopia (nearsightedness). The globe is elongated. The lens is able to focus rays from near objects, but rays from distant objects converge in front of the retina, blurring the retinal image. **C.** Hyperopia (farsightedness). The globe is foreshortened. The lens is able to focus rays from distant objects but rays from near objects converge behind the retina, blurring the retinal image. **D.** Presbyopia (distant rays). With age, the lens stiffens and can no longer change shape (thicken) to focus rays from near objects to converge on the retina. Rays from near objects converge behind the retina, blurring the image. **E.** Astigmatism. Irregular curvature of the cornea misfocuses images: some converge in front or behind the retina, blurring the image, and others are focused off-center, creating overlapping images.

7 o'clock line should be the same for the line through the cornea from 4 o'clock to 10 o'clock, and so on for every other line across the cornea. If the curvature is not uniform, the image is properly focused in some areas and blurred in others, a condition called **astigmatism** (Fig. 20.6E).

The Clinical Side, "Seeing the Big E," discusses the common eye chart test of visual function. Refractive disorders are correctable by eyeglasses, contact lenses, or surgical reshaping of the cornea. Corneal reshaping compensates for a globe that is too long or too short or for a lens that no longer focuses properly. This and other forms of eye surgery are discussed in *The Clinical Side*, "Surgery for Refractive Errors, Glaucoma, and Cataracts," later in this chapter.

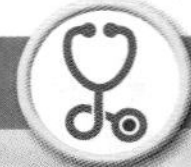

The Clinical Side

SEEING THE BIG E

The most common test of eye function is the familiar eye chart test, which tests visual acuity or sharpness.

The usual chart is a *Snellen chart*, named for 19th-century Dutch ophthalmologist Hermann Snellen (1834–1908), who came up with the idea. It is imprinted with block letters that decrease in size from the top line to the bottom line. The top line ("the big E") is the 200 line, which can be read by a normal person standing 200 feet away. The bottom line is the 10 line, which can be read by a normal person standing 10 feet away.

The test is administered with the patient standing 20 feet away. Therefore, if a patient standing 20 feet away can read only the "big E" (the 200 line) at the top, the patient's vision is 20/200, which is very poor. On the other hand, if a patient standing at 20 feet can read the smallest line (the 10 line) at the bottom, the patient's vision is 20/10, which is excellent.

Case Notes

20.8 Madelyn had worn glasses for reading since she was a child. Did she have presbyopia? If not, what condition did she have?

20.9 Without glasses, were Madelyn's images focused in front of or behind the retina?

Pop Quiz

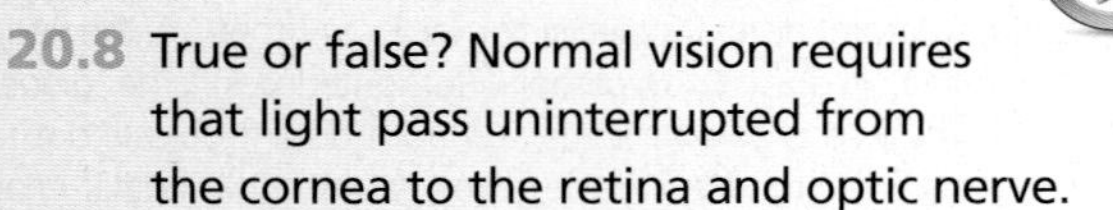

20.8 True or false? Normal vision requires that light pass uninterrupted from the cornea to the retina and optic nerve.

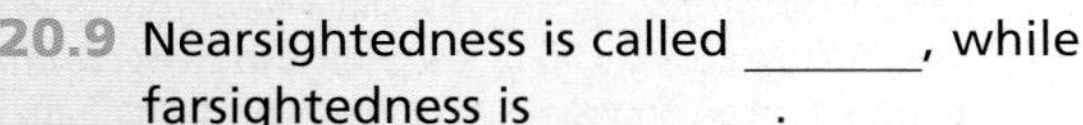

20.9 Nearsightedness is called _______, while farsightedness is _________.

Disorders of the Eyelid, Conjunctiva, Sclera, and Lacrimal Apparatus

The most common disorders or the eyelid, conjunctiva, sclera, and lacrimal apparatus are infections and inflammatory disease (Fig. 20.7).

Conjunctivitis Is Common

Inflammation of the conjunctiva (**conjunctivitis**) is common, mild, and usually bacterial, viral, or allergic. Numerous allergens can be responsible. Sometimes dust, sand, or other irritants are responsible. Viral or bacterial conjunctivitis is often contagious, sometimes highly so. Newborns are vulnerable to gonococcal or nongonococcal sexually transmitted infective conjunctivitis obtained by passage through an infected vaginal canal. The risk of *neonatal conjunctivitis* associated with maternal venereal infection with *Neisseria gonorrheoeae* or *Chlamydia trachomatis* is so great that all neonates receive prophylactic antibiotic eye drops immediately after delivery, which has almost completely eliminated the problem.

Conjunctivitis is one of the more common reasons for visits to a pediatrician. In children conjunctivitis is usually viral or bacterial, contagious, and is colloquially referred to as "pink eye. Since it can be highly contagious, parents are advised to keep their children home from daycare or school until the condition resolves, and caregivers must use precautions against transmission.

The sclera and the underside of the lids are affected. Symptoms include vascular congestion, photophobia, irritation, tearing, and an inflammatory discharge that crusts

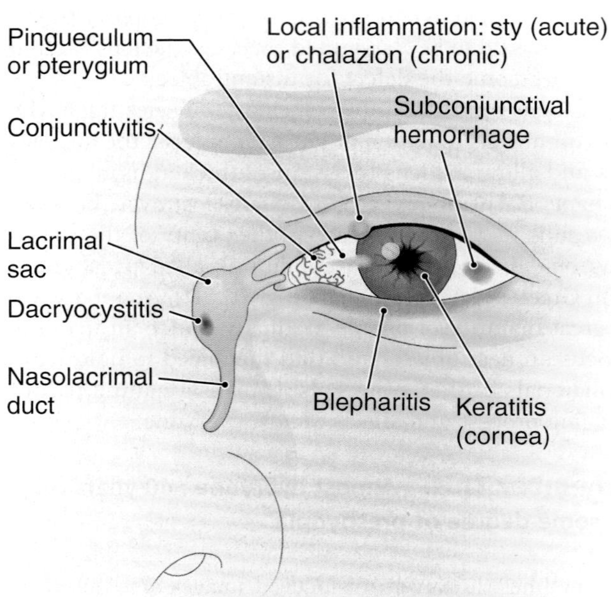

Figure 20.7 **Disorders of the eyelid, conjunctiva, sclera, and lacrimal apparatus.**

on the lids overnight. Plentiful discharge and preauricular lymphadenopathy suggest bacterial etiology, but the differential diagnosis between viral and bacterial infection can be difficult.

Incubation time is about 5–10 days. Typically, infection begins in one eye and spreads to the other in a few days. Diagnosis is clinical. Culture may be helpful. Treatment for bacterial infection is topical antibiotics. For severe viral infection, steroids may be used with caution and only after specialist examination has ruled out herpesvirus infection, which accelerates if treated with steroids.

In developed nations, most adult conjunctivitis is caused by seasonal allergies. It is also somewhat common in people who wear contact lenses and fail to change or clean them as directed. In developing nations, however, chronic conjunctival infection with *Chlamydia trachomatis* (**trachoma**) is a major cause of blindness—conjunctival scarring and contraction turns the eyelids inward (*entropion*) so that with every blink the cornea is scratched. Eventually, it becomes scarred. Diagnosis is by simple observation of the conjunctiva by a trained observer. Treatment is oral and intraocular antibiotics.

Other Conditions Are Less Common

Sty (*hordeolum*) is localized inflammation, sometimes a small abscess, of the eyelid resulting from bacterial infection of the sebaceous glands in the lid. Like sty, **chalazion** is a local inflammatory reaction of sebaceous glands except that it is a long-lasting condition characterized by chronic granulomatous inflammation.

Diffuse inflammation of the eyelids is called **blepharitis** (from Greek, *blefaros* = eyelid), which tends to be most severe at the lateral lid margins and mainly involves the external, nonconjunctival margin of the lid. It is common and usually caused by *Staphylococcus* infection, seasonal allergy, or skin conditions such as acne or seborrheic dermatitis. Treatment depends on the cause.

Inflammation of the lacrimal apparatus is called **dacryocystitis** (from Greek *dakryos* = tear) and may obstruct the flow of tears and predispose the patient to infection. The duct may be obstructed congenitally, or it may become obstructed at its drainage point in the nose owing to nasal conditions such as polyps or allergic rhinitis. Unrelieved obstruction may lead to bacterial infection of the lacrimal sac, scarring, and permanent ductal damage or obstruction. Irrigation, probing, and antibiotics are usually effective but some cases may require surgery to reestablish normal flow.

Keratoconjunctivitis sicca is a clinical syndrome of chronic dry eyes that can usually be attributed to insufficient tear formation, but it may alternatively be caused by poor tear quality and excessive evaporation. It may be caused by dry, cold air and therapeutic drugs, but often the cause is not detectable. When combined with dry mouth (*xerostomia*) it is called *Sjögren syndrome* (Chapter 3), which is usually caused by autoimmune inflammation of lacrimal and salivary glands. Treatment with ocular cyclosporine (an immunosuppressant) is often effective in restoring tear production.

Subconjunctival hemorrhage, or bleeding under the conjunctiva, is very alarming to patients because it is so sudden and dramatic—the white sclera suddenly becomes blood red. It may occur at any age and often without apparent cause, but it most often occurs in association with trauma, sneezing, or coughing. It is rarely of clinical significance.

Pinguecula and *pterygium* are lumps of yellowish fibrovascular tissue that grow in the sclera on either side of the cornea as a result of sun exposure. **Pinguecula** is the most common and is usually seen as a small lump on the nasal side of the cornea in an elderly person. **Pterygium** (from Greek *pterus* = wing) is less common, larger, and shaped like an insect wing; it becomes increasingly common with advancing age. It may grow over the outside edge of the cornea—pinguecula does not—but does not cross into the field of vision. Either pinguecula or pterygium may be excised for cosmetic reasons.

Tumors of the eyelids are rare; the most common is *basal cell carcinoma* of eyelid skin. Neoplasms of the conjunctiva and sclera are also very rare.

Pop Quiz

20.10 True or false? Neonatal conjunctivitis is most commonly caused by *Neisseria gonorrheoeae or Chlamydia trachomatis.*

20.11 True or false? Blepharitis is inflammation of the eyelids.

20.12 Chronic dry mouth that occurs with Sjogren syndrome is called __________, while dry eyes are called _________.

20.13 What is the most common tumor (cancer) of the eyelids?

Disorders of the Cornea

The most common problem of the cornea is abnormal shape, which is associated with the refractive problems discussed earlier.

As the most anterior part of the globe, the cornea is more exposed to the environment than are other parts of the eye and therefore more subject to injury and other environmental influences. Corneal abrasions (also discussed earlier) are common and usually minor.

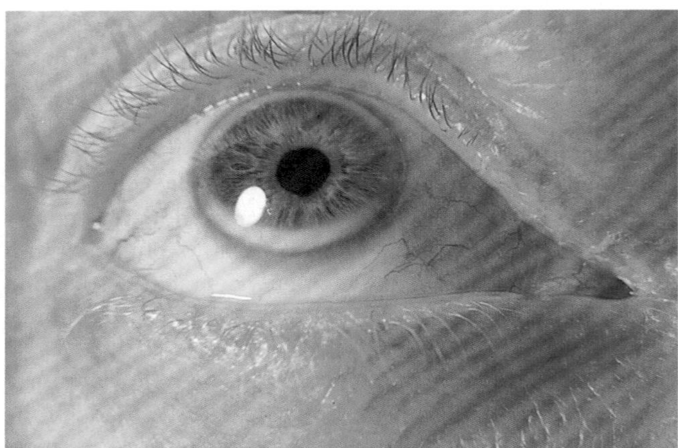

Figure 20.8 **Arcus senilis.** Whitish-yellow arc at the edge of the cornea may indicate abnormally high levels of blood lipids. (Reproduced with permission from Tasman W. *The Willis Eye Hospital Atlas of Clinical Ophthalmology.* 2nd ed. Philadelphia, PA: Lippincott Williams and Wilkins; 2001.)

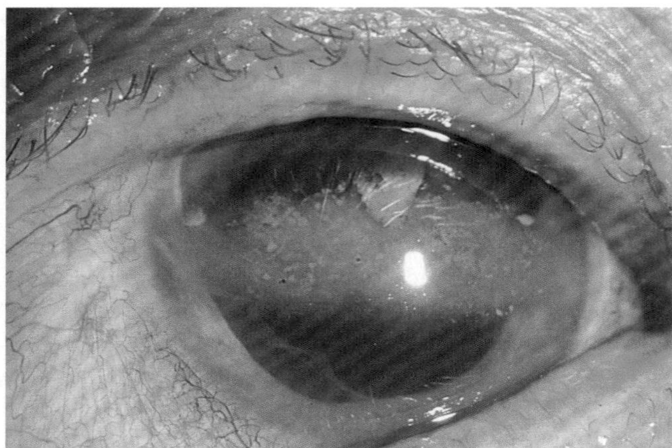

Figure 20.9 **Band keratopathy.** Corneal calcium deposits in sun-exposed cornea may be associated with many eye and systemic disorders. (Reproduced with permission from Tasman W. *The Willis Eye Hospital Atlas of Clinical Ophthalmology.* 2nd ed. Philadelphia, PA: Lippincott Williams and Wilkins; 2001.)

Arcus senilis, illustrated in Figure 20.8, is a white arc of lipid deposited around the edge of the cornea. It is usually, but not invariably, seen in older persons who have abnormally high blood lipid levels.

Inflammation of the cornea is called **keratitis**. Virtually any type of infectious agent can be responsible. *Herpesvirus infection* (with either herpes simplex virus or varicella-zoster virus) may cause particularly severe inflammation and ulceration, which, as with cold sores or shingles, may be recurrent. It may involve the iris. Symptoms and signs include foreign body sensation, tearing, photophobia, and conjunctival hyperemia. Recurrences are common and may lead to ulceration and scarring. Diagnosis is usually based on the characteristic branching corneal ulcer. Treatment is with topical (and occasionally systemic) antiviral drugs. Steroids are contraindicated.

In addition to herpes and shingles, corneal ulcer may be caused by bacterial infection (typically *Staphylococcus* or *Streptococcus*). It may also be caused by wearing a contact lens for an extended time without removal, by inadequate sterilization of a contact lens, by trauma, or by a foreign body in the cornea.

Corneal inflammation and scarring associated with trachoma (discussed above with conjunctival disease) is an important cause of blindness in the developing world. *Onchocerciasis* is a disease caused by a parasitic worm spread by the bites of black flies in Africa and South America. Larval worms invade the cornea and other anterior segment tissues, causing inflammation and blindness.

Keratopathy is noninflammatory disease of the cornea. **Band keratopathy** (Fig. 20.9) is an opaque, horizontal band of calcium deposits across the cornea that usually affects only one eye and may be associated with a variety of systemic conditions including hypercalcemia and inflammatory diseases of the anterior segment of the globe.

Corneal dystrophy (also called *stromal dystrophy*, Fig. 20.10) is a bilateral noninflammatory clouding of the cornea, usually as a result of a genetic defect. There are many varieties, and all affect one or more layers of the cornea. The result is gradual corneal clouding and loss of visual acuity, which may lead to blindness. **Fuchs endothelial dystrophy** is a variety of dystrophy that is a leading cause for corneal transplant in the United States. Endothelial cells degenerate and allow aqueous humor from the anterior chamber to diffuse into the cornea, clouding it. The etiology is unknown.

Keratoconus is a misshaped cornea that is conical instead of spherical. It affects about 1 in 2,000 persons. About 10% of cases are hereditary. It is usually bilateral

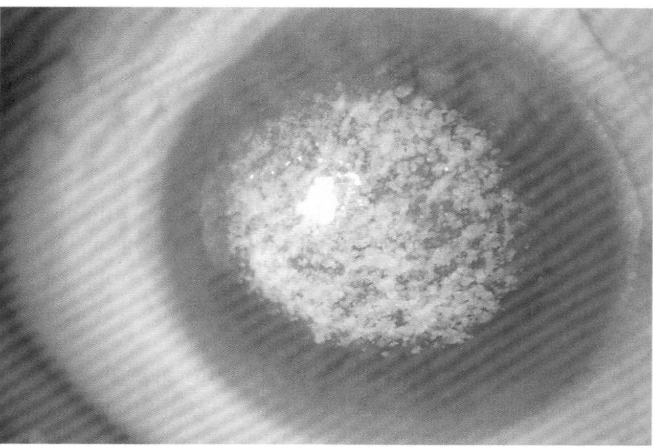

Figure 20.10 **Corneal dystrophy.** Most cases are hereditary. (Reproduced with permission from Tasman W. *The Willis Eye Hospital Atlas of Clinical Ophthalmology.* 2nd ed. Philadelphia, PA: Lippincott Williams and Wilkins; 2001.)

and characterized by progressive bulging and thinning of the cornea. The abnormal shape distorts vision and is difficult to correct with glasses. Rigid contact lenses may provide effective refraction. Corneal transplant is effective if contact lenses fail.

Pop Quiz

20.14 True or false? Inflammation of the cornea caused by viruses or bacteria is called keratitis.

20.15 What dystrophy is a leading cause for corneal transplant in the United States?

20.16 Conical distortion of the cornea is called ________________.

Disorders of the Lens

A **cataract** (Fig. 20.11) is a clouded lens. Cataracts are a major cause of poor vision and blindness around the world. In the United States, most cataracts are caused by age-related degeneration of lens fibers, which breaks the fibers into molecules small enough to exert an osmotic effect that attracts water into the lens, which interferes with light transmission.

Cataracts can be caused by a variety of other conditions. Foremost among them is diabetes, in which excessive blood sugar seeps into the lens and is converted into sorbitol, a molecule with high osmotic power that attracts water. Other causes of cataracts include hereditary disease, glaucoma, chronic steroid therapy, congenital rubella infection, and many more. *The Clinical Side*, "Surgery for Refractive Errors, Glaucoma, and Cataracts," describes surgery for cataracts as well as for refractive errors and glaucoma.

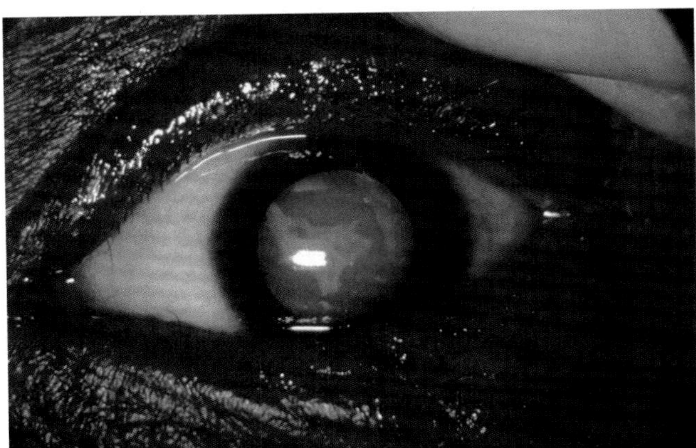

Figure 20.11 **Cataract.** This lens is completely opaque. (Reprinted with permission from Rubin E. *Pathology.* 4th ed. Philadelphia, PA. Baltimore, MD: Williams and Wilkins; 2005.)

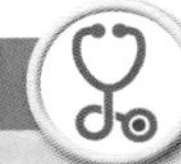

The Clinical Side

SURGERY FOR REFRACTIVE ERRORS, GLAUCOMA, AND CATARACTS

In the United States, refractive errors, cataracts, and glaucoma are the most common disorders of the eye for which people seek professional help.

Refractive errors can be corrected in many people by surgical reshaping of the cornea by *laser-assisted in situ keratomileusis (LASIK)*. In this procedure, a highly precise surgical instrument is used to cut a flap of the outer layer of the cornea. The flap is raised, and a computer-guided laser precisely shapes the middle layer of the cornea by burning away tissue to correct the refractive error. The flap is folded back in place, and the wound heals quickly. The procedure takes only a few minutes, vision recovers quickly, and postoperative pain is minimal.

Lasers can also be used in the treatment of glaucoma in patients whose intraocular pressure is not well controlled by eye drops. In laser *trabeculoplasty*, a laser beam is guided into the lateral angle to burn holes so that aqueous humor can flow into the canal of Schlemm. This procedure, too, takes only a few minutes and is usually pain free.

Cataracts are typically removed by *phacoemulsification* (Greek *phacos* = bean). In this procedure, a tiny (~3 mm) incision is made in the sclera near the edge of the cornea and an ultrasonic probe is inserted into the lens. The lens is liquefied by high-frequency sound waves, sucked out, and replaced by an artificial lens. The procedure is associated with mild postoperative discomfort.

In neglected cases, the cataractous lens may degenerate so markedly that debris escapes. Because lens proteins are normally sequestered from the immune system, they are viewed as nonself once they have escaped the confines of the eye. An autoimmune inflammatory reaction may be incited, owing to the fact that the autoimmune antibodies thus created can attack both the affected eye and the opposite eye.

Case Notes

20.10 Madelyn had a cataract. What was the most likely cause?

Pop Quiz

20.17 True or false? Cataracts lead to glaucoma.

Disorders of the Uveal Tract

Recall that, in the posterior segment, the vascular tunic is called the choroid and in the anterior segment it forms the ciliary body and the iris. Recall further that the *uveal tract* consists of the *choroid*, the *ciliary body*, and the *iris*, all of which are richly vascular. Inflammation of the uvea is called **uveitis**. For practical purposes, uveitis is the only significant disorder of the uvea.

Uveitis may occur in any part of the uvea (Fig. 20.12). **Iritis** is inflammation of the iris only; **iridocyclitis** is inflammation of the iris and ciliary body. **Choroiditis** is inflammation of the choroid and may or may not be associated with iritis or iridocyclitis.

Lens or corneal surgery or trauma to the anterior segment may cause iritis or iridocyclitis. Uveitis is frequently associated with rheumatoid arthritis, juvenile idiopathic arthritis, ankylosing spondylitis, and other autoimmune diseases (Chapters 3 and 18). Uveitis is also often caused by infectious agents, especially in patients with AIDS or other immune deficiency. Toxoplasma, syphilis, cytomegalovirus, and herpesvirus are the most common infectious

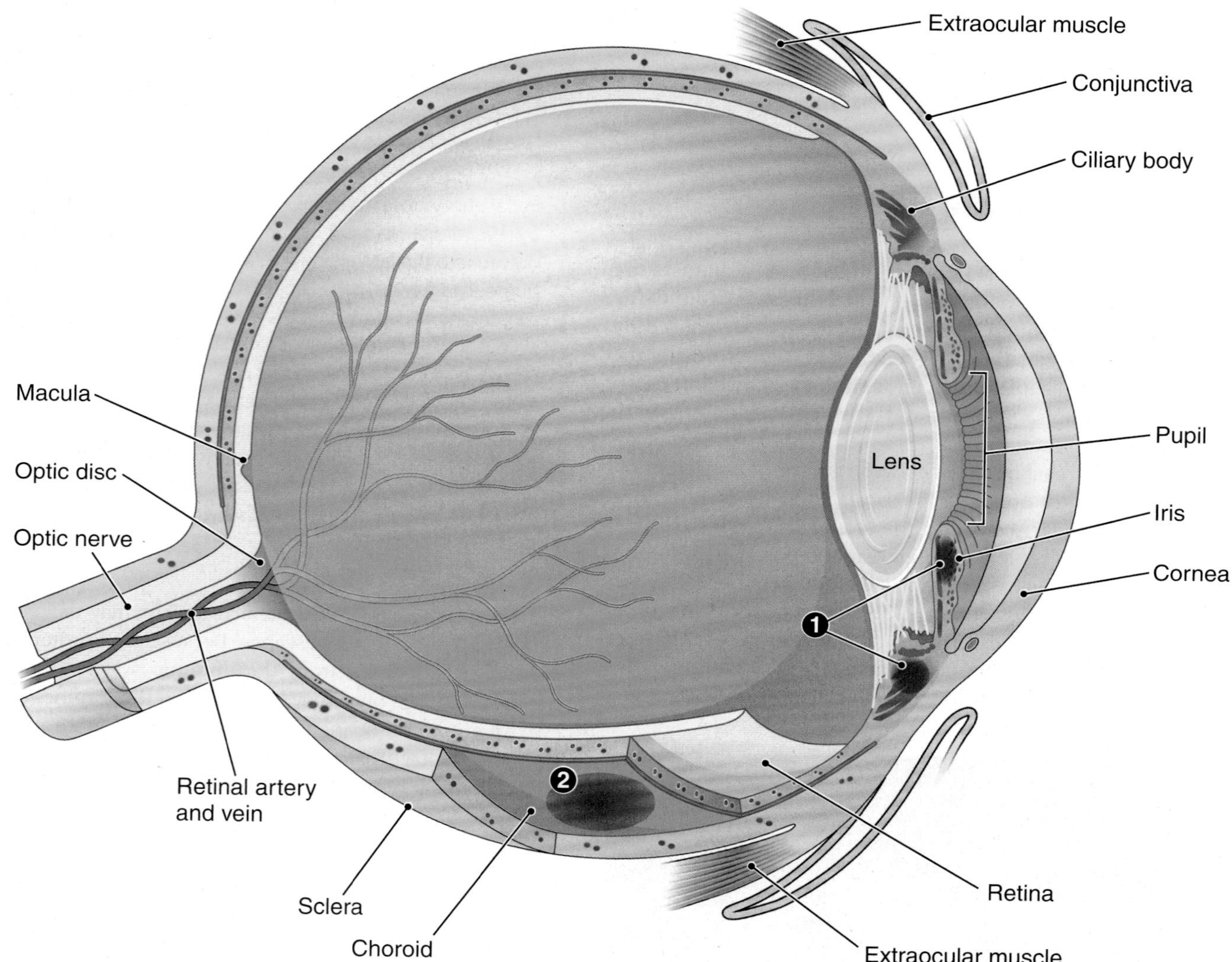

1 Anterior uveitis (iritis and iridocyclitis)

Acute
- Idiopathic
- Trauma/surgery
- Virus or *Chlamydia* infection

Chronic
- Juvenile idiopathic arthritis and related autoimmune conditions
- Sarcoidosis
- Herpesvirus infection
- Syphilis
- Sympathetic (autoimmune) ophthalmitis

2 Posterior uveitis (choroiditis)

Any of 1 plus:
- Diabetic retinopathy
- Opportunistic infections (toxoplasmosis, cytomegalovirus) in patients with AIDS or other immune deficiency

Figure 20.12 **The uveal tract and causes of uveitis.** Types of anterior uveitis (1) and posterior uveitis (2).

agents. About one-third of patients with sarcoidosis (Chapter 10) have uveitis.

Uveitis may have severe consequences, including adhesions (*synechiae*) between the iris and the lens or cornea and obstruction to the flow of aqueous humor with resultant glaucoma, cataract, detached retina, and retinal neovascularization, any of which can cause blindness.

Sympathetic ophthalmitis is an autoimmune uveitis involving the entire uveal tract that occurs after a latent period (a few weeks, months, or years) in response to eye injury. The reaction is caused by traumatic liberation (unmasking) of retinal antigens not previously exposed to the immune system. The immune system reacts to these antigens as if they are alien, not native, and incites an autoimmune reaction (Chapter 3) in either or both eyes.

Pop Quiz

20.18 True or false? Uveitis is the only clinically important disorder of the uvea.

20.19 What is the term for an autoimmune attack on the uvea after trauma to the globe?

Disorders of the Vitreous Humor and Retina

Normally, the vitreous humor is lightly but securely adherent to the retina, but with age the connection becomes less secure, and the vitreous can become detached, usually in the posterior half of the posterior segment. **Vitreous detachment** is not a problem and does not interfere with vision, but in some instances it can pull the retina away (*retinal detachment*), which is very serious. Sometimes vitreous protein may condense to form bits of condensed material that appear as "*floaters*" in the field of vision. Although floaters are not a threat to vision, they can be a forerunner of retinal detachment and call for careful examination of the retina by an eye specialist.

Vitreous hemorrhage is a consequence of some other condition, most often diabetic retinopathy (discussed below). Other causes include trauma and retinal detachment. Blood in the vitreous humor impairs vision because it blocks light transmission; but more importantly, blood is toxic to the retina and may cause permanent retinal damage with visual loss.

Retinal Detachment Causes Blindness

Retinal detachment is a peeling away of the retina from the retinal pigmented epithelium. Retinal detachment is a medical emergency. Separated retina is sightless; however, sight can usually be restored with reattachment.

There are two types of detachments (Fig. 20.13)—those associated with tears of the retina and those without. When no tear is present, the retina may be pulled away from the wall of the globe by abnormalities that occur in the vitreous humor. For example, inflammatory conditions or infections in the vitreous may create adhesions to the retina that pull the retina away as the adhesions mature and retract. In other circumstances inflammatory conditions deep in the retina or choroid may cause inflammatory fluid to seep into the potential space beneath the retina and lift the retina away.

Retinal tears are the most common cause of retinal detachment. They are often caused by trauma or age-related shrinking of the vitreous, which may pull on the retina and tear it. Tears allow fluid from the vitreous humor to seep under the retina and lift it away from its attachment.

Surprisingly, full thickness traumatic penetrations of the wall of the globe are not associated with retinal detachment even though they can cause very large retinal tears.

Retinal detachment usually becomes evident due to loss of part of the field of vision or due to painless visual disturbances such as large numbers of floaters or flashes of light. Treatment is surgical.

Retinal Vascular Disease Is Common

Retinal vascular disease is a frequent and serious complication of two of the most common diseases of humans: hypertension and diabetes (Fig. 20.14).

Hypertensive Retinopathy

The basic lesion of **hypertensive retinopathy** is *arteriolosclerosis* (Chapter 8). Hypertensive retinopathy occurs in direct proportion to the severity of hypertension. Normal retinal arteries (actually arterioles) appear somewhat broad and red, but as retinal arteriolosclerosis progresses, the vessels change to stiff, hard, shiny, narrow vessels that create a glossy "copper wire" (or "silver wire") effect visible in the retina by funduscopy. At points where these stiff arterioles cross veins, they narrow (nick) the veins (A-V nicking). Other findings include flame-shaped hemorrhages, yellow exudates, and white "cotton wool" patches of ischemic retina. In malignant hypertension with cerebral edema, the optic nerve may be pushed forward by the bulging brain, a condition known as *papilledema*, which is a feature common to any condition associated with markedly increased intracranial pressure. Diagnosis is clinical. Treatment is blood pressure control.

Diabetic Retinopathy

The most common and serious retinal vascular disease is **diabetic retinopathy**. The eye is profoundly affected by diabetes—cataracts, glaucoma, retinal detachment, and choroiditis are common. Diabetic retinopathy is present

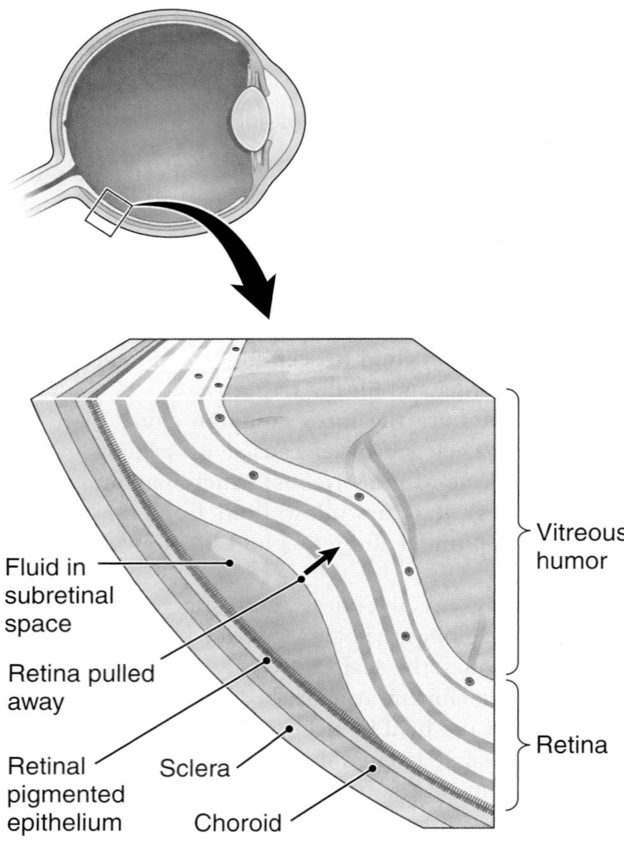

A Retinal detachment without tear

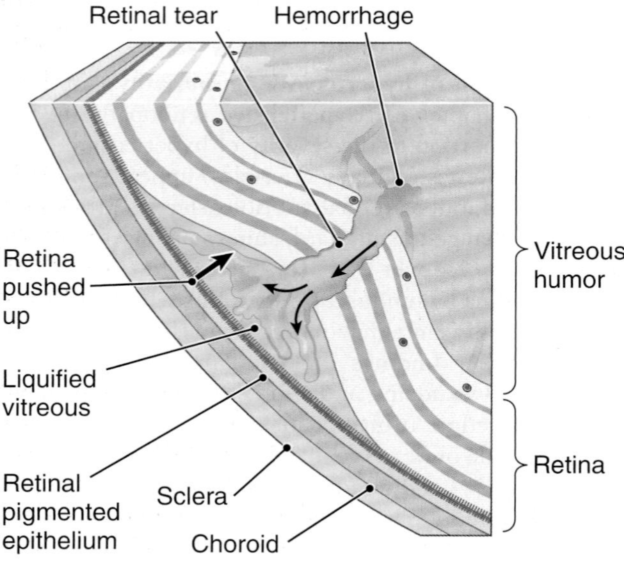

B Retinal detachment owing to tear

Figure 20.13 **Retinal detachment. A.** In detachment without tear, the retina is pulled away by conditions in the vitreous humor. **B.** In detachment with tear, the tear allows seepage of liquefied vitreous humor, which accumulates beneath the retina and pushes it away.

in about one-third of patients with diabetes at the time diabetes is first diagnosed. Moreover, virtually all patients with diabetes develop some form of detectable retinopathy within 10–15 years of diagnosis.

The characteristic findings of *early diabetic retinopathy* (also called "background retinopathy" or "nonproliferative retinopathy") are retinal arteries that develop microaneurysms and leak plasma or blood, creating retinal exudates and hemorrhages (Fig. 20.15A). After many years, early diabetic retinopathy progresses to *proliferative retinopathy*, a much more severe condition (Fig. 20.15B). Delicate new blood vessels, which bleed easily and obscure vision, begin to sprout among the hemorrhages and exudates. They first appear at the optic nerve and grow on the surface of the retina and into the vitreous humor. A film of reactive gliosis (neural scar as the retina is composed of neurons) develops in the retina and obscures vision. These scars may retract as they mature, causing retinal detachment and blindness. Blindness in a patient with diabetes is an ominous development because it usually indicates long-standing, severe, poorly controlled disease that is associated with high mortality from cardiovascular and renal disease.

Remember This! The eye is profoundly affected by diabetes.

Diagnosis of diabetic retinopathy is clinical. Treatment is prevention by blood glucose control. Nevertheless, large, persistent vitreous hemorrhages or preretinal inflammatory membranes may be removed surgically.

Retinal Occlusive Vascular Disease

Blockage of either the central retinal artery or vein (**retinal occlusive vascular disease, ROVD**) may be caused by thrombosis, embolism, vasospasm, or external compression. For example, ROVD may be a consequence of *temporal arteritis* (Chapter 8). Occlusion of the central retinal artery causes death of retinal light-sensing cells and permanent blindness unless the ischemia lasts less than a few minutes. Occlusion of the central retinal vein causes hemorrhage and edema in the retina and may produce obscured vision, but blindness rarely occurs despite the dramatic appearance of the retina. The ischemia produced by retinal vein occlusion frequently causes glaucoma secondary to inflammation and scarring in the anterior chamber.

Case Notes

20.11 Madelyn had evidence of nonproliferative diabetic retinopathy. Was this expected or unusual for someone with a 15-year history of diabetes?

20.12 Did Madelyn have retinal evidence of hypertension? If yes, what kind?

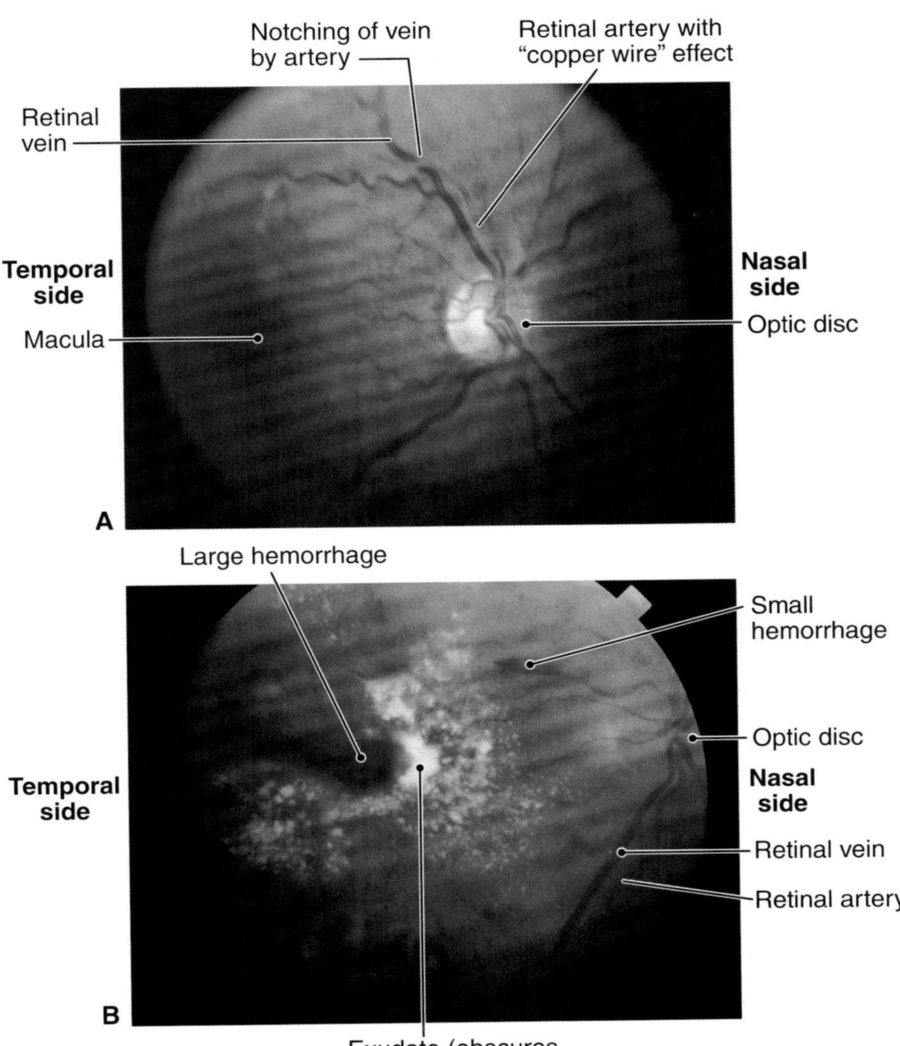

Figure 20.14 **The retina in hypertension (right eye). A.** Arteriolosclerosis of retinal arterioles creates a "copper wire" effect and notching of vein at points where arteries cross veins (A-V nicking). **B.** Hemorrhages and exudates are evident.

Degenerative Retinal Disease Is a Common Cause of Blindness

Especially common is **age-related macular degeneration (ARMD)**, deterioration of the macula, the central part of the retina with the greatest concentration of rods and cones and the most detailed central vision. It usually affects both eyes and is the most common cause of blindness in the United States, affecting about 8% of the U.S. population >75 yrs. Most cases are thought to be due to inherited genetic risk factors, but only a few defective genes have been identified. It is more common in African Americans than other racial groups in the United States. Smoking is an important acquired risk factor.

Patients with ARMD lose their central vision, progressing to legal blindness (vision of 20/200 or worse) despite having good peripheral vision. About 90% of patients have "dry" ARMD, which features retinal atrophy. The remaining 10% develop "wet" ARMD, which features growth of a neovascular membrane from the choroid onto the surface of the retina. New blood vessels, exudates, and hemorrhage interfere with vision. Diagnosis requires retinal examination by a specialist. Treatment options are limited and not very effective. They include dietary supplements, direct injection of antivascular drugs, laser photocoagulation, and newer experimental therapies.

Retinitis pigmentosa (RP) is a misnomer because the condition is not inflammatory. The name retinitis pigmentosa derives from the fact that, as the disease progresses, pigment escapes from degenerating cells in the retinal pigmented epithelium. The pigment then migrates to the surface of the retina and discolors it a deep brown. RP is a group of related, inherited conditions that feature bilateral, progressive retinal degeneration resulting in night blindness (an inability to see clearly in dim light) and constricted visual fields (tunnel vision). Later, the macula becomes involved, and complete blindness ensues. About half of patients have a positive family history for the

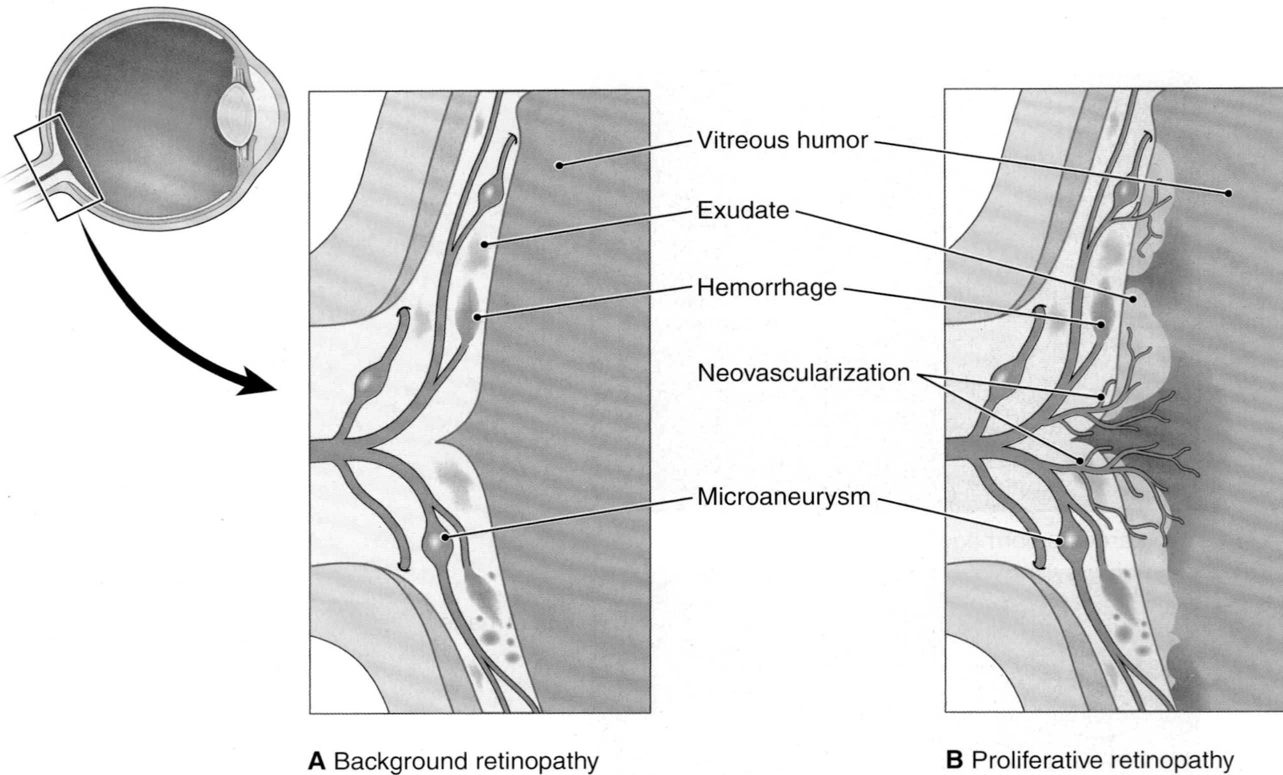

Figure 20.15 **The retina in diabetes. A.** Background (early, nonproliferative) retinopathy is seen in most diabetics at the time of the original diagnosis. No new growth of blood vessels (neovascularization) is present. **B.** In proliferative retinopathy (a late complication of diabetes), new blood vessels sprout in areas of hemorrhage and exudate.

disease. Multiple genetic defects have been identified. Diagnosis is clinical. Treatment is supportive.

"*Retrolental fibroplasia*" is an old term applied to **retinopathy of prematurity**, a condition induced in premature infants by oxygen treatment after birth. Until the relationship to oxygen was discovered in the mid-20th century, it was the leading cause of blindness in infants. High concentrations of oxygen destroy the immature blood vessels of the premature retina, prohibiting further retinal development. The name derives from the fact that the retina becomes scarred and detaches and shrinks into a ball of fibrous tissue behind the lens.

Pop Quiz

20.20 True or false? RP is inflammation of the retina which causes discoloration.

20.21 True or false? ARMD is one of the most common causes of blindness in the United States.

20.22 What are the two most common causes of retinal vascular disease?

Disorders of the Optic Nerve

Glaucoma is a disease of the optic nerve that causes progressive vision loss. It is usually associated with increased intraocular pressure. It features an optic disc that is enlarged, cupped (depressed), and pale. Among African Americans and Hispanics in the United States, it is the leading cause of blindness. Among Anglos it is second to macular degeneration. Nevertheless, it is the leading cause of preventable blindness in the United States. About 3 million people in the United States have increased intraocular pressure and are at risk, but perhaps half of them do not know it. It may occur at any age but is most common in people >60 years old.

Remember This! Glaucoma is the leading cause of preventable blindness in the United States.

Glaucoma Is Usually Associated with Ocular Hypertension

Glaucoma is usually, *but not always*, associated with increased intraocular pressure (**ocular hypertension**). Strictly speaking, glaucoma is a disease of the optic nerve; it is not synonymous with increased intraocular pressure.

Nevertheless, it is common, even among professionals, to speak of increased ocular pressure as glaucoma.

The etiology is congenital or acquired obstruction of the drainage of aqueous humor in the anterior segment of the globe. Some patients, however, develop glaucomatous optic nerve damage but have normal intraocular pressure, presumably because they are unusually sensitive to even normal levels of intraocular pressure. Conversely, some patients with increased intraocular pressure do not develop optic nerve damage and, therefore, do not have glaucoma despite having ocular hypertension. It is common, but erroneous, to refer to patients with increased intraocular pressure as having glaucoma even if they do not have nerve damage.

Remember This! Glaucoma and increased intraocular pressure are not synonymous.

As Figure 20.16 illustrates, the anterior segment of the globe encompasses the cornea, iris, lens, and related structures, and is divided into an anterior chamber between cornea and iris and a posterior chamber between iris and lens. Aqueous humor is secreted into the posterior chamber by the ciliary body, flows into the anterior chamber through the pupil, and flows outward into the lateral angle of the anterior chamber, where it is absorbed into blood via the canal of Schlemm. The production of aqueous humor contributes to the maintenance of intraocular pressure, which normally is 11–21 mm Hg. As mentioned above, however, the eyes of some people are very sensitive to intraocular pressure and may be damaged by pressures that by definition are normal, and conversely there are others whose optic nerves remain healthy even though they have abnormally high intraocular pressure. Nevertheless, the primary risk factor for glaucoma is increased intraocular pressure.

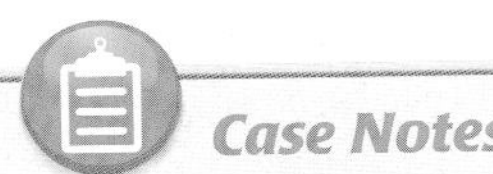

Case Notes

20.13 Did Madelyn have ocular hypertension on her emergency examination?

There Are Several Types of Glaucoma

Congenital glaucoma is caused by developmental abnormalities that interfere with aqueous drainage. It may or may not be evident at birth. When inherited, it most often occurs as an X-linked defect in males. Several defective genes have been identified.

Primary glaucoma develops in patients without underlying eye disease (Fig. 20.16 A, B, C). It is usually bilateral, though it may develop in one eye before the other is affected. There are two varieties of primary glaucoma: *open-angle* glaucoma and *closed-angle* glaucoma, referring to the sharpness of the lateral angle between the iris and the edge of the cornea.

Primary Open-Angle Glaucoma

Primary open-angle glaucoma (POAG) features normal anatomy, but flow out of the anterior chamber is impeded and intraocular pressure rises (Fig. 20.16B). About 15% to 20% of patients with glaucoma have POAG and normal intraocular pressure. POAG is the most frequent type of glaucoma and a major cause of blindness in the United States. Diabetes and myopia (Fig. 20.6B) are acquired risk factors. Some cases are genetic, and many gene defects have been identified.

POAG is a chronic disease that is clinically asymptomatic. Patients usually do not have pain, blurred vision, or other symptoms, despite progressive loss of peripheral vision. In patients with glaucomatous damage to the optic nerve, the optic disc is enlarged, pale, and cupped (depressed). Other findings can include symptoms of an acute attack, as described above, and loss of peripheral vision.

Diagnosis is usually made by an eye specialist in the course of a visit for an unrelated eye problem. By the time the patient becomes aware of visual field loss, optic nerve damage is severe, and the lost vision cannot be recovered. Treatment is reduction of intraocular pressure by local drugs and iridotomy.

Remember This! POAG is a silent destroyer of vision.

Primary Closed-Angle Glaucoma

Primary closed-angle glaucoma (PCAG) features a narrow lateral angle (Fig. 20.16C). PCAG affects people with a shallow anterior chamber. Hyperopia (Fig. 20.6C) is a risk factor. PCAG usually occurs in people over age 40 because the anterior chamber becomes shallower and the angle narrower with advancing age. When the pupil is constricted (Fig. 20.16C, left), the iris is stretched and flow is normal. In the mid-range or with a dilated pupil (e.g., at night or in dim light), however, the iris bunches at the angle, flow becomes obstructed (Fig. 20.16C, right), and pressure rises. Intraocular pressure may be normal between attacks.

PCAG usually presents as an acute eye emergency. Treatment must begin in the first 24–48 hours if blindness is to be avoided. As Figure 20.16C (right) illustrates, dilation of the pupil, as occurs at night or in a darkened theater, accentuates the problem because, as the pupil dilates, the iris gathers thickly around the edges and further obstructs flow of aqueous humor. An attack usually features severe pain in the eye (or forehead above the affected eye), tearing, redness, blurred vision, and puffy eyelids.

Acute medical therapy usually consists of eye drops to constrict the pupil and restore flow followed by peripheral iridotomy as soon as inflammation has subsided. PCAG may become symptomatic in one eye many years before the other eye is affected, but both eyes usually become affected eventually. Hence, iridotomy is usually performed on both eyes at the time the first eye becomes symptomatic.

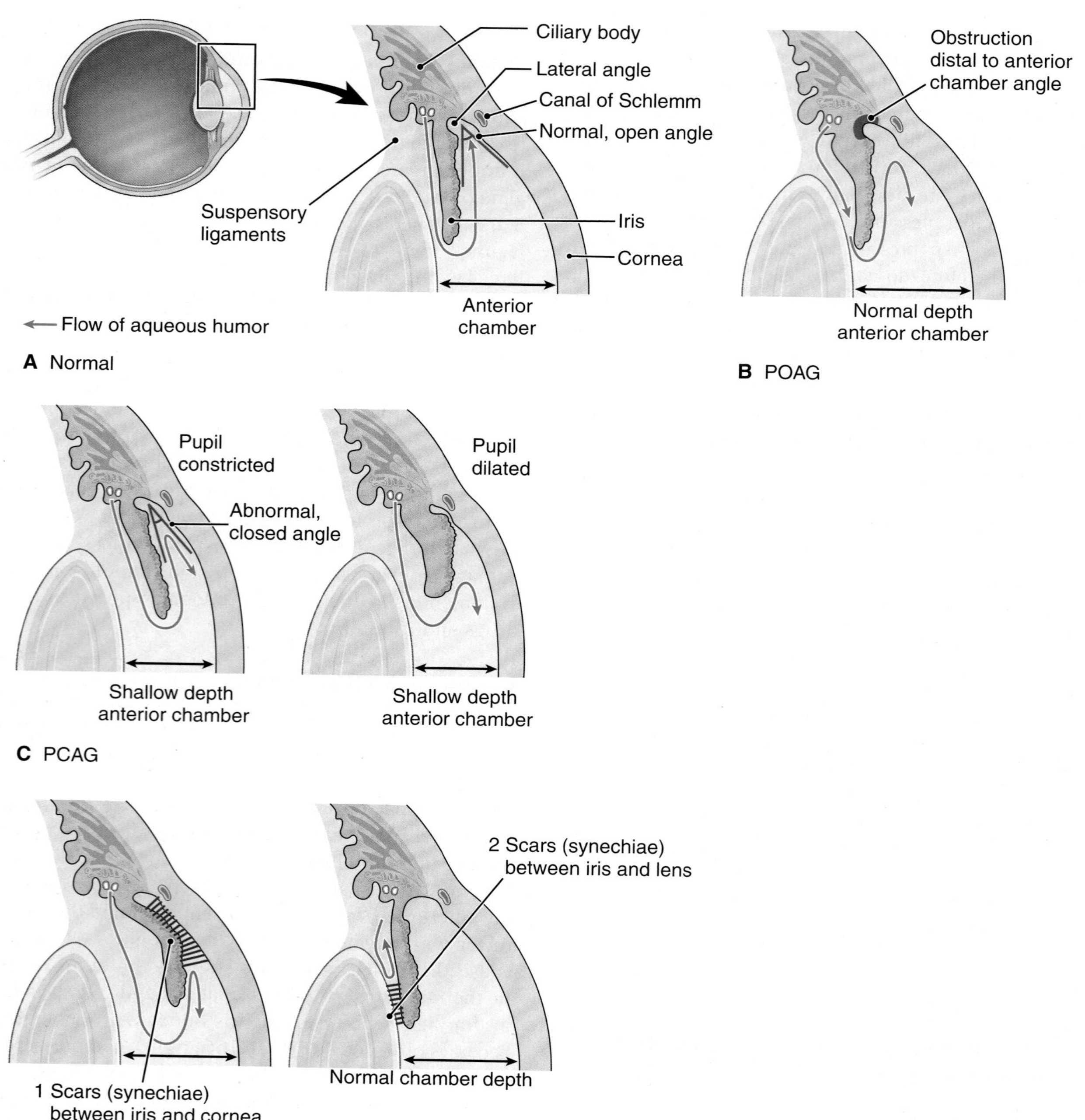

Figure 20.16 **The eye in glaucoma. A.** Normal flow of aqueous humor. **B.** POAG. The angle between iris and cornea is wide. Flow is obstructed at the canal of Schlemm. **C.** PCAG. In part 1 (left), the pupil is constricted, and the iris-corneal angle is narrow, impeding flow. In part 2 (right), the pupil is dilated. The iris retracts to open the pupil, and "piles up" in the angle, acutely obstructing flow. **D.** Secondary glaucoma. In part 1 (left), scars (synechiae) between the iris and cornea obstruct the flow of aqueous humor. In part 2 (right), scars between the iris and the lens obstruct flow.

Secondary Glaucoma

Secondary glaucoma is a disease of many causes. Red cells from intraocular hemorrhage or white cells from inflammation may plug the openings into the canal of Schlemm, or scars (synechiae) may bind the iris to the lens or cornea (Fig. 20.16D). In most instances it is unilateral. Treatment is local or systemic drugs to lower intraocular pressure. It may be necessary to perform surgery (iridotomy) to open holes in the iris as an alternative drainage pathway.

Primary Care Screening for Glaucoma Is Not Feasible

Primary care screening for glaucoma by routine measurement of intraocular pressure is not recommended because about half of patients with glaucoma have normal pressure at a single measurement. Measurement of intraocular pressure, visual examination of the optic disc, and testing peripheral vision provide clues but are too difficult and expensive to be used widely in primary care settings. The job of detecting increased intraocular pressure and early glaucoma is best left in the hands of eye specialists, who can integrate these measurements into patient visits for eyeglasses, contact lenses, or other ocular needs, with special attention to high-risk people: African Americans and Hispanics older than 40, Anglos older than 65, and patients with a family history of glaucoma or a personal history of diabetes or severe myopia.

Case Notes

20.14 Why was Madelyn's glaucoma called primary rather than secondary?

20.15 What common glaucoma risk factors did Madelyn have?

20.16 Madelyn's optic discs were normal, but we never learn if she had evidence of visual field loss. If she did not have visual field loss, could it be said truly that she had glaucoma?

Other Disorders of the Optic Nerve Are Uncommon

Papilledema is edema of the head of the optic nerve where it enters the globe at the optic disc. It may occur unilaterally following compression of the optic nerve by a neoplasm or other mass, but most often it is bilateral and caused by increased intracranial pressure. Papilledema is not associated with visual loss, but it is a sign of serious underlying disease that requires immediate diagnosis. Among the most common causes of papilledema are malignant hypertension and primary brain diseases such as brain tumor, hemorrhage, abscess, or encephalitis.

Ischemic optic neuropathy is caused by diminished blood flow (ischemia) in the optic artery, which can be caused by atherosclerotic obstruction, arteritis, or embolism, and which can cause necrosis of part or all of the optic nerve, with permanent loss of vision.

In daily clinical language, **optic neuritis** describes loss of vision owing to demyelination of optic nerve fibers, preventing transmission of nerve signals from the retina to the brain. Despite the name, however, inflammation may not be present. The causes of optic neuritis are many and varied and include multiple sclerosis, syphilis, lead or methanol poisoning, vitamin deficiency (especially in alcoholics), viral infection, therapeutic drugs, and hereditary disease. Nevertheless, the most common cause of optic nerve disease is glaucoma.

Pop Quiz

20.23 True or false? Glaucoma always causes increased intraocular pressure.

20.24 True or false? Eye drops which dilate the pupil improve the symptoms of PCAG.

20.25 Glaucoma is primarily a disease of the ________.

20.26 Glaucoma may be primary, secondary, or ________.

20.27 True or false? The most common cause of optic nerve disease is infection.

Ocular Neoplasms

The eye contains a wide variety of tissues, any of which may become malignant. Nevertheless, most ocular neoplasms arise from immature retinal neurons and melanocytes in the uveal tract.

The most common malignancy in the eye of an adult is *metastatic cancer*, which usually lodges in the rich vascularity of the uveal tract.

The most common primary ocular neoplasms, however, are nevi and melanoma of the uveal melanocytes. As in skin, uveal nevi are common and occur in about 10% of people. They are not premalignant and usually do not require treatment. **Ocular malignant melanoma** is very rare. There are no lymphatics in the eye, so spread is exclusively vascular, mainly to the liver. Approximately 50% of patients with ocular melanoma will develop metastases within 10–15 years after diagnosis, and a small percentage will develop metastases as late as 20–25 years after their initial diagnosis. Metastatic disease is universally fatal. Diagnosis requires biopsy. Treatment is surgical, usually removal (enucleation) of the globe.

Retinoblastoma is the most common primary ocular malignancy in children. It is a tumor of primitive neuronal cells in the retina and may be an inherited genetic defect (40% of cases) or a spontaneous mutation (60% of cases). It may be unilateral or bilateral. Most patients are diagnosed at about age three to four, when a parent catches a glimpse of something white in the pupil instead of the usual blackness. It may metastasize or invade the brain via the optic nerve; however, 90% of cases can be cured if detected while confined to the globe. A few cases regress spontaneously. Treatment is surgery or radiotherapy. Sometimes treatment spares some or most vision, but loss of sight is common.

Pop Quiz

20.28 True or false? Retinoblastoma is the most common malignancy of the eye in children.

20.29 Malignancies that metastasize to the eye generally lodge in the blood vessels of the ________.

Case Study Revisited

"I'm having a terrible headache." The case of Madelyn Q.

Madelyn developed an acute, severe headache over her right eye and eye symptoms. Pain from acute intraocular hypertension is usually referred to the brow above the affected eye. Madelyn had classic symptoms of acute glaucoma: headache or eye pain, redness, blurred vision or halos around lights at night, headache, nausea, and vomiting. She also had typical physical findings: tearing, puffy eyelids, cloudy cornea, fixed-dilated pupil, and conjunctival redness.

For experienced physicians, the diagnosis is easy, and fortunately so, because without treatment acute intraocular hypertension leads to optic nerve damage (glaucoma) and irreversible blindness within days. Madelyn was appropriately treated with drugs to lower ocular pressure. Treatment was rapidly effective and when she returned the next day her eye was no longer inflamed and a complete eye exam could be performed. Happily, no glaucomatous damage was noted in the optic disc of either eye, though she did have clear evidence of mild diabetic retinopathy and hypertensive retinopathy. Bilateral iridotomy was performed on both eyes. Iridotomy in the right eye provided a permanent solution to the current crisis. In the left eye, the iridotomy was prophylactic because the chances were high that her left eye would have suffered a similar crisis in the future.

In a certain sense, Madelyn was fortunate. First, she had acute PCAG, which called attention to her shallow anterior chambers and narrow lateral angles. Patients with POAG lose their sight without symptoms, hence the importance of regular eye examinations. Second, she had immediate access to expert care.

Section 2: Disorders of the Ear

Deafness: a malady affecting dogs when their person calls them and they want to stay out.

SOURCE: THE FIRST AND MOST COMMON DEFINITION FOUND IN AN INTERNET SEARCH FOR THE DEFINITION OF DEAFNESS, 2005

Case Study

"She has a fever." The case of JuJu F.

Chief Complaint: Fever.

Clinical History: JuJu F. was a six-month-old girl brought in the morning to a pediatrician's office by her mother, who said, "She has a fever." She added that JuJu had been irritable and "feverish" for several days because of "a cough and a runny nose." She became especially concerned the night before when JuJu became increasingly irritable, vomited, and began pulling at her left ear. She took JuJu's temperature with an electronic

"She has a fever." The case of JuJu F. (continued)

ear thermometer and found it to be 102°F. JuJu had no previous medical problems. She had received no medicine at home other than acetaminophen.

Physical Examination and Other Data: Physical examination revealed a healthy infant girl crying in her mother's arms. Temperature was 101.8°F. Heart rate and respirations were rapid but not unusual for a child with fever. Crusted mucus was present around the nostrils and the child was mouth breathing. The chest was clear, and cardiac sounds were not remarkable. The neck was supple, and the anterior fontanel was small, soft, and flat. The right ear was normal, but the left tympanic membrane was bulging, dull and red.

Clinical Course: The pediatrician made a diagnosis of acute otitis media (AOM) and wrote a prescription for an oral antibiotic. A follow-up visit was scheduled in two weeks. The office PA made a follow-up call the following morning. JuJu's mother reported that JuJu's temperature was 99°F and her appetite had improved. On follow-up two weeks later, JuJu was found to be happy and asymptomatic, but she had serous effusions in both middle ears. The pediatrician explained that effusions frequently occur but are not serious unless they persist for several months. Another follow-up visit was scheduled in six weeks. When she returned, the effusions had disappeared and she seemed perfectly normal.

The Normal Ear

The ear has two functions—*hearing* and *equilibrium*. **Hearing** is the detection of sound waves by the ear and integration into consciousness. **Equilibrium** is our sense of balance. It informs us of our position in space relative to the force of gravity and whether or not we are in control of our movements. Being in equilibrium does not mean being still; it means being in control.

The ear is divided into three anatomic parts: the *external*, the *middle*, and the *inner* ear (Fig. 20.17). Each part is involved in hearing; only the inner ear is involved in balance.

The External Ear Collects Sound Waves

The **external ear** consists of the **auricle** (*pinna*), a flap attached to the side of the head, and the **external auditory canal**. The auricle is covered by skin and is composed of elastic cartilage, fat, and fibrous tissue. The external auditory canal is lined by skin that contains sebaceous glands that secrete cerumen (ear wax). The canal leads from the auricle to *the middle ear*, which is embedded in the *temporal bone*. The external half of the auditory canal is surrounded by soft tissue, and the internal half is encased in the temporal bone. The auricle collects sound waves and channels them into the canal, which conveys them to the middle ear.

The Middle Ear Transmits Sound Vibrations to the Inner Ear

The **middle ear** begins with the **tympanic membrane** (*eardrum*), which stretches across the canal like the head of a drum. It is hollowed out of temporal bone. Its outer wall is the tympanic membrane, which vibrates in response to sound waves. On the inner side of the tympanic membrane is the **tympanic cavity**, an air-filled space in the temporal bone that is lined by simple cuboidal epithelium. Crossing the tympanic cavity from the eardrum, three tiny bones (**ossicles**)—the malleus, incus, and stapes—connect medially to the *oval window*, which marks the juncture of the middle ear and the inner ear. The facial nerve (cranial nerve VII) passes through the temporal bone very near the tympanic cavity and is separated from it only by a very thin layer of bone. Disease of the middle ear can, therefore, affect the facial nerve.

The Inner Ear Converts Sound Vibrations and Equilibrium Sensing into Nerve Signals

Deepest in the temporal bone is a cavity that contains the **inner ear**, which consists of the *cochlea* (for hearing) and the *vestibular apparatus* for equilibrium. All are hollowed out of bone, filled by fluid, and lined by ciliated sensory cells that connect to the brain via the **vestibulocochlear nerve** (cranial nerve VIII, often called the *auditory nerve*).

The **cochlea** is a hollow tube coiled upon itself like a snail shell. It joins the tympanic cavity of the middle ear via two openings—the **oval window** and the **round window**. Sound vibrations transmitted through the ossicles to the oval window are transformed into pressure waves in cochlear fluid. These pressure waves radiate up the cochlear spiral on one side of a membrane and down the cochlear spiral on the other side of the same membrane to the round window, which vibrates sympathetically much like one end of a drum vibrates in response to the other. The round window acts as a relief mechanism for vibrations that are transmitted to it by the ossicles. Without this mechanism, it would be impossible to create significant pressure waves in cochlear fluid.

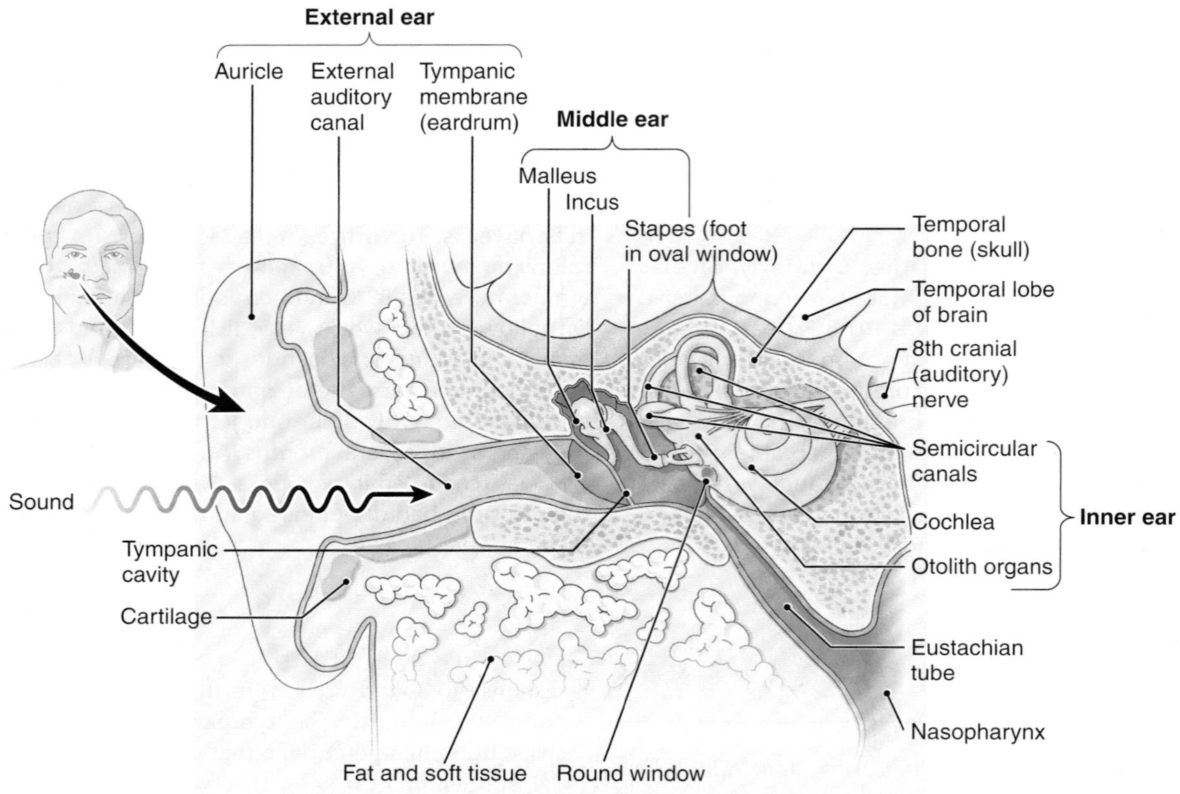

Figure 20.17 **The anatomy of the ear.** The diagram details the external ear, middle ear, and inner ear.

These fluid waves radiate into the cochlear spiral and disturb cochlear cilia, which are distributed along a cochlear membrane that is "tuned" to vibrate at this point or that according to the pitch of the incoming vibration and to vibrate more or less according to the volume of sound. Louder sound creates more ciliary motion and more signals at the particular point. Each point on the cochlear membrane is connected to its own nerve fibers. Therefore, disturbance of the cochlear membrane by sound of one pitch excites sensory nerve fibers distinct from every other pitch. These signals are relayed to the auditory cortex, which "hears" different pitches in different volume according to which sensory fibers were excited and by how much they were excited.

The second element of the inner ear is the **vestibular apparatus**, which is composed of the *otolith organs* and *semicircular canals*. The **otolith organs** are a sac that senses the orientation of the head relative to gravity and linear acceleration. The **semicircular canals** are tubular arcs that arise from the otolith organ sac. Each is set at a 90° angle to one another, like the sides of a box corner, such that each is oriented in one major anatomic plane of the body—horizontal, sagittal (vertical through the nose), and coronal (vertical through the shoulders). The semicircular canals sense *angular (rotational) acceleration*. The vestibular apparatus is filled with fluid and lined by ciliated sensory cells connected to the vestibulocochlear nerve. Consider a gymnast at the head of the vaulting runway. She knows "which way is up" from the signals from her otolith organs. As she accelerates into her run, the otolith organs tells her how rapidly she is gaining speed. As she vaults into a flip and twist, her semicircular canals sense her turns. The combination enables a safe landing.

The tympanic cavity of the middle ear is indirectly connected to the air outside the body via the Eustachian tube, which runs from space of the middle ear to the back of the nasal cavity (nasopharynx). This connection equalizes atmospheric pressure on both sides of the eardrum: pressure on the outside via the external auditory canal is matched by pressure on the inside via the Eustachian tube. For example, unequal pressure on the eardrum can occur during an elevator ride in a tall building if a stuffy nose has occluded the nasal end of the Eustachian tube. As the elevator rises, air pressure declines and air trapped in the middle ear expands, creating tension on the eardrum that temporarily impairs hearing because the added tension on the drum inhibits its ability to vibrate. In severe cases, it can be very painful or cause rupture of the eardrum.

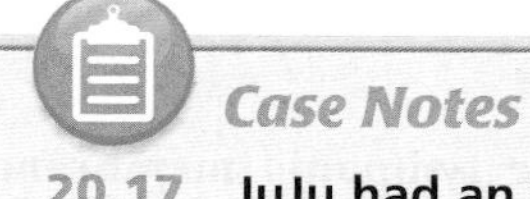

20.17 JuJu had an infection of the middle ear. What forms the lateral edge of the middle ear? The medial edge?

Pop Quiz

20.30 True or false? There are two semicircular canals within the inner ear that sense acceleration.

20.31 True or false? A stuffy nose impedes hearing by decreasing vibrations of the tympanic membrane.

20.32 What inner ear structure is responsible for hearing?

20.33 The middle ear consists of the tympanic membrane, tympanic cavity, and ________.

Disorders of the External Ear

Figure 20.18 shows some of the diseases affecting the ear. Many of these can impair hearing.

Most conditions affecting the auricle are diseases of skin. Auricular skin may be affected by virtually any skin disease, particularly *atopic dermatitis* (Chapter 21). The superior surface of the auricle is exposed to direct sunlight and in older persons is frequently the site of basal cell and squamous cell carcinomas (Chapter 21), which behave no differently on the ear than on skin elsewhere. In genetically susceptible persons (usually of African ancestry), the earlobe is a common site for *keloids*, a benign, exaggerated repair reaction subsequent to ear piercing or any other cause of laceration/wound.

The auditory canal is also lined by skin and it, too, may be affected by almost any skin disease or infection. Attempts by patients to clean the canal with toothpicks or cotton swabs, for example, usually do more harm than good—earwax or debris is typically pushed further into the canal, the skin may be irritated or cut, or the eardrum may be perforated. **Impacted cerumen** may accumulate on the tympanic membrane and impair its ability to vibrate, or large accumulations may block much or all of the external auditory canal. In either case, hearing is impaired. Manual removal by suction or blunt curette is the preferred treatment.

Otitis externa is inflammation of the external ear and usually comes to medical attention because of inflammation in the ear canal. The most common cause is bacterial infection, often associated with swimming and water in the ear canal (*swimmer's ear*). Otitis externa is also more common in people whose ears are affected by a skin condition such as psoriasis or atopic eczema; it is usually caused by bacterial infection. Because the inner half of the canal is constricted by bone and has little room to swell, otitis externa may be extremely painful.

Pop Quiz

20.34 True or false? Otitis externa is usually caused by viral infection, and therefore antibiotics are ineffective.

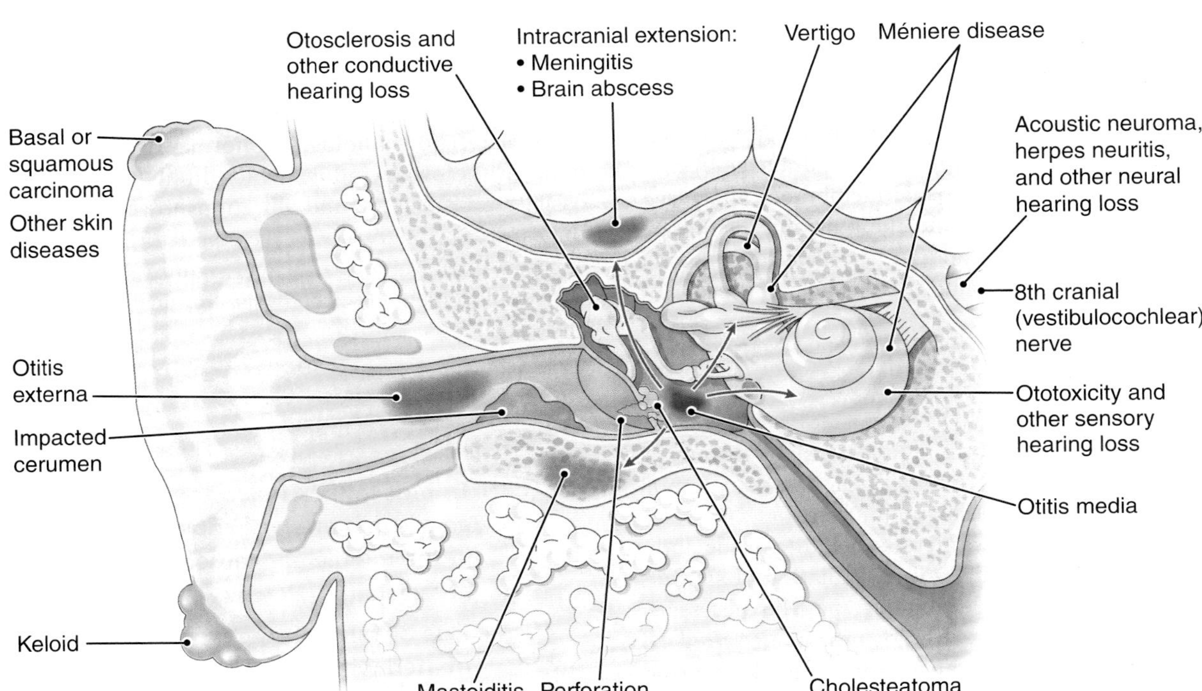

Figure 20.18 **Common diseases of both the external and internal ear.**

Disorders of the Middle Ear

Because it is exposed to the environment, the tympanic membrane is subject to direct trauma, either from objects or from sound waves so strong that the membrane ruptures. Small perforations usually heal quickly and spontaneously, but larger ones may require surgery.

Acute Otitis Media Is a Common Infection in Children

Acute otitis media (AOM), acute inflammation of the middle ear, may be either viral or bacterial. It is often secondary to an upper respiratory infection that causes nasopharyngeal edema and blockage of the Eustachian tube.

All varieties of otitis media occur almost exclusively in young children. About 10% of infants have three episodes before their first birthday. The susceptibility at this age is both anatomical and physiologic: the Eustachian tube in infants and toddlers is more narrow and more level than in adults, making it more difficult for fluid to drain out of the ear. In addition, a child's immature immune system may allow an infection to persist longer than it would in adults.

Patients have ear pain and fever and the tympanic membrane is bulging, red, and dull—it does not reflect the glare of the otoscope light (loss of light reflex). Most cases (~80%) resolve without treatment within a few days, but, in the United States, antibiotic treatment is standard for patients under age two. Complications of purulent otitis media can be severe: chronic otitis media (COM), septicemia, meningitis, or invasion of the mastoid process of the temporal bone (*mastoiditis*).

Secretory otitis media (SOM) is an effusion in the middle ear that results from incomplete resolution of AOM or from obstructed drainage (without infection) through the Eustachian tube. A skillful observer can usually see fluid through the membrane. In older children, there may be a complaint of ear fullness or loss of hearing acuity. If fluid remains for two to three months, surgical drainage by *myringotomy* (lancing of the tympanic membrane) and placement of drainage grommets into the tympanic membrane may be required. In older children, *adenoidectomy* may be helpful to reduce obstruction of the Eustachian tube.

Chronic Otitis Media Is Associated with Hearing Loss and Complications

Chronic otitis media (COM) is persistent (> six weeks) suppurative drainage into the auditory canal through a perforated tympanic membrane. Hearing loss is common and can impair language skills in children.

Diagnosis is clinical. Treatment is cleaning of the auditory canal several times daily with installation of steroids and antibiotics. Systemic antibiotics may be necessary. Middle ear reconstructive surgery may be required. If untreated, it may result in destruction of the ossicles and severe deafness.

Case Notes

20.18 Why did JuJu develop AOM?

20.19 What was the name of the condition that followed her AOM?

Complications include osteomyelitis of the temporal bone, facial nerve paralysis, meningitis, and inflammation of the vestibulocochlear apparatus with vertigo and related problems. A **granulation tissue polyp** is a vascular growth that prolapses through the perforation into the auditory canal. It is treatable by chemical cautery or surgery. **Cholesteatoma** is an accumulation of keratin debris in the middle ear caused by ingrowth of keratinizing squamous epithelium from the ear canal through the perforation. Despite the name, it is not a neoplasm nor does it have anything to do with cholesterol. The name derives from the glossy, yellow–white keratin debris, which looked to original observers like an accumulation of cholesterol in the tympanic cavity of the middle ear. It requires surgical removal, intensive irrigation, and local and systemic antibiotic therapy for the infection that is also usually present. Cholesteatoma tends to recur and may require multiple surgeries. Patients often respond favorably to surgical insertion of drainage tubes in the tympanic membrane, which is removed after infection has cleared and polyps or cholesteatoma has been cleared.

Otosclerosis Is a Common Cause of Deafness in Adults

Otosclerosis is a major cause of hearing loss in adults. It is much more common in Anglos than in African Americans, and about twice as common in women as in men. Both ears are usually affected, and there is strong familial influence. The pathologic abnormality is deposition of bone in the oval window, which limits the ability of the ossicles to transfer sound vibrations to the inner ear from the eardrum. In advanced cases the entire stapes becomes encased in new bone and may require surgical excision with replacement by prosthesis. Surgical results are usually excellent.

Pop Quiz

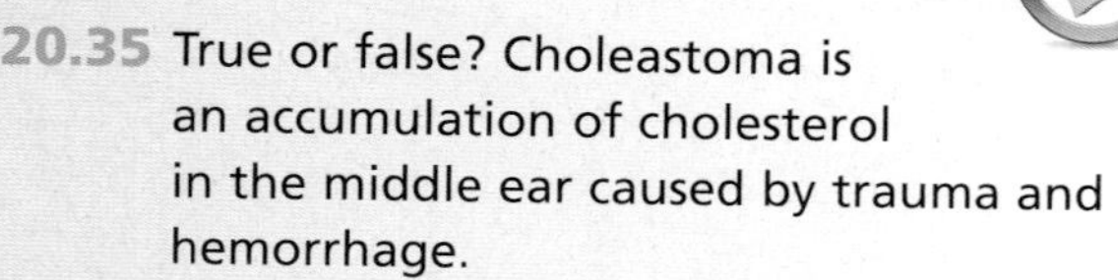

20.35 True or false? Choleastoma is an accumulation of cholesterol in the middle ear caused by trauma and hemorrhage.

20.36 True or false? Otosclerosis can be easily treated with surgery.

Disorders of the Inner Ear

Inasmuch as the inner ear is composed of the cochlea, which senses sound, and the vestibular apparatus, which senses body orientation and movement, diseases of the inner ear produce either impaired hearing or dizziness (vertigo) or both.

Vertigo Is a Symptom of Inner Ear Disorders

Vertigo is a false sensation of movement of self or the environment. It is a symptom, not a diagnosis. Patients with vertigo often say they are dizzy, but *dizziness* is an imprecise term that patients often use to describe other sensations, such as faintness, light-headedness, unsteadiness, or a vague "spaced out" disconnect from normal reality. Nausea and vomiting, and difficulty with balance or gait may accompany both sensations.

Sorting out the clinical problem underlying these symptoms can be one of medicine's most difficult diagnostic challenges. Causes of dizziness without true vertigo include orthostatic hypotension after suddenly rising from a reclining or sitting position, the effect of medication, hypoxia, and hypoglycemia. Dizziness with true vertigo usually relates to the vestibular apparatus, but can be caused by CNS disease or body movement such as spinning in a chair. The presence of *nystagmus* suggests true vertigo.

Many conditions can cause vertigo—too many to detail here. The most common example is **Meniere syndrome**, a clinical triad of *vertigo*, *fluctuating hearing loss*, and *tinnitus* (ringing in the ears). When the etiology is unknown, as it usually is, the triad is called **Meniere disease**. When the triad is secondary to some known cause, it is called Meniere *syndrome*. The underlying pathologic abnormality appears to be an increase in the amount of fluid filling the vestibular apparatus and cochlea. Why this occurs is not known. Meniere disease usually occurs in middle-aged adults and is marked by clustered episodes of vertigo, nausea, and vomiting for about 12–24 hours, followed by recovery. Nystagmus is usually present. Vertigo becomes less frequent with time, but hearing eventually becomes permanently impaired. A low-salt diet and diuretics may have some beneficial effect by lowering the amount of fluid in the cochlea.

Some patients suffer attacks of vertigo for which no cause is ever clearly determined:

- Viral infection of CN VIII is believed to be responsible for a clinical condition known as **vestibular neuritis**, which is characterized by severe, weeklong nausea and vertigo in adolescents and young adults. Multiple attacks occur over 12–18 months but eventually disappear. There is no associated tinnitus or hearing loss.
- *Herpes zoster* infection of CN VIII is associated with severe ear pain, hearing loss, vertigo, and facial nerve paralysis.
- Certain drugs, which are sometimes prescribed if serious disease leaves no less risky choice, are ototoxic and can damage the cochlea, prompting vertigo. Notable ototoxic drugs include antibiotics (among them streptomycin, vancomycin, gentamicin), the diuretic furosemide, and the antimalarial quinine and related compounds. Large doses of aspirin may cause tinnitus and hearing loss that is usually temporary.
- Neuromas (Chapter 19) of the vestibulocochlear nerve account for about 7% of intracranial tumors and may be associated with vertigo and hearing loss.

Deafness Is a Very Common Condition

Deafness is hearing loss that interferes with speech perception. About 10% of the U.S. population has some degree of deafness. Most deafness arises slowly, but sudden deafness does occur. There are three broad categories:

- *Conductive* deafness is interference with transmission of sound to the tympanic membrane or of sound vibrations beyond the footplate of the stapes (where vibrations enter the cochlea). In the elderly, impacted cerumen is a common culprit. Among children, COM may be the cause. Perforation of the tympanic membrane may be responsible. The most common form of deafness that cannot be ascribed as secondary to an underlying disorder is **presbycusis**, a slowly progressive, age-related decline of hearing acuity caused by otosclerosis (discussed earlier).
- *Sensory* deafness is interference with cochlear conversion of vibrations into sensory nerve signals. Noise trauma is a common cause, either from workplace noise or prolonged exposure to loud music. Sometimes the cause is genetic or due to ototoxic drugs such as high doses of aspirin or therapeutic doses of vancomycin or related antibiotics. Recent studies suggest that one in five teens have slight hearing loss caused by loud music played through headphones or earbuds. The loss is enough to impair their ability to hear a whisper or rustling leaves.
- *Neural* deafness is interference with sensory nerve signals in the vestibulocochlear nerve or from lack of cortical integration of sensory signals into consciousness. Causes include neuroma of the vestibulocochlear nerve, demyelinating disease such as multiple sclerosis, or CNS trauma that damages the neural pathway or cortex.

Sensory and neural are often lumped together as *sensorineural* hearing loss.

Diagnosis depends upon audiology techniques. Imaging may be necessary. Treatment first depends on eliminating the cause, be it loud music or a therapeutic drug. Most hearing loss is permanent and cannot be reversed. Treatment is with hearing aids. Hearing aids can be very helpful, but must be carefully tailored to the cause of the loss.

Case Notes

20.20 If JuJu's otitis media had caused hearing loss due to destruction of middle ear structure, which type of loss would it be: conductive, sensory, or neural?

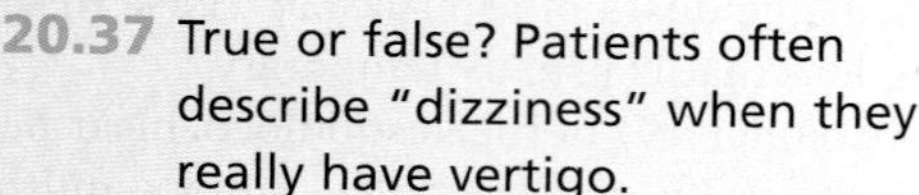

Pop Quiz

20.37 True or false? Patients often describe "dizziness" when they really have vertigo.

20.38 The three primary categories of deafness are ________, ________, and ________.

Case Study Revisited

"She has a fever." The case of JuJu F.

JuJu had a classic case of AOM—an acute middle ear infection that occurred in a young child after an otherwise unremarkable upper respiratory viral infection. Her pharyngeal and adenoidal edema blocked drainage from the Eustachian tube, which caused accumulation of fluid in the middle ear. This fluid became a culture medium for local bacteria, which proliferated to cause purulent infection. She exhibited classic signs and symptoms of purulent otitis media: fever, ear pain (tugging at the ear), irritability, and vomiting. The pediatrician's examination documented the signs of AOM: a bulging, dull, red tympanic membrane. The pediatrician also was appropriately careful to ensure, to the extent reasonable in an office examination, that she did not also have a related condition such as pneumonia or meningitis. Her chest was clear, indicating no concomitant pneumonia; her neck was supple, and her anterior fontanel was soft and not bulging, indicating that meningitis was not present. Like most children, she responded well to oral antibiotics, but, as many do, she developed bilateral SOM in the aftermath of the acute infection. In addition, as most cases do, the SOM resolved without further therapy.

Please review our Chapter 1 case, *"My daughter has a fever and an earache." The Case of Anne M.*, and compare it with this case.

Section 3: Disorders of Other Senses

A little learning is a dangerous thing; Drink deep, or taste not the Pierian spring.

ALEXANDER POPE (1688–1744), ENGLISH POET, ESSAY ON CRITICISM

Guests, like fish, begin to smell after three days.

BENJAMIN FRANKLIN (1706–1790), AMERICAN FOUNDING FATHER AND SCIENTIST

This section discusses the remaining special senses (taste and smell) and the somatic senses (touch, pressure, temperature, pain, and proprioception).

Normal Taste and Smell

Taste (*gustation*) is sensed by chemoreceptors on the tongue and throat that respond to chemicals (*tastants*) in food and drink. All tastes are a combination of five tastes, and each taste has specific type of receptor. The five tastes are *sour*, *salty*, *sweet*, *bitter*, and *umami*. *Umami* is a Japanese word for "savory" or "meaty" and refers to the taste imparted by glutamate and aspartate amino acids in meats and cheeses; hence the regular use of monosodium glutamate as a taste enhancer in oriental cuisine. Tastant signals are relayed by cranial nerves VII, IX, and X to the gustatory cortex in the temporal lobe. *Perception of taste is greatly influenced by smell.*

Smell (*olfaction*) is sensed by chemoreceptors, located high in the nasal cavity immediately beneath the cranium, that respond to volatile chemicals (odorants) in air. Not all molecules stimulate olfactory receptors: oxygen, nitrogen, water, and many other molecules are odorless; otherwise, they are all we could smell. Unlike taste, there is no five-letter "alphabet" for smell. The human nose can distinguish about 10,000 different odors based on the peculiar molecular mix of each. Odorant signals travel through the olfactory nerves (CN I) to multiple areas of the brain. One path goes to a special region of the cerebral cortex for recognition. Another path runs through the limbic system where emotional content is added. The latter accounts for the powerful ability of odors to stimulate memory of events associated with the odor.

Disorders of Taste and Smell

Ageusia is inability to taste. *Hypogeusia* is decreased ability to taste. *Dysgeusia* is distorted taste. Dysfunction of taste may be due to peripheral (conductive) interference with signal transport or with cortical interpretation of the signal. Much of what is perceived as defective taste is actually defective smell.

The intensity of taste signals decline with age. Other than dysfunctional smell, the most frequent causes of taste dysfunction are prior upper respiratory infection and head injury. Less commonly, cranial nerve conditions may diminish signals or CNS injury may damage the taste cortex.

Many conditions are capable of impairing taste: *xerostomia* (dry mouth), poor oral hygiene, and malnutrition. Both zinc deficiency and use of zinc lozenges can reduce or distort taste. Defective genes may account for failure of taste buds to develop or for an inability to detect certain tastes. Many times, however, the cause is unknown.

Diminished ability to smell, either temporary or permanent, is common. *Anosmia* is inability to detect odors. *Hyposmia* is diminished ability. *Dysosmia* is distorted detection: either an altered sense, usually unpleasant (*parosmia*); perception of odor without an odorant present (*phantosmia*); or an inability to identify the odor (*agnosmia*). Dysfunction of smell may be due to peripheral (conductive) interference with signal transport or with cortical interpretation of the signal.

The intensity of smell signals declines with age. Conductive defects are usually due to nasal inflammation—the odorant never reaches the sensor either because airflow is diverted through the mouth due to nasal congestion or the sensors are injured and covered with mucus (sinusitis, upper respiratory infections, allergies, and snorting cocaine or other substances). Some over-the-counter nasal spray cold remedies may interfere with the sensation of smell, especially those containing zinc. Lozenges containing zinc have also been implicated. CNS diseases such as Alzheimer disease or Parkinson disease may also interfere with smell.

Pop Quiz

20.39 What cranial nerve is responsible for olfaction?

20.40 True or false? Umami refers to the smell of meat.

20.41 True or false? Intensity of smell declines with age.

20.42 CNS diseases such as Parkinson disease and ____________ may interfere with the sense of smell.

Normal Somatic Senses

Somatic senses are detected by *receptors* in virtually every millimeter of skin, muscle, bones, joints, tendons, and other tissues.

Tactile receptors detect touch and pressure. They are among the most numerous sensory receptors, and are found in skin, muscle, joints, and internal organs. Anatomically, they consist of the tips of neuron dendrites, some of which are bare nerve endings while others are fitted with special sensing apparatus.

Temperature is sensed by **thermoreceptors**—free nerve endings located mainly in skin, although some are present in the upper digestive tract, the cornea of the eye, and the urinary bladder.

Pain is sensed by free sensory nerve endings called **nociceptors** (Latin *noci-* = harmful), which exist in every body tissue but the central nervous system. Nociceptors can be activated by physical deformation, such as that resulting from a cut or puncture wound, as well as by temperature extremes, oxygen deprivation, or by chemicals such as histamine that are released in response to tissue damage. Pain is difficult to define, to study, and to describe because it is so subjective.

We experience two types of pain: *fast* and *slow*, because we have two types of nociceptive sensory neurons. Consider the sensations when you step on a nail or a tack. **Fast pain** is perceived within a fraction of a second and rises almost instantly to peak intensity. Fast pain signals are carried by *myelinated* neurons. **Slow pain** begins more than one second after the stimulus, and rises to a peak over several seconds or minutes. Slow pain signals are carried by *unmyelinated* neurons and are the throbbing, aching, sometimes burning sensations that typically arise from an injured site (your foot) as the initial sharp pain subsides. Slow pain signals also characteristically arise from inflamed tissue, such as with infection or arthritis, as well as the rapid, marked stretching of visceral organs, such as the stretching of the cervix in childbirth or the stretching of a ureter with the passage a kidney stone.

Proprioception is the sensing and perception of the position of body parts *relative to one another*. Proprioception tells us, for example, whether our left leg is bent or straight, and whether our facial muscles are contracted into a smile or slack with boredom. The word derives from Latin *proprius* = one's own + *recipere* = to receive, therefore to receive information about one's self. Proprioceptive sensory receptors, called **proprioceptors**, sense the degree of muscle stretch or contraction and the angle of body joints, data that the brain integrates and interprets as the position of body parts relative to one another.

Proprioceptors are located in muscles and connective tissue. Skeletal muscle proprioceptors are formed from modified muscle fibers that detect skeletal muscle length. Muscle spindles protect against excessive muscle stretch. As stretch becomes ever greater, they activate a reflex that causes the muscle to contract and oppose or reduce the amount of stretch.

Similar receptors are located in collagen strands within tendons, near the point where they merge with muscle fibers. Golgi tendon organs protect against potentially damaging muscle tension that might tear muscle or tendon by use of excess force; their activation causes the muscle to relax, decreasing the tension. Other proprioceptors located in joint capsules and ligaments relay information about joint positions and angles.

Disorders of Somatic Senses

By and large, the somatic sensory disorders are neurologic disorders of the CNS. There is considerable overlap among the various conditions.

Disorders of Touch Often Involve Defective Proprioception

Primary **tactile disorders** consist of an inability to discriminate basic sensing information. Symptoms include the loss of pressure sensitivity, impaired ability to discriminate between one point touch and two point (two-point discrimination) touch, loss of vibratory sense, and proprioceptive deficit. Some individuals are born with diminished sensitivity to pain owing to genetic defects in the nociceptive neurons of the peripheral nervous system. Nevertheless, most tactile disorders arise after injury to the sensory cortex. These primary deficits can lead to problems in tactile object recognition such as an inability to distinguish between the key and the coin in your pocket.

Higher-order tactile disorders are failures to integrate tactile/proprioceptive sensations into conscious recognition. There are many such disorders, all a consequence of brain damage. For example, *tactile agnosia* is an inability to recognize an object by touch even though touch and proprioceptive sensors are intact.

Phantom limb phenomenon is a related sensory disorder not due to brain damage but to cortical interpretation of sensory signals. It features the persistent experience of the postural and motor aspects of a limb after its physical loss. Signals generated at the nerve stump are interpreted as if they arose from the limb itself. Patients may even feel itching or pain in a particular finger or toe. It occurs in 95% of patients who have lost a limb.

Pain Disorders May Involve Touch and Temperature

Pain disorders are discussed in detail in Chapter 24. A **pain disorder** consists of pain severe enough to warrant medical attention and to cause disruption of the patient's normal social or occupational function. Emotional factors have an important role, but the pain is not intentionally produced or feigned. Some patients may recall an initial stimulus that produced acute pain. Heightened sensitivity to touch and/or temperature may be part of the problem. *Fibromyalgia* (Chapter 18) appears to be such a condition.

Pop Quiz

20.43 True or false? Sensing requires conscious awareness of the thing being sensed.

20.44 True or false? Temperature is sensed by nociceptors.

20.45 What is the term for sensing your body position or body parts relative to each other (e.g., your leg is bent or straight)?

20.46 Are tactile disorders more likely to be primary or secondary to sensory cortex damage?

20.47 True or false? Ninety-five percent of amputees experience pain or itching of a phantom limb.

20.48 True or false? Fibromyalgia is an intentionally produced pain syndrome.

Chapter Challenge

CHAPTER RECALL

1. Which of the following forms the posterior side of the anterior chamber?
A. Ciliary body
B. Retina
C. Choroid
D. Iris

2. A 60-year-old African American male presents to his primary care physician complaining of "being unable to see what's right in front of him." His past medical history is remarkable only for a lengthy smoking history and benign prostatic hypertrophy. His eye exam is notable for normal peripheral vision but loss of central vision. From what condition does he likely suffer?
A. RP
B. ARMD
C. Ischemic optic neuropathy
D. Glaucoma

3. Which of the following can cause proptosis?
A. Chronic inflammation and infection
B. Hemangiomas and lymphomas
C. Lacrimal gland adenomas and Grave disease
D. All of the above

4. A 21-year-old Caucasian male is brought to the emergency room by his girlfriend on his birthday. She says he has been complaining of a headache and dizziness and she is concerned about the amount of alcohol he drank. His physical exam is notable for slurred speech and a rapid, repetitive, rhythmic horizontal beating motion of both eyes when he gazes to the right or left. What is this motion called?
A. Nystagmus
B. Amblyopia
C. Diplopia
D. Strabismus

5. What receptors protect against excessive force within muscles?
A. Proprioceptors
B. Muscle spindles
C. Golgi tendon organ
D. Nociceptors

6. A 45-year-old Hispanic woman comes to the clinic complaining of episodes of dizziness, nausea, and vomiting that last about a day. A review of systems reveals hearing loss and ringing in both ears, but it is otherwise unremarkable as is her past medical history. Her physical exam is only notable for nystagmus. You advise reduced salt intake and a trial of diuretics. What is your diagnosis?
A. Ménière syndrome
B. Meniere disease
C. Vestibular neuronitis
D. Aspirin overdose

7. When your mother advises you to turn down your music, she is trying to prevent what type of hearing loss?
A. Conductive deafness
B. Presbycusis
C. Neural deafness
D. Sensory deafness

8. A 16-year-old Caucasian female is seen by her pediatrician for complaints of difficulty hearing. She reports a recent upper respiratory infection that resolved a week ago. She denies fever, ear pain, and symptoms of congestion. An otoscopic exam demonstrates fluid behind the tympanic membranes. What is your diagnosis?
A. SOM
B. AOM
C. COM
D. Cholesteatoma

9. The main function of the Eustachian tube is which of the following?
A. To drain fluid from the middle ear
B. To collect sound waves for conversion to nerve signals
C. To equalize air pressure on both sides of the tympanic membrane
D. To aid in maintaining body orientation and balance

10. Your patient, a 53-year-old African American male, returns to the clinic for his yearly vision check. A fundoscopic exam demonstrates copper wire vessels with A-V nicking as well as flame-shaped hemorrhages, yellow exudates, and white "cotton wool" patches. What treatment do you recommend?
A. Blood pressure medication
B. Better sugar control
C. Iridotomy
D. Intraocular antibiotics

11. What is the inability to recognize an object by touch, even though touch and proprioceptive sensors are intact and visual recognition is unimpaired, called?
A. Fibromyalgia
B. Tactile apraxia
C. Tactile hyposensitivity
D. Tactile agnosia

12. A 14-year-old Caucasian male presents to the emergency clinic complaining of a foreign body sensation in his right eye. He believes his contact lenses must have scratched his eye. An ophthalmologic exam demonstrates inflammation of the lid margins (most notable at the lateral edges). The conjunctiva is not involved, and no scratches are seen with fluorescein dye. What is the likely diagnosis?
    A. Corneal abrasion
    B. Hyphema
    C. Conjunctivitis
    D. Blepharitis
13. Which of the following statements concerning glaucoma is true?
    A. Glaucoma is always associated with ocular hypertension and can be diagnosed through routine measurement of intraocular pressure.
    B. Patients with POAG usually do not have pain, blurred vision, or other symptoms, despite progressive loss of peripheral vision.
    C. Secondary glaucoma in most instances is bilateral and can be caused by hemorrhage or synechiae.
    D. Primary close-angle glaucoma features a narrow lateral angle, and is the most frequent type of glaucoma and a major cause of blindness in the United States.
14. A 35-year-old Caucasian female presents to the clinic for continued follow-up of an ocular disease she was diagnosed with as an adolescent; her family history is positive. Her conical misshaped corneas have been progressively bulging and thinning over the last several years, and her rigid contact lenses are no longer providing sufficient relief. You recommend she undergo corneal transplants for which of the following diseases?
    A. Keratopathy
    B. Keratitis
    C. Keratoconus
    D. Arcus senilis
15. Iridocyclitis is inflammation of which of the following?
    A. Part of the uveal tract
    B. The cornea
    C. The retina
    D. The lacrimal apparatus
16. True or false? The primary causes of cataracts in the United States are aging and diabetes.
17. True or false? Scleral pinguecula and pterygium can grow into the field of vision.
18. True or false? Each pitch excites sensory nerve fibers in the cochlear spiral distinct from every other pitch, and the louder the sound, the more ciliary motion at that particular point.
19. True or false? Conductive hearing loss is caused by impaired conduction of sound by the vestibulocochlear nerve.
20. True or false? The most common malignancy in the eye of an adult is metastatic cancer, which usually lodges in the rich vascularity of the uveal tract.
21. True or false? Conditions that affect the skin can affect the external auditory canal.

CONCEPTUAL UNDERSTANDING

22. Explain the cause of myopia, hyperopia, and presbyopia.
23. What are the complications of AOM?
24. What are the two causes of retinal detachment?

APPLICATION

25. Why is a diagnosis of papilledema an emergency?
26. Your friend, a 25-year-old African American female, pushes her lunch away from her while in her favorite restaurant. She complains that things just don't taste the same lately. You observe your friend's raw red nose, sniffles, and Kleenex sticking out her purse. What questions should you ask?

CHAPTER 21

Disorders of the Skin

Contents

Chapter Objectives

After studying this chapter, you should be able to complete the following tasks:

NORMAL SKIN

1. Differentiate between dermis, epidermis, and subcutis using architecture, function, and the elements contained within each.

GENERAL CONDITIONS OF SKIN

2. Using examples from the text, classify the general conditions of skin according to their underlying etiology and provide their accompanying signs and symptoms.

INFECTIONS, INFESTATIONS, BITES, AND STINGS

3. Discuss the infections and infestations that affect the skin.

DISORDERS OF HAIR FOLLICLES AND SEBACEOUS GLANDS

4. Describe the differences between acne and rosacea.

DERMATITIS

5. List and classify the types of dermatitis as acute or chronic, noting the clinical characteristics, underlying etiology, and treatment options where applicable.

DISEASES OF THE DERMIS AND SUBCUTIS

6. Compare and contrast scleroderma with panniculitis.

BLISTERING DISEASES

7. Categorize the blistering diseases according to the skin layer in which they are formed, and discuss their clinical and pathological features.

DISORDERS OF PIGMENTATION AND MELANOCYTES

8. Describe the etiology, clinical features, and treatment (as applicable) of vitiligo, albinism, freckles, and lentigos.
9. Discuss the spectrum of melanocytic lesions; pay particular attention to the diagnostic and prognostic features of melanoma.

NEOPLASMS OF SKIN NOT INCLUDING MELANOMA

10. List several neoplasms or neoplasm-like lesions of the dermis, catalog them as hyperplastic, premalignant, or malignant, and explain their pathogenesis.

DISORDERS OF HAIR AND NAILS

11. Provide a differential diagnosis for hair loss.
12. Compare and contrast onychogryphosis, onycholysis, paronychia, and onychomycosis.

Case Study

"She fries like bacon." The case of Brianna K.

Chief Complaint: Skin lesion

Clinical History: Brianna K. was a 25-year-old woman, a fashion model with striking red hair and fair skin. She appeared in a dermatologist's office with her husband. "I can't see it very well because it's back here," she said, reaching her right hand behind her neck to point out a lesion just below her collar. "A doctor friend saw it two weeks ago at a picnic. There was blood on the back of my blouse and she took a peek at it. She said people like me with fair skin tend to suffer more from sun exposure than others and this could be related and I should have a dermatologist look at it. It surprised me a lot because I get regular checkups with my gynecologist, but she never mentioned it."

When questioned about how long the lesion had been present, neither Brianna nor her husband could be sure. "It's in an area that's usually under my collar where I can't see it," she said.

"I've noticed it but never really paid any attention," her husband added. "It's hard for me to believe this could be related to sun exposure. She is very careful about her skin and appearance because it's so important in her job. If she gets a little too much sun, she fries like bacon."

Brianna added, "I turn red as a beet. I even blistered a time or two when I was a child."

Further medical history revealed the usual childhood illnesses and excellent general health. She had never been hospitalized and her only physician visits were for an annual gynecologic exam. She had a son two years old. Her parents were living and in good health.

Dermatologic history revealed that she was allergic to poison ivy and reported that she was "allergic" to household cleaning fluids. "If it involves cleaning with some kind of detergent, I leave it to him," she said, pointing to her husband. "My hands become ugly red in an instant if I don't. But fortunately it goes away quickly." The dermatologist asked other questions, which revealed her hands to be red, dry and without blisters.

When questioned about other skin complaints, she laughed and said, "I'm in fashion and my pale skin and red hair are my best assets. Photographers love my freckles, even this mole on my cheek," she said pointing to a small dark mole. "But good skin is a fragile thing. Most girls I know can model for a while when they are pregnant but my face turned blotchy brown. My husband and I laughed about me finally getting a tan. Thank goodness it went away after our son was born."

Physical Examination and Other Data: Vital signs were normal. She was thin and appeared in good health. Her face was freckled and she had numerous small, pink or lightly pigmented skin lesions scattered over her torso and upper arms and thighs, the largest of which was the one on her back. The dermatologist examined the lesion, took a close photograph, and recommended excisional biopsy, which was performed by a plastic surgeon the following week.

Clinical Course: Several days after surgery the following pathology report was sent to the dermatologist.

> ***Gross description:*** *The specimen is an ellipse of pale skin 3.5 x 2.5 x 0.5 cm. In the center is a roughly circular lesion 0.8 cm in diameter. The periphery is flat, irregular, and unevenly pigmented—some areas nearly black, others light tan to pink. In the center is a small, smooth, raised pink–brown nodule 0.4 cm in diameter. The remainder of the lesion varies from pink, shiny and smooth, to rough and black. Several*

"She fries like bacon." The case of Brianna K. (continued)

pigmented satellite lesions are present around the periphery of the main lesion.

Microscopic study: *The main lesion is a nodular mass of melanocytes with considerable variation of nuclear size and shape. Occasional mitotic figures are present and many cells have a large, eosinophilic nucleolus. Spreading outward from the main mass are clusters of atypical melanocytes at the dermal-epidermal junction, some of which form small satellites at the edge of the main growth. The surface of the tumor is focally ulcerated. Tumor extends to the junction of the papillary and reticular dermis (Clark level III). Minimal lymphocytic reaction is present. Breslow maximum tumor thickness is 2.0 mm. No lymphatic, perineural or vascular invasion is present. The margins of resection are free of neoplasm.*

Diagnosis: Nodular malignant melanoma, Breslow tumor thickness 2.0 mm; Clark level III.

Clinical Course: Further detailed family research revealed that the patient had an uncle in Ireland who had died of malignant melanoma.

At a follow-up appointment, the dermatologist made a careful photographic survey of Brianna's skin. She was found to have dozens of moles. Four of these proved to be dysplastic nevi and were excised. Each showed melanocytic atypia, but there was no evidence of advancement to malignant melanoma. She was referred to an oncologist for supervision of further care. Physical examination and multiple imaging studies show no enlarged lymph nodes or other evidence of metastasis.

The biopsy site was reexcised. No residual tumor was identified. Brianna was treated according to an experimental immunotherapy protocol. In her third year of follow-up, liver metastases were found. Brianna died 44 months after diagnosis, a few days after her 29th birthday.

All the beauty of the world, 'tis but skin deep.

RALPH VENNING (1620–1673), ENGLISH CLERGYMAN, FROM HIS BOOK OF DEVOTIONS, ORTHODOX PARADOXES. *VENNING'S MOST FAMOUS QUOTATION IS "BETTER LATE THAN NEVER."*

Skin is the largest human organ and is supremely important psychologically and physiologically. The appearance of skin is of supreme social importance. It is the natural canvas of life, revealing details of our personal histories and lifestyle choices. We spend liberally to improve its appearance—we moisturize it, paint it with cosmetics, lighten or darken it with chemicals, decorate it with jewelry and tattoos, and reshape it with surgery. But at the same time, many of us abuse it: years of smoking and excessive sunlight exposure are reflected in marked premature wrinkling. Even minor skin diseases sometimes assume outsized importance in our lives. Neither acne nor baldness threatens death or debility, but they can be very distressing.

Though appearance is important, it pales in comparison to skin's role as the protective covering that separates us from the environment. The barrier function depends mainly on the surface layer, the epidermis, which is formed of dead, dry cells that are mainly composed of an indigestible protein (keratin, the stuff of hair and nails). It is literally tough as leather, and yet it is easily damaged: in most areas, the epidermis is only a few tenths of a millimeter thick. Its vulnerability and its importance is indicated in cases of severe burns, when an early complaint of many patients is "I'm thirsty" and "I'm cold," because they are losing heat and fluid rapidly. Later, loss of the barrier function makes burn patients hospitable to microbes and vulnerable to massive infection.

But skin is ever so much more than a barrier. A complex organ composed of multiple cell types and specialized structures, skin is critical in body temperature control and immunity. When our internal temperature rises excessively, skin vessels dilate to deliver warm blood to the surface to radiate excess heat, and sweat glands bathe the skin surface for evaporative cooling. And skin is active immunologically: it contains a special type of immune cell (Langerhans) that plays a key role in environmental defense and in allergic and immune disease.

Skin comes into daily contact with countless environmental substances and conditions and is afflicted with more disease than any other organ. About one-third of the population of the United States develops a skin condition each year, and skin complaints account for about 10% of annual physician office visits. Many diseases, such as psoriasis, are primary in skin. Others are a secondary effect of systemic disease—the rashes typical of many infectious diseases, Kaposi sarcoma in AIDS, rheumatoid nodules in rheumatoid arthritis, and so forth.

Figure 21.1 defines and illustrates the most common terms. Also, detailed understanding of skin disease requires a grasp of microscopic pathology, a skill not usually required for clinical practitioners to understand diseases of other organs. Numerous special terms are used in the microscopic pathology of skin disease; they will be used

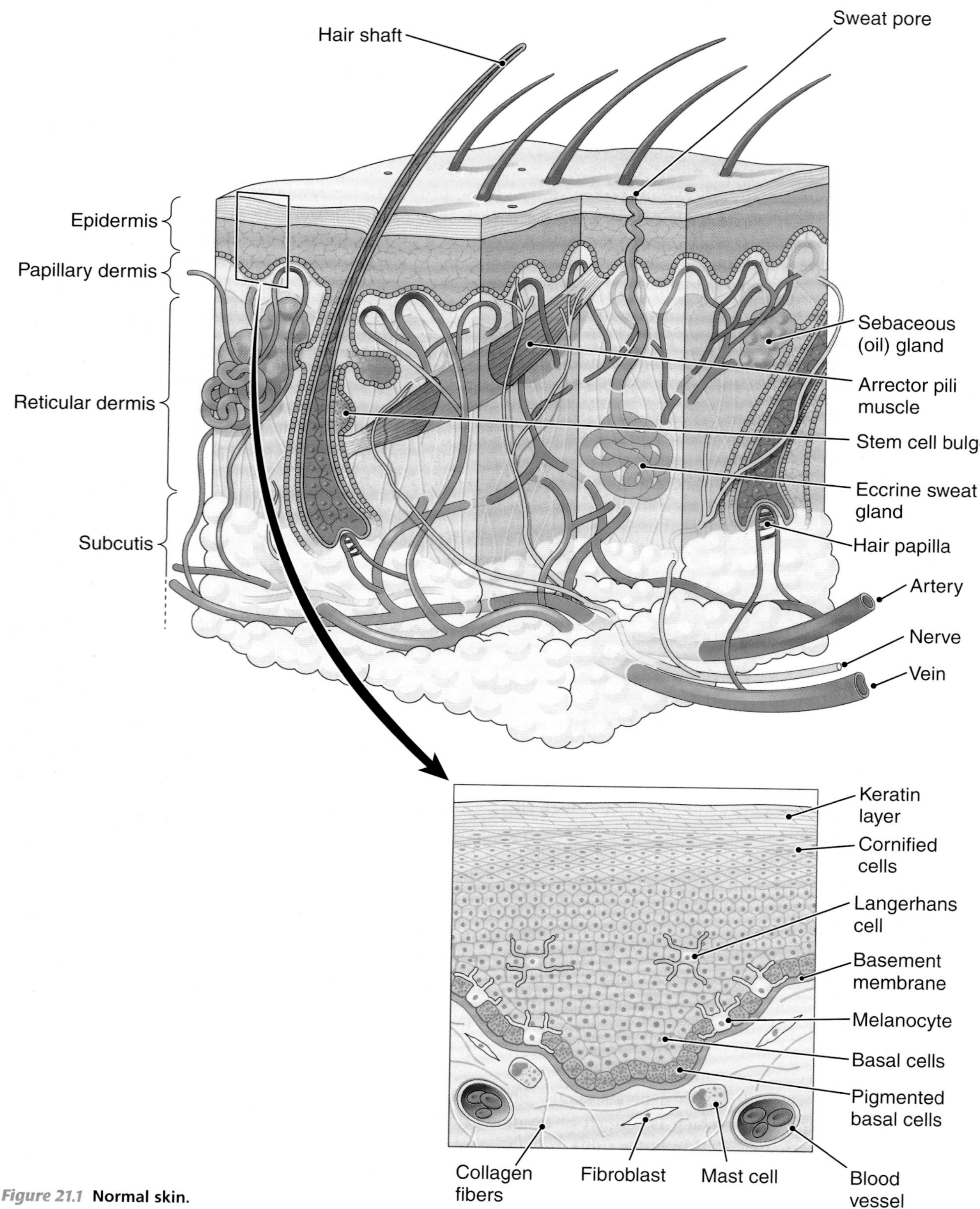

Figure 21.1 **Normal skin.**

sparingly in this discussion. Finally, the etiology and pathogenesis of many skin diseases are unknown.

Despite abundance, visibility, and easy access, skin disease is a mystery to many in healthcare for several reasons. Learning a discipline, be it carpentry or dermatology, requires learning the specialized language of the field. This is especially true for skin diseases, where words are used regularly that are uncommon elsewhere in medicine—try finding *lichenified* in your average medical textbook index (it is illustrated and defined in Fig. 21.3). But we cannot avoid using clinical dermatologic terms because, for skin disease, gross pathology and clinical description are one and the same.

Normal Skin

Anatomically, normal skin (Figs. 21.2 and 21.3) is composed of two layers—epidermis and dermis—and rests on a bed of subcutaneous fat (the subcutis or panniculus).

The **epidermis** is the surface layer. It is composed of keratinocytes, which produce keratin, a stiff protein. The cells of the epidermis are pancake-like and are called **squamous cells** (from Latin *squama* = scale), and are layered upon one another like the shingles of a roof. The deepest layer is composed of **basal cells** (*epidermal stem cells*), from which new squamous cells are formed and pushed upward by newer cells forming below. As they rise and mature, epidermal cells flatten and accumulate keratin to form the *stratum corneum*, a layer of dry, acidic, dead cells; these cells are inhospitable to microbes and are shed daily as they are replaced from below.

The epidermis rests on a *basement membrane*, a thin, acellular film of protein, which separates the epidermis from the dermis below and which plays an important role in skin physiology and disease. The epidermis does not contain blood vessels, nerves, or glands, and it gets its nourishment by diffusion across the basement membrane. In most areas, the epidermis is very thin—10 to 20 cells thick or about 0.1 mm. It is considerably thicker on the palms and soles because of the extra thickness of the surface layer of dead cells of the stratum corneum.

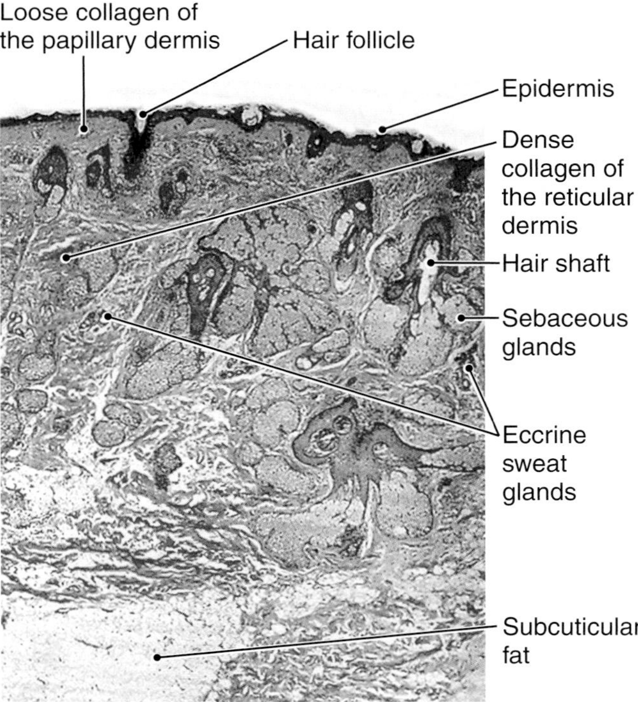

Figure 21.2 **Normal skin** (low-power photomicrograph). (Adapted with permission from Mills SE, *Histology for Pathologists*. 3rd ed. Philadelphia, PA: Lippincott Williams & Wilkins; 2007.)

The epidermis also contains **melanocytes**. These specialized cells, derived from the embryonic nervous system, lie among the basal cells on the basement membrane. They produce melanin pigment and deliver it into nearby basal cells. Skin color is determined by the amount of melanin (a dark brown pigment) deposited in basal cells.

Case Notes

21.1 Brianna's skin was fair, meaning she had relatively little melanin pigment in the ________ cells of her epidermis.

Also present among the basal cells of the epidermis are **Langerhans cells** (*dendritic cells*). These specialized immune system cells are voracious phagocytes. They trap microbes and other alien material that manage to cross the basement membrane. Langerhans cells then present captured antigen to immune system lymphocytes (Chapter 3).

The **dermis** is a framework of fibrous and elastic tissue that lies below the basement membrane and is home to nerves, specialized sensory nerve endings, blood vessels, and skin appendages (adnexa), such as sweat and sebaceous glands and hair follicles. The dermis is usually about 1–2 mm thick, much thicker than the epidermis. The superficial dermis is called the **papillary dermis**; it is less dense than the reticular dermis. The **reticular dermis** is the deepest part of the dermis. It is dense and tough (the stuff in animal skin that becomes leather) and is home to hair follicles and skin glands. It is less often involved in skin disease than other layers of the dermis.

The main cell in the dermis is the fibroblast (or fibrocyte), which produces the collagen and elastin fibers that account for skin toughness and resiliency. Also present in the dermis are dermal dendritic cells, which are similar to epidermal Langerhans cells.

Below the dermis is a pelt of fatty **subcutaneous tissue** (the subcutis), which serves as insulation and cushioning and which is home to some hair follicles. Below subcutaneous fat is a layer of dense fascia that sheaths the entire body and covers bone, muscle, and other deep structures.

Pop Quiz

21.1 True or false? The deepest cell layer of the epidermis is composed of basal cells.

21.2 What is the deepest part of the dermis?

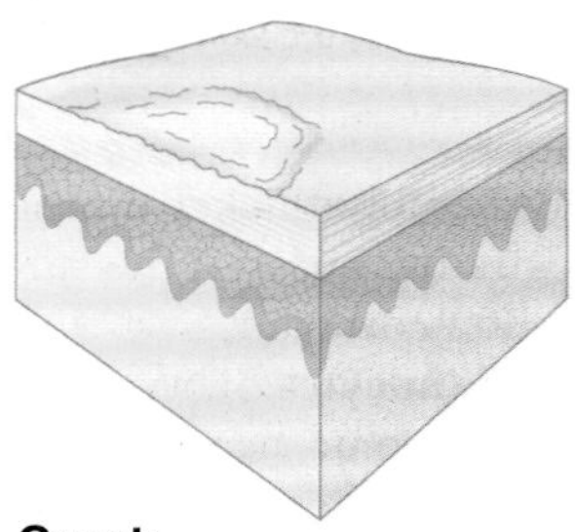

Crust:
A surface collection of dried serum and cell debris (see also Fig. 21.12)

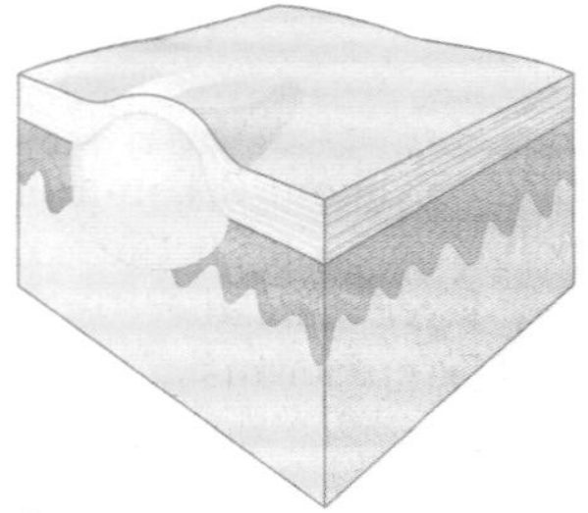

Cyst:
A closed space beneath the epidermis that contains fluid or semisolid material (see also Fig. 21.42)

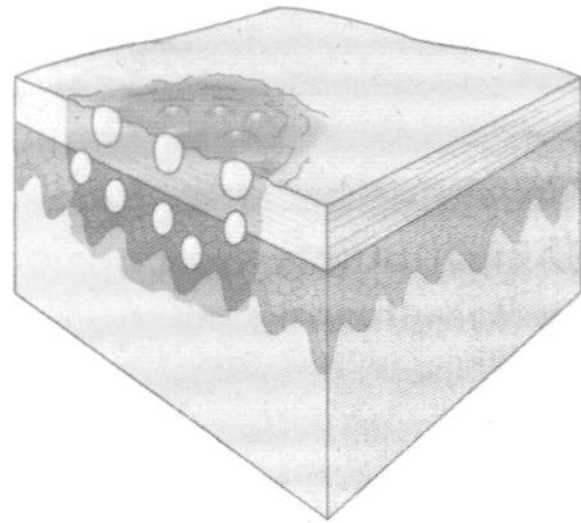

Eczema:
Inflamed, crusted skin with vesicles (see also Fig. 21.22)

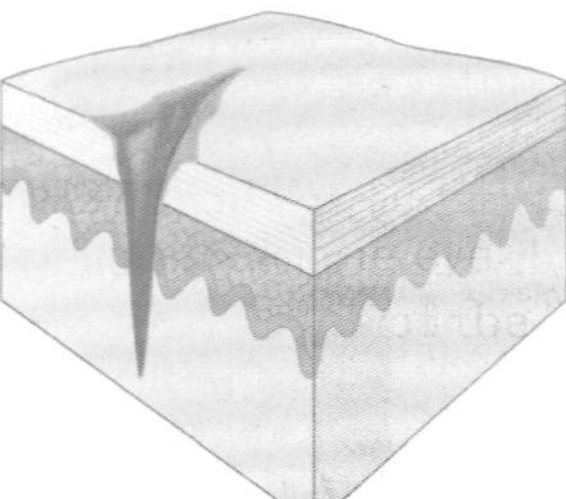

Fissure:
A groove or crack-like lesion

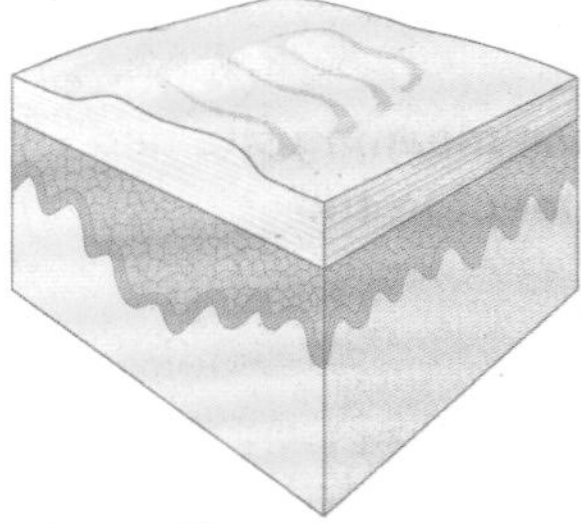

Lichenified:
An area of skin with thickening of epidermis and exaggeration of normal skin lines caused by chronic rubbing or scratching (see also Fig. 21.28)

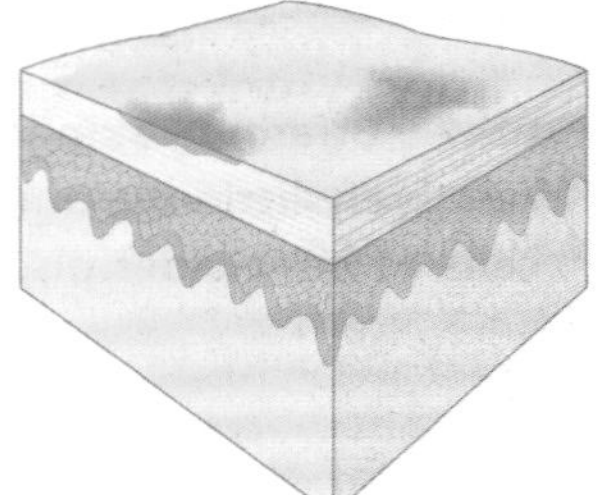

Macule:
A flat, discrete, discolored lesion <1.0 cm (see also Fig. 21.36)

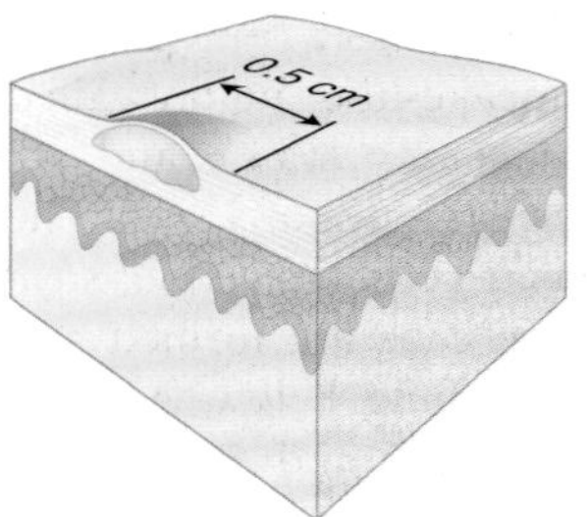

Papule:
A raised, domed superficial lesion <0.5 cm (see also Fig. 21.31)

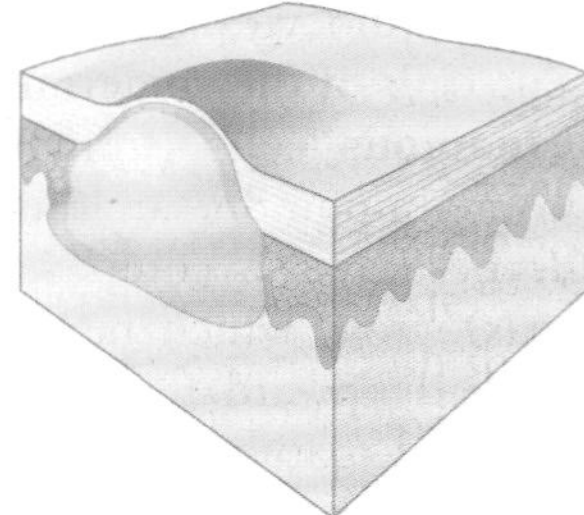

Nodule:
A firm, raised lesion; larger and deeper than a papule (see also Fig. 21.8)

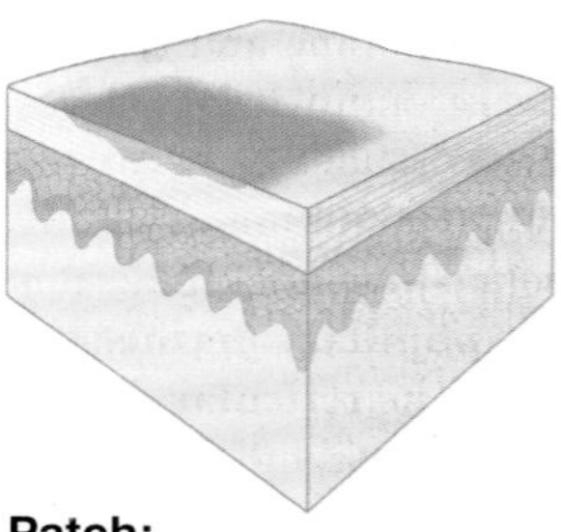

Patch:
A flat, discrete, discolored lesion larger than a macule (see also Fig. 21.36)

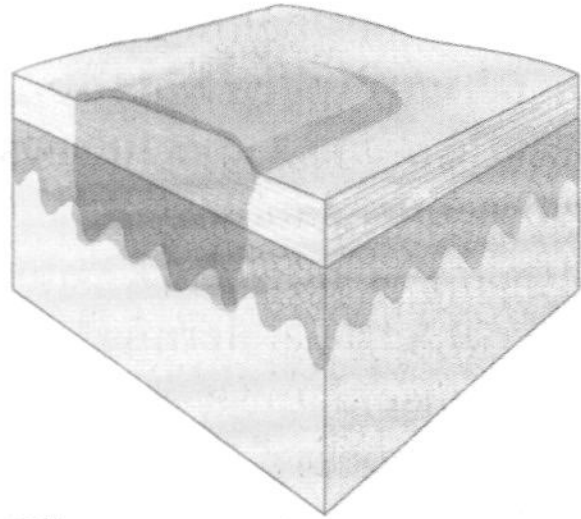

Plaque:
A raised, flat-topped superficial lesion larger than a papule (see also Figs. 21.7, 21.29)

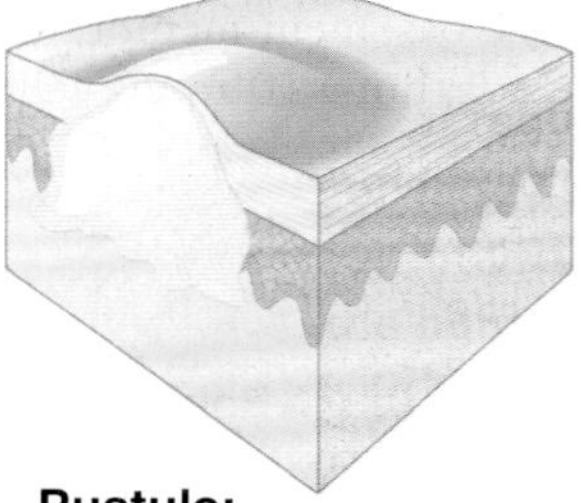

Pustule:
A small superficial abscess

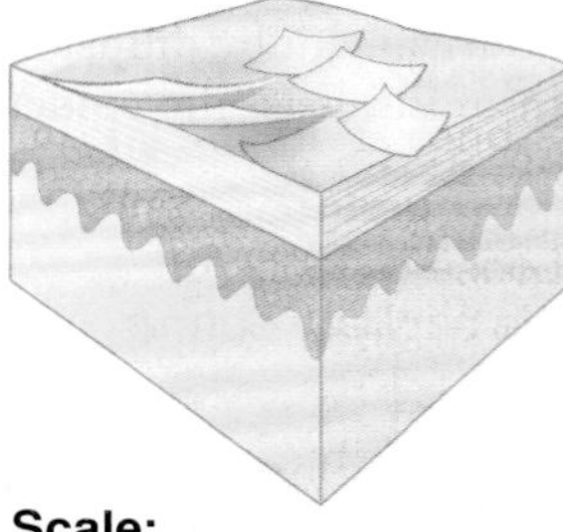

Scale:
A superficial, thin, plate-like flaking off of shedding epidermal cells (see also Figs. 21.11, 21.29)

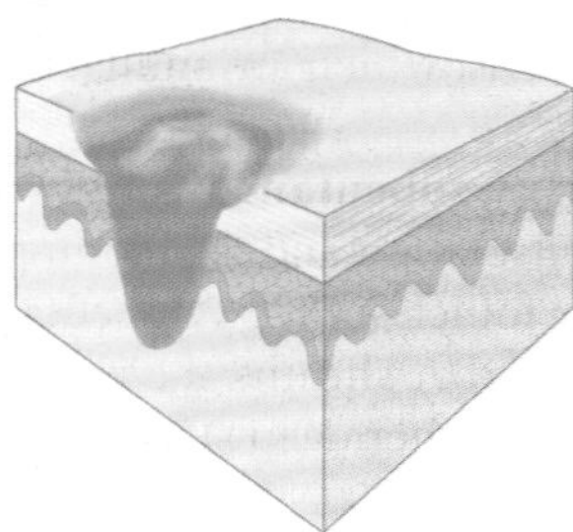

Ulcer:
A cavity not covered by epidermis (see also Fig. 21.6)

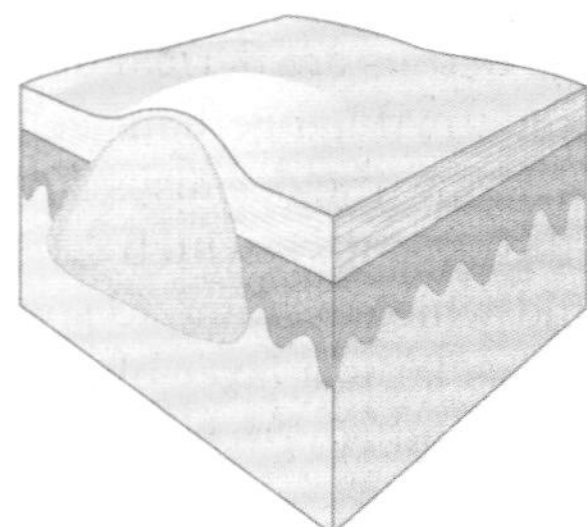

Vesicle/bulla:
A blister filled with fluid; a vesicle is small (<0.5 cm) whereas a bulla is larger (see also Fig. 21.15)

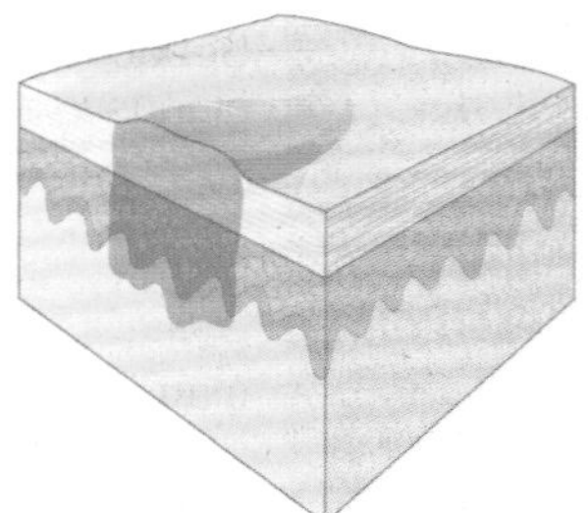

Wheal:
A smooth, slightly elevated lesion that is reddish or pale and usually itchy (see also Fig. 21.21)

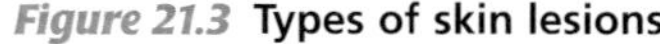

Figure 21.3 **Types of skin lesions.**

General Conditions of Skin

Skin occupies an outsized place of importance in human affairs because it contributes so strongly to appearance, and people care greatly about their appearance. Skin color, uniformity, smoothness, dryness, oiliness, hairiness, and other features are crucial to self-image, so much so that even medically minor skin disease may cause severe patient distress.

Skin Color May Be a Sign of Disease

The most important contributor to skin color is the amount of pigment in the basal layer, which in turn is governed by the number and activity of melanocytes. The degree of pigmentation is very low in people of northern European heritage, for example, and very high in those of African heritage. Much is made of race and skin color, but defining race based on skin color is not scientifically valid. Disorders of pigmentation are discussed below.

The second most important contributor to skin color is the redness of skin imparted by blood, which is influenced by 1) the amount of blood flowing through skin capillaries (dilated capillaries bring blood to the surface to lose heat; sunburned or otherwise injured skin is red from inflammatory vasodilation); 2) the amount of hemoglobin in blood (anemic blood is pale); and 3) the degree to which arterial blood is oxygenated (well-oxygenated blood is bright red, poorly oxygenated blood is bluish red). Poorly oxygenated blood imparts to skin a bluish cast called "cyanosis," which may be a clue to heart or lung disease.

Substances in blood can also affect skin color. Patients with high bilirubin, as in some hemolytic (Chapter 7) or liver (Chapter 12) disease, have yellow skin (*jaundice*, Chapter 12, Fig. 12.3). In *carbon monoxide poisoning* (Chapter 23, Fig. 23.6) carbon monoxide binds to hemoglobin, displacing oxygen and imparting a cherry red color to skin. An excessive consumption of carrots or carrot juice can turn skin orange; silver poisoning imparts a blue–gray hue.

Skin Changes Are Common in Pregnancy

Pregnancy can affect skin; some of these effects are so common they are considered normal and most disappear after childbirth. **Striae** (stretch marks) are common on the abdomen and breasts and are superficial dermal scars from the stress of stretched skin. **Melasma** ("the mask of pregnancy," Fig. 21.4) is a temporary darkening of facial skin caused by increased melanin pigment. High blood levels of estrogen in pregnancy can produce **spider angiomas**—small vascular lesions on the face or upper body that have a small, central arteriole and tiny radiating capillary spokes (Fig. 21.5). Spider angiomas also may be present in patients with severe liver disease because the liver does not metabolize estrogen properly. Pregnancy may also cause mild, temporary hair loss (*alopecia*) or excess facial or body hair (*hirsutism*).

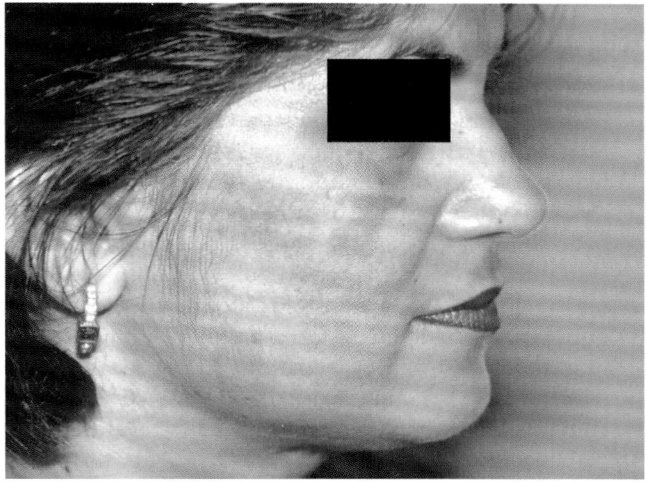

Figure 21.4 **Melasma** (the mask of pregnancy). Pigmentation fades after birth. (Reproduced with permission from Goodheart HP. *Goodheart's Photoguide of Common Skin Disorders*. 2nd ed. Philadelphia, PA: Lippincott Williams & Wilkins; 2003.)

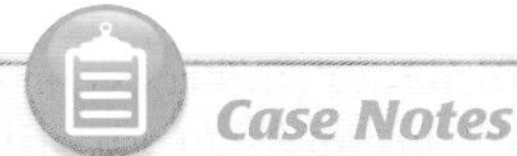

Case Notes

21.2 **What is the name of the change that occurred to Brianna's face during her pregnancy?**

Skin Is Often Affected by Systemic Disease

Many nonskin diseases have skin manifestations, far too many to mention here, but it is safe to say that the clinician who knows basic dermatology will be a more astute

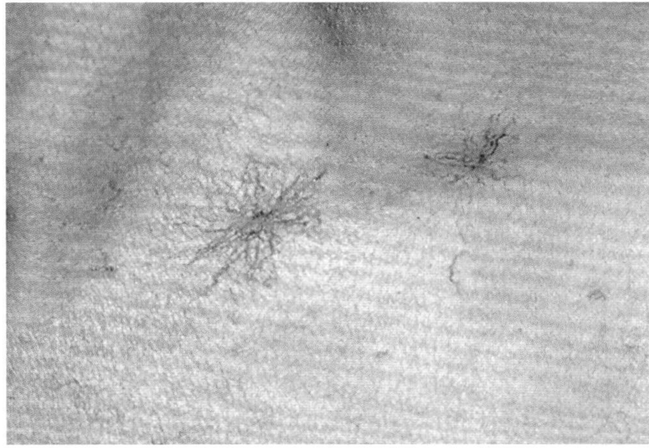

Figure 21.5 **Spider angiomas.** They occur in conjunction with sustained high estrogen levels such as pregnancy and cirrhosis. These are on the upper chest of a pregnant woman. (Reproduced with permission from Goodheart HP. *Goodheart's Photoguide of Common Skin Disorders*. 2nd ed. Philadelphia, PA: Lippincott Williams & Wilkins; 2003.)

practitioner than one who does not. Below is a short list of some common systemic conditions that often affect skin:

- *Diabetes*. It is an epidemic in the United States and becoming much more prevalent around the world. It is associated with several important skin conditions. Two worthy of specific mention are *Candida* fungal infections of skin, especially of or near the genitals, and diabetic skin ulcers (Fig. 21.6) at pressure points. Candida skin infection usually produces a raw, painful, red rash on the genitals or in skin folds around the genitals or buttocks. Diabetic ulcers are especially common in the foot and are caused by poor blood flow secondary to diabetic peripheral microvascular disease (Chapter 13) combined with impaired pain sensation resulting from diabetic neuropathy, which allows patients to repeatedly traumatize an area that otherwise would prove painful.
- *Thyroid disease* (Chapter 14). It affects skin because thyroid hormone has a profound influence on dermal and epidermal cell growth. Overproduction of thyroid hormones is associated with warm, moist, velvety skin, hair loss, changes in finger and toenails, increased skin pigmentation, and waxy translucent plaques over the anterior lower leg (*pretibial infiltrative dermopathy*). Underproduction of thyroid hormones features coarse, yellowish, dry skin; dry, brittle hair; and hair loss (including loss of lateral eyebrow hair).
- *HIV infection* (Chapter 3). Acute HIV infection is associated with a measles-like rash. Skin infections are common in AIDS, especially virus infections such as herpes simplex and herpes zoster. Kaposi sarcoma (Fig. 21.7) is an AIDS-defining vascular neoplasm of skin caused by a type of herpesvirus. It occurs typically as dark red macules, papules, or nodules on the nose, genitals, and extremities. Some AIDS patients may develop severe generalized dermatitis, such as seborrheic dermatitis and psoriasis.
- *Blood lipid abnormalities* (Chapter 8). Skin *xanthomas* are distinctive yellowish deposits of lipid. Very high levels of plasma triglyceride (usually above 2,000 mg/dL) may cause eruptive xanthomas—dozens of small, yellow-red papules on extensor surfaces (the back of the forearms or the shins) and pressure points such as the elbows, feet, or buttocks. High levels of total plasma cholesterol (usually above 300 mg/dL) may be associated with nodular xanthomas (Fig. 21.8)—nodular deposits of cholesterol crystals that appear over the elbow, on the palms or soles, or in the Achilles tendon. High cholesterol levels may also be associated with *xanthelasma*, a flat, bright yellow cholesterol xanthoma in the skin of the eyelids near the nose.
- *Autoimmune disease* (Chapter 3). Patients with systemic lupus erythematosus can be photosensitive and may also have the classic butterfly skin lesion on their cheeks (Fig. 21.9). Skin disease is prominent in systemic sclerosis (scleroderma)—skin progressively becomes waxy, stiff, and shiny, and so tight that the tips of fingers and toes may ulcerate (Chapter 3, Fig. 3.13).

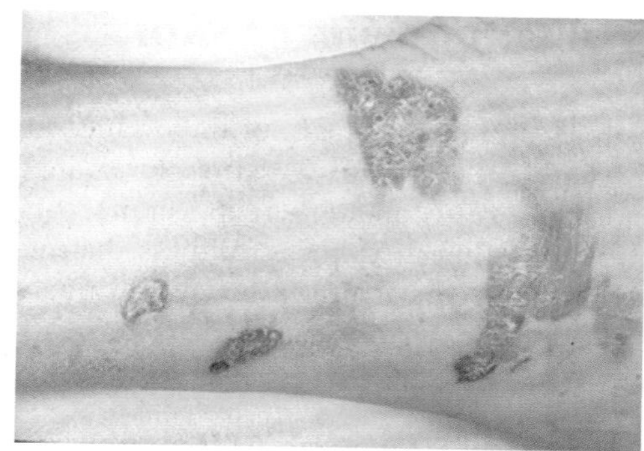

Figure 21.7 **Kaposi sarcoma**. Confluent plaques on the ankle of a patient with AIDS.

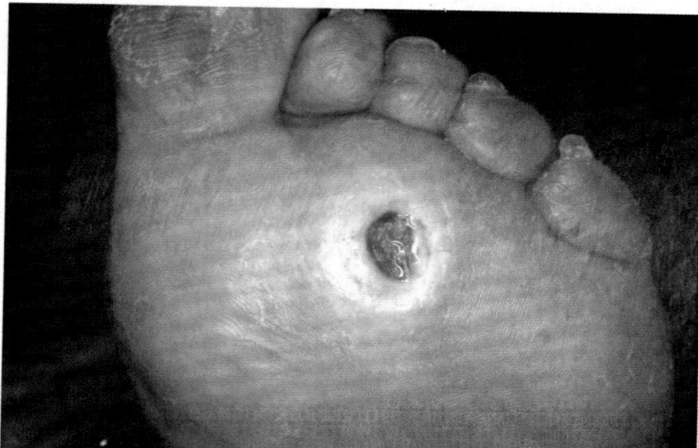

Figure 21.6 **Diabetic ulcer**. They tend to occur at pressure points.

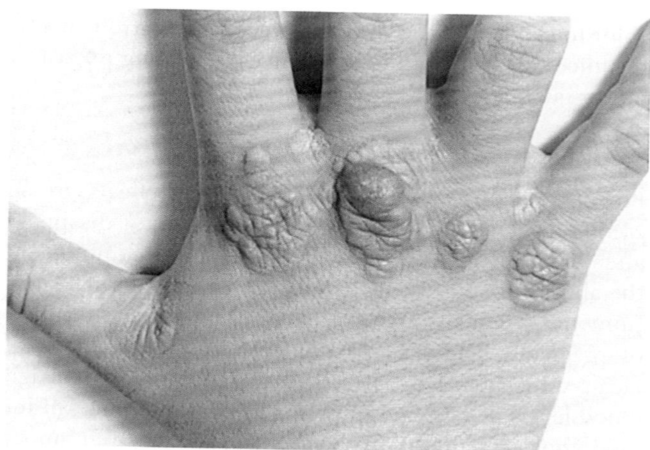

Figure 21.8 **Nodular xanthomas.** They are deposits of cholesterol in patients with abnormally high cholesterol and tend to occur on the knuckles, elbows, and knees. (Reproduced with permission from Rubin E, Farber JL. *Pathology*. 3rd ed. Philadelphia, PA: Lippincott-Raven; 1999.)

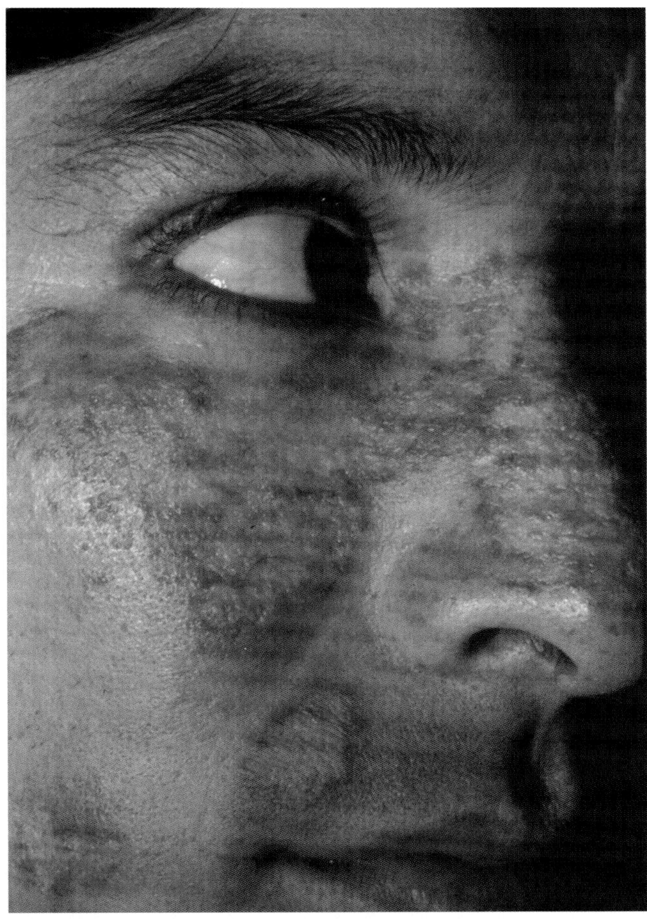

Figure 21.9 **Systemic lupus erythematosus**. Erythematous macules form a butterfly rash on the cheeks and across the bridge of the nose.

- *Sarcoidosis* (Chapter 10). It is a systemic disease most common in African Americans that features chronic granulomatous inflammation, chiefly in the lungs and mediastinal lymph nodes. Lesions in skin are small papules or plaques that occur mainly around the nose, lips, and eyes (Fig. 21.10).
- *Blood diseases*. Those that cause low platelet counts (<50,000) can cause tiny skin hemorrhages (*petechiae*, Chapter 6, Fig. 6.12). Coagulation defects can cause larger skin hemorrhages.
- *Neurocutaneous syndromes*. These are genetic neurologic syndromes with skin manifestations. They are exemplified by **neurofibromatosis**, a syndrome of peripheral nerve cell tumors (Chapter 19, Fig. 19.38A) accompanied by clusters of large, light brown skin macules called *café au lait* (coffee with milk) spots.

Sunlight Is Necessary for Good Health but Can Damage Skin

A certain amount of sunlight is necessary for good health. Among other things, it regulates sleep patterns, and most

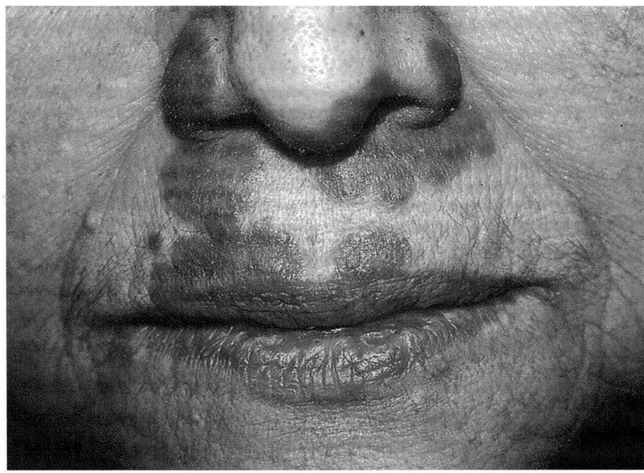

Figure 21.10 **Sarcoidosis**. Violaceous, confluent plaques. (Reproduced with permission from Goodheart HP. *Goodheart's Photoguide of Common Skin Disorders*. 2nd ed. Philadelphia, PA: Lippincott Williams & Wilkins; 2003.)

of our vitamin D supply depends on sunlight conversion of metabolic precursors into vitamin D. Recent studies indicate that 40% of the U.S. population has below-normal blood levels of vitamin D, much of which owes to poor exposure to sunlight. For African Americans and Hispanics, the figure is close to 75%.

Visible light is but one type of electromagnetic radiation, which also includes X-rays, radio waves, the radiation from decay of unstable elements such as uranium and cosmic rays, any of which can be damaging to any organism, including humans. The ultraviolet (short, bluish) wavelengths of sunlight contain higher energy levels than the red, longer wavelengths, although both can cause acute as well as chronic skin damage. Acute excessive exposure produces **sunburn**, which is very much like a mild burn produced by a hot water scald. Most sunburn results in a *superficial burn* (erythema only), but severe exposure can produce *partial thickness burns* (burns with blisters). Chronic sunlight overexposure produces photoaging, an excessive wrinkling and sagging.

Case Notes

21.3 Brianna said she blistered from sunburn as a child. What type of burn did she have?

Thermal injuries of skin (burns and frostbite) are discussed in Chapter 23.

Chronic overexposure to sunlight has an adverse effect on skin; it causes cancers of the epidermis and damages dermal collagen. Microscopically, dermal collagen is fragmented, as if it had been run through a kitchen blender.

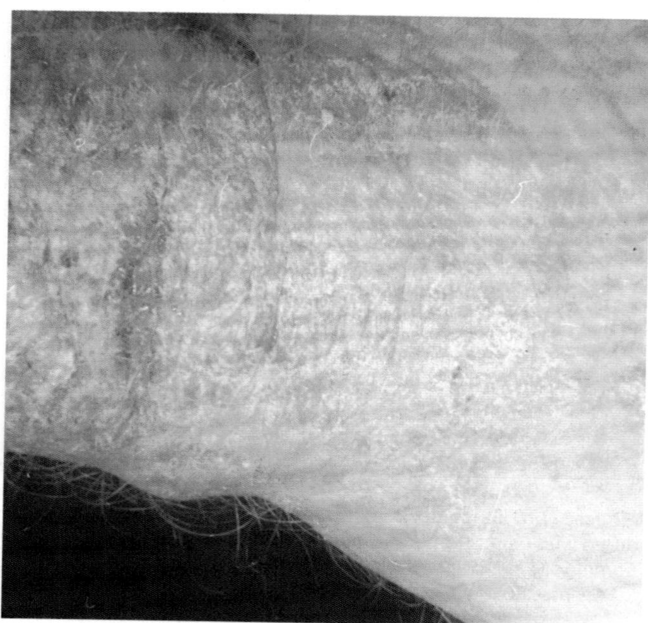

Figure 21.11 **Photoaging.** This wrinkled, leathery, scaly skin is on the dorsum of the right wrist of a farmer.

Too much sun for too long pulverizes the dermis and produces photoaging (Fig. 21.11). Skin over-exposed to sunlight becomes wrinkled, leathery, and scaly. It is home to premalignant keratoses and carries a marked increased risk for skin cancer. Photoaging is exaggerated by smoking.

Photosensitivity (phototoxicity) is an exaggerated reaction to sunlight. It may require only a few minutes of exposure. It is attributable to an underlying condition, such as lupus erythematosus (Chapter 3); to medication such as certain antibiotics (tetracycline, especially), diuretics, or over-the-counter drugs; or to local use of perfumes, cosmetics, or ointments. It may be expressed as almost any type of skin reaction—urticaria (allergic swelling), vesicles (blisters), or erythema. Patients with systemic lupus erythematosus may develop sunburn in a few minutes, or patients applying a new cosmetic may develop an acute skin reaction when the area is exposed to sunlight.

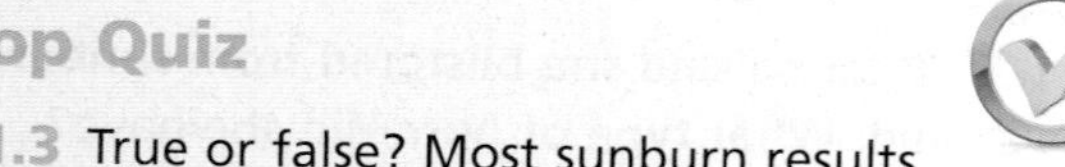

Pop Quiz

21.3 True or false? Most sunburn results in a partial thickness burns (burns with blisters).

21.4 ____________ are distinctive yellowish deposits of lipid.

21.5 Which poisonous agent imparts a cherry red color to the skin? A blue–gray hue?

Infections, Infestations, Bites, and Stings

Impetigo (Fig. 21.12) is a common, highly contagious, superficial skin infection common in healthy preschoolers. Staphylococcus and streptococcus are the usual infective organisms. Impetigo appears first as small pustules that quickly form into small blisters (vesicles) that soon unroof to form erythematous patches that are "honey-crusted" with dried exudate. It is usually asymptomatic and heals without scarring in a few weeks, even without treatment. Systemic infection and complications are rare. Topical therapy and systemic antibiotics are standard treatment.

Erysipelas (Fig. 21.13) is a superficial skin infection usually caused by *Staphylococcus pyogenes* or certain types of streptococci. The initial lesion is small, but it soon blossoms into a bright red, intensely painful, swollen area on the leg or face that may feature small blisters. As infection spreads to the lymphatic system, it causes fever, malaise,

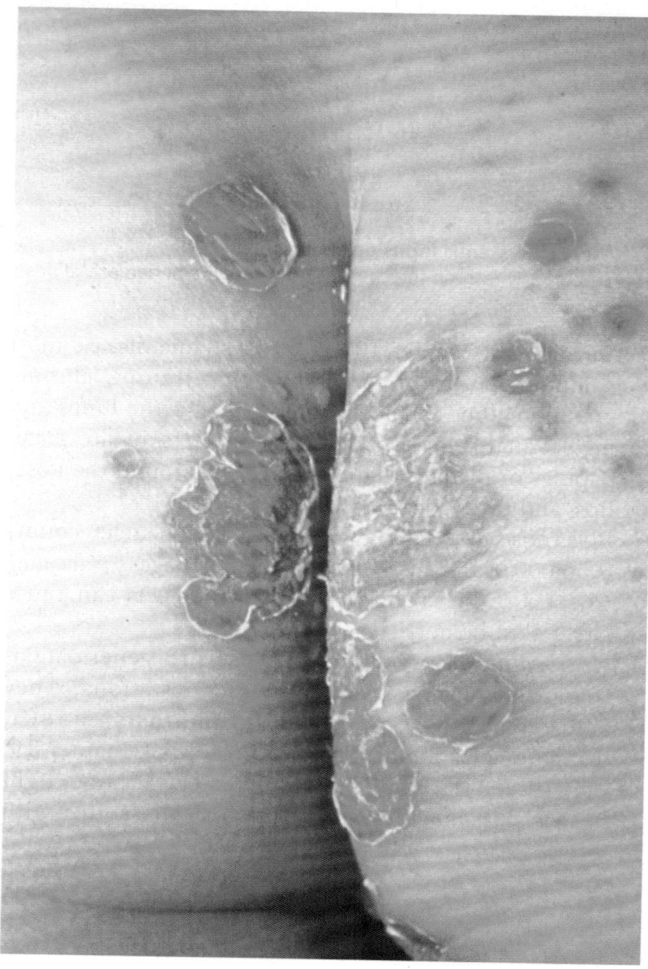

Figure 21.12 **Impetigo** (gluteal cleft in a child). The confluent erythematous patches of denuded vesicles and bullae have crusted rims.

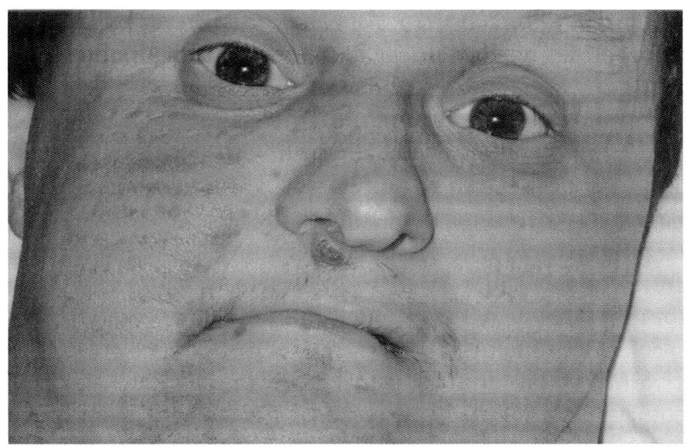

Figure 21.13 **Erysipelas.** Bright red, painful patches. Most cases owe to superficial skin infection by staph or strep. (Reproduced with permission from Berg D, Worzala K. *Atlas of Adult Physical Diagnosis*. Philadelphia, PA: Lippincott Williams & Wilkins; 2006.)

and enlarged, tender, local lymph nodes. Antibiotic treatment is effective.

Dermatophytosis is a common superficial skin, hair, and nail infection caused by a group of fungi that metabolize keratin. Dermatophytosis includes "athlete's foot," "jock itch," and "ringworm" (Fig. 21.14). The infectious agents are *Tinea* species fungi that have evolved an ability to digest keratin in the dead surface cells of the cornified layer of the epidermis, and in nails and hair. Positive diagnosis requires microscopic identification of fungi in scrapings from infected skin (see *The Clinical Side*, "The Potassium Hydroxide [KOH] Test"). Infections respond well to topical antifungals with the exception of nail infections, which may be difficult to eradicate even with prolonged oral antifungal drug therapy if the infection has spread deep under the nail.

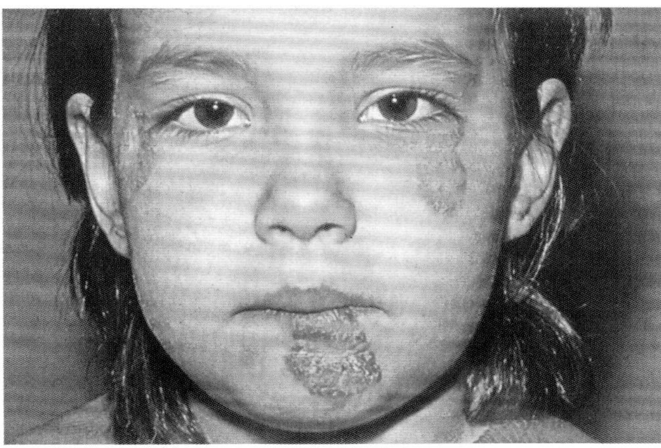

Figure 21.14 **Ringworm** (skin infection by *Taenia sp.* fungi). (Reproduced with permission from Engleberg NC, Dermody T, DiRita V. *Schaecter's Mechanisms of Microbial Disease*. 4th ed. Baltimore, MD: Lippincott Williams & Wilkins; 2007.)

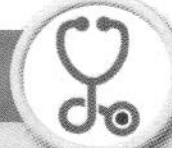

The Clinical Side

THE POTASSIUM HYDROXIDE (KOH) TEST

The KOH test is used in the diagnosis of dermatophytes (skin fungi). The test consists of microscopic examination of hair, skin, or nail scrapings. Skin specimens are collected by scraping at the active edge of the lesion. Nail scrapings are best obtained from beneath the nail edge with a curette or blade. Hair and associated scale are best obtained with a toothbrush.

A thin layer of specimen is placed on a glass slide. A small drop of KOH is added and covered by a glass coverslip. The KOH is heated by a small flame (a match will do) until bubbling begins. The reaction dissolves skin cells and debris, but does not dissolve any fungi that may be present because fungal cell walls contain cellulose, which resists digestion. The preparation is then examined microscopically for fungi (see figure). When performed by an experienced clinician, the KOH test is very accurate.

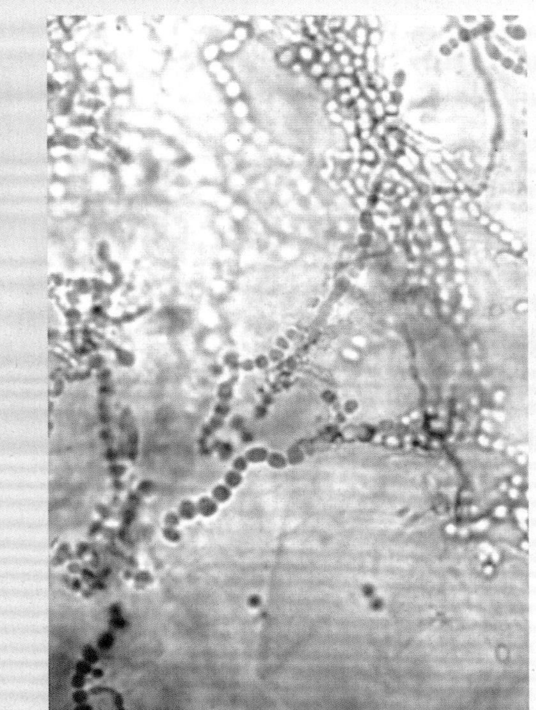

Dermatophyte fungi (*Tinea sp.)* in KOH skin scrapings from a case of ringworm. (Image © LWW.)

Herpesvirus infection causes common cold sores and genital infections (Chapter 4). Cold sores (Fig. 21.15) are painful eruptions of vesicles at the oral mucocutaneous border (where lip mucosa meets lip skin). Typically they are induced by stress, excess sun exposure, or dry, cold air.

Warts (common skin wart, *verruca vulgaris*) are common papillary growths of epidermis (Fig. 21.16) caused

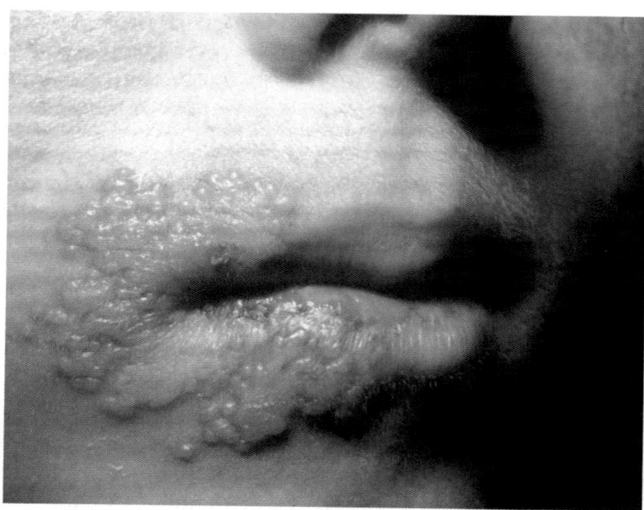

Figure 21.15 **Cold sores** (oral herpesvirus). This patient has an unusually large crop of confluent vesicles.

by certain types of *the human papillomavirus* (HPV). Warts are especially common in children and in patients with AIDS or other immunodeficiency. They are transmitted by casual skin-to-skin contact. In children, they usually disappear spontaneously, but, in adults, they usually persist and may be difficult to eradicate. Over 100 types of HPV have been identified, some of which cause *condyloma acuminatum* and cancers of the genitalia in men (Chapter 16) and women (Chapter 17). Treatment usually is with a topical salicylic acid, but electrocautery or surgical excision may be necessary.

Molluscum contagiosum is a common, self-limited contagious viral disease caused by one variety of the poxvirus. It is often transmitted by sexual contact (Chapter 4). Lesions often occur on the genitals or nearby skin, but may occur on the face, lips, or eyelids. They are small, firm, dome-shaped, white–pink nodules a few mm in diameter (Fig. 21.17). They contain a semisolid cheesy white material. Microscopic study of this material usually shows diagnostic large inclusion bodies (*molluscum bodies*).

Insects can transmit disease (e.g., malaria by mosquitoes, Lyme disease by deer ticks), but a more common problem is bites by mosquitoes, lice, fleas, mites, bedbugs, and ticks. Typically, the bite causes a small maculopapular lesion that itches. The reaction owes to substances injected by the insect. Topical steroids and oral antihistamines are effective treatment.

Mites are exceedingly small insects, almost invisible to the unaided eye, which cause pruritic rashes. The most common variety of mite bite, and the most intensely pruritic, is caused by the **chigger**, which is found outdoors in warm, dry climates. Diagnosis is clinical. Treatment is symptomatic with topical steroids and oral antihistamines.

Scabies is an obligate human parasite that is easily contagious. It is caused by infestation by *Sarcoptes scabiei*. Particularly severe and widespread infection can occur opportunistically in AIDS and other immunocompromised

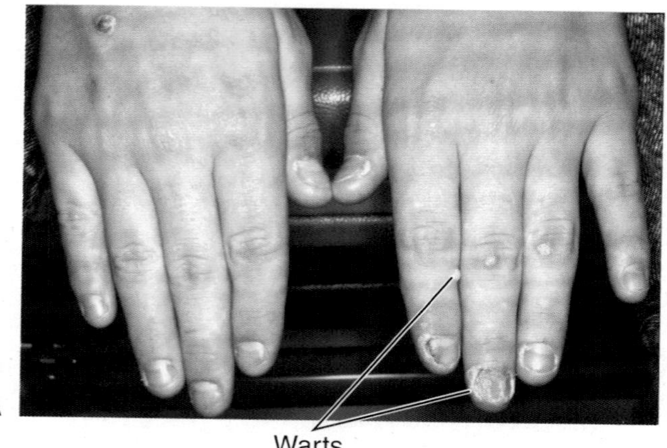

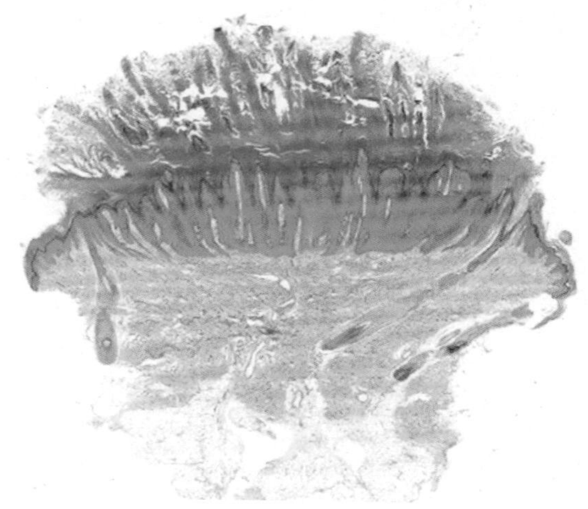

Figure 21.16 **Verrucae vulgaris** (warts). **A.** The multiple papules shown here occurred on the hands of a child. **B.** The microscopic study shows a markedly hyperplastic, jagged overgrowth of epidermis.

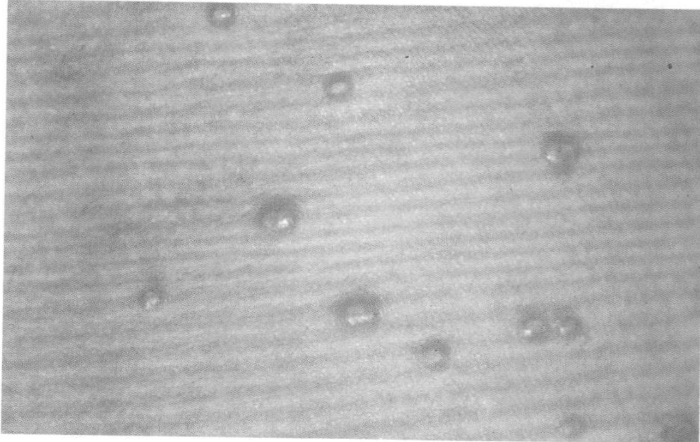

Figure 21.17 **Molluscum contagiosum.** These small nodules contain a semi-solid, cheesy white material. (Reproduced with permission from Goodheart HP. *Goodheart's Photoguide of Common Skin Disorders*. 2nd ed. Philadelphia, PA: Lippincott Williams & Wilkins; 2003.)

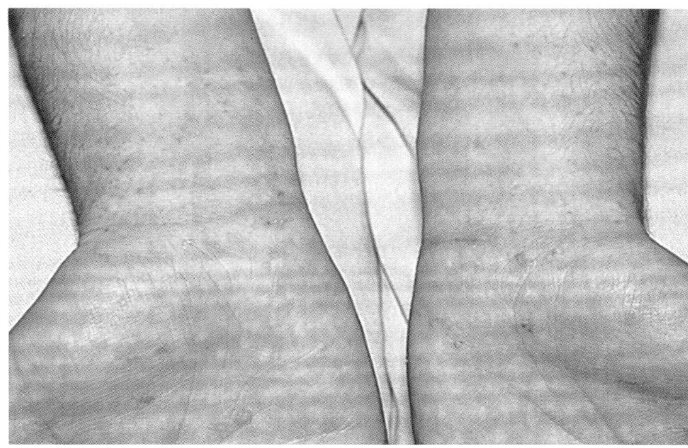

Figure 21.18 **Mite bites** (*scabies*). (Reproduced with permission from Goodheart HP. *Goodheart's Photoguide of Common Skin Disorders*. 2nd ed. Philadelphia, PA: Lippincott Williams & Wilkins; 2003.)

patients. Mites burrow into skin and are so small that they are barely visible to the naked eye. Infestation tends to occur in the web of the fingers or toes, wrist (Fig. 21.18), waistline, and genitals. The reaction is intensely pruritic. Diagnosis is clinical, but may be confirmed by finding the insect in skin scrapings. Special antiscabies ointment is the preferred treatment.

Infestation by **lice** is called **pediculosis**. Lice are wingless, bloodsucking insects that cling to hair or fabric threads. The three varieties of pediculosis—head lice, body lice, and pubic lice—are each caused by a different species.

- *Head lice* live on scalp hair and are transmitted by close contact. They are most common in girls ages 5 to 11. There is no association between head lice and poor hygiene or low socioeconomic status. Diagnosis is by finding larvae (*nits*) on scalp hair (Fig. 21.19). Treatment is hair wash and wet combing with a special medication.

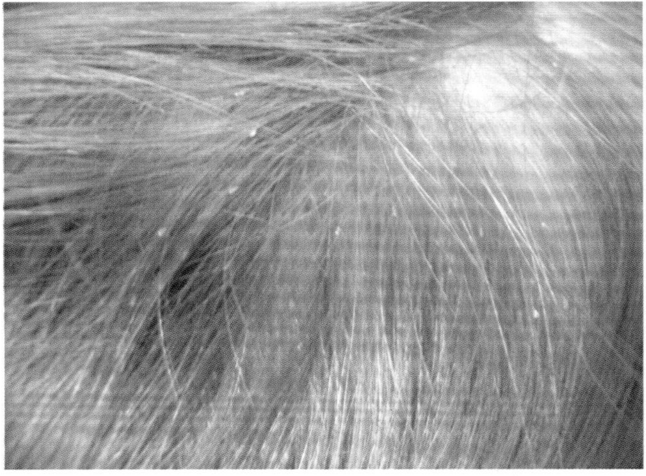

Figure 21.19 **Nits** (larvae) ***of head lice***. (Reproduced with permission from Goodheart HP. *Goodheart's Photoguide of Common Skin Disorders*. 2nd ed. Philadelphia, PA: Lippincott Williams & Wilkins; 2003.)

- *Body lice* live on bedding and clothing, not on people, and usually occur in crowded conditions such as college dormitories or military barracks. Nevertheless, they feed on human flesh. Diagnosis is by finding nits in bedding or clothing. Treatment of bites is symptomatic. Elimination is by thorough cleaning of bedding and clothing.
- *Pubic lice* ("crabs") live in coarse genital hair or sometimes on eyelashes or beards. They are transmitted by sexual or nonsexual intimate family contact. Treatment is washing with a special medication.

Bedbugs are another insect variety, which live in bedding and cloth-covered furniture and feed on blood. Their bites are pruritic like other insect bites. Though they can contain human pathogens, no study has shown them capable of transmitting human disease. Diagnosis is by finding the insect. They can be difficult to find and to eliminate. Treatment is symptomatic.

Pop Quiz

21.6 True or false? Bedbugs are capable of transmitting a wide variety of human diseases.

21.7 What virus causes painful eruptions of vesicles at the oral mucocutaneous border?

Disorders of Hair Follicles and Sebaceous Glands

Acne (Fig. 21.20) is an infectious disease associated with the bacterium *Propionibacterium acnes*. Nevertheless, it is best understood as a disease of hair follicles and sebaceous glands. It primarily affects adolescents and is characterized by red papules and pustules that can lead to unsightly scars.

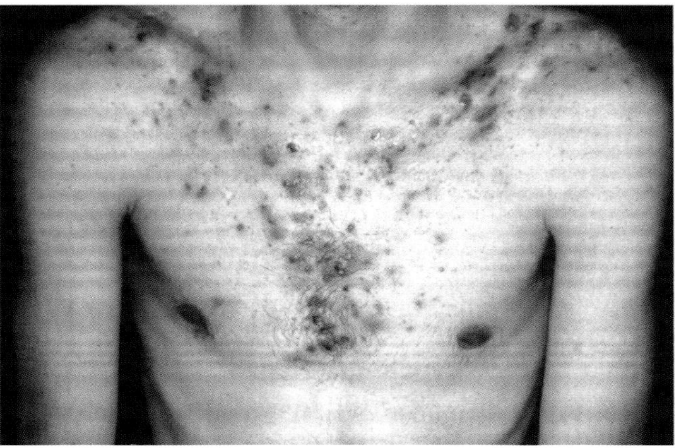

Figure 21.20 **Acne**. Confluent, erythematous papules, patches, and pustules on the chest of a teenager.

Although it is usually a disorder of teenagers, it may persist into adulthood. It is mainly a disease of Caucasians, has a strong genetic component, and begins when hair follicles become plugged by epidermal cells as they are shed. The plugged follicle fills with oily sebaceous gland secretions (*sebum*) to form a noninflammatory plug called a *comedo*. There are two types of comedos—*whiteheads*, pores that have small, tight openings, and *blackheads*, pores that have large openings, revealing a surface layer of dark, oxidized melanin (not dirt). Oily skin produces more and larger comedos, which are hospitable to growth of *Propionibacterium acnes*, a bacterium that colonizes sebum and causes rupture of the comedo and an inflammatory reaction in the surrounding skin. Inflammation may be caused by a direct irritant effect of sebum and keratin, an immune reaction to *P. acnes*, or a direct result of *P. acnes* infection. The result is collections of red papules and pustules over the face and upper chest and back. Treatment is complex. Topical retinoids (part of the vitamin A family) are a mainstay: they inhibit development and reduce inflammation; however, they carry a risk of fetal damage during pregnancy. Oral antibiotics may be useful in severe cases.

Postadolescent acne may arise in adult women, but it seldom occurs in men. Its appearance is related to hormone fluctuations associated with the monthly menstrual cycle. It is less severe than acne vulgaris and is less associated with comedo formation. Lesions appear and disappear quickly as red papules or pustules on the face. When men are affected, the lesions usually appear on the chest and back and are longer lasting.

Rosacea (formerly *acne rosacea*) is an inflammatory disorder of hair follicles and sebaceous glands that is frequently mistaken for acne. Nevertheless, it is confined mainly to fair-skinned women aged 30 or older and of northern European descent; it is not associated with comedos, and it has no relationship to hormonal status. Lesions are red papules and pustules on the face, which are not severe enough to cause scarring. Rosacea may be induced by sun exposure or chronic steroid therapy, but the cause is usually unknown. Treatment is topical, but oral antibiotics may prove useful in difficult cases.

Pop Quiz

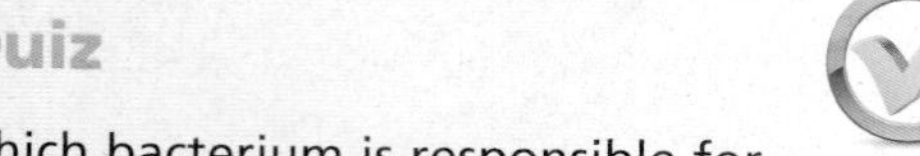

21.8 Which bacterium is responsible for acne?

Dermatitis

Dermatitis is inflammatory skin disease. Most dermatitis is characterized by inflammatory cell infiltrates of superficial skin. It tends to be superficial and involve the epidermis and papillary dermis rather than the deeper reticular dermis and subcutis. Thousands of types and causes have been described. The more common inflammatory dermatoses are discussed below.

Acute Dermatitis Lasts a Few Days or Weeks

Acute dermatitis usually lasts a few days or weeks. Skin is erythematous and often itchy. The inflammatory cell infiltrate is composed of lymphocytes and macrophages instead of neutrophils, usually involves both epidermis and dermis, and is accompanied by vasodilation and edema.

Urticaria

Urticaria (hives) is a localized, acute allergic reaction (*atopy*, Type I hypersensitivity, Chapter 3) that causes local vasodilation, increased vascular permeability, and local edema. The reaction produces short-lived, pale or pink, firm, itchy streaks and papules (Fig. 21.21) that quickly rise and fade in a few hours after exposure to an antigen to which the patient has been previously sensitized. **Angioedema** is similar but affects the deep dermis and subcutis and produces nodular, soft swellings up to several centimeters in diameter. The skin lesions of urticaria are usually innocuous, but they can be associated with systemic anaphylaxis that can be life threatening: anaphylactic vascular collapse or asphyxiation from bronchospasm or laryngeal edema. Urticaria and angioedema occur most frequently between the ages of 20 and 40 years. Treatment consists of avoidance of the offending antigen or administration of antihistamines or steroids.

Acute Eczema

Eczema (Fig. 21.22) is a general term for an acute inflammatory reaction in skin characterized by itchy, weepy, crusted, red lesions. Eczema is a *descriptive term*, not a diagnosis. It is applied to lesions having a certain appearance and says nothing of etiology. The word derives from Greek: *ek* = "out" and *zema* = boiling; hence a "boiling out," which offers a vivid indication of the clinical findings in acute eczema—a hot, bubbly (vesiculated) skin eruption.

Remember This! Eczema is a descriptive term, not a diagnosis.

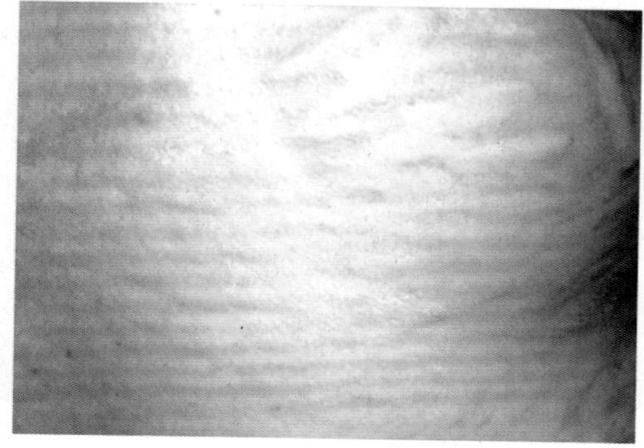

Figure 21.21 **Urticarial wheals**. These pale, pink, itchy streaks occurred in a patient with atopy.

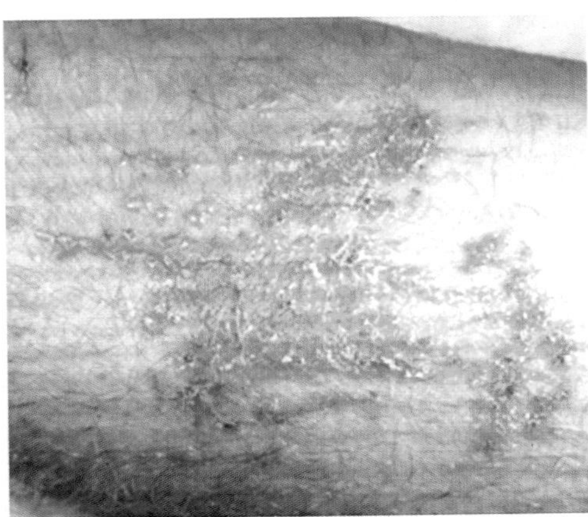

Figure 21.22 **Allergic contact eczema** (Type IV delayed T cell hypersensitivity). A case of allergic contact dermatitis (poison ivy) has produced a weeping, crusted, erythematous collection of vesicles and papules.

Atopic eczema (Fig. 21.23) is a very common dermatitis caused by Type I (atopic) hypersensitivity (Chapter 3) in genetically susceptible persons. It affects about 5% to 10% of the U.S. population. Patients almost always have other atopic conditions such as asthma or hay fever. In infants and children, atopic eczema tends to produce acute, weepy, crusted eruptions on the cheeks, scalp, chest, and extensor surfaces (Fig. 21.24). Children often outgrow the disease. Regardless of age, the lesions are usually itchy (pruritic), and symptoms wax and wane with the intensity of the patient's hay fever or other allergies. In adults, atopic dermatitis may be worse in winter months, when the air is dry; however, usually no precipitating agent can be identified. Topical antihistamines and steroids are mainstays of treatment.

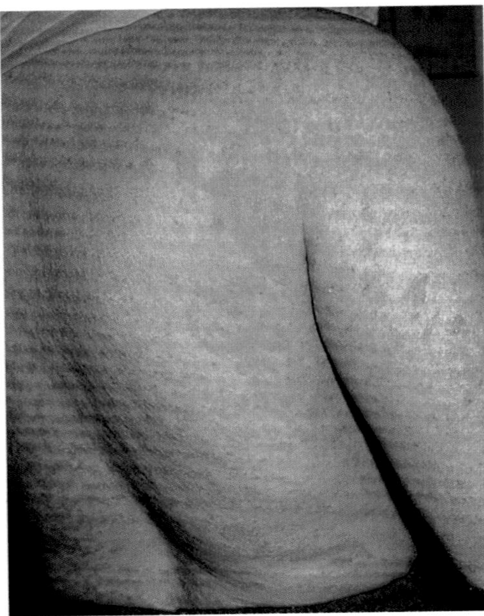

Figure 21.23 **Atopic eczema** (Type I hypersensitivity). This patient had other atopic symptoms (hay fever and asthma). (Reproduced with permission from Goodheart HP. *Goodheart's Photoguide of Common Skin Disorders*. 2nd ed. Philadelphia, PA: Lippincott Williams & Wilkins; 2003.)

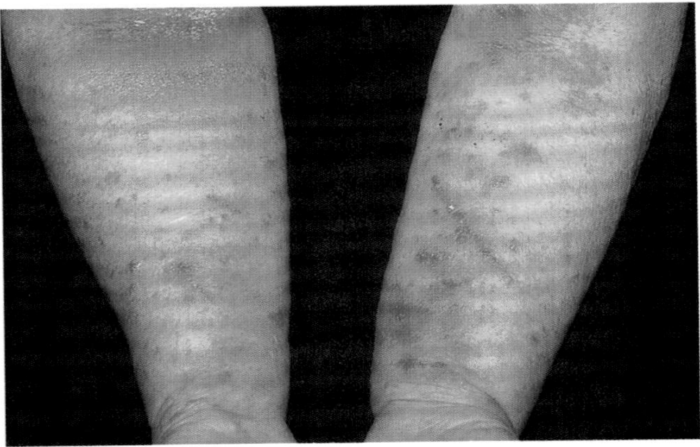

Figure 21.24 **Atopic eczema.** Extensor surfaces are often involved. (Reproduced with permission from Goodheart HP. *Goodheart's Photoguide of Common Skin Disorders*. 2nd ed. Philadelphia, PA: Lippincott Williams & Wilkins; 2003.)

Case Notes

21.4 Regarding Brianna's problem with household detergents: Is it likely she has atopic eczema?

Allergic contact eczema is a delayed-type immune reaction (*delayed*, T-cell–mediated hypersensitivity, Chapter 3) caused by contact with a sensitizing agent. Often the offending agent is a *hapten*, a small molecule that is not capable of stimulating an immune response unless attached to a large protein molecule. For example, the sensitizing agent in poison ivy is a hapten. Upon skin contact, the hapten attaches to an epidermal protein. The combination becomes antigenic, which stimulates a T-cell immune reaction. Within a few days, sensitized T cells proliferate and travel to the point of contact to incite an inflammatory reaction. The list of sensitizing agents is almost limitless—topical antibiotics, metals (such as nickel or gold in jewelry), cosmetics, nail polish, latex gloves, perfume, chemicals in leather, and so on.

Case Notes

21.5 Is it likely Brianna's detergent problem is allergic contact eczema?

Irritant contact eczema is skin inflammation caused by direct skin contact with some environmental substance. It is a very common skin problem. Given the number of things in daily contact with skin, it is somewhat of a miracle we do not have more of it, but the dry, dead cells in the stratum corneum offer little reactivity. It is caused by the direct toxic effect certain chemicals exert upon contact with the skin—no allergy is involved. Common offenders include soaps, solvents, acids, and alkalis found in the home and workplace. The lesions are itchy red, scaly papules and patches, but affected skin tends to be dry, not weepy, because vesicles are less common than in allergic contact dermatitis. The irritant effect of the offending chemical is aggravated by friction or rubbing—"dishpan hands" is one example. "Diaper rash" (Fig. 21.25) is another, which is caused by chafing diapers, soaps, and prolonged exposure to the wet environment of urine and feces. Treatment is by avoidance of the offending substance and by topical therapy with steroids and soothing ointments.

Case Notes

21.6 Is it likely Brianna's detergent problem is irritant contact eczema?

Drug-related eczema is a generalized, symmetric eczema that begins days or weeks after exposure. The list of drugs responsible is almost endless, but penicillin and sulfonamide antibiotics are a frequent cause. *Fixed drug eruptions* are reactions that occur at a single site and recur in the same site with reexposure. Treatment is avoidance.

Photosensory eczema is the development of eczema with sun exposure of skin upon which some cosmetic, perfume, ointment, or other substance has been applied.

Erythema Multiforme

Erythema multiforme (Fig. 21.26) is an acute, self-limited, allergic (Type II hypersensitivity) skin reaction in which antibody attacks cells in the basement membrane

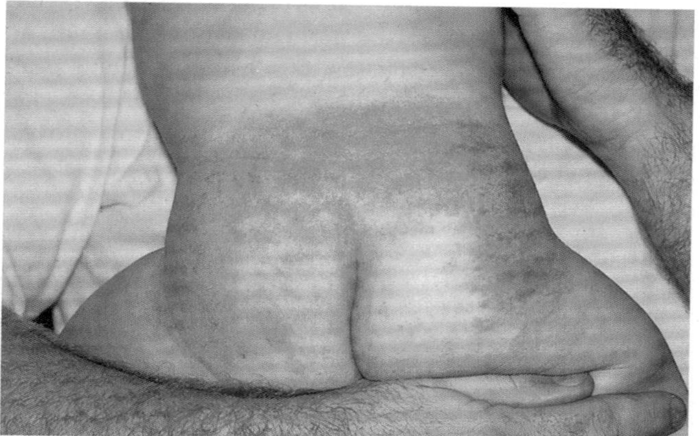

Figure 21.25 **Irritant contact eczema** (diaper rash). (Reproduced with permission from Goodheart HP. *Goodheart's Photoguide of Common Skin Disorders.* 2nd ed. Philadelphia, PA: Lippincott Williams & Wilkins; 2003.)

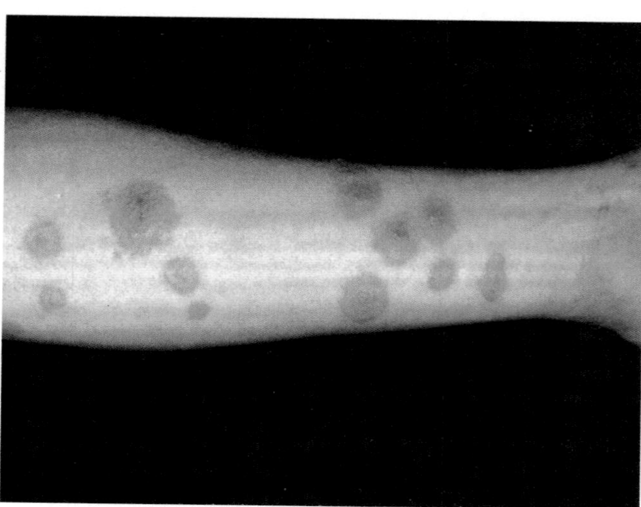

Figure 21.26 **Erythema multiforme** (Type II hypersensitivity). (Reproduced with permission from Roche Laboratories. Sauer GC, Hall JC. *Manual of skin diseases.* 7th ed. Philadelphia, PA: Lippincott-Raven; 1996.)

zone of the epidermis. It is a fairly common, self-limited disease, usually seen on the lips and palms of children or young adults as acute eruptions of round target-like red macules with a dark red or black center. The majority of cases are an autoimmune reaction stimulated by herpesvirus infection elsewhere, usually cold sores. Nevertheless, a long list of drugs and vaccines can also be responsible. Treatment is supportive. Systemic antiviral therapy may be required in severe or recurrent cases.

Stevens-Johnson Syndrome and Toxic Epidermal Necrolysis

Stevens-Johnson syndrome (SJS) and **toxic epidermal necrolysis (TEN)** (Fig. 21.27) differ only in extent: SJS if <10% of skin surface is involved; TEN if involvement is >30%. Most cases are related to drug hypersensitivity, especially sulfa antibiotics and antiseizure medications. The exact mechanism is unknown, but it may be that the drug acts as a hapten that binds to skin protein to produce a combination that stimulates a hypersensitivity reaction in the fashion of poison ivy. It begins as a febrile illness and skin lesions a week or two after exposure. Epidermal blisters appear and progress to necrosis and denuded skin. In its most severe form (TEN), the lesions widen and coalesce to produce skin damage analogous to an extensive burn, in which case fluid management and infection control are paramount concerns. Diagnosis is clinical. Treatment varies with severity. TEN may require hospitalization in a burn unit. Treatment is supportive and eliminating or avoiding known causes.

Chronic Dermatitis Tends to Last for Years

Chronic dermatitis tends to last for years. Acute dermatitis tends to be moist and crusted with exudate, but

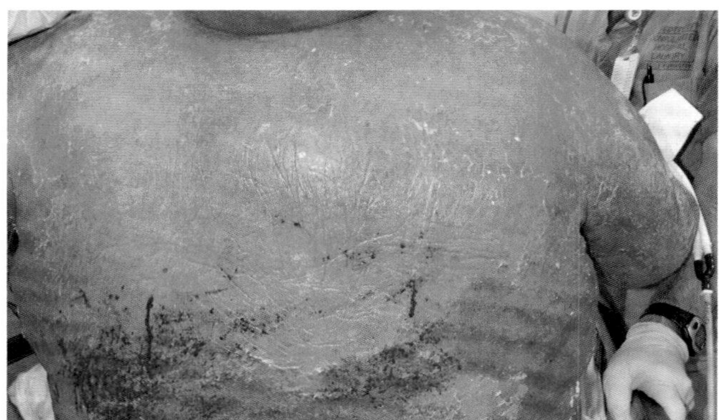

Figure 21.27 **Stevens-Johnson syndrome and toxic epidermal necrolysis.** More than 30% of this patient's skin was involved, so the diagnosis is toxic epidermal necrolysis. (Reproduced with permission from Mulholland MW, Maier RV et al. *Greenfield's Surgery Scientific Principles and Practice*. 4th ed. Philadelphia, PA: Lippincott Williams & Wilkins; 2006.)

chronic lesions are usually dry, scaly, and rough. The epidermis is usually thickened due to epidermal hyperplasia caused by the underlying disease, or by chronic rubbing or scratching.

Just as *eczema* is a descriptive term and not a diagnosis, so **lichen simplex chronicus** (Fig. 21.28) is a pattern of skin reaction that occurs as a common feature of many chronic inflammatory dermatoses. It can occur with any itchy skin disease (usually chronic atopic dermatitis) and is caused by repeated rubbing or scratching. The result is overgrowth (hyperplasia) of the epidermis, producing thick, rough skin with exaggeration of normal skin lines. Lesions are usually solitary, thick plaques on the back of the neck, scalp, forearm, ankle, inner thigh, or lower leg. Diagnosis is clinical. Treatment is aimed at interrupting the itch-scratch-itch cycle by covering the lesion or by use of topical steroids (see *The Clinical Side*, "Topical Steroid Therapy") or oral antihistamines.

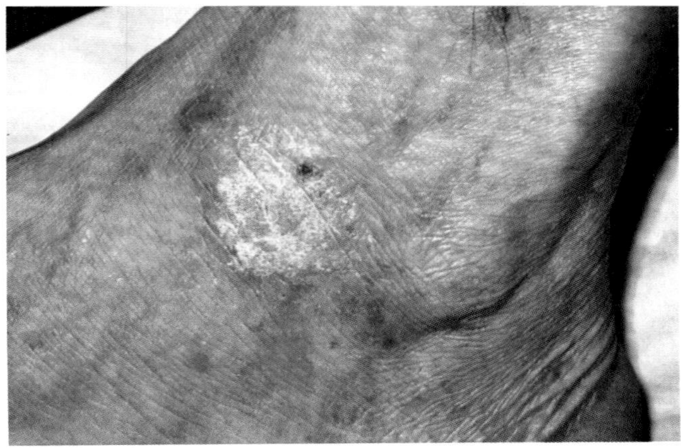

Figure 21.28 **Lichen simplex chronicus**. Shown here is the lateral aspect of the patient's left ankle, the skin of which is thickened and rough from rubbing and scratching subsequent to itching associated with chronic atopic dermatitis.

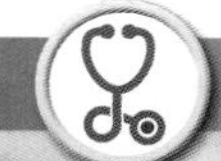

The Clinical Side

TOPICAL STEROID THERAPY

Because of their powerful antiinflammatory effect, topical steroids are widely used in the treatment of skin disease. Topical steroids are divided into classes according to potency: Class I are the most powerful and are synthetic compounds requiring physician prescription; betamethasone and dexamethasone are examples. Class IV are the weakest; over-the-counter hydrocortisone cream is an example. In any given class, little, other than price, recommends one over the other. Steroid ointment is more potent than steroid cream, but it is oilier and messier. Potency dramatically increases when skin is covered with dressings such as bandages or gloves.

Chronic topical steroid therapy causes skin to become thin and fragile. Elderly persons with thin skin should be advised to be careful and use topical steroids sparingly, and all patients should be so advised when applying steroids to thin skin such as the face, scrotum, or vulva. Although absorption into blood occurs, ill effects, such as diabetes or hypertension, are very rare.

Psoriasis

Psoriasis is an acquired proliferative disease of the epidermis characterized by epidermal hyperplasia that forms salmon-colored, dry, scaly, sharply delineated plaques (Fig. 21.29). It affects about 1–2% of the U.S. population and usually appears first in teenagers or young adults. Lesions most often occur bilaterally and with remarkable symmetry on the elbows, knees, and knuckles, but they may spread to involve the low back, scalp, cleft between the buttocks, glans penis, and nails. The patient's main concern usually is the unsightly nature of the lesions. The cause is unknown, but there is a strong genetic component—one-third of patients have a family history of psoriasis. Evidence suggests an autoimmune phenomenon that stimulates excess epidermal growth and is also responsible for the arthritis that occurs in 10–25% of patients. Enteropathy, myopathy, and other autoimmune phenomena may also occur.

Diagnosis is clinical. Skin lesions are treated by methods to slow cell reproduction, such as chemotherapy or immune agents. Less severe cases are treated with topical tar compounds, steroids, or ultraviolet light.

Seborrheic Dermatitis

Dandruff is white flakes of dead skin. When accompanied by inflammation, the diagnosis is **seborrheic dermatitis** (Fig. 21.30), a dermatitis that affects up to 3% of the U.S. population. It occurs in skin with a high concentration of sebaceous glands: scalp, forehead (especially between the

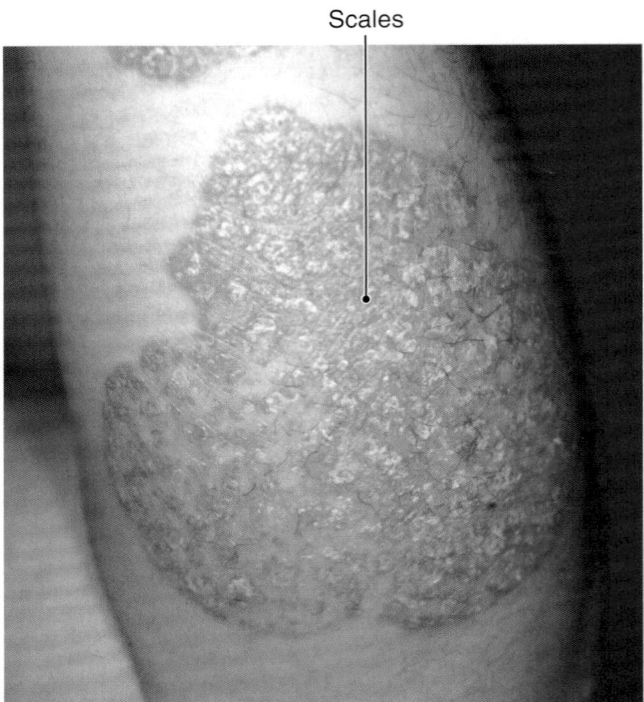

Figure 21.29 **Psoriasis.** A large, scaly, erythematous plaque.

eyebrows), the external auditory canal, behind the ears, in the nasolabial folds, and in the presternal area. Typical lesions are oily, scaly, red patches that shed dandruff. The cause is unknown. Men are more often affected than women. It may affect newborns (cradle cap), children, or adults. For unknown reasons, patients with Parkinsonism and other neurologic disorders may develop severe seborrheic dermatitis. In HIV-positive patients, an outburst of seborrheic dermatitis may be a clue that HIV infection has become serious enough to warrant a diagnosis of AIDS. Diagnosis is clinical. Therapy is topical.

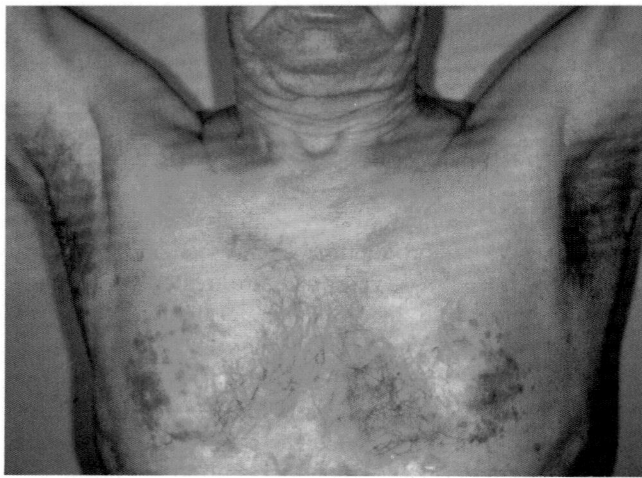

Figure 21.30 **Seborrheic dermatitis**. This severe case is composed of confluent papules and plaques in the oily skin of the chest and axillae. The face and scalp were also involved.

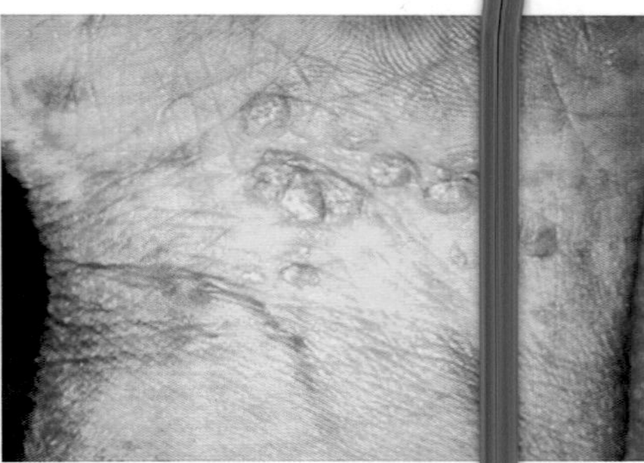

Figure 21.31 **Lichen planus.** These pruritic, pu[illegible]e, polygonal, planar papules and plaques are on the volar surface of[illegible]e wrist.

Lichen Planus

Lichen planus (Fig. 21.31) is a chro[illegible] disease of unknown cause that affects skin or the or[illegible] mucosa. Lesions are characterized by "the six Ps": prurit[illegible] purple, polygonal, planar papules and plaques of the [illegible]ists, ankles, and penis. In most cases, the lesions spo[illegible]aneously regress within a year or two. Oral lesions appe[illegible] as white-capped plaques (leukoplakia), which may pers[illegible] for many years. It occurs with greater frequency in pati[illegible]ts with other autoimmune diseases such as systemic lu[illegible]s erythematosus or ulcerative colitis. Therapy is usually [illegible]ot necessary.

Stasis Dermatitis

Stasis dermatitis accompanies severe [illegible]aricose veins in the legs. Sluggish blood flow causes [illegible]cal hypoxia and skin injury. Typically affected skin is [illegible]ollen, firm, and hyperpigmented. The epidermis frequ[illegible]tly is itchy, red, and scaly. Severe cases may progress [illegible] ulceration and infection. Lesions are most notable ove[illegible]the medial ankle and heel (Fig. 21.32). Diagnosis is cli[illegible]cal. Treatment is directed at improving blood flow and [illegible]eventing the occurrence or progression of ulcers.

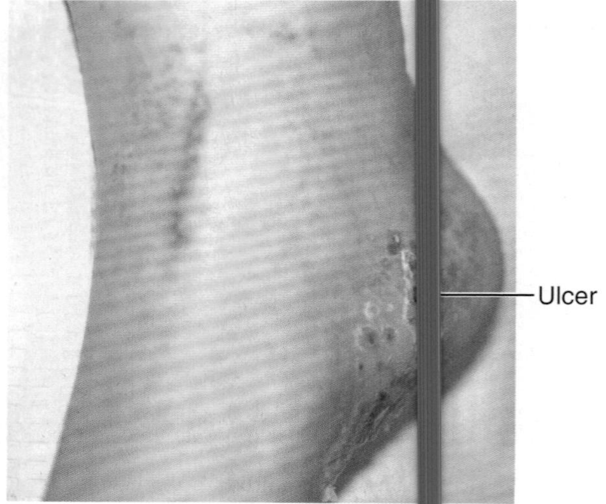

Figure 21.32 **Chronic stasis dermatitis.** The a[illegible]phic, ulcerated skin shown here is on the medial aspect of the an[illegible] of a patient with severe varicose veins (not evident).

Pop Quiz

21.9 True or false? Allergic contact eczema is a Type I (atopic) hypersensitivity reaction.

21.10 Stevens-Johnson Syndrome is diagnosed if less than ______% of skin surface is involved, while toxic epidermal necrolysis is diagnosed if greater than ________% of skin surface is involved.

21.11 Which lesion is characterized by "the six Ps": pruritic, purple, polygonal, planar papules and plaques of the wrists, ankles, and penis?

Diseases of the Dermis and Subcutis

Whereas dermatitis tends to be superficial and nonfibrotic, other conditions affect deeper layers of skin and are mainly fibrotic.

Scleroderma (*systemic sclerosis*) is a chronic systemic autoimmune disease that occurs most often in women, especially young women. It is characterized by microvascular damage and fibrosis of intercellular tissue in many organs. The gastrointestinal tract, lungs, kidney, heart, and skeletal muscle also may be affected. In skin, the dermis is dense and sclerotic to a degree that may be deforming (Chapter 3, Fig. 3.13). The normal loose, interwoven character of dermal collagen is replaced by dense bands of collagen that destroy hair follicles and other structures, leaving skin tight and smooth and devoid of hair follicles, sebaceous glands, or sweat glands. Raynaud phenomenon (Chapter 8) is almost always present. Diagnosis is clinical with laboratory confirmation of certain autoimmune antibodies in blood. No generalized treatment has proved effective, though some organ-specific therapies may prolong life.

Panniculitis is a subacute to chronic inflammatory and fibrotic disease of subcutaneous tissue (panniculus). The lower legs are most often affected. The most common form is **erythema nodosum**, an acute disease, probably due to autoimmunity, that is characterized by red, extremely tender nodules of chronic inflammation and fibrosis in the subcuticular tissue on the anterior aspect of the lower legs (Fig. 21.33). It is most common in young adult women and most often occurs 1) in patients with infections (such as streptococcal infections or tuberculosis), 2) in patients taking certain drugs (sulfonamide antibiotics, oral contraceptives), or 3) in patients with certain illnesses (sarcoidosis, inflammatory bowel disease, and some malignancies). Nevertheless, in many instances, no associated condition is identifiable. It usually begins as a febrile illness followed by tender skin nodules a few days later. Diagnosis is usually clinical but in some instances

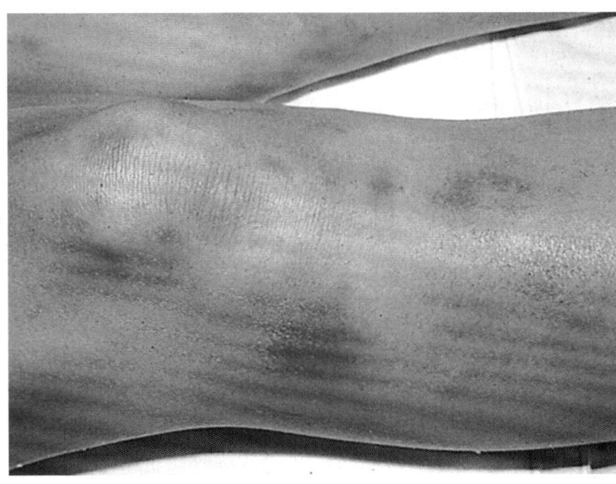

Figure 21.33 **Erythema nodosum**. Lesions are usually on the anterior aspect of the lower leg. (Image © LWW.)

biopsy may be required. Most cases resolve spontaneously within a few weeks. Treatment is supportive.

Weber-Christian disease is widespread panniculitis. It is a rare condition characterized by skin nodules, fever, fatigue, nausea, vomiting, weight loss, and joint pain. It is often associated with other conditions such as pancreatitis, pancreatic carcinoma, infections, or autoimmune disorders. Sometimes Weber-Christian disease appears as a paraneoplastic syndrome (Chapter 5) associated with an undiagnosed (hidden, occult) visceral cancer.

Pop Quiz

21.12 True or false? Scleroderma causes tightening of the skin, which is otherwise architecturaly unchanged.

Blistering Diseases

Bullous diseases of skin are mainly characterized by blisters, which can be small (*vesicles*) or large (*bullae*). They are classified according to the skin layer in which they form. *Subcorneal blisters* form beneath the surface cornified layer of the epidermis. *Suprabasal blisters* form immediately above the layer of basal cells. *Subepidermal blisters* form at the basement membrane, beneath the epidermis and dermis. Skin biopsy is usually required to make a diagnosis.

Inflammatory Blistering Diseases Are Autoimmune

Pemphigus (from Greek *pemphix* = bubble) is a serious blistering disease that features intraepidermal and

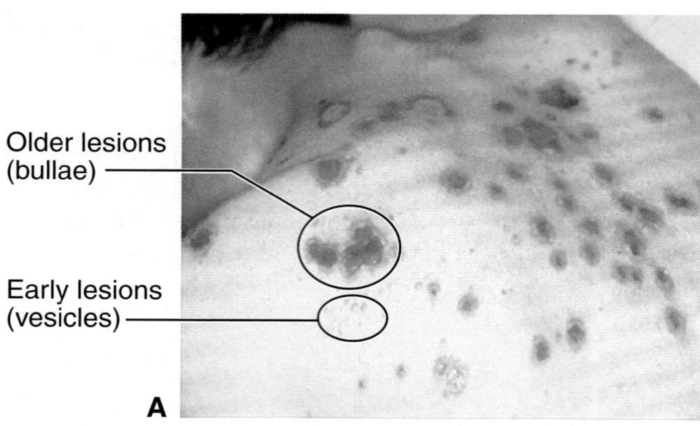

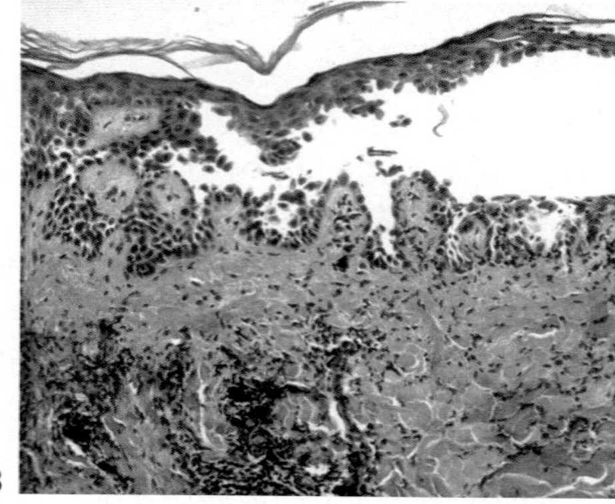

Figure 21.34 **Pemphigus. A.** Fresh lesions are small, intact vesicles. Older lesions are large, unroofed bullae that are now shallow ulcers. **B.** Microscopic study shows separation of epidermal layers. (**B.** Reproduced with permission from Rubin E, Farber JL. *Pathology*. 3rd ed. Philadelphia, PA: Lippincott Williams & Wilkins; 1999.)

suprabasilar blisters. Though rare, its pathogenesis offers valuable insights. It is caused by autoimmune antibody attack on intercellular connections (desmosomes), which bind epidermal cells to each other. It is most common in middle-aged adults and occurs most often in people of Mediterranean heritage. Skin (Fig. 21.34A) is the primary target, but the oral mucosa is often affected, sometimes in advance of skin. As epidermal cells come unglued (Fig. 21.34B), fluid accumulates in intraepidermal blisters (small vesicles or large bullae), which rupture to leave weeping, crusted, inflamed patches. Pemphigus usually begins in mature adults and affects the trunk, face, neck, and scalp, sparing the extremities. Skin infection is a frequent complication. Diagnosis is clinical. Severe cases can be fatal. Immunosuppressive agents are mainstays of treatment.

Bullous pemphigoid is a chronic blistering disease resulting from an autoimmune autoantibody attack against the basement membrane; fluid seeps into the loosened space to form subepidermal blisters. It is clinically similar to pemphigus, hence the name pemphigoid. Most cases are mild and disappear without therapy, but severe cases may be fatal if not treated. Diagnosis is clinical. Systemic steroid therapy is effective.

Dermatitis herpetiformis is an autoimmune disease. Most cases are associated with subclinical gluten-sensitive enteropathy (celiac sprue, Chapter 11). IgA-gluten immune complexes deposit in the superficial dermis and cause acute inflammation, which loosens the attachment of basement membrane and epidermis and allows accumulation of fluid as blisters. It presents as a chronic, pruritic (itchy) eruption of papules, clusters of vesicles (which look like herpes, hence "herpetiformis"), and urticarial wheals. These lesions gradually appear on the elbows, knees, buttocks, sacrum, and back of the head in middle-aged adults. Diagnosis is clinical. In gluten-related cases, a gluten-free diet is effective. Some cases can be managed by use of sulfonamide antibiotics (the mechanism is unknown).

Non-Inflammatory Blistering Diseases Are Genetic

Epidermolysis bullosa is a group of rare, blistering diseases caused by genetically defective binding of epidermis to dermis at the basement membrane. There are many dozens of genetic variants, all of which share a tendency to cause the formation of blisters at sites of pressure or minor trauma, usually on the hands and feet. Most varieties of epidermolysis bullosa are cosmetically disturbing but manageable; however, some can be fatal.

Porphyria is a group of inherited disorders of porphyrin metabolism. Porphyrins are pigments normally present in hemoglobin and myoglobin. The five major clinical types are caused by upwards of 250 different genetic defects. Signs and symptoms are bewilderingly variable. Among the most common problems are abdominal pain and neurologic defects. Skin lesions include urticaria and subepidermal blisters that are exacerbated by sunlight and that heal with scars.

Pop Quiz

21.13 True or false? Most cases of dermatitis herpetiformis are associated with subclinical gluten-sensitive enteropathy.

21.14 True or false? Epidermolysis bullosa forms blisters at sites of pressure or minor trauma, usually on the hands and feet.

Disorders of Pigmentation and Melanocytes

The most noticeable attribute of skin is its color (see discussion above). The degree of skin pigmentation is perhaps the most important distinguishing attribute of a healthy person, and it has profound social implications in all cultures. Normal skin color is shaded from very dark brown–black to light tan in infinitely small increments from one person to the next, depending on the amount of melanin in it.

Melanin is a dark brown pigment made by **melanocytes** located in the lower epidermis. After synthesis, it is distributed to nearby basal cells of the epidermis, so that most skin pigment is located in the basal cell layer. Pigmentary disorders, therefore, may result from decreased or increased numbers of melanocytes, or greater or lesser melanin production.

General darkening of the skin may appear as a manifestation of other disease or as a result of drug treatment. In Addison disease (Chapter 14), the adrenals fail and the pituitary secretes large amounts of ACTH in response. Metabolic breakdown of ACTH produces melanocyte-stimulating hormone (MSH), which causes increased melanin production in skin. For example, President John Kennedy's famous tan was not obtained at the beach—Kennedy had Addison disease. Rarely, dark skin is caused by increased levels of other compounds, most notably iron deposits in the skin associated with hemochromatosis (Chapter 12).

Vitiligo and Albinism Are Diseases of Depigmentation

Vitiligo (Fig. 21.35) is a common, acquired disorder characterized by white macules that may coalesce into large patches of bone-white, utterly depigmented skin. Melanocytes are absent in affected areas. It usually begins about age 20, but people of all ages are affected. It is seen especially in people with diabetes, Addison disease, thyroiditis, or pernicious anemia, or after head trauma. The cause is unknown, but an autoimmune reaction is suspected—other autoimmune disease is often present, including Hashimoto thyroiditis, Graves disease, Addison disease, and inflammatory bowel disease. Systemic phototherapy is successful in stimulating cosmetic repigmentation in a majority of cases.

Albinism is a very rare, genetic lack of melanin pigment owing to an inability of melanocytes to produce melanin pigment. Patients have very white skin and pink eyes (because they lack iris pigment).

Case Notes

21.7 **Brianna had noticeably pale skin. Did she have albinism or vitiligo?**

Freckle and Lentigo Are Non-Neoplastic Pigmentary Lesions

A **freckle** (ephelis) is a small macule of increased pigment in basal cells of the epidermis. It is caused by localized increased sensitivity of melanocytes to sunlight; the number of skin melanocytes is normal. Freckles appear or darken in summer and fade in winter according to sun exposure.

Lentigo (Fig. 21.36) is also characterized by patches of dark skin, but differs from freckles and melasma—lentigo is caused by a localized hyperplasia of melanocytes in skin. Lentigo is not neoplastic. Lesions are usually larger and more deeply pigmented than freckles; and freckles

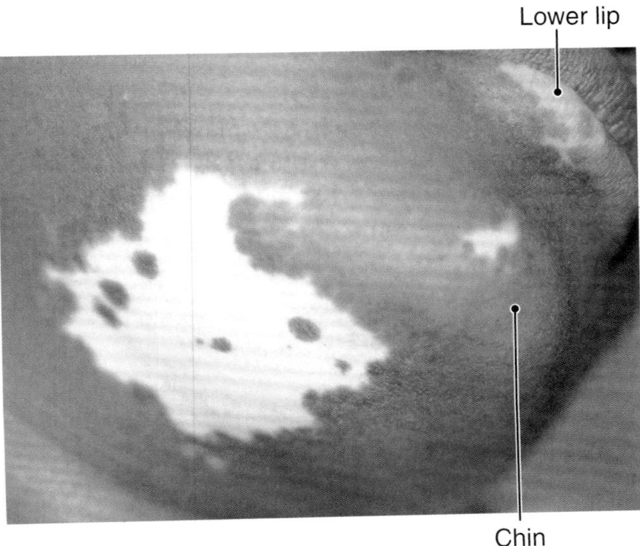

Figure 21.35 **Vitiligo.** These confluent macules and patches are on the chin and lower lip of an African American boy.

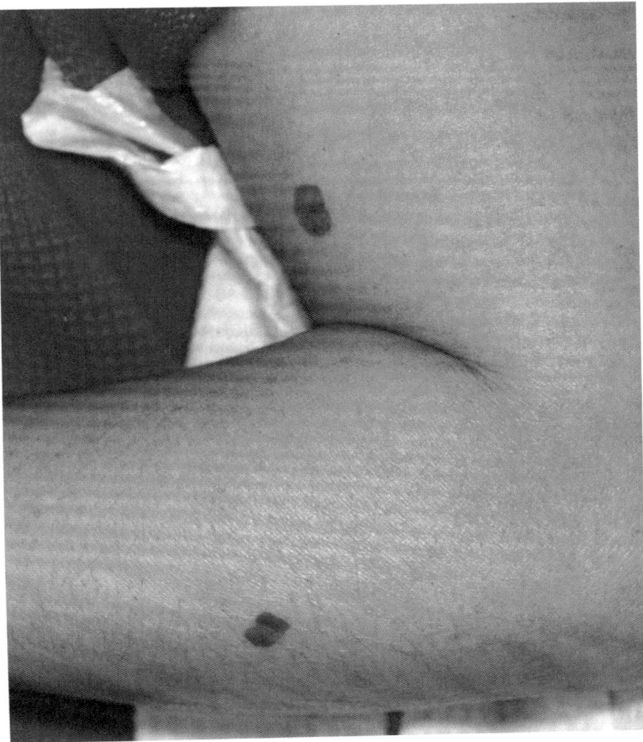

Figure 21.36 **Lentigo.** The flat, brown patches shown here are typical.

darken with sun exposure, whereas lentigo does not. The common pigmented mole is also composed of a localized collection of melanocytes; however, moles are nodular, and lentigo is macular (flat, nonpalpable).

Case Notes

21.8 Brianna had freckles. In the freckles, were there too many melanocytes?

Melanocytic Nevi Are Benign Tumors of Melanocytes

Melanocytic nevus (*pigmented nevus, pigmented mole,* Fig. 21.37) is an acquired benign tumor of melanocytes. There are several histologic varieties, some of which can be confused microscopically with malignant melanoma. Nevi are common and usually benign, appearing before age 20. They arise as a brown papule about 1 mm in diameter and slowly enlarge and become darker. They usually stop growing before they reach 5 mm in diameter, and, after many years, they tend to become pale and flat. In most people, the number of nevi gradually declines with age. They may darken and grow with pregnancy, but involute after birth. They are most common in persons with white skin who were exposed to significant amounts of sunlight in childhood. People with deeply pigmented skin rarely develop nevi. A clear relationship exists between the amount of sun exposure, the development of nevi, and the development of malignant melanoma. As a rule, a person with a large number of nevi (e.g., many dozens) is more likely to develop malignant melanoma than a person with a few nevi; however, because nevi are so common, the risk is very small that any given nevus will become malignant. Diagnosis is clinical. Some nevi are removed for cosmetic purposes.

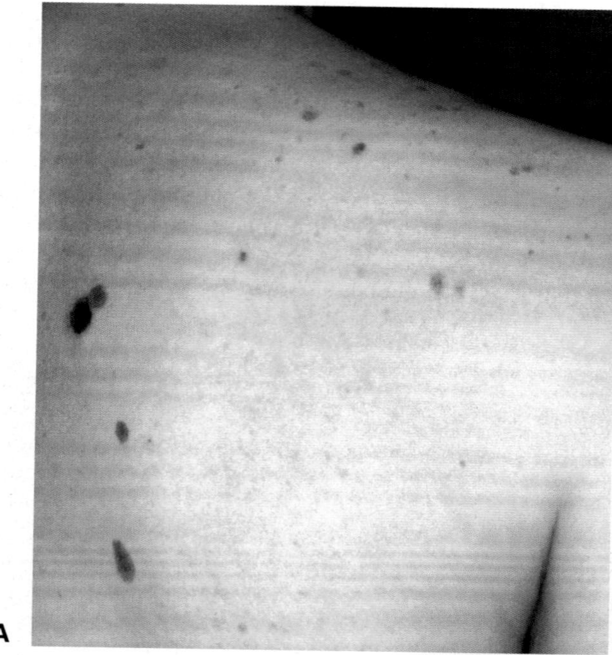

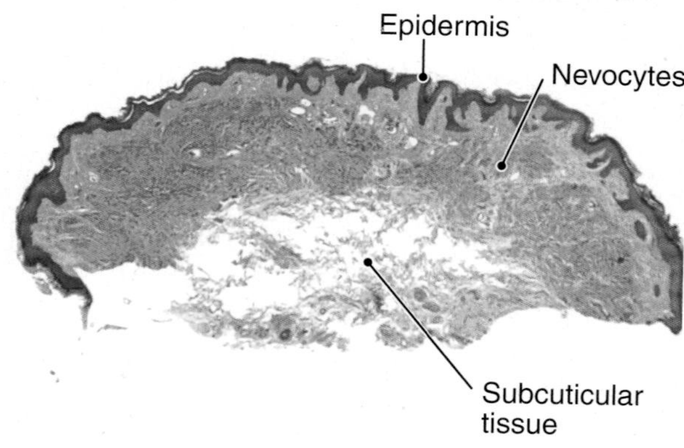

Figure 21.37 **Melanocytic nevi. A.** The multiple pigmented small (papules) and large (plaques) lesions on the back. **B.** In this microscopic study, nevus cells (benign melanocytes) are present in the dermis.

A **dysplastic nevus** is a distinctive clinical lesion worthy of note because of its relationship to malignant melanoma. Dysplastic nevi are usually larger (6–15 mm) than a common nevus and are surrounded by a slowly enlarging collar of irregularly pigmented skin. Dysplastic nevi are controversial. Though they are premalignant, they do not often become malignant, so it is debatable how much alarm should be attached to each individual one. Nevertheless, this much seems clear: people with large numbers of dysplastic nevi are at a much greater risk of developing malignant melanoma than people with one or two dysplastic nevi. Patients with multiple dysplastic nevi and a family history of malignant melanoma may have a genetic condition, *heritable melanoma syndrome*, which is associated with a very high risk for malignant melanoma. These people should have their skin examined by a dermatologist every year.

Case Notes

21.9 Brianna had several dysplastic nevi. Did this put her at risk for melanoma?

21.10 Did Brianna probably have heritable melanoma syndrome?

Melanoma Is a Malignant Tumor of Melanocytes

Melanoma (or *malignant melanoma* [MM]) (Fig. 21.38) is a malignant neoplasm of melanocytes. It is by far the most dangerous skin cancer and the most common malignancy of any kind occurring in women ages 25–29.

Remember This! Melanoma is the most common malignancy in women ages 25–29.

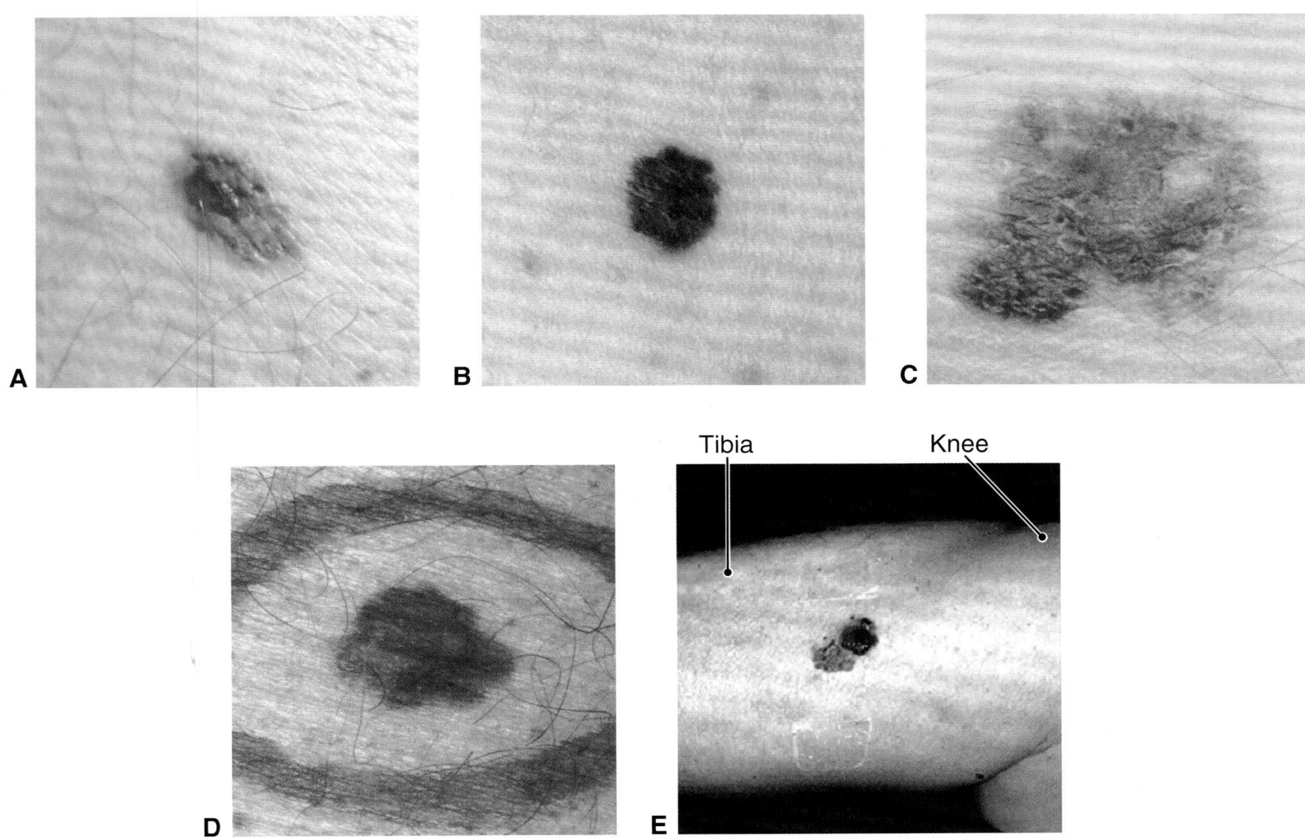

Figure 21.38 **Melanoma**. Important clues in each of these lesions are as follows: **A.** The irregular border of the lesion and the variation of pigmentation. **B.** The deep black pigmentation and the irregular border. **C.** The very irregular border and the variation of pigmentation. **D.** The pinkish area and the irregular border. **E.** The large size, pinkish area, variation of pigmentation, and irregular border of this neglected lesion on the lower leg.

The great majority of melanomas arise in skin, but some develop on mucosal surfaces of the vagina, oral cavity, and anus, and others in the eye or the meninges, each of which normally contain melanocytes. These diverse sites seem odd until one recalls that melanocytes are neuroectodermal cells, having common ancestry with nerves. MM occurs most often on sun-exposed skin, and light-skinned persons are more at risk than those with darker skin. About 75% of MM arise spontaneously and the remaining 25% arise from preexisting nevi (common moles). A fact worthy of special note: one of the most important signs of early melanoma is change in the appearance of a common mole.

Case Notes

21.11 Brianna was 29 when she died of melanoma. Of malignancies in women near her age, what is the most common one?

Grading and Staging

MM begins as a proliferation of melanocytes in the basal cell layer of the epidermis near the basement membrane. This initial malignant stage is *melanoma in situ*—growth is confined to the epidermis and has not broken through the basement membrane to invade the dermis, where it can gain access to blood vessels and lymphatics. After penetrating the basement membrane, it invades the upper few tenths of a millimeter of superficial dermis (microinvasion) and spreads outward in the radial growth phase called *superficial spreading melanoma* (Fig. 21.39A). In the radial growth stage, melanoma rarely metastasizes. Nevertheless, with time, the tumor enters the vertical growth phase and becomes much more dangerous, as it penetrates deeper into the dermis and forms a mass (*nodular malignant melanoma*, Figs. 21.39B and 21.40).

Case Notes

21.12 Was Brianna's melanoma a melanoma in situ?

MM spreads by lymphatic and vascular invasion. One of the most fearsome features about melanoma is its tendency for vascular invasion while still small. Vascular

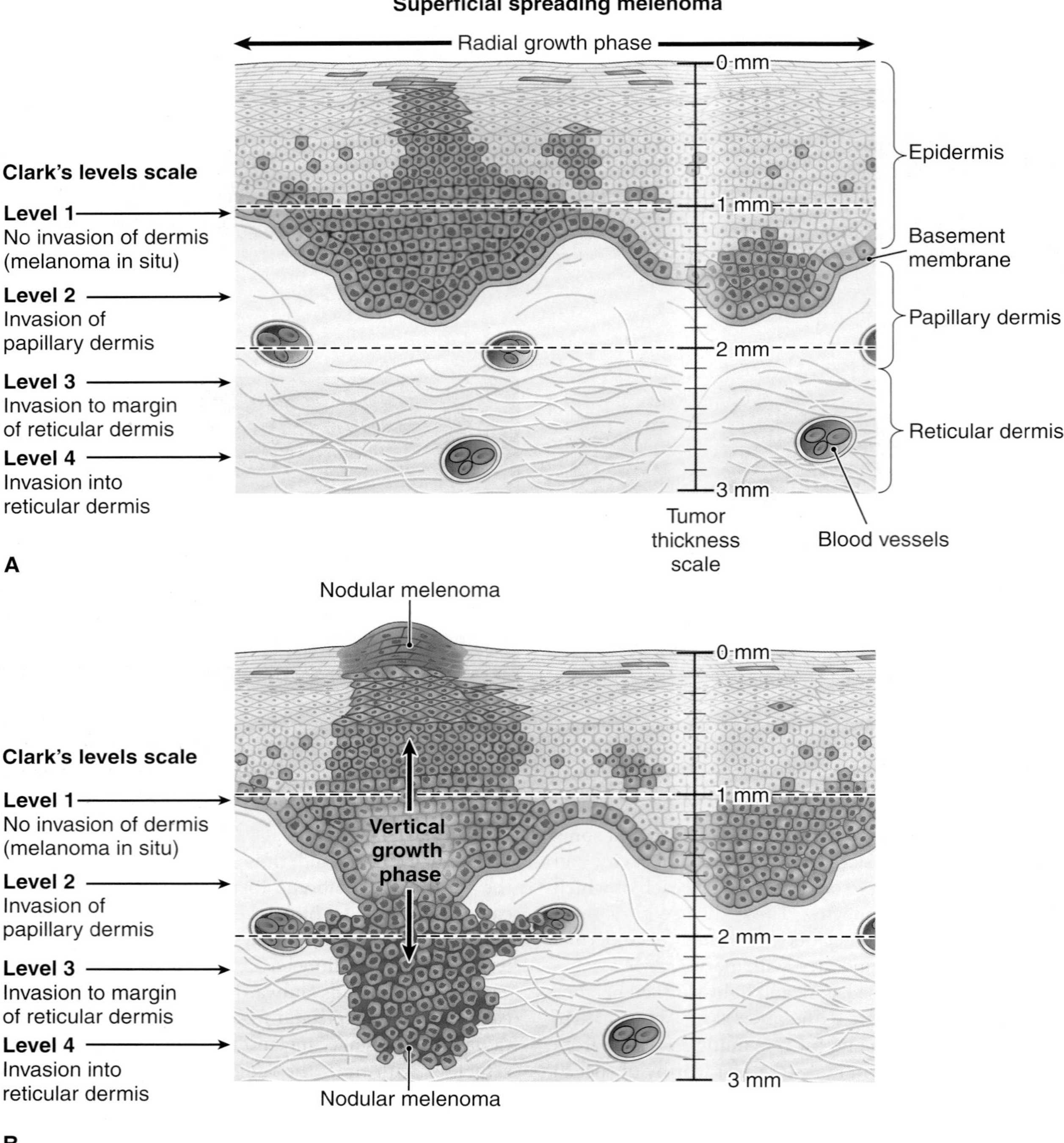

Figure 21.39 **The growth of melanoma. A.** Radial growth phase (superficial spreading melanoma). **B.** Vertical growth phase (nodular melanoma).

metastases usually appear first in the brain and lungs. Lymphatic metastases also occur but are not as dangerous.

The metastatic potential of any given melanoma can be estimated by careful microscopic measurements of the tumor, a process known as "microstaging." There are two methods:

- *Clark* method defines four levels (Levels 1–4) according to the deepest invasion of the tumor as indicated by the microscopic anatomy of the epidermis and dermis (Fig. 21.39).
- *Breslow* method is a simple measure of the maximum thickness of the tumor. The five-year survival rate for tumors that have less than 1.0 mm of dermal invasion is 95+%; 1–2 mm, 80–95%; 2.1–4 mm, 60–75%; and >4 mm, 35–50%.

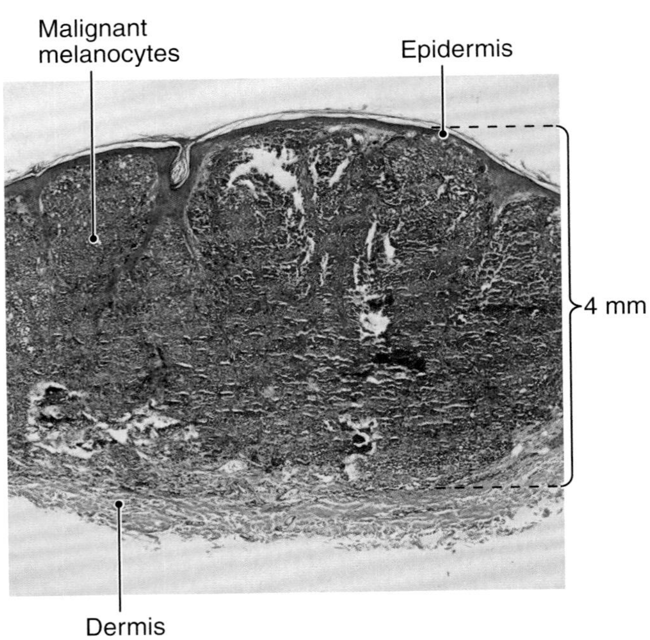

Figure 21.40 **Nodular melanoma**.

More recently, the American Joint Committee on Cancer (AJCC) has implemented a TNM (Chapter 5) staging method that incorporates microstaging and other features such as the presence or absence of tumor ulceration, lymph node metastasis, and distant metastasis. At whatever depth, the survival rate for women is somewhat better than for men.

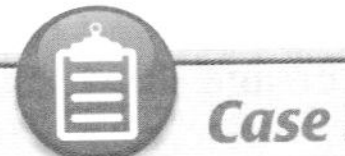

Case Notes

21.13 What was the Breslow thickness of Brianna's melanoma?

21.14 What was the Clark level of Brianna's melanoma?

Signs and Symptoms

The typical MM is a pigmented plaque about 1 cm in diameter with irregular borders and varying degrees of pigmentation (Fig. 21.38). Some melanomas may have areas of very dark tissue and others of light tan or pink, unpigmented tissue.

The most important clinical alarm signals for melanoma are the following:

1. Rapid enlargement of an existing pigmented lesion
2. A nodule in an otherwise flat pigmented skin lesion
3. Itching, pain, or bleeding in a previously asymptomatic pigmented lesion
4. Development of a new pigmented lesion in adult life
5. Irregular borders of a pigmented lesion
6. Satellite areas of pigmentation around a pigmented lesion
7. Varied coloration in a pigmented lesion, especially spots of pink or gray decoloration or spots that are much blacker than the rest of the lesion

Case Notes

21.15 From the nearby list of alarm signals, which ones did Brianna's lesion show for certain?

If a pigmented lesion looks suspicious, it warrants excisional biopsy—the entire lesion should be excised, because excision may prove curative. This also allows evaluation of the entire lesion and avoids disturbing the tumor by cutting directly into it.

Diagnosis and Treatment

Diagnosis requires biopsy. The medical community and general public have become better informed about melanoma in recent decades. As a result, lesions are now detected earlier and survival rates have improved substantially.

Treatment is surgical excision, chemotherapy, and immunotherapy, including vaccination. Research on a melanoma vaccine is at the forefront of cancer research and relies on the idea of injecting melanoma-related antigens to stimulate the immune system to fight the melanoma, either directly or by upregulating existing immune surveillance anticancer mechanisms (Chapter 3). Short-term results are encouraging, but their capacity to increase long-term survival is uncertain.

Pop Quiz

21.15 True or false? Albinism is a very rare, genetic lack of melanin pigment due to the inability of melanocytes to produce melanin pigment.

21.16 True or false? Freckles are characterized by localized hyperplasia of melanocytes in skin.

21.17 True or false? People exposed to relatively large amounts of sunlight in childhood are more likely to develop nevi.

21.18 True or false? Twenty-five percent (25%) of MM arise spontaneously and the remaining 75% arise from preexisting nevi.

Neoplasms of Skin Not Including Melanoma

Nonmelanoma skin neoplasms are classified according to the tissue or cells from which they arise:

- Tumors of the epidermis, which includes keratoses, epidermoid cysts, and basal and squamous carcinoma
- Tumors of the dermis, which includes tumors of sebaceous and sweat glands and other adnexal structures
- Tumors of the dermis and subcutaneous tissues, which includes lipoma (a tumor of fat), dermatofibroma (a tumor of fibrous tissue), hemangioma (a tumor of blood vessels), and neurofibroma (a tumor of nerves)
- Cellular migrants to skin, including immune system cells

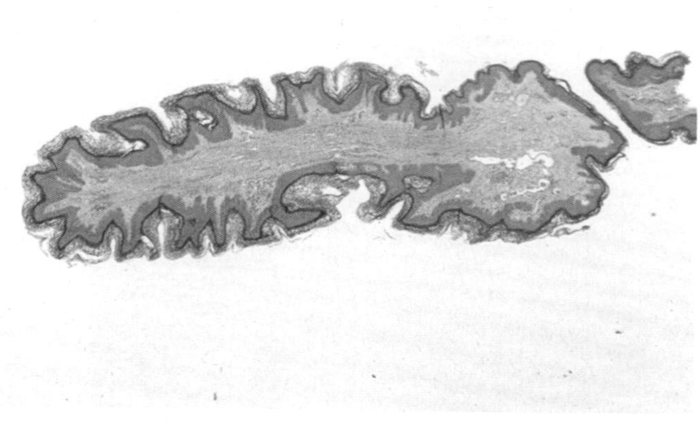

Figure 21.41 **Skin tag** (fibroepithelial polyp, microscopic study). The epidermis and fibrous core are plainly visible.

Tumors of the Epidermis Are Common and Usually Harmless

Benign and malignant tumors that arise in the epidermis are exceptionally common. Apart from malignant melanoma, they are, with rare exception, tumors of epidermal squamous cells and are famously indolent and rarely, if ever, metastasize. With the exception of malignant melanoma, they are not included in cancer statistics.

Benign Epidermal Tumors

Two of the most common skin growths are not actually neoplasms, but are tumors only in the broadest sense of the word—that is to say, they are masses.

Skin tags (Fig. 21.41) are innocent polypoid growths, usually a few millimeters but sometimes up to a centimeter or more. They have a simple core of blood vessels and fibrous tissue covered by unremarkable epidermis. They are often seen in the body folds of obese persons. Their cause is unknown. Skin tags are not associated with other conditions and rarely deserve treatment except for cosmetic purposes or if they become irritated.

Epidermoid cysts (*wens, epidermal inclusion* cysts) are not neoplasms. They form from occluded hair follicles or trapped pieces of epidermis that become cystic and grow as they fill with squamous cells and keratin debris (Fig. 21.42). Epidermoid cysts are innocuous and, like lipomas, are usually removed for cosmetic reasons; however, they can become infected and require surgical drainage.

Seborrheic keratosis (Fig. 21.43) is a very common lesion that usually appears in people over age 40. It is a

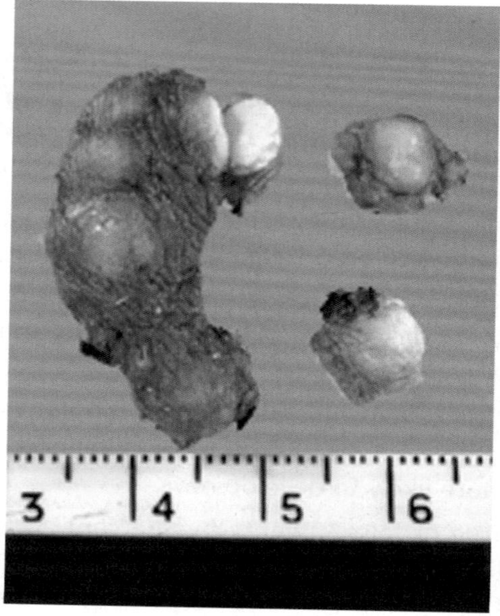

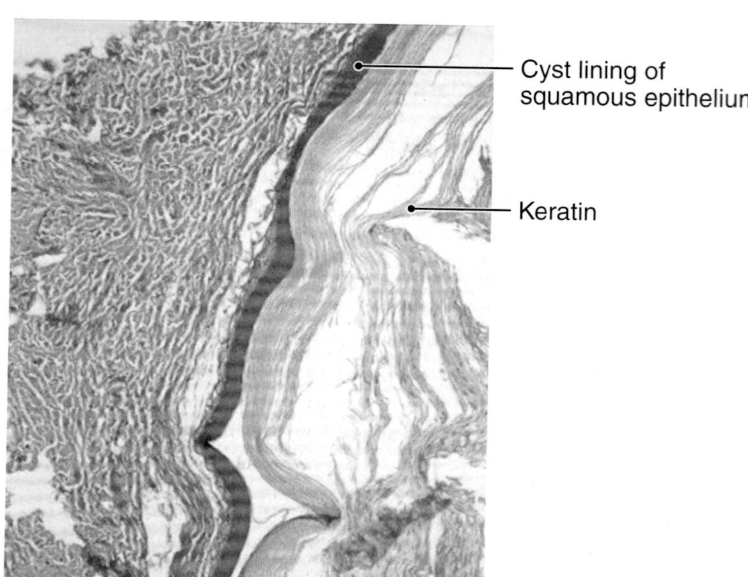

Figure 21.42 **Epidermoid cysts. A.** The multilobulated large cyst (left) has been opened to expose white, keratinaceous contents. **B.** The cyst's epidermal lining continues to grow and fills the cyst with dead epidermal cells.

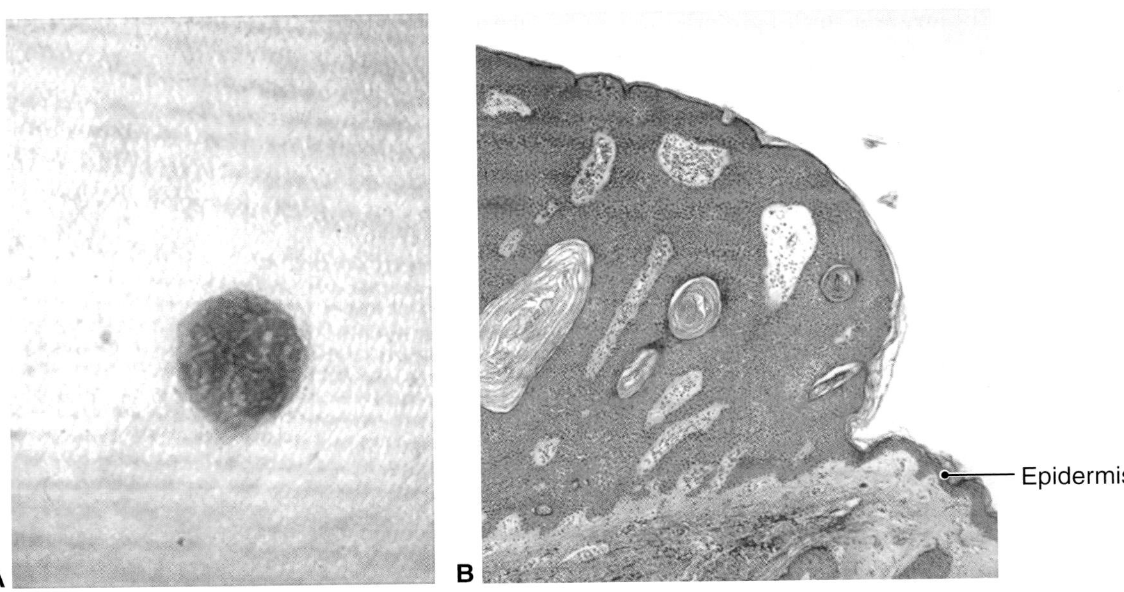

Figure 21.43 **Seborrheic keratosis. A.** This plaque is brown, dry, uniformly pigmented, sharply demarcated, and smoothly outlined. **B.** Superficial accumulation of basal cells with small keratin cysts.

pigmented, superficial, velvety, dry overgrowth of epidermal cells with a thick, loose layer of surface keratin. It is but one of many pigmented skin lesions (freckle, lentigo, nevus, malignant melanoma, and others). The cause is unknown; unlike most other keratoses, seborrheic keratosis is not premalignant, and it does not deserve treatment except for cosmetic improvement.

Because seborrheic keratoses (SK) are pigmented, sometimes very dark brown, they must be distinguished from malignant melanoma and other pigmented skin lesions. Some key differences are the following:

- SK is brown but not as dark as MM, which often contains black areas.
- SK has nearly uniform color, whereas MM often varies from brown to pink to black.
- SK has a dull, velvety surface and relatively uniform edges; MM is usually smooth and may have glossy areas, irregular borders, and small satellite pigmented spots.

Premalignant and Malignant Squamous Epidermal Tumors

There are two types of epidermal squamous malignancies—basal cell carcinoma (BCC) and squamous cell carcinoma (SCC). They have much in common: they arise from epidermis, occur principally in sun-exposed skin, grow slowly, may be locally aggressive, and metastasize only very rarely. If treated early, both are usually inconsequential. Nevertheless, neglected lesions near critical structures such as the nose, eyes, or ears can cause significant local problems. Also, keep in mind that SCCs of other organs, such as the lung, are much, much more aggressive than are SCCs of skin.

Actinic keratosis (AK) (from Greek *aktin* = ray; also known as **solar keratosis**) (Fig. 21.44) is very common and is an early precancerous forerunner of squamous cell

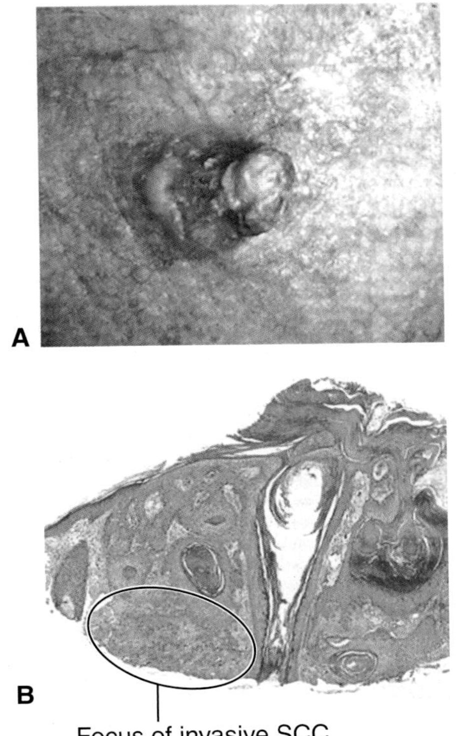

Figure 21.44 **Actinic (solar) keratosis. A.** The nodule is capped by a thick layer of keratin, while the adjacent skin shows a marked photoaging effect. **B.** This microscopic study shows epidermal hyperplasia with a thick cap of keratin. In the base of the lesion is a focus of invasive squamous cell carcinoma.

carcinoma of skin. It occurs as a small (<1 cm), discrete, rough, scaly patch or thickly cornified nodule in sun-exposed skin, especially on the face, back of the hand, and back of the neck. AK is especially common in people with lightly pigmented skin; people with deeply pigmented skin rarely are affected. AK often shows areas of squamous dysplasia and CIS and may progress to invasive squamous carcinoma. AKs can be removed safely by simple superficial methods such as curettage, lasering, topical chemotherapy, or freezing.

Squamous cell carcinoma (SCC) is a malignant tumor of epidermal cells that mature toward keratinizing squamous cells. SCC is the second most common skin cancer. It usually arises from a preexisting AK in sun-exposed skin of older persons. SCCs appear as scaly or ulcerated papules or plaques, or as hard, cornified nodules that grow slowly. Local destruction or excision is curative.

Keratoacanthoma (Fig. 21.45) is a rapidly growing squamous tumor of sun-exposed skin that can be alarming because it appears and grows so rapidly. Some consider it a variant of SCC of skin; others conceive of it as a benign tumor. The cause is unknown, but sun exposure is important. The typical lesion is volcano-like, with a central crater plugged with keratin, which rests on a base of malignant-appearing squamous cells. Most regress without therapy; however, those who view them as malignant treat them by excision.

Basal cell carcinoma (BCC) (Fig. 21.46) is the most common skin cancer and the most common invasive cancer in humans. It occurs most commonly in persons with fair skin. It arises from primitive basal cells located deep in the dermis along the basement membrane. BCC differs clinically from squamous carcinoma in four ways. BCC

- rarely appears on the back of the hand;
- may occur in skin not exposed to intense sunlight;
- may occur as a feature in some genetic disease syndromes;
- very rarely metastasizes (squamous carcinoma rarely metastasizes, but it does so more often than BCC).

Microscopically, BCC is composed of groups of round basal cells that contain no keratin, a contrast to squamous

A

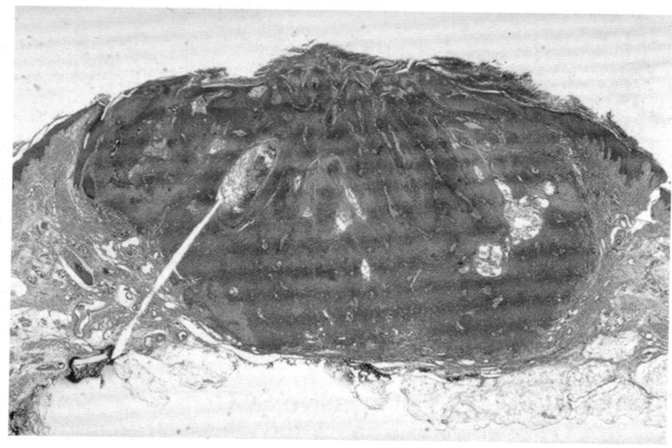

Figure 21.45 **Keratoacanthoma**. **A.** This rapidly growing nodule appeared on the sun-exposed dorsum of the wrist. Note its volcano-like appearance. **B.** The microscopic study shows hyperplasia of the epidermis and a central core of keratin.

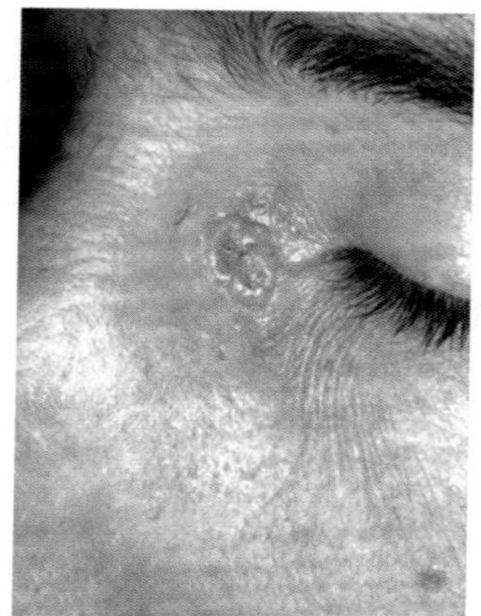

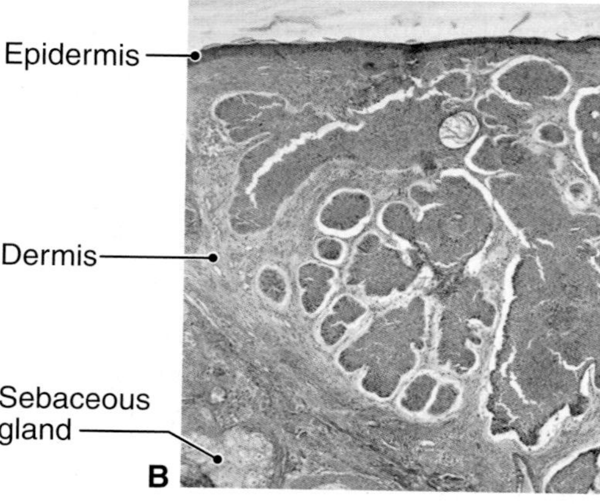

Figure 21.46 **Basal cell carcinoma**. **A.** A pearly plaque/nodule with raised, rolled edges. **B.** The microscopic study shows masses of small, dark basal cells invading the dermis.

carcinoma. Clinically, BCC appears as a pearly, semitransparent, shiny papule or nodule that has a raised, rolled margin, a central shallow crater, and tiny blood vessels arrayed across the surface. Local excision or destruction is curative.

Case Notes

21.16 Had Brianna lived longer, would she have been likely to develop actinic keratoses and skin cancers?

Non-Epidermal Tumors Are Diverse and Only Rarely Malignant

Beneath the epidermis are the dermis (which contains fibrous tissue, immune cells, blood vessels, and nerves), subcuticular fat, and skin appendages such as hair follicles, sebaceous glands, and sweat glands. Any of these tissues can become neoplastic. The great majority of these neoplasms are benign.

Lipomas are tumors of fat cells (Chapter 18, Fig. 18.21). They are rubbery, yellow, greasy, moveable subcutaneous masses in the subcuticular fat. They are not premalignant and are clinically distinctive enough not to warrant biopsy except under unusual circumstances.

Dermatofibromas (Fig. 21.47) are innocuous fibrous tumors that appear as small, brownish, sharply outlined, hard dermal nodules. They occur on the legs, arms, and trunk and they are most common in women over age 20. Treatment is not necessary.

Keloids (Chapter 2, Fig. 2.27) are nodular masses of exaggerated scar tissue that far exceed the degree of injury and the expected repair response. They occur in genetically susceptible persons, usually of African heritage. A common site is the earlobe after piercing.

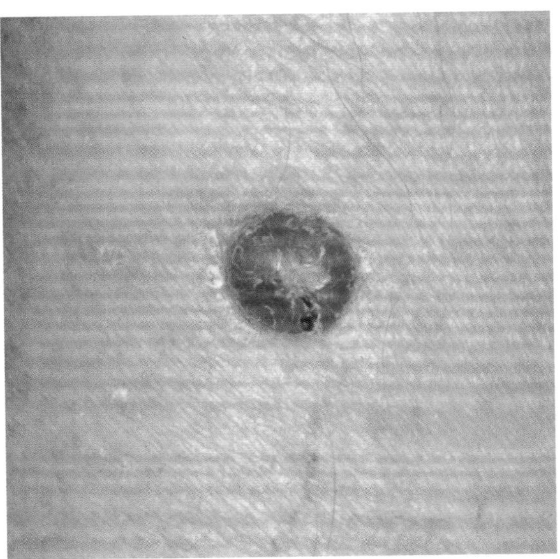

Figure 21.47 **Dermatofibroma**. The lesion in this patient is typical: a firm, sharply outlined, reddish-brown nodule.

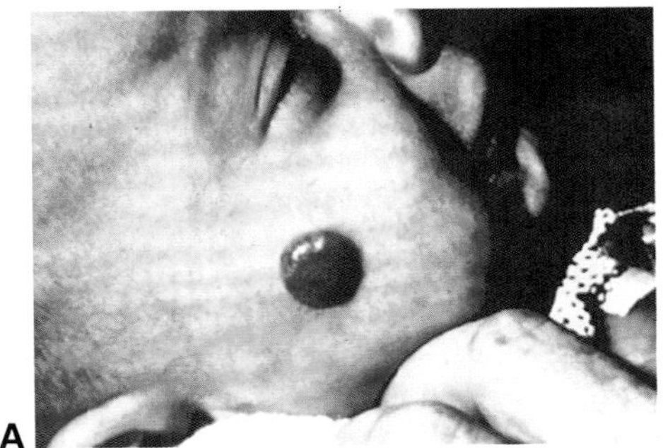

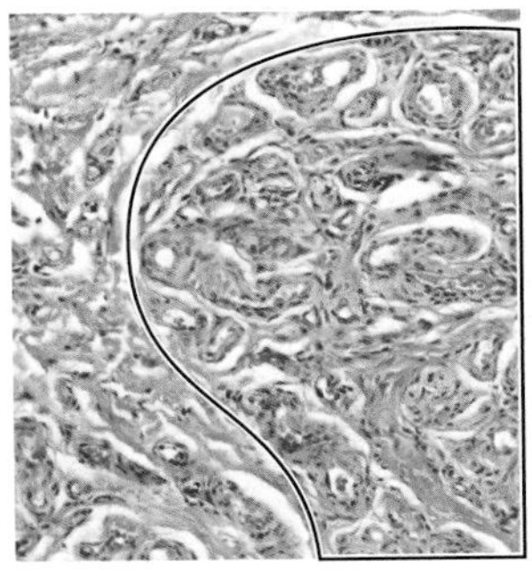

Figure 21.48 **Angioma** (hemangioma). **A.** The nodule on the cheek is a compact mass of blood vessels. **B.** A microscopic study shows an otherwise unremarkable mass of small blood vessels.

Angiomas (or *hemangiomas*, Fig. 21.48) are abnormal collections of blood vessels. They can occur anywhere in the body, but they are especially common in dermis, where they appear as small, reddish nodules or flat patches of discolored skin that vary from a few millimeters to several centimeters. Most are present at birth. It is not clear if angiomas are neoplasms or congenital anomalies; but it rarely matters because almost all are innocuous. Some are composed of small vessels (*capillary hemangioma*) and others of larger, thin-walled vessels (*venous hemangioma*). *Pyogenic granuloma* (Chapter 2) is an abnormal nodule of blood vessels that occurs in wound repair and for practical purposes is identical to a hemangioma. *Spider angiomas* (Fig. 21.5) were mentioned earlier in connection with skin changes in pregnancy. *Nevus flammeus* (*port wine stain*, Fig. 21.49) is a common congenital red or purple patch on the neck, scalp, or face. They can be quite large and are composed of small, dilated, dermal blood vessels. Some fade with time; others can be treated effectively with laser therapy.

Kaposi sarcoma (Fig. 21.7) is a malignant tumor of vascular endothelial cells caused by a certain type of herpesvirus. It is especially prevalent in people with an immunodeficiency, most notably patients with AIDS. It is discussed above in conjunction with HIV infection.

Adenomas of sweat or sebaceous glands are benign growths of specialized glandular epithelium. There are multiple varieties, all uncommon. Most appear as a small, smooth, tan skin nodule.

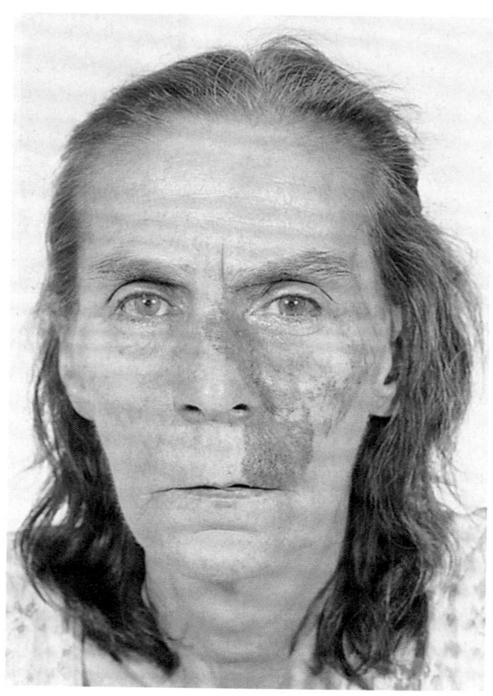

Figure 21.49 **Nevus flammeus**. (Reproduced with permission from Tasman W, Jaeger E. *The Wills Eye Hospital Atlas of Clinical Ophthalmology*. 2nd ed. Philadelphia, PA: Lippincott Williams & Wilkins; 2001.)

Neurofibromas are benign tumors of peripheral nerves usually seen in the dermis of patients with von Recklinghausen neurofibromatosis (Chapter 19, Fig. 19.38).

Tumors of blood and immune system cells may occur in skin. Most arise elsewhere as *lymphoma* or *leukemia* and involve skin secondarily. Some, however, originate in skin.

Mycosis fungoides is a T cell lymphoma primary in skin. It tends to remain in skin for years but a few may spread widely. Lesions typically begin as small patches or plaques and evolve into ulcerating nodules. Any area of skin may be affected. Diagnosis requires biopsy. Average survival is 7–10 years. Treatment is local surgery or radiation or sometimes systemic chemotherapy.

Histiocytosis X (*Langerhans histiocytosis*) arises as a malignancy of Langerhans dendritic cells and tends to spread widely. Most cases occur in children. Diagnosis requires biopsy. Prognosis is poor. Treatment is local irradiation or surgery or systemic chemotherapy.

Pop Quiz

21.19 True or false? AK, a precancerous forerunner of SCC of skin, is especially common in people with deeply pigmented skin.

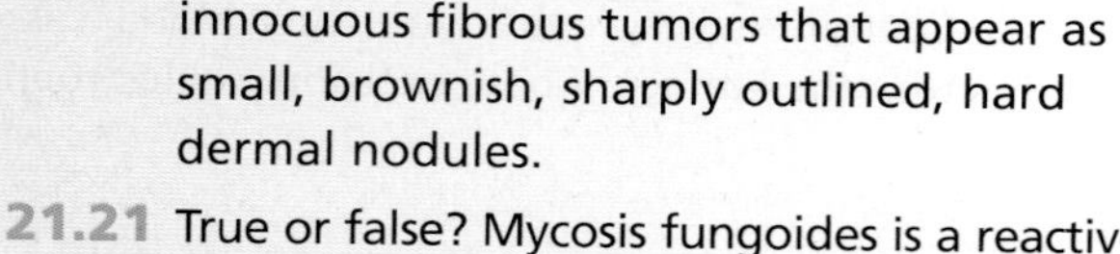

21.20 True or false? Dermatofibromas are innocuous fibrous tumors that appear as small, brownish, sharply outlined, hard dermal nodules.

21.21 True or false? Mycosis fungoides is a reactive T cell response caused by a fungal infection.

Disorders of Hair and Nails

Hair and nails are formed of exactly the same material: keratin. Just as hair grows from keratin-forming cells at the base of the hair follicle, nails grow from an arc of constantly dividing keratin-forming cells at the base of the nail.

Most Hair Disease Features Hair Loss

Fine hairs (*lanugo* hairs) cover the body at birth and are shed quickly and replaced by slightly darker, thicker hairs (*vellus* hairs) that cover the body from childhood onward. *Terminal* hairs, the thick hairs of the scalp and the male face, are usually deeply pigmented. Both vellus and terminal hairs go through a growth cycle, which varies from a few months (eyelashes) to several years (scalp).

The natural life cycle of hair growth has several phases. The growth phase (*anagen phase*) is the longest. It is followed by a very short transitional phase (*catagen phase*) before coming to the final resting phase (*telogen phase*), after which the hair is shed, and the cycle repeats. In the normal scalp, about 90% of follicles are in the growth phase, about 1–2% are in the transitional phase, and about 10% are in the resting phase.

Alopecia is abnormal hair loss. In almost all cases the cause is unknown, but stress seems to be involved. **Alopecia areata** is characterized by well-circumscribed areas of total hair loss, usually on the scalp (Fig. 21.50).

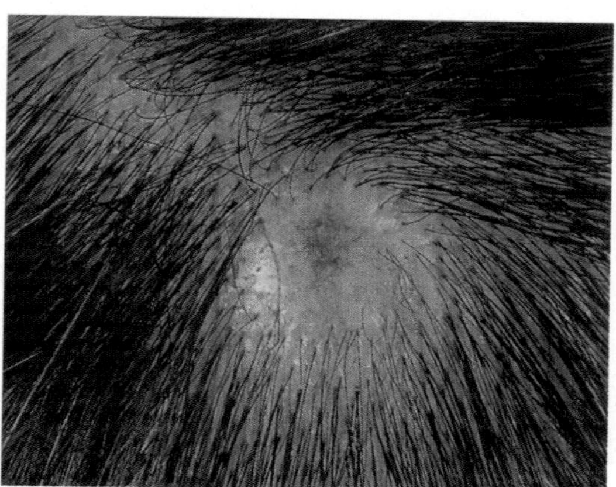

Figure 21.50 **Alopecia areata**.

Alopecia totalis is loss of all scalp hair. **Alopecia universalis** is loss of all body hair, including eyebrows, a condition that affected John D. Rockefeller Sr., perhaps the richest man in modern world history. Hair loss in these conditions may occur in conjunction with autoimmune disorders and thyroid disease. Recovery of hair growth sometimes occurs, but may be permanent.

Male pattern baldness is a natural consequence of aging attributable to male hormones (androgens), which act to shorten the growth (anagen) phase of hairs until, ultimately, no hair grows. No inflammation or scarring is involved. Women, too, naturally experience hair loss as they age, but it begins later and is less severe.

Other types of hair loss, however, are not permanent. **Telogen effluvium** is a sudden, diffuse shedding of resting (telogen) hairs (about 10% of all hairs) that occurs several weeks after severe illness, trauma, or emotional upset. Because telogen hairs comprise only about 10% of scalp hair, and because the loss has usually stopped by the time the patient is examined, the examining clinician usually cannot see much wrong despite the patient's complaint that "my hair is falling out." Much cancer chemotherapy is aimed at interrupting cell growth. Because the drugs act indiscriminately, one effect is interruption of hair growth. As a consequence roots become thin, and hair breaks away.

The etiology of hair loss is varied. Apart from male pattern baldness's relationship to male hormones, the most common causes of hair loss are drugs, especially chemotherapeutic agents; infections such as taenia capitis (ringworm); nutritional deficiencies; and autoimmune disorders such as lupus. Less commonly, heavy metal poisoning or rare skin diseases are responsible.

Diagnosis is by inspection. Complete evaluation and treatment usually requires a dermatologist. Treatment should focus on eliminating the cause, if one can be found. Certain drugs have limited ability to stimulate regrowth. Autologous scalp hair transplants are an option for those who are especially sensitive about baldness.

Hirsutism is the growth of dark, thick hair in women in locations where hair is normally minimal or absent. Hirsutism is one of the more common consequences of steroid therapy and of adrenal or pituitary disease (Chapter 14); Cushing syndrome is an example. Also, hirsutism is an integral part of polycystic ovary syndrome and certain hormone-secreting ovarian tumors (Chapter 17).

Nail Disorders Are Fairly Common and Usually Innocuous

Some nail deformities occur in newborns in connection with genetic defects. Other nail deformities and discolorations occur secondary to dermatologic conditions. Psoriasis is noted for nail deformities including irregular pits, discolored tan spots, nail loss, and thick, crumbling nails.

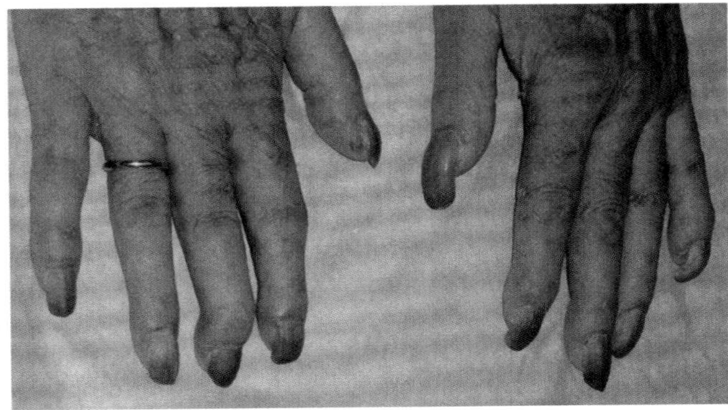

Figure 21.51 **Onychogryphosis.** (Reproduced with permission from Berg D, Worzala K. *Atlas of Adult Physical Diagnosis*. Philadelphia, PA: Lippincott Williams & Wilkins; 2006.)

Onychogryphosis (Fig. 21.51) is nail dystrophy. It usually occurs on the big toe in elderly people and features very thick, curved, deformed nails. Treatment is trimming.

Onycholysis is loss of the nail at the bed. Like hair loss, it can be a complication of cancer chemotherapy.

Bacterial infection of the cuticle is **paronychi**, which tends to occur in people who work with their hands in water, such as kitchen personnel.

Fungus infection of the nail is **onychomycosis**. Infection usually begins at the tip, burrows beneath the nail, and may eventually cause loss of the nail. Infected nails tend to be thick, yellow, and unsightly with ridges. Antifungal therapy is usually effective but must be continued for months until entirely new nail growth has completely replaced the infected nail. Nail trauma can cause bleeding beneath the nail, a tight space. Pain can be severe. Treatment is not necessary unless for pain relief, which can be obtained by creating a hole in the nail to drain the blood.

Pop Quiz

21.22 What hormone is responsible for causing male pattern baldness?

21.23 ____________ is nail dystrophy, which usually occurs on the big toe in elderly people and features very thick, curved, deformed nails.

21.24 Alopecia ____________ is loss of all body hair, including eyebrows.

Case Study Revisited

"She fries like bacon." The case of Brianna K.

As Brianna was quick to realize, her skin was an important asset in her fashion career but it was a major problem as well. She was allergic to poison ivy, had allergic contact dermatitis, and was extremely sensitive to the effect of sunlight. That she had four dysplastic nevi and an uncle who died of melanoma indicates she probably had heritable melanoma syndrome.

The "missing link" in this case is the primary care physician. Gynecologists are considered primary care providers and have a responsibility to care for the entire patient, not just their sex organs. Her gynecologist had ample opportunity to find this lesion but didn't. Inspection and assessment of all moles and pigmented lesions is an essential part of every history and physical examination. Close inspection of the skin of white patients at the time of first visit is a vital part of responsible patient care, as essential as measuring blood pressure—initial diagnosis (or suspicion) of melanoma is in the hands of primary caregivers. Look for large (>1 cm), dark brown lesions with irregular borders and variegated pigmentation and keep in mind the mnemonic: MMRISK, which stands for the following:

- **M**oles: many common moles. Brianna had many moles.
- **M**oles: dysplastic or unusual moles. Brianna had dysplastic moles.
- **R**ed hair or freckles. Brianna qualified.
- **I**nability to tan. Brianna qualified.
- **S**unburns, especially as a child. Brianna qualified.
- **K**indred: family history of melanoma. Brianna qualified.

In summary, Brianna almost certainly died of heritable melanoma syndrome, which could have been detected much earlier. Only a minority of melanomas arise from preexisting nevi. Even so, annual examination by a dermatologist likely would have spotted early any melanomas arising de novo and any nevus that became dysplastic could have been excised. Had her skin been examined regularly, it seems likely she could have enjoyed a normal life span.

Chapter Challenge

CHAPTER RECALL

1. A 42-year-old Hispanic female visits her primary care physician for early menopause. She denies changes in her menstrual cycles but reports hot flashes. A physical exam is notable for warm, moist, velvety skin, with hair loss and waxy translucent plaques over her anterior lower legs. What is the underlying etiology of her skin findings?
   A. An excess of thyroid hormone
   B. A deficiency of thyroid hormone
   C. Diabetes
   D. Blood lipid abnormalities

2. Lichen simplex chronicus is caused by which one of the following?
   A. Autoimmunity
   B. Chronic rubbing or scratching
   C. Sun exposure
   D. None of the above

3. A 40-year-old Caucasian female, with fair skin, is referred to a dermatologist for a skin rash. You observe red papules and pustules on the face, and note an absence of scarring. She confirms she is of northern European descent. What disease is responsible for her skin findings?
   A. Acne
   B. AK
   C. Rosacea
   D. SK

4. Which of the following can cause photosensitivity?
   A. Lupus erythematosus
   B. Tetracycline
   C. Perfume
   D. All of the above

5. A seven-year-old African American female is brought to the pediatrician's office by her father, who is concerned about her recent onset of fever. Several days ago, she developed a small lesion on her lower leg, which has rapidly progressed to a bright red, painful, swollen area that now features small blisters. What is your diagnosis?
   A. Impetigo
   B. Erysipelas
   C. Dermatophytosis
   D. Molluscum contagiosum

6. Which of the following lesions is characterized by red, extremely tender nodules of chronic inflammation and fibrosis in the subcuticular tissue on the anterior aspect of the lower legs?
A. Scleroderma
B. Impetigo
C. Erythema nodosum
D. Erysipelas

7. Your 15-year-old cousin asks to borrow a long-sleeved shirt while at your house. He is embarrassed by "his rash," and would like to hide it. He shows you several sharply delineated dry, scaly, salmon-colored plaques on his elbows. You recognize the lesions present there and on his lower back and tell him that there are several treatments available, including tar compounds or steroids. What skin disorder do you believe he has?
A. Psoriasis
B. Seborrheic dermatitis
C. Lichen planus
D. Atopic eczema

8. Which of the following is the most common malignancy of skin?
A. Malignant melanoma
B. Basal cell carcinoma
C. Melanocytic nevus
D. Squamous carcinoma

9. A two-year-old Hispanic female is seen in the clinic for acute, weepy, crusted eruptions on her cheeks, scalp, chest, and extensor surfaces. You diagnose her with Type I (atopic) hypersensitivity and warn her mother that she might develop what disease later in life?
A. Gluten-sensitive enteropathy
B. Hyperthyroidism
C. Irritable bowel disease
D. Asthma

10. Which of the following is bacterial infection of the cuticle occurring in people who work with their hands in water?
A. Onychogryphosis
B. Onycholysis
C. Paronychia
D. Onychomycosis

11. A 36-year-old African American male with a past medical history significant for AIDS presents to the clinic concerned about an intensely pruritic rash present on the webs of his fingers and toes, as well as his wrists. A physical exam demonstrates burrows so small they are barely visible to the naked eye. What agent is responsible for his "rash?"
A. Scabies
B. Lice
C. Bedbugs
D. Chiggers

12. A middle-aged Mediterranean woman presents for her initial patient visit at a dermatology clinic through which you are rotating. Her physical exam is remarkable for small vesicles as well as large bullae, some of which have ruptured to leave weeping, crusted, inflamed patches on her trunk, face, neck, and scalp. Notably, her extremities are spared. You recognize the disease, which is caused by an autoimmune antibody attack on the intercellular cement that binds epidermis. What is your diagnosis?
A. Epidermolysis bullosa
B. Pemphigus
C. Bullous pemphigoid
D. Dermatitis herpetiformis

13. True or false? SK are premalignant.

14. True or false? The epidermis has its own supply of blood vessels, nerves, and glands.

15. True or false? About one-third of the population of the United States develops a skin condition each year.

16. True or false? Hair and nails are formed of exactly the same material: keratin.

17. True or false? Langerhans histiocytosis arises as a malignancy of cutaneous dendritic cells.

18. True or false? A papule is a small, solid, raised lesion less than 0.5 cm in diameter.

CONCEPTUAL UNDERSTANDING

19. What is the characteristic finding of erythema multiforme?

20. List the causes of vitiligo.

APPLICATION

21. A freshman college student comes to clinic concerned about her hair loss. You suggest that she receive counseling. Why?

22. If you could ask the pathologist only one question about his/her diagnosis of malignant melanoma, what would it be?

PART

3

Disorders of the Stages and States of Life

Chapter 22 Congenital and Childhood Disorders
- Cystic fibrosis and selected other Mendelian disorders
- Down syndrome and other cytogenetic disorders
- Respiratory distress syndrome, hyperbilirubinemia, and other conditions of prematurity
- Measles, chickenpox, diphtheria, other childhood infections; sudden infant death syndrome
- Wilm's tumor, retinoblastoma, and other tumors peculiar to children

Chapter 23 Disorders of Daily Life
- Burns, heat stroke, frostbite, environmental pollution
- The effects of tobacco use; alcohol and drug abuse
- Malnutrition, obesity
- The cardiovascular risks of the metabolic syndrome

Chapter 24 Aging, Stress, Exercise, and Pain
- Cellular senescence and the effects of age
- Stress and its effect on health
- Athletic injuries, immobility, exercise and its effect on health
- Neuropathic pain syndromes, the perception of pain

CHAPTER 22

Congenital and Childhood Disorders

Contents

Chapter Objectives

After studying this chapter, you should be able to complete the following tasks:

NORMAL PREGNANCY AND GESTATION

1. Describe the timeline of embryonic and fetal development throughout a normal pregnancy.

OVERVIEW OF CONGENITAL DEFECTS

2. Compare and contrast malformations, deformations, and disruptions.

DEFECTS CAUSED BY ENVIRONMENTAL FACTORS

3. Describe the environmental factors responsible for causing congenital malformations including: nutrient deficiencies, radiation, teratogens/drugs, and infections.

GENETIC DISORDERS AN INTRODUCTION

4. Describe different types of mutations and how they affect the genetic code.

DISORDERS CAUSED BY SINGLE-GENE DEFECTS

5. Using examples from the text, describe the different modes of inheritance, and the different types of genes that may be mutated.

DISORDERS INFLUENCED BY MULTIPLE GENES

6. Using examples from the text, define the pathogenesis of multifactorial diseases.

DISORDERS CAUSED BY LARGE-SCALE CHROMOSOME ABNORMALITIES

7. Describe the signs, symptoms, and cytogenetic changes found in Turner, Klinefelter, and Down syndromes.

GENETIC DIAGNOSIS

8. Understand the indications for genetic screening, and the tests available.

PERINATAL AND NEONATAL DISORDERS

9. Describe the changes that take place after an infant's birth, including pulmonary, cardiovascular, hemoglobin production, immune system, renal function, and liver function (glucose metabolism and metabolism of bilirubin).
10. Discuss the problems that arise in premature infants.
11. Know the infectious processes that present in the perinatal/neonatal period.

INFECTIONS OF INFANTS AND CHILDREN

12. Be able to recognize the presentation of the following diseases:
    a. RSV, bronchiolitis, whooping cough, croup, diphtheria, epiglottitis, mono
    b. Acute otitis media
    c. Chickenpox
    d. Measles, mumps, rubella
    e. HIV/AIDS

SUDDEN INFANT DEATH SYNDROME (SIDS)

13. Be able to name the risk factors associated with SIDS.

TUMORS AND TUMOR-LIKE CONDITIONS IN CHILDREN

14. Answer the following questions: What are the differences between choristoma, hamartoma, and teratoma? What are the most common tumors, by tissue, in children?

Case Study

"I'm going to have a baby." The case of Natasha V.

Chief Complaint: Labor pains

Clinical History: Natasha V. was a 24-year-old, obviously pregnant and equally obviously intoxicated woman who presented in the emergency room in labor saying, "I'm going to have a baby."

Clinic records revealed that Natasha smoked heavily and chronically abused both alcohol and illicit drugs. One prior pregnancy had ended with an early spontaneous abortion. Natasha's intoxicated state made it difficult to obtain a recent medical history but she was able to recall the date of her last menstrual period, which put her pregnancy at 36 weeks.

Physical Examination and Other Data: Natasha was 5′4″ tall and weighed 162 lb. Vital signs were

(continued)

"I'm going to have a baby." The case of Natasha V. (continued)

unremarkable. She was having hard uterine contractions every five minutes and smelled of alcohol, but otherwise her physical exam was unremarkable.

A complete blood count revealed that her hemoglobin, white cell count, and platelet count were normal. Urinalysis was unremarkable.

Clinical Course: Labor progressed rapidly. Natasha delivered a 1,525 gm (3 lb, 6 oz) boy with an Apgar score of 3. He scored 1 point for heart rate <100; 1 point for irregular, gasping respiratory effort; 0 point for flaccid muscle tone; 0 point for no cry in reaction to insertion of nasal catheter; and 1 point for color (body pink with blue extremities). The infant's small head and facial features suggested he suffered from fetal alcohol syndrome.

Natasha recovered quickly and was discharged home on the third hospital day with instructions to return to obstetric clinic in seven days.

The newborn, however, was hospitalized for seven weeks. His initial problem was respiratory distress: rapid, labored respirations that required ventilatory assistance and respiratory inhalant medication. He also failed to thrive and weighed less on discharge than at birth. In the months following discharge, his development continued to be slow and he remained underweight. At three months of age, he began experiencing seizures. These progressed in frequency and severity, and he died before his first birthday.

Life is a flame that is always burning itself out, but it catches fire again every time a child is born.

GEORGE BERNARD SHAW, IRISH PLAYWRIGHT (1856–1950)

In the long, slow arc of life we progress, if we are lucky, from conception through embryonic and fetal growth, birth, childhood, adolescence, adulthood, and old age before we die. Along the way, we experience the joys and the sorrows—especially the diseases—that living inevitably brings. The previous chapters dealt with adult diseases. Now it is time to turn our attention to the earlier stages of life. The catalog of congenital and pediatric disease, however, is too vast for us to do much more than skim the surface. Still, we'll review the basics of embryonic and fetal development, genetics, and newborn physiology before we touch on the most common diseases of newborns and children.

Recall from Chapter 1 that all disease is due, to a greater or lesser extent, to the interplay of genetic and environmental forces. In the embryo, fetus, and growing child, the evidence of these forces tends to be more plainly visible than in adults because growth magnifies their effect.

Remember This! All disease involves the interplay of genetic and environmental forces.

Normal Pregnancy and Gestation

Pregnancy (*gravidity*) begins with fertilization (*conception*) and ends with birth. During gestation, the fertilized human ovum begins as an embryo whose initial appearance is remarkably similar to the embryos of reptiles, birds, and other animals, but each differentiates differently to form a particular life form.

Pregnancy Is Divided into Three Trimesters

In humans, the length of normal pregnancy is 40–42 weeks, or 280–294 days, measured from the beginning of the *last menstrual period* (LMP). Measurements in pregnancy typically begin from the LMP because most women recall it easily. Nevertheless, conception usually occurs two weeks after that date, so the actual length of gestation is about 266–280 days.

Pregnancy is divided into three **trimesters**, each about 13 weeks. Certain physiologic signs and symptoms characterize each:

- In the **first trimester**, about three-fourths of women will experience nausea, which is called *morning sickness* though it may last all day. The breasts become fuller and the nipples darken. Pelvic examination reveals a soft, bluish cervix and enlarged uterus. Ultrasonography detects an amniotic sac at about 4–5 weeks, heart motion a week later, and fetal heart sounds at about 8–10 weeks.
- About the beginning of the **second trimester**, the dome of the uterus has grown above the rim of the pelvis. Women feel fetal movement at about 16–20 weeks, but occasionally much later. The uterus reaches the umbilicus at about week 20.
- The **third trimester** is characterized by continuing growth of the uterus, which reaches near to the xiphoid process by week 36. Late in this period, the fetus "drops down" as the fetal head descends into the pelvis and engages the cervix as birth nears.

Gravidity and **parity** are terms used to describe, respectively, the number of a woman's pregnancies and the number of pregnancies that have reached 24 weeks, the age at which 50% of fetuses will survive outside the womb. A woman is a *primigravida* with her first pregnancy, and a *multigravida* with her second and subsequent pregnancies. Thus, a woman pregnant for the third time who gave birth twice previously after 24 weeks would be gravida 3, para 2. Some notation systems record the number of abortions, number of living children, and so on.

The diagnosis of pregnancy is usually made by simple home or office test of urine for the presence of **chorionic gonadotropin**, a hormone secreted by the developing placenta as soon as the fertilized ovum implants in the endometrium. Diagnosis also can be made clinically by a combination of sexual and menstrual history and physiologic changes in the patient or by ultrasonographic detection of a gestational sac in the uterus.

Case Notes

22.1 In which trimester was Natasha when she appeared in the emergency room?

22.2 True or false? When she arrived in the emergency room, Natasha was gravida 2, para 0.

Embryonic and Fetal Development Is Controlled by DNA

From the moment of conception, the development of new human life is controlled by genes and influenced by the uterine environment provided by the mother.

For the first eight weeks, the developing human is called the **embryo;** afterward, it is called the **fetus.** About four to five days after fertilization, embryonic cells form a hollow structure called the *blastocyst* (Fig. 22.1), which has three components:

- The blastocyst wall is composed of *trophoblast* cells, which develop into the fetal portion of the placenta.
- The *inner cell mass* is a nodule of cells on in the inner wall of the cyst. It develops into the fetus and amniotic sac.
- The *blastocyst cavity* is a hollow cavity that eventually shrinks and disappears as the fetus enlarges from the inner cell mass.

The blastocyst implants in the uterine endometrium between 7 and 10 days after fertilization. Cell division continues, and by days 10–14, the cells of the inner cell mass have begun to differentiate into the three **primary germ layers**—endoderm, mesoderm, and ectoderm—identified in Chapter 2. Together, these layers are referred to as the **embryonic plate**.

By week 4, the germ layers have begun to develop into distinct tissues and organs in a meticulously timed sequence. The embryonic plate grows, stretches, and folds into a series of chambers (e.g., the heart and the cerebral ventricles) and tubes (e.g., the intestines, bronchi, gland ducts, and spinal canal). Many of these spaces begin originally as grooves that become tubes as the groove rims grow upward and fold over and join to form an enclosed space. Failure of these spaces to close is the cause of many congenital defects.

Simultaneously, the amniotic sac develops: it is composed of a tough but flexible membrane that completely surrounds the embryo and is filled with amniotic fluid. Added to amniotic fluid is fetal urine and a small amount of fluid and cell debris issuing from the fetal bowel. Both are, of course, sterile. The fetus "breathes" amniotic fluid during its time in the uterus. The amniotic sac provides room for movement and growth and cushions the fetus against abdominal trauma to the mother.

The **placenta** is a temporary organ of pregnancy that at maturity is a disc about 9 inches (23 cm) in diameter and 1 inch (2.5 cm) thick in the center. It serves as an exchange device for transfer of nutrients and oxygen from mother to fetus and waste materials from fetus to mother. Blood travels between the embryo/fetus and the placenta via the **umbilical cord**.

It is helpful to think of the placenta as the functional equivalent of fetal lungs, intestines, and kidneys. The placenta keeps maternal and fetal blood from mixing, but allows substances to diffuse back and forth. Two umbilical arteries carry deoxygenated blood and metabolic waste from the fetus to the placenta, where the blood picks up oxygen and nutrients and drops off carbon dioxide and metabolic waste. The single umbilical vein carries nutritious, freshly oxygenated and waste-free blood back to the fetus.

Remember This! The placenta functions as the fetus's lungs, digestive system, and kidneys.

The placenta is composed of an outer layer maternal and an inner layer of fetal tissue. The maternal portion is **decidua**, uterine endometrium that is thickened and modified by the effect of progesterone. The fetal part arises from the wall of the blastocyst and forms into **chorionic villi**, finger-like projections containing fetal blood vessels that extend into lakes of maternal blood in the decidua.

Case Notes

22.3 How did alcohol ingested by Natasha reach her infant?

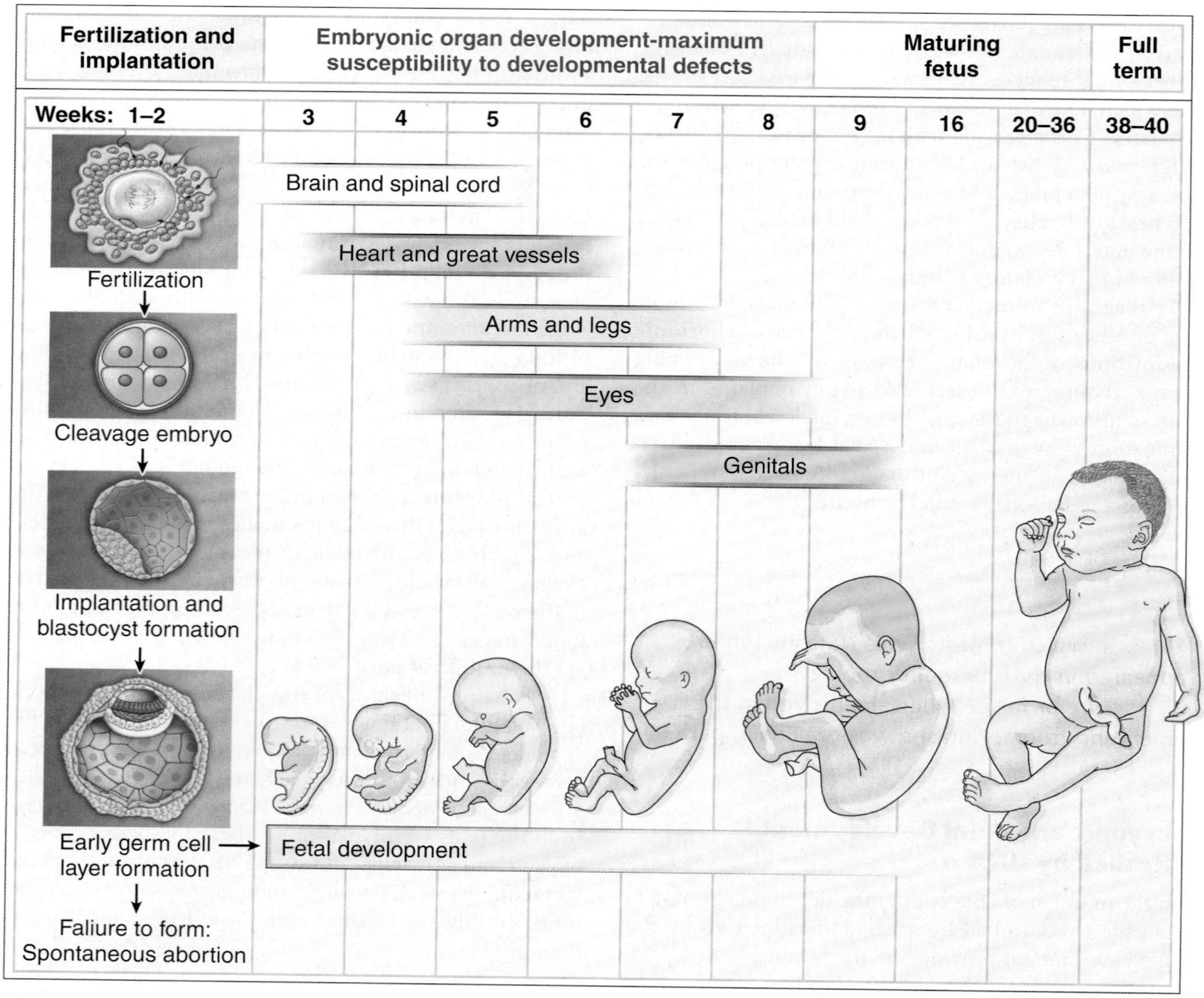

Fertilization and implantation | Embryonic organ development-maximum susceptibility to developmental defects | Maturing fetus | Full term

Weeks: 1–2 | 3 | 4 | 5 | 6 | 7 | 8 | 9 | 16 | 20–36 | 38–40

Brain and spinal cord

Heart and great vessels

Arms and legs

Eyes

Genitals

Fertilization

Cleavage embryo

Implantation and blastocyst formation

Early germ cell layer formation → Fetal development

Faliure to form: Spontaneous abortion

Figure 22.1 **Critical stages of embryo development**. Important congenital malformations are most likely to occur in early pregnancy (weeks 3–9), when organs are first developing. Maternal exposures to microbes, usually virus infection, and chemical abuse (drugs and alcohol) are the most common identifiable causes. Serious exposures before or near the time of endometrial implantation usually lead to spontaneous abortion. Exposures to infections, toxins, and other forces have less effect after the ninth week. (Portions of this image adapted with permission from McConnell TH, Hull KL. *Human Form Human Function: Essentials of Anatomy & Physiology*. Baltimore, MD: Wolters Kluwer Health; 2011.)

If all goes well, by the end of the embryonic period (weeks 1–8), the embryo has typically reached a length of about 3 cm (1.2 inches) and is identifiable as human (Fig. 22.1). Most of the major organs are formed, but are not mature. From week 9 through 13, the fetal face becomes more distinct, limbs appear with fingers and toes, and spontaneous movements occur.

The second trimester is a period of rapid growth, differentiation, and maturation of body tissues and organs. In the third trimester, the nervous system begins regulating body functions, the respiratory system matures, and sexual development is completed. In general, this is a "polishing" stage during which final birth weight is achieved and organs complete their maturation.

Pop Quiz

22.1 How long is a normal pregnancy?

22.2 What are the names of the three embryonic germ layers?

22.3 True or false? Most major organs are formed by the end of the eighth week of gestation.

22.4 Name the fetal and maternal parts of the placenta.

Overview of Congenital Defects

*"Find out the cause of this effect,
Or rather say, the cause of this defect,
For this effect defective comes by cause."*

WILLIAM SHAKESPEARE (1564–1616),
ENGLISH PLAYWRIGHT, HAMLET (II, II)

A **congenital defect** (*congenital anomaly*) refers to an abnormality present at birth. Defects may or may not be *detectable* at birth; however, it is common practice to use the term to refer to those that are. Defects may be due to the following:

- *Mechanical* factors: normal intrauterine development is distorted. These defects are called *congenital deformations*. Clubfoot is an example—the fetal foot becomes trapped and twisted and cannot develop properly.
- *Genetic* factors: defective genes or chromosomes are responsible for some diseases. Defects caused by genetic factors are called *congenital malformations* or *developmental defects*. For example, sickle cell disease is caused by a defect on one region of a single gene. By contrast, Down syndrome is caused by the presence of an entire extra chromosome.
- *Environmental* (maternal) factors: dietary deficiency, infection, drugs, and other factors can distort embryologic development. Defects caused by environmental factors are also *congenital malformations* or *developmental defects*. For example, maternal alcohol abuse can cause characteristic physical defects as well as mental deficiencies.
- Some congenital conditions are *multifactorial* and due to a mix of genetic and environmental influences. Cleft lip (Fig. 11.6) is an example.

In 2012, there were about 3.958 million births in the United States, down from a peak of 4.317 in 2007. About 125,000 (3%) had significant birth defects. The figure is higher if minor abnormalities are included. For about 75% of defects the cause will never be discovered; 20% are due to identifiable genetic factors; about 5% are due to identifiable maternal or environmental factors. These figures, however, understate the problem because about half of spontaneously aborted fetuses have chromosome abnormalities, indicating that many of these defects are lethal in utero.

In developed nations, congenital defects are responsible for about half of newborn and childhood deaths. By contrast, in underdeveloped nations, infectious diseases, malnutrition, and other environmental factors are responsible for the great majority of newborn and childhood deaths.

Congenital Deformations Are Caused by Mechanical Factors

Congenital deformations are caused by maternal mechanical factors that distort the fetus. The two most common deformations (and their approximate birth incidence) are the following:

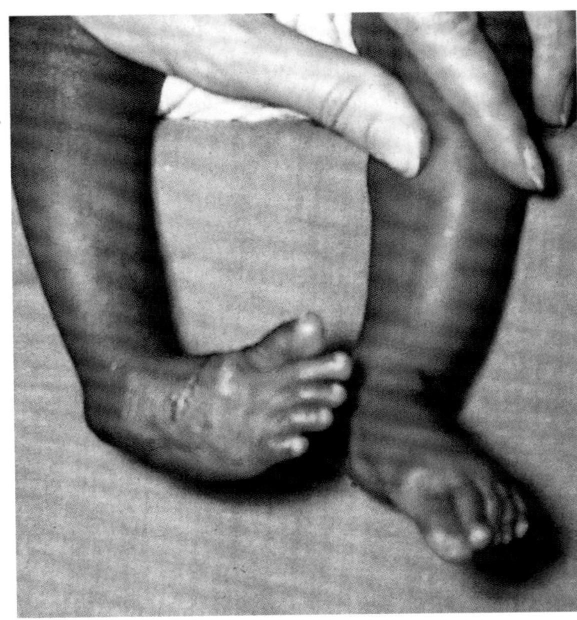

Figure 22.2 **Clubfoot**. The cause is malposition of the foot in the uterus, which does not allow room for it to grow properly. (Image courtesy of J. Adams).

- Clubfoot (~1:400) (Fig. 22.2), a twisting inward or outward of the foot so that the sole is not flat to the ground
- Hip dislocation (~1:1,100), a failure of the head of the femur to rest in its socket in the pelvis

Deformations usually arise in the 35th–38th weeks of pregnancy when the growth of the fetus exceeds the growth of the uterus, filling it to the point that there may not be enough amniotic fluid surrounding the fetus to provide cushioning and room for movement. Maternal factors include a malformed uterus owing to large leiomyomas (benign tumors of the uterine wall), the crowding of multiple pregnancy, and oligohydramnios, a condition of decreased amniotic fluid caused by lack of fetal urine production. Fetal urine is a major component of amniotic fluid. Lack of fluid gives the fetus less room to maneuver and may cause mechanical problems in development.

Congenital Malformations Are Caused by Environmental or Genetic Factors

Congenital malformations are fetal defects that owe to environmental or genetic factors that interfere with the intricate and delicate process that transforms a few cells into an embryo and then a fetus.

Most birth defects originate in the first trimester, especially the first eight weeks (the embryonic period). The fetus is much less vulnerable after the first trimester because the complexities of organ formation are completed.

Defects typically arise from the following failures of embryogenesis:

- *Failure of an embryologic space to close properly*. For example, the *neural tube* is an embryonic structure from which arise the brain and spinal cord and their meninges. It begins as a furrow, the edges of which grow together to form a tube. Normally, the bony vertebral body and arch of the spinal vertebrae contain the spinal cord and its meninges (Fig. 22.3A). But if the neural tube fails to close, the bony vertebral arch will remain open posteriorly, usually in the lower back, causing *spina bifida* and related conditions.
- *Failure of embryologic tissue to divide*. For example, fingers and toes must divide from one another; if division is erroneous, digits may be fused (*syndactyly*) or may be too numerous (*polydactyly*).
- *Failure of an embryologic structure to disappear normally*. For example, the thyroid gland is formed by cells budding from a temporary embryonic duct that arises from the base of the tongue (the thyroglossal duct). If the duct fails to involute normally, it may accumulate fluid to form a *thyroglossal duct cyst*.
- *Failure of tissue or organ to differentiate or grow (agenesis)*. For example, the drug thalidomide, a sedative no longer prescribed for pregnant women, prevented normal limb development in children of mothers taking the drug.

Remember This! Most birth defects originate in the first eight weeks of pregnancy.

Pop Quiz

22.5 Distinguish between congenital deformation and congenital malformation.

Defects Caused by Environmental Factors

Ordinarily, the intrauterine environment is a safe, warm, nutritious place to grow. But it does not completely shield the developing fetus from harm. This rule usually applies: whatever happens to mother happens to child.

Harmful environmental influences are of two types: the *absence* of a dietary necessity like vitamins or minerals, or the *presence* of some abnormal factor like a toxin or infection. The opposite of deficiency, a **teratogen** (from Greek *teraton* = monster) is an environmental force that causes a congenital malformation. Teratogens can be *physical* (e.g., radiation), *chemical* (e.g., alcohol, therapeutic drugs) and *microbial* (e.g., viruses, bacteria).

The most common congenital malformations are listed below (approximate birth incidence is in parentheses):

- *Hypospadias* (~1: 300), an abnormal opening of the urethra on the ventral surface of the penis
- *Patent ductus arteriosus* (~1: 600), a persistent open connection between the pulmonary artery and the aorta, which normally closes at birth
- *Ventricular septal defect* (~1: 900), an opening between the left and right ventricles of the heart
- *Cleft lip* (~1: 1,100), a malformation of the upper lip that features a slit extending from the margin of the lip up to the base of the nose (A more severe deformity is cleft palate, in which the defect extends through the palate and into the nasal cavity.)
- *Spina bifida* (~1: 2,100) and anencephaly (~1: 3,200), neural tube defects discussed previously
- *Atrial septal defect* (1: 5,900), an opening between the right and left atria of the heart, which should close shortly after birth

Case Notes

22.4 Is fetal alcohol syndrome a fetal deformation or malformation?

Nutrient Deficiency Can Cause Congenital Malformations

During the first few weeks of embryonic development, the nervous system is vulnerable to vitamin and mineral deficiencies in the mother's diet. For example, maternal iodine deficiency can impair the ability of the fetal thyroid to produce thyroid hormones. Severe mental and physical defects may result.

Adequate levels of folate, a B vitamin, are essential for proper closure of the embryonic neural tube. Normally, the bony vertebral body and arch of the spinal vertebrae contain the spinal cord and its meninges (Fig. 22.3A). If the neural tube fails to close, the bony vertebral arch will remain open posteriorly, usually in the lower back, causing *spina bifida* and related conditions. Occult spina bifida, or *spina bifida occulta* (Fig. 22.3B), is common and innocuous. Nevertheless, in more severe defects (Figs. 22.3C and 22.3D), the meninges or spinal cord protrude through the defect in the spinal column and are associated with infection and neurologic defects, especially paralysis in the legs and loss of bowel and bladder control. In the severest type of neural tube defect, almost all of the brain and spinal cord fail to form, a condition known as *anencephaly* (Fig. 22.3E). *The Clinical Side*, "Preventing Birth Defects," discusses an important public health measure to reduce the incidence of neural tube defects.

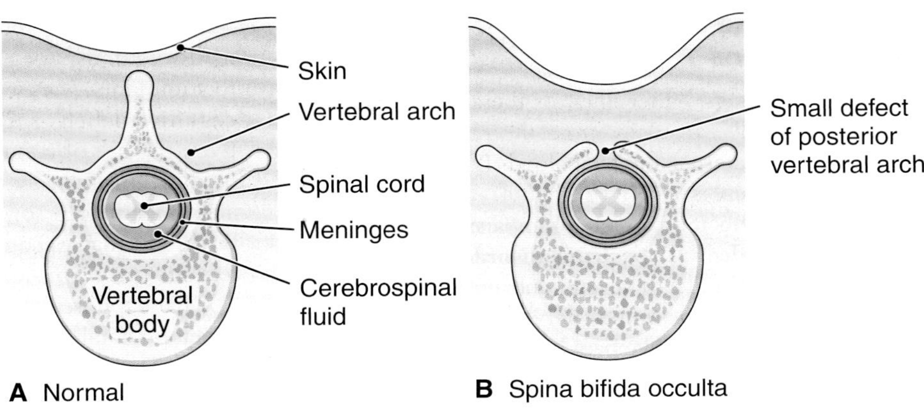

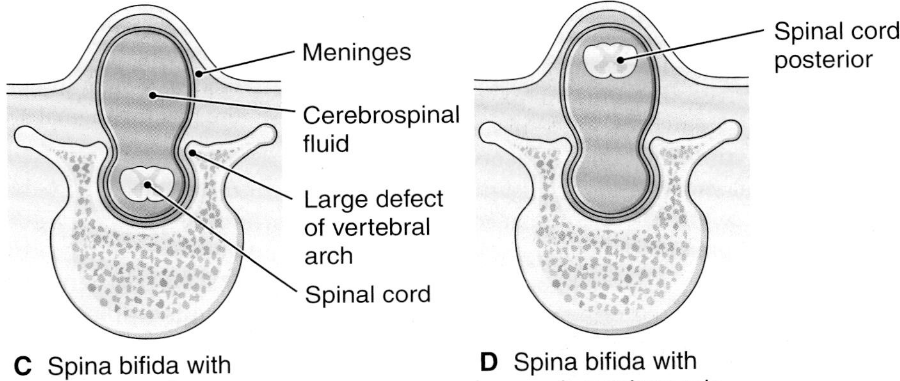

Figure 22.3 **Neural tube defects**. Cross-section studies of spine. **A.** Normal vertebra and spinal cord. **B.** In occult (minimal) spina bifida (spina bifida occulta), the posterior vertebral arch fails to form. It is usually asymptomatic. **C.** In spina bifida with meningocele, the meninges protrude through the defect. **D.** In spina bifida with myelomeningocele, the meninges and spinal cord protrude through the defect.

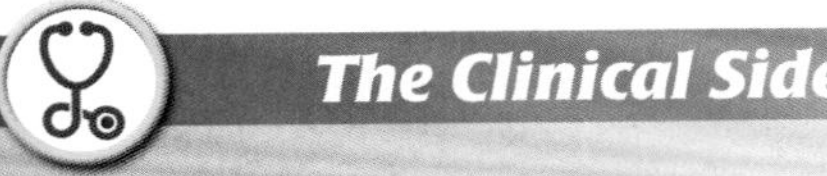

PREVENTING BIRTH DEFECTS

The cause of most birth defects is unknown, but known causes include smoking, alcohol or other drug abuse, poor nutrition, poorly controlled diabetes, and a wide variety of other maternal factors. In pregnancy alcohol should be avoided. Diabetes, if present, should be tightly controlled, and pregnant women should never take any medication without supervision.

Because folate, one of the B vitamins, is important for normal development of the nervous system in the first few weeks after conception, there is universal agreement that, *before becoming pregnant, women of childbearing age should take a daily multivitamin containing folic acid* (the form of folate found in most supplements). Daily consumption of the amount of folic acid in most multivitamin tablets reduces by about 60% the number of infants born with neural tube defects such as spina bifida. Despite this dramatic benefit, only about 25% of women of childbearing age take a multivitamin supplement. In the United States, certain basic food products (e.g., breads, breakfast cereals, and enriched flour) have supplemental folic acid added.

Vitamin A functions in the formation of the heart, limbs, eyes, and ears; a deficiency can lead to congenital malformations, low birth weight, and premature birth. Because vitamin A is fat-soluble and can readily build up in tissues, a woman's needs increase by just 10% during pregnancy. Excessive vitamin A supplementation is teratogenic, however, increasing the risk of craniofacial malformations, including cleft lip and palate, as well as heart defects and central nervous system abnormalities.

Ionizing Radiation Can Cause Congenital Malformations

Ionizing radiation (e.g., X-rays) can pass through the mother's tissue to harm ovarian germ cells or the developing fetus by damaging DNA. Damaged ovarian germ cells are destined to produce a defective fetus. On the other hand, an originally normal fetus may develop a defect if the irradiation occurs in early pregnancy when very complex genetic instructions are being executed. For example, the atomic bomb explosions in Hiroshima and Nagasaki, Japan, which ended World War II, released ionizing radiation that resulted in an increased number of birth defects in the following months and years. X-ray imaging of pregnant women should be kept to a minimum.

Chemicals and Drugs Can Cause Congenital Malformations

Chemicals and *drugs*, either illicit or therapeutic, that enter the mother's body can easily cross the placenta and make their way from maternal into fetal blood. The most important chemical teratogen is alcohol (ethanol). Alcohol abuse in pregnancy accounts for a variety of impairments collectively known as **fetal alcohol spectrum disorder**. These impairments range from mild to severe, and include intrauterine fetal growth restriction, central nervous system abnormalities, and distinctive facial characteristics (Fig. 22.4). The full-blown syndrome occurs in about 1 in 1,000 live births in the general population, usually to a mother who is a chronic alcoholic. A more common result, however, is less severe maternal alcohol abuse that causes mild childhood mental deficiency and behavioral problems. According to the U.S. Surgeon General, there is no known safe level of alcohol consumption in pregnancy. The best practice is total abstinence.

Smoking deprives the fetus of oxygen and exposes it to toxins. It is known to cause tissue damage to the fetal lungs and brain, and some evidence suggests a link between maternal smoking and cleft lip. Smoking is also thought to increase the risk for spontaneous abortion, low birth weight, and premature birth.

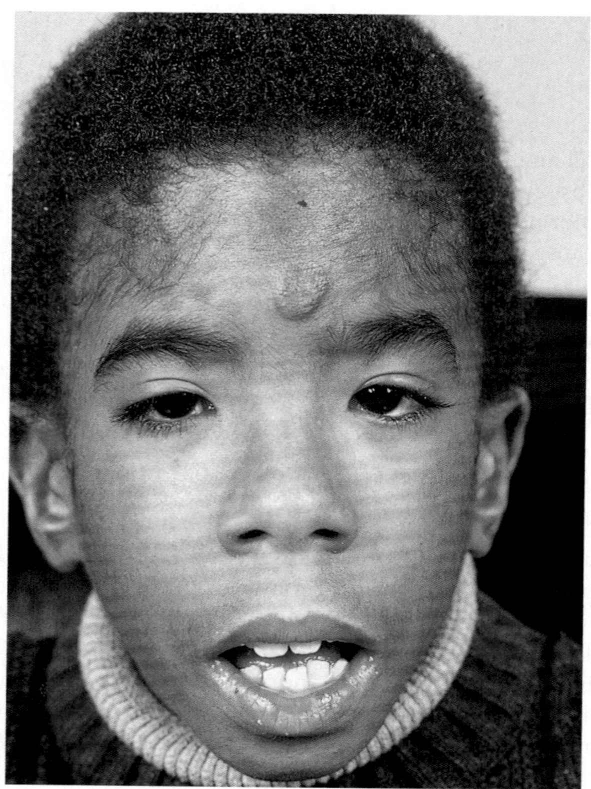

Figure 22.4 **Fetal alcohol spectrum disorder.** Note long, flat philtrum (upper lip below nose), telecanthus (wide-set eyes), flat face, mild ptosis (drooping upper eyelids). (Reproduced with permission from Gold DH, Weingeist TA. *Color Atlas of the Eye in Systemic Disease.* Baltimore, MD: Lippincott Williams & Wilkins; 2001.)

Maternal drug abuse is also associated with congenital malformations. All classes of illicit drugs—from opioids to stimulants—cause growth deficiencies, and many cause cognitive deficits and facial or other physical deformities. Even the use of certain prescription and over-the-counter medications can be harmful. The effects of moderate alcohol, tobacco, or drug use may not be noticeable at birth, but may become apparent later when behavioral or learning problems appear.

That supposedly safe therapeutic drugs can cause severe developmental defects is illustrated by the thalidomide calamity. *Thalidomide* is a sleeping pill introduced in the 1950s and prescribed abundantly to pregnant women with insomnia. An epidemic of children with short, deformed limbs resulted. Another prescription medication, diethylstilbestrol (DES), a synthetic form of estrogen used to prevent miscarriage, was prescribed from 1938 until 1971, when it was determined to interfere with development of the fetal reproductive system in both males and females. It also increases the risk for vaginal and cervical cancer ("DES daughters").

Case Notes

22.5 When was Natasha's infant most vulnerable to the influence of alcohol?

22.6 Is fetal alcohol spectrum syndrome considered a congenital defect?

22.7 What is the name of the environmental forces that cause congenital defects?

Microbes Can Cause Congenital Malformations

Microbial infection of the mother also can cross the placenta to infect the developing embryo/fetus. Infection occurs in 1–5% of live-born infants in the United States. The greatest damage results if infection occurs during the third to ninth week, the critical period of gestation when fetal organs are formed. Infection before three weeks often induces abortion; infections after nine weeks produce milder disturbances, including mental impairment.

The most common infectious teratogens are the so-called **TORCH teratogens**, discussed later in this chapter:

- Toxoplasmosis
- Other (syphilis, hepatitis B, AIDS virus, many others)
- Rubella
- Cytomegalovirus
- Herpesvirus

The effects of TORCH infections are usually not distinguishable from one another and produce a similar set of signs and symptoms (the *TORCH syndrome*). Affected infants exhibit some, but not all, of the following characteristics (see

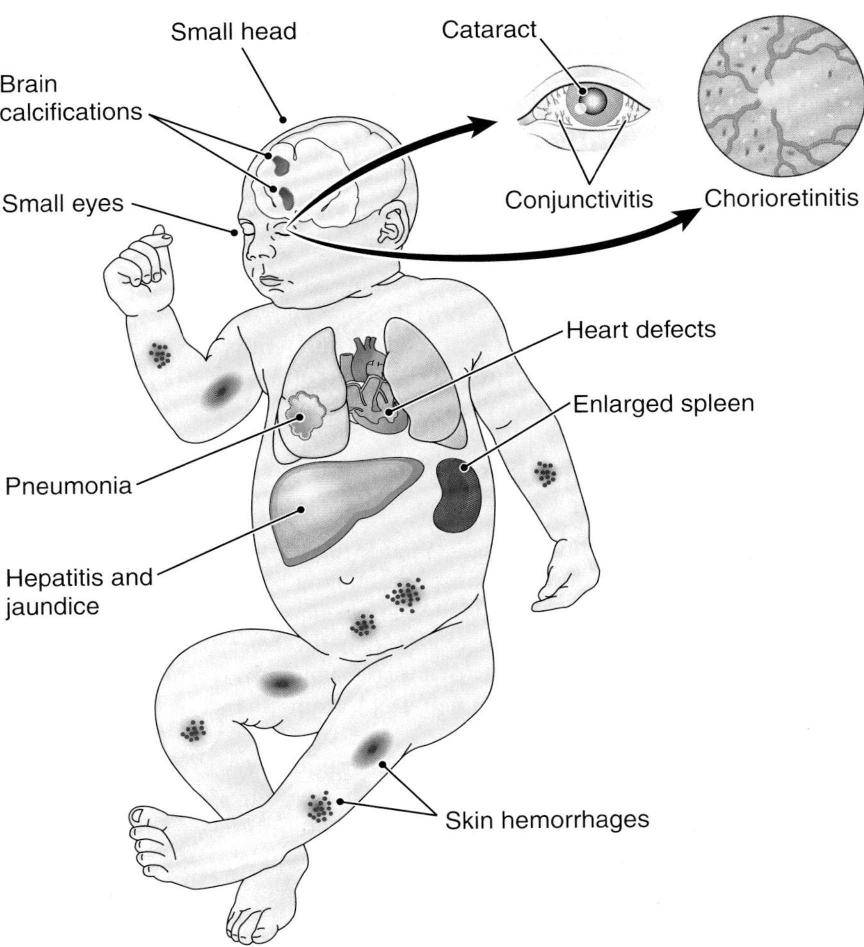

Figure 22.5 **TORCH infections.** Fetuses infected in the first trimester by Toxoplasma, rubella, cytomegalovirus, herpesvirus, or many other microbes have similar clinical findings as those illustrated in this figure.

Fig. 22.5): microcephaly (small skull), mental retardation, brain calcifications, microphthalmia (small eyeballs), cataracts (opacified lenses), chorioretinitis (inflammation of the retina and iris) and conjunctivitis, deafness, congenital heart defects, pneumonia, hepatitis and jaundice, splenomegaly (enlarged spleen), and skin hemorrhages.

Infection by cytomegalovirus or herpesvirus may produce severe fetal damage as late as the third trimester. Congenital rubella infection can be prevented by maternal vaccination. A vaccine for herpes is gaining acceptance, but there are no vaccines for other TORCH infections.

Maternal syphilis and AIDS virus (HIV) infections can also pass from mother to infant. Most pregnant women who have untreated primary or secondary syphilis pass the infection to the fetus. Latent and tertiary syphilis, however, are not transmitted. **Congenital syphilis** is a highly distinctive clinical syndrome characterized by severe brain, bone, dental, and ophthalmic problems. In contrast, **congenital HIV infection** develops in children in much the same way it does in adults and is characterized by opportunistic infections and malignancies. Congenital defects usually do not occur because the fetus does not become infected until just before or at delivery.

Transplacental infection is not the only manner of fetal infection. Infection can ascend upward into the uterus from the vagina, usually following a break in the amniotic membrane that may be heralded by an amniotic fluid leak. A broken amniotic membrane usually leads promptly to labor and delivery, with little time for infection, but, if labor is delayed, amniotic infection, and infection of the fetus, may follow. For example, fetal pneumonia may occur, although developmental abnormalities rarely occur.

Pop Quiz

22.6 True or false? Failure of the embryonic neural tube to close properly may result in failure of spinal and brain tissue to form.

22.7 Define teratogen.

22.8 Name the three varieties of teratogens.

22.9 Name two ways that smoking harms a developing embryo/fetus.

Genetic Disorders An Introduction

Insanity is hereditary; you get it from your children.

SAM LEVENSON (1911–1980), AMERICAN COMEDIAN

The mechanism of inheritance lies within the structure of **DNA (deoxyribonculeic acid)**, a very long molecule packed into the *nucleus* of every body cell. Some DNA is also present in *mitochondria* and is inherited far differently from DNA. Before we discuss the role of DNA in congenital disorders, let's review some basics of human genetics.

The Sequence of Nucleotide Bases in DNA Is the Genetic Code

DNA is constructed of nucleotides, organic molecules that contain a sugar, one or more phosphates, and a base. There are four bases: *adenine* (A), *cytosine* (C), *thymine* (T), and *guanine* (G) (see Fig. 22.6C). Notice that the base is the only part of the nucleotide that varies, but this variation in bases distinguishes human DNA from that of other animals, and your DNA from that of your best friend. That's because, despite such a limited "alphabet" of four chemical "letters," nucleotides can combine into sequences of different lengths containing a nearly infinite variety of letter combinations. For example, one snippet of DNA might "read" GGATTTCCATCAT.

Do *all* such "words" convey a meaning? The answer to this question is evolving. We currently recognize that only about 2% of human DNA is partitioned into about 23,000 **genes**, relatively short segments, each of which instructs the cell in how to make a particular protein made by no other gene (see Figs. 22.6B and 22.6C). The instructions for protein synthesis are encoded in the base sequence of the gene. In other words, the sequence of nucleotide bases in coding DNA is the **genetic code**. Cells use the code like a set of recipes for building the proteins they need. Proteins then do the work of cells.

About 95% of human DNA is noncoding; that is, its base "letters" do not instruct cells in the synthesis of proteins. Certain segments of this noncoding DNA, referred to as *switches*, are clearly regulatory: they "turn on" or "turn off" the activity of one or more genes. In other words, genetic switches determine whether or not a given gene is *expressed* as a protein to be synthesized according to the gene's instructions.

In the nucleus of a cell, DNA is spread among 23 distinctive pairs of **chromosomes**, each of which is a packet containing a unique set of genes not present in the other pairs. There are 22 pairs of **autosomes**, chromosomes not involved in sex determination. There is one pair of **sex chromosomes**, which determine the sex of the fertilized ovum as well as some other characteristics. There are two types of sex chromosomes, X and Y. Males have one X and one Y; females have two Xs.

A **karyotype** is a photographic or drawn display of chromosomes (Fig. 22.6A). Notice that the 22 pairs of autosomes are displayed according to size from the largest (1) to the smallest (22), plus the sex chromosomes (either XX or XY) are pair 23.

The human body has two types of cells:

- Specialized **germ cells** in the ovary and testis produce ova and sperm.
- **Somatic cells** form all other tissues and organs.

Somatic cells contain 46 chromosomes (23 matched pairs)—a set of 23 inherited from one parent and another set of 23 from the other parent. Germ cells are a bit more complicated. In their resting state in the ovary or testis, they have 46 chromosomes like somatic cells. When they become ova or sperm, however, they halve their chromosomes so that each has a single set of 23. All ova have 22 autosomes plus an X sex chromosome. Sperm have 22 autosomes; half have an X sex chromosome and the other half a Y. The **chromosomal notation** for a normal male is 46,XY; a normal female is designated 46,XX. An individual's genetic makeup is his or her **genotype**. The **phenotype** is the *physical traits* (female) produced by the genotype (XX).

Only germ cells can transmit the genetic code from one generation to the next. As we'll see shortly, defective genes cause disease; however, a parent's defective genes can be transmitted to a child only via germ cells. For example, smoking damages genes in lung (somatic) cells to cause lung cancer, but the cancer is not transmissible because germ cells in the ovary or testis are unaffected. In contrast, if an agent such as radiation were to damage testicular or ovarian germ cells, the defect would become a transmissible disease.

Remember This! Only germ cells (ova or sperm) can transmit defective DNA code from one generation to the next. Defective DNA in somatic cells, as in cancers, cannot be transmitted.

Case Notes

22.8 Are the defects of fetal alcohol syndrome in the fetus's somatic or germ cells?

A Mutation Is a Permanent Change in DNA

A **mutation** is a permanent change in DNA. Mutations are "typographic" mistakes—a wrong letter, missing letter, inserted letter, or a combination of errors. They can be caused by errors in the DNA replication machinery, or chemical or radiologic damage. Any such damaging force is said to be *mutagenic* (causing mutations). Again, mutations in germ cells of the ovary or testis are transmissible; those in all other (somatic) cells are not.

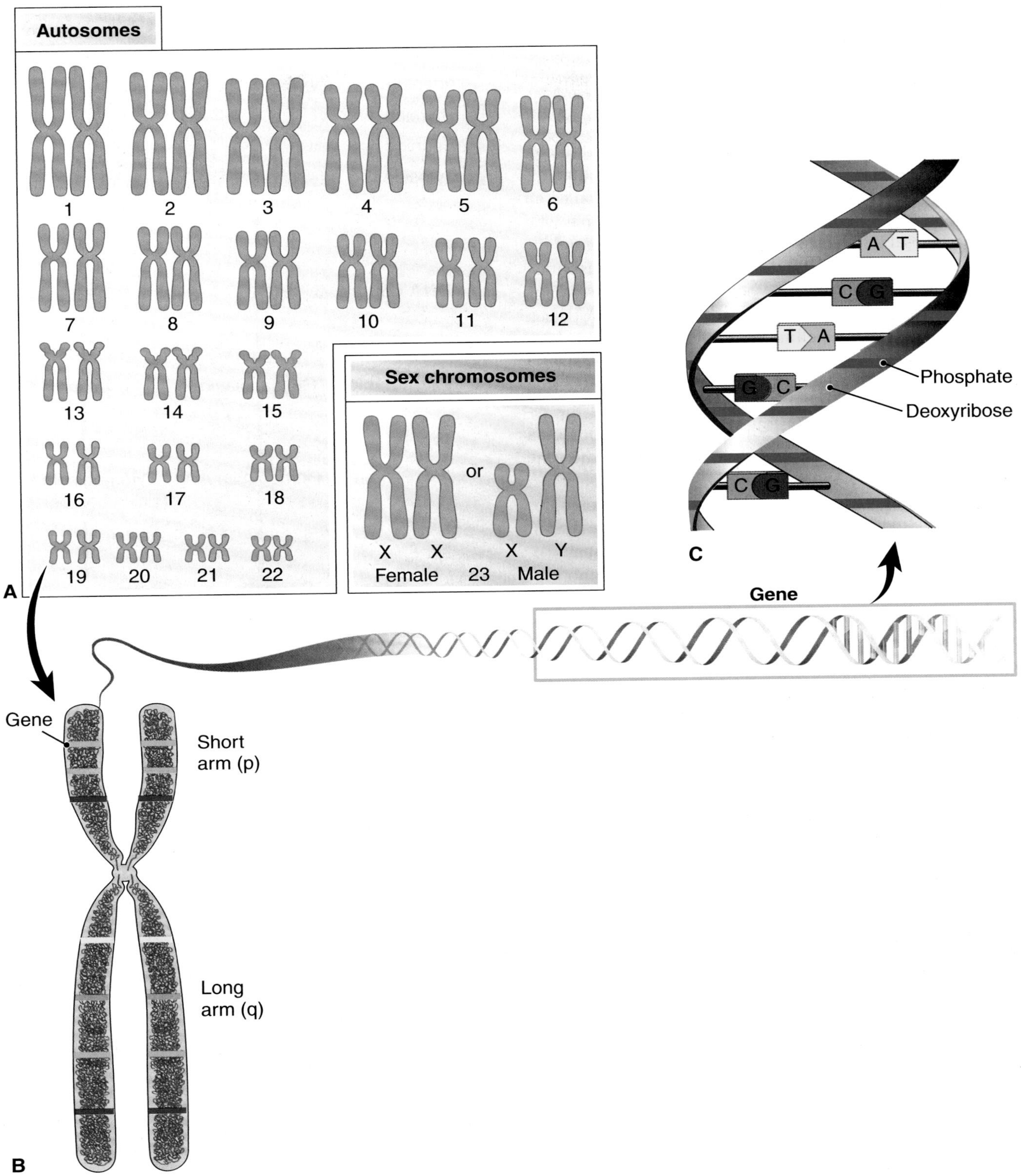

Figure 22.6 **Chromosomes, Genes, and DNA. A.** A normal set of 46 chromosomes for somatic cells (liver, lungs, muscle, etc.) is 44 autosomes and two sex chromosomes (X + Y for males; X + X for females. Genetic notation for males = 46,XY; for females = 46, XX). **B.** Image of a chromosome from a dividing cell. The chromosome has duplicated itself but is still attached at the waist to its identical partner. Final separation yields two identical chromosomes, one for each new cell. **C.** Each gene is composed of long strand of DNA containing thousands of bases (A,C,T,G). (**C.** Reproduced with permission from McConnell TH, Hull KL. *Human Form Human Function: Essentials of Anatomy & Physiology*. Baltimore, MD: Wolters Kluwer Health; 2011.)

Mutations can occur in utero. Those in embryonic *somatic* cell genes produce noninheritable congenital defects. An example is a first- trimester maternal rubella virus infection that invades the developing fetus. It damages embryonic somatic cell genes in the heart, eyes, brain, and so on and can produce severe congenital defects.

Some in utero mutations occur in *germ* cells of the embryonic ovary or testis. Although most germ cell mutations are inherited from one or both affected parents, some can arise spontaneously in the ovaries or testes of people who are not themselves affected. Most new cases of *achondroplasia* (short-limb dwarfism) arise due to new spontaneous mutations in germ cells of a parent who does not have the disease. A minority of cases are inherited as an autosomal gene defect.

When the DNA "spelling" error involves the *replacement* (substitution) of one base by another, it is called a **point mutation** (Fig. 22.7). For example, a sequence that should read GAG becomes GTG. This is actually the error responsible for sickle cell disease: thymine (T) occurs where adenine (A) should be at a single point in the gene that controls hemoglobin synthesis. This error is called the *sickle mutation*. In the production of normal hemoglobin A, the affected segment of DNA codes for the amino acid *glutamic acid*. In the presence of the sickle mutation, however, the code causes the production of the amino acid *valine*. The net result is that red cells synthesize hemoglobin that has a valine where glutamic acid ought to be. This abnormal hemoglobin is called *hemoglobin S*, the behavior of which is the underlying defect in sickle cell disease.

Many other types of spelling errors exist. **Insertion errors** are those in which one or more bases are *inserted*. (Note! Insertion and substitution, above, are not the same. Insertion *adds* an extra link or links in the chain; substitution *replaces* a link.) In the simplest example, one base is *substituted* for another (e.g., ATA becomes AT<u>C</u>A). Addition of the extra base (or bases) is added and the others *shift* to make room. **Deletion** errors are those in which one or more bases are missing (ATACC becomes AACC). Nearby bases *shift* to fill the empty space. Because DNA code is read in sets of three-base frames ("words"), insertion or deletion errors that shift sets of bases right or left are called **frameshift errors**. For example, in the sequence ACTCAT, the first "word" is ACT and the second is CAT. But if a new G is inserted to make GACTCAT, the ACTCAT sequence is shifted to the right. Now the first word is GAC, the second is TCA, and the first letter of the third word is T. This spells genetic trouble.

There Are Three Categories of Genetic Effect in Disease

Genes influence the development of some diseases and are the direct cause of others. The three categories of genetic effect are the following:

- *Monogenic (single-gene) defects*. **Monogenic diseases** are passed down by strict rules of inheritance from parent to child. An example is sickle cell disease.

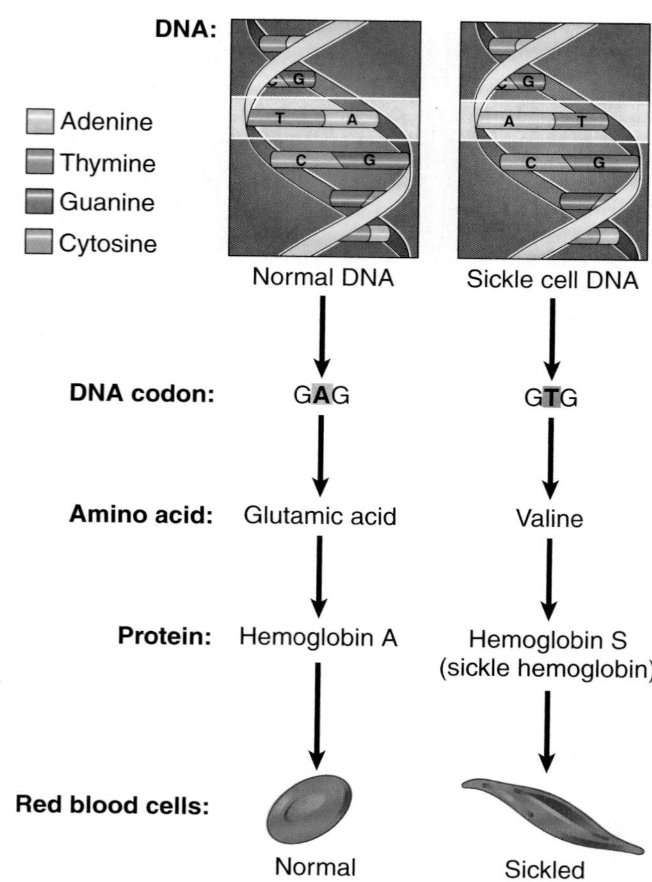

Figure 22.7 **Point mutation: the DNA mutation in sickle cell disease**. In the gene hemoglobin synthesis, the DNA contains adenine at a certain point, which causes production of normal hemoglobin A, which contains glutamic acid at a corresponding point. In sickle cell disease, the gene undergoes a mutation in which thymine (T) is *substituted* for the adenine (A), so that the normal code GAG becomes GTG. This in turn causes production of hemoglobin containing valine at a point where glutamic acid should be. This abnormal hemoglobin is called "hemoglobin S," or "sickle hemoglobin," because it is less soluble than normal hemoglobin A and tends to crystallize and deform red blood cells.

- *Polygenic (multi-gene) influence*. **Multifactorial diseases** develop under the polygenic influence of multiple genes as they interact with environmental factors, such as obesity. An example is Type II diabetes, which occurs almost exclusively in obese patients. Physical traits such as facial features and body shape are also determined by the effect of many genes, mutations of which can prompt (or predispose to) a disease.
- *Cytogenetic defects*. Cytogenic defects reflect large-scale abnormalities of chromosomes. **Cytogenetic diseases** are caused by extra or absent whole chromosomes, or structural dislocations of chromosome parts, such as pieces of chromosomes that *translocate* (switch) from one chromosome to another. These defects arise downstream as germ cells differentiate into ova or sperm (gametogenesis) and do not exist in the original germ cell. Therefore, *most* cytogenetic disorders are not inheritable. Nevertheless, there are exceptions. For

Table 22.1 Genetic Influence in Human Disease

Category of Genetic Effect	Genetic Features	Disease
POLYGENIC (ENVIRONMENTAL INFLUENCE REQUIRED)	Combined influence of multiple genes	Type II diabetes
Monogenic (single-gene defect)	Mutation in gene 19 at locus p13	Familial hypercholesterolemia
Cytogenetic	Extra chromosome 21	Down syndrome

example, there are certain rare defects of chromosome 21 that are responsible for inheritable Down syndrome.

Table 22.1 compares these three varieties of genetic influence on human disease.

Pop Quiz

22.10 Name the two types of chromosomes.

22.11 Name the two types of human cells.

22.12 Define mutation.

22.13 What are the three ways genetic material may influence the development of disease?

22.14 True or false? Cytogenetic disease is caused by a point mutation in a single gene.

Single-Gene Defects Transmitted According to Mendel's Rules

DNA analysis has identified thousands of diseases caused by single-gene (monogenic) defects, almost all of which are inherited according to strict rules and characterized by specific and predictable abnormalities. The three inheritance mechanisms for single-gene characteristics were first worked out in the 1860s by Austrian monk Gregor Mendel and are called **Mendel's rules**. They are rules of inheritance for 1) autosomal dominant; 2) autosomal recessive; and 3) sex-linked recessive genes. A few genetic defects are transmitted in nonmendelian fashion and are discussed later.

A Defective Gene Is Not Always Expressed as Disease

Of every pair of chromosomes, one is from the father and carries the genetic code for his traits, and one is from the mother and carries the genetic code for her traits. The two chromosomes in each pair are structurally similar, each carrying particular genes for particular traits—for example, type of hemoglobin. The matching genes are called **alleles**. You might think of alleles as somewhat like two earrings, one given by the father and the other by the mother. The alleles are said to be **homozygous** if they are identical; that is, if they code for exactly the same trait, say normal hemoglobin A. If the alleles are not identical, however, the condition is said to be **heterozygous**. For example, if one allele codes for hemoglobin A and its partner codes for hemoglobin S, the offspring is heterozygous for that trait (type of hemoglobin).

Either allele may behave in a **dominant** or in a **recessive** (submissive) manner. Dominant genes have greater power of **expression** (greater effect) than do recessive genes. Thus, if a person has one dominant and one recessive gene for the same characteristic, the trait carried by the dominant gene is expressed. If a dominant *healthy* allele from one parent is paired with a *defective* recessive allele from the other parent, the dominant healthy trait is expressed. The normal overpowers the recessive, and the person does not develop disease. The patient is healthy but carries the recessive trait, and is therefore called a **carrier**. This principle can be observed in the inheritance of cystic fibrosis (CF), discussed below.

Although a particular gene codes a particular trait, that trait may not be manifested at all, or it may be manifested only mildly. **Penetrance** is the percentage of individuals with the disease allele that actually have the disease. Some genes are relatively weak—they have low penetrance—and as a result, they affect fewer patients. **Expressivity** is the manner of manifestation of the disease. Certain genetic diseases vary in their expressivity. For example, some patients with cystic fibrosis have severe lung disease, whereas others have mild lung disease, but more pancreatic trouble.

Over 5,000 single-gene disorders have been identified, and new ones are discovered regularly. They occur in about 0.5% of the population and account for about 1% of hospital admissions. Most humans carry about six to eight defective genes, but almost all are recessive and therefore not expressed.

Expression of Autosomal Dominant Disorders Requires Only One Copy of the Defective Gene

An autosomal trait is expressed by a gene located on one of the 44 autosomes. A gene on an autosome is **autosomal dominant** (Fig. 22.8) if the trait or disease is expressed phenotypically (physically), even if the matching allele is normal. Marfan syndrome (Chapter 18) is an example.

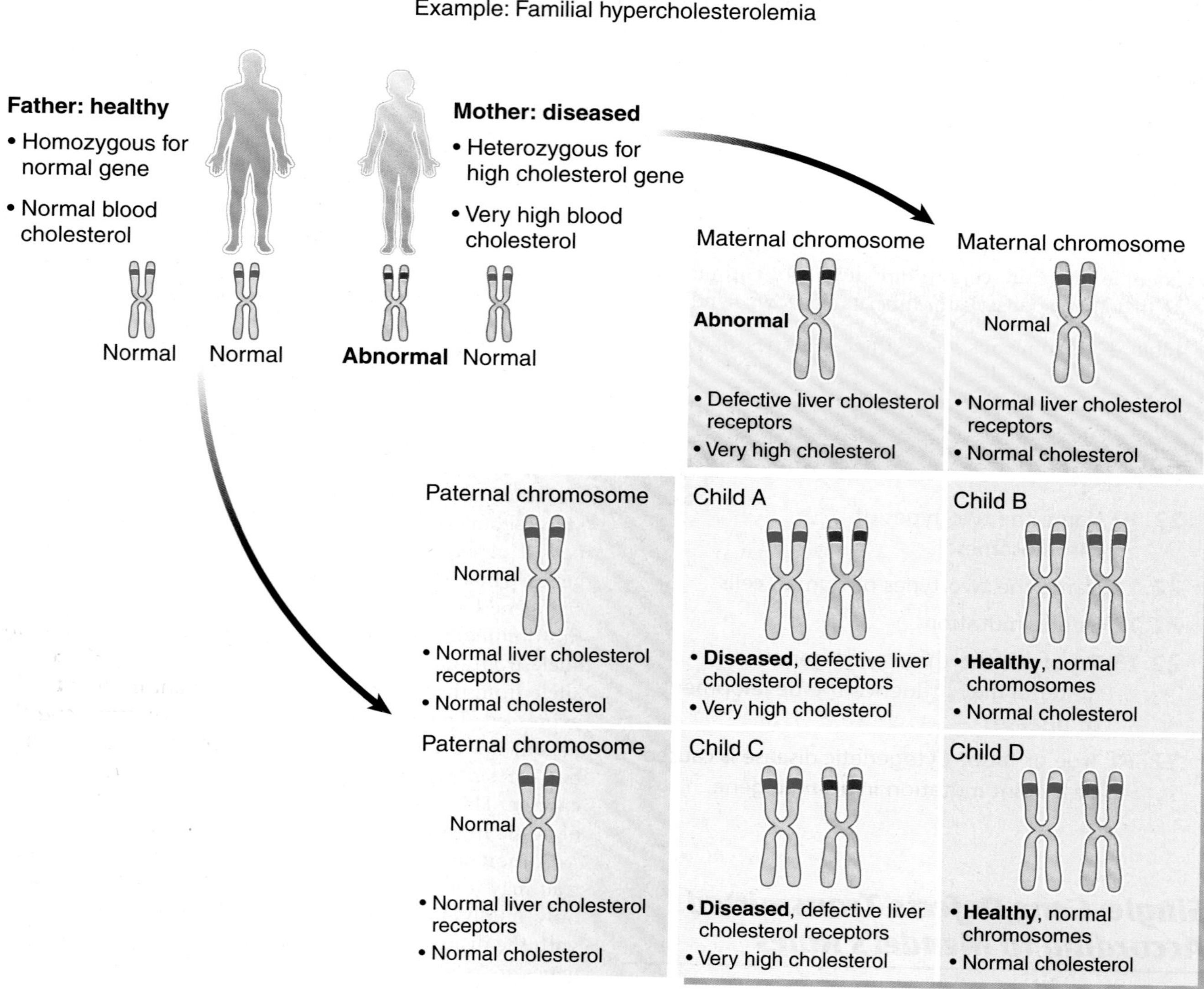

Figure 22.8 **Autosomal dominant inheritance: familial hypercholesterolemia.** The dominant allele is present in one affected (diseased) parent. Half of the children will carry the defective allele and have the disease. The other half will not have the allele and will be unaffected.

The rules of autosomal dominant disease inheritance are the following:

- The gene is physically expressed, even if only one defective allele is present in a pair of chromosomes.
- An affected parent has a 50% chance of passing the gene to a child.
- Inheritance of the defective gene ensures physical expression of the defect.

Not all mutant genes are inherited from affected parents; some arise as a new mutation in the *germ* cells of the ovary or testis of a parent and are then passed down the generations as a new defect. For example, about half of all new cases of neurofibromatosis (multiple tumors of nerves) occur when new mutations arise in chromosome 17 in the germ cells in the ovary or testis of a parent.

Expression of Autosomal Recessive Disorders Requires Two Copies of the Defective Gene

A gene on an autosome is **autosomal recessive** (Fig. 22.9) if the trait or disease is expressed phenotypically (physically) only if both alleles are defective: one from the mother and one from the father. CF, discussed below, is an example.

The rules of autosomal recessive inheritance are the following:

- The gene is physically expressed only if both chromosomes of a pair carry the defective allele (the homozygous state).
- If a child carries two copies of the defective allele, each parent necessarily has at least one copy of the defective allele.

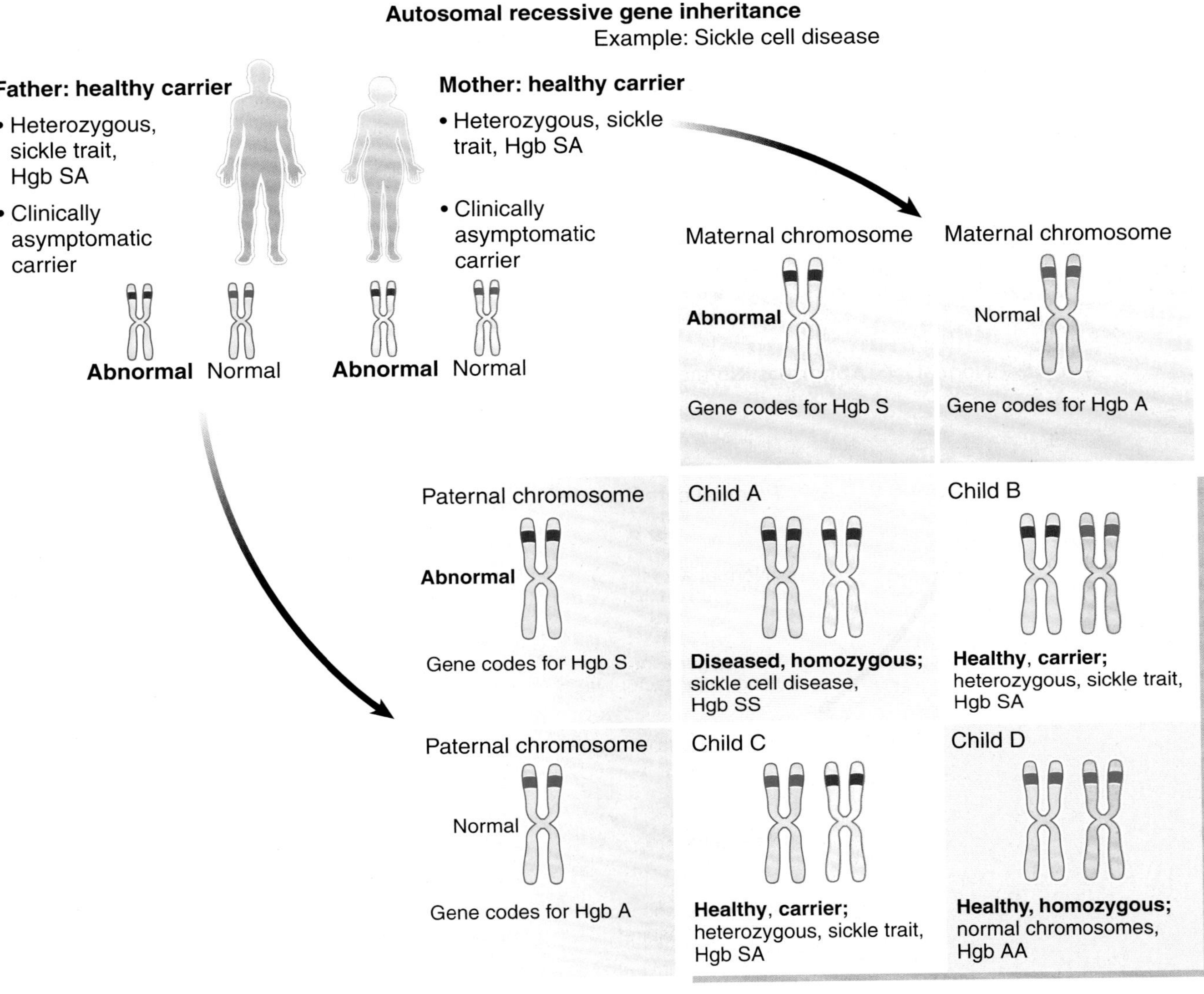

Figure 22.9 **Autosomal recessive inheritance: sickle cell disease.** The recessive allele is present in both parents, who are unaffected carriers. Half of the children will carry the defective allele as carriers, one-fourth will carry both copies and have sickle cell disease, and one-fourth will not inherit the allele and will not be carriers or have sickle cell disease.

- A parent with two copies of the defective allele mated with a parent not having the defective allele will produce offspring with a 50% chance of being a carrier of the defective allele, but none of the offspring will be physically affected.
- Two parents, each of whom has a single copy of the defective allele, will produce offspring with a 25% chance of being homozygous for the defective allele and therefore physically affected; a 50% chance of inheriting a single copy of the defective allele and being an asymptomatic carrier (the heterozygous state); and a 25% chance of inheriting two normal alleles (the normal homozygous state) and being neither affected nor a carrier.

Genes for autosomal recessive disorders are much more common than are those for autosomal dominant ones. Nevertheless, they are physically expressed only in the homozygous state, and it is rare that two people mate who are carrying the same gene.

Recessive Alleles on Sex Chromosomes Are Expressed

Patterns of inheritance are different for mutations of sex (X and Y) chromosomes. Recessive alleles (normal or defective) on sex chromosomes are expressed phenotypically if the allele is present on the X chromosome of a male (XY) or, very rarely, on both X chromosomes of a female (XX). This pattern owes to the fact that in males there are no normal alleles on Y to compensate for a defective X allele. Thus, as Figure 22.10 illustrates, a recessive allele on one of the mother's two X chromosomes is transmitted in Mendelian

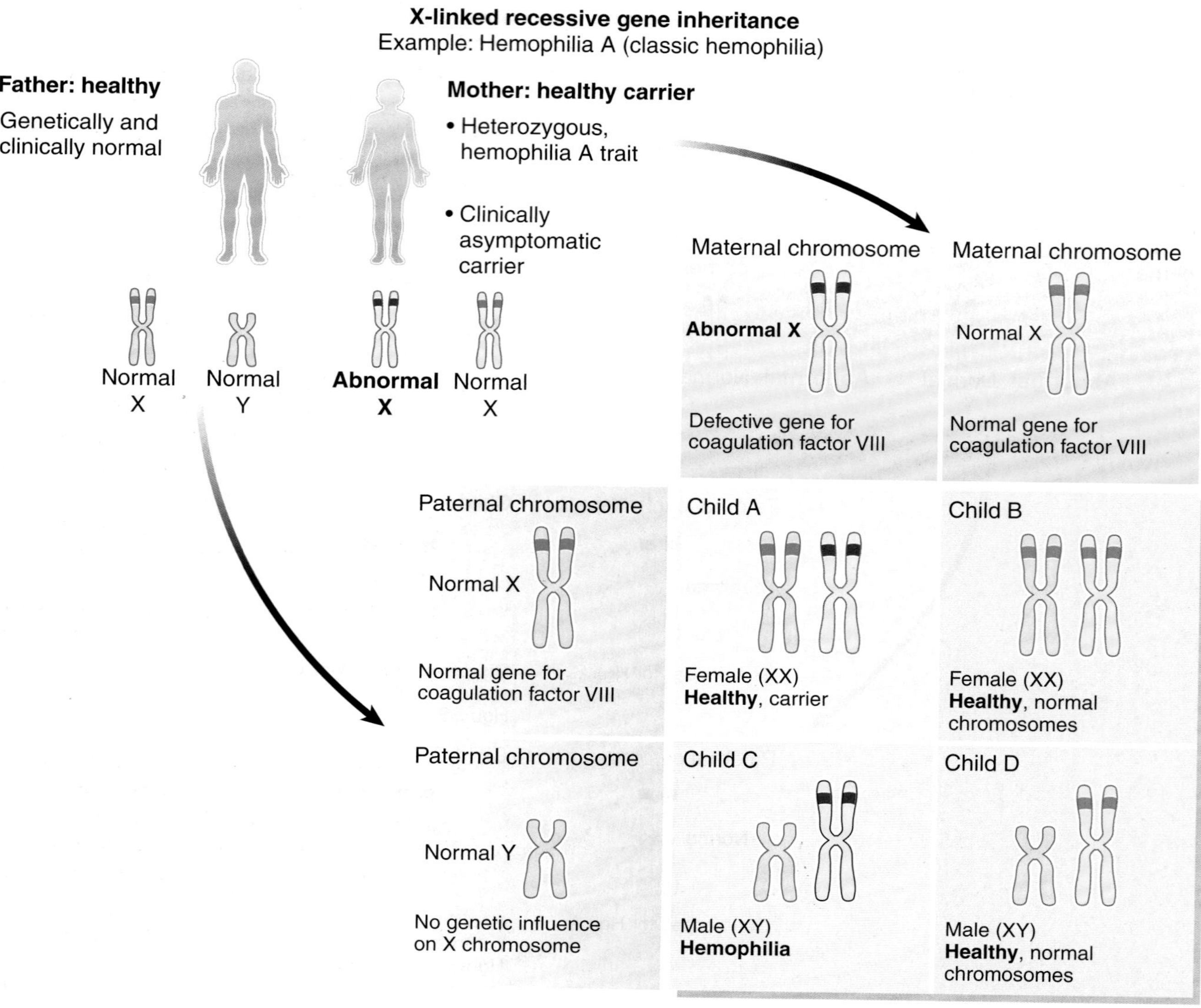

Figure 22.10 **X-linked recessive gene inheritance: classic hemophilia (hemophilia A).** The defective allele on the X chromosome is expressed in males only because the Y chromosome contains no matching normal allele to offset the effect of the defective X allele.

fashion to half of her offspring (either male or female), but *disease occurs only in sons* as an **X-linked recessive** defect. There is an exception, however: daughters may be affected if both parents carry the defective allele. This is more likely to occur in closely intermarried clans. An example is red–green colorblindness: the daughter of a colorblind father and a carrier mother has a 50% chance of being colorblind herself. Classic *hemophilia* (hemophilia A) and *Duchenne muscular dystrophy* are inherited as X-linked recessive diseases: diseased males are offspring of carrier mothers. Figure 22.11 illustrates these and other X-linked recessive diseases and the location of their alleles on the X chromosome.

The same rules of inheritance apply to genes on the Y chromosome, but Y-related defects are rare and are related mainly to infertility caused by defective sperm.

Single-Gene Defects Are Clinically Expressed according to the Type of Defective Protein

The protein coded by a gene can be one of four types:

- Enzymes and proteins that regulate enzyme activity
- Membrane receptor and transport proteins
- Proteins that regulate cell growth
- Structural, coagulation, and other proteins

Every disease resulting from a single-gene defect falls into one of these categories.

Defective Enzymes and Proteins That Regulate Enzyme Activity

Enzymes are proteins that accelerate chemical reactions. They act on a substance called a *substrate* and convert it

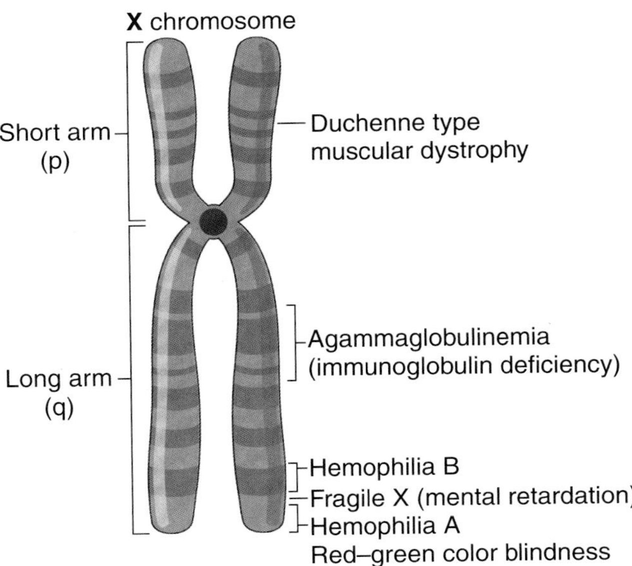

Figure 22.11 **The X chromosome.** The allele locations of some X-linked recessive inherited diseases.

into a *product*. Therefore, enzyme defects cause either an accumulation of upstream (substrate) material and/or a deficit of an end (downstream) product, much like a dam on a stream results in an accumulation of water upstream and a lack of it downstream.

Gaucher disease is an example of an autosomal recessive disease caused by accumulation of unmetabolized substrate. It results from a defect in the gene that codes for an enzyme that metabolizes *glucocerebroside*. Unmetabolized glucocerebroside accumulates in macrophages throughout the body, especially in the brain, bone marrow, lymph nodes, and spleen.

Sometimes, deficiency of an end product is the cause of disease. *Glycogen storage disease* is a genetic condition in which the affected enzyme normally converts muscle glycogen into glucose. The defect causes an accumulation of glycogen and a shortage of glucose that result in severe muscle cramps and muscle cell necrosis.

Alpha-1 antitrypsin (AAT) deficiency is an autosomal recessive disorder of enzyme regulatory proteins. AAT, a blood protein synthesized by the liver, permeates tissues to protect against *excess* effect of proteolytic enzymes released by neutrophils recruited to sites of tissue injury and inflammation. Deficiency of AAT is associated with excessive tissue digestion by inflammatory reactions. This is particularly noticeable in the lungs of affected patients, especially smokers. The inflammatory reaction caused by cigarette smoke is not lessened by AAT, which results in severe autodigestion of alveoli. The result is emphysema.

Defective Genes of Membrane Receptor and Transport Proteins

Some proteins are designed to attach to other molecules. When a protein attaches to and carries a molecule from one place to another, it is called a **transport protein**. If the receptor is defective, the message (signal) cannot be transmitted. For example, *Wilson disease* is an autosomal recessive disorder of copper metabolism that is characterized by toxic accumulations of copper in many tissues, especially brain and liver. The defective gene on chromosome 13 codes for a copper transport protein, without which copper cannot be normally removed from cells.

Receptor proteins attach to chemical messenger molecules and relay messenger instructions. For example, receptors in the liver capture low-density lipoprotein (LDL) during the process of converting cholesterol into bile salts for excretion into bile. Thus, a genetic defect resulting in too few LDL receptors would manifest with high levels of blood cholesterol. *Familial hypercholesterolemia* is a result of such a genetic defect. It is an autosomal-dominant defect of liver receptor proteins for LDL and is the most common, serious Mendelian disorder, affecting about 1 of every 500 people. It assumes special significance because high LDL cholesterol levels in blood are associated with accelerated atherosclerosis. Nevertheless, most cases of high cholesterol result from poor dietary habits, not a genetic defect.

Defective Genes of Growth Control Proteins

Proto-oncogenes are normal genes that promote cell growth in a normal physiologic setting. They are opposed by **tumor suppressor genes**, which inhibit cell growth. Normal cell growth depends on proper balance between these opposing forces. Mutations in these genes are the cause of some malignancies. They can be thought of metaphorically as the gas pedal (proto-oncogenes) and the brakes (tumor suppressors) of a vehicle.

When a mutation occurs in a proto-oncogene, it is then called an oncogene. The oncogene is capable of "stepping on the gas": driving cells to undergo unlimited replication and also allowing the cells to escape the control of a tumor suppressor "brakes."

A defective tumor suppressor, on the other hand, fails to suppress activity of a proto-oncogene, which also results in uncontrolled growth. For example, *neurofibromatosis Type I (von Recklinghausen disease*, Chapter 19) is an autosomal recessive disorder of a tumor suppressor gene. Patients with neurofibromatosis have peripheral nerve and other tumors that may become malignant.

Defective Genes for Structural, Coagulation, and Other Proteins

Structural proteins provide support for cells and tissues. For example, fibrillin, a structural protein synthesized by fibroblasts, is an important component of the extracellular matrix. A genetic defect of fibrillin synthesis produces *Marfan syndrome*, an autosomal dominant disease characterized by the defects illustrated in Figure 22.12. Marfan

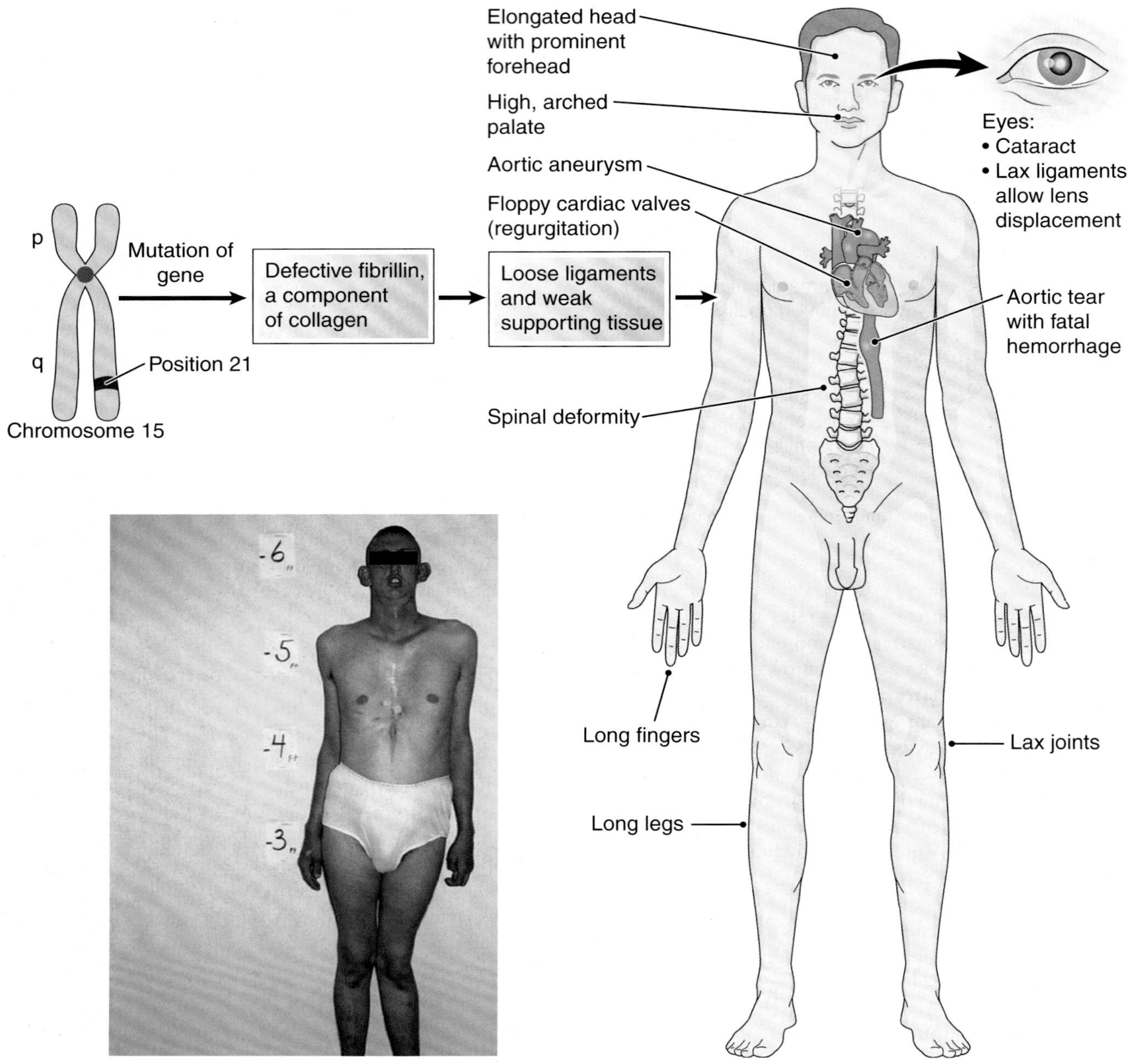

Figure 22.12 **Marfan syndrome.** The defective gene at position 21 on the long (q) arm of chromosome 15 causes production of defective collagen, which results in clinical findings known as "Marfan syndrome." **Photo inset**: The sternal scar is from surgical repair of an aortic aneurysm.

disease is rare, affecting about 1 in 10,000. Moreover, the genetic defect has decreased penetrance and often fails to manifest. Because of his tall, lanky habitus, some speculate that Abraham Lincoln had Marfan syndrome; however, most experts think it unlikely.

Classic hemophilia (hemophilia A) is an X-linked recessive disorder of factor VIII, an important blood *coagulation* protein. Males with hemophilia A lack enough factor VIII for normal clotting.

Cystic Fibrosis Is a Common and Frequently Fatal Genetic Disease

Cystic fibrosis (CF) is an autosomal recessive genetic disease of exocrine glands that primarily affects the lungs and gastrointestinal tract. It leads to chronic lung disease and infection, pancreatic insufficiency with attendant intestinal symptoms, and high sweat chloride. CF is the most common fatal genetic disease of Caucasians, occurring in about 1 in 3,300 live Caucasian births. Rates in other ethnic groups are much lower. The defect occurs on chromosome 7 and is carried by about 3% of the Caucasian population.

Pathogenesis

CF can be caused by any one of thousands of mutations in a single gene, the cystic fibrosis transmembrane regulator (CFTR). The most common mutation is one that deletes a set of three bases that code for the amino acid phenylalanine, one of the many amino acids in the protein made by the CFTR gene. Loss of this single amino acid causes all of the symptoms seen in CF.

The genetic defect affects the transport of chloride (Cl^-) across epithelial cell membranes of gland ducts. Nearly all exocrine glands are affected. Because sodium and chloride are transported across the cell membrane together, glandular secretions have decreased sodium and chloride and low osmotic pressure. As a result, they are unable to attract water. The consequence is thick secretions that obstruct bronchial and intestinal mucus gland ducts, pancreatic ducts, hepatic bile ducts, and the vas deferens.

Signs and Symptoms

The signs and symptoms of CF vary according to the organs affected. They also vary in severity and onset: diagnosis is made early in some patients, whereas in others the disease may not manifest itself for several years.

Accumulations of thick mucus in pancreatic ducts prevent digestive enzymes from reaching the GI tract. The result is chronic pancreatitis, gastrointestinal malabsorption, and malnourishment. In the fetus or newborn, intestinal mucus may be so thick that it causes intestinal obstruction (*meconium ileus*). Obstruction of hepatic bile ducts causes chronic inflammation and widespread liver scarring (*cirrhosis*). Obstruction of the vas deferens causes low sperm count and infertility in 98% of affected males. Thick mucus from bronchial glands obstructs small bronchi, impairs respiration, and promotes infection.

In certain patients, intestinal malabsorption symptoms predominate, and patients have large, fatty, smelly stools; malnutrition; and abdominal distention. In most patients, however, severe bronchitis and recurrent pneumonia are the biggest problems. Pulmonary infections account for the great majority of CF deaths.

Diagnosis and Treatment

The glandular secretions in CF patients are characterized by low levels of sodium and chloride. In sweat gland ducts, however, the chloride transport defect has the opposite effect: sweat sodium and chloride levels are abnormally high. This characteristic finding is the basis for the sweat chloride test, a common diagnostic test for CF.

Treatment for lung disease consists of intensive pulmonary therapy along with mucus-thinning and bronchodilating drugs, with antibiotics as needed to control infection. Malabsorption syndrome is treated by careful attention to caloric need, pancreatic enzyme supplements, and fat-soluble vitamins to replace those lost in stool fat. In some patients, a feeding tube is surgically implanted to deliver additional nutrition during sleep. In the past, CF was routinely fatal during childhood. With improved treatment, median life expectancy is now about 35 years.

Single-Gene Defects Transmitted According to Non-Mendelian Rules

Three categories of single-gene defects do not obey Mendel's rules:

- *Triplet repeat mutation* is characterized by several hundreds or thousands of repeating DNA bases. The most common is **Fragile X syndrome**: familial mental retardation owing to excess repeats of the CGG triplet. Discussion of the manner of inheritance is beyond the scope of this text.
- *Genomic imprinting* is a poorly understood process that defies the long held notion that the parental origin of a gene makes no difference: it should behave the same no matter its origin. A few diseases have been identified in which a single-gene defect behaves differently according to whether it was inherited from mother or father.
- *Mitochondrial gene mutations* are very rare. Mitochondrial DNA is passed to both male and female offspring by the mother, but is transmissible to the next generation only by females. This occurs because sperm, in their development, shed virtually all of their mitochondrial DNA to slim down for easy travel. By contrast, an ovum packs in four cells' worth of mitochondrial and cytoplasm to sustain the metabolism of the zygote until it implants in the endometrium. **Wolf-Parkinson-White syndrome** is an example of a *mitochondrial gene mutation*. It features an accessory bundle of conductive tissue between the atria and ventricles, which causes paroxysms of tachycardia.

Pop Quiz

22.15 Name the three Mendelian categories for the inheritance of single-gene defects.

22.16 Distinguish between expressivity and penetrance.

22.17 True or false? Two copies of a gene are required for expression of an autosomal recessive trait.

22.18 Which type of protein is affected if a gene defect causes an excess or a deficit of a substance?

22.19 Which type of protein is affected if a gene defect causes growth of a tumor?

22.20 What type of body tissue is primarily affected by CF?

22.21 The function of which organs is most affected by CF?

manner, some ethnic groups show unique tendencies to have certain diseases—African Americans are much more likely to develop high blood pressure than are people of European extraction. Nevertheless, in any individual patient, the degree of genetic influence is less certain and usually outweighed by environmental factors.

In addition to obesity and Type II diabetes mentioned above, other notable examples of multifactorial disorders are cleft lip, congenital heart disease, gallstones, gout, and mental retardation. Cardiovascular disease, arthritis, osteoporosis, many forms of cancer, and an array of other common, chronic diseases are also known to be multifactorial.

Disorders Influenced by Multiple Genes

Our *genotype*, the sum of all of our genes, influences the development of many diseases, but typically requires a partner in crime*: environmental factors*, such as alcohol abuse, smoking, radiation, or overeating. In Chapter 1, we called such disease *multifactorial*. We said that DNA is like a genetic soil into which the seed of injury can be planted: genetically susceptible soil will sprout disease in response to a particular environmental condition. For example, plant enough fast food calories in the genetic soil of one population group and you may get a bumper crop of obesity and Type II diabetes, whereas in another group, you may get far fewer cases. This point is illustrated by some southwestern tribes of American Indians, who have very high rates of obesity and diabetes when compared to other populations eating a similar diet.

Remember This! Most diseases are multifactorial: they are a product of genetic influence and environmental factors.

The inheritance risk in multifactorial disorders can only be estimated. Most epidemiologists suggest that genetic susceptibility equates to an approximate 5–10% increase in risk for the disease in question. We also know little about exactly which of the 23,000 genes may be responsible for any given disease. It may be that, like adverse drug interactions, the genes themselves are normal but in some way they produce an undesirable result when combined. In Type II diabetes, for example, about 40 genes governing glucose metabolism and body weight have been identified that appear to play a role. In other diseases, a genetic effect (predisposition) becomes apparent only in studies of large populations. For example, cancer of the esophagus is much more common in Iran than in the United States. Diet may explain some of the difference but genetic factors are most important. In like

Pop Quiz

22.22 Other than the influence of multiple genes, what factor is required to produce multifactorial disease?

22.23 Provide an example of a multifactorial disease.

Disorders Caused by Large-Scale Chromosome Abnormalities

As noted earlier, cytogenetic disease results from abnormalities involving large parts of chromosomes or entire chromosomes. These abnormalities arise during the production of ova and sperm from ovarian and testicular germ cells. Division of an ovarian or testicular germ cell into ova or sperm (meiosis, or reduction division) requires separation of the 44 autosomes and two sex chromosomes (46,XX or 46,XY) into equal sets of 22 autosomes plus one sex chromosome (23,X or 23,Y). Misallocation (unequal division) of chromosomes between the two new ova or sperm is the cause of most cytogenetic disease. For example, one ovum may get both chromosomes 21 (24,X+21) and the other gets none (22,X-21). If the 24,X+21 is fertilized, the sperm adds a third copy of chromosome 21. The result in a female is 47, XX,+21 (trisomy 21, or *Down syndrome*).

Cytogenetic disorders may affect any chromosome. The three most common defects are

- one or more extra chromosomes;
- a missing chromosome;
- a structural abnormality of chromosomes, such as missing parts (deletion), parts that have been moved from one chromosome to another (translocation), or parts that detach and reattach upside down (inversion). The chromosomes are otherwise normal.

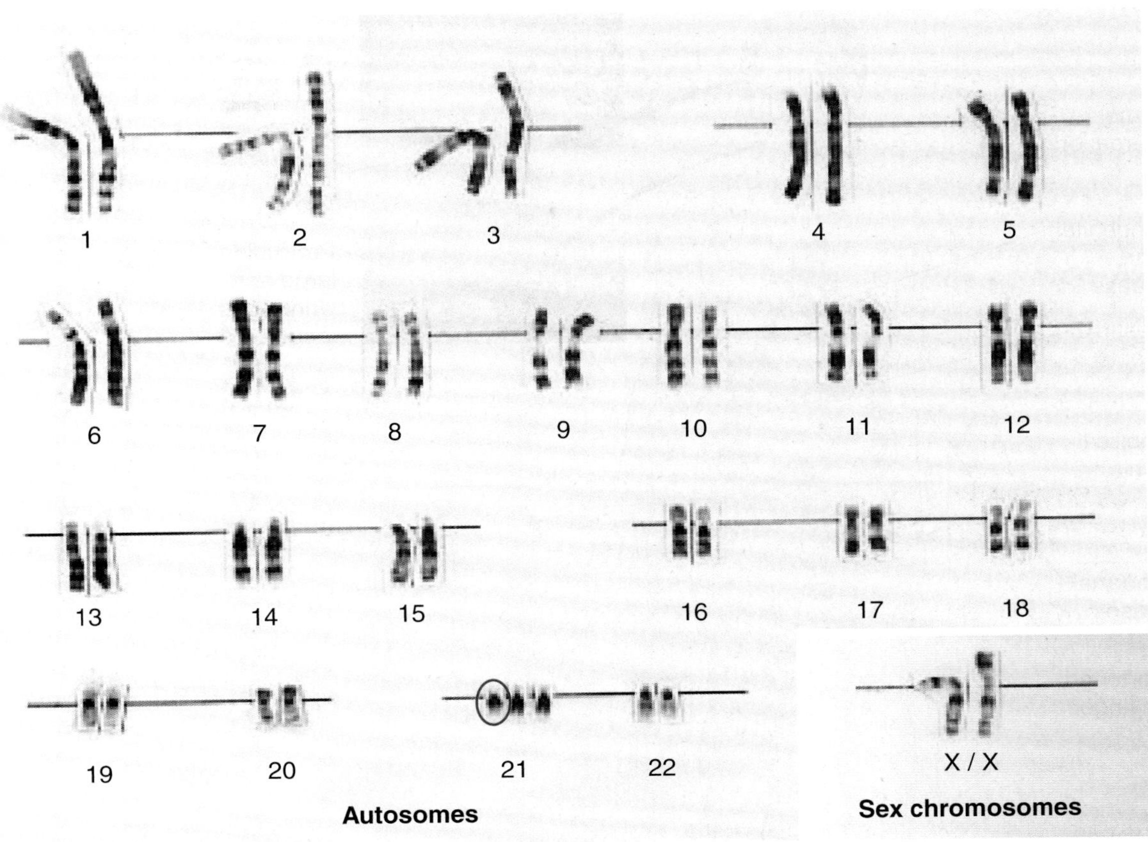

Figure 22.13 **Karyotype of Down syndrome**. A photographic display of the chromosomes of a female (XX) patient with Down syndrome reveals three copies of chromosome 21 (trisomy 21) instead of the normal two.

The basic tool of cytogenetic investigation is the karyotype. Creating a karyotype enables geneticists to identify extra or missing chromosomes and other abnormalities. Figure 22.13 is an example of a karyotype of a female patient with Down syndrome. Notice that there are three copies of chromosome 21. Additionally, chromosomes may be stained to reveal patterns of alternating dark and light bands that enable definitive identification of each chromosome and some of its internal detail. About 1 in 200 newborns has some detectable cytogenetic abnormality (although most are innocuous). About 50% of spontaneous first-trimester abortions have chromosome abnormalities.

Some Cytogenetic Diseases Are Due to Abnormal Numbers of Autosomes

The loss of an autosome, which leaves the embryo with only one copy of the chromosome instead of the normal pair, is called *monosomy*, a condition that is not compatible with life and results in spontaneous abortion. An extra copy of an autosome, so that the patient has three copies of a particular chromosome, not two, is *trisomy*. Most autosomal trisomy results in spontaneous abortion; however, some fetuses survive, especially those with trisomies of chromosomes number 13, 18, or 21, each of which is associated with significant mental and physical problems.

Trisomy 21 (Down syndrome) is the most common cytogenetic disorder in the United States and the single most common cause of mental retardation. Overall, it occurs in about 1 in 1,000 births; however, it is strongly influenced by maternal age, occurring in about 1 in every 1,500 births to women under age 30, but in about 1 in 25 births to women over age 45.

A Down syndrome fetus possesses three copies of chromosome 21 (Fig. 22.13), rather than the normal two. The usual cause is a defective ovum that contains two number 21 chromosomes, rather than one; fertilization by sperm adds the third copy.

Infants with Down syndrome are mentally retarded; however, the degree of impairment can vary from mild to severe. Physical signs include a flat face with epicanthal folds and abnormalities of the hands and feet, as Figure 22.14 illustrates. They also may have cardiac and intestinal malformations, as well as immune deficiencies and associated infections, and have an increased risk of leukemia.

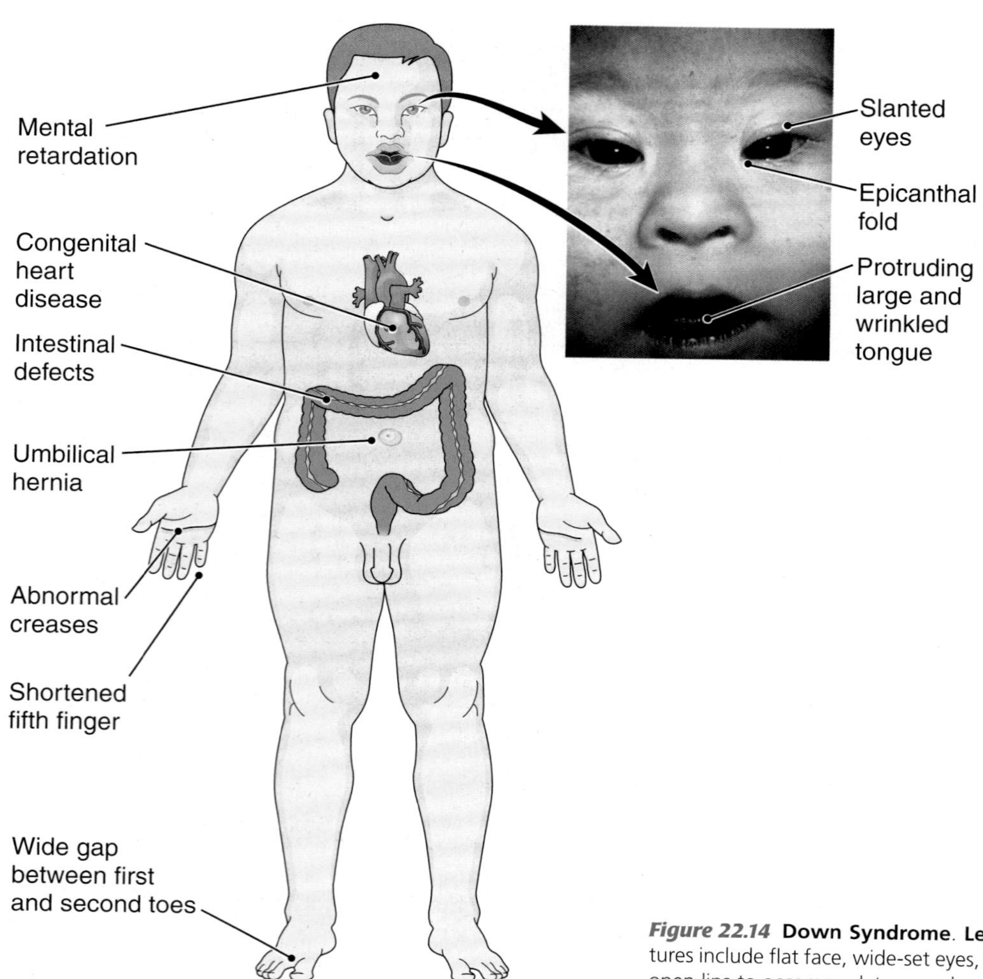

Figure 22.14 **Down Syndrome**. **Left**: Clinical features. **Right**: Facial features include flat face, wide-set eyes, low nasal bridge, epicanthal folds, and open lips to accommodate an enlarged tongue.

Although there is no cure for children born with Down syndrome, supportive therapies can greatly increase quality of life. Some patients require surgery to correct heart and other organ defects. Behavioral training and special education are important. With appropriate care, many patients live productive and meaningful lives. Although early death is not uncommon, the lifespan of people with Down syndrome is increasing: many live beyond age 50, although they often develop a form of early Alzheimer disease.

Case Notes

22.9 Keeping in mind that karyotyping was not done on Natasha's infant, what is his probable genotype?

Some Cytogenetic Diseases Are Due to Abnormal Numbers of Sex Chromosomes

The most common cause of sex chromosome cytogenetic disease is faulty ovarian or testicular meiosis that produces ova or sperm with an extra sex chromosome or none. For example, if an ovum contains an extra X chromosome (24,XX instead of 23,X) and is fertilized by a normal sperm (23,Y) the result is 47,XXY, which is recognized clinically as **Klinefelter syndrome** (Fig. 22.15). A typical patient is tall and effeminate, with long arms and legs, a small penis and atrophic testicles, scant pubic hair, no beard, and female-like hip shape. Some patients may also have enlarged breasts (gynecomastia).

By way of further example, abnormal sperm or ovum can be the cause of cytogenetic disease. For example, a normal sperm is either 23,X or 23,Y. Nevertheless, rarely a sperm will be 22,0; that is, it has neither X nor Y. If such a sperm with no sex chromosome fertilizes a normal (23,X) ovum, the genotype is 45,X0, which is recognized clinically as **Turner syndrome**. These patients clinically appear to be females who are sexually immature, infertile, have short stature, a wide, webbed neck, a low hairline on the back of the neck, a broad, flat chest (with no breast development) and with widely separated nipples, scant pubic hair, and multiple pigmented skin lesions (nevi). They do not have menstrual periods, and their ovaries are rudimentary streaks. Congenital cardiac malformations are common.

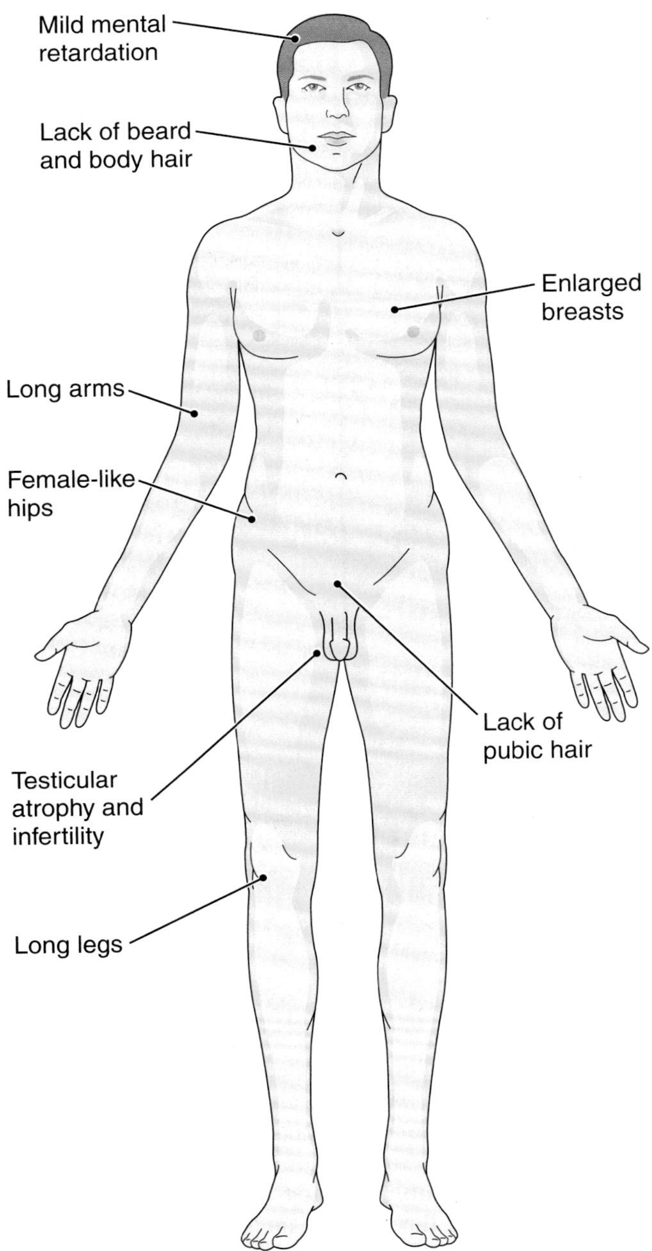

Figure 22.15 **Clinical features of Klinefelter syndrome (47,XXY).**

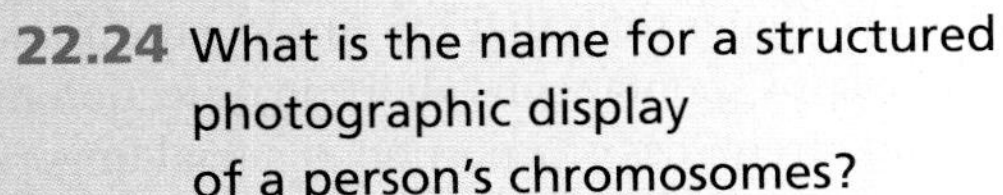

Pop Quiz

22.24 What is the name for a structured photographic display of a person's chromosomes?

22.25 Name the specific chromosomal defect in Down syndrome.

Genetic Diagnosis

Prenatal genetic diagnosis is important for three main reasons. Genetic diseases: 1) are transmissible down the generations; 2) can create lifelong burdens for parents, families, and the affected child; and 3) consume large amounts of health resources per patient. Diagnosis of genetic disorders usually requires expert advice by a geneticist and laboratory examination of maternal and/or fetal chromosomal material.

Preconception and Prenatal Testing Are Available

Prior to the arrival of molecular techniques, genetic disorders were diagnosed during infancy by clinical study or by detection of abnormal accumulations of substances in blood, urine, or tissue. Observation of mental retardation as a component of certain diseases is an example of the former; detection of hemoglobin S by a sickle cell test on blood is an example of the latter. Now, however, direct examination of DNA is possible both for preconception testing (of both partners' DNA) and for prenatal testing (of fetal DNA).

Indications for genetic testing include the following:

- Mother 35 years or older
- Parents who already have a child with a known genetic disease
- Other family history of genetic problems
- Parents from ethnic group with increased incidence of a particular genetic disorder

Prenatal genetic screening should be offered to all pregnant patients early in their pregnancy, and specific tests should be advised for those with known risk factors for carrying a fetus with a particular genetic disease (Fig. 22.16). For example, all pregnant women over age 35 should be offered screening for chromosomal trisomies.

Preconception counseling and testing are available for patients at high risk for conceiving a child with a serious genetic disease. For example, women and their partners who are of French Canadian, Cajun, or Ashkenazi Jewish descent should receive counseling and screening to rule out the possibility that they may be carriers of the gene for Tay Sachs disease, a rare but always fatal autosomal recessive disorder more common in these populations.

Non-Invasive Methods Include Maternal Blood Tests and Ultrasound

Currently, maternal blood for genetic screening can be obtained as early as the 15th week of pregnancy. Commonly called the *triple test*, this screening looks for levels of two types of hormones and a fetal protein that may indicate an increased risk for genetic abnormalities. The test, however, is 70% sensitive (it misses 30% of defects) and the false-positive rate is 5%. A positive test therefore simply

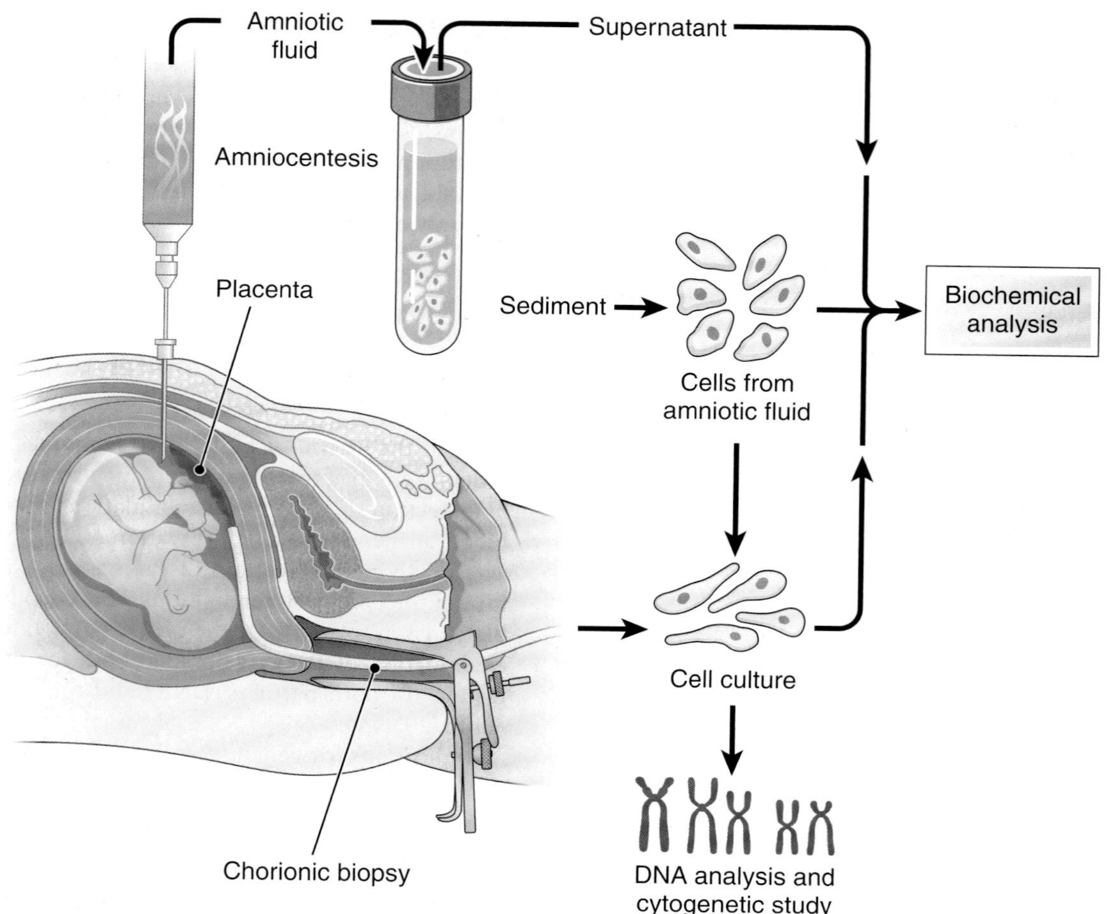

Figure 22.16 **Prenatal specimen collection for genetic diagnosis.** Amniocentesis obtains fluid and fetal cells from amniotic fluid. Chorionic biopsy obtains fetal cells. Both specimens are subject to genetic and biochemical analysis.

indicates that further testing is needed, usually collection of fetal cells by one of the techniques discussed below.

Some fetal cells find their way into maternal blood and can be harvested for fetal RNA and DNA analysis. The technique is new, and preliminary data suggest that the procedure test is reliably accurate for detecting chromosomal trisomies.

Ultrasound may also be used to examine the fetal head for size and general anatomical development; however, it cannot be used to assess for congenital anomalies until fetal structures have developed sufficiently, usually by 18 weeks.

Fetal Cell Sampling Methods Carry Risks

Cell sampling tests are, of course, invasive, and therefore carry risks of injury to the fetus. Nevertheless, they are highly accurate and can provide information earlier in the pregnancy than ultrasound imaging.

Fetal cells may be obtained by needle aspiration of the amniotic sac or placental biopsy (Fig. 22.16). Needle aspiration of amniotic fluid is called **amniocentesis**. Fetal cells line the amniotic sac and can be collected from centrifuged sediment and subjected to molecular, genetic, or chemical analysis. The test can be performed as early as 15 weeks, and is usually reliable in detecting certain genetic defects. Risks include amniotic fluid leakage, infection, and fetal death in about 1 in 1,500 cases.

As noted earlier, the placenta includes fetal tissue. Placental biopsy (**chorionic villus sampling, CVS**) carries more risk but can be employed earlier than amniocentesis, an advantage if the genetic risk is higher. After 10 completed weeks of pregnancy, the clinician inserts a catheter into the cervix and, guided by ultrasound, aspirates a sample of cells from the placental edge. These cells can be studied biochemically for evidence of abnormal substances; chromosomes can be studied by karyotype, and DNA can be analyzed for defects. The risk of complications from CVS is higher than that for amniocentesis, and includes a 3% risk for spontaneous abortion, infection in 1 in 200 cases, and rarely, loss of a portion of a fetal finger or toe. It is therefore important for the clinician and patient to weigh the risks and benefits, considering carefully why the test is being performed and what will be done with the information obtained.

Postnatal genetic analysis of fetal or parental cells may be indicated after the mother has had two or three spontaneous abortions, or after a child is born with multiple congenital anomalies, Down syndrome, or other recognizable clinical cytogenetic or genetic disease. Fetal cells are often obtained immediately after birth from a sample of umbilical cord blood. Infertile patients also may require genetic diagnosis.

Pop Quiz

22.26 What is the primary drawback of the triple test?

22.27 How can fetal cells be obtained for analysis before birth?

Perinatal and Neonatal Disease

Teach your children well, . . .
And feed them on your dreams
The one they pick 's, the one you'll know by.

GRAHAM NASH (B. 1942), OF CROSBY, STILLS & NASH, AMERICAN ROCK GROUP, TEACH YOUR CHILDREN (1970)

Listed below are definitions of some important terms in perinatal and neonatal medicine. All dates are calculated from the first day of the last menstrual period (LMP):

- The **perinatal period** is the time from the 28th week of pregnancy to the seventh day after birth.
- The **neonatal period** is the first month after birth.
- **Gestational age** is length of time the fetus has been in the womb. It is about two weeks longer than the actual age, however, because fertilization usually occurs about two weeks after the first day of the LMP.
- **Full-term pregnancy** is a pregnancy that passes beyond the last day of the 37th week (259 days).
- **Premature** infants are those born before the end of the 37th week (258 days or less); sometimes these infants are called *preterm*.
- **Post-term** infants are those born after 42 weeks.
- **Normal birth weight** is 3,500 gm (7 lb, 12 oz).
- **Low birth weight** infants weigh less than 2,500 gm (5 lb, 8 oz)

Case Notes

22.10 Was Natasha's infant premature?

The Fetal Transition to Extrauterine Life is Stressful

The sudden change from intrauterine dependence on the mother to independent life is uniquely stressful and accounts for certain diseases of newborns. Consider the important physiologic changes that must occur. Prior to birth, the mother eats, digests, and delivers nutrients; she inhales oxygen and exhales carbon dioxide; and she collects and eliminates fetal metabolic waste in maternal urine. But at birth, the placenta is lost and everything changes. With its first breath, a newborn must rely on its own lungs, not its mother's; and when the umbilical cord is cut, it must rely on its own digestive and urinary tracts. *Of the phenomena discussed below, prematurity, infection, low birth weight, or fetal injury or stress may amplify any of them into an illness.*

Apart from the particulars of gestational age, birth weight, and other factors, it is useful to assess the overall condition of the infant immediately after birth, using a tool known as the **Apgar score** (after its originator, pediatric anesthesiologist Virginia Apgar). A numerical assessment of an infant's condition immediately after birth, the Apgar score is a useful method for clinical assessment of the vigor of a newborn infant. Low scores correlate directly with neonatal illness and death. Table 22.2 presents scoring and interpretation details.

Neurological Challenges

The brain is the least mature organ at birth. It is especially vulnerable to birth-related hemorrhage as the skull deforms as it passes through the birth canal. Respiratory effort may lack vigor because of an immature respiratory center; the suckling reflex may not be vigorous; and the temperature control center may not be mature enough to prevent hypothermia.

Respiratory Challenges

Before birth, the lungs are filled with a mix of amniotic fluid and surfactant. During passage through the birth canal, much of this fluid is squeezed out, clearing the way for the air of first breath. In utero, the lungs mature rapidly between 28 and 32 weeks, as Type II pneumocytes begin secreting surfactant, a slick, soapy fluid that decreases surface tension of intra-alveolar fluid and decreases the effort required to keep alveoli open after birth. If not enough surfactant is present, often the case in premature infants, alveolar fluid keeps alveolar walls stuck to one another by capillary action similar to the capillary action that keeps the lungs stuck to the inner surface of the rib cage. Lack of surfactant is the cause of the foremost respiratory challenge: *respiratory distress syndrome (RDS) of the newborn.*

Gastrointestinal Challenges

Necrotizing enterocolitis, a severe inflammatory condition of the gastrointestinal tract, occurs in about 10% of

Table 22.2 The Apgar Score

	Apgar Points		
Sign	0	1	2
HEART RATE	Absent	Below 100	Over 100
Respiratory effort	Absent	Slow, irregular	Good, crying
Muscle tone	Limp	Some flexion of extremities	Active motion
Response to catheter inserted in nostril	No response	Grimace	Cough or sneeze
Color	Blue, pale	Body pink, extremities blue	Completely pink

Application and Interpretation

- The purpose of the Apgar test is to determine quickly whether a newborn needs urgent attention. It is not intended to make long-term predictions of a child's health.
- The test is usually performed at one and five minutes after birth, and may be repeated if the score remains low. Scores depend on physiologic maturity, maternal perinatal condition, and fetal cardiovascular, respiratory, and neurologic condition.
- A score of 7–10 at 5 min is considered normal; 4–6, moderately low; and 0–3, critically low. A low Apgar score is not by itself diagnostic of anything.
- A one-minute score of 10 is uncommon due to the prevalence of transient hypoxemia and cyanosis in the extremities as the infant adjusts to its new environment.
- A low score on the one-minute test may show that the neonate requires attention but is not necessarily an indication that there will be long-term problems, particularly if there is an improvement by the stage of the five-minute test.
- A low score at 10 minutes or beyond predicts increased risk of mortality in the first year of life.

newborns weighing less than1,500 gm (3.3 lb). The cause is unknown. The findings are distinctive: intestinal mucosal hemorrhage with bloody diarrhea and shock. Surgical excision of affected bowel is often required. Mortality is high.

Cardiovascular Challenges

Cardiovascular changes are also dramatic. In the fetus, intrapulmonary pressure is high and blood is shunted around the lungs—it travels from the right atrium to the left through the foramen ovale and from the pulmonary artery to the aorta through the ductus arteriosus (Chapter 9). With the first breath, however, as the lungs fill with air, intrapulmonary pressure falls and blood surges into the lungs. The foramen ovale and ductus arteriosus usually close slowly, but sometimes they may remain open or may reopen, pathologic conditions responsible for certain congenital heart disease.

Hemoglobin production slows markedly. Before birth, fetal blood oxygen is relatively low, which encourages oxygen flow across the placenta. With birth, however, fetal blood oxygen soars, which causes fetal erythropoietin to fall. With it, hemoglobin synthesis and red blood cell production fall and remain low for about six to eight weeks. Mild anemia is the result.

Immune Challenges

At birth, the fetus loses passive transfer of maternal immunoglobulins across the placenta. What's more, the fetal immune system is not fully mature relative to that of an adult. Although immune factors in breast milk can compensate partially, full immunologic maturity does not arrive until about age 10. Infants, especially premature or ill ones, are vulnerable to *infection* as a result.

Metabolic Challenges

Renal function in infants does not reach full capacity until about two years of age. Function may be further compromised in prematurity. Inability to excrete fixed acids (metabolic acids) may cause long-term growth failure, which may be further aggravated by acid byproducts derived from high protein content in some infant formulas.

Birth deprives the infant of glucose from maternal blood and the infant must immediately generate glucose from its own glycogen stores in the liver. The neonatal liver, however, does not metabolize glucose well. Failure to convert hepatic glycogen stores to glucose can cause severe *hypoglycemia*.

All neonates develop high blood bilirubin (*physiologic jaundice*) for a few days as bilirubin metabolism shifts from mother to infant. Usually no harm occurs, but prematurity or illness may exaggerate the phenomenon and cause **neonatal hyperbilirubinemia**. Sometimes the result is **kernicterus**, a syndrome of severe brain damage due to accumulation of unconjugated bilirubin in the brain. High bilirubin is treatable in two ways. For most infants, *phototherapy* is sufficient. For a few hours a day, the infant is exposed to intense light, which penetrates deep enough into skin to interact with bilirubin in superficial blood vessels and converts it into a form more easily handled by the infant's immature liver. A second treatment, reserved for the severest cases, is *exchange transfusion*. In this procedure, small amounts of infant blood are repeatedly withdrawn and replaced each time with fresh donor blood or plasma that, of course, has little bilirubin in it. Thanks to modern prenatal and neonatal care, kernicterus is now very rare in developed nations.

Case Notes

22.11 Though not mentioned in the case study, is it likely that Natasha's infant developed physiologic jaundice?

The Birth Process Can Be Hazardous

About 1 in 5,000 live-born infants suffer an injury directly traceable to the birth process. Considering the contortions and forces of vaginal passage, it is surprising infants are not injured more often. **Dystocia** is an abnormal or difficult childbirth. For example, the anterior fetal shoulder may not be able to pass under the symphysis pubis. Dystocia can become a life-threatening emergency if the umbilical cord becomes compressed in the birth canal. Complications include fetal death, respiratory depression, or hypoxic brain damage.

The most common injuries are, in descending order: fractured clavicle, facial nerve injury with facial paralysis, brachial plexus injury with paralysis of an upper extremity, skull fracture or intracranial injury, and fracture of the humerus. Intracranial hemorrhage is the most severe injury and can produce immediate problems or death; or it may become manifest later as cerebral palsy.

Cerebral palsy is a broad clinical term for a nonprogressive syndrome of motor impairment due to brain damage. Risk factors include prematurity, low birth weight, and small size for gestational age. Most cases arise from unknown prebirth conditions. Some arise from damage suffered after birth: brain or meningeal infections, hyperbilirubinemia, automobile accidents, falls, or child abuse. Cerebral palsy is characterized by varying degrees of motor difficulty including paralysis, uncontrollable movement, and inability to coordinate movement, problems that may not be evident at birth but reveal themselves as development progresses. Mentation and sensation are not affected.

Prematurity Is Early Birth

Prematurity is birth before the first day of the 38th week of gestation. Most premature infants are of low birth weight, too, but the most critical aspect is time: it takes time for organs to mature. About 5–10% of pregnancies produce premature infants. Usually the cause is unknown.

The major known causes of prematurity are preterm rupture of the amniotic sac ("rupture of membranes"); intrauterine infection; multiple gestation (twin pregnancy); structural abnormalities of the uterus, cervix, or placenta (e.g., leiomyomas of the uterine wall); placental hemorrhage; abnormal location of the placental implantation in the wall of the uterus (*placenta previa*); or a relaxed cervix that opens too early (*incompetent cervix*).

The hazards of prematurity are many and most relate to immature organ systems. Premature infants have immature organs regardless of birth weight and are at substantial risk for brain damage, RDS, and hyperbilirubinemia. Those that are small for their gestational age are at even greater risk.

Respiratory distress syndrome (RDS) of the newborn (*hyaline membrane disease*) is a condition that occurs almost solely in premature infants. It stems from a lack of surfactant in immature infant lungs. RDS is a disease of prematurity that affects about 25% of infants born between 32 and 36 weeks and more than 50% of those born before 28 weeks. Keeping alveoli open requires intense respiratory effort, and some infants die because they suffocate as their muscles tire. The typical case is a premature, low birth weight infant whose mother has diabetes or some other complication of pregnancy. Shortly after birth, the infant's breathing becomes labored and blood oxygen falls. Hypoxia causes alveolar and pulmonary vascular damage, and fluid exudes into the alveoli. Water evaporates with each breath, but protein in the exudate cannot be absorbed, and condenses into a glue-like material, which forms a thick membrane (the *hyaline membrane* that coats the alveolar walls and further impairs oxygen transfer, Fig. 22.17). Surviving infants may suffer hypoxic brain damage. Oxygen and surfactant inhalation may be effective treatments.

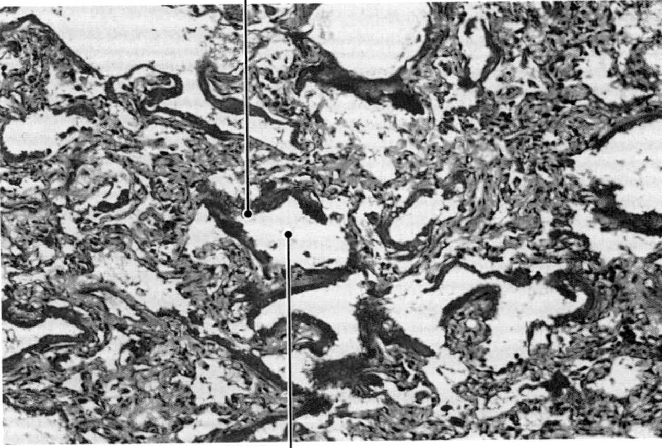

Figure 22.17 **Hyaline membrane disease.** (Adapted with permission from Rubin E, Farber JL. *Pathology.* 3rd ed. Philadelphia, PA: Lippincott Williams & Wilkins; 1999.)

Oxygen therapy can be lifesaving in many circumstances. Nevertheless, in newborns, and especially in premature infants, it must be administered with special care. Inhalation of high concentrations of oxygen can result in **retinopathy of the newborn** ("oxygen blindness") caused by the toxic effect that high blood oxygen can have on the neonatal retina. A similar toxic effect on bronchial mucosa causes scarring of the bronchi and lungs (*bronchial dysplasia*). Oxygen blindness is rare, but bronchial dysplasia occurs in about half of infants weighing less than 1,000 gm who are treated with oxygen.

Case Notes
22.12 What is the cause of Natasha's infant's RDS?

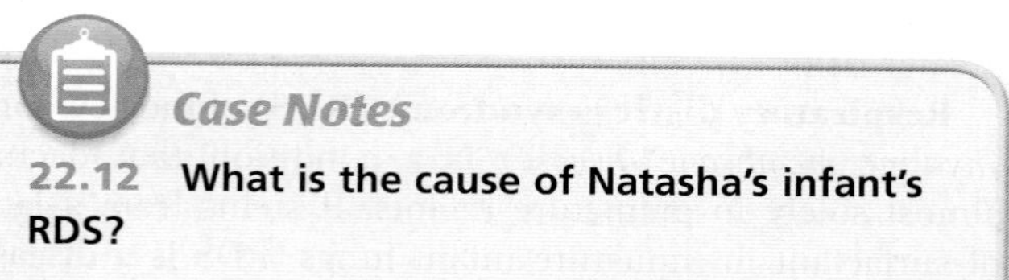

Remember This! Prematurity is a significant neonatal health risk.

Some Newborns Are Small or Large for Gestational Age

In normal pregnancy, duration of gestation, birth weight, and organ maturity go hand-in-hand (Fig. 22.18). Most term infants have normal birth weight and organs that are mature and ready for life outside the womb. Infants with low birth weight and shorter gestational age have less mature organs, however, and suffer higher mortality and morbidity than do full-term infants. It is helpful to classify newborn infants according to a system that takes into account both birth weight and gestational age:

- **Small for gestational age (SGA)** infants are those whose birth weight is below the 10th percentile for gestational age (Fig. 22.18). The condition is sometimes referred to as *intrauterine growth restriction (IUGR)*. If otherwise free of disease, the SGA infant has normal physiology for gestational age, including normal suckling reflex, alertness, and cry. An infant may be small for genetic reasons: small parents may have small children. Or the infant may have a genetic disease. But the most common culprits are maternal factors: drug abuse, heavy smoking, malnutrition, infection, and placental insufficiency owing to maternal small vessel disease. *Fetal alcohol syndrome* is a common cause of SGA.
- **Appropriate for gestational age (AGA)** infants are those weighing as much as expected at any given gestational age.
- **Large for gestational age (LGA)** infants are those whose birth weight is above the 90th percentile for gestational age (see Fig. 22.18). By far, the most common cause is maternal diabetes. Fetal blood glucose parallels maternal glucose. High fetal glucose stimulates high fetal blood insulin, which stimulates tissue growth. Vaginal birth may be difficult and there is increased risk for birth injury. Early birth risks respiratory distress syndrome. Infants of diabetic mothers may develop severe hypoglycemia due to high blood insulin levels.

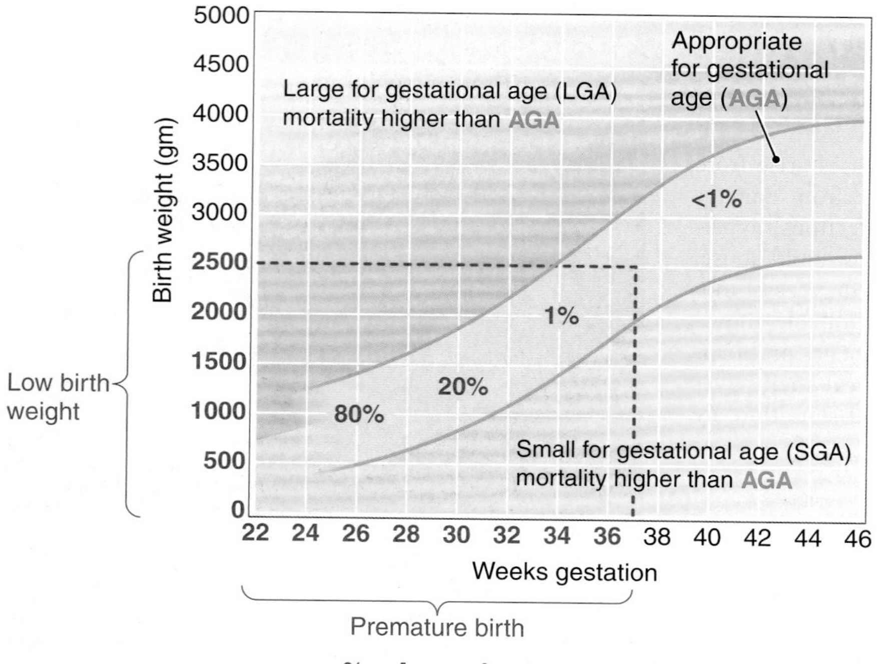

Figure 22.18 **Neonatal mortality risk**. Fetal death rate (percent) as a function of birth weight and gestational age. Normal gestation is 38–40 full weeks. Prematurity is gestational age less than 37 full weeks. For example, the mortality is <1% for term infants that weigh appropriately for gestational age (AGA), but it is about 20% for infants born weighing under 1,500 gm and born at about 30 weeks gestational age.

Let's consider a few examples. According to Figure 22.18, an infant born at 32 weeks should weigh near 1,500 gm. An infant born at 32 weeks that weighs 2,500 gm is LGA but is very premature. It is sure to have immature organs and is at high risk for complications of prematurity, especially RDS (discussed below). Nevertheless, an infant born at 36 weeks and weighing 1,500 gm, though SGA, is at relatively less risk for complication because its organs are more mature.

Case Notes

22.13 Natasha's infant was SGA. Why?

Neonatal Infections Can Be Fatal

Infections in neonates differ from infections in infants and children because the newborn immune system is less mature, and the source of infection, the behavior of the disease, and the infecting microbes differ. Infections of various organ systems are discussed in the pertinent chapters.

Some fetal infections cross the placenta from the mother. Many of these infections can cause congenital defects, as discussed earlier.

Neonatal infection can be acquired as the fetus passes through the vaginal canal. Bacteria can also ascend through the cervix to infect the amniotic fluid (*amnionitis*), usually late in pregnancy, particularly if there is an amniotic fluid leak. Infected amniotic fluid is inhaled by the fetus and may cause premature labor and *fetal pneumonia* or other infection.

Herpes simplex virus may be a serious fetal threat if a pregnant woman suffers an outbreak of genital herpes at the time of delivery. The threat is so serious that Caesarean section may be required in mothers with active genital herpes who are near term. Neonatal herpes infection may be confined to skin, eyes, or mouth, but may disseminate to cause fatal encephalitis, hepatitis, and pneumonia. Diagnosis is by viral culture and other complex laboratory procedures. Therapy is parenteral antiviral drugs.

Neonatal conjunctivitis is a purulent inflammatory reaction of the conjunctiva. It occurs in about 1–2% of births, and is most often caused by *Chlamydia trachomatis*, gonorrhea, or another sexually transmitted infection acquired from the mother. Diagnosis is clinical and by culture or microscopic study of exudate. Installation of antibiotic ointment is preventive.

Neonatal sepsis is systemic infection spread by the bloodstream. Symptoms are varied and include lethargy, jaundice, failure to suckle, apnea, bradycardia, temperature instability, respiratory distress, vomiting, and diarrhea. Risk factors include low birth weight, male sex, and maternal risk factors such as premature rupture of membranes, toxemia of pregnancy, or infection. Diagnosis is supported by blood culture, but in the end the diagnosis is clinical and depends on experienced professional judgment. Sepsis should be suspected in any infant with risk factors who deviates from the norm. Mortality rates vary from 10% to 40%. Antibiotic therapy is required and should be begun upon suspicion of the diagnosis.

The differential diagnosis of elevated neonatal bilirubin is difficult because almost all newborns, premature infants in particular, have temporary physiologic jaundice. Severe or prolonged hyperbilirubinemia associated with other causes is often termed **neonatal cholestasis** or **neonatal hepatitis** until a definitive cause can be determined. Actual obstruction of bile flow (cholestasis) usually results from bile duct obstruction due to failed development (*primary biliary atresia*) or inflammatory scarring. Prompt differential diagnosis is important because extrahepatic bile duct obstruction is sometimes surgically correctible, and prolonged obstruction can cause severe liver disease or death.

Of the many causes of *neonatal hepatitis*, the most commonly identifiable offender is *hepatitis B virus*. Infants are infected with hepatitis B during vaginal birth by their infected mothers. Transplacental infection is uncommon. Symptomatic neonates typically have jaundice, dark urine, light stools, and an enlarged liver, but most infections are asymptomatic. Diagnosis depends on detection of hepatitis B antigen or antibody in blood. Treatment is supportive.

Pop Quiz

22.28 Define prematurity.

22.29 How is gestational age calculated?

22.30 True or false? All infants develop physiologic jaundice.

22.31 The lack of what substance in premature lungs is the cause of neonatal RDS?

22.32 What activity of the nervous system is affected by cerebral palsy?

22.33 What is the most common cause of neonatal conjunctivitis?

22.34 Define neonatal sepsis.

Infections of Infants and Children

Childhood infections are the most common causes of childhood illness. Most infections are viral. Many of them cause acute upper respiratory illnesses featuring fever, cough, and rhinorrhea. Diagnosis is usually by clinical observation and does not require use of laboratory tests or imaging. In most of these diseases, the illness is short, the prognosis is good, and treatment is symptomatic and supportive.

Pediatric Viral Infections Can Be Mild or Severe

Pediatric cases account for about 1% of HIV infections in the United States, and maternal transmission accounts for almost all cases. From 10% to 40% of infected mothers infect their fetus. In pediatric HIV/AIDS, the natural history and behavior of the infection is much the same as in adults; however, the type of antiviral drug therapy differs.

Respiratory syncytial virus (RSV) is a common virus that causes a syndrome of acute bronchitis, bronchiolitis, and bronchopneumonia characterized by respiratory distress and asthma-like wheezing. RSV infection usually presents clinically as **bronchiolitis**, a winter epidemic syndrome of low-grade fever, wheezing respiration, and shortness of breath. Secondary bacterial pneumonia may develop, but most cases resolve in 7–10 days with supportive therapy.

Croup is an acute inflammatory disease of the upper airway of children, usually age three or younger, associated with *parainfluenza* viral infection. It causes inflammation of the larynx, trachea, or bronchi. The most dangerous aspect is laryngitis, which features laryngeal edema that causes a crowing sound (stridor) on inspiration and a hoarse, brassy, barking cough. Diagnosis is clinical. Most cases resolve spontaneously, but a neglected case can cause fatal suffocation. Treatment is supportive but may require steroids to combat swelling and inflammation and epinephrine for bronchial relaxation.

Measles (*red measles, rubeola*) is a highly contagious respiratory virus best known for the skin rash it produces and similar lesions of the oral mucosa (Koplik spots). In well-nourished, healthy children it is usually not much more than a rite of passage, but in malnourished children it can cause fatal pneumonia, accounting for over one million deaths per year worldwide. Vaccination is effective. Diagnosis is clinical and by detection of blood antibodies; treatment is supportive.

Rubella (*German measles, three-day measles*) is caused by the rubella virus and presents as sore throat, skin rash, and enlarged lymph nodes. It is much shorter in duration and is a less serious condition than rubeola. Nevertheless, maternal rubella infection in early pregnancy is a threat to the fetus, and can cause especially severe and deforming disease or fetal death. Vaccination is effective. Diagnosis is clinical, supported by virus culture and antibody studies; treatment is supportive.

Mumps virus causes acute inflammation of the parotid salivary gland (*parotitis*), and it occasionally causes inflammation of the testes (*orchitis*), pancreatitis, or encephalitis. It has been virtually eliminated by vaccination. Diagnosis is clinical; treatment is supportive.

Chickenpox is caused by the *varicella-zoster* virus, which causes an acute febrile illness characterized by vesicular skin eruptions that may leave unsightly scars. Diagnosis is clinical, supported by detection of distinctive cells in wound scrapings (Tzanck smear) and by culture and antibody studies; treatment is supportive.

Infectious mononucleosis is a self-limited (disappears without treatment), mild syndrome of fever, sore throat, listlessness, lymphocytosis, and splenomegaly, which typically occurs in late adolescence or early adulthood. It is caused by the *Epstein-Barr virus (EBV)* and almost always is passed in saliva during kissing. Transmission by sexual contact is rare. Transmission by shared eating and drinking utensils is uncommon. Diagnosis requires finding distinctive large lymphocytes (atypical lymphocytes) in the peripheral blood and characteristic antibodies (*heterophil antibodies*) in blood. Treatment is supportive.

Some Bacterial Infections Can Be Fatal

One of the most common bacterial diseases of children is **acute otitis media**, discussed in detail in Chapter 20. *Streptococcus pneumoniae* and *Haemophilus influenzae* are the most common bacteria involved.

Whooping cough (WC) is a contagious disease that may occur in unvaccinated populations. It is caused by *Bordetella pertussis*, a Gram-negative bacillus that produces a syndrome of intense inflammation in the larynx, trachea, and bronchi. Severe cases can cause fatal asphyxia, especially in infants. It gets its name from severe spasms of coughing and the sharp, inspiratory barking sound (stridor, or whoop) that is characteristic of the disease. Typically, it runs a course of several weeks that begins with mild cough and upper respiratory symptoms and evolves into severe coughing spasms and asphyxia. Fever is uncommon. Diagnosis is confirmed by culture of the organism. Antibiotic therapy is effective. Vaccination is effective. WC causes hundreds of thousands of deaths in unvaccinated children in developing nations. US reported cases surged from about 2–4000/yr in 1970–90 to over 41,000 in 2012. Dozens of children die. There are several causes, among them parents who refuse to vaccinate their children.

Diphtheria is caused by a gram-positive bacillus, *Corynebacterium diphtheriae*, which produces a pharyngitis and laryngitis associated with a thick, obstructive gray inflammatory membrane that can cause death by suffocation. Moreover, the bacillus secretes an exotoxin that can damage the heart, kidney, and brain. Diphtheria now has been almost eliminated in developed nations by effective vaccinations. Treatment is antibiotics and antitoxin.

Acute bacterial **epiglottitis** is a disease of school-aged children caused by *H. influenzae* and marked by hoarseness and painful swallowing and drooling. The epiglottis and nearby pharyngeal tissues are severely inflamed, narrowing the airway and sometimes causing critical airway obstruction. Vaccination has virtually eradicated epiglottitis in developed nations, but misplaced public concerns about potential vaccine side-effects have allowed it to make a comeback. Diagnosis is clinical. Airway examination can be hazardous because asphyxia may result. Prior to examination, the examiner should be prepared to intubate the patient if necessary. Treatment is airway protection and antibiotics.

Pop Quiz

22.35 True or false? Most infections of infants and children are caused by bacteria.

22.36 True or false? The natural history and behavior of HIV/AIDS in neonates and children is much the same as it is in adults.

22.37 True or false? Whooping cough and diphtheria can be fatal.

Sudden Infant Death Syndrome (SIDS)

Sudden infant death syndrome (SIDS) is the abrupt and unexpected death of an infant between two weeks and one year of age in which an autopsy fails to reveal the cause of death. SIDS, formerly referred to as *crib death*, is characterized by its epidemiology:

- Age generally under six months
- Sleep in the prone position
- Prematurity or low birth weight
- Male sex
- Maternal age <20 years
- Maternal smoking (Babies whose mothers smoke are about three times as likely to die from SIDS.)
- Maternal drug abuse
- African American and American Indian ethnicity (genetic? socioeconomic?)
- Overly hot or cold sleeping conditions
- Bulky, soft bedding, and blankets
- Sibling of SIDS' victim

The cause is unknown. Pathologic findings at autopsy are scant. Defective brain respiratory control is suspected. About 5% of victims have prolonged apnea spells preceding the death. There is slight familial tendency. The American Academy of Pediatrics recommends infants be placed in a supine position for sleep (the so-called "Back to Sleep" campaign) and care be taken to avoid overheating (hot room, too much cover) or a cold room. Some US jurisdictions ban sale of soft crib bumpers. Infants should sleep in the same room as their parents, though not the same bed.

Pop Quiz

22.38 What is suspected as the probable cause of SIDS?

Tumors and Tumor-Like Conditions in Children

In children, benign tumors and tumor-like masses are much more common than malignant ones. The following are the most common types:

- An **ectopic rest** (*choristoma*) is a common benign nodule of *normal* tissue in an *abnormal* location. For example, a fairly common one is a patch of embryologically misplaced but otherwise normal pancreas found in the stomach wall. Most are innocuous and do not warrant treatment.
- A **hamartoma** is a benign neoplastic growth composed of tissue elements *normally found at that site*, but which are growing in a disorganized mass. An example is *bronchial hamartoma,* a small, disorganized mass of normal bronchial cartilage, epithelium, blood vessels, and lymphoid tissue. Congenital benign collections of blood vessels called *hemangiomas* are also hamartomas. Although the ovary and testis are the most common location of hamartomas in adults, these are not common locations in newborns. Most are innocuous and do not warrant treatment.
- A **teratoma** is a neoplastic growth of tissue *not normally found at the site*—skin in an ovarian teratoma, for example. By definition, teratomas include components derived from each of the three embryonic layers: ectoderm, endoderm, and mesoderm. They are thought to arise from embryologic remnants. The most common in newborns is **sacrococcygeal teratoma** (Fig. 22.19), typically a mass several centimeters in diameter located at the base of the spine.

Although malignant neoplasms are not common in children, they are still the second most common cause of childhood death—exceeded only by fatal accidents. Many of these tumors also occur in adults, but some are unique to childhood. According to the National Cancer Institute, the distribution of childhood (age <20 years) cancer is as follows:

- *Leukemia and lymphoma*: 40%. The most common of these is *acute lymphocytic leukemia* (Chapter 7).
- *Brain and other intracranial*: 17%. The most common of these are *astrocytomas* (Chapter 19).
- *Soft tissue and bone*: 14%. These are many and varied. Most are benign. The most common is *nonossifying fibroma* (Chapter 18).
- *Peripheral nervous system*: 5%. The most common is **neuroblastoma**, a malignancy of primitive neural cells that is unique to children. It is the most common solid, extracranial tumor of children and the most common malignancy of infants. It usually arises in the adrenal gland or in the ganglia of the sympathetic chain. It features a wide array of clinical behavior: some disappear spontaneously, some mature and stop growing,

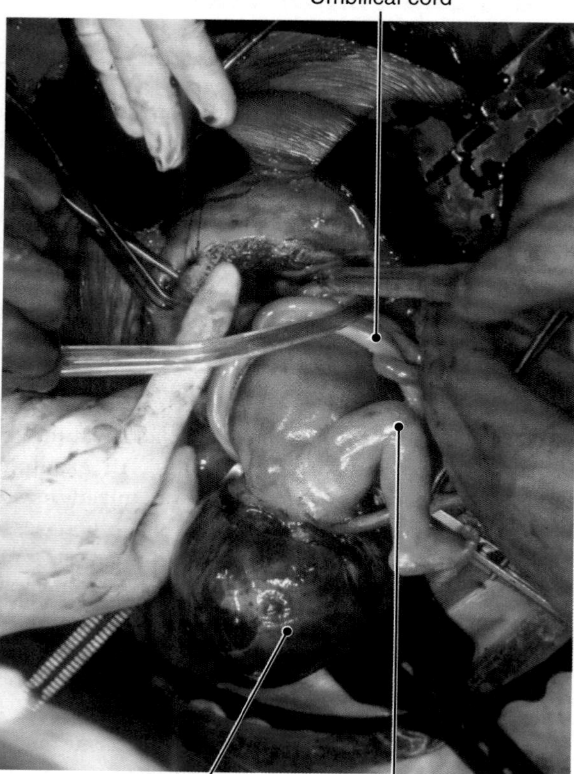

Figure 22.19 **Neonatal sacrococcygeal teratoma**. (Reproduced with permission from Mhairi G, MacDonald, MM, Seshia K, et al. *Avery's Neonatology Pathophysiology & Management of the Newborn*. 6th ed. Philadelphia, PA: Lippincott Williams & Wilkins; 2005.)

and others are frankly malignant. Five-year survival for malignant ones is about 40%.

- *Renal*: 4%. The most common of these is **Wilms tumor**, a malignancy of the kidney that arises from embryologic renal cells and is unique to children. About 5–10% are bilateral. Some may be caused by an inheritable genetic defect. Five-year survival varies from 60% to 90% depending on microscopic type.
- *Germ cell tumors (GCTs)* and a variety of others: 20%. GCTs develop from primitive germ cells, which migrate to the gonads during embryogenesis. Most are mature teratomas, described above and in Chapter 5, but aggressive and malignant varieties also occur. Most GCTs arise in midline sites (i.e., sacrococcygeal, mediastinal, and retroperitoneal).

In the varied group of other tumors is **retinoblastoma**, a rare, ophthalmic, malignant tumor of retinal neurons usually diagnosed in children younger than age two. It is attributed to a genetic defect in the RB gene on chromosome 13. About half are inherited defects, and the remainder are spontaneous mutations. About one-fourth are bilateral. Five-year survival is 90% for children with tumors that have not spread beyond the eye at time of diagnosis.

Compared to adult malignancies, those in children are more often associated with genetic abnormalities, congenital malformations, and a tendency to spontaneously regress or mature into a less malignant neoplasm. They have a better survival rate, often because they are more responsive to therapy.

Pop Quiz

22.39 True or false? Malignant neoplasms are the most common cause of childhood death.

22.40 True or false? The most common lymphoma/leukemia of childhood is acute granulocytic leukemia.

Case Study Revisited

"I'm going to have a baby." The case of Natasha V.

This case is a clear example of the dangers of substance abuse, especially during pregnancy, and most especially in the first eight weeks of gestation when embryonic organs are forming.

Natasha was intoxicated with alcohol at the time she appeared in the emergency room. Her medical record revealed a history of chronic alcohol and other drug abuse that made it likely she abused alcohol during the critical first eight weeks of gestation. Adding to the problem, she was also a smoker. Heavy cigarette smoking is also associated with fetal birth defects.

That a previous pregnancy ended in a spontaneous abortion suggests that the aborted fetus may have been more adversely affected than the current one.

Natasha's infant was premature (36 weeks gestation). The lungs of premature infants typically lack enough surfactant to keep alveoli open and blood adequately oxygenated, so it is not surprising that he developed RDS.

The infant's low Apgar score (3 on a scale of 10) and unusually low birth weight (SGA) is consistent with his prematurity, fetal alcohol syndrome, and placental ischemia from maternal smoking. Mortality and the risk of severe neurologic morbidity are increased in infants with low scores.

Finally, the infant's failure to thrive, seizure disorder, and early death are proof positive of the devastating effects of maternal alcohol abuse and fetal alcohol syndrome.

Chapter Challenge

CHAPTER RECALL

1. Mesoderm gives rise to which of the following?
   A. Bone, muscle, blood cells, kidneys, gonads, heart and blood vessels, dermis, and connective tissues
   B. Epithelial lining of the intestinal and respiratory tracts, the endocrine glands, and the liver and pancreas
   C. Epidermis, tooth enamel, and nervous tissue
   D. All of the above

2. The decidua is which of the following?
   A. Endometrium that is thickened and modified by the effect of progesterone
   B. Fetal urine and a small amount of fluid and cell debris issuing from the fetal bowel
   C. A maternal blood vessel that serves as an exchange device for transfer of nutrients and oxygen
   D. Composed of finger-like projections containing fetal blood vessels that extend into lakes of maternal blood

3. Conditions caused by mechanical factors that distort an otherwise normal fetus are known as which of the following?
   A. Inherited defects
   B. Malformations
   C. Genetic mutations
   D. None of the above

4. Which of the following time points is correct?
   A. An infant is premature if born before 36 weeks.
   B. Most birth defects occur in the first trimester, usually within the first eight weeks.
   C. A fetus is post-term after week 42.
   D. The perinatal period is from the 28th week of pregnancy until birth.

5. Which of the following organisms is not included in the TORCH infections?
   A. Toxoplasmosis
   B. Cytomegalovirus
   C. HPV
   D. Herpesvirus
   E. Rubella

6. Which of the following statements about Down Syndrome patients is correct?
   A. Down syndrome patients have a decreased likelihood of developing Alzheimer disease.
   B. It is the most common cause of mental retardation.
   C. It is always caused by three copies of chromosome 21, 2 paternal copies, and 1 maternal copy.
   D. Infants are at increased risk for cardiac and intestinal manifestations, but have no increased risk of malignancy.

7. Which of the following is true of Gaucher disease?
   A. It results from a defect in the gene that codes for an enzyme that metabolizes *glucocerebroside*.
   B. It is a genetic condition in which the affected enzyme normally converts muscle glycogen into glucose.
   C. It is an autosomal dominant disease.
   D. In conjunction with cigarette smoke, it results in severe autodigestion of alveoli, which in turn results in emphysema.

8. Which of the following is the most common cause of prematurity?
   A. Unknown
   B. Rupture of membranes
   C. Multiple gestations
   D. Relaxed/incompetent cervix

9. Thirty-six hours after birth, an infant presents with lethargy, jaundice, failure to suckle, vomiting, and diarrhea. You suspect he has which of the following?
   A. Neonatal conjunctivitis
   B. Neonatal sepsis
   C. Neonatal hepatitis
   D. Neonatal cholestasis

10. True or false? An embryo becomes a fetus at seven weeks.

11. True or false? Teratogens can be physical, chemical, and microbial.

12. True or false? All cells in the human body are made of up 23 pairs of chromosomes: 22 pairs of autosomes and 1 set of sex chromosomes.

13. Match the following infectious agents to their symptoms.
    i. Measles
    ii. *H. influenza*
    iii. *Bordetella pertussis*
    iv. Epstein Bar virus
    v. Rubella
    vi. Mumps
    vii. Diphtheria
    A. Severe coughing spasms with inspiratory barking sound (stridor, or whoop)
    B. Sore throat, skin rash, and enlarged lymph nodes
    C. A highly contagious respiratory virus best known for the skin rash it produces that may cause fatal pneumonia in malnourished children
    D. Parotitis, orchitis, pancreatitis, encephalitis
    E. Pharyngitis and laryngitis associated with a thick, obstructive gray-colored inflammatory membrane that can cause death by suffocation
    F. Mild syndrome of fever, sore throat, listlessness, lymphocytosis, and splenomegaly
    G. Acute bacterial epiglottitis marked by hoarseness and painful swallowing

CONCEPTUAL UNDERSTANDING

14. Describe the purpose of the amniotic sac, the placenta, and the umbilical cord.

15. What are the mechanisms of genetic inheritance? Give examples.

16. What are the four types of proteins? Give examples in each of these categories.

17. Define small and LGA.

18. Compare and contrast choristoma versus hamartoma.

APPLICATION

19. A 17-year-old woman presents to your office complaining of amenorrhea (she has never had a period). On physical exam, you note her short stature, her webbed neck, and a broad, flat chest with widely separated nipples. What syndrome is this patient suffering from?
    A. Turner syndrome
    B. Klinefelter syndrome
    C. Down syndrome
    D. CF

20. A patient describes to you a family history of a disease. She has it, as does her father and grandfather. Several uncles and aunts also have this disease, as does her sister. She has another sister and brother who do not have the disease. She worries that she will pass this disease on to her own children. What is the inheritance pattern if this disease is monogenic, and what is the likelihood that her daughter also has this familial disease?
    A. Autosomal dominant, 25%
    B. Autosomal recessive, 25%
    C. X-linked recessive, 100% in boys
    D. Autosomal dominant, 50%

21. A mother presents with prolonged rupture of membranes and a fever. Discuss the sequence of events that led to her presentation with amnionitis.

22. How do the actions of tumor suppressors and proto-oncogenes/oncogenes differ in causing neoplasms?

23. Identify the indications for genetic counseling and testing, and the methods available in genetic diagnosis.

24. Compare and contrast expressivity and penetrance. Consider these terms in the context of CF.

25. What physiologic changes does an infant undergo at birth? Discuss cardiovascular, pulmonary, hemoglobin production, immune system function, glucose metabolism, maternal metabolism of bilirubin, and renal function.

26. Describe the complications faced by premature infants.

27. What are the risk factors associated with SIDS?

CHAPTER 23

Disorders of Daily Life

Contents

Chapter Objectives

After studying this chapter, you should be able to complete the following tasks:

INJURY FROM PHYSICAL AGENTS

1. Name several of the most common causes of death in the United States, and discuss the environmental aspects.
2. Distinguish between the grades and types of injury that occur with burns (including electrical) and cold and heat exposure; describe the potential complications of each.
3. Discuss the manifestation of, and the variables that influence, radiation injury.

TOXIC EXPOSURE

4. Using examples from the text, briefly discuss the clinical presentations and findings of occupational pollutant, toxin, and drug exposure; include asbestos, silica, ozone, second hand smoke, carbon monoxide, organophosphate, lead, mercury, arsenic, cadmium, and iron.
5. Discuss the risks associated with the following therapeutic agents: hormone replacement therapy, oral contraceptives, anabolic steroids, aspirin, and acetaminophen.

TOBACCO USE

6. Name several diseases other than lung cancer that are related to cigarette smoking.

ALCOHOL USE AND ABUSE

7. Name several conditions associated with alcohol abuse.

DRUG ABUSE

8. List the complications of drug abuse, and explain why intravenous use is especially risky.

NUTRITIONAL DISORDERS

9. Explain the potential consequences of diets containing a calorie deficiency or excess, and be able to calculate body mass index.
10. Using examples from the text, discuss how the differences between fat-soluble and water-soluble vitamins are reflected in vitamin deficiency and toxicity.

Case Study

"I think he's having a heart attack." The case of Marvin B.

Chief Complaint: Chest pain and shortness of breath

Clinical History: Marvin B. was a 58-year-old obese man who was brought to the hospital by his wife and son. The son told the triage nurse, "He has had heart trouble for a long time. I think he's having a heart attack."

He was obtunded and groaning and not capable of responding to questions. Interviewing his wife and son revealed that he began having crushing substernal pain and shortness of breath an hour earlier. He was under the care of a physician for diabetes, high blood pressure, chronic lung disease, and chronic heart disease.

Physical Examination and Other Data: Marvin was of average height and markedly obese. Temperature was normal. Blood pressure was 158/92, heart rate 86, respiratory rate 20. His lungs were "wet" with rales and rhonchi and expiratory wheezes. An electrocardiogram suggested a myocardial infarct. Cardiac troponin levels in blood were increased.

Clinical Course: Marvin suffered cardiac arrest and could not be resuscitated. His wife, a medical records librarian, asked for an autopsy. "I would like to know how much damage he has done to his body by being so fat, by drinking like he did, and by smoking," she said. "I've been after him for years to quit his drinking and smoking. It ruined our marriage. I want our children to read the report so they can learn a lesson."

Postmortem interview with his wife revealed Marvin drank a six-pack of beer or more each night and had been recently put on leave from his job as a truck driver after he was ticketed for driving his truck while intoxicated. "I was hoping," his wife said, "that he would use the time to recover his senses and let his knees heal. They were so worn out he could barely climb into the truck." He had been smoking "about a pack and a half a day" since he was a teenager. Among the drugs he took were a daily aspirin, a statin to lower cholesterol, two antihypertensives, nitroglycerin for chest pain, a bronchodilator for wheezing, a hypoglycemic agent for diabetes, and pain medication for his aching knees. He was 5" 9" tall, weighed "nearly 300 pounds," and wore size 46 pants. Tests on blood collected before death revealed LDL cholesterol 145 mg/dL, HDL cholesterol 42 mg/dL, and triglyceride 447 mg/dL.

An autopsy was performed. Final diagnoses in the autopsy report were:

- Severe generalized and coronary atherosclerosis
- Thrombosis of right coronary artery with acute posterior myocardial infarction
- Chronic alcoholic hepatitis and steatosis ("steatohepatitis")
- Moderate pulmonary emphysema and chronic bronchitis (COPD)
- Cor pulmonale (right ventricular hypertrophy with COPD)
- Moderate dysplasia of left mainstem bronchial mucosa
- Severe arteriolar nephrosclerosis
- Morbid obesity
- Clinical metabolic syndrome
- Clinical hypertension
- Clinical diabetes mellitus
- Clinical osteoarthritis

For thy sake, Tobacco, I would do anything but die.

CHARLES LAMB (1775–1834), ENGLISH ESSAYIST, A FAREWELL TO TOBACCO

This chapter focuses on disorders that arise from the more or less regular routines and exposures of daily life: the air we breathe, the water we drink, the food we eat, and our work, recreation, and personal habits.

An important influence on how we live is the environment in which we live. In our study of genetic disease (Chapter 22), we used the term *environment* in the broadest sense to refer to any nongenetic influence. In this chapter, however, "environment" has a much narrower definition, referring to the effects of 1) physical forces and extremes of temperature; 2) air and water pollution; 3) occupational exposures; 4) personal exposures to chemicals, radiation, and drugs, legal and illegal, including alcohol and tobacco; and 5) too much or too little food.

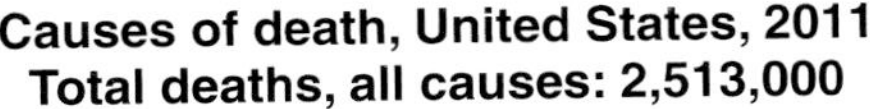
Remember This! Personal habits are the most important factor in the majority of U.S. deaths.

Most environmental disease is the result of personal habits—cigarette smoking, alcohol and other drug abuse, and consuming more energy than we expend. Environmental disease is an important factor in most deaths in the United States (Fig. 23.1). Smoking and overeating, for instance, are major risk factors in deaths associated with heart disease. Smoking directly accounts for most chronic lung disease and almost every lung cancer; and smoking, alcohol abuse, and overeating all increase the risk for cancers in other organs. Accidents are the only purely environmental category, and they claim in excess of 100,000 lives per year.

Case Notes

23.1 Is Marvin's heart attack related more to genetics or environment?

23.2 In Figure 23.1, into which slice does Marvin fall?

Injury from Physical Agents

Trauma is any injury to the body caused by sudden violence or accident, usually physical force associated with accidents, suicide, or homicide. **Blunt trauma** (without an open wound) is the leading cause of traumatic death in the United States. A **contusion** is a blunt force injury that results in local hemorrhage in any tissue. Most blunt injuries are caused by motor vehicle accidents; falls are the second most common cause of blunt injury death. In this discussion, we include accidental acute toxic exposures (poisonings) as injuries in order to separate them from chronic toxic exposures. Figure 23.2 illustrates the causes of accidental death in the United States.

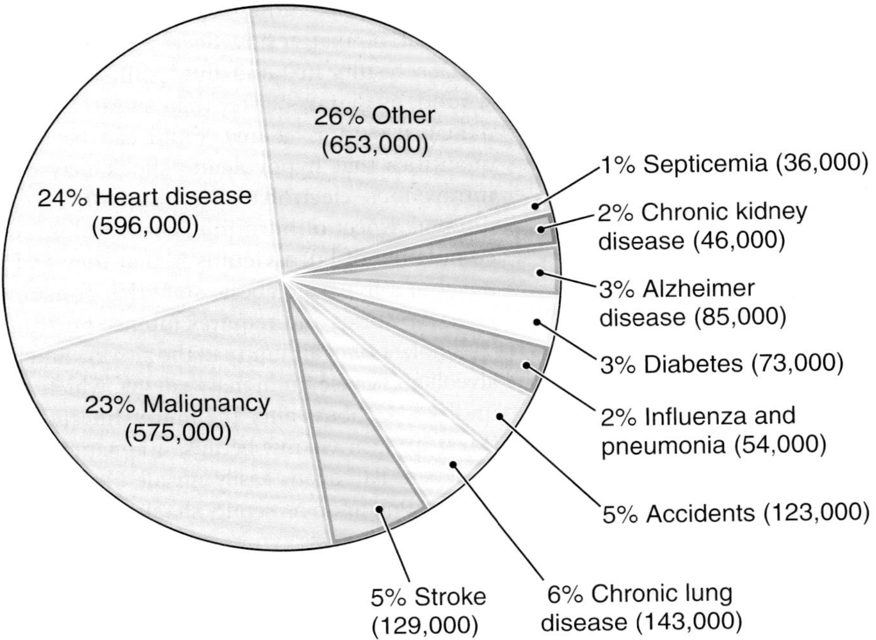

Figure 23.1 **Causes of death in the United States, 2011.** Environmental factors are important in many categories but are not listed separately. For example, cigarette smoking is an important cause of heart disease, malignancy, stroke, and chronic lung disease. Lack of exercise is important in heart disease and stroke. Alcohol abuse plays an important role in accidents. (Adapted from Centers for Disease Control, National Vital Statistics Report, 2007.)

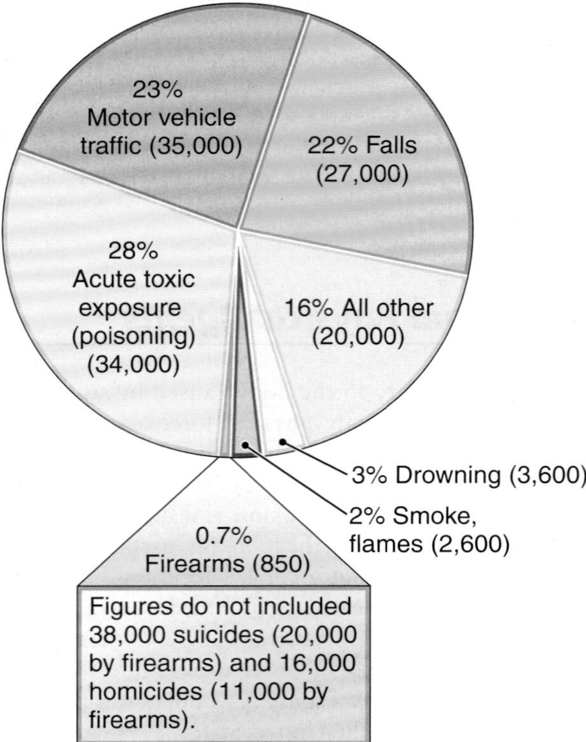

Figure 23.2 **Deaths from accidents in the United States, 2011.** Deaths from the direct effect of alcohol are not included, though alcohol plays a role in many categories. For example, alcohol is implicated in 40% of motor vehicle traffic deaths. Most gunshot deaths are suicide or homicide. (Adapted from Centers for Disease Control, National Data on Injuries, 2011.)

Thermal Burns Are a Serious Problem

In 2010 in the United States, about 500,000 people needed medical treatment for thermal burns, 45,000 were hospitalized, and 3,500 died of their injury.

Clinical Assessment

The clinical significance of a burn depends on the following factors:

- Burn depth
- Percentage of body surface affected
- Lung injury from hot or toxic gas
- Promptness of therapy, especially fluid replacement and infection prevention and control: delayed treatment makes any burn more serious

Skin burns are classified according to whether or not necrosis is present, and, if so, how deep it extends (Fig. 23.3A).

- *Superficial burns* (formerly *first-degree* burns) are those confined to the epidermis. Sunburn is an example. They are red and blanche with pressure, indicating blood flow is intact. Accumulation of dermal edema fluid may make the area swell. They are dry and painful, and heal without scarring in less than a week.
- *Partial thickness burns* (formerly *second-degree* burns) are those in which injury extends into the dermis. Blisters usually form quickly. They usually do not blanche to pressure, a clue that dermal blood vessels are damaged. Edema is always present. They are red, wet, painful, and usually heal with scarring.
- *Full thickness burns* (formerly *third-degree* burns) are those in which injury extends completely through the dermis and into fat, muscle, or bone beneath. Skin may be charred or translucent, with coagulated vessels visible through it. The most severely burned areas are insensate from nerve destruction. Pain arises from partial thickness burns at the edges. They do not heal on their own and require skin grafting. Severe scarring is common.

The *rule of nines* (Fig. 23.4) is a convenient way to estimate the percentage of body surface burned. The front and the back of the legs are 9% each (total 36%); the front and back of the torso are 18% each (total 36%); the front and the back of the arms are 4.5% each (total 18%); the head, neck, and face are 9%. The genitalia account for 1%. The greater the percentage of the body that is burned, the greater the threat to the patient; however, burn location is important, too. Burns to the face, neck, and chest may interfere with breathing. The social importance of the face and its complex anatomy add to the significance of facial burns.

Complications

Shock, sepsis, and respiratory failure are the greatest threat to life. Burns exceeding 40% of body surface area are usually fatal, no matter how deep. Any burn over 20% of body surface results in rapid fluid shifts: fluid seeps from the wound, evaporates faster than sweat, and is absorbed into damaged skin as edema. Fluid can be lost in such large quantities that hypovolemic shock may develop. Intense intravenous electrolyte fluid support is critical. An additional aspect of burn injury is heat loss (one of the first complaints of burn victims is that they feel cold) and the onset of a hypermetabolic state that consumes huge numbers of calories and requires intense nutritional support.

Smoke or hot air injury to the airways and lungs can injure alveoli and cause pulmonary edema, which may not develop until 24–48 hours after the injury. Infections are a constant threat in burn victims because the natural barrier of skin is breached. Pathogens easily invade blood vessels and spread widely. Pneumonia, septic shock, renal failure, and acute respiratory distress syndrome are common consequences of blood infection (septicemia) associated with burns.

Treatment

Most superficial burns may be handled with analgesia and supportive care, but large superficial burns and all partial or full-thickness burns require specialized care.

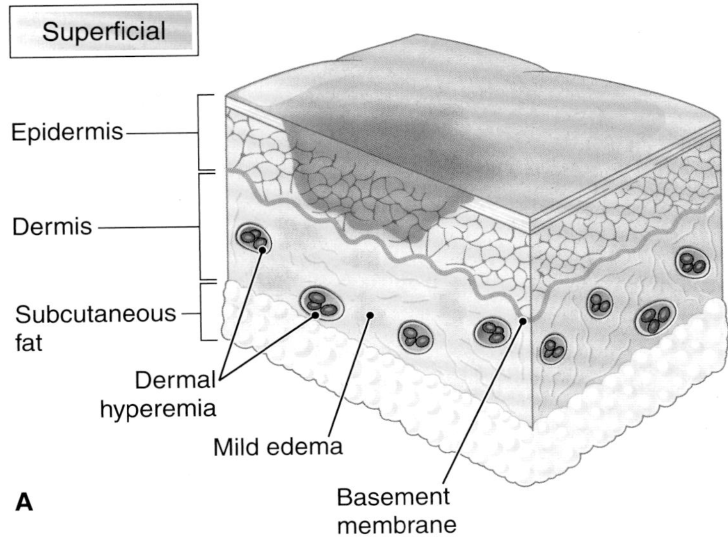

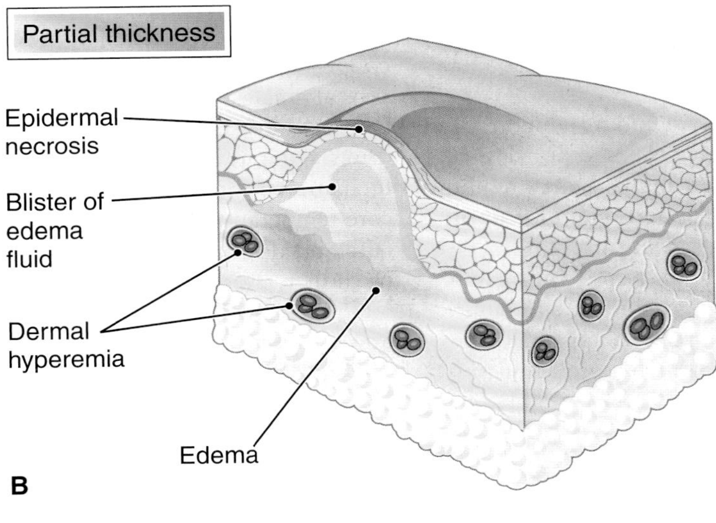

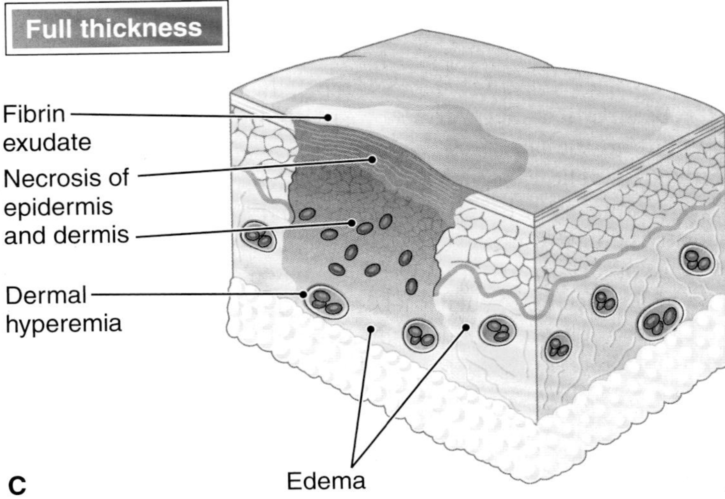

Figure 23.3 **The pathology of skin burns. A.** Superficial burn shows only dermal hyperemia and mild edema. No blistering or necrosis is present. **B.** Partial thickness burn shows epidermal necrosis, blister formation, and dermal hyperemia and edema. **C.** Full thickness burn shows necrosis of the full thickness of the epidermis and dermis.

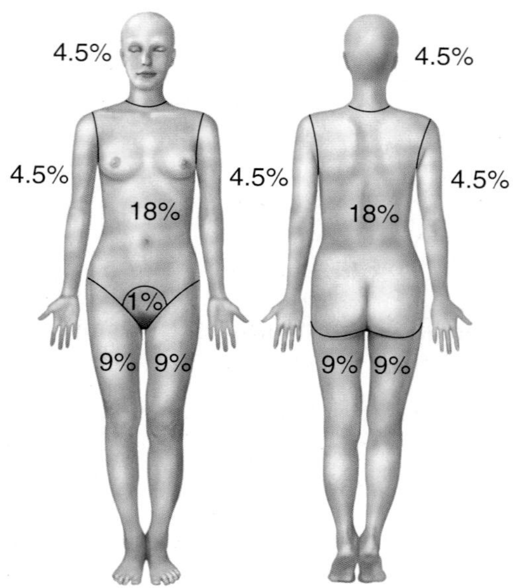

Figure 23.4 **Burns: the rule of nines.** (Adapted with permission from McConnell TH, Hull KL. *Human Form Human Function: Essentials of Anatomy & Physiology*. Baltimore, MD: Wolters Kluwer Health; 2011.)

Intravenous fluid support is of paramount importance for burns >10% of body surface area (BSA). For example, a 250 lb man burned over 40% of his BSA may require 10–20 liters of intravenous fluid support, half of it in the first eight hours. Soap and water cleansing and surgical debridement of the wound are necessary to prevent or limit infection and require analgesia or anesthesia. Antibiotics should be used only if infection becomes apparent. Skin grafting and other specialized treatments are frequently required.

Cold Injury Can Be Fatal or Disfiguring

Susceptibility to cold injury is increased by drug or alcohol use, hunger, dehydration, and impaired cardiovascular function. Wet clothing and high wind speed also increase the risk.

Frostnip (first-degree frostbite) involves freezing of superficial skin, somewhat similar to a superficial burn. It is characterized by firm, white patches on the face, ears, fingers, or toes and results in mottled red, yellow, or blue splotches that peel or blister on rewarming. Pain is variable. Long-term hot-cold hypersensitivity may result.

Frostbite is cold injury to dermis or deeper tissues. Affected areas are hard and white and lack feeling. When warmed, the lesion becomes swollen, red, blistered, and painful, very similar to a scald with hot fluid (Fig. 23.5). Blisters (bullae) may form and fill when blood flow returns. Some lesions may heal without tissue loss, but deep frostbite always results in gangrene and requires skin grafting or amputation. Treatment is by gradual warming in water, supported by analgesia and anti-inflammatory drugs. Anticoagulants and vasodilators may be indicated. Infection is a risk.

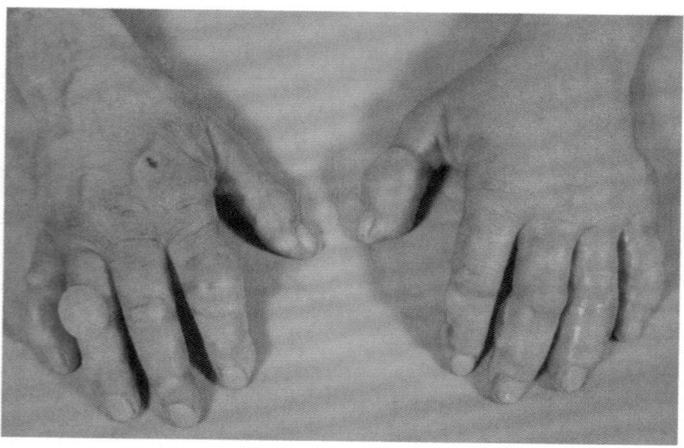

Figure 23.5 **Frostbite.** On the left is a scald with bullae. On the right is frostbite with bullae. (Reproduced with permission from Berg D., Worzala K. *Atlas of Adult Physical Diagnosis*. Philadelphia, PA: Lippincott Williams & Wilkins; 2006.)

Hypothermia (exceptionally low body temperature) results in a slowing of all physiologic functions. It is caused by low temperatures, high humidity, wet clothing, and the peripheral vasodilation caused by ingestion of alcohol—a combination common in homeless people. Persons at greatest risk are the very old, the debilitated, those with cardiovascular disease, and those abusing alcohol or drugs. Symptoms are lethargy, clumsiness, confusion, hallucinations, and slow respiratory and heart rate. At body core temperature of about 90°F, loss of consciousness occurs and death may follow, owing to cardiac arrhythmia or cardiac arrest. Treatment is complex and difficult, and requires immediate and expert care.

Heat Illness Can Be Life-Threatening

Heat affects many bodily functions and may cause dehydration. Effects range from cramps to fainting, heat exhaustion, and heat stroke. Body temperature may or may not be elevated. People with dehydration may have rapid heart and respiratory rate and low blood pressure. Mental dysfunction suggests *heat stroke*, the most serious problem.

Typically, heat illness occurs when the heat produced by strenuous exertion combines with factors that limit heat loss. Work or athletic clothing limits convection loss, and high humidity limits evaporative loss. Obese patients are at risk because managing and maintaining their bulk requires more energy, which generates more heat. Drugs may play a role: some medications impair sweating (e.g., antihistamines) and some act to increase heat production (e.g., stimulants such as amphetamine).

Heat cramps are spasms of voluntary muscle caused by electrolyte loss, most often following vigorous exercise. Rest and intake of a rehydration fluid such as a sports beverage is recommended.

Heat exhaustion, a more serious condition, is characterized by profuse sweating and sudden weakness and disorientation or fainting owing to the inability of the cardiovascular system to compensate for water loss. Body temperature may rise to near 102°F, but after a brief period of instability, homeostasis is reestablished. If body temperature continues to rise, heat stroke may occur. Rest, relief from the hot environment, and fluid replacement are necessary to avoid continued rise of body temperature and heat stroke.

Heat stroke is hyperthermia that causes multiple organ dysfunction. Signs and symptoms include temperature >104°F and altered mental status. Sweating is typically absent. Because sweating has stopped, the patient's skin is flushed from peripheral vasodilation as the body attempts to shed heat through the skin. The person may experience an intense headache, nausea and vomiting, rapid respirations and pulse, muscle weakness or rigidity, and loss of consciousness. Hypotension and shock are common. Other problems include cardiac arrhythmias or cardiac arrest, seizures, coma, and disseminated intravascular coagulation. Skeletal muscle necrosis may liberate massive amounts of myoglobin, causing kidney failure.

Heat stroke is a medical emergency. Immediate action is necessary. Treatment includes rapid external cooling, either with ice packs on the head, neck, armpits, and groin, or by continuously misting the body with cold water. Clinical treatment includes continued cooling, administration of cold IV fluids, and support as needed for organ failures. Even with treatment, death occurs in half of patients whose temperature rises above 106°F.

Malignant hyperthermia is a rare autosomal dominant genetic condition in which certain anesthetics and anesthesia-related drugs induce skeletal muscles to burn energy at an extraordinarily high rate, far above the body's ability to supply oxygen or get rid of the CO_2 and heat generated. During anesthesia, the first sign is rising blood CO_2 despite good ventilation. Treatment is with dantrolene, which blocks the molecular mechanism of muscle energy production.

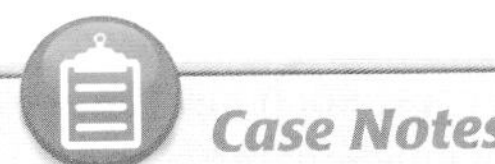

Case Notes

23.3 Is Marvin more likely, equally likely, or less likely than a nonobese person to have a heat-related illness?

Electrical Injury

Electricity injures by two means: heating tissue until it burns (in the same way that it causes a griddle to heat), or disrupting critical processes that depend on orderly electrical activity such as heartbeat, skeletal muscle contraction, and the transmission of nerve signals.

The severity of injury depends on the following factors (the relationship among them is complex and beyond the scope of this review):

- *Type of current* (direct, DC; or alternating, AC). Household current is AC; battery power is DC. AC is many times more dangerous and powerful than DC in most settings.
- *Strength of current* (voltage and amperage). Higher voltage and amperage increase injury.
- *Duration of exposure*. Longer exposure increases injury.
- *Resistance of tissue*. High resistance increases heat production. Thick, calloused, dry skin is the most resistant of all tissues and the most likely to burn.
- *Pathway of current*. For example, current traveling from one hand to another is likely to flow through the heart and cause cardiac arrhythmia.

Low-strength current produces nothing more than an unpleasant "shocked" feeling. The pathology of high-strength current includes hemolysis, blood coagulation, skin burns, and necrosis of muscle and other tissues. Seizures, muscle tetany, or cardiac arrhythmias (including fatal ventricular fibrillation) may occur with little associated tissue damage.

Electrical injuries are often fatal. Muscle spasms may produce involuntary grasping of the source, which prolongs contact and increases risk of death or severe burn. Higher voltage (lightning or power lines) increases the risk of severe burns and respiratory arrest.

Treatment includes cardiopulmonary resuscitation for cardiac arrest, analgesia, cardiac monitoring, and wound care. Burns may be severe and are managed as described above.

Ionizing Radiation

Radiation can be classified into two groups. *Low-energy radiation* includes visible light, radio waves, and radar, none of which packs enough punch to cause ionization of tissue molecules. *High-energy (ionizing) radiation* includes ultraviolet (UV) light, X-rays, and gamma rays. These rays possess enough energy to convert stable molecules into unstable ions, which react with other molecules, injuring them. An important aspect of ionizing radiation damage is that it cannot be repaired and thus is *cumulative over a lifetime*. Unlike toxins, which usually can be cleared from the body, radiation damage is forever, and each new dose adds to the burden.

The effect of radiation depends upon several variables, including the following:

- *Field size*. The body can survive high doses to small areas, an advantage in radiation treatment of cancer, whereas a smaller dose delivered to the entire body may be fatal.
- *Rate of cell proliferation*. DNA is vulnerable to ionization, especially during cell division. This is a double-edged sword: the very features that make it dangerous also make it useful for radiation therapy. Tissues with rapid cell division (labile tissues)—bone marrow, lymphoid tissues, gonads, respiratory and GI mucosa, and epidermis—are most susceptible to radiation, an advantage in radiation treatment of certain malignancies, and a disadvantage in radiation of healthy tissues.

- *Tissue oxygenation*. Well-oxygenated tissue is most vulnerable because radiation creates reactive oxygen species and free radicals, which enhance the damage. The centers of rapidly growing tumors are often hypoxic, which limits the effectiveness of radiation therapy.

The most common form of radiation exposure is the invisible UV spectrum of sunlight. UVA waves are high frequency, high energy, waves that damage skin cell DNA, and can induce malignancy or excess wrinkling (photoaging) in chronically over-exposed skin.

Apart from sunlight, medical radiation carries the most risk. Some exposure to the more powerful energy of X-rays is a necessary hazard for medical professionals and patients. Modern diagnostic radiographic techniques, however, have reduced the dosage to very low levels, so that the exposure for most diagnostic tests is less than that obtained from a day at the beach. Nevertheless, other body parts, the gonads in particular, should be shielded during X-ray studies.

Patients receiving high doses of radiation over a short period of time suffer short- and long-term effects. **Acute radiation sickness (ARS)** follows intense exposure and is characterized by severe infections, owing to bone marrow and lymphoid (immune) system failure, and by severe diarrhea and intestinal infections due to damage to the intestinal mucosa. Long-term radiation injury is associated with scarring (e.g., bone marrow fibrosis) and increased cancer risk. The Chernobyl nuclear power plant disaster in Ukraine in 1986 produced over 100 cases of ARS, of whom about one-fourth died in a short time. Long-term effects remain under study. Increased numbers of thyroid cancer, leukemia, and other malignancies are present among those who were living in the contamination zone at the time of the accident.

Pop Quiz

23.1 True or false? Heart disease is the leading cause of death in the United States.

23.2 Define laceration.

23.3 A red, wet, painful burn with blisters is a __________ burn.

23.4 At about what core temperature does a person suffering from hypothermia lose consciousness?

23.5 A marathon runner is transported to the emergency room. His skin is flushed and he feels hot to the touch, but he is not sweating. What is he suffering from?

23.6 What type of tissue is the most susceptible to ionizing radiation?

Toxic Exposures

A **toxin** is any substance that is injurious to health or dangerous to life. "Toxin" and "poison" mean much the same thing; however, "poison" is often used to connote deliberate acts; in this discussion "toxin" will be used because it carries a broader meaning.

Almost any substance is capable of being toxic in the right set of circumstances. Even the most innocuous substances can be injurious if taken in large quantity over a short period of time. For example, forced ingestion of very large amounts of water, as in a college hazing prank, can produce fatal brain edema, and prolonged therapeutic use of inhaled oxygen can cause direct damage to the lungs.

Moreover, exposure to toxins can occur at anytime, anywhere. **Occupational disease** often develops because of long-term exposure to toxins. For example, lung cancer is associated with asbestos inhalation in asbestos miners, and bladder cancer is associated with occupational exposure to aniline, a toxic chemical used in the manufacture of dyes, rubbers, and other products. Although the most common workplace disorders are associated with repeated trauma—for example, arthritis in the hands of persons operating vibrating equipment—the second most common are skin diseases due to allergy or irritation from contact with solvents, acids, or alkalis. Moreover, workplace exposures can be fatal. Overall, occupational disorders claim about 6,300 lives per year, and although about 90% of them are due to physical trauma, the remaining 10% are due to fatal exposures to toxic substances. Table 23.1 offers a brief list of some of the more important occupational toxic exposures.

Air Pollution Can Occur Outdoors or Indoors

A **pollutant** is a substance in air or water that can injure those exposed to it. Pollutants may have short-term effects, such as the acute toxicity of carbon monoxide (CO) poisoning from incomplete burning of fuel in a faulty room heater. They can also have long-term effects, such as the lung cancers and vascular diseases that plague cigarette smokers.

Air pollution is a problem in industrial societies. For example, average pulmonary function is permanently impaired in people who live downwind of factories that put pollutants into the air; people living upwind are unaffected. Both outdoor and indoor air can become polluted.

Outdoor air pollution is produced by combustion of fossil fuels, coal- or oil-fired power plant emissions, waste incinerators, and industrial plants. Inhaled *particulate matter* (soot) can be dangerous, especially if the particles are small. Large particles are removed by the upper airway, but small ones reach the alveoli and damage the lungs. On hot days, some air pollutants undergo photochemical reactions to produce ground-level *ozone* (O_3, a powerful oxidant), which can damage lungs directly or aggravate pre-existing asthma or emphysema. Even low levels can be dangerous, especially

Table 23.1 Occupational Toxic Exposures and Disease

System	Toxins	Effect
RESPIRATORY	Asbestos, rock dust (silica), arsenic, chromium, nickel	Lung cancer
	Grain dust, coal dust, rock dust (silica), asbestos, cobalt, beryllium, cadmium	Chronic pulmonary disease
NERVOUS	Mercury, lead, arsenic, solvents	Peripheral neuropathy
	Mercury, toluene, solvents, aldehydes, ketones	Brain toxicity
URINARY	Benzidine, naphthylamines, aniline dyes, rubber products	Bladder cancer
REPRODUCTIVE	Lead, cadmium, mercury, polychlorinated biphenyls (PCB)	Infertility, teratogenesis
HEMATOPOIETIC	Benzene, uranium	Leukemia

when combined with other pollutants. In contrast to this ground-level ozone, the ozone of the upper atmosphere is naturally produced and serves to protect the earth from excessive exposure to UV light.

Indoor air pollution accumulates in poorly ventilated spaces. The most important worldwide indoor pollutant is from indoor solid fuel usage or open fires for cooking inside the home, primarily in third-world countries where electricity or natural gas is not available. This leads to an increase in respiratory infections, chronic obstructive pulmonary disease (COPD), lung cancer, CO exposure (see below), and other problems.

Tobacco smoke is a significant source of air pollution. **Secondhand smoke**, also known as "passive smoke," is a mixture of two forms of smoke from burning tobacco products. Smoke flowing into the air from the tip of a burning cigarette is called *sidestream smoke*. Smoke inhaled and exhaled by a smoker is *mainstream smoke*. Sidestream smoke contains twice the tar and higher levels of many of the other toxins in mainstream smoke because it has not been filtered by being drawn through the cigarette. The U.S. Surgeon General reports that there is no risk-free level of exposure to secondhand smoke. Passive smoke inhalation increases the risk of lung cancer, heart attack, and other diseases. Risk for lung cancer increases 30% in those chronically exposed to passive smoke, and evidence suggests that about 10% of heart attacks can be attributed to passive smoke inhalation. Passive smoke inhalation also increases the number of respiratory infections and asthmatic attacks in children, the risk of sudden infant death syndrome (SIDS) and middle ear infections in young children, and the number of low birth weight infants born to exposed mothers.

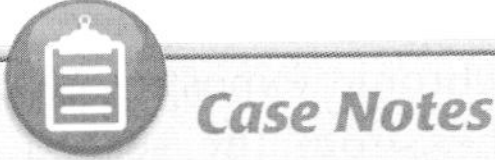

Case Notes

23.4 Two of Marvin's three children are smokers. Is the third free of tobacco-related risk?

Carbon monoxide (CO) is a colorless, odorless, nonirritating gas product of incompletely burned fuels. Accidental poisoning usually arises in a confined space from CO emissions from gas space heaters, furnaces, stoves, or internal combustion engines. For example, 5% of auto exhaust is CO and gas from burning charcoal has high CO content. In well-ventilated spaces it is little threat, but it is very dangerous in confined spaces because of its great affinity for hemoglobin. CO is the leading cause of accidental poisoning death in the United States. CO combines permanently with hemoglobin to form carboxyhemoglobin, a bright red form of hemoglobin to which oxygen cannot attach. The result is anoxia despite adequate pulmonary ventilation. CO poisoning can prove rapidly fatal. The bright red color of carboxyhemoglobin provides an important clinical or postmortem clue to the problem: the patient's skin is cherry red, even in death (Fig. 23.6). Note that CO is a component of secondhand smoke, and can harm nonsmokers, especially those already suffering from respiratory disease.

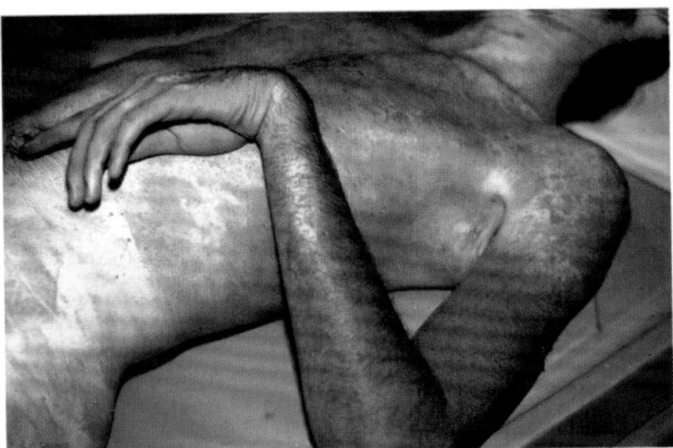

Figure 23.6 **Carbon monoxide (CO) poisoning.** A faulty natural gas room heater caused this fatal poisoning. The characteristic cherry-red coloration of skin persists in death. CO binds irreversibly with hemoglobin to produce bright red hemoglobin, which retains its color even though no oxygen is present.

Exposure to Toxic Chemicals Is a Widespread Hazard

About 10 million natural and synthetic chemicals are known to exist. Most toxic exposures derive from a group of about 2,500 of them.

Toxicity depends on the properties of the chemical and the amount (*dose*). Some toxins work slowly and even in large doses may not necessarily be life—threatening. A few milligrams of some other substances can be fatal. About 30,000 people in the United States die each year of acute exposure to toxins. Eighty percent of those deaths are attributed to drug overdose, primarily overdose of illegal drugs. Alcohol, however, is commonly the agent. To cause fatal respiratory arrest requires upwards of 100 grams of pure *ethanol*, the rough equivalent of quick ingestion of about five to six shots of distilled spirit such as bourbon. But in drinking games and other behaviors involving binge drinking—in men five drinks, in women four, in less than two hours—many people expose themselves to this life-threatening level of alcohol.

U.S. National Poison Data Center data for 2010 show about 2.4 million episodes of poisoning. Children under age three accounted for nearly 40% of cases. The most common agents among children were cosmetics and personal care products. Among adults the most common agents were analgesics. Oral medications and cleaning products were commonly involved. The most serious incidents were usually in the home.

Vitamins, minerals, and other dietary supplements, such as iron, are not toxic in recommended doses; however, overdose can be very serious. *Iron overdose* is especially harmful to children. By law in the United States, no dietary supplement tablet may contain more than 30 mg of iron per tablet; nevertheless, 20 such tablets can contain enough iron (600 mg) to cause fatal iron poisoning in a child. Acute iron toxicity is one of the leading causes of accidental poisoning death in children, usually from curious toddlers who think pills are candy. Death occurs due to hemorrhagic gastroenteritis, metabolic acidosis, cardiovascular collapse, or coma. Chronic iron overload is *hemochromatosis* (Chapter 12), which may be genetic, due to repeated blood transfusions, or due to increased intestinal absorption in alcoholics. Iron deposits in and damages the heart, liver, and pancreas.

Occupational exposure to chemicals is usually more intense than is casual, everyday exposure, because in the workplace, potentially toxic substances are in active use in high concentration. There are large numbers of hazardous workplace chemicals, some of which are listed in Table 23.1.

Volatile organic compounds (VOCs) and *petroleum products* are used in industry and at home. They are an important ingredient in solvents, glues, paint remover, and charcoal lighter fluid, and they may be abused (e.g., glue sniffing). Acute exposure can be associated with dizziness, unsteady gait, confusion, and nausea. In severe cases, coma and death may occur. Chronic exposure includes risk for liver toxicity, neuropathies, bone marrow suppression, and leukemia.

Agricultural chemicals may prove acutely toxic or fatal to farm workers. These include pesticides, fertilizers, and veterinary products. Some of these chemicals tend to accumulate in water and soil; they pose a long-term threat to wildlife and humans. Others are acutely dangerous. Organophosphates (such as parathion) are insecticides that are easily absorbed through skin or lungs and have their effect by blocking nerve signal transmission at synapses. The result is paralysis, including respiratory muscles. Acute toxicity causes sweating, blurred vision, constricted pupils, salivation, bronchospasm, muscle twitching (fasciculation), paralysis, and respiratory arrest. Chronic, low-level exposure such as pesticide residue on foods may harm children or a developing fetus. Other exposures may harm children working or playing in the outdoors.

Some Metals Are Hazardous

Certain metals are toxic. High-dose exposure can cause acute illness, whereas long-term exposure can increase the risk of neurological disorders, cancer, and other diseases.

In 1977, federal regulations banned the use of **lead** in paints, but lead toxicity still occurs. Older urban homes and factories may contain large amounts of flaking lead-based paint. In some developing nations, lead may be present in earthen cookware or lead-based paint may be used to decorate souvenir plates and cups bought by tourists. Soils may still be contaminated with lead from paints and gasoline.

Acute lead toxicity produces anemia, kidney disease, abdominal cramps, headache, memory loss, numbness and pain in the arms or legs, and distinctive bone deposits visible by X-ray imaging. Long-term exposure to low levels of lead may not cause detectable clinical symptoms, but can be damaging, especially to children. Exposed children suffer subtle neurologic and behavioral problems and lower intelligence, which persist into adult life.

Mercury poisoning may be acute or chronic. Mercury is found in many products, including batteries, and is important in many industrial processes. Acute exposure is rare and may cause coma, renal failure, and death. Acute poisoning features tremors and bizarre behavior of the type exhibited by the Mad Hatter in *Alice's Adventures in Wonderland*, whose author, Lewis Carroll, based the characterization on fact: 19th-century hat makers used a solution containing mercury to treat felt for hats. Inhaling the toxic fumes in poorly ventilated workshops led to mercury poisoning. Modern chronic exposure comes mainly from mercury that leaches from the seabed or industrial sites into ocean water and concentrates in large carnivorous fish like swordfish and shark. Levels are not high enough to cause problems for most people who eat such fish; however, mercury is exceptionally toxic to the brain of a developing fetus. Pregnant women are therefore advised to limit their intake of swordfish and other sea carnivores. There also has been much alarm in the public media regarding *thiomersal* (also known as *thimerosal*), a mercury-based preservative in some vaccines, as a potential cause of autism. Numerous large, reputable scientific studies have found no such relationship.

Arsenic poisoning has a long and colorful history as "the poison of kings and the king of poisons" because it was readily available, odorless, and tasteless. It acts by blocking basic metabolic processes. Acute symptoms include headaches, confusion, and diarrhea. Acute poisoning is rare today, but as recently as 2003 an episode of deliberate poisoning occurred due to spiked coffee at a church in Maine. Chronic exposure nowadays may be found in parts of Bangladesh, China, and Chile, where groundwater and soil contain enough arsenic to cause increased risk for skin and lung cancer.

Cadmium poisoning is a modern phenomenon. Cadmium is used in mining and electroplating and in nickel-cadmium (NiCad) batteries, which find their way into garbage and landfill sites and thence into the food chain by water contamination. Chronic exposure leads to lung and kidney disease.

Many Therapeutic Drugs Have Adverse Effects

Adverse reaction to therapeutic drugs is common. Acute reactions, such as allergy or accidental overdose, are uncommon. The most frequent problems occur in patients on long-term therapy. Of these, the most commonly involved substances are hormone replacement therapy (HRT) and oral contraceptives in women; anabolic steroids, mainly in men; and aspirin and acetaminophen.

Hormone replacement therapy consists of long-term estrogen and progesterone administration mainly to postmenopausal women for relief of postmenopausal hot flashes and prevention of osteoporosis. Although once administered almost routinely, careful studies have highlighted the benefits and risks in such a way that HRT is now used much more selectively.

- HRT increases the risk for breast cancer, but only after five to eight years.
- HRT has a protective effect against cardiovascular disease, but only in women who start therapy at a relatively young age. It has no benefit for women over age 60.
- HRT increases the risk of venous thromboembolism and stroke.

Nevertheless, HRT is very effective at relieving disabling postmenopausal hot flashes, and it continues to be prescribed in selected circumstances.

After many years of uncertainty, it is now clear that **oral contraceptives** are safe and effective. Regarding their contraceptive value, it is wise to recall that pregnancy itself can be a hazard. Moreover, oral contraceptives appear to provide protection against endometrial and ovarian cancer. Still, oral contraceptive use is associated with the following risks:

- *Venous thrombosis and pulmonary thromboembolism.*
- *Cardiovascular disease in women who smoke.* Women over age 35 who smoke and take oral contraceptives have a 10-fold increased risk of heart attack and stroke.
- *Hepatic adenoma.* Older women who have been taking oral contraceptives for a long time are at risk for developing a benign liver tumor, which can rupture and cause life-threatening bleeding.

Anabolic steroids are synthetic versions of testosterone. They have become popular with athletes to increase muscle mass and improve performance; however, they are illegal in the United States, and their use is banned by all major collegiate and professional sports organizations. They are usually taken by injection in doses 10–100 times higher than therapeutic doses. The side effects of steroid use include testicular atrophy and gynecomastia in men; acne; stunted growth in adolescents; and excess facial hair and abnormal menstruation in women. Users are also at risk for psychological problems, including uncontrollable anger, and for heart attacks and certain forms of cancer. Oral administration has similar risks plus the risk for liver disease.

Aspirin is the most widely used medicine in the world because it is cheap and effective as a pain reliever and fever reducer. It also inhibits platelet activity and is widely used in small doses to prevent thrombosis, mostly in populations at risk for heart attack or stroke. A side effect is a slight bleeding tendency with injury or surgery.

Ingestion by a child of 10–20 standard tablets (325 mg per tablet) can be toxic, while in adults acute aspirin toxicity requires 30–100 standard tablets (sometimes less than a full bottle). Acute toxicity stimulates respiration and causes respiratory alkalosis (Chapter 6), which is followed by metabolic acidosis from interference with metabolism. Patients also commonly complain of tinnitus, that is, ringing in the ears. Childproof containers have almost completely eliminated accidental overdose among children, which at one time was common. Aspirin use in children for treatment of fever associated with a viral syndrome is no longer recommended because of its possible association with liver toxicity in *Reye syndrome* (Chapter 12).

Chronic aspirin toxicity (**salicylism**) may occur in patients taking more than 10–12 tablets per day, usually for pain control associated with chronic disease, such as rheumatoid arthritis. Doses in this range can cause gastrointestinal problems (including irritation and ulceration of the stomach), dizziness, tinnitus, deafness, and mental problems. Bleeding may occur, because aspirin inhibits platelet "stickiness," an effect achievable by a single tablet. Because of this effect, long-term low-dose aspirin therapy has been found effective in prevention of heart attacks and strokes.

Case Notes

23.5 A nurse noticed that, before his death, Marvin was bleeding from the puncture wound made when an intravenous line was inserted. What is the likely reason?

At recommended dosages, **acetaminophen**, the active ingredient in Tylenol®, has fewer side effects than aspirin and has largely replaced aspirin as a pain reliever and fever reducer in the United States. Nevertheless, toxicity is common because of its widespread use and the unwarranted presumption that, because it is used for minor illnesses, it is safe to take at doses larger than recommended. Acetaminophen is also a common ingredient in other household medicines, which accounts in part for the fact that about 50,000 patients are treated in US emergency rooms each year for acetaminophen toxicity. The liver is most affected by acetaminophen: half of all cases of acute liver failure are due to acetaminophen, frequently in conjunction with alcohol abuse. Despite acetaminophen widespread use, it is arguable that it would not be approved were it a new drug seeking federal approval today.

Pop Quiz

23.7 True or false? Oral contraceptive use is associated with ovarian or uterine cancer.

23.8 True or false? Mainstream smoke contains more tar than sidestream smoke.

23.9 What compound is responsible for the bright red skin color of a patient suffering from CO poisoning?

23.10 What is occupational disease? Give an example.

23.11 Define toxin.

23.12 Name two over-the-counter medications that commonly cause toxicity.

Tobacco Use

In the United States, tobacco use, mainly cigarette smoking, causes more than 440,000 deaths per year, most of which can be attributed to lung cancer or cardiovascular disease. That figures does not include the estimated 50,000 deaths in nonsmokers due to inhalation of secondhand smoke. Snuff and chewing tobacco are also harmful and are important risk factors for oral cancer.

Smoking is arguably the most corrosive, health-destroying, individual habit ever adopted by humankind. Tobacco smoke accelerates disease in almost every organ system, and it is not much of a stretch to say that, for any given disease, smokers have more of it than those who do not smoke. Smokers have higher rates of lung cancer, other kinds of cancer, emphysema, chronic bronchitis, heart attack, stroke, atherosclerosis, hypertension, gastric ulcers, and many other diseases. About 50% of smokers die from the habit. Whereas about 70% of nonsmokers will live to age 75, only about 40% of smokers will do so, and their shortened life will be filled with more disability and disease. Smoking is the most preventable cause of death. Figure 23.7 offers a summary of the ill effects of smoking.

Remember This! Stopping smoking is the single most important action the average person can take to improve his or her health and prolong life.

Cigarette smoke contains over 60 known carcinogens, plus toxic metals and formaldehyde. Adding to the damage is the effect of CO, which has a 200 times greater affinity for hemoglobin than oxygen does and deprives tissue of oxygen by occupying red blood cell space where oxygen belongs. All of these effects are dose related; that is, they are directly proportional to the number of cigarettes smoked in a lifetime. Figure 23.8 illustrates the close relationship between the number of new lung cancers diagnosed per year in smokers and the number of cigarettes smoked per day. In the medical community, the standard measure of consumption is **pack-years**: the number of packs per day multiplied by the number of years smoking.

Case Notes

23.6 Which of Marvin's illnesses can be associated with smoking?

The ill effects of cigarette smoking are *not* associated with **nicotine**. Nicotine is a stimulant that is responsible for *addiction* to tobacco. It is arguably the most addictive of all substances, but it has little pathologic effect compared to the tars, phenol, benzopyrene, formaldehyde, and hydrocarbons found in smoke. The latter cause cancer by damaging bronchial DNA; others irritate the bronchial mucosa, causing chronic inflammation, excess mucus production, and paralysis of bronchial cilia, which inhibits their cleansing sweep.

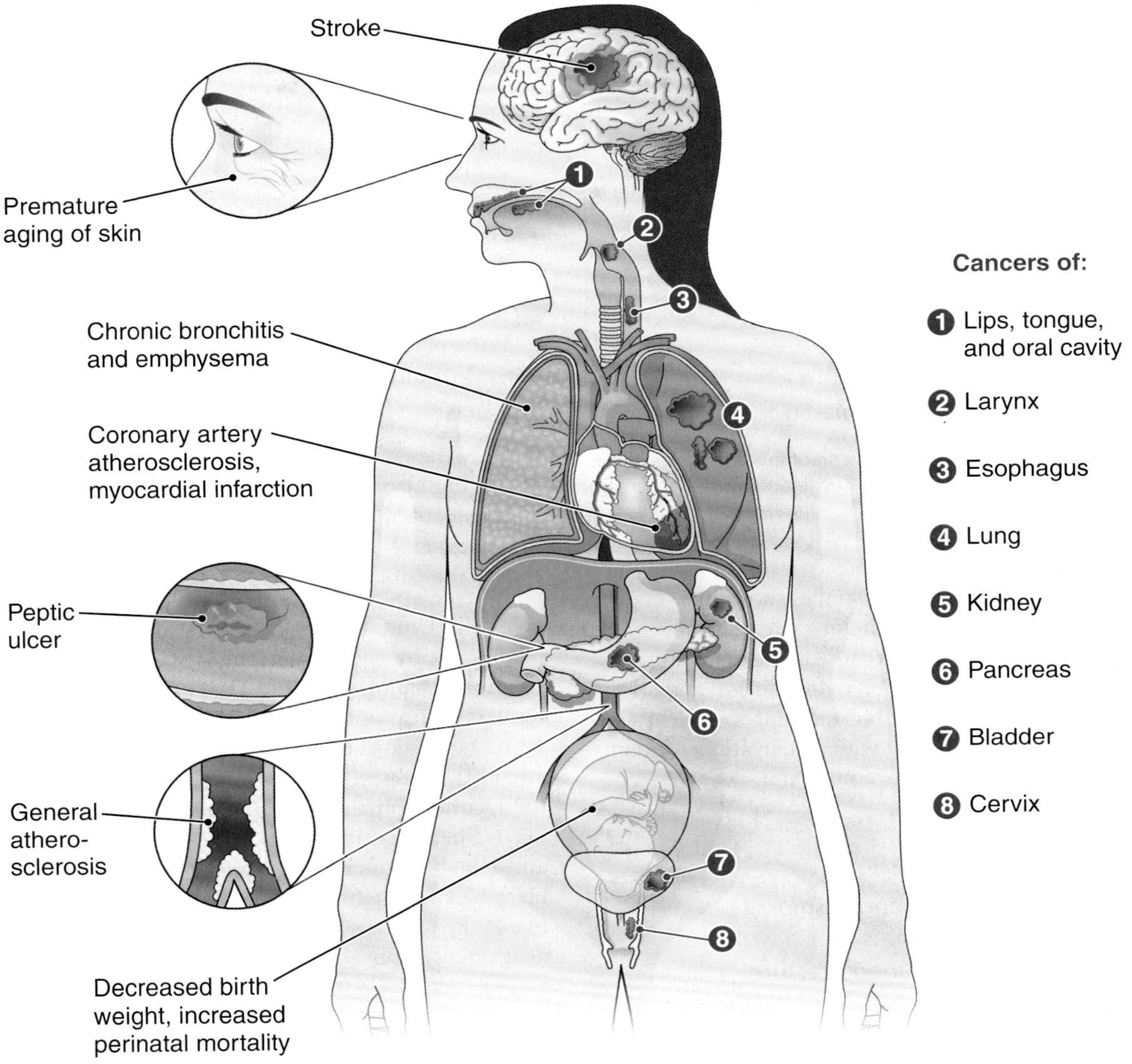

Figure 23.7 **The effects of smoking.**

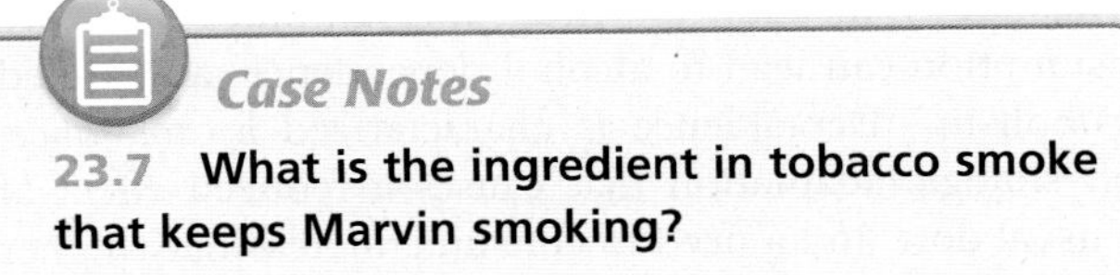

Case Notes

23.7 What is the ingredient in tobacco smoke that keeps Marvin smoking?

Fetuses are vulnerable to the effects of maternal smoking. Smoking half a pack a day causes fetal hypoxia, low birth weight, and prematurity. Smokers are at increased risk of abnormal implantation of the placenta, placental bleeding, abortion, and early rupture of amniotic membranes. Mothers who quit smoking while pregnant, however, do not suffer these risks.

The life expectancy of smokers who quit before age 30 is approximately that of people who have never smoked, but older smokers who quite also benefit. After one year of not smoking, smoking-related cardiovascular risk decreases 50%. Cancer risk fades more slowly than cardiovascular risk does, falling to near nonsmoker risk after 15–20 years. For those who find it impossible to quit, even smoking fewer cigarettes can help: recent evidence indicates that, for heavy smokers, smoking half as many cigarettes significantly reduces lung cancer risk. This has led to the common misperception among young adults that a few cigarettes a week ("social smoking") is harmless. This is not true. There is no safe level of smoking, only degrees of risk.

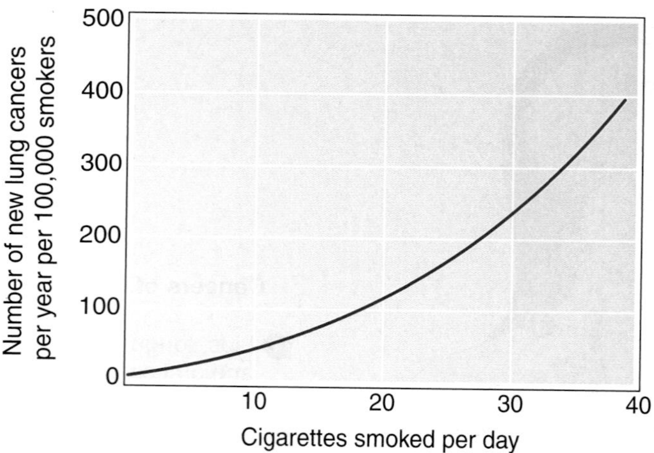

Figure 23.8 **The relationship between smoking and lung cancer.** The number of new lung cancers increases directly with the number of cigarettes smoked per day. A similar relationship exists between the number of new lung cancers and the number of years smoking.

Most smokers want to quit, but studies show three-fourths of high school smokers are still smoking five years after graduation. Quitting is difficult: it can cause intense craving, anxiety, depression, headache, insomnia, drowsiness, and a long list of other complaints. Counseling and drug treatment with nicotine or nicotine substitute or with certain antidepressants is most effective, but relapses are common.

Pop Quiz

23.13 True or false? Cigarette smokers have an increased risk for gastric ulcers and high blood pressure.

23.14 Fill in the blank. ___________ is the addictive ingredient in tobacco.

Alcohol Use and Abuse

For all of the headlines about illicit drug abuse, alcohol, a legal substance, is the greater hazard. In discussing alcohol, it is important to distinguish between *use* and *abuse*.

Each year, alcohol *use*—at any level—is associated with about 75,000 deaths, the majority of which are alcohol-influenced motor vehicle accidents. Studies over many years have shown that even low levels of alcohol consumption can impair driving skills, and statistics bear this out: alcohol is a contributing factor in 40% of motor vehicle deaths. It is also a contributing factor in other types of accidental deaths, including drowning, falls, and deaths in fires.

About 20,000 deaths each year are directly due to alcohol *abuse*. **Alcohol abuse** is a chronic disease in which people fail to stop drinking even though it causes neglect of important family and work obligations. About 5% of drinkers are abusers. The *CAGE questionnaire* is a convenient diagnostic tool if the patient is cooperative. It asks:

- Have you ever felt a need to Cut down on drinking?
- Have people Annoyed you by complaining about your drinking?
- Have you ever felt Guilty about drinking?
- Have you ever felt the need to have a drink first thing in the morning (an Eye opener) to steady your nerves or to get rid of a hangover?

If the patient is not available or is uncooperative, someone who knows the patient can be asked the following questions:

- Does the patient drink when it is dangerous (e.g., while driving or operating equipment)?
- Has alcohol caused difficulties with family, friends, or coworkers?
- Has the patient had legal problems related to drinking?

In the United States, the legal definition of drunkenness is set by each state, but is widely defined as blood alcohol (**ethanol**) 80 mg/dL (0.08%) or higher. To produce legal intoxication in a 140 lb person takes about three 12-oz bottles of beer, three 1-oz shots of 100 proof (50% ethanol) whiskey, or two-thirds of a bottle of wine, with the alcohol consumed in a short period of time. Women may experience intoxication at levels lower than these, and heavy drinkers can typically consume higher levels before experiencing intoxication. Blood alcohol of 200 mg/dL is associated with severe drunkenness; coma and death may occur at 300–400 mg/dL.

Case Notes

23.8 Does Marvin's alcohol consumption make him a user or an abuser?

Alcohol is an addictive drug, and chronic, excessive consumption can lead to alcohol dependence, also called "alcoholism." Dependence is characterized by *tolerance*, a physiologic adaptation that causes a reduced effect at the usual dose and a need to consume increasingly higher amounts to experience the effect desired. Dependence also prompts *withdrawal symptoms*, such as nausea, sweating, tremors, and anxiety when the person attempts to go without alcohol. Even in the absence of dependence, heavy drinking can cause disease in almost any organ. Most commonly, it affects the liver, gastrointestinal tract, cardiovascular system, and nervous system (Fig. 23.9):

- *Liver*. The liver is most severely affected. All chronic alcoholics have fatty livers (Fig. 23.10) and about 15%

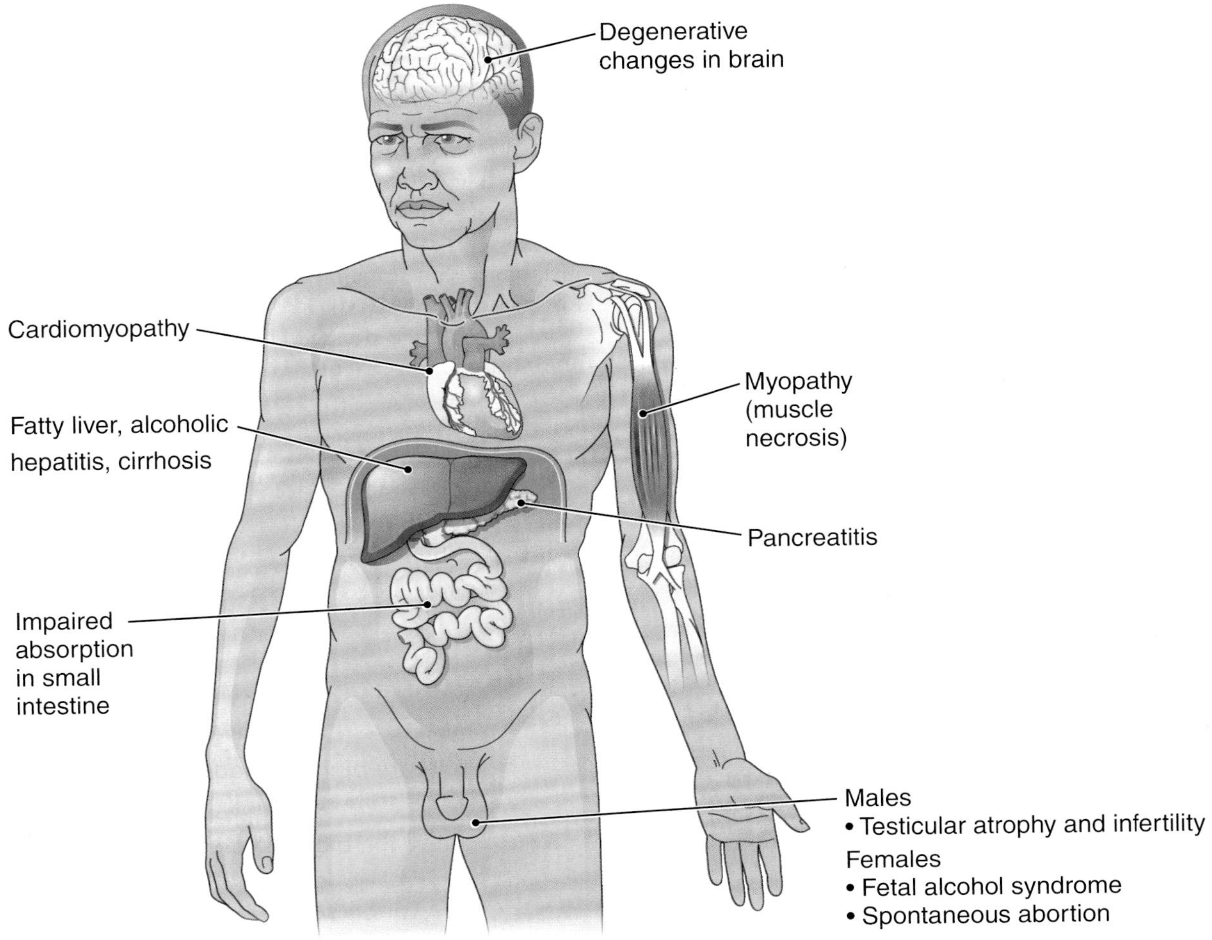

Degenerative changes in brain
Cardiomyopathy
Myopathy (muscle necrosis)
Fatty liver, alcoholic hepatitis, cirrhosis
Pancreatitis
Impaired absorption in small intestine
Males
• Testicular atrophy and infertility
Females
• Fetal alcohol syndrome
• Spontaneous abortion

Figure 23.9 **The effects of chronic alcohol abuse.**

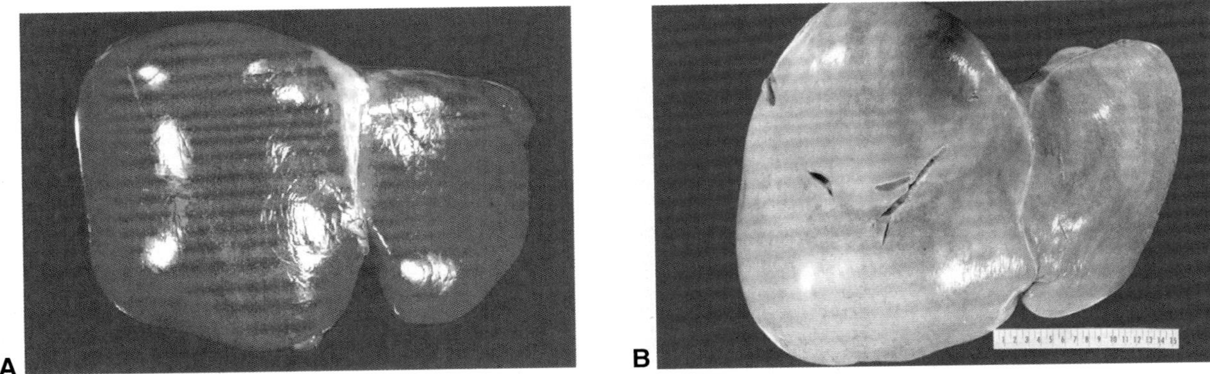

Figure 23.10 **Fatty liver of chronic alcoholism. A.** Normal liver. **B.** Fatty liver in a chronic alcoholic. The cuts are postmortem artifacts.

develop cirrhosis (severe scarring), which is associated with liver failure, intestinal hemorrhage, and liver cancer.

- *Gastrointestinal tract and pancreas.* Alcohol abuse is associated with gastritis, gastric and esophageal ulcers, fatal intestinal bleeding, and increased risk for cancers of the mouth and esophagus. Smoking further escalates cancer risk. Alcohol abuse is second only to gallstones as a cause of acute and chronic pancreatitis.
- *Cardiovascular system.* Alcohol abuse is associated with dilated cardiomyopathy and increased risk of

cardiovascular disease. By contrast, moderate social consumption of alcohol is protective (see below).

- *Nervous system*. Alcohol abuse affects both the brain and the peripheral nervous system. Chronic alcohol abuse severely affects the brain, most notably *cerebellar degeneration* (Fig. 23.11), which causes severe motor incoordination and stumbling gait. Other effects on the brain are attributable to alcoholic nutritional deficiencies—alcohol supplies calories only, no vitamins or other nutrients. One of the most noteworthy deficiencies is thiamine (vitamin B_1) deficiency, a disease known for hundreds of years as **beriberi**; it is characterized by peripheral neuropathy, cardiac failure, and either or both Wernicke encephalopathy or Korsakoff psychosis. *Wernicke encephalopathy* features severe neurologic dysfunction that may proceed to coma and death. *Korsakoff psychosis* features impaired recent memory, confusion, and rambling speech.
- *Pregnancy*. Even small amounts of alcohol have an adverse effect on the fetus. *Fetal alcohol syndrome* (Chapter 22) may be the result.

Formal diagnosis of alcoholism requires clinical assessment and questionnaire aids available from a variety of sources, such as the National Institute of Alcohol Abuse and Alcoholism. Treatment of immediate physical problems comes first, followed, if possible, by enrollment in an inpatient rehabilitation program, outpatient counseling, self-help groups, and consideration of drug treatment.

So much for the bad news. It is now abundantly clear that moderate alcohol intake appears to be beneficial, but the balance of benefit versus harm depends on age, sex, weight, and genetic and other factors. *Moderate use* is considered to be about two 150 ml glasses of wine, two beers, or two cocktails per day for males, and one per day for females. Many studies have documented the benefit of moderate consumption of alcohol—it decreases risk of developing cardiovascular disease and Type II diabetes. The positive cardiovascular effect is attributed to increases in HDL cholesterol and decreases of fibrinogen levels and platelet agglutination. The latter two are important in thrombus formation, which is important in the pathogenesis of heart attack and stroke. Nevertheless, *any* amount of ethanol can impair physical and mental performance for a short time, and few, if any, healthcare professionals would encourage nondrinkers to start drinking in moderation for cardiovascular or antidiabetic benefits.

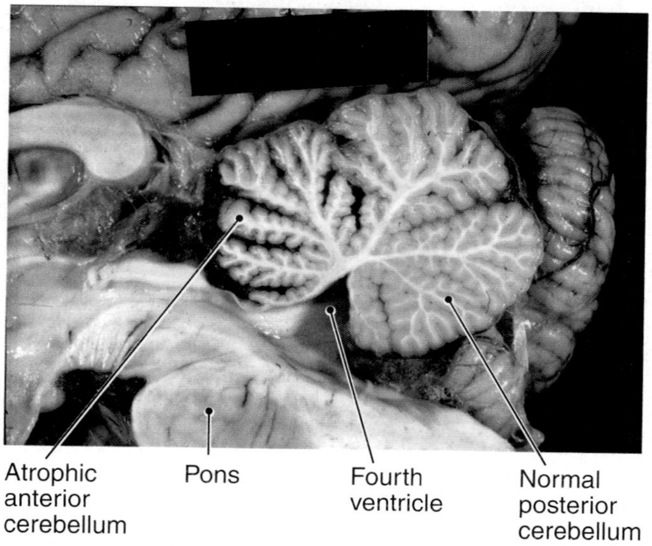

Atrophic anterior cerebellum
Pons
Fourth ventricle
Normal posterior cerebellum

Figure 23.11 Cerebellar atrophy of chronic alcoholism.

Case Notes

23.9 Which of Marvin's systems were most affected by alcohol?

Pop Quiz

23.15 True or false? Heavy drinkers can tolerate higher blood alcohol levels than nondrinkers can.

23.16 Fill in the blank. A deficiency of ____________ is responsible for anemia in alcoholics.

Illicit Drug Abuse

In this discussion, **illicit drug abuse** refers to any substance other than alcohol and nicotine (legal; i.e., licit drugs) that is used in excess to achieve an altered mood. In 2011 a federal study of students in grades 9-12 found that 23% used marijuana in the prior month. Hard drugs were also commonly abused, but less often. Each year, drug abuse accounts for about 20,000 deaths in the United States.

Drug abuse is associated with suicide, homicide, assaults, motor-vehicle injury, HIV infection, pneumonia, mental illness, hepatitis, and sudden death from cardiac disease or coma. In addition, as with tobacco and alcohol, illicit drug use commonly leads to addiction—an uncontrollable, chronic compulsion to use. Addiction can be psychological, physical, or both. Psychological addiction is self-explanatory. In physical addiction, body systems become physiologically dependent on the drug and withdrawal may produce physical effects ranging from anxiety to seizures and death. With chronic use comes tolerance. Abstinence from the drug decreases tolerance, a feature that can be dangerous. Many overdose deaths occur in relapsing users, who give themselves a big dose calculated for their tolerant body and die when the dose overwhelms their intolerant systems. Drug abusers also frequently abuse more than one drug at a time, such as an illicit drug and alcohol, expecting to enjoy the different effects simultaneously without realizing that adverse effects, like respiratory depression, may be additive. Death is sometimes the result.

Drug abuse in pregnancy is dangerous for the fetus. Like maternal alcohol use, maternal drug use may be associated with prematurity and birth defects. Some infants are also born addicted, and must be weaned from the drug slowly.

Drugs can be ingested, sniffed or inhaled, or injected. Ingestion produces less of the desired effect because intestinal absorption is slow. Greater effect is produced by injection or by sniffing or inhaling (including smoking) for quicker absorption into the bloodstream. Intravenous injection is particularly risky (Fig. 23.12). Shared needles and other unsanitary practices can lead to injection of microbes and foreign material. The most common infections obtained by injection are HIV (the virus that causes AIDS), hepatitis virus, and bacterial infections, including bacterial endocarditis. Injected foreign material can also stimulate formation of antigen-antibody complexes (circulating immune complexes, Chapter 3) that lodge in the glomeruli to produce chronic kidney disease. Some foreign substances, such as talc (used to dilute the drug dose), lodge in the lungs to produce "narcotic lung," characterized by inflammatory nodules and scarring.

Illegal drugs fall into four main categories: depressants, stimulants, narcotics, and hallucinogens. In the United States, the most popular illegal drug is marijuana, followed by prescription opioids and cocaine.

Treatment for acute overdose is a medical emergency that requires high-level medical intervention. Treatment for addiction and abuse requires long-term counseling and other interventions similar to those for alcohol addiction.

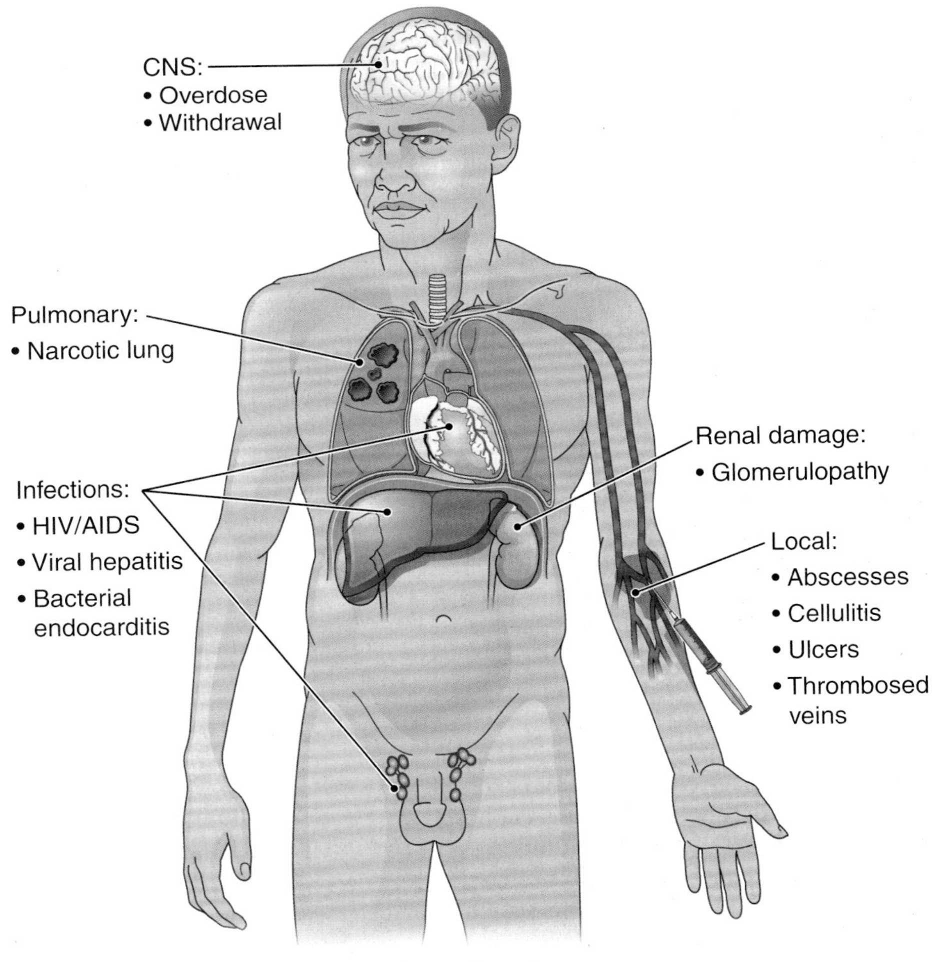

Figure 23.12 **The effects of intravenously injected illegal drugs.** Illegal drugs affect the lungs, kidneys, and brain, cause a variety of infections, and produce local effects such as vein thrombosis and abscess.

Depressants Have a Calming Effect

Depressants have a sedative or calming effect and include *ethanol*, *barbiturates*, and *benzodiazepines*. At low doses, they loosen inhibition, but at high doses, they can produce coma and death by respiratory paralysis. *Barbiturates* are sedatives that relieve anxiety. Barbiturate tolerance develops quickly, and abrupt withdrawal may be accompanied by seizures and death. *Benzodiazepines* are antipsychotic drugs that, when abused, have similar depressive effects.

Stimulants Produce Euphoria

Stimulants enhance one's sense of awareness and produce euphoria. The most popular illegal stimulant drug is **cocaine**. In the US in 2012, 5% of US 12th graders admitted using cocaine at least once, 1% having done so in the last month. The stimulating effects of cocaine are so seductive that it is one of the most addictive and destructive of all illegal drugs. Cocaine produces its euphoria by causing repeated firing of neurons in the brain centers responsible for feelings of pleasure. Cocaine use also stimulates excess peripheral catecholamine production, which causes hypertension, cardiac arrhythmias, and sudden cardiac death. Acute overdose of cocaine can produce seizures and cardiorespiratory arrest. Chronic abuse is also associated with premature atherosclerosis, coronary spasm, heart attack, and stroke. Finally, cocaine use during pregnancy is associated with spontaneous abortion, fetal growth retardation, congenital anomalies, and permanent brain damage.

Amphetamines are widely abused stimulants as well. Overdose produces delirium, convulsions, cardiac arrhythmias, coma, and death. Inappropriate use of attention deficit hyperactivity disorder (ADHD) stimulant (and nonstimulant) prescription drugs is a growing problem, especially among youth.

Narcotics Are Derived from Opium

The word **narcotic** (from Greek *narkosis* = numbing) originally referred to a variety of substances that induce sleep and relieve pain. The federal Drug Enforcement Administration, however, defines *narcotics* as "opioids"—drugs such as morphine that are derived from the opium poppy plant and that bind opiate receptors, as well as synthetic drugs that have a similar morphine-like effect. This can be confusing because cocaine, discussed above, is derived from opium but has a stimulant effect, though it is classified as a narcotic.

The most abused nonprescription narcotic is **heroin**. More powerfully addictive than cocaine, heroin crosses quickly into the brain to produce an intense euphoria followed by sedation. About 2% of young adults report having used heroin at least once, and heroin abuse is in the background of up to 25% of inmates in state and federal prisons. It creates psychological and *physical* addiction associated with an agonizingly painful withdrawal syndrome that can prove fatal. On a case-by-case basis, heroin is more dangerous than cocaine, because heroin is often taken intravenously, and accidental overdose can prove fatal, usually owing to respiratory depression or cardiac arrhythmias. Intravenous use is associated with the constant threat of hepatitis, HIV/AIDS, staphylococcal abscesses, bacterial endocarditis, and other infections. Pulmonary edema and renal disease occur regularly.

In the past decade, abuse of prescription narcotics has surged ahead of heroin abuse. In US in 2011, 2.7% of the population were using prescription pain relievers, sedatives, tranquilizers or stimulants for non-medical purposes. These drugs are legally manufactured and available in limited quantity by prescription to be used for medical treatment; however, they find their way onto the black market, typically via physicians who overprescribe and patients who obtain prescriptions from multiple providers. Moreover, the ready availability of such narcotics—morphine, fentanyl, meperidine (Demerol®), oxycodone (OxyContin®), and others—makes their abuse a particularly common problem among healthcare workers.

Hallucinogens Distort Reality

A **hallucinogen** is a drug that distorts reality or produces altered sensory experiences. Hallucinogens such as mescaline, LSD, and phencyclidine (PCP) are, in general, less physically dangerous than the drugs mentioned above, but their power to distort reality may lead to lethal behavior. **Marijuana** rarely causes hallucinations, but is classified as a hallucinogen. It is the most widely abused of all illegal drugs. Year in and year out, about 15% of teenagers and young adults report marijuana use within the past month. Usage declines to about 5% in older adults. Marijuana is usually smoked and distorts sensory perceptions in a way that users find novel and pleasing. At the same time, it impairs memory, concentration, motor coordination, and problem-solving skills. These effects fade in a few hours. Marijuana smoke contains many of the same toxins and carcinogens as cigarette smoke and chronic use is associated with respiratory damage. Though medical use is a hotly debated topic, there is evidence that marijuana is effective in relieving nausea associated with cancer chemotherapy, relief of chronic pain, and in the treatment of glaucoma (Chapter 20). Indeed, a few states currently permit the use of "medical marijuana" even though use is prohibited by federal law. Experience shows that access is likely to be abused.

Pop Quiz

23.17 True or false? Heroine is the most widely abused narcotic.

23.18 Define drug tolerance.

23.19 Fill in the blank. __________ is an illicit drug that stimulates peripheral catecholamine production, which causes hypertension, cardiac arrhythmias, and sudden cardiac death.

Nutritional Disease

Diet has been alleged to have a role in, or be the salvation for, almost every condition known to humankind. Although many "diet cure" regimens are more imaginary than real, there is no doubt that diet plays an important role in some diseases. The character of diet varies culturally and geographically. A comparison of the typical diet of American and other Western nations to that of Mediterranean nations is a useful example. The Mediterranean diet contains more fresh fruit, vegetables and whole grains, unsaturated vegetable oil, and less refined sugar. To the surprise of most, the Mediterranean diet contains slightly more fat than the American diet; however, the Mediterranean dietary fat is mainly fish and vegetable oils, especially olive oil, which are low in atherosclerosis-inducing saturated fat. In contrast, American dietary fat is high in saturated fat obtained from beef and other animals. The American diet is also high in salt (sodium), a fact linked to the high prevalence of hypertension and the cardiovascular disease that accompanies it. In Mediterranean nations, there are lower rates of both cardiovascular disease and cancer. Nevertheless, it is difficult to prove a *causative* relationship between the precise content of the diet and many of these conditions. For example, people living in Africa eat a diet high in fiber content and have low rates of colon cancer, whereas people living in the United States eat a diet containing relatively little fiber and have a high rate of colon cancer. Even so, studies prove conclusively that low dietary fiber does not *cause* colon cancer.

A useful tool in the evaluation of nutrition is **body mass index (BMI)**, a measure of the ratio of body weight to height as expressed by body weight in kilograms divided by the square of the height in meters. *The Clinical Side*, "Body Mass Index (BMI)," details classification of BMI categories.

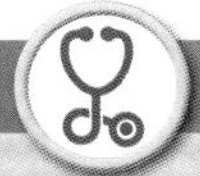

The Clinical Side

BODY MASS INDEX (BMI)

By widely accepted agreement, people are classified as underweight, normal, overweight, or obese according to their BMI, a calculation that relates body weight and height.

The kilograms and meters formula for BMI is:

[weight in kilograms] ÷ [height in meters]^2

The pounds and inches formula is:

[weight in pounds × 704.5] ÷ [height in inches]^2

The BMI for a person 6 feet tall (72 inches), weighing 200 lb is calculated thus:

200 (weight in lb) × 704.5 = 140,900

72 (height in inches) × 72 = 5,184

140,900 ÷ 5,184 = 27.18, which rounds to BMI = 27

The table below displays the prevalence of various BMI categories in the United States according to the most recent U.S. National Health and Nutrition Examination Survey (NHANES III).

Prevalence (%) of Various BMI Groups in the United States (NHANES Study)2008

Category	BMI	Prevalence (%)
Malnutrition	<16	Very low
Underweight	16–18.4	2%
Normal	18.5–24.9	31%
Overweight	25–29.9	33%
Obese	30–39.9	34%*

* Includes 6% with BMI ≥40 who are extremely (morbidly) obese

For example, for a person 5′ 8″ tall:

- 104 lb is malnutrition
- 121 lb is underweight
- 175 lb is overweight
- 198 lb is obese
- 263 lb is morbidly obese

Some athletes are heavy because of large muscle mass, and they have lower body fat than most others with the same BMI.

Undernutrition Is Hazardous

Undernutrition is insufficient dietary intake or intestinal absorption of protein or calories.

In children, definitions vary because malnutrition stunts growth. The *Gomez criteria* for children compare actual weight to predicted normal weight for age. For example, an average three-year-old should weigh 31 lb; 27 lb would be mild malnourishment; 18 lb would be severe. As used here, "undernutrition" does not imply vitamin-mineral deficiency, which will be discussed separately.

Undernutrition can be the result of the following:

- *Eating disorders*, such as *anorexia nervosa* and *bulimia*
- *Poverty*
- *Ignorance*
- *Disease*, such as chronic alcoholism or gastrointestinal malabsorption syndrome

Protein-Energy Malnutrition

Undernutrition is clinically referred to as **protein-energy malnutrition (PEM)**. Children are particularly susceptible to PEM because their growing bodies need an ample supply of calories (energy) and protein. PEM is widespread in poor nations, but not absent in wealthy ones. In any particular individual, the effect may be as devastating as death or as subtle as mildly impaired intelligence.

In addition to calories, the body needs protein to maintain the tissues of its two protein compartments: the somatic compartment, mainly skeletal muscle, and the visceral compartment, mainly the liver. Diets deficient in protein are almost always deficient in calories, and vice versa, so that protein and energy deficiencies usually go hand-in-hand. Deprivation of *both* protein and calories leads to **marasmus**, a widespread condition in some developing nations, especially among refugees from famine or war. Marasmus is characterized by skeletal thinness, particularly in the limbs. Muscles waste away, but the liver and other viscera are initially spared, and the abdomen bulges. Blood albumin remains normal or nearly so. These children also have an aged, wrinkled appearance because their bodies shrivel to the point that their skin no longer "fits."

If the diet contains some calories from carbohydrate but is very low in protein, the child develops **kwashiorkor** (from the Niger-Congo language of Ghana, in West Africa). Kwashiorkor typically develops after children are weaned from breast milk and begin consuming a watery cereal that provides little protein. This form of PEM affects the liver and other viscera (Fig. 23.13). Intestinal villi atrophy and cannot absorb food properly, and the child experiences diarrhea. Blood albumin also falls dramatically. Low albumin causes decreased intravascular osmotic pressure, resulting in extravascular accumulations of fluid as tissue edema and ascites. This accumulation of fluid gives the patient a puffy appearance that can mask underlying skeletal thinness. Hair, composed of keratin, a protein, loses its color and becomes sandy or reddish, and epidermis, also composed partially of keratin, develops splotches of white depigmentation and other skin disease. The typical clinical picture of kwashiorkor is a toddler near death with a potbelly, puffy face, red or sandy discolored hair, skin lesions, thin arms and legs, and swollen feet.

Therapy is refeeding, usually oral. Children may need to be refed slowly to avoid diarrhea.

Cachexia (Fig. 23.14) is a variety of PEM that occurs as a complication of patients with certain types of advanced cancer or AIDS. It occurs in about half of patients with advanced lung, pancreatic, or gastrointestinal cancer. Clinical findings include severe wasting, anemia, anorexia, and edema. The cause is thought to be a cytokine called *tumor necrosis factor (TNF)* and possibly other tumor-produced factors as well. Cachexia accounts for about one-third of deaths in patients with advanced cancer.

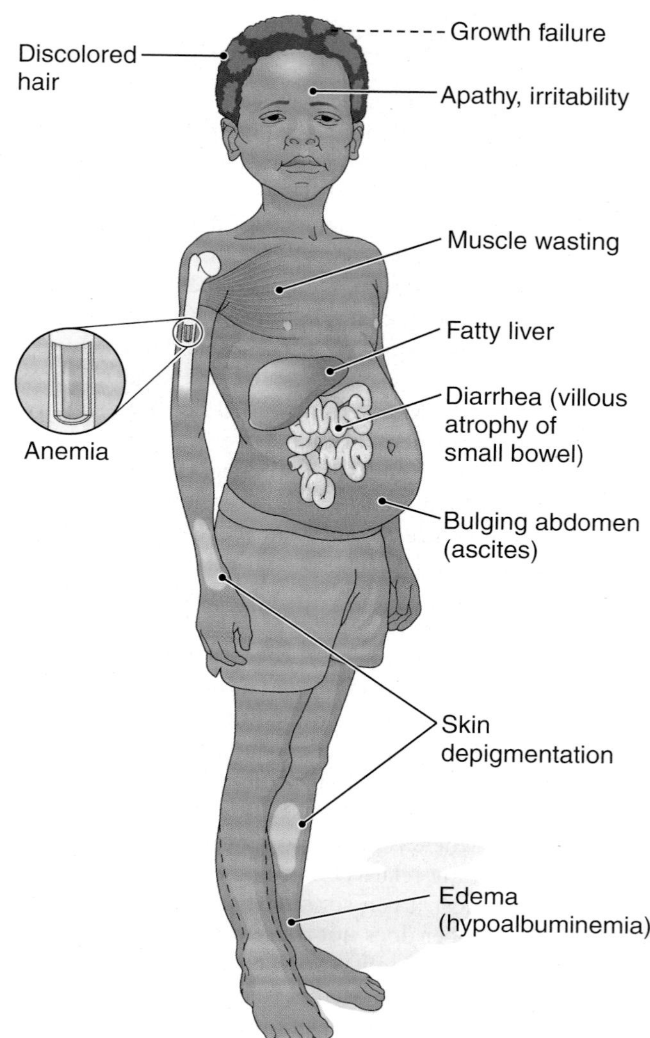

Figure 23.13 **Kwashiorkor.**

Eating Disorders

Anorexia nervosa is self-induced starvation and weight loss, which usually occurs in young women who become obsessed with an unreasonably thin self-image; indeed, much of their behavior (e.g., strict willingness to eat only a limited amount of certain foods, occasional binging, bulimia and purging) is obsessive-compulsive.

Anorexia nervosa is the most fatal of psychiatric disorders, more so than depression. The cause is unknown, but psychosocial factors are thought to play an important role. The clinical picture is similar to severe PEM. Endocrine effects are most severe, and amenorrhea is nearly universal. Anemia and impaired immune function are common. Thyroid hormone secretion falls and accounts for slowed heart rate, constipation, and dry skin. Dehydration and electrolyte imbalance account for cardiac arrhythmias, some of which may be fatal.

Patients with **bulimia** are usually young women who regularly engage in binge overeating and then purge themselves by induced vomiting. PEM is usually not part of the picture. Amenorrhea occurs in about half of these women, but other endocrine and immune functions are not often affected. Nevertheless, there are serious hazards.

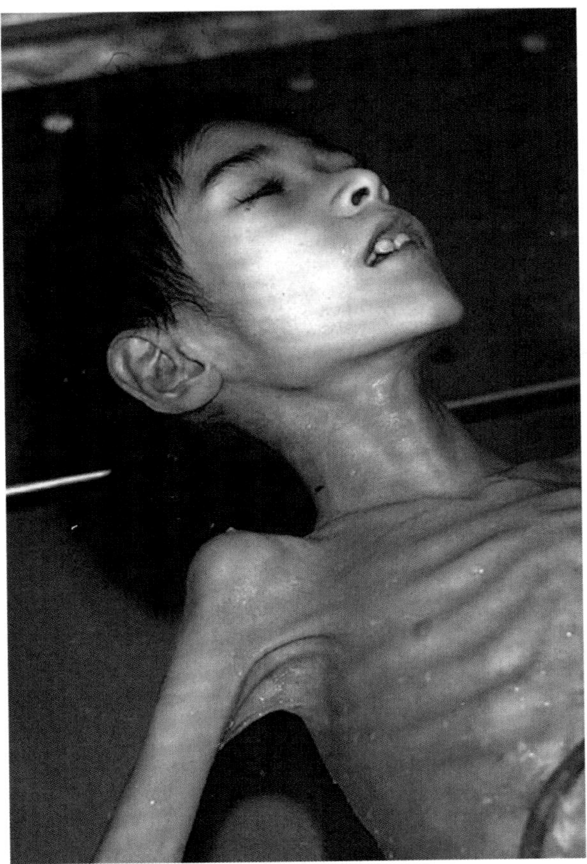

Figure 23.14 **Cachexia.** This patient died of pancreatic cancer. The wasting away is not entirely a matter of lost appetite.

Electrolyte imbalance may cause hypokalemia, cardiac arrhythmia, and death. Vomitus may be aspirated into the lungs, resulting in pneumonia or abscess, and tears of the stomach or esophagus may cause severe hemorrhage or infection.

Treatment of eating disorders is difficult and may involve hospitalization, long-term counseling, drugs, and group therapy.

Vitamin and Trace Mineral Deficiency and Toxicity

Vitamins are organic substances essential in minute amounts for every aspect of human physiology. With the exceptions of vitamins D and K, vitamins are not synthesized by the body and must be obtained through a person's diet: Vitamin D is synthesized in skin upon exposure to sunlight, and intestinal bacteria synthesize vitamin K. An adequate dietary supply of all vitamins is necessary for good health.

Four vitamins (A, D, E, and K) are *fat soluble*; vitamin C, the B vitamins, niacin and folate are *water soluble*. The distinction is important. Fat-soluble vitamins are carried into the body in dietary fat and are stored in body fat. This means that they can become depleted in intestinal fat malabsorption syndromes. In healthy people, fat stores of these vitamins means that they are less likely to become depleted by short-term inadequate intake. The concern then becomes vitamin toxicity, because fat solubility makes it easier for the body to accumulate a toxic amount. By contrast, excess amounts of the water-soluble vitamins are quickly excreted in stool or urine, so toxicity is not typically a concern, but deficiency is more common. The exception is vitamin B_{12}, for which deficiency is rare because it is stored in the liver in large amounts.

Remember This! With the exception of vitamin B_{12}, deficiencies of water-soluble vitamins can develop after a few months of poor nutrition. Deficiencies of fat-soluble vitamins take more than one year to develop because of body fat stores.

In developed countries, deficiencies result mainly from poverty, food faddism, alcoholism, drug abuse, or long-term intravenous (parenteral) feeding. Mild vitamin deficiency also goes hand-in-hand with PEM in the institutionalized elderly. For pregnant women, children who are picky eaters, and older adults on a limited income, diet alone may not provide adequate amounts of some vitamins, and a daily multivitamin supplement may be recommended. In developing nations, deficiency usually occurs in conjunction with malnutrition.

Vitamin deficiency syndromes are too numerous to be discussed fully here. Among the more important syndromes are folic acid deficiency, which can cause neural tube defects in developing fetus (Chapter 22), the anemia of B_{12} deficiency (Chapter 7), the coagulation defect and bleeding tendency of vitamin K deficiency (Chapter 6), and the bony deformities of *rickets*, a syndrome of vitamin D deficiency in children (Chapter 18).

Historically important, but now uncommon, deficiencies are *scurvy* (vitamin C deficiency) and *beriberi* (thiamine, or vitamin B_1, deficiency). Both plagued sailors on long voyages.

- Vitamin C deficiency was determined to be due to lack of fresh fruits and vegetables. Symptoms include depression, fatigue, gingivitis, petechiae, rash, intestinal bleeding, and impaired wound healing. In children, bone growth may be impaired. Diagnosis is clinical. Treatment consists of oral vitamin C.
- Beriberi was found to be due to thiamine deficiency owing to a narrow diet of polished rice without other foods. Nowadays, it may be found in some developing nations, but rarely occurs in developed nations except in chronic alcoholics—about one-fourth of chronic alcoholics admitted to hospitals are thiamine deficient. Diagnosis is clinical. Treatment is oral thiamine.

Again, vitamin toxicity can occur, but it is almost always associated not with foods, but with supplements.

Despite lack of reputable scientific proof of any benefit, many people take megadoses of vitamin supplements. Toxicity from chronic overdoses of vitamin A can be fatal. Vitamin D toxicity causes hypercalcemia, as too much calcium is pulled from bone. Excessive vitamin B_6 supplementation can lead to neurological impairment, and niacin toxicity can damage the liver. Vitamin C toxicity can cause nausea and diarrhea.

Trace minerals are elements —chromium, copper, fluoride, iodine, iron, manganese, selenium, and zinc—that account for a tiny fraction of body weight but have an outsize role in metabolism. By far, the most common *deficiency* is iron deficiency, a common cause of anemia discussed in Chapter 7. Iodine deficiency can cause hypothyroidism (Chapter 14). Though hypothyroidism is a common ailment, in developed nations few cases are due to iodine deficiency because of supplemental iodine added to table salt. Deficiencies of other trace minerals are exceptionally rare and usually due to unusual circumstances.

With the exception of iron, trace metal *toxicity* is uncommon. Some cases are due to environmental (mainly industrial) exposures or accidents; others owe to dietary supplement excesses. Iron toxicity is the most common (see above).

Obesity Is Excess Body Fat

Obesity is excess body fat. It is a psychological and physical burden. The physical consequences depend on the amount of fat and its location: abdominal obesity is especially harmful. Complications are numerous, especially cancer, stroke, coronary artery disease, hypertension, and diabetes.

Remember This! One in every eight deaths in the United States is caused by an illness directly related to overweight and obesity.

As the *History of Medicine*, "French Food, Fast Food, Fat Food," relates, obesity was rare anywhere in the world until about 200 years ago. As recently as 1980, only 5% of children and teenagers were obese; by 2010, 17% were. In the United States, the prevalence of obesity in adults was 13% in 1960; in 2010, it was 33%.

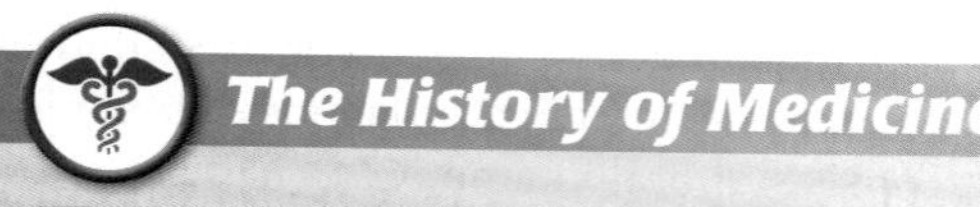

FRENCH FOOD, FAST FOOD, FAT FOOD

For most of human history, the average person ate to satisfy hunger; eating for pleasure was unknown except to kings, queens, and tyrants, among whom obesity occurred because only they could afford cooks and inventories of food. The average person's meal was simple and was determined more by availability than choice. Travelers staying overnight at an inn could obtain drink, but food was only what the innkeeper was having for supper—if there was some to spare. There was no such thing as a restaurant (as we know it) until 1765 in Paris, when Monsieur A. Boulanger opened a business that was not an inn but specialized in prepared food. Thinking to trade on the idea of food as a cure (like chicken soup for a cold), the sign above the door said "Restaurants," French for "restoratives." Politics, however, made his experiment short lived and thus, the first-ever restaurant, was closed.

In 1782, the first truly luxury restaurant was opened in Paris, but the idea of restaurants did not really catch on until 1789, when the French Revolution destroyed French royalty and nobility and emptied kitchens of hundreds of chefs, many of whom opened places to eat, which they also called "restaurants." Monsieur Boulanger was among them, and his restaurant became the first to offer a menu with a choice of dishes. By 1804, Paris had more than 500 restaurants, and the concept swept the world.

Restaurants were slow to come to America. The first true American luxury restaurant was Delmonico's, which opened in 1827 in New York City. Americans, however, always wanting more of everything faster and cheaper, soon invented fast food. Some food historians consider that the first fast-food restaurant was established in 1891 when the YWCA of Kansas City, Missouri, established a cafeteria—a place where prepared food was set on display and sold by the dish. Others suggest that fast food had its origins in San Francisco in 1849 during the California gold rush, when prepared food was set out on open-air tables and sold by the dish to the "forty-niners" who flocked to California to make their fortune.

With the coming of the automobile in the early 1900s, restaurants began to serve patrons in their cars. After World War II, with the development of the American interstate highway system and the idea of franchising pioneered by the Holiday Inn motel chain, "fast-food" restaurants spread across America. McDonald's began in 1955, Kentucky Fried Chicken in 1956, and Pizza Hut in 1958; each followed the burgeoning interstate highway system.

About the same time, the U.S. government began to subsidize corn production, which brought down the cost of processed food. All of these developments—cheap corn sugar, standard quality, and easy access—made "fast-food" calories cheap and readily available.

In 1950, there was no state in the United States with *more* than 10% of the population overweight. By the year 2000, a mere 50 years later, there was no state with *less* than 60% of the population overweight: an entire nation became fat in 50 years.

Defining Obesity

To identify obesity with scientific rigor requires body composition analysis, which is cumbersome and expensive. Nevertheless, because excess fat is responsible for weight gain in most people, a very good substitute for body fat measurements is BMI: a BMI of 30 or greater constitutes obesity. *Morbid obesity*, which dramatically increases the risk for severe health problems, is a BMI of 40 or greater.

Abdominal obesity can occur in people who are overweight but not clinically obese. It is defined as a man with a 40" waist or a woman with a 35" waist. Waist size is properly measured horizontally, across the fat part of the belly, not below it. The majority of American adults over age 55, regardless of race, exceed these measurements; that is to say, the average American over age 55 is centrally obese.

Case Notes

23.10 Does Marvin have abdominal obesity?

Factors Contributing to Obesity

The risk for obesity increases with age: roughly twice as many adults are obese as teenagers. Genetics is also important: about two-thirds of children of obese parents will be obese. Among identical twins reared separately, if one is obese, the other very likely is, too. African Americans are more likely to be obese (44%) than whites (32%).

Nongenetic factors also play a role: low-income Americans, for example, are more likely to be obese than affluent Americans. In addition, although regulation of body weight is exceptionally complex and not thoroughly understood, multiple hormones have been identified as playing a role in body weight and fat deposition. These hormones work in homeostatic fashion with the autonomic nervous system to maintain body weight and fat content at a "set point." It is difficult to reset: dieters can lose weight but >90% of them regain their weight because the set point remains unchanged.

Consequences of Obesity

Being obese is bad for health (Table 23.2). As a result of housing and job discrimination, poor body image, and low self-esteem, obese people are at greater risk for social, economic, and psychological problems, including diagnosed mental illness. For example, obese people are more often poor and less likely to be employed. What's more, the ill effects of obesity are pervasive and appear in unexpected ways. Obese people are more prone to home accidents because they are less fit and unable to manage their bulk; on average, they are twice as likely to suffer from hearing loss, poor eyesight, and mobility disorders of the arms or legs.

The physical consequences of obesity are the following:

- *Insulin resistance and Type II diabetes.* Weight loss is effective treatment.
- *Hypertension.* Though the mechanisms are not clear, obesity and hypertension go hand in hand. Weight loss lowers blood pressure.
- *Dyslipidemia.* Obesity is associated with low blood HDL cholesterol and high triglyceride; both are risk factors in coronary artery disease.
- *Fatty liver.* Excess liver fat is toxic and may lead to cirrhosis.
- *Gallstones.* Obese people are six times more likely to develop gallstones.
- *Hypoventilation.* The bulge of abdominal fat and the thick pelt of fat on the chest and breasts limit ventilation. Chronic hypoxia causes vasoconstriction in the systemic and pulmonary circulation, causing high blood pressure, pulmonary hypertension, and right heart failure.
- *Osteoarthritis.* Joints bearing the excess weight wear out.
- *Cancer.* In men, obesity is strongly associated with increased risk for cancers of the esophagus, thyroid, colon, and, kidney. In women, the risk is for cancer of the endometrium, gallbladder, and kidney.

Case Notes

23.11 List Marvin's conditions related to his obesity.

Abdominal (central) obesity, a "beer gut" in American slang, is especially perilous, as is indicated in the discussion below of *metabolic syndrome*. Abdominal obesity is not

Table 23.2 *Relative Risk for Cancer, Cardiovascular Disease, and Diabetes in People with Various Body Mass Indices (BMI)*

Body Mass Index Classification	Weight of a Person 5′ 8″ tall (lb)	Increased Cancer Risk	Increased Cardiovascular Risk	Increased Diabetes Risk
18.5–24.9 Normal	122–164	None	None	None
25–29.9 Overweight	165–196	10%	20%	100%
30–40 Obese	197–263	30%	90%	250%
≥ 40 Morbidly obese	>263	70%	140%	550%

merely a convenient measure. Large abdominal girth caused by abdominal fat is much more of a health hazard than is the same amount of extra fat stored elsewhere. Apart from other risk factors, waist size is an independent risk factor for Type II diabetes, hypertension, coronary artery disease, gallstones, stroke, cancer (especially of the endometrium and breast), pulmonary disease, and osteoarthritis.

Morbidly obese patients are even more vulnerable to health problems than are those who are merely obese. Morbidly obese patients are especially at increased risk for the following:

- Obstructive sleep apnea and chronic hypoventilation, which is associated with hypoxia and CO_2 retention
- Pulmonary hypertension and right heart failure (cor pulmonale)
- Esophageal reflux
- Urinary incontinence
- Irregular menses and infertility
- Osteoarthritis

The morbidly obese can suffer from **fatty heart syndrome**, a condition in which heart muscle accumulates fat and loses contractile power. Heart failure and other problems may result.

Case Notes

23.12 Calculate Marvin's BMI. Is he morbidly obese?

The Metabolic Syndrome Conveys Grave Cardiovascular Risk

Obese persons may develop **metabolic syndrome**. Definitions vary slightly; Figure 23.15 outlines a widely accepted one. It is important to note that, while most patients with metabolic syndrome are obese, elevated BMI is not a necessary requirement for the diagnosis—waist size is a key measure. Nevertheless, one-fourth of obese people have metabolic syndrome.

Individuals with metabolic syndrome typically eat a high carbohydrate diet and have a sedentary lifestyle. Exact criteria vary for diagnosis. A commonly accepted requirement for a diagnosis of metabolic syndrome is the presence of at least three of the following:

- *Abdominal obesity:* waist measurement 40" or more in men, 35" or more in women

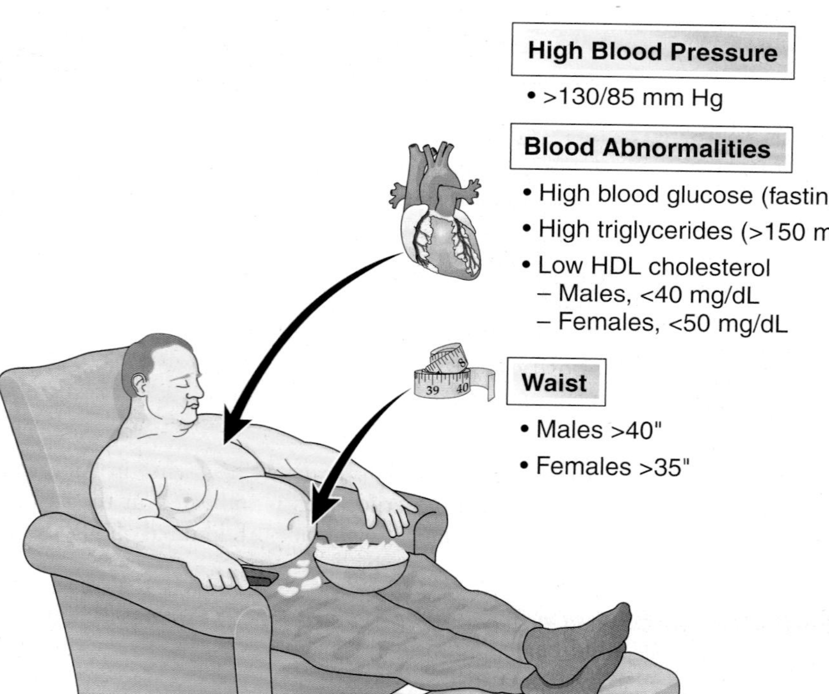

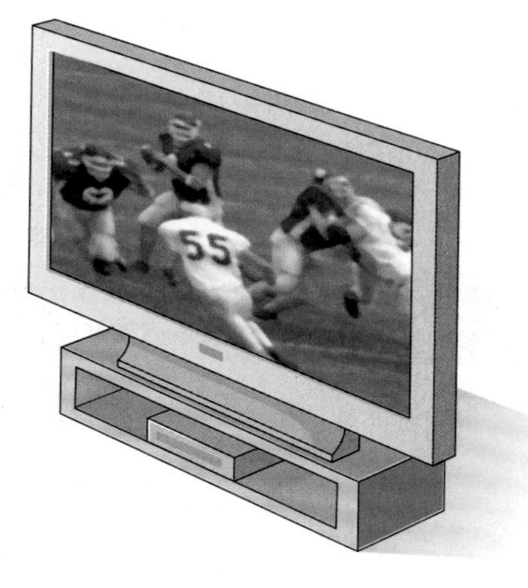

Figure 23.15 **The metabolic syndrome.** As the figure illustrates, people with this syndrome typically have abdominal obesity, do not get enough exercise, and eat a high carbohydrate diet. They are at grave risk for cardiovascular disease.

- *Abnormal glucose metabolism:* fasting blood glucose level >100 mg/dL
- *Abnormal plasma lipids (dyslipidemia)*: triglyceride level >150 mg/dL; or HDL cholesterol <40 mg/dL in men, or <50 mg/dL in women
- *Hypertension:* blood pressure > 130/85 mm Hg

About 70% of patients with Type II diabetes and 40% of patients with abnormal glucose metabolism (but who are not frankly diabetic) have metabolic syndrome.

There is a distinct genetic tendency to develop metabolic syndrome. In the United States, Hispanics and Americans Indians are especially vulnerable.

Metabolic syndrome is associated with grave cardiovascular risk. For example, compared to people with no metabolic syndrome factors, patients with two of the required diagnostic factors in the list above are twice as likely to die of coronary artery disease; patients with three factors are three-and-a-half times more likely to die of coronary artery disease.

Weight loss and exercise reduce the risk dramatically. Exercise alone (without weight loss) reduces risk significantly, but not to the level of nonobese patients.

Case Notes

23.13 Does Marvin suffer from metabolic syndrome?

Pop Quiz

23.20 True or false? Water-soluble vitamins are most commonly responsible for vitamin toxicity.

23.21 True or false? Abdominal girth is a health risk factor independent of weight.

23.22 Fill in the blank. __________ is a deficiency of both protein and calories, characterized by thinness, muscle wasting, normal blood albumin, and wrinkled skin.

23.23 Metabolic syndrome is characterized by the presence of which factors (name at least three)?

Case Study Revisited

"I think he's having a heart attack." The case of Marvin B.

Among healthcare professionals, cases like Marvin B. are sometimes referred to as "a heart attack waiting to happen." His is a cautionary tale about the ill effects of personal habits.

We know he had "been smoking since he was a teenager," or at least 40 years, more than enough time for the damaging effects of tobacco smoke to work their trouble. He had severe generalized and coronary atherosclerosis, and he died of an acute myocardial infarct. Smoking also accounted for the chronic pulmonary disease and precancerous dysplasia found in his bronchial tree, never mind the increased cancer and cardiovascular risk associated with obesity.

Alcohol abuse added to his problems. Although moderate alcohol use is protective, abuse is associated with increased cardiovascular risk. Alcohol abuse had ruined his marriage, may have been about to cost him his job, and had given him severe alcoholic liver disease that, had he survived a few more years, could have progressed to cirrhosis and liver cancer. Though the autopsy does not mention examination of the mouth, throat, and tongue, it would be no surprise had an exam found dysplasia or cancer: tobacco use and alcohol abuse combined create great risk for oropharyngeal and esophageal cancer.

Piled on top of this was obesity, and not just mere obesity, but morbid obesity with abdominal obesity, each a risk factor. Obesity is a strong risk factor for diabetes, itself an independent risk factor for cardiovascular disease. That he was morbidly obese added even more difficulty. It easily explains the problems he had with his knees. Had X-ray images been available, they surely would have shown osteoarthritis from the crushing effect of his bulk. Though we do not know from the history whether or not he suffered hypoventilation and sleep apnea, the autopsy finding of right ventricular hypertrophy suggests that he was hypoventilating and probably had pulmonary hypertension. Smoking compounded the problem.

Marvin's profile fits metabolic syndrome, a particularly toxic combination of abnormalities with great risk for cardiovascular disease. Finally, he had severe arteriolar nephrosclerosis, a fingerprint of hypertension. Smoking and obesity, especially morbid obesity, are strongly linked to hypertension.

Chapter Challenge

CHAPTER RECALL

1. A 15-year-old Caucasian female presents to the emergency room complaining of abdominal pain, nausea and vomiting, dizziness, and ringing in her ears. Her physical exam is significant for hyperventilation only. What toxic exposure has most likely caused her symptoms?
   A. Acetaminophen
   B. Aspirin
   C. CO
   D. Lead

2. Which of the following organs is most affected by exposure to radiation?
   A. Heart
   B. Brain
   C. Intestine
   D. Skin

3. While on a medical mission trip, you evaluate a six-year-old African boy who presents to the clinic with a large goiter, fatigue, low body temperature, and mental retardation. You correctly diagnose his disorder, which is uncommon in developed nations due to a salt additive. Deficiency of what trace element has caused this child's symptoms?
   A. Iron deficiency
   B. Selenium deficiency
   C. Zinc deficiency
   D. Iodine deficiency

4. A 17-year-old Hispanic male is brought to the ER in custody. Police picked him up after they found him staggering down the sidewalk. He is laughing uncontrollably throughout the exam and demonstrates impaired memory and coordination. His other symptoms include sensory distortion and increased appetite. He is likely suffering from intoxication of which drug?
   A. Marijuana
   B. Barbiturates
   C. Alcohol
   D. Opioid

5. Intravenous drug abuse predisposes to which of the following?
   A. Hepatitis C virus (HCV)
   B. Lung scarring
   C. Bacterial endocarditis
   D. All of the above

6. A 63-year-old African American male presents to the clinic for a physical. His past medical history is significant for morbid obesity, hypertension, hyperlipidemia, and diabetes. He admits to smoking a pack a day, being a couch potato, and drinking two six-packs of beer per week. Which of his habits is arguably the most detrimental to his overall health?
   A. Alcohol abuse
   B. Cigarette smoking
   C. Fast food
   D. Not getting enough exercise

7. A 54-year-old Caucasian male is brought to the clinic by his wife for evaluation. While you are interviewing him in the presence of his wife, he repeats comments and questions several times. He also answers questions regarding daily activities with long rambling stories that his wife reports are untrue. You recognize the symptoms of Korsakoff psychosis due to chronic alcoholism. Which of the following vitamin deficiencies is responsible for the patient's findings?
   A. Vitamin B_1 deficiency
   B. Vitamin A deficiency
   C. Vitamin B_{12} deficiency
   D. Vitamin E deficiency

8. A 40-year-old Hispanic female presents to your clinic for assistance in smoking cessation. She reports that she has tried to quit several times but each time she resumes smoking again a few weeks later. Which compound is responsible for her addiction?
   A. Tobacco tar
   B. Phenol
   C. Nicotine
   D. Formaldehyde

9. A 32-year-old Hispanic male farmer is brought to the ER. His physical exam is positive for sweating, constricted pupils, salivation, fasciculation, and a flaccid paralysis. These symptoms are hallmark for which toxin exposure?
   A. Mercury
   B. Silica
   C. Organophosphate
   D. Volatile organics

10. A 25-year-old African American female marathon runner presents to the clinic with nausea, vomiting, and abdominal pain. She reports a normal "healthy" diet with several daily vitamin supplements. Her labs reveal elevated blood calcium, likely caused by ________________ toxicity.
    A. Vitamin A
    B. Vitamin E
    C. Vitamin C
    D. Vitamin D

11. True or false? Acetaminophen is the most common cause of acute liver failure.

12. True or false? Alcohol consumption in moderation has no positive effects on health.

13. True or false? Metabolic syndrome is characterized by abdominal obesity (>40 in), abnormal glucose metabolism (fasting glucose >100 mg/dL), abnormal plasma lipids (high triglycerides or low HDL), and hypertension (BP >130/85 mm Hg).

14. True or false? Cocaine produces both euphoria and sedation.

15. True or false? Patients with bulimia are usually young women who regularly binge and purge.

16. Matching: hot/cold/burn
    i. first-degree burns
    ii. second-degree burns
    iii. third-degree burns
    iv. Electrical burns
    v. Frostnip
    vi. Frostbite
    vii. Hypothermia
    viii. Heat cramps
    ix. Heat exhaustion
    x. Heat stroke
    A. Dry painful burns of the epidermis that are red and blanche with pressure
    B. Temperature >104°F, altered mental status, absence of sweating, flushed skin, headache, nausea/vomiting, rapid respirations and pulse, muscle weakness or rigidity, and loss of consciousness
    C. Burns extending completely through the dermis with charred, translucent skin and coagulated vessels (painless except at the edges; healing with scarring) (Skin may be charred or translucent, with coagulated vessels visible through it.)
    D. Superficial skin freezing, with firm white patches, resulting in mottled red, yellow, or blue splotches that peel or blister on rewarming
    E. Burns extending into the dermis characterized by blisters (nonblanching, red, wet, and painful)
    F. Cold injury to dermis or deeper with hard white areas lacking feeling (bullae form: when warmed, the lesion becomes swollen, red, blistered, and painful)
    G. Spasms of voluntary muscle caused by electrolyte loss
    H. Profuse sweating and sudden weakness and disorientation with a body temperature that may rise to near 102°F
    I. Muscle spasms that may produce involuntary grasping
    J. A slowing of all physiologic functions characterized by lethargy, clumsiness, confusion, hallucinations, and slow respiratory and heart rate

CONCEPTUAL UNDERSTANDING

17. Using examples from the text, discuss the primary causes of death and disease in children. How does this differ from the primary causes of death and disease in adults?

18. Compare and contrast kwashiorkor and marasmus.

19. Briefly explain the costs and benefits of therapeutic drugs.

APPLICATION

20. An intravenous drug abuser presents to the clinic with shortness of breath. He admits to abusing heroin; however, he has no signs of intoxication at this time. He says that his shortness of breath has been going on for a long time. He denies being a cigarette smoker. The physicians are concerned about a chronic lung disease. A lung biopsy is performed which shows inflammation and scarring in the lung tissue, with refractile angulated material trapped in small blood vessels. A polarizing filter placed on the microscope shows that fragments of the material are polarizable. What is the likely source and nature of material, and why is it found in the lungs?

21. A patient brought in to the ER is barely breathing. A new intern takes one look at the patient and diagnoses him with alcohol intoxication. You, however, observe track marks along the patient's arm. What alternative diagnosis is possible? Why is it important to distinguish between the two?

22. What are some ways for healthcare workers to do a better job of reducing death and disease and promoting health?

CHAPTER

24

Aging, Stress, Exercise, and Pain

Contents

Chapter Objectives

After studying this chapter, you should be able to complete the following tasks:

AGING AND THE DECLINE OF BODY FUNCTIONS

1. Explain the role of telomere length, reactive oxygen species (free radicals), environmental toxins, and apoptosis in cellular aging.
2. Compare the form and function of different body systems between young and older adults.

STRESS

3. Describe the three phases of the stress response.
4. Compare and contrast the effects of cortisol and the sympathetic nervous system during the stress response.
5. Describe the deleterious effects that occur with stress exhaustion.
6. List some stress-related diseases and disorders affecting different body systems.

EXERCISE

7. Explain how exercise training improves the functioning of different body systems.
8. Identify the three main types of sports injuries, and be able to give examples of each.
9. Describe the effects of immobility of different body systems.

PAIN

10. Understand the subjective nature of pain and be able to describe types of pain.

Case Study

"She thought it was a wasp." A Multigenerational Family Goes Hiking.

To celebrate his 71st birthday, Tom treated his children and grandchildren to a family vacation at a mountain dude ranch. After a picnic lunch, he decided to take his granddaughter Kate, 7, and her mother, Lea, 38, on a hike up to a nearby mountain meadow to see the wildflowers.

"There won't be any yellow jackets, will there, Mommy?" Kate asked.

"No," Lea said. "Wasps don't live this high up in the mountains." To her dad she added, "A yellow jacket stung her last week."

As the trail led upward, Kate scampered ahead, while Tom and Lea lagged behind. Soon Tom became short of breath, his respirations deep and fast. He said to Lea, "Let's take a little break. There was a time I could have done this all day, but not any more."

Lea called for Kate, who frolicked back with a smile and no noticeable shortness of breath.

"Look at her, Dad. She doesn't even know it's 10,000 feet," Lea said. "I think of myself as fit, but even I'm a bit winded at this altitude."

After a quick gulp of water, Kate began tugging Lea ahead to the meadow. Soon they had disappeared over the next rise, leaving behind Tom, who had to take frequent stops to catch his breath. Despite a regular exercise regime incorporating weights, he was finding the climb difficult.

Upon reaching the meadow, Lea enjoyed the view while Kate picked some flowers. The placid scene was broken by a wild shriek from Kate, who began clawing at her hair and screaming about a wasp. Lea rushed to Kate's side and immediately saw a small, yellow butterfly tangled in Kate's long, curly hair. While working to free the insect, she tried to explain to Kate that it was merely a butterfly, but Kate, still clutching a cluster of red wildflowers, was screaming and thrashing so frantically that it was several moments before her mother succeeded. Finally, the butterfly floated away and Lea took Kate in her arms and comforted her.

Meanwhile, Tom had heard the screams and broken into a run. With his first step he twisted an ankle, but rushed on. He quickly found himself at his limit, but fearing that something terrible might have happened to Kate, he pushed until he finally reached the top.

"She's okay, Dad," Lea said. "Poor thing, a butterfly got caught in her hair. She thought it was a wasp. She got so scared I could feel her heart pounding as if it was about to leap out of her chest, and she was breathing harder than you are now."

Tom, still gasping for air, could only nod his head to signal that he understood, and inspect his twisted ankle, which was painful. After a minute of rest he was able to say a few words of comfort to Kate, who had become calmer and was breathing easier, too.

Age is an issue of mind over matter. If you don't mind, it doesn't matter.

ATTRIBUTED VARIOUSLY TO MARK TWAIN, SATCHEL PAIGE, JACK BENNY, AND OTHERS.

Courage is grace under pressure.

ERNEST HEMINGWAY, AMERICAN AUTHOR (1899–1961)

It is exercise alone that supports the spirits, and keeps the mind in vigor.

MARCUS TULLIUS CICERO (106–43 BCE), ROMAN STATESMAN AND PHILOSOPHER

Prior chapters focused on particular systems and diseases, each of which occurs in a person of a particular age, who may or may not be under stress, and who has a certain pattern of physical activity. In this chapter, we turn our attention to aging, stress, exercise, and pain. Previously, we likened our genetic makeup to the soil in which the seed of disease is planted —some soils sprout the weed of disease. Age, stress, and exercise can be soil additives that kill the seed of disease or encourage its growth.

Aging and the Decline of Body Functions

Humans are usually at their physical and intellectual peak in early adulthood. It is not merely a coincidence that competitive athletic records are held almost entirely by youth or young adults. Sexual function in males peaks in the late teens, and fertility in females begins to decline before age 30. In addition, the most brilliant and revolutionary flights of human genius, especially in science and mathematics, have throughout history been the province of young brains: Einstein had his greatest insights in his late 20s, Newton in his late 20s and early 30s, and so on. But if you're over 30, there's no need for dismay: our ability to act thoughtfully and with good judgment improves well into advanced age. Although Alzheimer disease and other forms of dementia rob some people of memory and cognition, many people find emotional fulfillment in the wisdom accumulated in a long life.

As a rule, populations worldwide are growing older. A commonly accepted definition of **old age** is anyone 65 or older. The *young old* are 65–74; *middle old* are 75–84; and *old old* are 85+. In 1900, people over 65 accounted for 4% of the U.S. population. In 2009, that figure was about 13%, and in 20 years it is expected to be over 20%. Caring for the elderly (*geriatrics*) will be an increasingly important part of medicine.

Bear in mind that aging is simply the process of growing older. It's not restricted to the elderly—even infants are aging. Still, after several decades have gone by, the physical and mental limitations associated with advancing years begin to interfere with physical performance and the quality of life. These age-related deteriorations, which are technically known as **senescence**, are associated with the following:

- Reduced *physiologic capacity*. That is, organs and systems no longer function optimally. Muscles contract with less force and ears hear less acutely. Healing is slower.
- Diminished *adaptability*. Older adults cannot easily adjust to environmental changes. For example, reduced ability to control body temperature makes older persons more vulnerable (e.g., temperature) to heatstroke and hypothermia.
- Increased disease *susceptibility*. Illnesses that are minor in younger adults (e.g., a respiratory infection) can be life threatening in the elderly because complications occur with greater frequency and severity.

Remember This! **Senescence differs from aging.**

Case Notes

24.1 What is Tom's old age classification?

24.2 Simply based on their age, who is at greater danger of heatstroke—Tom or Lea?

Declining Endocrine Function Is Responsible for Some Senescence

Central to many age-related deteriorations is the decline of the endocrine system. Growth hormone (GH) secretion, for instance, can be as low in an elderly person as it is in a younger person who is symptomatic from GH deficiency. Decline in the production of sex steroid hormones is also important. In older women, the decline of estrogen can prompt postmenopausal hot flashes and increase the fragility of bones. In men, the decline of testosterone production accounts for increasing abdominal girth due to belly fat deposits, declining sex drive, and loss of muscle mass and strength.

Case Notes

24.3 Could endocrine decline partially explain Tom's loss of muscle mass? Explain.

Senescence Reflects Cellular Changes

An older adult's reduced function reflects cell senescence. There are two interrelated problems with aging tissues and cells. First, cells become damaged and no longer function normally. Second, cells lose the ability to replicate; therefore, damaged cells are not replaced as readily. For example, hair cells in the inner ear convert sound vibrations into nerve impulses. Their senescence is one cause of hearing loss.

Cellular Damage

Scientists now agree that aging is the result of accumulating damage to the molecules that make up our cells (especially proteins, lipids, and nucleic acids), and certain genetic programs (apoptosis and telomeres, discussed later). As molecules are damaged, cell function becomes less robust. As cell function declines, our tissues and organs do not perform as well, and soon our health begins to deteriorate. Moreover, DNA damage causes DNA mutations, and mutations in key genes may result in cancer or impaired cell function. But what causes the damage? As discussed in Chapter 23, tobacco smoke tops the list. Although cigarettes and other environmental villains are obvious candidates, equally important are the adverse consequences of normal cellular processes and everyday necessities such as oxygen.

Reactive Oxygen Species

Without oxygen we die quickly. There is, however, the other side of the coin: the metabolic reactions necessary for life also produce **reactive oxygen species (ROS)**, molecules containing an oxygen atom with an unpaired electron. Examples include superoxide (O_2^-), the hydroxyl radical (OH^-), and hydrogen peroxide (H_2O_2).

ROS are a type of **free radical**—a general term describing any molecule or atom with an unpaired electron. Free radicals are unstable: they need another electron to make a stable pair. When an electron is removed from a molecule, the molecule is said to be *oxidized*. Free radicals, therefore, are *oxidants* and can oxidize and damage important biomolecules like DNA, proteins, and lipids, causing them to stop performing their normal function.

ROS are a natural part of body chemistry and play a role in certain enzymatic reactions. If uncontrolled, however, they can cause considerable damage. For example, when ROS damage DNA, the DNA accumulates mutations that can lead to the development of cancer.

Cells control ROS production and action by the use of natural **antioxidants**, which include compounds such as vitamins C and E. Because there is evidence that excess free radicals damage cells, it is natural to think that increasing our antioxidant defenses can help humans live longer. For example, science has proven that fruit flies genetically engineered to clear away free radicals live 50% longer than normal fruit flies. *But do antioxidants delay aging and prevent human disease?* We don't know for sure. Someday, an antioxidant strategy might be developed that prolongs life and reduces the prevalence of chronic diseases, but currently, no such magic elixir exists. Still, many researchers advise consuming at least five servings of antioxidant-rich fresh fruits and vegetables daily. In contrast, antioxidant supplements may paradoxically promote oxidation and are not recommended.

Case Notes

24.4 Whose DNA is more likely damaged by free radicals: Tom's or Lea's?

Telomere Length Limits Cell Replacement

Cells with damaged molecules frequently stop dividing. Nevertheless, even undamaged old cells eventually lose their ability to reproduce. The key to this behavior is a structure at the end of each chromosome—the **telomere**, a region of DNA that loses a few nitrogenous bases with every cell division. It appears that when a cell runs out of telomere, it "retires." After cells divide about 50 times, they quit the hard work of dividing and leave the task to other cells. Of course, organs with many retired cells don't function as well as others. Proof of this point is that our organs shrink as we age. Compared to a healthy young adult, a late adult brain is 5–15% smaller, the liver weighs 35% less, and the respiratory capacity of the lungs is about 50% less.

Case Notes

24.5 Tom's chromosomes are minutely smaller than Kate's chromosomes. Why?

Abnormal Apoptosis Hastens Aging

Recall that cells have a natural life span, and after living out their life of a few days, a few months, or a human lifetime, they die by "natural suicide" in a carefully regulated, orderly process called **apoptosis**. Science now has evidence that some degenerative diseases, especially Alzheimer disease and other diseases of the nervous system, are caused by excessive apoptosis. Therefore, in a sense, Alzheimer can be considered abnormally rapid aging of the brain.

Progerias Are Disorders of Accelerated Aging

Proof that DNA and telomeres are important for aging is provided by the *progerias*, a family of genetic diseases associated with premature aging (Fig. 24.1). In the severest type, children begin to lose their hair as early as age 12 months and tend to develop the adult form of diabetes (Type II) during early childhood. The average life expectancy of these children is about age 13, though some live to be 19 or 20. Most die as a result of cardiovascular disease.

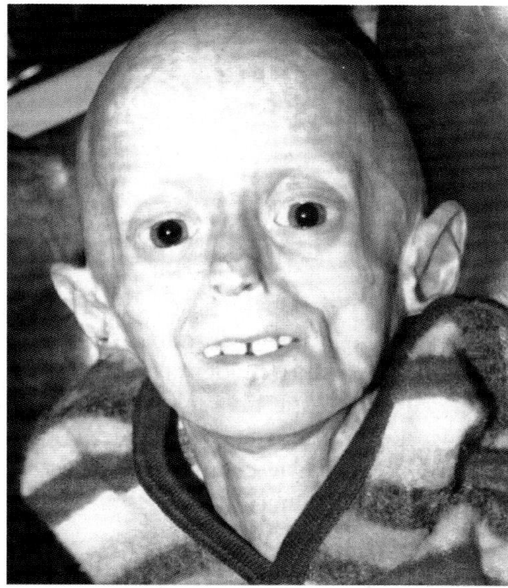

Figure 24.1 **Progeria.** This 10-year-old girl shows the typical signs of premature aging associated with progeria, such as hair loss; thin, wrinkled skin; and the loss of subcutaneous adipose tissue. (Reproduced with permission from Rubin R, Strayer DS. *Rubin's Pathology: Clinicopathologic Foundations of Medicine*. 5th ed. Philadelphia, PA: Lippincott Williams & Wilkins; 2008.)

Werner syndrome is a type of progeria in which patients lack a protein that participates in DNA replication, telomere maintenance, and DNA repair. Without this protein, DNA replication frequently stalls, new cells are not produced to replace retiring ones, and aging accelerates. Because Werner syndrome patients also lack normal DNA repair, mutations go unrepaired and cancers tend to occur. People with Werner syndrome are also prone to cardiovascular disease and diabetes mellitus. They usually die at about age 40.

Remember This! DNA plays a critical role in senescence.

Senescence Affects Every Body System

The age-related decrease in quality of life and increase in death rate reflects changes in every body system. These age-related changes are summarized in Figure 24.2.

Certain conditions are found much more commonly in the elderly:

- Almost exclusively in the elderly:
  - Urinary incontinence
  - Accidental hypothermia
  - Normal pressure hydrocephalus
- Much more common in the elderly:
  - Skin cancers other than malignant melanoma
  - Pressure sores of skin
  - Degenerative arthritis (osteoarthritis)
  - Osteoporosis
  - Hip fracture
  - Falls with injury
  - Multiple myeloma
  - Chronic lymphocytic leukemia
  - Prostate cancer
  - Dementia
  - Parkinson disease
  - Stroke

Skin Changes

Skin changes are the most obvious sign of aging. Hair grays and thins. Gravity tugs relentlessly: buttocks and breasts droop, and skin sags. Skin wrinkles and sags due to loss of subcutaneous fat and elastic fibers that keep it robust and smooth. Aging skin is thinner, more easily wounded, and slower to heal. Accumulated sunlight damage produces wrinkling, mottled pigmentary changes, and skin cancers. The sum is a bonanza for plastic surgeons and cosmetic sales.

Case Notes

24.6 Tom has some dark spots on the back of each hand. What is the likely cause?

Musculoskeletal Changes

Because of decreased estrogen, bone mineral density declines precipitously in many postmenopausal women. In this condition, called *osteoporosis*, bones fracture more easily and the vertebral column may assume an abnormal curvature. An excessive forward thoracic curve, *kyphosis (dowager's hump)*, is especially common. Note that osteoporosis develops in older males, too: by age 70, men have the same rate of bone *loss* as women although on average men's bones remain more robust. Bones must have weight-bearing stress to remain dense and strong. Recalling our case, Tom limits reduction of bone mineral density by regular weight-bearing exercise; however, Tom's bone density is still lower than Lea's or Kate's, rendering him more susceptible to fractures.

Degenerative changes in the joints, called *osteoarthritis*, also limit mobility. A herniated intervertebral disc, especially in the lower back, may press on a spinal nerve, most often resulting in pain or numbness radiating into the leg or foot, or muscle weakness. Flexibility also declines as ligaments become less compliant.

Even with frequent exercise, muscle mass decreases with age. Tom's muscle mass is probably only about half of what it was when he was younger. Since muscle fiber number and size is a determinant of power development, his muscles have also lost strength. To strengthen the muscles he relies on to recover from missteps, Tom's trainer regularly includes exercises that require balancing.

Case Notes

24.7 Is it likely that Tom's bone density is lower than Kate's?

Cardiovascular Changes

Cardiovascular performance declines as we advance into adulthood. Maximum heart rate, a reliable measure of capacity, declines. The maximum expected rate is roughly 220 minus the person's age in years. That is, someone 30 years old can reach about 190 beats/min and someone 70 years old can reach about 150. Cardiac output is limited by the decreasing size and number of cardiac muscle cells, which are permanent cells and cannot be replaced as they die. Cardiac output also may be limited by coronary artery disease.

Hypertension is very common in the elderly. Nevertheless, the main change is atherosclerosis, which leads especially to myocardial infarcts, stroke, kidney disease, and vascular insufficiency of the lower limbs.

Respiratory Changes

Respiratory capacity declines with age and may further limit cardiorespiratory performance. The average 70-year-old has 30–40% less vital capacity than at his or

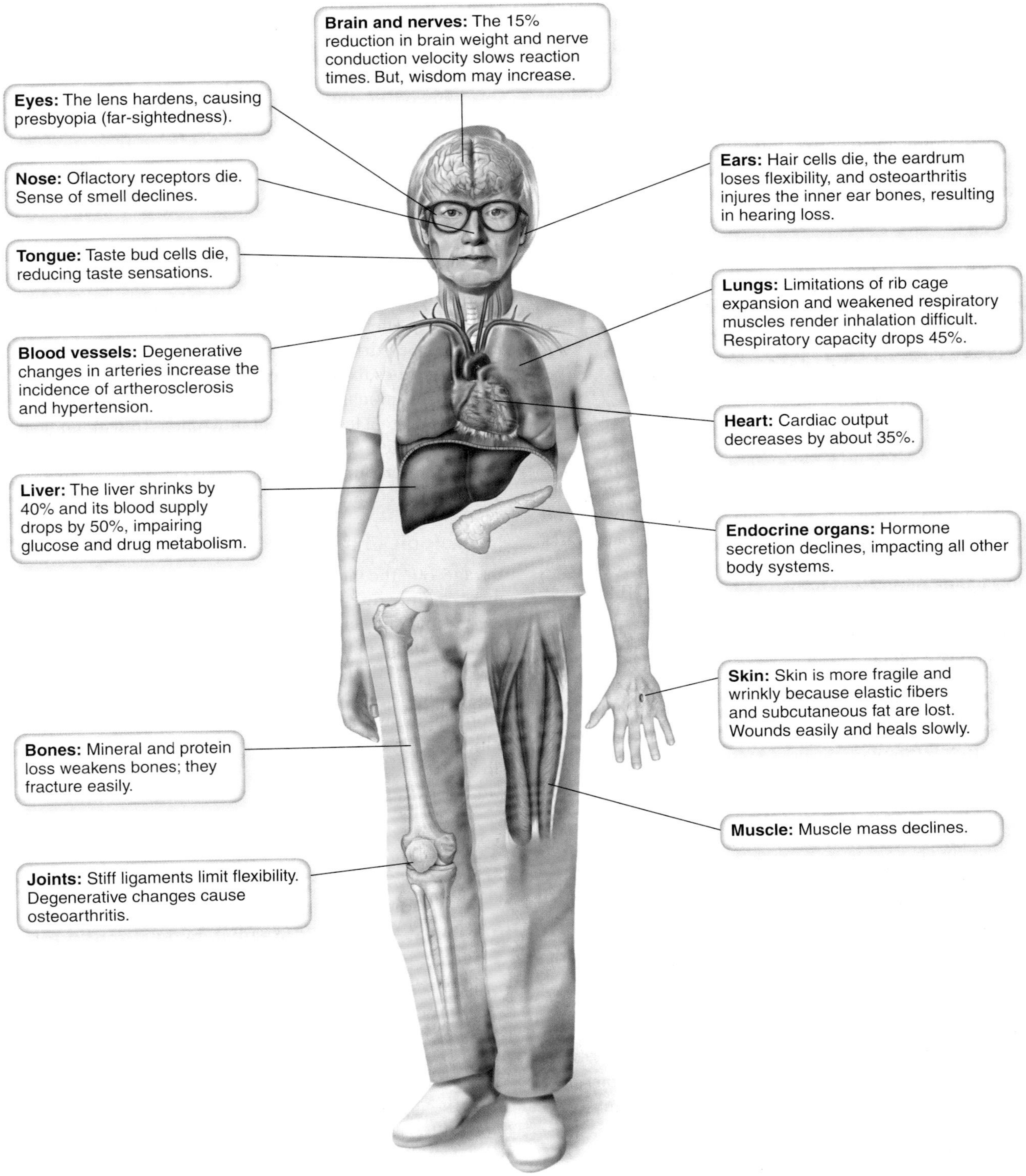

Figure 24.2 **Senescence and body systems.** Cell death (or lack of cell replacement) and impaired neural/endocrine communication negatively impact every body system. (Modified with permission from McConnell TH, Hull KL. *Human Form Human Function: Essentials of Anatomy & Physiology*. Baltimore, MD: Wolters Kluwer Health; 2011.)

her physical peak in young adulthood. A number of factors contribute to this decline. The lungs are not as easily distensible to bring in air; that is, compliance decreases. Rib joints do not move as easily, limiting chest expansion. Inspiratory muscles weaken, and spinal deformities, especially kyphosis, may further limit chest expansion. Finally, chronic obstructive pulmonary disease is more common in the elderly and may further limit respiratory function.

Case Notes

24.8 About how much less lung capacity does Tom have as compared to his peak as a young adult?

Digestive and Nutritional Changes

With age, liver size and blood flow decline. This limits the ability of the liver to store glycogen and convert it to glucose, thereby reducing its ability to correct low blood glucose. Because the liver metabolizes and inactivates many drugs, some medications can persist in the blood for a longer time period and at higher levels than in younger patients. Thus, medication monitoring is essential in older patients, and dose adjustment may be necessary to avoid toxicity.

Poor nutrition is common. Loss of smell dulls appetite, loss of saliva makes chewing and swallowing difficult, and dental disease and ill-fitting dentures compound the problem. Moreover, dementia robs some patients of the ability to organize a meal or even remember to eat.

Constipation and dehydration are also common. Lack of dietary fiber, poor intestinal peristalsis (often due to drug side effect), and lack of adequate fluid intake are the usual culprits. Age dulls thirst, and dehydration is usually due to a basic failure to drink enough water. Dehydration is often the hidden cause of fainting in the elderly. In older adults with dementia, the cognitive deficits interfere with the simple act of finding water or asking for it.

Kidney and Urinary Changes

The kidneys gradually shrink (*nephrosclerosis*) and the glomeruli can become progressively scarred (*glomerulosclerosis*). The kidneys lose about 20–25% of their mass by age 75, and the glomerular filtration rate, a key measure of renal function, declines as well, falling to about half its peak. Slow renal excretion of medications may require dosage adjustment in older patients. Ability to react to rapid changes in blood pH or electrolyte content may compound other problems like diabetic ketoacidosis or dehydration.

In women, loss of urinary control may cause increased frequency, nocturia, and incontinence. Pelvic tissues weaken and sag and decreased estrogen levels lead to decreased urethral resistance, length, and decreased ability to tightly close the voluntary sphincter. Bladder capacity declines, the ability to restrain the impulse declines, involuntary bladder contractions occur more often, and bladder contractility is impaired. It becomes more difficult to "hold it" and the bladder does not empty completely, which means it refills sooner, requiring frequent trips to the bathroom. Men may develop similar problems due to urinary retention caused by prostate enlargement.

Reproductive Changes

Reproductive capacity declines with age. Women cease ovulating at menopause, which usually occurs about age 50. In men, fertility declines but does not cease so abruptly. Sex drive, at its peak in the late teens and twenties, continues to decline owing to a variety of psychological and hormonal changes, especially lower testosterone in men and to a lesser extent in women. In women, loss of vaginal lubricity or vulvar atrophy may cause dyspareunia (painful intercourse). In men, erectile dysfunction can be a problem.

Neurologic Changes

By age 80, the brain has lost about 5–15% of its peak mass, mainly due to loss of neurons, which, because they are permanent cells, generally cannot be replaced. Some decline of mental function affects every person living beyond age 70. Though it may not be evident in daily life, mental agility tests in older adults show a slowing of problem-solving ability; nerve conduction velocity slows, which slows reflexes; and voluntary motor movements slow. Dementia, especially Alzheimer disease, and Parkinson disease take their toll.

Case Notes

24.9 Tom is humorously known in his family as "WGLA" (world's greatest living authority) because of his broad fund of information. How does the current size of Tom's brain compare to when he was in college?

Changes to the Special Senses

Our ability to taste declines with age. Remember, however, that most of the sense of taste is attributed to our sense of smell, which also fades with age. Indeed, some elderly people lose nearly all of their sense of smell and with it lose their appetite.

The lens of the eye begins to stiffen around age 40, which reduces the ability to focus on close subjects (*presbyopia*). Other ocular problems increasingly common with aging include cataracts, glaucoma, and macular degeneration.

High pitch deafness is almost universal among the elderly. Middle ear function declines, too. Decay of the vestibular apparatus makes older persons less able to maintain their balance. Often it is the case that an older person with a cane or walker is not using the device to make up for a sore knee or weak hip. Rather, they depend on the device to steady their balance. When unsteady, they may lack reflexes fast enough or muscles strong enough to recover, resulting in falls and the breaking of already weakened bones.

Pop Quiz

24.1 What is the difference between senescence and aging?

24.2 Many older adults wear hearing aids. What is this an example of?

24.3 As an adult ages, respiratory function decreases due to multiple aging factors. What common disease often further impairs respiratory function?

24.4 Identify the role of ROS in DNA mutations.

24.5 Do telomeres lengthen or shorten as we age?

25.6 Lea, aged 38, wants to train for endurance exercise. What is her target heart rate?

Stress

Stress is difficult to define, but the origin of the word offers some insight: stress derives from Latin *strictus*, which means "drawn tight." Stress can be helpful (*eustress*; e.g., exercise) or harmful (*distress*; e.g., death of a loved one).

Stress occurs in response to a *stressor*, which is anything that causes stress. Stressors can be physical, such as lifting more weight, running longer distances, or being deprived of food or water. Stressors can also be emotional or psychological, such as beginning or ending a relationship or watching a scary movie.

Stress involves perception. That is, stressors differ between individuals and over time in the same individual. Stressors are not always unpleasant—weddings and job promotions can be stressful and the stress they bring can have harmful effect. Stress depends on viewpoint. For example, on a Saturday afternoon in a football stadium, the final score of the game brings joy to some and distress to others. Or consider Kate's stress response to the butterfly in her hair. She perceived a fluttering insect in her hair as a threat, based on her previous experience with a yellow jacket. Kate's stress was entirely due to her viewpoint: she thought it was going to sting her. A child with a different viewpoint may have been charmed to the point of giggling at having a butterfly in her hair.

Remember This! Stress can be beneficial or detrimental.

Case Notes

24.10 Kate and Tom are stressed by the butterfly episode. How does their stress differ?

The Stress Response Includes Three Phases

The stress response includes three phases: alarm, adaptation, and exhaustion. These are not necessarily sequential events. If alarm continues without adaptation, exhaustion will occur. Adaptation is a learned behavior that increases with familiarity to the perceived threat.

Alarm Phase

The first response to a stressor is called the "alarm phase" (Fig. 24.3). It has two components: the sympathetic nervous system and hormones, especially epinephrine (adrenaline) and cortisol.

The sympathetic nervous system reaction to a stressor is immediate, and affects many body systems. When Kate interpreted the butterfly as a threat, sympathetic nerves stimulated epinephrine release from the adrenal medulla, which increased her heart rate, respiratory rate, and blood pressure to support the "fight or flight" reaction. Kate was ready to fight or escape from the threat—which was real to her.

The autonomic (sympathetic) nervous response is quick while the endocrine reaction is slower but longer lasting. In the butterfly incident, Kate's brain stimulated pituitary ACTH release. ACTH circulated to the adrenal cortex, stimulating a flood of cortisol into Kate's blood. This second, endocrine arm of the alarm phase is devoted to a longer, sustainable reaction to stress. It is useful when a stressor persists—if Kate and her mother had had to flee from a bear, for example.

Case Notes

24.11 Kate's heart rate was high when Tom reached her. Does increased heart rate reflect the actions of epinephrine or cortisol?

Adaptation Phase

As Kate matures and understands her butterfly encounter, she will become less alarmed by insects. That is, she will enter the second phase of the stress response—*adaptation*. The sight of a yellow butterfly or a yellow jacket will not be quite so stressful and will not necessarily activate her

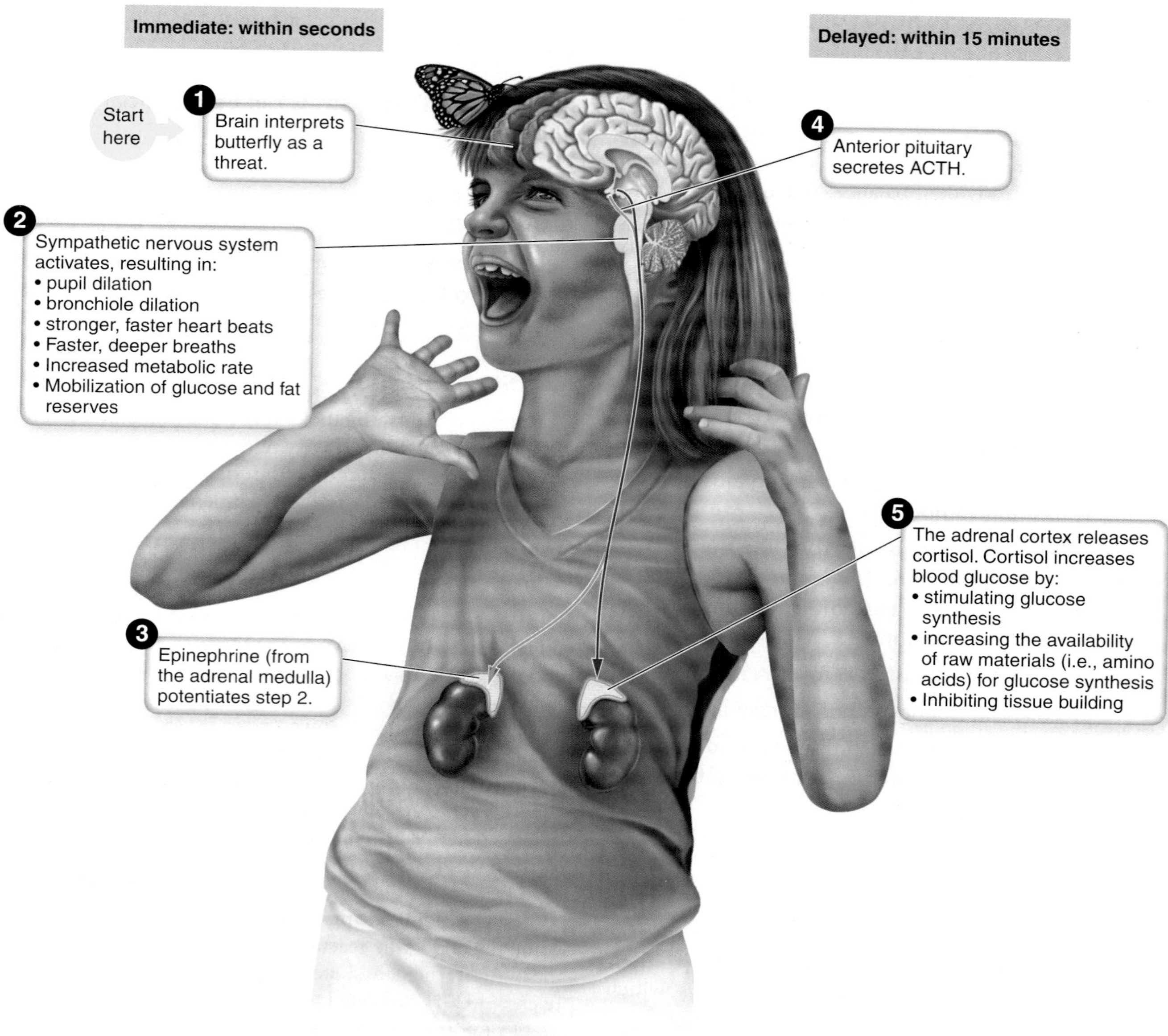

Figure 24.3 **Stress: the alarm phase.** The alarm phase uses the sympathetic nervous system, adrenal epinephrine, and cortisol to improve the chances of escaping a physical stressor. (Modified with permission from McConnell TH, Hull KL. *Human Form Human Function: Essentials of Anatomy & Physiology*. Baltimore, MD: Wolters Kluwer Health; 2011.)

sympathetic nervous system and adrenal cortex. Insects aren't likely to change, but Kate's perception is. We also adapt to physical stressors. For example, the improved fitness that comes with regular exercise is a physical adaptation to physical stress.

Exhaustion Phase

If adaptation fails—if we do not adapt to the stressor, or if the threat is ongoing and real, then we enter the third phase: *exhaustion*. In this phase, cortisol secretion stays high for a time. Eventually, however, it ceases. The detrimental effects of stress become manifest, and disease or death can result.

Stress Exhaustion Harms Cells and Systems

The stress response evolved as a means of coping with physical stressors, such as food deprivation and predators. Yet most modern stressors are psychological and often of long duration. When we do not adapt to these chronic stressors, we experience stress exhaustion, which is linked to three deleterious changes:

1. *Chronic inflammation*: Stress induces inflammation, which in turn damages tissues, especially blood vessels. Stress is a prime factor in atherosclerotic vascular disease.
2. *Accelerated cellular aging*: Chronic stress may inhibit DNA repair, which increases the frequency of unrepaired mutations in genes and also accelerates telomere shortening causing cells to age faster.
3. *Increased oxidative stress*: Stress increases free radical production and the DNA and other cell damage that attends it.

The steps linking stress to these three changes are not well understood, but may reflect long-term elevations in cortisol. In any case, the results of chronic stress exhaustion are clear. The immune system atrophies. Resistance to infection is diminished. Though evidence is not conclusive, some studies suggest that anticancer immune surveillance is weakened and cancers are more common and more aggressive. High cortisol also induces insulin resistance and high blood sugar, which in turn causes widespread damage of the type associated with diabetes. Cortisol coupled with insulin resistance leads to abdominal obesity—a factor that some researchers think helps explain the link between the stress of poverty and an increased risk for obesity. Excess abdominal fat releases all sorts of hormones and inflammatory mediators that prompt or exacerbate disease.

Apart from these physical effects are mental effects, which are no less real. Chronic stress plays a major role in interpersonal discord, divorce, child abuse, drug abuse, and other social ills. Two types of acute psychological stress disorders are recognized. *Acute stress disorder* follows an acute psychological trauma. It features a few days of terrifying recollection, avoidance of stimuli that recall the event, a feeling of numbness and detachment, and dazed behavior. Most people recover spontaneously within a few days. Some require psychoactive drugs. On the other hand, *post-traumatic stress disorder* is a longer-term syndrome (> 1 month) of similar symptoms. It may be disabling. Nightmares, flashbacks, and feelings of helplessness are common. Treatment consists of controlled exposure to triggering stimuli and psychoactive drugs.

It is important to remember that disease itself is a stressor. Chronic disease can have deleterious effects on the rest of the body. For example, chronic disease of any sort can often lead to anemia (anemia of chronic disease, Chapter 7). Of course, there are important psychological consequences of chronic disease as well, including anxiety and depression. The negative effects of chronic disease on society are enormous (think about obesity!).

Table 24.1 summarizes some of the effects of stress exhaustion on different body systems. Of note is how many stress-related disorders have an immune component.

Table 24.1 Diseases and Conditions Related to Stress

Body System	Disease or Condition
Immune	Decreased mass of lymphoid tissue*
	Infections*
	Cancers?*
Gastrointestinal	Ulcers (oral, gastric, etc.)
	Irritable bowel syndrome
	Diarrhea or constipation
Skin	Eczema*
	Acne
Cardiovascular	Heart rhythm disturbances (arrhythmias)
	Coronary artery disease
	Hypertension
	Stroke
Respiratory	Asthma*
	Hay fever, other allergies*
	Frequent respiratory infections*
Endocrine	Diabetes mellitus
Reproductive	Erectile dysfunction
	Infertility
	Amenorrhea (absence of menstrual periods)
Nervous	Migraines
	Fibromyalgia, other pain disorders
	Multiple sclerosis*
	Depression
	Insomnia or sleepiness
	Posttraumatic stress disorder
	Appetite changes
	Learning difficulties
Musculoskeletal	Backache, muscle spasms
	Rheumatoid arthritis*

*Immune component

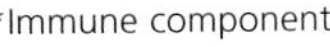

Case Notes

24.12 **Afterward, Tom and Lea discuss stress. Lea reports that a neighbor's child has been bullied at school for most of the year. Is the child likely to have increased or decreased cortisol production?**

Pop Quiz

24.7 True or false? Virtually anything can be a stressor.

24.8 During the alarm phase of the stress response, which hormone is secreted first: epinephrine or cortisol?

24.9 Which substance increases heart rate: cortisol or epinephrine?

24.10 Name three immune-related disorders that are also stress related.

24.11 Ms. M has been running three miles daily for four years. While the run was difficult at first, she now finds the run very comfortable, and her pace hasn't changed for the past two years. Ms. M is in which phase of the stress response?

24.12 What are the three deleterious effects that occur with stress exhaustion?

Exercise

We've seen how our physical, and to a certain extent our mental, abilities begin to decline as soon as our organs are fully mature. Distress adds to this burden. Eustress, however, can be beneficial, and exercise is a special form of beneficial eustress.

Exercise Improves Health

Exercise is part of a healthy lifestyle at every age. If we don't "use it," we will indeed "lose it"; that is, we'll lose the capacity to perform even the modest activities of daily life. Healthy young adults take for granted the ability to run for a bus, carry a small child, dance at a party, or simply climb a flight of stairs, yet many adults lack the basic physical ability to perform these tasks comfortably. People who lead sedentary lives quickly begin to lose their physical capacity. Muscles lose mass and strength; joints stiffen; bones lose calcium and become easily fractured; blood flow becomes sluggish and venous thrombi may form. Even cognitive function begins to decline.

The remedy is exercise—and surprisingly little pays a big bonus. For example, the 1996 U.S. Surgeon General's report on physical activity stated that Americans need to accumulate only 30 minutes of physical activity on most days of the week to optimize their health. What's more, the exercise need not be performed all at once: a brisk 10-minute walk three times a day is enough. More recent studies suggest that even less time may have nearly as much effect. Even for wheelchair-bound patients in nursing homes, a program of regular arm lifts of small weights has a positive effect on health and well-being.

Regular exercise has many benefits (Fig. 24.4), including the following:

- *Improved vascular function.* Regular exercise increases maximal cardiac output and the ability to deliver oxygen to tissues, which improves endurance. Exercise decreases the incidence of atherosclerosis in two ways. First, it improves lipid profiles, increasing the proportion of "good" high-density lipoprotein (HDL) cholesterol and reducing the proportion of "bad" low-density lipoprotein (LDL) cholesterol. It also decreases resting blood pressure, which lessens the accelerating effect of high blood pressure on atherosclerosis and nephrosclerosis.
- *Improved flexibility and strength.* Flexibility and strength are not only for athletes, they are required for easy performance of daily tasks as simple as walking up a flight of stairs, lifting a bag of groceries, reaching or bending to grasp, and dozens of other activities, the limitation of which makes living less of a joy.
- *Decreased body fat.* Endurance exercise can reduce body fat, and resistance exercise increases muscle mass. The improvement in lean body mass (that is, body mass minus fat mass) reduces the incidence (or severity) of obesity and many of the disorders associated with obesity, including Type II diabetes, heart disease, stroke, sleep apnea, some cancers, infertility, and degenerative joint disease.
- *Enhanced psychological well-being and improved ability to cope with stress.* Regular endurance or resistance training improves our sense of well-being, often to the same extent as antidepressant medication, and helps prevent stress exhaustion from psychological stressors.

Remember This! **Exercise is good for health.**

Case Notes

24.13 Based solely on Tom's exercise habits, how might his blood pressure and blood lipids differ from someone who does not exercise?

24.14 Since he began weight lifting, Tom's body weight has increased despite his consistent eating habits. Do you think weight lifting increased or decreased his risk of obesity-related disorders?

Certain Types of Injuries Occur with Exercise or Athletics

For those who exercise regularly, especially those in competitive sports, injury is common (Fig. 24.5). Many sports

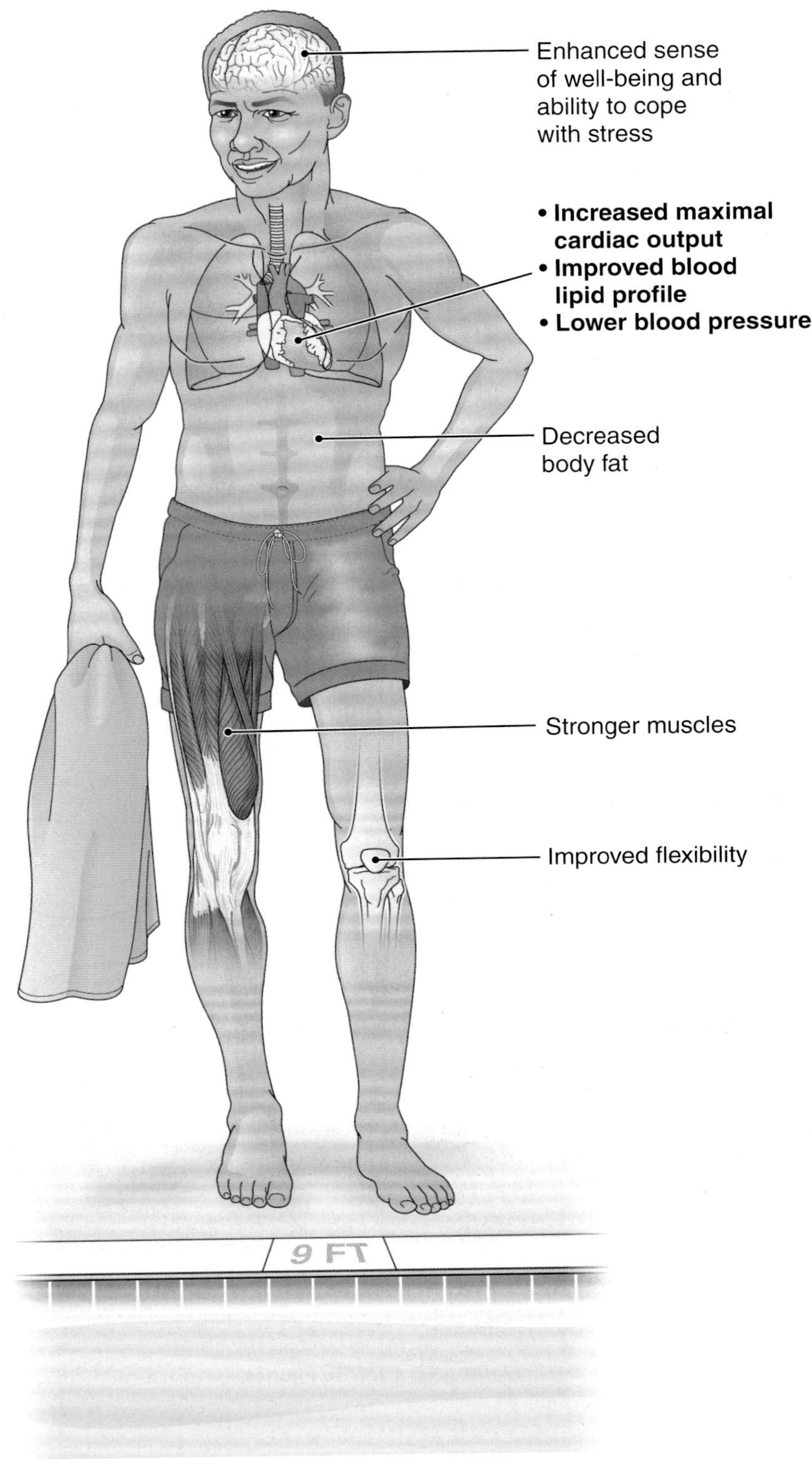

Figure 24.4 **The benefits of exercise.**

injuries are not unique to athletics—fractures, joint dislocations, and concussions can occur in any setting. Generally, sports injuries are due to overuse, blunt trauma, and acute soft tissue strains and sprains.

Overuse injury is one of the most common and can involve bones, ligaments, tendons, cartilage, fascia, and bursae in any combination. Runners are prone to overuse injury, especially with increased intensity

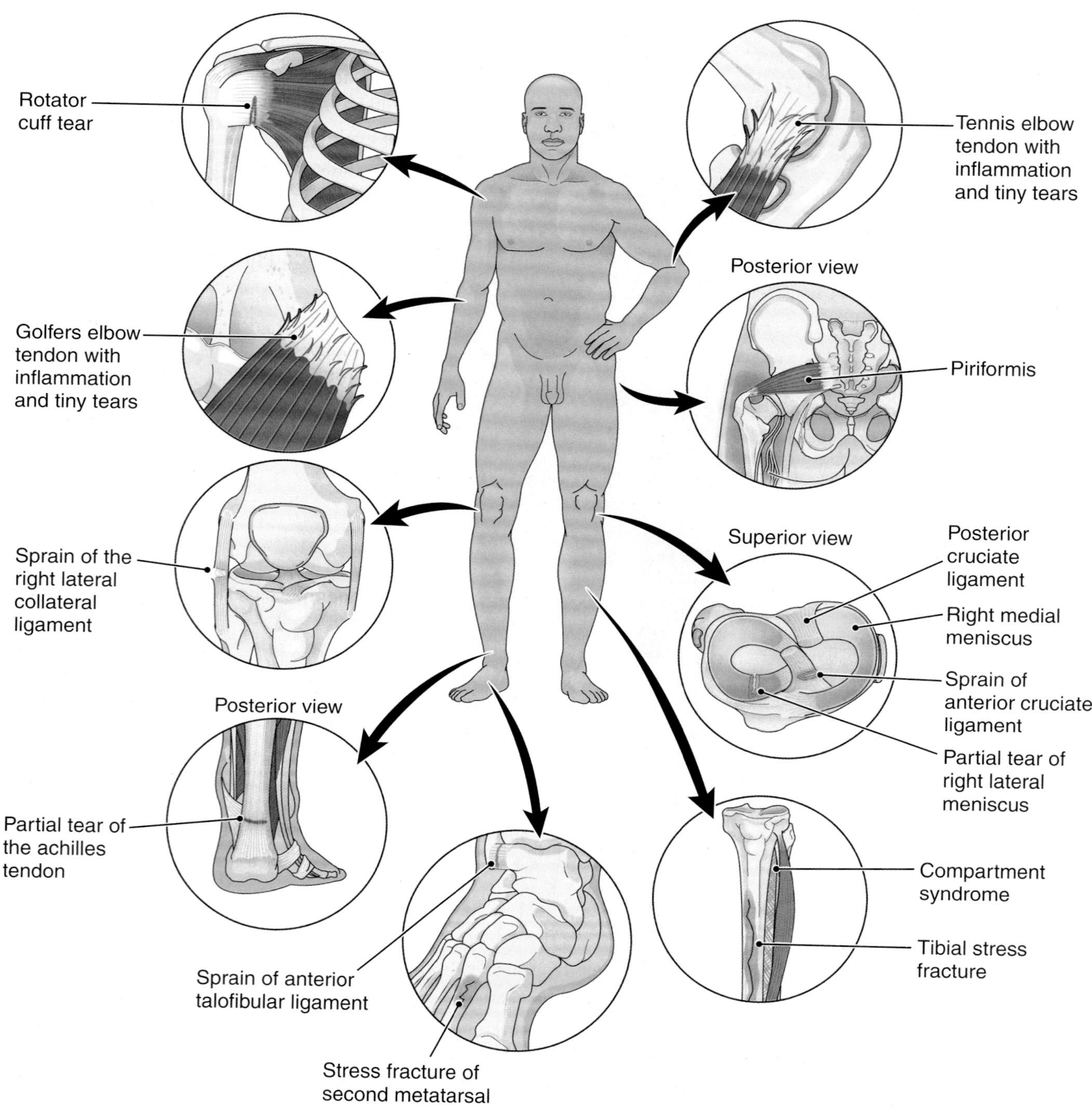

Figure 24.5 **Exercise injuries.**

or duration of workouts. Whatever the cause, the treatment of most athletic injury is *RICE: rest, ice, compression, and elevation.* In addition, nonsteroidal anti-inflammatory drugs (NSAIDs), like ibuprofen, are often used to reduce inflammation and pain. NSAIDS, aspirin in particular, carry a slight risk of increased bleeding.

The rotator cuff consists of four shoulder muscles that hold the humeral head in the glenoid fossa of the scapula. **Rotator cuff injury** (Fig. 24.5A) occurs with repeated overhead motion of throwing, swimming, weightlifting, and racket sports. Perhaps 50% of adults have some degree of rotator cuff dysfunction, some caused by injury, some by age-related degeneration. Rest and muscle strengthening exercises are usually effective treatment. Ligament tears require surgery.

Tendinitis (inflammation of tendons) is also common. **Tennis elbow** (Fig. 24.5B) is pain due to inflammation and microtears in the tendons of the extensor muscles of the forearm where they attach to the lateral epicondyle of the humerus. RICE treatment and NSAIDs are usually effective. Steroid injection may be required for prolonged or severe pain. Surgery is rarely necessary.

Golfer's elbow (Fig. 24.5C) is pain due to inflammation and microtears in the tendons of the flexor muscles of the forearm where they attach to the medial epicondyle of the humerus. It is much less common than tennis elbow. Treatment is similar.

Piriformis syndrome (Fig. 24.5D) is compression of the sciatic nerve by the pyriformis muscle, which crosses over the nerve as it travels from the sacrum to the greater trochanter of the femur. Symptoms are chronic ache or pain, and numbness or tingling in the buttock, which may extend down the back of the thigh and calf. Low back pain is absent and helps distinguish pyriformis syndrome from a herniated intervertebral disc. Rest is the best treatment, but steroid injections may help severe or prolonged cases. Surgery is rarely warranted.

Knee injuries (Fig. 24.5E) are very common and usually involve the ligaments that bind the head of the femur to the tibial plateau, or the cartilages (menisci) that cover the tibial plateau. The knee has four main ligaments. The *medial and lateral collateral ligaments* join the medial and lateral ends of the femur and tibia and lie beneath the skin, outside the joint capsule. The *anterior and posterior cruciate (cross-like) ligaments* lie inside the joint. They form a cross in their path from tibia to femoral head. Some injuries arise from direct impact, but most involve excessive torque from twisting, quickly stopping, or landing from a jump. Torn ligaments often require surgery. The knee has two cartilages, the *medial and lateral menisci*. They are inward-facing lemon-wedge shapes. The outer edges are thick, the inner margins thin. Tears tend to occur in the thin, inner part of the cartilage and may be caused by sudden force or by chronic stress. Impaired joint motion may be due to loose fragments (joint mice), or curled pieces that project into the joint. Surgery is often required. An alternative to surgery in some patients may be intra-articular injection of the patient's own platelet-rich plasma, which contains growth factors that promote healing.

Medial tibial stress syndrome (commonly called *shin splints*) (Fig. 24.5F) is pain along or posterior to the tibia. It occurs during physical activity, especially running. Although it has many causes, about half of cases are due to tibial stress fracture. *Compartment syndrome* is another common cause. It occurs when the perfusion pressure of blood falls below tissue pressure in a closed anatomic space (such as one enclosed by bone and fascia). The result is diminished blood supply, tissue ischemia, and painful cramps. The usual treatment is to stop the activity until it can be resumed without causing pain; however, some cases may require surgical decompression to avoid severe and irreversible muscle damage.

Ankle injuries (Fig. 24.5G) are also quite common. The ankle is a very complex joint that is bound together by multiple ligaments, most of them on the medial and lateral aspects. The most common injury is sprain of one or more of the lateral ligaments when the foot is extended (plantar flexion) and rolls to the side, sole inward (inversion). Most injuries occur on uneven surfaces. RICE treatment suffices for minor injuries, but a cast or surgery may be indicated for more severe injuries.

Achilles tendon injuries (Fig. 24.5H) are common to runners and include inflammation and tears. Inflammation features pain and tenderness in the tendon. Treatment is RICE and NSAIDs. Tears may be complete or partial. Although less common than inflammation, they are much more serious. They are usually sudden, associated with extreme pain, and prevent ambulation. Surgery is usually required.

Metatarsal stress fractures (Fig. 24.5I) are small fractures caused by repeated weight-bearing stress as opposed to a sudden force, such as a fall. They are most common in runners. The second metatarsal is most often affected. Risk factors include high arch, uncushioned shoes, and osteoporosis. Typically, arch pain occurs gradually and at first it disappears with rest. With continued activity, however, the pain worsens and lengthens. X-rays may be normal until callus formation begins after several weeks. Treatment usually includes a special shoe or crutches. Recovery may take months.

Case Notes

24.15 Tom had tennis elbow years ago. Which part of the elbow was involved?

Immobility Is Unhealthy

Immobility is the "lose it" part of "use it or lose it." As exercise is good for health, immobility is unhealthy. As exercise strengthens muscles and limbers joints, immobility weakens muscles and stiffens joints. As exercise improves cardiovascular health, immobility degrades it. As exercise sharpens the spirit, immobility dulls it. And so on through every body system.

Immobility is a sizeable and underappreciated problem. Nursing homes are filled with elderly people, many of whom are bedfast or who can escape bed only by sitting in a chair. The more confining and the longer the limitation to movement, the more damaging it is to health.

Under some circumstances, after surgery for example, even a few hours of immobility can have serious consequences. For example, deep vein thrombi can arise quickly, one of the reasons surgery patients are treated with heparin (or another anticoagulant) and serial leg compression devices after surgery and ambulated as quickly as possible.

Treatment of immobility is movement. Active movement is best. For a patient recovering from surgery, sitting up in bed or standing by the bed is worthwhile. A short walk down the hall is better. For the weak or paralyzed, passive movement by a therapist has significant benefit.

Remember This! Immobility is bad for health.

Musculoskeletal Effects

Inactive muscle atrophies quickly and, with prolonged disuse, may undergo fibrosis. Because flexor muscles are usually stronger than extensors, an unused limb may flex and scar into an irreversible deformity, a **flexion contracture** (Fig. 24.6). Even for short-term immobility, such as wearing a cast while a fracture heals, muscles lose strength and joints become stiff.

Skin Effects

Decubitus ulcers (pressure sores, from Latin *decumbrere* = to lie down, Fig. 24.7) represent the effect of immobility on skin. Unrelieved pressure deprives skin of blood. Skin first turns red, and then necrosis occurs, followed by inflammation and ulceration. Infection is common. Most vulnerable are bony prominences: sacrum, elbows and heels when lying on the back, ischial tuberosities and elbows while sitting, greater trochanter while lying on one side. Lack of body fat, a common problem in malnourished elderly patients, adds to the risk. Poor circulation, especially in the lower limbs of diabetics, is another risk. Finally, skin is meant to be dry, so moisture from perspiration or urine is a risk factor. Prevention, which requires strict attention to turning, padding, and good hygiene, is of paramount importance because most ulcers heal very slowly.

Cardiovascular Effects

Recall that venous return from the legs depends on the massaging action of contracting muscles on veins.

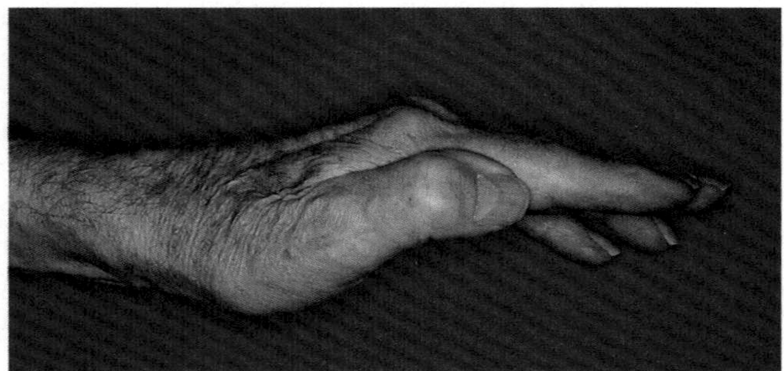

Figure 24.6 **Flexion contracture**. Contraction of metacarpophalangeal joints after joint surgery. (Reproduced with permission from Strickland JW, Graham TJ. *Master Techniques in Orthopeadic Surgery: The Hand*. 2nd ed. Philadelphia, PA: Lippincott Williams & Wilkins; 2005.)

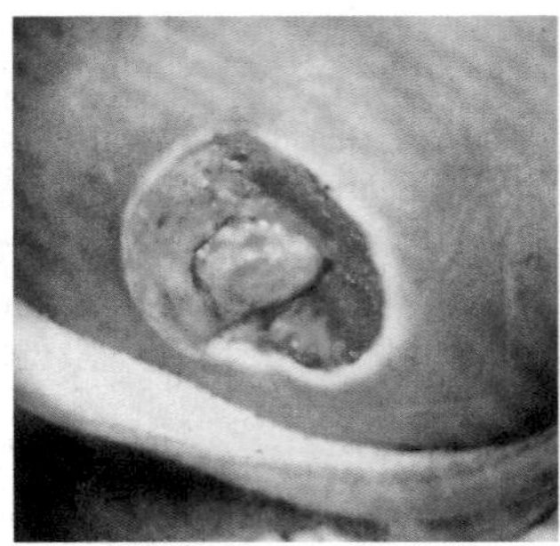

Figure 24.7 **Decubitus ulcer.** (Reproduced with permission from Nettina, SM. *The Lippincott Manual of Nursing Practice.* 7th ed. Philadelphia, PA: Lippincott Williams & Wilkins; 2001.)

Immobility in the recumbent position increases the risk of deep vein thrombosis and can cause pulmonary thromboembolism and infarction. Some can be fatal. Even the immobility of a long plane flight can be enough to prompt thrombus formation. Effective treatment consists of in-bed or in-seat leg exercises, elastic stockings, or for hospitalized patients, automatic massage leggings.

Immobility while recumbent shifts blood from the extremities to the chest and abdomen. Ventral venous pressure increases, which may cause *orthopnea*, an aggravation of the breathlessness associated with congestive heart failure. Prolonged recumbency also dulls vascular pressure sensors, which normally act to constrict leg blood vessels to maintain standing blood pressure. Standing up after prolonged recumbency may cause blood pooling in the legs, which can result in plummeting blood pressure and potential fainting (syncope).

Pulmonary Effects

Immobility means less demand for oxygen and shallower respirations. What's more, breathing and coughing are more difficult in the recumbent position because the chest is less expandable—abdominal viscera press upward on the diaphragm and body position limits chest wall movement. Additionally, many patients are also on drugs such as opiates that further suppress cough and respiration. The net effect is to encourage retention of secretions, which in turn favors pneumonia and atelectasis. Respiratory therapy may be required.

Gastrointestinal Effects

Immobility's main gastrointestinal effect is constipation. The reduced demand for energy and the dull appetite that comes with illness means that immobile patients generally drink less fluid, eat less food, and get less fiber. Many pain-killing drugs (i.e., opiates) directly decrease intestinal motility. When transit time through the bowel is longer, the result is increased water absorption and compacted, hard stools. Defecation is more difficult—bedpans are awkward and undignified, and patients are weak.

Elderly patients are especially vulnerable. Supplemental fiber, laxatives, or stool softeners may be indicated. In *impaction*, stool is not passable with laxative or enema and must be manually removed.

Urinary Effects

The urinary effect from immobility is urinary stasis. When upright, the flow of urine from kidneys to bladder is aided by gravity, an effect denied in the recumbent position. What's more, complete emptying of the bladder is difficult when using a bedpan. Retained urine and stasis promote kidney stone formation and infection. This is especially true in patients paralyzed by spinal cord injury. The effect is long term and the injury often interrupts autonomic innervation of the ureters, paralyzing ureteral peristalsis.

Case Notes

24.16 Tom frequently takes transoceanic airplane trips. He makes a point to get out of his seat and walk about the cabin several times. Why?

Pop Quiz

24.13 True or false? All of the following are risk factors for decubitus ulcers: lack of body fat, poor circulation, and dry skin.

24.14 Tina, a 25-year-old athletic female, has increased the intensity of her training, running up to 20 miles per day. Which of the three types of athletic injuries is she most likely to suffer from?

24.15 Which of the following would be higher in a resting athlete than in a resting couch potato—stroke volume or heart rate?

24.16 Which type of lipoprotein increases in response to regular exercise: LDL or HDL?

24.17 What nerve is compressed in piriformis syndrome?

24.18 John recently underwent surgery to repair a large ventral hernia. He was doing well postoperatively until he became short of breath. What complication of immobility did John likely suffer from?

Pain

Pain is an unpleasant sensation that all of us know when we feel it. Beyond that, it is famously difficult to describe and therefore equally difficult to assess because it is so singularly personal. No examiner can experience it, nor can the examiner see it, touch it, measure it with an instrument, or characterize it in any way other than by trying to understand the patient's description of it and observing the effect the pain has on the patient. Trying to describe pain is almost as difficult as describing color to a patient blind from birth, which is, of course, impossible.

Pain is the most common reason patients seek medical care. It has both sensory and emotional components.

When pain from tissue damage at a particular anatomic area appears to be coming from somewhere else, the pain is said to be **referred pain**. If you cut your finger, it is the finger that hurts, but if you are having a heart attack, the pain may appear to come from—be referred to—your left jaw, neck, or left arm. Referred pain occurs when visceral sensory fibers from an affected organ enter the spinal cord along with sensory fibers from another part of the body, and both fiber types converge, carrying signals to a single point in the cerebral cortex.

Pain Can Be Classified in Two Primary Ways

Pain is typically classified by duration:

- *Acute pain* is pain accompanying acute tissue injury. It disappears with healing, and in any case lasts for less than one month. It is usually associated with anxiety and hyperactivity of the sympathetic nervous system: increased heart rate and blood pressure, rapid breathing, and so on.
- *Chronic pain* is longer lasting and will be discussed in detail below. It is usually associated with fatigue, depressed mood, loss of appetite, and other vegetative signs.

Clinicians also classify pain according to the type of injury:

- **Nociceptive pain** arises from injury and activation of tissue pain receptors (*nociceptors*, Latin *nocere* = to harm), which send signals up special nerve fibers into the spinal cord and on to the brain. It may be somatic or visceral. Somatic nociceptors are located in skin, connective tissue, bone, and joints, and the pain is usually acute, sharp, and localized. Visceral nociceptors are located in most viscera, and pain is usually dull, aching or cramping, and not well localized.
- **Neuropathic pain** results from injury to or dysfunction of the nervous system rather than stimulation of nociceptors.

Acute pain is always nociceptive, whereas chronic pain can be either nociceptive or neuropathic.

Psychological factors may be important in pain of any kind. Purely psychological (delusional) pain is rare, but psychological factors play an important role, sometimes the main role, in chronic pain. Many pain syndromes are multifactorial and may have nociceptive, neuropathic, and psychological elements. Some chronic low back pain seems to be this way.

Case Notes

24.17 What type of pain receptors was activated when Tom sprained his ankle?

Several Mechanisms May Provoke Chronic Pain

Chronic pain is pain that persists for more than three months, or for more than one month after resolution of an acute injury, or pain that accompanies a chronic disease or unhealed injury. The usual causes are chronic diseases such as cancer, rheumatoid arthritis and other autoimmune disease, diabetic peripheral neuropathy, and injuries such as herniated intervertebral disc or joint injury.

How does pain become chronic? Diseases that repeatedly stimulate pain pathways can sensitize neural circuits to a degree that, though the original stimulus has lessened or disappeared, pain may persist or worsen, even with slight provocation. Similarly, factors specific to the patient may affect the brain in a way that alters pain perception. Thus, what seems a minor provocation to an observer may evoke severe pain. This may account for the pain-relieving ability of antidepressants, anticonvulsants, and some other CNS-active drugs that are not usually used for pain treatment. *Fibromyalgia* (Chapter 18), for example, is a common chronic pain syndrome of unknown cause that features generalized aching and tenderness of muscles and periarticular tendons and soft tissues. Joints are not involved. Muscle stiffness, fatigue, and insomnia are common. No physical, lab, or imaging abnormalities are present. Diagnosis is clinical. Many patients respond to antidepressants.

Case Notes

24.18 Was the throbbing pain in Tom's ankle in the days after the injury chronic pain?

Neuropathic Pain Involves Nervous System Damage or Dysfunction

Neuropathic pain results from damage to or dysfunction of the nervous system. Nociceptor stimulation is not involved. Peripheral nerve injury or dysfunction is the most common cause. Nerve compression by a herniated intervertebral disc and diabetic peripheral neuropathy are two common examples. Less common is phantom limb pain: pain perceived to originate in an amputated limb (phantom pain, Chapter 20).

Complex regional pain syndrome is a special variety of chronic neuropathic pain. The cause is not clear. *Type I (reflex sympathetic dystrophy)* follows crushing soft tissue or bone injury. *Type II (causalgia)* is similar to Type I except that overt nerve damage is present. Both types persist long after damage is healed. Damage is usually to the hand or foot, but may follow myocardial infarct, stroke, or cancer, or have no apparent cause. Young adults, women especially, are most affected. The sympathetic nervous system is more involved in Type II. The involved part may sweat or alternately blanch from vasoconstriction or redden and swell with vasodilation. Burning or aching pain is the main symptom. Depression and anger are common. Treatment varies across the spectrum from drugs to injection of a portion of the sympathetic chain with local, long-lasting anesthetic (sympathetic blockade). Prognosis is difficult because the cause is unknown and treatment may not be effective.

Signs and Symptoms of Pain Are Individualistic

Pain should be evaluated on the following factors:

- *Quality*: Assessment of the quality of pain (burning, cramping, deep, shooting, etc.) can be especially difficult because it is dependent on the linguistic skill of the examiner and, especially, the patient.
- *Severity*: Several scales can be offered to the patient to describe their pain. For example, on a 1–10 scale pain level 1 is no pain, 5 is moderate pain, and 10 is the worst possible pain. Another scale (1–5) depends on a description of the degree pain interferes with life: 1 is no interference, 3 is some interference but patient can use the phone or watch TV, and 5 prevents verbal communication.
- *Location*: Where is it and is it superficial or deep?
- *Radiation*: Does the pain spread down an arm or leg, or from one region to another?
- *Duration*: How long does each pain last, or is it continuous?
- *Pattern*: Is there a pattern, and how does it change with time?
- *Other factors*: What makes it better or worse?

Apart from these factors, social factors are also relevant. Does the patient gain anything from the pain, such as a disability payment or time off? Might the patient be manipulating someone, a spouse or employer, for example, by being in pain?

Options in Pain Treatment Are Largely Pharmacologic

Pain relief is **analgesia** (Greek *an-* = without + *algos* = pain). The best way to relieve pain is to remove the offending stimulus. But often it is not possible. Some cancers, for example, are painful and cannot be removed. Neither can inflammation, whether from a chronic condition such as arthritis, or an acute injury such as a sprained ankle. That's where pharmacologic pain relievers come in. Anti-inflammatory drugs like aspirin, for example, block formation of local inflammatory chemicals that increase the sensitivity of pain receptors. Other drugs, especially opiates such as morphine, work in the nervous system at two levels: 1) in the spinal cord they block some signals from reaching the brain; and 2) in the cerebral cortex they alter the quality of pain perception—the pain doesn't go away, but the patient doesn't care about it as much.

Anesthesia (Greek *aisthesis* = feeling) is loss of all sensation, either locally or generally, not just the sensation of pain. **General anesthesia** is a drug-induced, coma-like state in which there is a loss of all sensation owing to the effect of drugs on the brain. Sensory signals reach the brain, but the brain does not register them. **Local anesthesia** is drug-induced loss of all sensation in the distribution of a peripheral nerve or nerves. Sensory signals are blocked and do not reach the CNS.

The treatment mainstay for pain is opioid (narcotic) and nonopioid drugs. *Opioids* are opiumlike compounds, many of them synthetic, which attach to opioid receptors in the brain and spinal cord. Opioids are tightly regulated because of the hazard of addiction. Controversy surrounds this regulation. According to pain specialists, the threat of addiction among pain patients is overstated and leads to widespread undertreatment of severe pain. On the other hand, the resources of law enforcement agencies have become severely strained over the last decade by the surge in criminal activity prompted by widespread addiction to prescription opioids obtained illegally or from "pill mills" run by unscrupulous practitioners who prescribe large quantities to anyone who walks in.

The most widely used *nonopioids* are the 20 or so drugs known as **nonsteroidal anti-inflammatory drugs (NSAIDs)**. These drugs relieve pain by reducing inflammation and interfering with the production of local factors that increase nerve sensitivity. The most popular NSAIDs are aspirin and ibuprofen. All NSAIDS, especially aspirin, have a tendency to promote bleeding and should be used accordingly. Acetaminophen is also a popular nonopioid that does not have an antiinflammatory effect but shares some of the other pain-relieving mechanisms of NSAIDS. It does not promote bleeding.

Nonpharmacologic approaches to pain treatment include anesthetic and steroid nerve blocks or other injections, physical therapy, or psychotherapy.

Pop Quiz

24.19 True or false? Some pain originates without tissue injury.

24.20 Name the two types of pain.

24.21 What type of pain follows an acute injury?

Case Study Revisited

"She thought it was a wasp." A Multigenerational Family Goes Hiking.

As they made their way up the mountain trail, Kate, 7, scampered ahead, oblivious of the altitude. Her mother, Lea, 38, lagged behind. Bringing up the rear was grandfather Tom, 71, who exercised regularly but could not keep up with the other two. Each of the three is healthy and fit. The differences in their cardiorespiratory performance owes solely to age. Everyone's heart, lungs, and muscles were performing as they should, but Lea's and Tom's organs contained more senescent, less robustly functional cells than Kate's. Though anyone can stumble on rough terrain, Tom's aging nervous system, inner ear equilibrium apparatus, and relatively weaker muscles may have contributed to his ankle sprain.

At the meadow at the top of the trail, Kate mistakenly thought the yellow butterfly was a wasp. Fearful of wasps because of a prior sting, she became acutely stressed by the harmless butterfly, a perfect example of the importance of perception in stress. In the initial (alarm) phase of stress, Kate's heart rate, blood pressure, and respiratory rate instantly increased due to stimulation by the sympathetic nervous system. Her brain also signalled the pituitary to release ACTH, which stimulated her adrenal cortex to secrete steroid hormone (cortisol) to sustain the alarm phase over a longer period of time, enough time to flee far away from the threat. Kate's stress was relieved by the comfort of her mother and grandfather and by the fact that the butterfly flew away. As she matures and understands the difference between wasps and butterflies, Kate will adapt (the second phase of stress) and will not be stressed by butterflies. Kate did not enter the third (exhaustion) phase of stress, which occurs only with unrelieved, chronic stress.

Hiking up the mountain trail was good exercise for each of the three. Tom exercised regularly, which enabled him at age 71 to keep fairly close to Kate and Lea, though they were much younger.

As with any type of exercise, injuries can occur. Tom sprained his ankle in his rush to come to Kate's aid. It produced sharp, superficial, localized pain below the right lateral malleolus from nociceptive sensors in the sprained ligament. He limped down the trail later and back at their cabin took an NSAID tablet to reduce inflammation and limit the production of local inflammatory molecules that increase nerve sensitivity. He also applied RICE therapy. Treatment was effective. Over the next few days, he continued NSAID therapy and the pain was reduced to a dull throb; Tom was able to go along on other outings though he didn't do much walking. The pain and swelling disappeared in a week.

Case Notes

24.19 Tom took NSAIDs for his pain. What is the mechanism of NSAIDs?

Chapter Challenge

CHAPTER RECALL

1. A 67-year-old male is diagnosed with prostate cancer. In addition to surgery, he will receive antiandrogen (antitestosterone) therapy. What side effects (similar to those of aging) can be expected due to this therapy?
   A. Muscle wasting
   B. Decreased libido
   C. Abdominal adiposity
   D. All of the above

2. Aging is due in part to the accumulation of cellular damage. Which of the following is an important cause of cellular damage?
   A. Accelerated DNA repair
   B. Decreased telomerase activity
   C. Free radicals
   D. All of the above

3. An 88-year-old African American female experiences urinary frequency and incontinence. Urinary cultures to assess for urinary tract infection are negative. What is the most likely cause of her symptoms?
   A. Increased bladder capacity
   B. Increased bladder contractions
   C. Increased estrogen
   D. Increased urethral resistance

4. Heritable mutations in DNA-associated proteins can cause different types of pathology including predisposition to cancer and premature aging (progeria).

Which disease or syndrome is associated with progeria?
A. Lynch syndrome
B. Werner syndrome
C. Sick sinus syndrome
D. Wegener granulomatosis

5. A 73-year-old Hispanic female presents to the ER after falling down a flight of stairs. Which of the following conditions increases the likelihood that a bone fracture has occurred with this trauma?
A. Lordosis
B. Osteoporosis
C. Osteoarthritis
D. Kyphosis

6. What is the best term for aging at the cellular level?
A. Obsolescence
B. ROS
C. Senescence
D. Senility

7. A 25-year-old African American male visits his primary care physician complaining of pain in his left elbow. He is an avid athlete, playing tennis, golf, and baseball at least once per week as part of his exercise regimen. His physical exam is normal, except for pain centered over the lateral epicondyle of his humerus. You prescribe NSAIDs for treatment of his pain, and recommend that he abstain from sports for the next month. What injury does he suffer from?
A. Rotator cuff injury
B. Tennis elbow
C. Golfer's elbow
D. Piriformis syndrome

8. Aging predisposes to which of the following?
A. Increased elastin production in the skin
B. Improved healing after falls
C. Urinary continence
D. Increased cerebrospinal fluid pressure

9. A 34-year-old, thin, Caucasian female presents for an annual checkup. What is one recommendation that can be made to help prevent loss of bone density as she ages?
A. Vitamin A supplementation
B. Vitamin C supplementation
C. Weight-bearing exercises
D. Oral contraceptives

10. A 75-year-old Hispanic male is prescribed a drug that is normally metabolized by the kidney at a lower dose than would be prescribed to a younger patient. What are the likely percent changes in kidney mass and kidney function, respectively, in this older patient?
A. 50% and 25%
B. 50% and 50%
C. 25% and 25%
D. 25% and 50%

11. A 44-year-old Caucasian female visits her physician. She complains of generalized aching, muscle tenderness and stiffness, fatigue, and insomnia. After a physical exam, you diagnose her with fibromyalgia. Which of the following statements regarding her disease is true?
A. No physical, lab, or imaging abnormalities are present.
B. Peripheral nerve injury or dysfunction is the most common cause.
C. Treatment includes injection of a portion of the sympathetic chain with local, long-lasting anesthetic (sympathetic blockade).
D. The treatment of choice is an NSAID.

12. True or false? The first phase of a stress response is the exhaustion phase.

13. True or false? Stress causes increased oxidative stress in cells leading to DNA damage.

14. True or false? The U.S. Surgeon General recommends one hour of daily exercise for optimal health.

15. True or false? Athletic injuries should often be treated with SPICE (steroids, painkillers, ice, compression, and elevation).

16. True or false? NSAIDs carry a risk of increased gastrointestinal bleeding.

CONCEPTUAL UNDERSTANDING

17. Using examples from the text, discuss the consequences of immobility including the major categories of complications.

18. Compare and contrast acute and chronic pain.

19. Briefly describe the attributes of pain that are clinically useful.

APPLICATION

20. A 75-year-old Caucasian male presents to your office for his annual checkup. He reports that he has no complaints, but that his wife says he is losing his hearing. What explanation might you offer?

21. Explain the statement: Oxygen is a necessary poison.

22. Your friend, a graduate student, complains of fatigue and recent weight gain. The symptoms started two months ago after she found out her lab was closing. Normally a very active person, her long hours in the lab have made it difficult for her to find the time to work out. What are you concerned about, and what advice might you offer?

Index

Page numbers in *italics* indicate figures. Page numbers followed by "t" indicate tables. Words in bold indicate diseases or conditions.

B

D

G

H

I

M

S

T

U

V